Perioperative Transfusion Medicine

Perioperative Transfusion Medicine

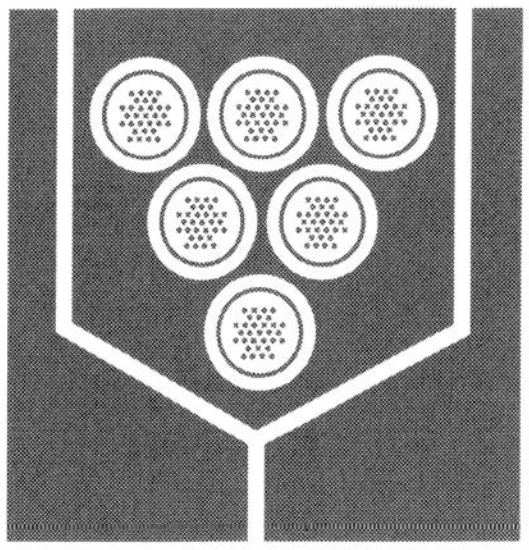

BRUCE D. SPIESS, MD

Associate Professor
Chief, Division of Cardiothoracic Anesthesia
University of Washington School of Medicine
Seattle, Washington

RICHARD B. COUNTS, MD

Professor of Medicine
University of Washington School of Medicine
Executive Director
Puget Sound Blood Center
Seattle, Washington

STEVEN A. GOULD, MD

Professor, Department of Surgery
University of Illinois College of Medicine
Chicago, Illinois
President
Northfield Laboratories, Inc.
Evanston, Illinois

SANS TACHE

Williams & Wilkins
A WAVERLY COMPANY

BALTIMORE • PHILADELPHIA • LONDON • PARIS • BANGKOK
BUENOS AIRES • HONG KONG • MUNICH • SYDNEY • TOKYO • WROCLAW

Editor: Sharon R. Zinner
Managing Editor: Tanya Lazar
Marketing Manager: Diane M. Harnish
Production Coordinator: Cindy Park
Book Project Editor: Karen M. Ruppert
Designer: Artech Graphics II
Illustration Planner: Ray Lowman
Cover Designer: Artech Graphics II
Typesetter: Peirce Graphic Services, Inc.
Printer/Binder: The MapleVail Book Manufacturing Group

351 West Camden Street
Baltimore, Maryland 21201-2436 USA

Rose Tree Corporate Center
1400 North Providence Road
Building II, Suite 5025
Media, Pennsylvania 19063-2043 USA

Printed in the United States of America

First Edition,

Library of Congress Cataloging-in-Publication Data

Perioperative transfusion medicine / [edited by] Bruce D. Spiess,
Richard Counts, Steven A. Gould.
p. cm.
Includes index.
ISBN 0-683-07892-5
1. Hemostasis, Surgical. 2. Blood—Transfusion. I. Spiess, Bruce D.
II. Counts, Richard. III. Gould, Steven A.
[DNLM: 1. Blood Transfusion. 2. Intraoperative Care. 3. Preoperative Care.
4. Postoperative Care. WB 356 P4449 1997]
RD33.3.P47 1997
615′.39—dc21
DNLM/DLC
for Library of Congress 97-4138
CIP

98 99 00
2 3 4 5 6 7 8 9 10

This volume is dedicated to the following three groups of people:

Ann G. Spiess, Phillip B. Spiess, and Erica A. Spiess:
A warm family who has endured far too many days and nights
of my absence while I was actively making transfusion decisions.

Ronald Faust, MD, Joseph Messick, MD, and Ronald McKenzie, DO:
Valued teachers at the Mayo Clinic who provided inspiration and the
groundwork for my career in transfusion-related issues.

Luretta D. Spiess, PhD, and Eliot B. Spiess, PhD:
Parents who unknowingly imparted the value and excitement of research
and teaching to a son who swore he would never write an academic paper.

B.D.S.

Preface

It is said that medicine is changing at an ever-accelerating pace. Those of us who trained even 15 years ago are baffled by the expanse of the knowledge base. What seemed an insurmountable information base to be mastered in medical school has now been expanded many-fold. Basic research in immunology, endothelial cell biology, the human genome, and imaging technology—to name a few—has expanded the capability of diagnosis and disease understanding exponentially. In the surgical subspecialties, whole new therapies are now available that a generation ago were thought of only in science fiction. Solid organ transplantation has been taken from experimental trials with poor success rates to liver, heart, and lung transplantation programs that not only are widespread but also have very acceptable long-term (5-year) success rates.

The surgical population is aging, as is the general populace, and the procedures being performed are increasingly complex for older and progressively more critically ill patients. Laparoscopic surgery is now applied to all types of surgery, including cardiovascular surgery. Alongside these revolutions in research and applied surgical therapy, the specter of cost containment has been driven by the national/international political and economical climates. Thus, today we are operating on sicker, more elderly patients undergoing more complex operations for which expectations of superb outcomes are the norm; and, lastly, these are expected to be performed for the least cost. These complex issues are constantly affecting the decision making of practitioners in today's surgical perioperative care.

One generation ago, blood transfusion for the surgical subspecialist was a relatively simple topic. The classic teaching was that patients were to be transfused to maintain a 10 gm/dL hemoglobin concentration. That "magic 10" was a milepost that interns learned to have their patients above prior to anesthesia or surgery, and for those intraoperatively and postoperatively, it was rare to let a patient fall much below this number. Those patients undergoing progressive or continuous blood loss intraoperatively were transfused when 15 to 20% of projected blood volume was lost. Again, a teaching point that was easily assimilated, that required little physiological analysis on a patient-by-patient basis, and that certainly affected transfusion behavior. Unfortunately, these teachings of a generation ago were based on a small amount of animal research, driven by inadequate understanding of the difference between hypovolemia and euvolemic anemia, and passed from text to text quoting earlier learned and esteemed founders of the surgical field. Transfusion concerns for this earlier generation of surgical subspecialists were not so much critically examining the decision to transfuse as they were concerned with whether enough blood was available to meet demand. Concerns today are considerably different.

If medicine at large has undergone an information explosion and research and politicization, then the field of transfusion is a prime example of those complex changes. It is so often said today that "the blood supply is the safest we have ever had." This statement is indeed true, but it is at the expense of massive outlays of research dollars and extreme pressures brought on medicine by the acquired immunodeficiency syndrome (AIDS) crisis of the 1980s and 1990s. New blood tests have been developed, and political organizations have made public calls for a zero-risk blood supply. A zero-risk blood supply is impossible, but the pressure exerted has certainly improved the statistics on viral transmission in blood. These public crises have raised consciousness both outside and inside medicine such that blood transfusion is a very timely topic. *Perioperative Transfusion Medicine* is written in direct response to the radical changes that have occurred in the field of transfusion medicine.

When initially undertaken, the vision was to create an extensive reference text for the surgical practitioner regarding all aspects of the management of patients and blood therapy. Today, more than 60% of blood products are transfused in the perioperative period. Cardiovascular surgery alone accounts for approximately 18 to 20% of all blood products used in the United States, and hepatic transplantation has provided significant pressure on blood services to increase supply and maintain an adequate inventory. To the editors of this text, at its inception it appeared that although many books were available on transfusion medicine, those texts focused on blood banking, laboratory medicine, internal medicine, and oncology. Each existing volume had mentions of the use of blood in surgery, but were often limited to one or two chapters. Often such summary chapters were not authored by surgeons or anesthesiologists—the physicians making the transfusion decisions. Therefore, it appeared that although excellent information was available, this information was neither directed toward surgical subspecialists nor likely to be widely read by such persons. The text we have created has drawn from the knowledge of a wide range of specialists. Internists and hematologists have contributed basic background information regarding history, basics of blood banking, and product preparation and storage. Topics applicable to all transfusion decisions are discussed by anesthesiologists and surgeons who have done internationally recognized research in each area. Transfusion issues regarding numerous key subspecialty situations are examined by surgeons and anesthesiologists. The transfusion decision is examined as an overview by the editors of this text.

The book is divided into three main sections. These do not stand alone; in many ways they interrelate and feed on the information presented in the other sections. The first seven chapters deal with a foundation of information key to blood banking, the risks of transfusion, and the interaction between the surgical services and blood services.

Chapter 1 is a summarized short history of blood banking. Surgical practitioners may not be widely interested in the details of the history of blood banking, but some of the highlights have paralleled developments in surgery as well as supported surgery's development. Chapter 2 examines what is needed for a blood bank to function normally to provide the support necessary for an active surgical service. Frustration can exist in the communication between surgical needs and the supply side of the blood services. If surgical practitioners can further understand the basic organization, mechanisms, limitations, and motivations of the blood banking system, positive interactions can be facilitated. Chapter 3 forms an up-to-date foundation for much of the remainder of this book. Earlier in this preface, the teachings of earlier generations regarding a "magic 10" were discussed. Chapter 3 looks at updated basic research regarding normal oxygen transport. Transfusion of red cell products should be driven solely by a desire to increase oxygen carrying capacity. Thus, Chapter 3 should be read by every surgery and anesthesia trainee.

Chapter 4 looks at the interaction of the blood bank and the surgeon/anesthesiologist even more closely than does Chapter 2. Those delivering the blood products may not wish to know all the details of compatibility testing; however, understanding the frequency of difficult crossmatches and the incidence of adverse events with such products as uncrossmatched blood, or type and screened blood, may provide the knowledge to make appropriate emergent decisions in the surgical patient with confidence. Platelet transfusion is the largest growth of product demand within the blood banking industry in the United States. Much of the demand for platelets has come from the growth of stem cell and bone marrow transplantation therapies. Yet, cardiac and liver transplantation surgeries certainly make substantial demands here as well.

Chapter 5 deals with platelet harvesting, and storage and physiology of those products that are available. Because of its limited shelf-life and the increased demand, the platelet product is a scarce resource. The surgical practitioner whose practice often or occasionally demands platelet transfusions would be well advised to read this chapter and understand how these products are obtained and assured available for his or her patients' use. Chapter 6 examines the normal physiology of hemostasis. Basic science research in this area has provided extensive new understanding, not only of the proteins and how they cascade to create fibrin but also of how these cascades interact with procoagulant cell lines. The research in cell adhesion proteins, particularly on platelet surfaces, has introduced a contemporary view of coagulation that is considerably different from the classically taught, mutually exclusive intrinsic and extrinsic cascades. Many physicians and other practitioners in the surgical subspecialties are understandably frustrated by the complexity of the coagulation systems. Perhaps some of the demand on blood banks for coagulation precursor products is the result of this lack of understanding. Those who specialize in areas in which coagulopathies are commonly encountered should avail themselves of this wonderful basic contemporary review of hemostasis.

To conclude the first section, Chapter 7 examines the timely subject of the infectious risks of transfusion. Perhaps this chapter will be outdated before long, as the development of new laboratory testing continues and as reports are published that look at series of donors and recipients regarding seroconversion for various viral transmissions. Although AIDS has created a whirlwind of political activity and changed transfusion forever, more importantly, hepatitis now is almost nonexistent as a risk of transfusion in the United States. In prior generations of physicians, hepatitis was widely known as a risk of transfusion, with the risk of transmission being approximately 10% of patients transfused. That is an astounding number, and today transfusion liberalization in the face of such a risk might be considered reprehensible. The reader should be cautioned, however, that although the blood supply is the safest it has ever been with regard particularly to viral transmission, those risks will never be zero, and other problems of transfusion have simply replaced viral transmission as being of key importance. Therefore, Chapter 7 is must reading for all who wish to be educated in transfusion and surgery. The readers should be cautioned that the data are, of course, relevant to the time at which the chapter was written (the late 1990s), and the seemingly wonderfully low risks of viral transmission should not be interpreted as reasons to liberalize transfusion practice.

The second group of chapters, 8–28, deals with issues that have a wide range of applicability through many surgical subspecialties. These chapters, perhaps more than any other group, relate this text to the rapid changes in transfusion medicine. Many of the topics are timely and represent new modes of harvesting, conserving, or applying blood transfusion. Chapter 8 looks at preoperative autologous donation of blood (predominately red cell products). Considerable controversy rages concerning which surgeries it is appropriate to store autologous blood for, how many units of blood should be stored, and their cost effectiveness. Autologous blood has been called the blood of choice, but as allogeneic blood has fewer viral risks, is the "need" for autologous blood as great?

Chapter 9 examines the use of erythropoietin as a drug therapy to increase the production of red cells. This drug's use in the perioperative period should not be limited to only those patients with decreased erythropoiesis from renal failure, but may be used in other groups with anemia such that autologous predonation now becomes available for them as well. Once again, issues of cost effectiveness and appropriate target groups for therapy are raised. Physicians and laymen alike have been pursuing the dream of a blood substitute—an artificial product that will get away from many of the limitations of banked blood supplies. Chapter 10 discusses the current progress of contemporary blood substitutes. These are hemoglobin-based products and totally man-made perfluorocarbon emulsions. It may surprise the reader to know that both are well along the way through United States Food and Drug Administration testing. However, and as the chapter points out, each type of blood substitute technology will have its limitations. Neither should be looked at as equivalent to, or replacing, the use of allogeneic blood completely. Indeed, these products should be thought of as pharmaceutical infusion products, and they may well have treatment applications for diseases in which transfusion has not traditionally played any role.

Chapter 11 looks critically at the issues surrounding patients who refuse blood transfusion. Often this refusal is based on religious grounds, and thus numerous ethical and legal problems exist. The surgical practitioner should have a working knowledge of the issues surrounding patients who refuse a therapy that they might otherwise view as life-giving or mandatory. Several legal cases are reviewed in this chapter as well as the arguments regarding the views held by Jehovah's Witnesses. The time to think of one's reaction as a practitioner is in advance of being confronted with such difficult moral and legal judgments, rather than at the last minute in an emergency surgical situation.

Chapter 12 follows the theme of legal and ethical standards already introduced in the preceding chapter. The quality control of transfusions and hospital practice regulations have increased dramatically as transfusion has become a national and international issue. Hospital transfusion care committees as well as blood bank quality control committees are now being asked to perform functions they previously did not perform. Some of these functions include not only providing accountability but also guiding the appropriateness of transfusion through regulation and feedback to practitioners. Considerable controversy exists regarding how to best accomplish some of these goals, as well as what should be the actions of these committees. Chapter 13 is written by two legal counselors well acquainted with the problems of transfusion and medicine. Not only are there legal considerations in dealing with patients who refuse transfusion, but some case law now exists regarding liability of medical practitioners and the complications of transfusion. Particular cases are discussed to illustrate certain points. In today's heightened medical-legal climate, this chapter is worthwhile and focused reading for a dose of reality regarding the impacts of the transfusion decision.

Chapter 14 looks at how one should resuscitate a bleeding patient. Clearly not all bleeding requires blood transfusion, and other interventions including judicious use of crystalloid and colloid volume infusions make a considerable difference before blood products are ever required. This chapter makes a point of providing a framework for how to approach a hemorrhaging patient, yet it does not attempt to settle once and for all the ongoing controversy of whether it is "better" to resuscitate with crystalloid or colloid infusions. Some patients have unique hemoglobin problems such as sickle cell disease, other hemoglobinopathies, polycythemia, and hemolytic anemias. Although surgical cure is not offered for these diseases, it may be relatively common for these patients to present to the operating room. If and when they do, there are often unanswered questions regarding transfusion decisions and the risks of certain therapies vis-à-vis their underlying disease. Chapter 15 looks at some of these very specific and difficult problems. All too often these disease states are rare enough that there are simply no outcome data to guide certain therapeutic decisions, but the explanations of the pathophysiology involved should help practitioners.

Although Chapters 5 and 6 lay wonderful groundwork regarding the physiological basis for coagulation, in terms of both platelet physiology and protein function, the application of that physiology to the hypo- and hypercoagulable patient in the operating room may be difficult. Chapter 16 goes further into the basis of coagulation and provides a rational (although not always widely practiced) series of approaches to coagulopathic patients. As noted before, all too often physicians struggle with the knowledge base necessary for understanding coagulation function. The tests and some of the effects on transfusion outcome are discussed when those tests are appropriately and timely applied. Patients may come to the operating room anticoagulated, and the decisions surrounding reversal of that anticoagulation or intervention in it are vexing.

Chapter 17 discusses the types of anticoagulation used both preoperatively and postoperatively. This chapter, although discussing heparin to some extent, does not focus greatly on large-dose heparin therapy for cardiopulmonary bypass, a complex subject dealt with in Chapter 28.

Chapter 18 should serve as a resource for surgical physicians faced with a rare or congenital coagulopathy. Very often these congenital abnormalities will be known to a family or patient. Since they may well be worked up in the preoperative period, a hematologist may be able to coordinate the perioperative care of such patients. However, the surgical caregiver should have a source of information regarding these relatively infrequently encountered coagulopathies. In keeping with the theme of anticoagulation and management of coagulopathies, there is a special chapter on what to do with patients entering surgery with known hypercoagulable states (Chapter 19). Considerable research in the areas of protein C and S deficiency or ineffectivity has recently been advanced. The effectivity of hypercoagulability probably goes far beyond simply congenital coagulopathies and may influence platelet adhesiveness (incidence of vascular atherosclerosis) and perioperative embolism, myocardial infarction, graft occlusions, and other adverse outcomes. Chapter 19 discusses some of the new research and thinking regarding these very difficult patients.

Chapter 3 gives a wonderful introduction into the physiology of oxygen supply and demand. In the operating room, that basic science is necessary, but techniques for measurement of these parameters must be applied to those patients who are critically ill. Chapter 20 discusses a little of the technologies involved but more extensively looks at some provocative research that suggests that matching supply or exceeding the demands can, in some critically ill patients, prove beneficial. This chapter has implications not only in the operating room but also in intensive care units. It stands alone as a chapter, the likes of which this editor has never before seen summarized. It asks the question, when is enough oxygen transport enough, and is too much even better? Like so many other chapters, it is timely but limited to the available research today.

Chapter 21 provides an overview of blood conservation techniques. Many methods exist to avoid allogeneic transfusion, but for surgical practitioners it is worth noting that many techniques that can be used in anesthesia and surgery actually lessen the bleeding and therefore the requirement for transfusion. One example is the use of regional anesthesia in certain procedures; another might be the use of deliberate ("controlled") hypotensive anesthesia. These techniques are not universally effective and may be contraindicated in some surgeries or with certain disease states.

Although conservation of blood loss through anesthesia techniques may be useful, these techniques cannot salvage blood intraoperatively, and Chapter 22 discusses acute normovolemic hemodilution, red cell salvage, and harvest of platelet-rich plasma. These techniques are constantly undergoing change, and new creative techniques, technologies, and applications are being introduced continuously. Debate now rages over whether certain of these autologous blood-saving techniques are as effective as or more effective than autologous predeposit. Furthermore, the timely question of cost effectiveness is important for each of these technologies, as well as the comparisons made between them.

Massive hemorrhage and therefore massive transfusion are an occasional event in the operating room and intensive care unit. The frequency of these events depends in some part on the nature of the caseload for which a given facility provides care. Undoubtedly transfusion in this setting is lifesaving, but there are numerous particular biochemical, pathophysiological, and coagulopathic abnormalities specific to massive transfusion. Chapter 23 discusses these idiosyncrasies of massive transfusion.

One of the problems with massive hemorrhage is hypothermia. In modern operating rooms, and particularly after cardiopulmonary bypass, core body temperature may be depressed. The effects of hypothermia may cause further blood loss that can compound the need for transfusion. One should remember that it may not be the core body temperature that is important for coagulation but the temperature at the wound edge, and often this is considerably below that measured in the esophagus or rectum. Chapter 24 focuses on the research performed with hypothermia and hemorrhage.

Fresh frozen plasma is perhaps the most overused or inappropriately transfused blood product. Today, it has no indication for volume replacement, and since most coagulation protein precursors are present in the plasma in great excess of their critical minimum levels, truly large amounts of blood loss can be tolerated before the effects of hemodilution require the transfusion of fresh frozen plasma. Because the viral transmission by blood products has been greatly reduced in the recent past, there is still no reason to liberalize the indications for fresh frozen plasma. Chapter 25 therefore forms a wonderful framework for understanding the indications and applications of fresh frozen plasma.

Aprotinin, DDAVP, and other lysine analogue drugs have been given to cardiopulmonary bypass patients and in hepatic transplantation, as well as in many other surgeries. The pharmacology of these drugs and their impact on blood loss and transfusion requirements are discussed in Chapter 26. The question of cost effectiveness with these drugs is, again, an important one.

Fibrin glues have been used in certain surgeries to decrease hemorrhage, and in the United States these glues are made from cryoprecipitate. Chapter 27 examines the use of and some recipes for making fibrin glue in the operating room. In some surgeries in which patients are at risk for microvascular bleeding, fibrin glue can be effective in halting oozing. But, like so many other events in surgery, planning ahead for this therapy is useful.

The third group of chapters, 28–36, examines the use of blood in certain surgical subspecialties. Again, the final chapter attempts to summarize a wide range of the information presented throughout the book with a careful look at how the physician actually arrives at the decision to transfuse a given patient.

A tremendously complex subject for which there has been much research, disagreement, and controversy is that of coagulation dysfunction—bleeding and transfusion in cardiac surgery. Because cardiovascular disease is the largest killer in the United States, and more than 400,000 patients undergo cardiopulmonary bypass procedures each year, changes in therapy in this group of patients have far-reaching effects. Chapter 28 is an expertly crafted summary of the basic science and therapeutic options. This chapter has complementary information in Chapter 26, as well as in the early chapters on platelet function (Chapter 5), the physiology of hemostasis (Chapter 6), and coagulation monitoring (Chapter 16). There is still no agreement on indications for transfusion in cardiac surgery, and the utilization of blood products is highly variable from one institution to another.

In one sense, peripheral vascular surgery patients are similar to ischemic cardiac disease patients in that their disease processes are probably caused by many of the same factors. But these patients may have transfusion triggers different from those undergoing cardiopulmonary bypass. Most will have coronary artery disease present that has not been bypassed or angioplastied; therefore, they may be less tolerant of even mild and moderate anemia, compared with those who have had a partial or total correction of their coronary disease. Also, because patients with peripheral vascular disease tend to be relatively hypercoagulable as a group, issues of graft thrombosis are of concern. The potential for massive blood loss is present with ruptured vascular lesions, and some of these concerns are discussed in Chapter 29.

Liver transplantation represents both an advance for care of end-stage hepatic disease and one of the most important pressures on the blood supply in the United States. Because these operations can result in unpredictable extreme hemorrhaging, institutions and cities where active transplant programs are underway are quite familiar with the demands that an active program can create. Other solid organ transplants are discussed in Chapter 30.

Blood demands and opportunities are unique for patients undergoing orthopedic surgery. Some procedures, particularly total hip arthroplasty, major pelvic surgery, and extensive spine surgery, may have extensive blood losses. For some of these procedures, the techniques that the anesthesia team can employ (as described in Chapter 21) may be applied to reduce the transfusion requirement. The use of autologous predonation of blood is uniquely suited for orthopedic surgery, as many of these cases are relatively elective, thereby giving time for blood to be harvested. Since autologous blood is so widely used in orthopedic surgery, this specialty's experience with it is extensive. Yet, considerable controversy rages over whether the indications for reinfusion of autologous blood should be the same as those for allogeneic blood, or somehow different and more liberal. The assessment of that controversy can be seen in the variability of reports that examine the appropriateness of transfusion in orthopedic surgery (Chapter 31).

Transfusion in obstetrical patients has unique features, in terms of both the ability for sudden and poorly controlled hemorrhage and in some of the central nervous system sequelae, as well as the risks of allo-immunization in this child-bearing age group. Patients undergoing major trauma and burns also have unique transfusion considerations. Some of these overlap with the discussion of massive transfusion, but there are considerable coagulation issues as well. The pediatric patient may be unable to tolerate anemia as well as an adult, and neonates compared with 2-year-olds have profoundly different physiologies. Considerations of transfusion volume, biochemistry, and hypothermia are therefore issues of great concern. The above-named subjects are covered in Chapters 32, 33, and 34. Chapter 35 examines the use of blood and risks for hemorrhage in neurosurgery. Specific concerns regarding brain oxygen supply/demand, uniqueness of the blood brain barrier, and vascular spasm are all discussed. The critical care postoperative setting is also a unique area wherein transfusion utilization may have many unique and not fully understood concerns. Anemia and the postoperative period are discussed in Chapter 36.

Lastly, and as a summary, Chapter 37 examines the actual decision to transfuse. This focuses mostly on the decision to infuse a red cell product. Often in the surgical arena, the decision to transfuse a unit of blood is based on an emotional uneasiness among practitioner decision makers. There is a view that transfusion of blood is a preventive measure rather than a treatment. There is no desire to wait until dire circumstances are encountered and the limits of human physiology are tested. One cannot find argument with that general philosophy regarding red cell transfusion, but it is interesting to consider all the potential information that could and perhaps should go into a decision to transfuse. Not only are the risks of transfusion important, but the relative consequences of transfusion or withholding blood should be considered. In a sense, all the information presented in the prior 36 chapters is important, weighing on that one instant when a decision is made to transfuse. Chapter 37 therefore examines how the decision is or should be made and takes perhaps a philosophical view that transfusion should not be an emotional decision, but one of risk and benefit.

In summary, this text is written in an attempt to provide information regarding blood utilization to the group of physicians and other health care practitioners who use the greatest amount of blood in the United States: the surgical subspecialist. The physiology is fascinating, the problems are complex, the solutions are varied and creative, and considerable controversy rages in and between many subspecialty areas regarding transfusion issues. As risks of transfusion change (viral transmission decreases, cost and immunosuppressive risks are better understood), the issues, controversies, and solutions are in a constant state of debate. What an exciting time to be involved with transfusion medicine. Perhaps this volume will make a difference in some patient's care!

Acknowledgment

The editors gratefully acknowledge the secretarial assistance of Donna J. Rowe and Marlys Bauer, who have provided support, organization, extensive communication, and other contributions all too innumerable to make this project possible.

B.D.S.
R.B.C.
S.A.G.

Contributors

Ronald J. Alvarez, MD
Resident
Department of Otolaryngology
Temple University School of Medicine
Philadelphia, Pennsylvania

Linda S. Barnes, BA
Manager
Quality Assurance/Regulatory Affairs
Puget Sound Blood Program
Seattle, Washington

Kenneth A. Bauer, MD
Associate Professor of Medicine
Harvard Medical School
Chief
Hematology-Oncology Section
Brocton-Westbury VA Medical Center
West Roxbury, Massachusetts

Simon Body, MD, MHB, MB, ChB
Instructor
Harvard Medical School
Director of Thoracic Anesthesia
Brigham & Women's Hospital
Boston, Massachusetts

Mark Brecher, MD
Associate Professor of Pathology
Transfusion Medicine Service
University of North Carolina Hospital
Chapel Hill, North Carolina

Oswaldo Castro, MD, FACP
Professor of Medicine and Pediatrics
Director, Sickle Cell Center
Howard University College of Medicine
Washington, District of Columbia

Edward Chen, MD
Instructor in Anesthesia
Harvard Medical School
Cardiac Anesthesia Group
Massachusetts General Hospital
Boston, Massachusetts

Keith D. Clancy, MD
Resident, General Surgery
Falk Research Fellow
Burn and Shock Trauma Institute
Loyola University Medical Center
Bolingbrook, Illinois

JA Cohen, BS, MS, MD
Chief Resident
Department of Pathology and
Laboratory Medicine
University of North Carolina Hospital
Chapel Hill, North Carolina

Philip Comp, MD, PhD, FACP
Associate Chief of Staff for Research
Oklahoma City Veterans Hospital
University Hospital
Oklahoma City, Oklahoma

Charles J. Coté, MD
Professor of Anesthesia and Pediatrics
Northwestern University Medical School
Vice Chairman
Department of Pediatric Anesthesia
Children's Memorial Hospital
Chicago, Illinois

Richard B. Counts, MD
Professor of Medicine
University of Washington School of Medicine
Executive Director
Puget Sound Blood Center
Seattle, Washington

Michael N. D'Ambra, MD
Assistant Professor
Harvard Medical School
Associate Anesthetist
Director, Cardiac Anesthesia Group
Massachusetts General Hospital
Boston, Massachusetts

Richard M. Dsida, MD
Instructor
Department of Anesthesiology
Attending Anesthesiologist
The Children's Memorial Hospital
Chicago, Illinois

Mark H. Ereth, MD
Assistant Professor of Anesthesiology
Mayo Medical School
Consultant in Anesthesiology
Mayo Clinic
Rochester, Minnesota

Richard L. Gamelli, MD, FACS
Professor of Surgery and Pediatrics
Loyola University
Chicago Stritch School of Medicine
Director, Burn and Shock Trauma Institute
Loyola University Medical Center
Maywood, Illinois

Thomas A. Gasior, MD
Associate Professor of Anesthesiology
University of Pittsburgh School of Medicine
Presbyterian University Hospital
Pittsburgh, Pennsylvania

Larry M. Gentilello, MD
Assistant Professor, Surgery
Associate Director
Surgical Critical Care Unit
University of Washington, Harborview Medical Center
Seattle, Washington

Steven A. Gould, MD
Professor
Department of Surgery
University of Illinois College of Medicine
Chicago, Illinois
President, Northfield Laboratories, Inc.
Evanston, Illinois

A. Gerson Greenburg, MD, PhD, FACS
Professor of Surgery
Brown University
Surgeon-in-Chief
The Miriam Hospital
Providence, Rhode Island

Douglas M. Hansell, MD, MPH
Assistant Professor, Anesthesia
Harvard University
Massachusetts General Hospital
Boston, Massachusetts

Jan Hemstad, MD
Chief
Division of General Anesthesia
Department of Anesthesiology
Providence Medical Center
Seattle, Washington

Robert S. Hillman, MD
Professor of Medicine
University of Vermont College of Medicine
Burlington, Vermont
Chairman
Department of Medicine
Maine Medical Center
Portland, Maine

Kaj H. Johansen, MD, PhD, FACS
Professor of Surgery
University of Washington School of Medicine
Seattle, Washington
Director
Surgical Education
Providence Medical Center

Yoogoo Kang, MD
Professor of Anesthesiology
University of Pittsburgh School of Medicine
Director
Hepatic Transplantation Anesthesiology
Presbyterian University Hospital
Pittsburgh, Pennsylvania

Agnes Kim, MD
Clinical Pathologist
New England Baptist Hospital
Boston, Massachusetts

Auda Kuo, AB
Medical Student
University of California San Francisco
San Francisco, California

Steven Labensky, Esq
Attorney at Law
Lewis & Roca
Phoenix, Arizona

Jerrold H. Levy, MD
Associate Professor of Anesthesia
Emory University School of Medicine
Division of Cardiothoracic Anesthesia and Critical Care
The Emory Clinic
Atlanta, Georgia

James MacPherson, AAS, BS, MS, MPH
Executive Director
Council of Community Blood Centers
Washington, District of Columbia

Joseph McCarthy, MD
Associate Clinical Professor
Orthopedic Surgery
Tufts University School of Medicine
New England Baptist Hospital
Boston, Massachusetts

Michael M. Millenson, MD
Assistant Professor of Medicine
Temple University School of Medicine
Director of Hematology and Associate Member
Fox Chase Cancer Center
Philadelphia, Pennsylvania

Antonio Morales, MD
Assistant Professor of Anesthesiology
Emory University School of Medicine
Division of Cardiothoracic Anesthesiology
The Emory Clinic
Staff Anesthesiologist
Crawford Long Hospital of Emory University
Atlanta, Georgia

Gerald S. Moss, MD
Michael Reese Hospital and Medical Center
University of Illinois College of Medicine
Chicago, Illinois

Cynthia M. Murray, MSA, MT(ASCP), SBB
Transfusion Service Manager
Puget Sound Blood Center
Seattle, Washington

Patricia O'Donnell, RN, BSN, ONC, CNOR, CCRN
New England Baptist Hospital
Boston, Massachusetts

William C. Oliver, Jr., MD
Assistant Professor of Anesthesiology
Mayo Medical School
Mayo Clinic
Rochester, Minnesota

Mick J. Perez-Cruet, MS, MD
Chief Resident
Department of Neurosurgery
Baylor College of Medicine
Houston, Texas

Lawrence D. Petz, MD
Professor
Department of Pathology
and Laboratory Medicine
UCLA
Director of Transfusion Medicine
UCLA Medical Center
Los Angeles, California

Mark A. Popovsky, MD
Adjunct Clinical Professor of Pathology and Laboratory Medicine
Boston University School of Medicine
and University Hospital
Medical Director
American Red Cross Blood Services
Dedham, Massachusetts

Thomas H. Price, MD
Professor
Department of Medicine
Division of Hematology
University of Washington School of Medicine
Medical Director and Chief Medical Officer
Puget Sound Blood Center
Seattle, Washington

Sohail Rana, MD, FAAP
Associate Professor
Director, Pediatric Hematology/Oncology
Howard University College of Medicine
Washington, District of Columbia

R. Lawrence Reed, II, MD
Associate Professor of Surgery and Anesthesiology
Duke University Medical Center
Director
Trauma Center and Surgical Care Unit
Durham, North Carolina

Alexander P. Reiner, MD
Senior Fellow/Acting Instructor
Department of Medicine
University of Washington School of Medicine
Director of Medical Education
Puget Sound Blood Center
Seattle, Washington

Paula J. Santrach, MD
Assistant Professor
Laboratory Medicine and Pathology
Consultant
Division of Transfusion Medicine
Director
Intraoperative Autotransfusion Team
Mayo Clinic
Rochester, Minnesota

Raymond Sawaya, MD
Professor and Chairman
Department of Neurosurgery
MD Anderson Cancer Center
Houston, Texas

Hansa L. Sehgal, BS
Northfield Laboratories, Inc.
Evanston, Illinois

Lakshman R. Sehgal, PhD
Northfield Laboratories, Inc.
Evanston, Illinois

Sherrill J. Slichter, MD
Professor of Medicine
Division of Hematology
University of Washington School of Medicine
Director
Research and Education
Puget Sound Blood Center
Seattle, Washington

Richard K. Spence, MD
Professor of Surgery
Cooper Hospital/University Medical Center
Assistant Dean for Education and Student Affairs
Robert Wood Johnson Medical School
Camden, New Jersey

Bruce D. Spiess, MD
Associate Professor of Anesthesiology
Chief, Division of Cardiothoracic Anesthesia
University of Washington School of Medicine
Seattle, Washington

Linda Stehling, MD, BSI
Vice President and Director
Medical and Regulatory Affairs
Blood Systems, Inc.
Scottsdale, Arizona

Arthur R. Thompson, MD, PhD
Professor of Medicine
University of Washington School of Medicine
Director
Hemophilia Program and Coagulation Laboratory
Puget Sound Blood Center
Seattle, Washington

Robert L. Thurer, MD
Associate Professor of Surgery
Harvard Medical School
Associate Cardiothoracic Surgeon
Beth Israel Hospital
Boston, Massachusetts

Roderick H. Turner, MD
Professor Emeritus
Orthopedic Surgery
Tofts University School of Medicine
Fort Myers, Florida

Robert G. Valeri, MD
Director
Naval Blood Research Laboratory
Boston University School of Medicine
Boston, Massachusetts

Mark A. Warner, MD
Associate Professor
Department of Anesthesiology
Mayo Clinic
Rochester, Minnesota

Robert M. Winslow, MD
Professor of Medicine
University of California at San Diego
Chief, Hematology/Oncology
Department of Veterans Affairs
Medical Center
San Diego, California

Ian Wright, MB, BS, MRCP, FRCA
Assistant Professor
Department of Anesthesiology
University of Washington
Seattle, Washington

Howard L. Zauder, MD, PhD
Professor Emeritus of Anesthesiology and Pharmacology
State University of New York
Health Science Center
Chief, Anesthesia Section
Carl T. Hayden Veterans Affairs Medical Center
Scottsdale, Arizona

Contents

SECTION IV OPERATIVE TRANSFUSION MANAGEMENT

SECTION V TRANSFUSION SURGICAL SUBSPECIALTY CONCERNS

Section I
Introduction

Chapter 1

A History of Transfusion*

The ancient Greeks believed that blood was formed in the heart and passed through the veins to the rest of the body, where it was consumed. Arteries were part of an independent system transporting air from the lungs. Although Erasistratus (circa 270 BC) had imagined the heart as a pump, his idea was ahead of its time. As long as veins and arteries were dead-end channels transporting blood and air, there was little need for a pump in the system. Although Galen (131–201 AD) finally proved that arteries contain blood, communication with the venous system was not suspected. Blood, formed in the liver, merely passed through the blood vessels and heart on its way to the periphery (1). These teachings remained in place for 1400 years until they were swept away in 1628 by Harvey's discovery of circulation.

The realization that blood moved in a circulating stream opened the way to experiments on vascular infusion. In 1642, George von Wahrendorff injected wine (2), and in 1656, Christopher Wren and Robert Boyle injected opium and other drugs (3) intravenously into dogs. The latter studies, performed at Oxford, were the inspiration for Richard Lower's experiments in animal transfusion.

THE FIRST ANIMAL TRANSFUSION

Richard Lower (1631–1691) was a student at Oxford when Christopher Wren and Robert Boyle began their experiments on infusion. In due course, Lower joined their scientific group and studied the intravenous injection of opiates, emetics, and other substances into living animals (4). In time, the transfusion of blood itself became the objective. The announcement of the first successful transfusion, performed by Richard Lower at Oxford in February 1665, was published as a notation (5) and as a full description (6, 7) in the *Philosophical Transactions of the Royal Society*.

These studies inevitably led to the transfusion of animal blood to humans. In England, this occurred on November 23, 1667, when Lower and Edmund King transfused sheep blood into a man named Arthur Coga (8). Described by Samuel Pepys as "a little frantic," Coga was paid 20 shillings to accept this tranfusion with the expectation that it might have a beneficial "cooling" effect. One week later, Coga appeared before the Society and claimed to be a new man, although Pepys concluded he was "cracked a little in the head" (7). However, this was not the first transfusion performed in humans. The credit for that accomplishment belongs to Jean Baptiste Denis (1635–1704), who had performed the first human transfusion several months earlier in Paris.

THE FIRST ANIMAL-TO-HUMAN TRANSFUSION

Denis probably read of Lower's experiments in the *Journal des Savants* on January 31, 1667, and he began his own studies about a month later (9, 10). The first human transfusion was then performed on June 15, 1667, when Denis administered the blood of a lamb to a 15-year-old boy (11).

Although discovery of circulation suggested the idea of transfusion, indications for the procedure remained uninformed. Transfusion was still thought to alter behavior and possibly achieve rejuvenation. The blood of young dogs

*Abstracted and modified from Rossi EC, Simon TL, Moss GS, Gould SA. Transfusion into the next millennium. In: Rossi EC, Simon TL, Moss GS, Gould SA, eds. Principles of transfusion medicine. 2nd ed. Baltimore: Williams & Wilkins, 1996.

made old dogs seem frisky; the blood of lions was proposed as a cure for cowardice (10); and 5 months later, Arthur Coga would be transfused with sheep blood for its presumed "cooling" effect. Denis used animal blood for transfusion because he thought it was "less full of impurities" (11):

> *Sadness, Envy, Anger, Melancholy, Disquiet and generally all the Passions, are as so many causes which trouble the life of man, and corrupt the whole substance of the blood: Whereas the life of Brutes is much more regular, and less subject to all these miseries. . . .*

It is thus ironic that the symptoms of the first transfusion recipient may have been explained in part by profound anemia, and that the single transfusion of lamb blood may have produced some temporary amelioration based on increased oxygen transport. Denis described the case as follows (11):

> *On the 15 of this Moneth, we happened upon a Youth aged between 15 and 16 years, who had for above two moneths bin tormented with a contumacious and violent fever, which obliged his Physitians to bleed him 20 times, in order to asswage the excessive heat.*
>
> *Before this disease, he was not observed to be of a lumpish dull spirit, his memory was happy enough, and he seem'd chearful and nimble enough in body; but since the violence of this fever his wit seem'd wholly sunk, his memory perfectly lost, and his body so heavy and drowsie that he was not fit for anything. I beheld him fall asleep as he sate at dinner, as he was eating his Breakfast, and in all occurrences where men seem most unlikely to sleep. If he went to bed at nine of the clock in the Evening, he needed to be wakened several times before he could be got to rise by nine the next morning, and he pass'd the rest of the day in an incredible stupidity.*
>
> *I attributed all these changes to the great evacuations of blood, the Physitians had been oblig'd to make for saving his life. . . .*

Three ounces of the boy's blood were exchanged for 9 ounces of lamb arterial blood. Several hours later he arose, and "for the rest of the day, he spent it with much more liveliness than ordinary." Thus, the first human transfusion, which was heterologous, was accomplished without any evident unfavorable effect.

Although the first two subjects transfused by Denis were not adversely affected, the third and fourth recipients both died. The death of the third subject was easily attributable to other causes. However, the fourth case initiated a sequence of events that put an end to transfusion for 150 years.

Anthony du Mauroy was a 34-year-old man who suffered from intermittent bouts of maniacal behavior. On December 19, 1667, Denis and his assistant, Paul Emmerez, removed 10 ounces of the man's blood and replaced it with 5 or 6 ounces of blood from the femoral artery of a calf. Failing to note any apparent improvement, they repeated the transfusion 2 days later. After the second transfusion, du Mauroy experienced a classic transfusion reaction (12):

> *His pulse rose presently, and soon after we observ'd a plentiful sweat over all his face. His pulse varied extremely at this instant, and he complain'd of great pains in his kidneys and that he was not well in his stomach.*

Du Mauroy fell asleep at about 10 o'clock in the evening. He awoke the following morning and "made a great glass full of urine, of a colour as black, as if it had been mixed with the soot of chimneys" (12). Two months later, the patient again became maniacal, and his wife again sought transfusion therapy. Denis was reluctant but finally gave in to her urgings. However, the transfusion could not be accomplished, and du Mauroy died the next evening.

The physicians of Paris strongly disapproved of the experiments on transfusion. Three of them approached du Mauroy's widow and encouraged her to lodge a malpractice complaint against Denis. She instead went to Denis and attempted to extort money from him in return for her silence. Denis refused and filed a complaint before the Lieutenant in Criminal Causes. During the subsequent hearing, evidence was introduced to indicate that Madame du Mauroy had poisoned her husband with arsenic. In a judgement handed down at the Chatelet in Paris on April 17, 1668, Denis was exonerated, and the woman was held for trial. The court also stipulated "that for the future no Transfusion should be made upon any Human Body but by the approbation of the Physicians of the Parisian Faculty" (13). At this point, transfusion research went into decline, and within 10 years it was prohibited in both France and England.

THE BEGINNINGS OF MODERN TRANSFUSION

After the edict that ended transfusion in the 17th century, the technique lay dormant for 150 years. Stimulated by earlier experiments by Leacock, transfusion was "resuscitated" and placed on a rational basis by James Blundell (1790–1877), a London obstetrician who had received his medical degree from the University of Edinburgh (14). Shortly after graduation, Blundell accepted a post in physiology and midwifery at Guy's Hospital. It was there that he began the experiments in transfusion that led to its rebirth. The frequency of postpartum hemorrhage and death troubled Blundell. In 1818 he wrote (15):

> *A few months ago I was requested to visit a woman who was sinking under uterine hemorrhage. . . . [H]er fate was decided, and notwithstanding every exertion of the medical attendants, she died in the course of two hours.*
>
> *Reflecting afterwards on this melancholy scene . . . [,] I could not forbear considering, that the patient might very probably have been saved by transfusion; and that . . . the vessels might have been replenished by means of the syringe with facility and promptitude.*

This opening statement introduced Blundell's epoch-making study, entitled "Experiments on the Transfusion of Blood by the Syringe" (15). Blundell described, in detail, a series of animal experiments. He demonstrated that a syringe could be used effectively to perform transfusion, that the lethal effects of arterial exsanguination could be reversed by the transfusion of either venous or arterial blood, that the injection of 5 drams (20 mL) of air into the veins of a small dog was not fatal, but that transfusion across species ultimately was lethal to the recipient (15). Thus, Blundell was the first to state clearly that only human blood should be used for human transfusion. This latter conclusion was confirmed in France by Dumas and Prevost, who demonstrated that the infusion of heterologous blood into an exsanguinated animal produced only temporary improvement and was followed by death within 6 days (16). These scientific studies provided the basis for Blundell's subsequent efforts in clinical transfusion.

The first well-documented transfusion with human blood took place on September 26, 1818 (17). The patient was an extremely emaciated man in his mid-30s who had pyloric obstruction caused by carcinoma. He received 12–14 ounces of blood in the course of 30 or 40 minutes. Despite an initial apparent improvement, the patient died 2 days later. The transfusion of women with postpartum hemorrhage was more successful. In all, Blundell performed 10 transfusions of which 5 were successful. Three of the unsuccessful transfusions were performed on moribund patients, the fourth was performed on a patient with puerperal sepsis, and the fifth was performed on the aforementioned patient with terminal carcinoma. Four of the successful transfusions were given for postpartum hemorrhage, and the fifth was administered to a boy who bled after amputation (14). Blundell also devised various instruments for the performance of transfusion. They included an "impellor," which collected blood in a warmed cup and "impelled" the blood into the recipient via an attached syringe, and a "gravitator" (18) (Fig. 1.1), which received blood and delivered it by gravity through a long vertical cannula.

The writings of Blundell provided evidence against the use of animal blood in humans and established rational indications for transfusion. However, the gravitator (Fig. 1.1) graphically demonstrated the technical problems that remained to be solved. Blood from the donor, typically the patient's husband, flowed into a funnel-like device and down a flexible cannula into the patient's vein "with as little exposure as possible to air, cold and inanimate surface" (18). The amount of blood transfused was estimated from the amount spilled into the apparatus by the donor. In this clinical atmosphere, charged with apprehension and anxiety, the amount of blood issuing from a donor easily could be overstated. Clotting within the apparatus then ensured that only a portion of that blood actually reached the patient. Thus, the amount of blood actually transfused may have been seriously overestimated. This may explain the apparent absence of transfusion reactions. Alternatively, reactions may have been

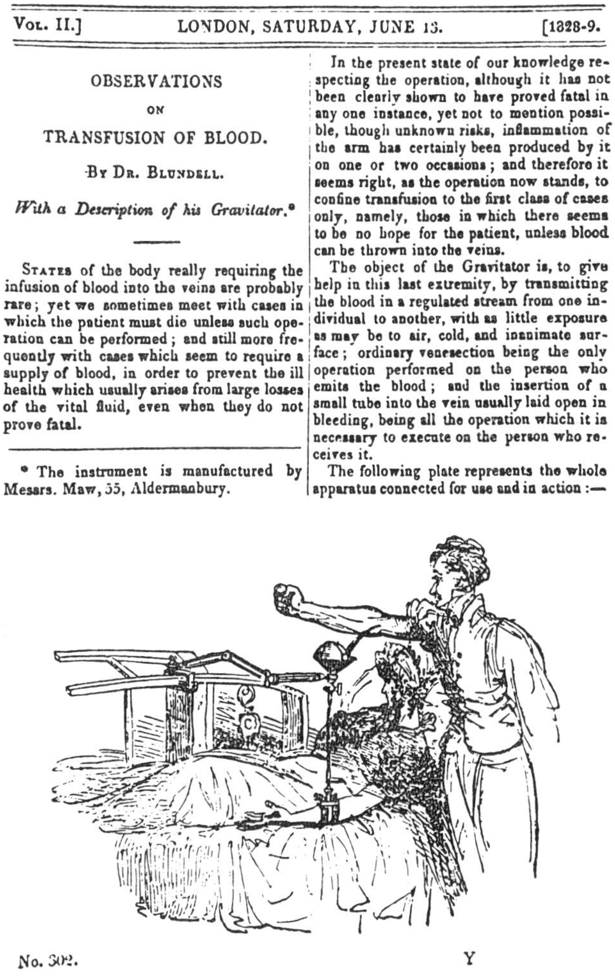
Vol. II.] LONDON, SATURDAY, JUNE 13. [1828-9.

OBSERVATIONS ON TRANSFUSION OF BLOOD.

By Dr. Blundell.

*With a Description of his Gravitator.**

States of the body really requiring the infusion of blood into the veins are probably rare; yet we sometimes meet with cases in which the patient must die unless such operation can be performed; and still more frequently with cases which seem to require a supply of blood, in order to prevent the ill health which usually arises from large losses of the vital fluid, even when they do not prove fatal.

* The instrument is manufactured by Messrs. Maw, 55, Aldermanbury.

In the present state of our knowledge respecting the operation, although it has not been clearly shown to have proved fatal in any one instance, yet not to mention possible, though unknown risks, inflammation of the arm has certainly been produced by it on one or two occasions; and therefore it seems right, as the operation now stands, to confine transfusion to the first class of cases only, namely, those in which there seems to be no hope for the patient, unless blood can be thrown into the veins.

The object of the Gravitator is, to give help in this last extremity, by transmitting the blood in a regulated stream from one individual to another, with as little exposure as may be to air, cold, and inanimate surface; ordinary venesection being the only operation performed on the person who emits the blood; and the insertion of a small tube into the vein usually laid open in bleeding, being all the operation which it is necessary to execute on the person who receives it.

The following plate represents the whole apparatus connected for use and in action:—

No. 302. Y

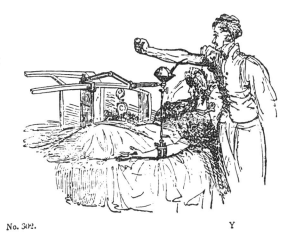

Figure 1.1. Blundell's "gravitator." (Reprinted with permission from Blundell J. Observations on transfusions of blood. Lancet 1828;2:321.)

unrecognized. Patients submitted for tranfusion were frequently agonal. As Blundell (18) stated, "it seems right, as the operation now stands, to confine transfusion to the first class of cases only, namely, those in which there seems to be no hope for the patient, unless blood can be thrown into the veins." Under these circumstances, "symptoms" associated with an "unsuccessful" transfusion might be ascribed to the agonal state rather than the transfusion itself. For a time, the problem of coagulation during transfusion was circumvented by the use of defibrinated blood. This undoubtedly increased the amount of blood actually transfused. However, there were numerous fatalities. Interestingly, these deaths were attributed to intravascular coagulation when in actuality they were probably fatal hemolytic reactions caused by the infusion of incompatible blood (19). Transfusion at the end of the 19th century, therefore, was neither safe nor efficient.

In the latter half of the 19th century, there were many attempts to render transfusion a more predictable and less arduous procedure. In 1869, Braxton-Hicks (20) performed a number of transfusions in women with obstetrical bleeding, using blood anticoagulated with phosphate solutions. Many patients were in extremis, and ultimately all died. Unfortunately, a detailed description of terminal symptoms was not provided (20). Some investigators attempted to rejuvenate animal-to-human tranfusion, and Hasse persisted in this approach despite obviously disastrous results. Studies by Ponfick and by Landois finally put an end to this practice. Ponfick, in carefully controlled studies, confirmed the lethality of heterologous transfusion and identified the resulting hemoglobinuria along with its donor erythrocytes by human serum in vitro (2).

Frustration with blood as a transfusion product led to even more bizarre innovations. From 1873 to 1880, cow, goat, and even human milk was transfused as a blood substitute (21). The rationale was derived from an earlier suggestion that the fat particles of milk could be converted into blood cells. Milk transfusion was particularly popular in the United States (21), where the practice of animal-to-human transfusion was recorded as late as 1890 (22). Fortunately, these astonishing practices were discontinued when saline solutions were introduced as "a life-saving measure" and "a substitute for the transfusion of blood" (23). A passage from an article written by Bull in 1884 (23) is particularly instructive:

> *[T]he danger from loss of blood, even to two-thirds of its whole volume, lies in the disturbed relationship between the calibre of the vessels and the quantity of the blood contained therein, and not in the diminished number of red blood corpuscles; and . . . this danger concerns the volume of the injected fluids also, it being a matter of indifference whether they be albuminous or containing blood corpuscles or not. . . .*

Mercifully, volume replacement with saline solutions deflected attention from the unpredictable and still dangerous practice of blood transfusion. Accordingly, transfusions were abandoned until interest was rekindled by the scientific and technical advances of the early 20th century.

THE 20TH CENTURY

The 20th century was ushered in by a truly monumental discovery. In 1900, Karl Landsteiner (1868–1943) observed that the sera of some individuals agglutinated the red cells of others. This study, published in 1901 in the *Wiener Klinische Wochenschrift* (24), revealed for the first time the celluar differences in individuals from the same species (25).

With the identification of blood groups A, B, and C (subsequently renamed group O) by Landsteiner and of group AB by Decastello and Sturli (26), the stage was set for the performance of safe transfusion. For this work, Landsteiner somewhat belatedly received the Nobel Prize in 1930. But even that high recognition does not adequately express the true magnitude of Landsteiner's discovery. His work was like a burst of light in a darkened room. He gave us our first glimpse of immunohematology and transplantation biology and provided the tools for important discoveries in genetics, anthropology, and forensic medicine. Viewed from this perspective, the identification of human blood groups is one of only a few scientific discoveries of the 20th century that changed all of our lives (25). And yet the translation of Landsteiner's discovery into transfusion practice took many years.

At the turn of the century, the effective transfer of blood from one individual to another remained a formidable task. Clotting was still uncontrolled, quickly occluded transfusion devices, and frustrated most efforts. Thus, in 1901 the methods used in transfusion were too primitive to demonstrate the importance of Landsteiner's discovery. Indeed, the study of in vitro red cell agglutination may have seemed rather remote from the technical problems that demanded attention. An intermediate step was required before the importance of Landsteiner's breakthrough could be perceived and the appropriate changes could be incorporated into practice. This process was initiated by Alexis Carrel (1873–1944), another Nobel laureate, who developed a surgical procedure that permitted direct transfusion via arteriovenous anastomosis.

Carrel (27) introduced the technique of end-to-end vascular anastomosis with a triple-threaded suture. This procedure brought the ends of vessels in close apposition and preserved luminal continuity, thus avoiding leakage or thrombosis. This technique paved the way for successful organ transplantation and brought Carrel the Nobel Prize in 1912. It was also adapted by Carrel (28) and others (29, 30) to the performance of transfusion. Crile (29) introduced the use of a metal tube to facilitate the placement of sutures, and Bernheim (30) used a two-piece cannula to unite the artery to the vein (Fig. 1.2). Because these procedures usually culminated in the sacrifice of the two vessels, they were not performed frequently. Direct transfusion was also fraught with danger. In a passage written two decades later, the procedure was recalled in the following manner (31):

> *[T]he direct artery to vein anastomosis was the best method available but was often very difficult or even unsuccessful. And, what was almost as bad, one never knew how much blood one had transfused at any moment or when to stop (unless the donor collapsed). (I remember one such collapse in which the donor almost died—and the surgeon needed to be revived.)*

Despite these many difficulties, direct transfusion via arteriovenous anastomosis, for the first time, efficiently transferred blood from one individual to another. In the process it also disclosed fatal hemolytic reactions that were undeniably caused by transfusion (32). However, the relationship of these fatal reactions to Landsteiner's discovery was not recognized until Reuben Ottenberg (1882–1959) demonstrated the importance of compatibility testing.

Ottenberg's interest in transfusion began in 1906 while an intern at German (now Lenox Hill) Hospital in New York. There, Ottenberg learned of Landsteiner's discovery and began pretransfusion compatibility testing in 1907 (33). He accepted an appointment at Mount Sinai Hospital the following year and continued his studies on transfusion. In 1913, he published the report that conclusively demonstrated the importance of preliminary blood testing for the prevention of transfusion "accidents" (34). This was not Ottenberg's only contribution. He observed the Mendelian inheritance of blood groups (35), and he was the first to recognize the relative unimportance of donor antibodies and, consequently, the "universal" utility of type O blood donors (36).

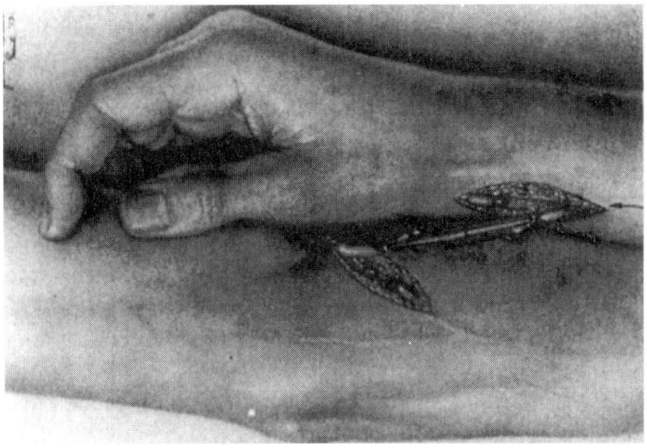

Figure 1.2. Direct transfusion by arteriovenous anastomosis via the two-piece cannula of Bernheim. (Reprinted with permission from Bernheim BM. Blood transfusion: hemorrhage and the anaemias. Philadelphia: J.B. Lippincott, 1917.)

Further advances in immunohematology were to occur in succeeding decades. The MNSs and P systems were described in the period between 1927 and 1947 (37). The Rh system was discovered in connection with an unusual transfusion reaction. In 1939, Levine and Stetson (38) described an immediate reaction in a group O woman who had received her husband's group O blood shortly after delivery of a stillborn fetus with erythroblastosis. This sequence of events suggested that the infant had inherited a red cell agglutinogen from the father that was foreign to the mother. At about the same time, Landsteiner and Wiener (39) harvested a rhesus monkey red cell antibody from immunized guinea pigs and rabbits. This antibody agglutinated 85% of human red blood cell samples ("Rh positive") and left 15% ("Rh negative") unaffected. When the experimentally induced antibody was tested in parallel with the serum from Levine's patient, a similar positive and negative distribution was observed, and the Rh system was discovered. Other red blood cell antigen systems were subsequently described, but when Rh immune globulin was introduced as a preventive measure for hemolytic disease of the newborn, it became one of the major public health advances of the century.

Despite the introduction of compatibility testing by Ottenberg, transfusion could not be performed frequently as long as arteriovenous anastomosis remained the procedure of choice. Using this method, Ottenberg needed 5 years to accumulate the 128 transfusions he reported in his study on pretransfusion testing (34). New techniques, such as Unger's two-syringe method introduced in 1915 (40) (Fig. 1.3), even-

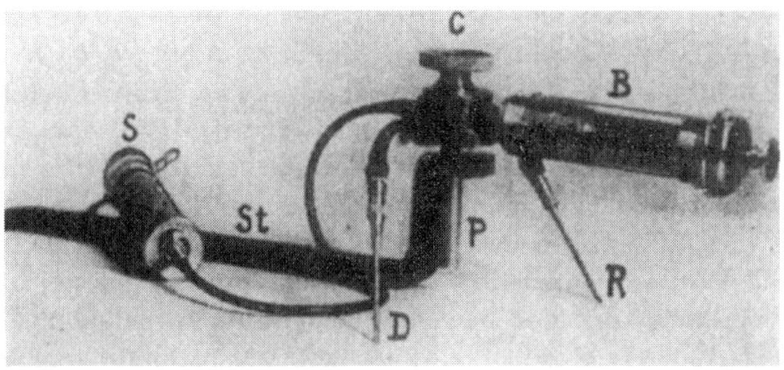

Figure 1.3. Unger's two-syringe, four-way stopcock method of indirect transfusion. (Reprinted with permission from Unger LJ. A new method of syringe transfusion. JAMA 1915;64:582.)

tually put an end to transfusion by arteriovenous anastomosis. However, transfusion did not become commonplace until anticoagulants were developed and direct methods of transfusion were rendered obsolete.

ANTICOAGULANTS, THE BLOOD BANK, AND COMPONENT THERAPY

The anticoagulant action of sodium citrate completely transformed the practice of transfusion. Early reports from Belgium (41) and Argentina (42) were followed by the work of Lewisohn (43) that established the optimal citrate concentration for anticoagulation. The work of Weil (44) then demonstrated the feasibility of refrigerated storage. Subsequently, Rous and Turner (45) developed the anticoagulant solution that was used during World War I (46). Despite its very large volume, this solution remained the anticoagulant of choice until World War II, when Loutit and Mollison (47) developed an acid-citrate-dextrose (ACD) solution used in a ratio of 70 mL of ACD to 450 mL of blood. ACD provided 3–4 weeks of preservation of a more concentrated red cell infusion. Thus, the two World Wars were the stimuli for the development of citrate anticoagulants and the introduction of indirect transfusions (48). For the first time, the donation process could be separated, in time and place, from the actual transfusion. Blood, drawn and set aside, now awaited the emergence of systems of storage and distribution. Again, it was the provision of medical support during armed conflict that stimulated these developments.

A blood transfusion service, organized by the Republican Army during the Spanish civil war (1936–1939), collected 9000 L of blood in citrate-dextrose anticoagulant for the treatment of battle casualties (49). At about that same time, Fantus (50) began the first hospital blood bank at Cook County Hospital in Chicago. His interest had been stimulated by Yudin's report (51) on the use of cadaveric blood in Russia. Apart from certain scruples attached to the use of cadaveric blood, Fantus reasoned that a transfusion service based on such a limited source of supply would be impractical. Accordingly, he established the principle of a "blood bank" from which blood could be withdrawn, provided it had previously been deposited. As Fantus (50) himself stated, "just as one cannot draw money from a bank unless one has deposited some, so the blood preservation department cannot supply blood unless as much comes in as goes out. The term 'blood bank' is not a mere metaphor." The development of anticoagulants and the concept of blood banks provided an infrastructure upon which a more elaborate blood services organization could be built. World War II was the catalyst for these further developments.

At the beginning of World War II, blood procurement programs were greatly expanded (48). In Great Britain, an efficient system had been developed through the organization of regional centers. When the war started, these centers, already in place, were able to increase their level of operation. In the United States, the use of plasma in the treatment of shock had led to the development of plasma collection facilities (52). The efficient long-term storage of plasma had been further facilitated by the process of lyophilization developed by Flosdorf and Mudd (53). In 1940, the United States organized a program for the collection of blood and the shipment of plasma to Europe. The American Red Cross, through its local chapters, participated in the project, which collected 13 million units by the end of the war (48).

The national program of the American Red Cross ceased at the end of the war. However, many local chapters continued to help recruit donors for local blood banks, and in 1948, the first regional Red Cross blood center was begun in Rochester, New York. By 1949–1950 in the United States, the blood procurement system included 1500 hospital blood banks, 1100 of which performed all blood bank functions. There were 46 nonhospital blood banks and 31 Red Cross Regional Blood Centers. By 1962, these numbers had grown to 4400 hospital blood banks, 123 nonhospital blood banks, and 55 American Red Cross Regional Blood Centers, and the number of units collected had grown to between 5 and 6 million per year (54).

During this time, blood was collected through steel needles and rubber tubing into rubber-stoppered bottles. After washing and resterilization, the materials were reused. On occasion, "vacuum bottles" were used to speed up the collection. However, the high incidence of pyrogenic reactions soon led to the development of disposable plastic blood collection equipment.

In a classic article written in 1952, Walter and Murphy (55) described a closed, gravity technique for whole-blood preservation. They used a laminar flow phlebotomy needle, an interval donor tube, and a collapsible bag of polyvinyl resin designed so that the unit could be assembled and ready for use after sterilization by steam. The polyvinyl resin was chemically inert to biological fluids and nonirritating to tissue. Shortly thereafter, Gibson and colleagues (56) demonstrated that plastic systems were more flexible and permitted the removal of plasma after sedimentation or centrifugation. In time, glass was replaced by plastic, and component therapy began to emerge.

Component and derivative therapy began during World War II when Edwin J. Cohn developed the cold ethanol method of plasma fractionation (57). As a result of his work, albumin, γ globulin, and fibrinogen became available for clinical use. As plastic equipment replaced glass, component separation became a more widespread practice, and the introduction of automated cell separators provided even greater capability in this area.

Clotting factor concentrates for the treatment of patients with hemophilia and other hemorrhagic disorders were also developed during the postwar era. Although antihemophilic globulin had been described in 1937 (58), unconcentrated plasma was the only therapeutic material until Pool and Shannon discovered that factor VIII could be harvested in the cryoprecipitable fraction of blood (59). This resulted in the development of cryoprecipitate, which was introduced in 1965 for the treatment of hemophilia. Pool and Shannon showed that cryoprecipitate could be made in a closed-bag system, and urged its harvest from as many donations as possible. The development of cyroprecipitate and other concentrates was the dawn of a "golden age" in the care of patients with hemophilia. Self-infusion programs, made possible by the technological advances in plasma fractionation, permitted early therapy and significantly reduced disability and unemployment. This golden age abruptly came to an end with the appearance of the acquired immunodeficiency syndrome (AIDS).

TRANSFUSION IN THE AGE OF TECHNOLOGY

In contrast to the past century's long ledger of lives lost because of the lack of blood, transfusion in the 20th century has saved countless lives. In 1937, during those early halcyon days of transfusion, Ottenberg (31) wrote the following:

> *Today tranfusion has become so safe and so easy to do that it is seldom omitted in any case in which it may be of benefit. Indeed the chief problem it presents is the findings of the large sums of money needed for the professional donors who now provide most of the blood.*

It is ironic that Ottenberg's statement should refer to paid donors and foreshadow difficulties yet to come. However, experience to that point had not revealed the problem of viral disease transmission. More transfusions would have to be administered before that problem would be perceived.

After the introduction of anticoagulants, blood transfusions were given in progressively increasing numbers. At Mount Sinai Hospital in New York, the number of blood transfusions administered between 1923 and 1953 increased 20-fold (60, 61) (Table 1.1). This increase was particularly notable after the establishment of blood banks. It was during this period that Beeson wrote his classic description of transfusion-transmitted hepatitis (62). He had been alerted to the problem by the outbreaks of jaundice that followed inoculation programs with human serum during World War II (63). Thus, we entered a new era. Blood components not only saved lives but also transmitted disease. The discovery of the Australian antigen (64) and the subsequent definition of hepatitis A (65) and B (66) still left residual non-A and non-B disease (67), a gap largely filled by the recent discovery of the hepatitis C virus (68). However, it was the outbreak of AIDS that galvanized public attention to blood transfusion.

TABLE 1.1. INCREASE IN THE NUMBER OF BLOOD TRANSFUSIONS AT MOUNT SINAI HOSPITAL, NEW YORK, 1923–1953

Year	No. of Transfusions
1923	143
1932	477
1935	794
1938	Blood bank started
1941	2097
1952	2874
1953	3179

Adapted from Lewisohn R. Blood transfusion: 50 years ago and today. Surg Gynecol Obstet 1955;101:362.

The AIDS epidemic was first recognized in the United States, and the first case of AIDS associated with transfusion was observed in a 20-month-old infant (69). Subsequently, the suspicion that AIDS could be transmitted by transfusion was confirmed (70); the human immunodeficiency virus was identified (71, 72) and an effective test to detect the human immunodeficiency virus antibody was developed (73).

CONCERN FOR BLOOD SAFETY: A GLIMPSE OF THE FUTURE

Since 1943, transfusion therapy has been shadowed by the specter of disease transmission. In that year, Beeson described posttransfusion hepatitis and unveiled a problem that has grown with time. As transfusion increased, so did disease transmission. In 1962, the connection between paid donations and posttransfusion hepatitis was made (74). A decade later, the National Blood Policy mandated a voluntary donation system in the United States. And yet, blood use continued to increase.

Concern about posttransfusion hepatitis was not sufficient to decrease the number of transfusions (75). Although the use

TABLE 1.2. TRANSFUSIONS IN THE UNITED STATES (IN MILLIONS OF UNITS)

	1971	1979	1980	1982	1984	1986	1987	1989
Whole blood and red cells	6.32	9.47	9.99	11.47	11.98	12.16	11.61	12.06
Platelets	0.41	2.22	3.19	4.18	5.53	6.30	6.38	7.26
Plasma	0.18	1.29	1.54	1.95	2.26	2.18	2.06	2.16
Total	6.91	12.98	14.72	17.60	19.77	20.64	20.05	21.48

Adapted from Surgenor DM, Schnitzer SS. The nation's blood resource—a summary report, National Institutes of Health (NIH) publication 85-2028, Bethesda, MD: U.S. Department of Health and Human Services, Public Health Service, NIH, 1985; Surgenor DM, Wallace EL, Hao SHS, et al. Collection and transfusion of blood in the United States, 1982–1988. N Engl J Med 1990;322:1646; Wallace EL, Surgenor DM, Hao HS, et al. Collection and transfusion of blood and blood components in the United States, 1989. Transfusion 1993;33:139.

of whole blood declined as blood components became more popular, total blood use in the United States doubled between 1971 and 1980 (76) (Table 1.2).

Improved donor screening and increased donation testing have greatly decreased the risk of disease transmission (77–79) and rendered the blood supply safer than it has ever been in the past (80). Nonetheless, the realization that transfusion can transmit an almost invariably fatal disease has had a chilling effect on the public (81). Two major changes in blood services have occurred in the aftermath of the AIDS epidemic. The Food and Drug Administration, using pharmaceutical manufacturing criteria not "tailored to . . . blood banks," has become more aggressive in regulatory actions against blood collection establishments (82). And, finally, blood use has begun to moderate. Through the 1980s, red blood cell and plasma transfusion peaked and began to stabilize (Table 1.2). Only platelet usage, driven by the demands of cancer chemotherapy, has continued to increase (83, 84). Educational programs to encourage more judicious use of blood have been initiated (85), and they have been favorably received by practicing physicians.

During the 1980s, innovative programs were developed to address educational needs, and *transfusion medicine* emerged as the term to describe these educational innovations. In Europe, the Committee on Blood Transfusion of the Council of Europe proposed the establishment of "blood transfusion centres" within teaching hospital complexes to serve as centers of excellence in transfusion medicine (86). In the United States, Transfusion Medicine Academic Awards granted by the National Heart, Lung, and Blood Institute provided a mechanism to introduce transfusion medicine curricula into undergraduate medical education (87). These initiatives, occurring independently on two continents, were mutually reinforcing and emphasized the importance of clinical training for the transfusion specialist (88) and of transfusion education for the future medical practitioner (89). Thus, there has been a transition from blood banking to transfusion medicine. This transition encourages the cooperation of clinical disciplines in studies of blood use. It also increases the emphasis on alternatives to homologous blood, such as autologous transfusion and the use of growth factors and other products of genetic engineering.

The emergence of transfusion-transmitted disease has added a clinical dimension to the laboratory discipline that brought transfusion from Karl Landsteiner's laboratory to its present stage of development. Laboratory progress must, of course, continue to provide ever safer and more effective blood components and derivatives. But as hemotherapy becomes more complex, the specialty of transfusion medicine (90, 91) must develop, *pari passu,* to ensure that the "life-giving force" of blood is always used wisely and sparingly.

REFERENCES

1. Majno G. The healing hand. Cambridge, MA: Harvard University Press, 1975:330–332.
2. Maluf NSR. History of blood transfusion. J Hist Med 1954;9:59–107.
3. Wren C. An account of the rise and attempts, of a way to conveigh liquors immediately into the mass of blood. Philos Trans R Soc Lond 1665;1:128–130.
4. Hollingsworth MW. Blood transfusion by Richard Lower in 1665. Ann Hist Med 1928;10:213–225.
5. Lower R. The success of the experiment of transfusing the blood of one animal into another. Philos Trans R Soc Lond 1666;1:352.
6. Lower R. The method observed in transfusing the blood out of one animal into another. Philos Trans R Soc Lond 1666;1:353–358.
7. Hoff EC, Hoff PM. The life and times of Richard Lower, physiologist and physician (1631–1691). Bull Hist Med 1936;4:517–535.
8. Lower R. An account of the experiment of transfusion practised upon a man in London. Philos Trans R Soc Lond 1667;2:557–559.
9. Brown H. Jean Denis and transfusion of blood. Paris 1667–1668. Isis 1948;39:15–29.
10. Hoff HE, Guillemin R. The first experiments on transfusion in France. J Hist Med 1963;18:103–124.
11. Denis J. A letter concerning a new way of curing sundry diseases by transfusion of blood. Philos Trans R Soc Lond 1667;2:489–504.

12. Denis J. An extract of a letter. . .touching a late cure of an inveterate phrenisy by the transfusion of blood. Philos Trans R Soc Lond 1668;3: 617–623.
13. Denis J. An extract of a printed letter. . .touching the differences risen about the transfusion of blood. Philos Trans R Soc Lond 1668;3: 710–715.
14. Jones HW, Mackmull G. The influence of James Blundell on the development of blood transfusion. Ann Hist Med 1928;20:242–248.
15. Blundell J. Experiments on transfusion of blood by the syringe. Med Chir Trans 1818;9:56–92.
16. Foreign Department. Transfusion and infusion. Lancet 1828;2:324–326.
17. Blundell J. Some account of a case of obstinate vomiting in which an attempt was made to prolong life by the injection of blood into the veins. Med Chir Trans 1819;10:296–311.
18. Blundell J. Observations on transfusion of blood. Lancet 1828;2:321–324.
19. Moss WL. A simple method for the indirect transfusion of blood. Am J Med Sci 1914;147:698–703.
20. Braxton-Hicks J. Cases of transfusion with some remarks on a new method of performing the operation. Guy's Hosp Rep 1869;14:1–14.
21. Oberman HA. Early history of blood substitutes—transfusion of milk. Transfusion 1969;9:74–77.
22. Schmidt PJ. Transfusion in America in the eighteenth and nineteenth centuries. N Engl J Med 1968;279:1319–1320.
23. Bull WT. On the intravenous injection of saline solutions as a substitute for transfusion of blood. Med Rec 1884;25:6–8.
24. Landsteiner K: Ueber Agglutinationserscheinungen normalen menschlichen Blutes. Wien Klin Wochenschr 1901;14:1132–1134 (English translation taken from Ref.12).
25. Dixon B. Of different bloods. Science 1984;5:65–67.
26. Decastello A, Sturli A. Ueber die Isoagglutinine im Serum gesunder und kranker Menschen. Muench Med Wochenschr 1902;49:1090–1095.
27. Carrel A. The transplantation of organs: a preliminary communication. JAMA 1905;45:1645–1646.
28. Walker LG Jr. Carrel's direct transfusion of a five day old infant. Surg Gynecol Obstet 1973;137:494–496.
29. Crile GW. The technique of direct transfusion of blood. Ann Surg 1907;46:329–332.
30. Bernheim BM. Blood transfusion: hemorrhage and the anaemias. Philadelphia: J.B. Lippincott, 1917:259.
31. Ottenberg R. Reminiscences of the history of blood transfusion. J Mt Sinai Hosp 1937;4:264–271.
32. Pepper W, Nisbet V. A case of fatal hemolysis following direct transfusion of blood by arteriovenous anastomosis. JAMA 1907;49:385–389.
33. Ottenberg R. Transfusion and arterial anastomosis. Ann Surg 1908:47: 486–505.
34. Ottenberg R, Kaliski DJ. Accidents in transfusion: their prevention by preliminary blood examination: based on an experience of 128 transfusions. JAMA 1913;61:2138–2140.
35. Epstein AA, Ottenberg R. A simple method of performing serum reactions. Proc NY Pathol Soc 1908;8:117–123.
36. Ottenberg R. Studies in Isoagglutination I. Transfusion and the question of intravascular agglutination. J Exp Med 1911;13:425–438.
37. Diamond LK. The story of our blood groups. In: Wintrobe MM, ed. Blood, pure and eloquent. New York: McGraw-Hill, 1980:690–717.
38. Levine P, Stetson RE. An unusual case of intragroup agglutination. JAMA 1939;113:126–127.
39. Landsteiner K, Wiener AS. An agglutinable factor in human blood recognized by immune sera for rhesus blood. Proc Soc Exp Biol Med 1940;43:233.
40. Unger LJ. A new method of syringe transfusion. JAMA 1915;64: 582–584.
41. Hustin A. Principe d'une nouvelle methode de transfusion. J Med Bruxelles 1914;12:436.
42. Agote L. Nuevo procediemento para la transfusion del sangre. An Inst Mod Clin Med (Buenos Aires) 1915;2:24–30.
43. Lewisohn R. A new and greatly simplified method of blood transfusion. Med Rec 1915;87:141–142.
44. Weil R. Sodium citrate in the transfusion of blood. JAMA 1915; 64:425–426.
45. Rous P, Turner JR. The preservation of living red blood cells in vitro. J Exp Med 1916;23:219–248.
46. Robertson OH. Transfusion with preserved red blood cells. Br Med J 1918;1:691–695.
47. Loutit JF, Mollison PL. Advantages of a disodium-citrate-glucose mixture as a blood preservative. Br Med J 1943;2:744–745.
48. Diamond LK. A history of blood transfusion. In: Wintrobe MM, ed. Blood, pure and eloquent. New York: McGraw-Hill, 1980:658–688.
49. Duran-Jorda F. The Barcelona blood transfusion service. Lancet 1939;1:773–775.
50. Fantus B. The therapy of the Cook County Hospital. JAMA 1937; 109:128–131.
51. Yudin SS. Transfusion of cadaver blood. JAMA 1936;106:997–999.
52. Strumia MM, McGraw JJ. The development of plasma preparations for transfusions. Ann Intern Med 1941;15:80–87.
53. Flosdorf EW, Mudd S. Procedure and apparatus for preservation in "lyophile" form of serum and other biological substances. J Immunol 1935;29:389–425.
54. Diamond LK. History of blood banking in the United States. JAMA 1965;193:40–45.
55. Walter CW, Murphy WP Jr. A closed gravity technique for the preservation of whole blood in ACD solution utilizing plastic equipment. Surg Gynecol Obstet 1952;94:687–692.
56. Gibson JG II, Sack T, Buckley ES Jr. The preservation of whole ACD blood, collected, stored and transfused in plastic equipment. Surg Gynecol Obstet 1952;95:113–119.
57. Cohn EJ. The separation of blood into fractions of therapeutic value. Ann Intern Med 1947;26:341–352.
58. Patek AJ, Taylor FHL. Hemophilia. II. Some properties of a substance obtained from normal human plasma effective in accelerating the coagulation of hemophilic blood. J Clin Invest 1937;16:113–124.
59. Pool JG, Shannon AE. Production of high-potency concentrates of antihemophilic globulin in a closed-bag system. N Engl J Med 1965;273: 1443–1447.
60. Lewisohn R. Blood transfusion: 50 years ago and today. Surg Gynecol Obstet 1955;101:362–368.
61. Rosenfeld RE. Early twentieth century origins of modern blood transfusion therapy. Mt Sinai J Med 1974;41:626–635.
62. Beeson PB. Jaundice occurring one to four months after transfusion of blood or plasma. JAMA 1943;121:1332–1334.
63. Editorial. Jaundice following yellow fever vaccination. JAMA 1942; 119:1110.
64. Blumberg BS, Alter HJ, Visnich S. A "new" antigen in leukemia sera. JAMA 1965;191:541–546.

65. Feinstone SM, Kapikian AZ, Purcell RH. Hepatitis A detection by immune electron microscopy of a virus-like antigen associated with acute illness. Science 1973;182:1026–1028.
66. Dane DS, Cameron CH, Briggs M. Virus-like particles in serum of patients with Australia-antigen associated hepatitis. Lancet 1970;1:695–700.
67. Feinstone SM, Kapikian AZ, Purcell RH, Alter HJ, Holland PV. Transfusion-associated hepatitis not due to viral hepatitis type A or B. N Engl J Med 1975;292:767–770.
68. Choo Q-L, Kuo G, Weiner AJ, Overby LR, Bradley DW, Houghton M. Isolation of a cDNA clone derived from a blood-borne non-A non-B viral hepatitis genome. Science 1989;244:359–362.
69. Ammann JA, Cowan MJ, Wara DW, et al. Acquired immunodeficiency in an infant: possible transmission by means of blood products. Lancet 1983;1:956–958.
70. Curran JW, Lawrence DN, Jaffe H, et al. Acquired immunodeficiency syndrome (AIDS) associated with transfusions. N Engl J Med 1984; 310:69–75.
71. Barre-Sinoussi F, Cherman JC, Rey F, et al. Isolation of a T-lymphotropic retrovirus from a patient at risk for acquired immunodeficiency syndrome (AIDS). Science 1983;220:868–871.
72. Popovic M, Sarngadharan MG, Read E, Gallo RC. Detection, isolation, and continuous production of cytopathic retroviruses (HTLV-III) from patients with AIDS and pre-AIDS. Science 1984;224:497–500.
73. Sangaharan MG, Popovic M, Bruch I, Schupbach J, Gallo RC. Antibodies reactive with a human T-lymphotropic retrovirus (HTLV-III) in the serum of patients with AIDS. Science 1984;224:506–508.
74. Allen JG, Sayman WA. Serum hepatitis from transfusion of blood. JAMA 1962;180:1079–1085.
75. Solomon JM. Human blood and social policy. Plasmapheresis 1989;3: 180–186.
76. Surgenor DM, Schnitzer SS. The nation's blood resource—a summary report. National Institutes of Health (NIH) publication 85–2028. Bethesda, MD: U.S. Department of Health and Human Services, Public Health Service, NIH, 1985.
77. Cumming PD, Wallace EL, Schorr JB, Dodd RY. Exposure of patients to human immunodeficiency virus through the transfusion of blood components that test antibody-negative. N Engl J Med 1989;321: 941–946.
78. Leitman SF, Klein HG, Melpolder JJ, et al. Clinical implications of positive tests for antibodies to human immunodeficiency virus type I in asymptomatic blood donors. N Engl J Med 1989;321:917–924.
79. Donahue JG, Munoz A, Ness PM, et al. The declining risk of post-transfusion hepatitis C virus infection. N Engl J Med 1992;327:369–373.
80. Dodd RY. The risk of transfusion-transmitted infection. N Engl J Med 1992;327:419–421.
81. Zeckhauser RJ, Viscusi WK. Risk within reason. Science 1990;248: 559–564.
82. Solomon JM. The evolution of the current blood banking regulatory climate. Transfusion 1994;34:272–277.
83. Surgenor DM, Wallace EL, Hao SHS, Chapman RH. Collection and transfusion of blood in the United States, 1982–1988. N Engl J Med 1990;322:1646–1651.
84. Wallace EL, Surgenor DM, Hao HS, An J, Chapman RH, Churchill WH. Collection and transfusion of blood and blood components in the United States, 1989. Transfusion 1993;33:139–144.
85. Salem-Schatz SR, Avorn J, Soumerai SB. Influence of clinical knowledge, organizational context, and practice style on transfusion decision making: implications for practice change strategies. JAMA 1990;264: 476–483.
86. Committee of Experts on Blood Transfusion and Immunohaematology. Final draft report. May 1984. Montpellier: Council of Europe, 1984.
87. Chernoff AI. Transfusion medicine: the maturing of a specialty. Transfusion 1988;28:509–510.
88. Committee of Ministers of Member States. On a model curriculum for the training of specialists in blood transfusion, March 1985. Montpellier: Council of Europe, 1985.
89. Simon TL. Curriculum Committee of the Transfusion Medicine Academic Award Group. Comprehensive curricular goals for teaching transfusion medicine. Transfusion 1989;29:438–446.
90. Klein HG. Transfusion medicine: the evolution of a new discipline. JAMA 1987;258:2108–2109.
91. Council on Transfusion Medicine of the ASCP Commission on Continuing Education. The expanded role of the pathologist in transfusion medicine. Lab Med 1988;19:672–673.

Section II
Blood Services Interaction With Surgical Care

Chapter 2

Transfusion Medicine in the Surgical Patient

RICHARD B. COUNTS

INTRODUCTION

A safe and adequate supply of blood components for transfusion is indispensable to a modern surgical service. Although transfusion therapy is almost always supportive rather than definitive treatment in surgical patients, many advances in surgery, such as trauma and burn care, cardiovascular surgery, and some organ transplants, are absolutely dependent on a ready supply of blood components. At one time or another, most major surgical procedures will require substantial transfusion support, even though considerable progress has been made to reduce the routine need for transfusions.

A great deal of attention has been given in the last 25 years to improving the safety of blood transfusion by reducing the risks of transfusion-transmissible infections (see Chapter 3). Earlier work that perfected our knowledge of red cell immunology led to the development of sensitive compatibility testing methods that have made serious transfusion reactions uncommon; the major causes of those that do occur are clerical errors rather than inadequacy of the tests. One important component of transfusion safety still beset with problems is adequate supply. This component cannot be ensured by the blood center or the transfusion service alone, but rather relies on volunteer blood donors and knowledge by physicians of appropriate ordering and transfusion practices. Although the importance of available blood for emergency use is obvious to most physicians, many people still have in mind the old image of appeals for blood donors after a disaster or donating to someone in an emergency. Since the 1970s, the time required for testing and other processing, advances in resuscitation, and the management of surgical emergencies have precluded waiting until a need is evident to ask for donors.

Even when the blood center has a supply that is continually adequate for the community need, ensuring that each patient's transfusion support is adequate and timely requires that the physician understand how the blood bank system works in their community and in their hospital, how to obtain blood components, the time required for compatibility testing and other preparation, where blood supplies are kept, and whom to talk to in order to resolve problems. This chapter describes the operation of blood centers and transfusion services, blood components commonly available, special processing and preparation that may be needed in certain clinical situations, and the logistics of transfusion support of surgical patients.

THE AMERICAN BLOOD SUPPLY

In the United States, virtually all blood components for transfusion are from volunteer unpaid donors. A significant amount of the plasma used for fractionation into albumin and clotting factor concentrates is from paid vendors. However, because of a Food and Drug Administration (FDA) regulation (21 CFR 606.121) instituted in the 1970s requiring that all blood components are labeled as to whether they are from a volunteer donor or a paid donor, the reluctance of doctors to transfuse, and of patients to receive, blood from paid donors has resulted in almost complete elimination of paid donors as a source of blood for transfusion. Some 13.8 million units of blood are donated each year in the United States. About 11.3 million units of red cells are transfused to 3.8 million patients (1). Approximately 45% of the total is collected by independent nonprofit regional community blood centers, an additional 45% is collected by the American Red Cross, and the remainder is collected in blood banks associated with transfusion services in individual hospitals.

All establishments that collect, test and process, and provide blood for transfusion do so under extensive federal regulation through the FDA. This regulation began in the late 1940s and early 1950s with the licensing of blood banks supplying blood and plasma for military use in Korea, expanded incrementally in the late 1960s and the 1970s with the development of new blood products and tests for hepatitis, and increased dramatically from 1989 to 1995 as a result of the acquired immunodeficiency syndrome (AIDS) epidemic and public concerns about transfusion safety. The principal sections of federal regulations applying to blood and blood establishments are in the following sections of title 21 of the Code of Federal Regulations, the volume pertaining to the FDA: parts 210 and 211 deal with general pharmaceutical good manufacturing practices and parts 600, 601, 606, 607, 610, and 640 deal specifically with blood and blood components. The regulations cover, inter alia, such matters as licensing, labeling, purity, potency, good manufacturing practices, donor selection, and mandatory testing of blood. As with many government regulations, they are often general and for practical application are supplemented by detailed FDA criteria for such things as licensing blood products, approving labels or donor questionnaires, or conducting inspections. As blood banks sought guidance on methods and standards for blood components and testing, various organizations, preeminently the American Association of Blood Banks (AABB), developed voluntary standards to which virtually all blood banks adhere (2). In addition to the FDA regulations and AABB standards, a textbook by Mollison et al. and the AABB Technical Manual are useful references for many standard procedures and techniques in blood banking and transfusion medicine (3, 4).

REGIONAL COMMUNITY BLOOD CENTERS

Most blood is collected and processed by regional blood centers. This has several advantages over collection of blood directly by hospital blood banks. Large referral hospitals, with large needs for blood components to support special procedures, have access to donors from a wide area, ideally corresponding to the referral area. Also, small hospitals are ensured a steady supply without excessive outdate rates. A uniform recruiting message can be given to volunteer donors, decreasing confusion, and usually there is some cost efficiency from larger size. The basic functions of the regional blood center are recruitment of donors, blood collection, testing and typing the blood, separation of various blood components such as platelets and cryoprecipitate, and distribution to the transfusion services in the region served. Commonly, a single regional center will provide the blood for a given geographical area, but this is not always the case. Two centers may compete, or hospital blood banks may compete with a regional center for donors. Recently, with the growth of large for-profit hospital chains, there has been some interest among hospitals in bidding out blood supply contracts. Although cost savings is the impetus for this, hospitals have found that care must be taken to ensure that a low bidder is able to provide a steady supply of blood components. Otherwise, the costs of canceled surgeries or disruption of oncology treatment programs could outweigh direct savings from an overextended supplier.

TRANSFUSION SERVICES

It is useful to distinguish between activities involved in collecting and processing blood components and those related to preparing the blood for transfusion. The latter are generally referred to as transfusion services. Although some regional blood centers also provide centralized transfusion services, in most communities, compatibility testing, pooling of components, and special component preparations are not done by the regional center but by hospital transfusion services located in each hospital. In the beginning, most hospital blood banks also collected blood but have largely given this up because of the greater efficiency of regional blood centers and have concentrated on the medical services related to transfusion. When cost reimbursement and fee-for-service were the rule, transfusion services were usually profit centers for a hospital; under managed care and DRGs, they have become cost centers. There is a tendency toward centralization of transfusion services, either among several hospitals or in regional blood centers. Although care must be taken to ensure that transportation time does not unduly delay the provision of blood in emergencies, there are a number of advantages of centralized transfusion services: cost efficiency of larger specialized laboratories; central records that allow ready reference even if a patient goes to several hospitals over a period of years; specialized staff training; and efficiency in standardization, quality assurance records, and procedures. A significant clinical advantage is that if a large quantity of blood is needed for emergencies—especially more than one at the same time—more people can be put to work on the problem in a larger laboratory. Finally, the centralization of a community's blood supply permits more effective management and support of critical patient needs in times of blood shortages than can be done if the blood is distributed in many small transfusion service inventories.

Ordinarily, services provided by a transfusion service include not only compatibility testing of red cells, but all the special modifications of blood components needed to prepare them for transfusion. These may include such things as washing red cells to remove plasma, irradiating cellular components to reduce the possibility of an unwanted graft in a severely immunosuppressed patient, or pooling platelets or cryoprecipitate to provide the desired dose for transfusion. In the event that a patient is found, on antibody screening or cross matching, to have an unexpected red cell antibody, the antibody must be identified to permit selection of compatible units. This antibody identification may be performed by the transfusion service, by a regional red cell reference laboratory associated with a large transfusion service, or by a regional blood center. Because in a civilian hospital population there is about a 1% chance that a patient needing a transfusion will have an unexpected red cell antibody (5), red cell antibody identification is usually centralized in a large laboratory.

Experience has shown that the lack of knowledge of blood-ordering procedures by physicians and nurses is a significant cause of delay and error in obtaining blood components for their patients, especially in emergency situations. Because blood bank and transfusion service organization vary between hospitals, it behooves physicians, especially surgeons and anesthesiologists who frequently place emergency orders, to familiarize themselves at once with the transfusion service procedures of any hospital in which they work. The assumption that one hospital has the same procedures as another can have tragic consequences.

SELECTION OF BLOOD DONORS: TRANSFUSION SAFETY

Because no substitute for red cells or platelets is available for clinical use, the blood donor is the sole source. For reasons of safety, almost all blood for transfusion is from altruistic volunteer donors. Many studies show that individuals who sell their blood have, as a group, much higher rates of hepatitis than volunteer blood donors (6). The collection of blood from volunteer donors is the first, and probably still the most significant, "layer of safety" for blood transfusion. Second, all donors are asked a lengthy series of questions about their health history. Some questions are general ("Are you in good health today?"), whereas others relate to particular infectious disease risks ("Have you been in a malaria area within the past year?" or "Have you had sex with another male since 1977?"). Since the AIDS epidemic, a number of questions related to AIDS risk have been added. Starting in 1983, most blood centers provided prospective donors with an information sheet concerning risk factors for human immunodeficiency virus (HIV) infection and asked whether any factors applied to the donor. After the screening test for anti-HIV became available in 1985, studies of donors who answered the questions negatively yet tested positive for anti-HIV showed that a number of the screening questions were misunderstood or misconstrued by high-risk donors. Out of these studies came revised requirements and recommendations by the FDA for donor screening questions. Although each blood center determines how each question is to be asked—within the FDA requirements—and there is some variation in questions other than AIDS and hepatitis risk questions, each licensed center's donor questions must be reviewed and approved by the FDA. A sample of donor screening questions is shown in Figure 2.1.

If the donor's history is satisfactory as to the lack of evident risk for bloodborne infections and as to factors that relate to the safety of the donor (e.g., freedom from clinically significant heart disease or arrhythmias), a brief assessment of physical signs is done. This usually includes temperature, pulse rate, blood pressure, and examination of arms for needle track scars and for skin infections overlying the antecubital veins, which might lead to contamination of blood. In addition, a screening test for an adequate level of hemoglobin is done. The most frequent test is a simple estimate of the density of a drop of blood using a copper sulfate solution. Microhematocrit measurements are usually not done because they take too long, and direct measurements of hemoglobin concentration are more expensive than the copper sulfate method. The method is sufficiently reliable as a screening test provided it is carefully calibrated, but consistent attention to quality control of the copper sulfate solutions and of the procedures is required.

The last layer of safety is provided by tests for infectious agents. At present, up to nine tests are performed on each unit of blood collected (Table 2.1).

Some of these tests have brought about tremendous improvements in transfusion safety. For example, the anti-HIV tests reduced the risk of exposure to HIV-1 from 1 in 2500 or higher in the period 1983 to 1984 (7, 8) to 1 in 600,000 in 1996 (9, 10); the tests for hepatitis C reduced the risk from about 4% in the 1970s to less than 1 in 10,000 in 1996. Other tests, mandated in the effort to reduce the risk of HIV transmission as close to zero as possible, give far smaller incremental improvements. For example, the HIV p24 antigen test was expected, on its introduction in 1996, to prevent perhaps five exposures a year in the United States by shortening the window period after infection during which the virus cannot be detected from 23 to 18 days (10).

	YES		NO
Are you in good health today?	☐	28	☐
Do you currently have a cold, sore throat or flu?	☐	29	☐
Have you donated whole blood in the last 8 weeks or have you donated plasma or platelets in the last 72 hours?	☐	27	☐
Have you ever had any problems donating blood?	☐	30	☐
Have you ever been told not to donate?	☐	60	☐
Do you weigh less than 110 pounds?	☐	33	☐
In the last 12 months have you had a direct exposure to blood or body fluids by an accidental needle stick or splatter into an open wound or mucous membrane?	☐	36	☐
In the last 12 months have you had (please circle): an injection, tattoo, blood transfusion, acupuncture, ears pierced, body piercing, vaccination/immunization, gamma globulin or organ/tissue transplant?	☐	37	☐
In the last 12 months were you exposed to anyone with hepatitis or yellow jaundice at the time of your exposure?	☐	38A	☐
In the last 12 months were you exposed to anyone who is a carrier of hepatitis?	☐	38B	☐
Have you ever had yellow skin or eyes, liver disease, hepatitis or a positive blood test for hepatitis?	☐	39	☐
Have you traveled outside the U.S./Canada in the past 3 years?	☐	40	☐
Are you currently taking any medications? If yes, please list:	☐	41	☐
Have you ever had (please circle): cancer, diabetes, blood disease, bleeding tendency, lung or heart disease, multiple sclerosis, strokes, seizures, malaria, Chagas disease or babesiosis?	☐	42	☐
Have you been hospitalized or under medical care in the past 12 months?	☐	43	☐
Have you ever taken Proscar, Accutane, Tegison?	☐	53	☐
Are you aware of a diagnosis of Creutzfeldt-Jakob Disease (CJD) in your family, or have you ever received a dura mater (brain membrane) transplant, or have you ever taken pituitary growth hormone of human origin?	☐	58	☐
In the last 12 months, have you been incarcerated in a correctional institution for more than 72 consecutive hours?	☐	59	☐

Questions below will be asked by interviewer:

Do you have AIDS or have you ever had a positive AIDS test?	52A ☐
Have you ever used needles for self injection of drugs not prescribed by a physician, even once?	52B ☐
Have you received clotting factor concentrates for a disorder such as hemophilia?	52C ☐
Have you taken money or drugs in exchange for sex anytime since 1977?	52D ☐
(M) Have you had sexual contact of any kind with another male, even once, since 1977?	52E ☐
In the last 12 months have you had sexual contact of any kind, even once, with:	
Anyone who has AIDS or positive AIDS test?	52F ☐
Anyone who has ever used needles for self injection of drugs?	52G ☐
Anyone who has received clotting factors?	52H ☐
Anyone who has taken money or drugs in exchange for sex since 1977?	52J ☐
(F) A male who has had sex with another male, even once, since 1977?	52K ☐
Do you understand that you should not give blood if you have engaged in any of the above activities *EVEN ONCE?*	52M ☐
Have you had or have you been treated for syphilis or gonorrhea within the last 12 months?	52L ☐
Do you understand that a person infected with the AIDS virus can feel well and show no symptoms of infection?	☐
Do you understand that you should not donate blood to get an AIDS test?	52N ☐
Do you understand that if you have engaged in high risk activity recently your blood may be infectious but your test for AIDS may be negative?	☐
Have you read and do you understand all the donor information presented to you, and have all your questions been answered?	☐
Apheresis Use Only Reviewed Apheresis Repeat Donor questions.	☐

CONSENT FOR TESTING

I read and understand the information provided to me regarding the spread of the AIDS virus by blood. To the best of my knowledge, I am not at risk for spreading the virus known to cause AIDS (HIV). I understand that my blood will be tested for antibodies to HIV and for other disease markers. If this testing indicates that I should no longer donate blood because of a risk of transmitting AIDS or other disease I will be notified, and my donor record will be coded to indicate that I am permanently deferred. ***(Apheresis Donors – I have read the Apheresis Information Sheet and consent to having the procedure performed.)***

Signature X 52Q

(Must be signed after the interview)

Donor meets all criteria? YES ☐ NO ☐ INITIALS OF SCREENER

PSB-000-01 (REV. 12/95)

Figure 2.1. Blood donor screening questions.

For a unit of blood to be released for transfusion, the collecting center must confirm that the donor's history is negative for the known infectious risk factors, that the viral screening tests have been done and are all nonreactive, that the donor is not listed on the center's permanent registry of donors who have been permanently deferred, and that the ABO and Rh blood groups of the unit have been accurately determined. The unit can then be labeled for blood group and released to the transfusion service.

BLOOD COMPONENTS AVAILABLE

Until the advent of plastic blood bags in the early 1960s, the separation of the components of blood was fraught with

TABLE 2.1. TESTS FOR INFECTIOUS AGENTS

Agent	Test Detects	Year Adopted
T. pallidum	Antibody	1939–1941
Hepatitis B	Viral antigen (HBsAg)	1971
HIV-1	Antibody to the virus	1985
Cytomegalovirus	Antibody to the virus	1985–1986
Non-A, non-B hepatitis	HBc Ab and ALT	1986–1988
HTLV-1	Antibody to the virus	1989
Hepatitis C	Antibody to viral proteins	1990
HIV-1 and 2	A combination test: antibodies to both viruses	1992
HIV	HIV p24 antigen	1996

practical difficulties. Centrifugation of the glass bottles was awkward, and the system could not be kept sterile because of the necessity of introducing air into the bottles when removing liquid. By the early 1970s, component fractionation technology had advanced to where components such as red cells, platelets, and plasma could be readily prepared aseptically and stored in concentrated form so that patients might be given only the cellular plasma component that they needed. This lowered costs, greatly increased the availability of components such as platelets, and literally made possible procedures such as bone marrow transplantation and extensive cardiopulmonary bypass operations that could not adequately be supported with transfusions of whole blood only. The commonly available components are described below along with a brief summary of common indications and certain precautions and contraindications.

MODIFIED WHOLE BLOOD

Although many blood centers now provide no whole blood because they tend to separate plasma from all units collected to send it for fractionation, there are certain clinical situations, notably massive transfusion, in which whole blood has clear advantages over the usual red cells supplemented with frozen plasma (11).

The official name, "modified whole blood," was applied because platelets, and sometimes cryoprecipitate, have been removed from the blood as concentrates. Modified whole blood, then, contains the red cells and most of the plasma (less than 60–70 mL if a platelet concentrate has been prepared) present in the original donated unit. This might be thought to impoverish the unit, and indeed the myth is widespread that modified whole blood contains no active clotting factors. On the contrary, it does contain near-normal levels of clotting factors, except for factor VIII (11). Any blood stored in the refrigerator at 4°C could properly be described as "modified," because when platelets are cooled to 4°C, dense granule contents leak out of the platelets and the platelets become nonfunctional. Therefore, no blood or red cell concentrate provided for transfusion has functional platelets. The volume of modified whole blood is approximately 425–450 mL. The levels of clotting factors after various periods of refrigerated storage are shown in Table 2.2 (11).

Indications

Modified whole blood is indicated for a patient who has large blood loss, equal to or exceeding one blood volume, or for large ongoing bleeding in which transfusions exceeding the patient's blood volume are expected. The advantage is that it provides, at the same time, red cells, volume, and most clotting factors from one donor.

The number of donors the patient is exposed to is thereby minimized, which increases safety; the cost is usually less than when giving separate components (e.g., red cells and plasma); and because it does not require thawing or separate handling, administration is usually faster and simpler. Studies of the use of modified whole blood in massive transfusion demonstrate that it prevents the dilution of clotting factors seen with the replacement of red cells alone or in cases of large-volume red cell salvage where blood is collected from the wound but plasma is removed by washing the red cells before reinfusion (11).

Precautions and Contraindications

Modified whole blood is not indicated for the correction of anemia except in an actively bleeding patient in which replacement of blood volume, plasma proteins, and red cells is necessary. Overtransfusion could lead to hypervolemia and

TABLE 2.2. CLOTTING FACTOR LEVELS

Clotting Factor	Levels in Blood Stored 21 Days (% of initial)
Fibrinogen	100
Prothrombin	70
VII	66
IX	97
X	85
XI	100
XIII	>90
VIII	<5
V	35

congestive heart failure, particularly if other fluids are being given and the volume of the plasma in modified whole blood is not taken into account. Because platelets are not present, modified whole blood cannot be expected to prevent or correct thrombocytopenia. In any massive transfusion situation, platelet counts should be monitored frequently and platelet concentrates should be used to prevent excessive dilution of platelets.

RED BLOOD CELLS

The usual component provided by blood banks contains the red cells from 450 mL of blood with enough plasma and anticoagulant with adenine-saline additive solution to give a hematocrit of around 60%. The total volume of each unit of red cells is approximately 300–350 mL. The additives in the anticoagulant extend the storage time of the red cell concentrate to 42 days. One advantage of some of the additive solutions for the blood center is that additional plasma may be removed from the unit for sale to pharmaceutical plasma fractionators. This makes little difference in the clinical use of red cells because the volume of plasma contained in red cell concentrates is not enough to be of use anyway. Another practical advantage is that the additional saline lowers the viscosity of the red cells so that the administration time can be somewhat less. In most cases, this is not a significant advantage. Red cell concentrates do not contain viable platelets nor significant amounts of albumin or plasma clotting factors.

Indications

Red cells are indicated for the prevention or treatment of anemia. Although the question of when red cell replacement is physiologically necessary is a complicated one (See Chapter 3), the main functions of red cells are oxygen transport and providing a significant part of the intravascular volume.

Precautions and Contraindications

Red cell concentrates, having no platelets and little plasma, are not indicated for the correction or prevention of thrombocytopenia or clotting factor deficiencies. Although red cell units have less volume than units of whole blood, the cells themselves are distributed intravascularly and, if their contribution to intravascular volume is not considered, can contribute to hypervolemia. If a patient requires transfusion greater than 1.0–1.5 blood volumes, plasma and platelets may need to be given to prevent excessive dilution of these components.

PLATELET CONCENTRATES

Each unit of platelets separated from a unit of donated blood contains a minimum of 5.5×10^{10} platelets in approximately 60 mL of plasma. Platelet concentrates may be stored at the blood center or transfusion service for 5 days or less. Over this period of time, the platelets retain 70% or more of their original viability and the clotting factors in the plasma, except for factor VIII, remain above 75–80% of their initial activity (12). Platelet concentrates contain traces (usually less than 0.3 mL) of red cells and, as they are prepared, contain $0.5–2.5 \times 10^8$ white cells, both granulocytes and mononuclear cells. Platelets must be stored at room temperature (20–24°C) to prevent loss of activity. Usually, several units of platelets are pooled to make a transfusion dose. Each unit of platelets can be expected to raise the platelet count of an average adult by 8,000–10,000/mL. Thus, in most clinical situations, a dose of four to eight units is appropriate, although this will vary depending on the size of the patient, the increment needed, and whether or not there is continuing consumption or dilution of platelets.

Indications

Platelet transfusions are indicated to correct clinically significant thrombocytopenia that is not caused by immune destruction. In cases of nonimmune platelet consumption (e.g., disseminated intravascular coagulation [DIC], vasculitis, consumption on an aortic balloon pump), the survival of transfused platelets, although shorter than normal, is long enough that one can maintain hemostatic levels for a period of hours at least. Whether effective platelet support can be given in such clinical situations must usually be determined empirically. If a patient has immune thrombocytopenia (ITP) or has developed alloantibodies from prior platelet transfusions, platelet transfusions usually will not raise the platelet count. If platelet transfusions are attempted in support of splenectomy for ITP, for instance, they should not be given until after the splenic pedicle is clamped and tied off. This practice will minimize the destruction of platelets and give the best chance of raising the count. Frequently, platelets given before clamping the spleen are destroyed in a matter of seconds or minutes and are merely wasted without being of any benefit.

Precautions and Contraindications

Platelet concentrates are of little use when the platelet survival is less than at least several hours. Because the concentrate contains a small number of red cells, Rh-positive platelet concentrates should not be given to Rh-negative patients, especially women of childbearing age. One prefers to give ABO and Rh type-specific platelets when they are available; however, although platelets have been shown to have some A-substance on their membranes, the survival of group A or B platelets in group O recipients is not appreciably shortened. Therefore, if platelets of the same group as a given patient are not available, substitution of another ABO group may readily be made. When platelets are pooled and sent for transfusion, they are no longer shaken. This decreases effective O_2 and CO_2 exchange through the plastic bag, and the pH begins to fall. For this reason and to decrease the risk of bacterial infection because they cannot be refrigerated, pooled platelets must be transfused within 4 hours of the time they are pooled. Therefore, platelets should only be ordered when there is a known need and not in anticipation of a possible later need.

Platelet concentrates, as prepared, contain white cells and may cause febrile reactions in multiply transfused recipients. However, because platelets are stored at room temperature, the potential for growth of any contaminating bacteria is also greater than with components stored refrigerated or frozen. Although the usual febrile reactions to white cell antigens consist of moderate fever (38–38.5°C) and mild to moderate chills, severe reactions, especially if associated with prostration or hypotension, should raise the suspicion of bacterial sepsis (13, 14). Although they are uncommon, cases of sepsis from *Yersinia enterocolitica* have been reported, evidently caused by platelets collected from donors with subclinical bacteremia.

PLATELETS COLLECTED BY APHERESIS

Platelets collected from a single donor by an apheresis procedure contain a minimum of 3×10^{10} platelets ordinarily suspended in 250–500 mL of plasma. The label of an apheresis platelet collection has the volume written on it and should be consulted if careful control of administered volume is important. A single apheresis collection is usually equivalent to six to nine units of pooled platelets prepared from whole blood. Unless collected by an available method that yields platelets with low levels of white cell, an apheresis platelet unit may contain 10^7–10^9 white cells. Recently, apheresis apparatus has been licensed that consistently gives apheresis platelets with less than 5×10^6 platelets per collection. Such units may be labeled "Platelets, Pheresis, Leukocytes Reduced," according to the FDA ("Recommendations and Licensure Requirements for Leukocyte-Reduced Blood Products," Memorandum to Registered Blood Establishments from FDA, May 29, 1996).

Apheresis platelets are stored up to 5 days; the limit is the same as that for platelets prepared from whole blood donations. It is likely that the plasma transfused with apheresis platelets contains near-normal levels of all but the most labile clotting factors.

Indications

The indications for the use of apheresis platelets are generally the same as for platelets prepared from whole blood. Because they can be collected from selected individual donors, however, there are some additional uses of apheresis platelets. Human leukocyte antigen (HLA)-matched or otherwise compatible donors may provide platelet support for patients who have become refractory to random platelet transfusions. Apheresis platelets do not require pooling and thus are available for transfusion in somewhat less time than that for pooled platelets. Because a transfusion dose can be obtained from a single donor rather than from four to eight donors, it has a correspondingly lower risk of transmitting infections.

Precautions and Contraindications

The precautions are essentially the same as those for platelets prepared from whole blood.

PLASMA

Plasma is the liquid part of blood from which the cells have been separated by centrifugation. It is distinguished from serum, clotted plasma, largely by the presence of fibrinogen and active factor V and factor VIII. To prepare fresh-frozen plasma, the cells are removed and the plasma frozen at a temperature below −20°C within 8 hours of the time the blood was collected. Each unit of plasma is prepared from a unit of donated blood and usually has a volume between 220 and 280 mL. Plasma contains all plasma proteins in their usual concentration but is not a concentrate of any. When stored frozen below −18°C, the clotting factor proteins retain their initial activity for a year. For transfusion, plasma is thawed at 37°C. This can be done in a circulating water bath or in other devices designed for the purpose. It takes 15–30 minutes to thaw a unit of plasma, depending on the method used. Because plasma for transfusion is stored frozen, it has no intact or viable white cells and is not known to transmit cytomegalovirus.

Indications

There are few proven indications for fresh-frozen plasma (15, 16). Millions of units are given to patients each year, usually merely by rote or out of conviction that something so nearly like fresh blood is bound to have the power to control bleeding. Unfortunately, this is often not the case, not because fresh-frozen plasma lacks clotting factors, but because the most common causes of microvascular bleeding in surgical patients are thrombocytopenia and consumption of fibrinogen, neither of which is readily correctable by plasma transfusion. Plasma can be effectively used to reverse clotting factor deficiencies resulting from warfarin anticoagulation; this is perhaps its major clinical indication. It is also indicated for the treatment of factor V deficiency, a rare congenital defect for which there is no effective factor concentrate. Plasma can often be used for the temporary treatment of clotting factor deficiencies in patients with liver failure, but because it does not contain the proteins in concentrated form, hypervolemia soon supervenes unless massive bleeding or plasma exchange prevents it. This limits the amount of plasma that can be given. Administration of plasma, either alone or in combination with apheresis plasma exchange, is used to treat thrombotic thrombocytopenic purpura, Guillain-Barré syndrome, myasthenia gravis unresponsive to other therapy, and certain other autoimmune disorders.

Precautions and Contraindications

Fresh-frozen plasma should not be used whenever more specific, or more effective, therapy is available. A diagnosis should be attempted even in emergency situations. Misguided faith in the efficacy of fresh-frozen plasma as a general procoagulant tonic too often leads physicians to give plasma without investigating the specific cause of bleeding. This shotgun approach, by delaying effective treatment, all too often allows excessive bleeding to continue longer than necessary, jeopardizes the success of the operation, increases morbidity and mortality, exposes the patient to an unnecessarily large amount of transfusion, wastes the surgeon's time, and increases the cost.

Plasma can cause anaphylactic reactions in patients with hypersensitivity to plasma proteins. This is a rare complication, usually seen only in people who have had many plasma or blood transfusions over a period of years (e.g., patients with congenital clotting factor deficiencies or people with IgA deficiency). Techniques for viral inactivation of fresh-frozen plasma with solvent detergent mixtures have been developed, but no such sterilized plasma is licensed at present in the United States. Thus, plasma carries the same risk of transfusion-transmitted infection as blood or red cells. Plasma should not be used as a volume expander or as a nutritional supplement; safer, more effective products are available for these purposes. Very rarely, a unit of plasma may be associated with the development of pulmonary edema not evidently related to hypervolemia or heart failure. This has been termed transfusion-related acute lung injury. The cause is thought to be antibodies in the transfused plasma against antigens on the recipient's white cells (17).

CRYOPRECIPITATE

Cryoprecipitate is prepared from single units of volunteer donor plasma by freezing the plasma at −80°C and then thawing the frozen plasma at 4°C, most efficiently in a circulating water bath (18). Most plasma proteins are soluble enough in the cold that they redissolve in the 4°C plasma, but factor VIII, fibronectin, and some of the fibrinogen remain as a precipitate. This "cold precipitate" is separated from the supernatant plasma by centrifugation; the supernatant is drained off and the cryoprecipitate refrozen and stored below −18°C. To prepare cryoprecipitate for use, it is thawed at 37°C in a water bath. In some blood centers, 20 mL of plasma is left with the cryoprecipitate for the purpose of redissolving the precipitate, whereas in others, the plasma is removed and 10–20 mL of saline added to each bag to reconstitute it. The number of bags needed is pooled into a single bag and sent for transfusion.

A unit (bag) of cryoprecipitate is prepared from one unit of donor blood. When cryoprecipitate was used mostly as a concentrate of factor VIII, there was frequently confusion between the terms "unit of cryoprecipitate" and "unit of factor VIII." One factor VIII unit is a unit of biological activity, being the mean amount of factor VIII clotting activity contained in 1.0 mL of normal plasma. It is less confusing, although less elegant, to speak of a given number of "bags" of cryoprecipitate. One bag of cryoprecipitate contains, on average, 80–120 factor VIII units of factor VIII clotting activity and approximately 150 mg of fibrinogen. It also contains von Willebrand factor and fibronectin. The reconstituted volume usually used for transfusion is 15–20 mL per bag of cryoprecipitate. The necessary number of bags is pooled into a single bag for transfusion. A typical dose for an adult, 10–15 bags , would thus have a volume of 200–300 mL.

Indications

Cryoprecipitate is primarily used today as a fibrinogen concentrate (19). It is the only concentrated form of fibrinogen available, because freeze-dried commercial fibrinogen concentrates were removed from the market by the FDA in the 1970s because of high rates of hepatitis. In estimating the dose, one can assume that one bag of cryoprecipitate provides 150–180 mg of fibrinogen. Therefore, 10–12 bags of cryoprecipitate, a typical adult dose, can be expected to contain 1.5–2.1 g of fibrinogen. Because the plasma volume of an average-sized adult is about 2700 mL, this dose would be expected to raise the plasma fibrinogen concentration by about 75 mg/100 mL. Because plasma contains fibrinogen at a concentration of 2 mg/mL, it would seem logical that a similar dose of fibrinogen could be given by administering three to four units of plasma (750–1000 mL). However, in practice, it is often difficult to raise a patient's fibrinogen level significantly by giving plasma, especially in consumptive states. The reason may be that the volume of plasma given limits the rate; more fibrinogen can be given in a shorter time with a concentrate such as cryoprecipitate. At any rate, cryoprecipitate is the most effective means of raising the fibrinogen in DIC or similar disorders of fibrinogen consumption. If consumption is continuing, the level may fall rapidly; repeated assays of plasma fibrinogen are necessary to guide therapy. Likewise, if cryoprecipitate is given to correct hypofibrinogen induced by streptokinase or other fibrinolytic agents, continued fibrinolysis may necessitate repeated doses of cryoprecipitate.

Cryoprecipitate also contains factor VIII and was formerly primarily used for hemophilia A treatment. However, it is impractical to apply viral inactivation procedures to cryoprecipitate because it is prepared from individual units of plasma. Therefore, heat-treated or solvent-detergent-treated factor VIII concentrates or recombinate factor VIII have largely displaced cryoprecipitate in hemophilia care and also for the treatment of von Willebrand's disease. Although the clinical indications, if any, for fibronectin are poorly defined, cryoprecipitate is a rich source of fibronectin also.

Cryoprecipitate is used by many surgeons as the substrate for preparing fibrin glue. For this purpose, it is important to have the fibrinogen concentration as high as possible, so the cryoprecipitate is usually dissolved in 10 mL of saline per bag. Thrombin is added just before use and the solution spread on the site desired. It is likely that cryoprecipitate will be replaced by commercial fibrin glue preparations that will have higher fibrinogen concentrations and are sterilized. Cryoprecipitate does have the advantage, however, that for planned surgery, autologous units may be prepared.

SPECIAL PREPARATIONS AND MODIFICATIONS OF BLOOD COMPONENTS

Before 1970, whole blood accounted for most transfusions given in the United States. As more complex and sophisticated procedures and treatments were developed (e.g., cardiopulmonary bypass operations and bone marrow transplants), the use of specific components of blood grew. Going beyond component therapy, certain clinical situations may require additional processing and modification of blood components beyond the basic separation or concentrate preparation. In some cases, such as leukoreduction, this may be done by the community blood center at the time of component preparation, by the transfusion service at the time of compatibility testing, or on the nursing unit at the time of administration. The preparation and use of common specially treated blood components are described.

LEUKOREDUCTION

The most commonly used method of reducing the number of white cells in blood components today is filtration through filters of cotton or synthetic fibers to which white cells, but not red cells or platelets, adhere. The filters on the market all cause the loss of some red cells or platelets (different filters are designed for use with each component); any filter used should consistently permit the recovery of at least 80% of the red cells or platelets in the unit being filtered while removing most of the leukocytes. The reduction of white cells required depends on the clinical goal. To prevent febrile transfusion reactions, white cells should be reduced below 5×10^8 white blood cells per unit. Studies have demonstrated that leukoreduction below 5×10^6 white blood cells per unit is as effective in preventing cytomegalovirus transmission as is the use of anti-cytomegalovirus-negative blood components (20, 21). There is a trend toward preparation of leukoreduced components at the time the components are prepared from whole blood by the blood center. This has several advantages, probably the most important being greater standardization and quality control. Several studies have found considerable variability in bedside filtration with a significant rate of failure to realize the necessary degree of leukoreduction. Newer apheresis techniques permit the collection of platelets having less than 5×10^6 white blood cells per dose without the necessity of filtering the unit (22).

Indications

The accepted indications for leukoreduced components are the prevention of febrile transfusion reactions and prevention of cytomegalovirus transmission to severely immunosuppressed recipients. A number of other uses have been proposed. Most are under investigation but so far have not been proven to be definitely effective. These suggested uses include prevention of alloimmunization to platelets, prevention of HLA alloimmunization, avoidance of possible transfusion-related immunosuppression, and prevention of reactivation of latent viral infections (e.g., cytomegalovirus or HIV).

Precautions and Contraindications

Leukoreduction is ineffective in preventing graft-versus-host disease (GVHD) and transfusion-related acute lung injury and must not be relied on for either. Blood components given to patients at high risk of GVHD should be irradiated. It should be kept in mind that some red cells or platelets are inevitably lost during leukoreduction by filtration. Thus, the procedure should not be applied unless there is an indication, particularly to platelets, as the dose of the blood component is decreased.

IRRADIATION

Treatment of blood components with gamma irradiation inactivates nucleated cells and prevents unwanted engraftment of lymphocytes that could cause GVHD. The recommended minimum radiation dose is 1500 cGy to any point in a blood component being treated. Irradiation is usually accomplished at the blood center using machines that deliver 2500 cGy or more in the midplane of the canister holding the component to be irradiated. If this service is not available from the blood center, a radiation therapy gamma source may be used provided that an adequate minimum dose may be reliably delivered to the blood component. Little data exist to indicate significant damage to red cells or platelets by the radiation doses used, although questions have been raised about damage to red cell membranes, leading to excessive potassium leakage (23). Therefore, the expiration date for irradiated red cells is set at no more than 28 days from the date of irradiation. Irradiation of platelet concentrates does not alter the expiration date.

Indications

The only indication for gamma irradiation of blood components is the prevention of GVHD. The patients known to be susceptible to GVHD, who should always receive irradiated allogeneic blood components, are recipients of bone marrow transplants and low-birthweight neonates. Most organ transplant recipients and chemotherapy patients do not require irradiated components. A further indication is transfusions from close (first-degree) relatives. There have been a number of reports of fatal GVHD in persons receiving direct donations from family members. Some have occurred even though the recipient was not immunosuppressed (i.e., in patients undergoing coronary artery bypass operations). The risk is higher when the donor and recipient share one HLA haplotype. The chance of GVHD in transfusions between unrelated individuals in the United States is so low that routine irradiation is unwarranted.

Precautions and Contraindications

Because gamma irradiation is not known to damage red cells other than shortening the storage time, there are not any absolute contraindications. Units that have been irradiated must have a label permanently affixed to them that indicates this. The main concern has been the possibility of high extracellular potassium, which suggests caution in the administration of irradiated red cells to oliguric infants.

REDUCTION OF THE VOLUME OF PLATELET CONCENTRATES

Platelets prepared from whole blood have a volume of 60–70 mL per individual unit. The total volume of a typical adult dose of six units is thus about 400 mL. Occasionally, patients who need platelet transfusions are also hypervolemic. In such cases, the volume of the platelet concentrate may be reduced by a centrifugation step to 15–20 mL (24). This procedure takes at least 45–60 minutes—the centrifugation requires perhaps 15 minutes and the platelets must be left to stand 30 minutes before they can be resuspended to reduce their tendency to clump together. It also causes the loss of some platelets. On average, the recovery of platelets after volume reduction can be as low as 50–60% of the platelets originally present. Thus, volume reduction is not necessarily an improvement over the standard platelet concentrate. The indication for volume reduction, thrombocytopenia in the presence of congestive heart failure, is relatively uncommon in acute surgical bleeding.

Indications

Volume-reduced platelet concentrates should be used only when a patient cannot tolerate the usual volume of platelet concentrates and other means of preventing or treating hypervolemia (e.g., diuretics are inadequate or ineffective).

Precautions and Contraindications

Some loss of platelets attends any volume reduction procedures. Volume-reduced platelets are not appropriate emergency treatment for patients with active blood loss caused by thrombocytopenia because of their long preparation time and their low platelet yield.

WASHING RED CELLS AND PLATELETS

Red cells, and less successfully platelets, may be washed with saline to remove most of the plasma. Saline is added to packed red cells and the bag is then centrifuged and the saline supernatant removed. The process is often repeated once. Rarely, cells may be washed several times in an attempt to remove as much residual plasma as possible. Saline washing does dilute the plasma proteins and removes most platelet microaggregates. It also removes a variable fraction of the white cells; however, washing is not a very efficient or consistent way of accomplishing leukoreduction. Automated equipment sometimes is used for cell washing. The machines are similar to the machines used for intraoperative cell salvage. It should be kept in mind that although modified whole blood has relatively normal levels of plasma clotting factors and packed red cells have relatively little, washed red cells and red cells recovered in intraoperative red cell salvage provide no clotting factors. Thus, transfusion of more than one blood volume of either component may lead to dilution of clotting factors.

Indications

There are few firm indications for washed red cells. The only use is in situations in which it is desired to avoid transfusing plasma proteins. Probably the best documented use is in patients with paroxysmal nocturnal hemoglobinuria, in which one seeks to avoid giving complement that might exacerbate hemolysis. Some have suggested that washing red cells may be of value in other situations (e.g., hemolysis associated with high-titer cold agglutinins), but in most cases there seems to be no real benefit. If one is faced with the necessity of transfusing a patient with marked hypersensitivity to plasma proteins (e.g., IgA-deficient patients) and compatible blood cannot be obtained, the red cells should probably be washed at least three times. Even so, it may not be possible to lower the plasma concentration enough to prevent anaphylactoid reactions.

Precautions and Contraindications

Although washing red cells has been recommended as a means of removing granulocytes to prevent febrile transfusion reactions, it is an inefficient way of doing so and should not be used for this purpose. Leukoreduction by filtration, or even by centrifugation and buffy coat removal, is far more effective. Likewise, the usual red cell washing procedure does not reduce the risk of hepatitis or other viral transmission, although some have suggested that the more extensive washing during deglycerolization of frozen red cells can decrease hepatitis risk. Washing does not result in the loss of many red cells from red cell concentrates because the cells are relatively dense and sediment quickly. However, washing platelet concentrates is associated with significant loss of platelets. Furthermore, there is likely to be some decrease in platelet function and viability with washing platelets. Therefore, washed platelets should be given only when absolutely necessary lest one trade a certain loss of efficacy for a mere hypothetical benefit.

LOGISTICAL CONSIDERATIONS IN ORDERING BLOOD

All blood components require a certain amount of time to prepare them for transfusion. Unlike a drug or saline solution that can be kept in the operating room or at the bedside for instant use, blood components almost always require some procedure to ensure biological compatibility, to pool concentrates that cannot be stored pooled, or to thaw frozen components. The surgeon should keep these necessary procedures in mind and try to anticipate a patient's need for blood. The approximate times needed for testing and processing are as follows:

- Emergency compatibility tests, 20 minutes;
- Pooling platelets (six units), 15–30 minutes;
- Thawing fresh-frozen plasma (two units), 20–40 minutes;
- Thaw and pool cryoprecipitate, 20–60 minutes;
- Leukofiltration, 15 minutes;
- Red cell or platelet washing, 20–30 minutes;
- Reduced-volume platelet concentration, 45 minutes.

To these process times, one should add the inevitable time it takes to transmit an order from the ward or the operating room to the transfusion service and to deliver the component.

PHYSICIAN'S ROLE IN THE COMMUNITY BLOOD PROGRAM

It is the community blood center's responsibility to ensure a constant, safe, reliable supply of blood at all times. This concept, generally accepted today, was not always accepted. In the early days of blood centers, one of the common models was that of money banking; that is, the blood bank would be an agent that made it possible for donors to make deposits to the community supply and then to draw against those deposits if they or their friends or relatives needed blood. The implication was that the blood center would facilitate transfusions but that the responsibility for the blood supply lay with individuals in the community. As cities have grown and transfusion needs have greatly increased, it is evident that central organization is necessary to coordinate donor recruitment and blood collection so as to ensure a constant supply.

Although it is generally recognized that the community blood center has the primary responsibility for recruiting and collecting blood, every physician who transfuses blood has a responsibility, not only to his or her patients but also to the community, to use blood components appropriately and prudently. In any given year, fewer than 5% of people donate blood. Although this is sufficient to provide the blood needed in the United States, maintaining an adequate supply every day in the face of the large day-to-day variations in use that occur in most communities has always been difficult. The difficulties can be minimized if each physician transfusing blood components takes care to avoid transfusion not only where it would be harmful or contraindicated, but also whenever it would simply be ineffective. Examples of ineffective uses are situations in which plasma is transfused when platelet concentrates or cryoprecipitate might be more effective (as in certain cases of ruptured aortic aneurysms). Prolonged transfusion support in cases where no definitive treatment is available and there is no hope of arresting bleeding is also inappropriate. The challenge of a hopeless situation cannot be met with arbitrary limits on transfusion support. It requires skill, wisdom, and judgment on the part of the physician and compassionate but honest communication with patients and family members. At all times it should be kept in mind that transfusions in actively bleeding surgical patients are, for the most part, supportive rather than definitive treatment. The prognosis depends on correction of the underlying cause of bleeding. As with other forms of life support, vigorous, even heroic, transfusion support is appropriate as long as there is realistic expectation for the patient's recovery. When that expectation vanishes, so does the rationale for continued transfusion. Although prolonged transfusion support of irremediable bleeding may sow the seeds of hope in the physician and family, false hopes often yield a bitter harvest.

REFERENCES

1. Wallace EL, Churchill WH, Surgenor DM, An J, Cho G, McGurk S, Murphy L. Collection and transfusion of blood and blood components in the United States, 1992. Transfusion 1995;35:802–812.
2. Standards for blood banks and transfusion services, 17th ed. Bethesda, MD: American Association of Blood Banks, 1996.
3. Mollison PL, Engelfriet CP, Contreras M. Blood transfusion in clinical medicine, 9th ed. Oxford: Blackwell Scientific Publications, 1993.
4. Technical manual, 11th ed. Bethesda, MD: American Association of Blood Banks, 1993.
5. Giblett ER. Blood group alloantibodies: an assessment of some laboratory practices. Transfusion 1977;17:299–308.
6. Aach RD, Szmuness W, Mosley JW, et al. Serum alanine aminotransferase of donors in relation to the risk of non-A, non-B hepatitis in recipients. N Engl J Med 1981;304:989–994.
7. Busch MP, Young MJ, Samson SM, Mosley JW, Ward JW, Perkins HA. Risk of human immunodeficiency virus (HIV) transmission by blood transfusion before implementation of HIV-1 antibody screening. Transfusion 1991;31:4–11.
8. Human immunodeficiency virus infection in transfusion recipients and their family members. MMWR 1987;36:137–140.
9. Busch MP, Kleinman SH, Williams AE, et al. Frequency of human immunodeficiency virus (HIV) infection among contemporary anti-HIV-1 and anti-HIV-1/2 supplemental test-indeterminate blood donors. Transfusion 1996;36:37–44.
10. Schreiber GB, Busch MP, Kleinman SH, Korelitz JJ. The risk of transfusion-transmitted viral infections. N Engl J Med 1996;334: 1685–1690.
11. Counts RB, Haisch C, Simon TL, Maxwell NG, Heimbach DM, Carrico CJ. Hemostasis in massively transfused trauma patients. Ann Surg 1979;190:91–99.
12. Simon TL, Henderson R. Coagulation factor activity in platelet concentrates. Transfusion 1979;19:186–189.
13. Morrow JF, Braine HG, Kickler TS, Ness PM, Dick JD, Fuller AK. Septic reactions to platelet transfusions: a persistent problem. JAMA 1991;266:555–558.
14. Wagner SJ, Friedman LI, Dodd RY. Transfusion-associated bacterial sepsis. Clin Microbiol Rev 1994;7:290–302.
15. Fresh-frozen plasma. Indications and risks. Report of an NIH Consensus Conference. JAMA 1985;253:551–553.
16. American Society of Anesthesiologists Task Force on Blood Component Therapy. Practice guidelines for blood component therapy. Anesthesiology 1996;84:732–747.
17. Popovsky MA, Chaplin HC, Moore SB. Transfusion-related acute lung injury: a neglected, serious complication of hemotherapy. Transfusion 1992;32:589–592.
18. Burka ET, Harker LA, Kasper CK, Kevy SV, Ness PM. A protocol for cryoprecipitate production. Transfusion 1975;15:307–311.
19. Ness PM, Perkins HA. Cryoprecipitate as a reliable source of fibrinogen replacement. JAMA 1979;241:1690–1691.
20. Bowden RA, Sayers MH, Gleaves CA, Banaji M, Newton B, Meyers JD. Cytomegalovirus-seronegative blood components for the prevention of primary cytomegalovirus infection after marrow transplantation. Transfusion 1987;27:478–481.
21. Bowden RA, Slichter SJ, Sayers MH, Weisdorf D, Cays M, Schoch G, Banaji M. A comparison of filtered leukocyte-reduced and cytomegalovirus (CMV) seronegative blood products for the prevention of transfusion-associated CMV infection after marrow transplant. Blood 1995;86:3598–3603.
22. Burgstaler EA, Pineda AA, Brecher MA. Platelet pheresis: comparison of platelet yields, processing time, and white cell content with two apheresis systems. Transfusion 1993;33:393–398.
23. Hillyer CD, Tiegerman KO, Berkman EM. Evaluation of the red cell storage lesion after irradiation in filtered packed red cell units. Transfusion 1991;31:497–499.
24. Simon TL, Sierra ER. Concentration of platelet units into small volumes. Transfusion 1984;24:173–175.

Chapter 3

A Physiological Basis for the Transfusion Trigger

ROBERT M. WINSLOW

INTRODUCTION

The nation's red cell supply is safer now than it ever has been. The number of days of life lost as a result of transfusions probably reached a minimum by 1990 as a result of improved testing and other blood bank procedures (1). However, it will always be impossible to specify the exact components in a unit of donated human blood, a desired and increasingly required standard of the pharmaceutical industry (2). Beyond the risks of infectious disease transmission are the risks of infectious complications after surgical procedures, possibly due to immunosuppressive effects of transfusion (3). Thus, we cannot deny that new, as yet undiscovered, dangerous infectious agents *might* be transmitted by blood transfusion, and we are obliged to endeavor, as clinicians, to transfuse only when there is a clear clinical indication.

To control and limit transfusion practice, hospitals now routinely empower transfusion committees to monitor the use of blood and blood products. For example, all transfusions of packed red blood cells in which the recipient's hemoglobin concentration is 8 g/dL or greater may be reviewed by peers, and if sufficient justification is not found, a letter of reprimand may be placed in the physician's credentialing file that documents unnecessary exposure to blood products. Adequate documentation in the patient's record of the rationale for transfusion would include hemodynamic instability, objective evidence of ischemia (ECG, etc.), or evidence or reasonable anticipation of uncontrolled bleeding. For example, a patient with actively bleeding esophageal varices with a hemoglobin over 8 g/dL would be an obvious candidate for red cell transfusion because of the possibility of overwhelming blood loss and the inaccuracy of hemoglobin concentration or hematocrit to track rapid blood loss.

The "transfusion trigger" is that event or set of events that result in a patient's receiving a red cell transfusion. Excellent recent discussions have been published regarding the transfusion trigger (4–6), and numerous conferences have been held to attempt to set up specific guidelines or algorithms whereby clinicians can make objective decisions regarding the use of red cells (7, 8). Nevertheless, no guidelines exist that would reliably serve a clinician who is not familiar with the basic principles of O_2 transport physiology.

For many years, an empirical transfusion trigger was a hemoglobin concentration of 10 g/dL. If the value was less, the patient received at least 2 units of packed red cells or whole blood, despite the well-known fact that many patients tolerate modest anemia quite well (9). The rationale for such transfusions was that an O_2 reserve needed to be maintained so that if unexpected (or expected) blood loss occurred during surgery, the patient would be in less danger of suffering deficient O_2 delivery to tissue. Guidelines for the transfusion of blood or packed red cells in the face of severe blood loss have been less well defined.

Physiologists and physicians have always been aware that hemoglobin concentration as a transfusion trigger is a gross oversimplification. But because the risks of blood transfusion were considered to be negligible, there was little concern about the possibility of overtransfusing. Now that finite risks of blood products are focused more clearly, the trigger must be re-examined. For example, if the normal male hematocrit ranges from 42 to 52%, is it logical that all patients should have the same trigger? Should males and females, young and old, and patients with ischemic coronary disease all have the same trigger? Probably not, but tools have not been available to sharply define individual transfusion triggers. There are, in general, two types of indication for transfusion of red blood cells: inadequate O_2 delivery (anemia) and acute blood loss (volume depletion). They are different, and there is no reason, a priori, to assume the triggers for transfusion should be the same in the two instances.

NORMAL ERYTHROPOIESIS

Red blood cells are produced in the bone marrow. These cells, like others produced in the marrow, derive from stem cells that differentiate as they divide under the influence of several growth factors, including erythropoietin, a hormone produced primarily in the kidney and transported to the marrow by the blood. In vitro, red blood cell maturation is not possible in the absence of erythropoietin, and this undoubtedly explains why anephric patients have chronic, often transfusion-dependent, anemia. In vivo, small amounts of erythropoietin may be produced in extrarenal sites.

The stages of maturation of immature red blood cells are defined by their morphology (Fig. 3.1). In normal erythropoiesis, the nucleus is extruded from the cell before it leaves the marrow, and the cell is released as a reticulocyte. The reticulocyte contains residual RNA in its cytoplasm and is still capable of some protein synthesis. The RNA gives this cell its characteristic bluish appearance on staining with Wright's stain. An increase in the absolute number of reticulocytes indicates accelerated erythropoiesis, and a failure to increase after blood loss suggests a limitation of normal erythropoiesis.

In normal humans, the average red blood cell exists in the circulation for approximately 120 days. Because destruction is random, this means that the half-life for the red cell mass is about 28 days. In cases in which red cells are broken down faster, as in hemolytic anemia, the red cell half-life can be much less. For example, in sickle cell anemia patients, the red cell half-life may be only a few days. If such patients experience even short periods of red cell aplasia, as they do with some viral infections, symptomatic anemia can develop extremely quickly.

Iron is required for normal erythropoiesis, and its deficiency is one of the most common causes of anemia. Normal men have approximately 50 mg/kg of iron and women 35 mg/kg in their body. This is present mainly as heme iron, contained not only in hemoglobin (about half) but also in myoglobin, other heme-containing proteins, and in various storage forms, including ferritin and hemosiderin. A small amount of free iron is present in the plasma bound to transferrin, and measurement of this protein and its degree of saturation is a useful way to assess the adequacy of body iron

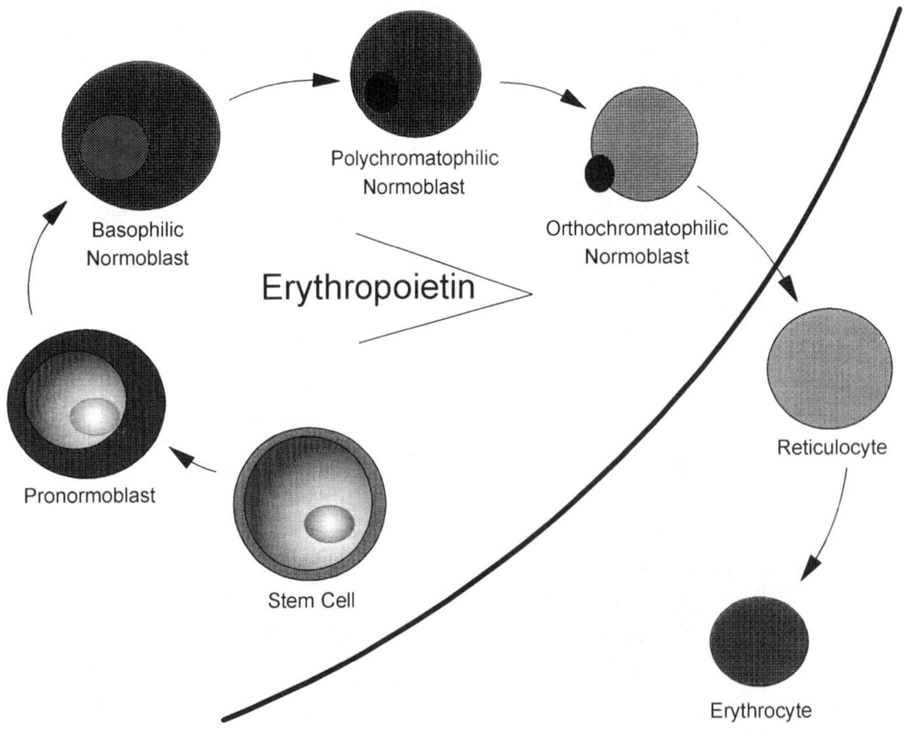

Figure 3.1. The stages of development of red blood cells.

stores. Iron enters the body via the gastrointestinal tract, mainly in the duodenum and upper jejunum. In addition to measurement of transferrin saturation and plasma free iron, direct examination of bone marrow after Prussian blue staining can help estimate the adequacy of the body iron stores for erythropoiesis.

Other common nutritional factors required for normal DNA synthesis (including erythropoiesis) are vitamins B_{12} and folic acid. Vitamin B_{12} deficiency is the underlying cause of pernicious anemia, a condition not encountered as frequently now as in years past. Vitamin B_{12} deficiency can result from a deficiency of gastric intrinsic factor (true pernicious anemia) or from prior surgical procedures in either the stomach, its site of production, or the small intestine, the site of absorption of intrinsic factor-B_{12} complex. Folic acid is also present in the normal diet, but vegetarians who overcook their food, alcoholics, and patients with chronic hemolysis are among those at risk for deficiency. Both B_{12} and folic acid deficiency lead to megaloblastic anemia, so called because the primary defect is in DNA synthesis and marrow erythroid cells do not divide normally, leaving cells in which cytoplasmic and nuclear maturation are discordant. Some of these cells are large, hence the name *megaloblastic*. A key difference between deficiencies of vitamin B_{12} and folic acid is that the former also leads to irreversible and characteristic nerve degeneration if not treated promptly.

Vitamin B_{12} and folate deficiencies are almost always *macrocytic*; that is, the mean cell volume (MCV) is greater than normal. Iron deficiency characteristically produces a microcytic anemia. The MCV is reported on all routine hematological screens, and abnormal values should always be taken seriously. Patients with abnormal MCV should be evaluated for treatable deficiencies.

Consideration of these principles of normal erythropoiesis is relevant to any consideration of the transfusion trigger. The physician must be able to assess each patient's capacity to regenerate red cells after surgical or traumatic loss, and this assessment will influence the decision to transfuse and the determination of the amount of red blood cells that will be needed.

PHYSIOLOGY OF OXYGEN TRANSPORT

DEFINITION OF TERMS

Global (sometimes called *convective,* as opposed to capillary or *diffusive*) O_2 transport is the product of the blood flow (cardiac output) and the difference between arterial and mixed venous blood O_2 content (Fig. 3.2). This relationship is simply a statement of the following well-known Fick equation:

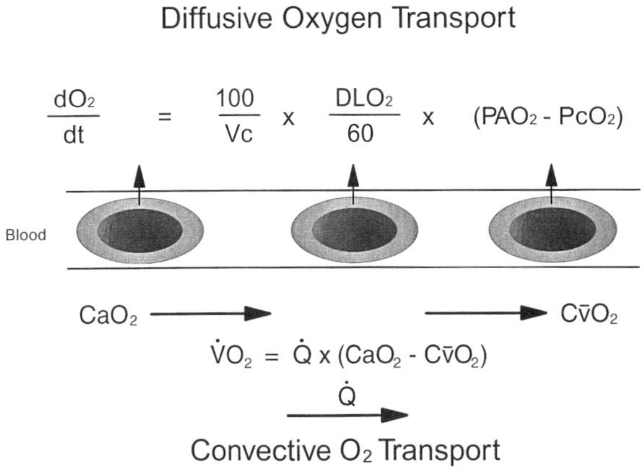

Figure 3.2. Convective and diffusive O_2 transport.

$$\dot{V}O_2 = \dot{Q} \cdot (CaO_2 - C\bar{v}O_2) \quad (1)$$

where $\dot{V}O_2$ is the O_2 used by the body, $\dot{Q}$ is the cardiac output, CaO_2 and $C\bar{v}O_2$ are the arterial and mixed venous O_2 contents, respectively.

Diffusive O_2 uptake in the lung (Fig. 3.2) is described by the following diffusion equation:

$$\frac{d(O_2)}{dt} = \frac{100}{V_c} \cdot \frac{DLO_2}{60} \cdot (PaO_2 - PcO_2) \quad (2)$$

In this equation, $d(O_2)/dt$ is the rate of O_2 diffusion into the capillary, PaO_2 is the alveolar PO_2, PcO_2 is the pulmonary capillary PO_2, DLO_2 is the diffusion coefficient for tissue, and V_c is the volume of capillary blood. Roughton and Forster (10) described the components of this coefficient:

$$\frac{1}{DLO_2} = \frac{1}{DMO_2} + \frac{1}{\Theta O_2 \times V_c} \quad (3)$$

In this equation, DMO_2 is the diffusion coefficient for the alveolar/capillary membrane interface and is proportional to the thickness of the membrane. ΘO_2 is the reaction rate constant of O_2 with hemoglobin.

These relationships are conceptually simple, but their numerical modeling is complex and iterative. For example, ΘO_2 is dependent on the hemoglobin saturation, which in turn is dependent on the position of the O_2-hemoglobin saturation curve (P_{50}), itself dependent on 2,3-diphosphoglycerate (2,3-DPG), pH, and $PCO_2 \cdot$ pH and PCO_2 are further interdependent, and both are affected by the buffering of hemoglobin. Each term in Equations 1–3 has a number of determinants that can vary in different physiological conditions and in disease or pathological states. Although complex, these variables can be accounted for using computer techniques, and, as shown in Figure 3.3, exchange curves for O_2 and CO_2 in the lung can be calculated (11). The situation in the tissues is slightly more

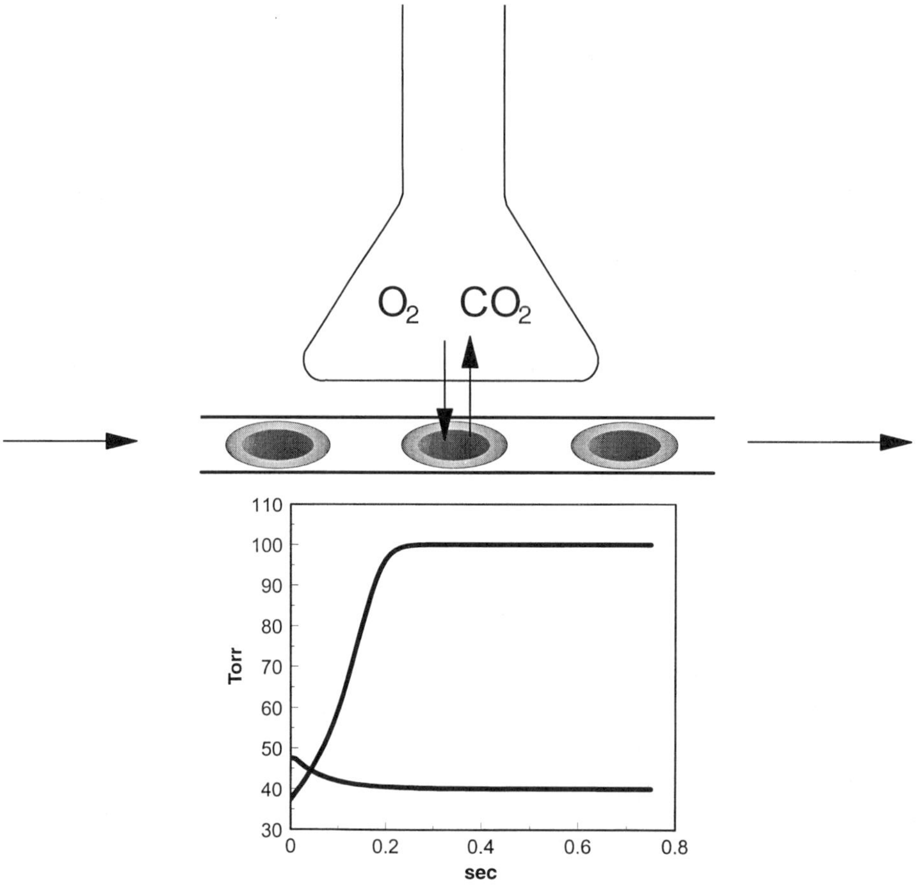

Figure 3.3. Diffusive exchange of CO_2 and O_2 in the lung. As venous red blood cells pass into pulmonary capillaries, they take up O_2 from plasma that is oxygenated by diffusion across the pulmonary capillary membrane, and CO_2 is released. The uptake curve for O_2 and release curve for CO_2 are shown in the lower panel, representing an example of normal red cells for a resting human. The average time of transit for a red cell under these conditions is approximately 0.8 seconds.

complicated, but in general represents the mirror image, and the principles governing the exchange of gases are the same.

Another, perhaps clearer, way to view the Fick relationship is shown graphically in Figure 3.4. Each figure panel is made up of two components: the hemoglobin-O_2 dissociation curve and the cardiac output. The numerical calculations, summarized in Table 3.1, for the three examples to follow were done based on data from patients and normal humans studied under different physiological conditions (10).

EXAMPLES

The examples to be discussed consider a number of variables that can alter overall O_2 transport individually. Using this approach, the cardiac output is determined by two factors: the O_2 requirement (Vo_2) and the blood viscosity (determined by the hematocrit). The regulation of these variables is well documented (12). The mixed venous Po_2 ($P\bar{v}o_2$) is calculated as the Po_2 that corresponds to the mixed venous O_2 content when all conditions in the Fick equation are satisfied. These calculations and the assumptions underlying them have been described in the literature (11). The following variables are considered in these examples:

1. Alveolar Po_2 (Pao_2) is assumed to be 100 Torr, corresponding to a normal sea level environment in a subject with normal ventilation.
2. Arterial Po_2 (Pao_2) is also assumed to be 100 Torr and assumes no alveolar-arterial diffusion gradient. In fact, a small gradient usually is present but does not affect the calculations because the blood is well-saturated even at 80 Torr.
3. Arterial Pco_2 ($Paco_2$) is assumed to be 40 Torr, the value found in normal resting persons with normal ventilation.
4. Arterial pH is assumed to be 7.4, a normal value.
5. The red cell 2,3-DPG:hemoglobin molar ratio. In a large number of normal volunteers studied in our laboratory, this value is 0.88 mol:mol (13). The 2,3-DPG:Hb ratio, pH, and Pco_2 are the principal determinants of the position of the blood

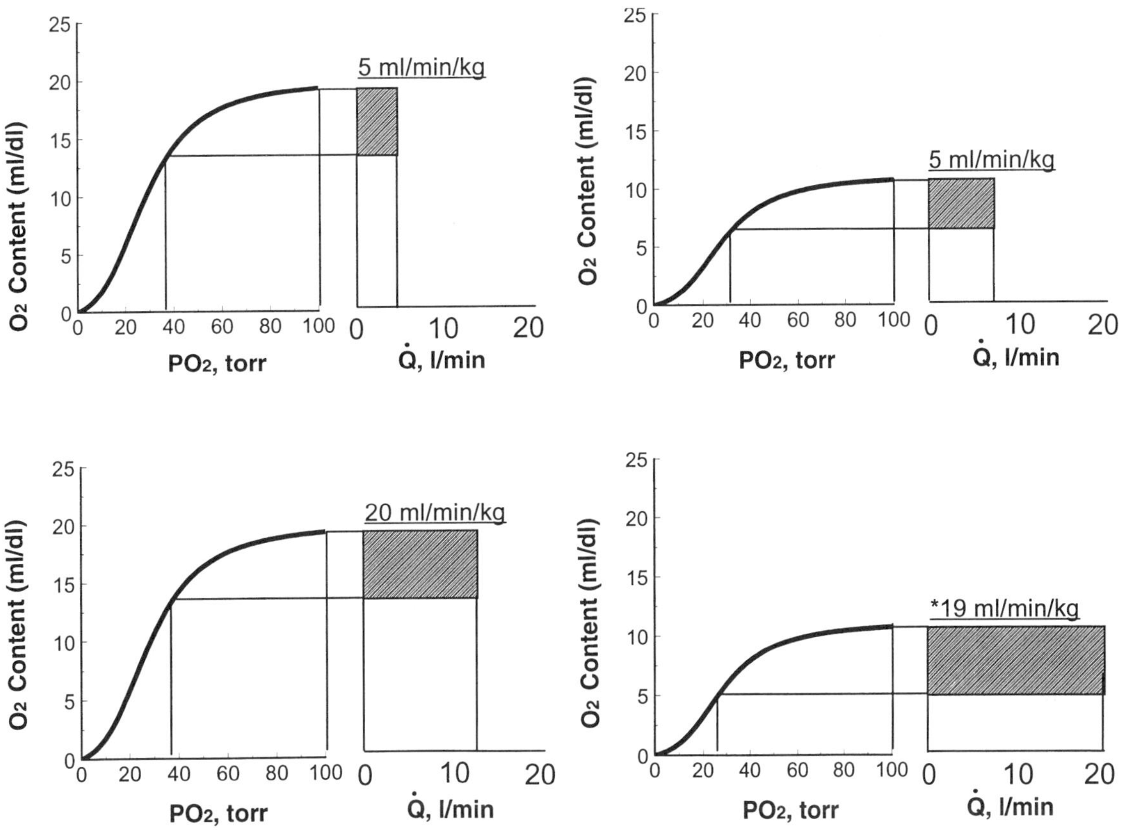

Figure 3.4. Graphical representation of the Fick equation. The examples are described in the text and include normal resting conditions (*top left*); anemia (*top right*); increased O_2 demand (*bottom left*), as in mild to moderate exercise; and the combination of exercise and anemia (*bottom right*). A numerical summary is provided in Table 3.1.

O_2-dissociation curve (P_{50}). These parameters are used to calculate a continuous curve for the given conditions used in the example calculations (14).

6. Pulmonary diffusing capacity (DMO_2) is assumed to be 40 mL/mL/mm Hg, as it is in normal persons. Alterations of this value will change the alveolar-arterial diffusion gradient (15).
7. The volume of pulmonary capillary blood (V_c) is a parameter of pulmonary diffusion (10) and in certain pulmonary diseases can increase the alveolar-arterial diffusion gradient. A value of 70 mL is used.

Normal Hematocrit and O_2 Demand

The first example is a normal resting human with a hematocrit of 45%. In this example, the O_2 utilization is approximately 5 mL/kg/min and the arterial O_2 content is about 18 mL/100 mL of blood. To satisfy the conditions that there is no base excess, that the O_2 dissociation curve is determined by the factors mentioned above, and that the cardiac output (as determined by hematocrit and VO_2) is 5.46 L/min, the arterial-venous O_2 content difference results in a $P\bar{v}O_2$ of 37.4 Torr. These calculations show that 34% of the arterial O_2 is extracted by tissue.

TABLE 3.1. OXYGEN EXCHANGE

	Rest	**Anemia**	**Exercise**	**Exercise + Anemia**
Pa50 (Torr)	28.6	28.6	28.6	28.6
SaO_2 (fraction)	0.961	0.961	0.961	0.961
CaO_2 (mL/dL)	18.85	10.61	18.85	10.61
BEBa (mEg/L)	−0.1	−0.1	−0.1	−0.1
pHv	7.365	7.367	7.340	7.353
$S\bar{v}O_2$ (fraction)	0.645	0.550	0.437	0.385
$C\bar{v}O_2$ (mL/dL)	12.44	5.89	8.43	4.12
$P\bar{v}50$ (Torr)	29.8	29.7	30.7	30.2
$P\bar{v}CO_2$ (Torr)	47.6	45.8	53.2	48.5
$P\bar{v}O_2$ (Torr)	37.4	32.0	27.8	25.1
OER (fraction)	0.34	0.44	0.53	0.61
Pulmonary transit time (sec)	0.77	0.57	0.31	0.22
$\dot{Q}$(L/min)	5.46	7.42	13.4	19.4

Anemia, Normal O_2 Demand

The second example considers holding all variables constant except that the hematocrit is dropped to 25%. As a result of this change, the cardiac output rises to 7.42 L/min by virtue of reduced blood viscosity and resistance to flow. This increased flow, however, does not completely compensate for the reduced arterial O_2 content, and a larger fraction of the arterial O_2 must be extracted (44%), resulting in a lower $P\bar{v}O_2$ (32.0 Torr). Still, however, the O_2 requirement (5 mL/kg) can be satisfied.

It should be appreciated that this example is a simplification, because in anemia, ventilation increases, raising PaO_2, lowering $PaCO_2$, and raising pH. In turn, the changes shift the O_2 dissociation curve to the left (increased affinity, lower P_{50}) that, in turn, affects ΘO_2. Furthermore, with time, this respiratory alkalosis becomes compensated by metabolic (renal) mechanisms.

Normal Hematocrit, Increased O_2 Demand

The third example illustrates still another variation on these variables: increased VO_2, as might be found in moderate (but aerobic) exercise. In this case, the VO_2 is placed at 20 mL/kg, but all other variables are held constant. The result is that the cardiac output is much higher (13.3 L/min), the mixed venous PO_2 is lower (27.9 Torr), but a larger fraction of the arterial O_2 is extracted (53%). Again, all conditions are satisfied, and O_2 requirements are met.

This, too, is a simplification of the actual situation; hyperventilation may increase PaO_2 and DMO_2 with resulting alkalosis, but muscular work will also produce lactic acid that drops pH with the effect of reducing hemoglobin O_2 affinity (increased P_{50}). Furthermore, raised cardiac output shortens the "dwell" time for a red cell in the pulmonary capillary and when raised to extreme values, can actually lead to reduced PaO_2 during heavy exercise.

OXYGEN UTILIZATION: DO_2, VO_2, AND THE "CRITICAL O_2"

A useful way to consider O_2 transport was introduced by Cain (16). He compared the delivery of O_2 (DO_2, cardiac output × arterial O_2 content) with O_2 utilization (e.g., cardiac output × (a-v)O_2 difference). This analysis led to the demonstration that as hematocrit is decreased (decreasing DO_2), there is no change in O_2 uptake (VO_2) until a "critical" DO_2 is reached, at which point VO_2 can no longer be sustained (Fig. 3.5). Thus, DO_2 has two components, called *diffusion limited* (above the critical DO_2) and *supply limited* (below the critical DO_2) O_2 delivery.

As discussed below, patients are in serious danger of organ failure if DO_2 is allowed to drop below the critical value,

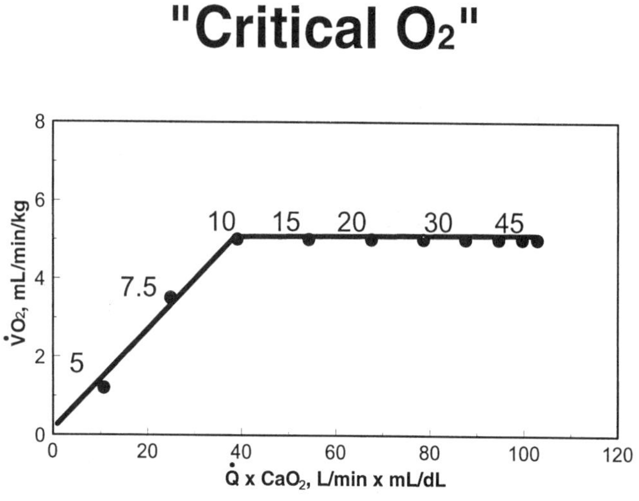

Figure 3.5. The critical DO_2 (Q × CaO_2). As the hematocrit is reduced in 5% steps, VO_2 is maintained by a combination of rising cardiac output and dropping $P\bar{v}O_2$. When these compensations no longer suffice, VO_2 falls, and tissue ischemia occurs. The goal of transfusion therapy is to maintain the O_2 reserve such that this point is not reached.

and the goal of transfusion (and other) therapy is to maintain DO_2 well above that value so that an appropriate reserve of O_2 is maintained should the patient require it because of blood loss or elevated VO_2.

THE "OPTIMAL" HEMATOCRIT

What is the "optimal" hematocrit? Obviously, there is no simple answer to this question and certainly none that would apply to all patients. But a review of the basic principles of this concept is useful to consider the optimal usage of red blood cells in transfusion therapy.

The bulk viscosity of blood increases exponentially with hematocrit, and increased viscosity raises resistance to blood flow, limiting cardiac output in the absence of compensatory mechanisms. As shown in Figure 3.6, as the O_2 capacity of the blood (hemoglobin or hematocrit) increases, cardiac output decreases, and over a wide range of hematocrit there exists an optimum, defined as the point of maximal DO_2. These principles have been studied theoretically (17), in animals (18), and in humans with extensions to high altitude polycythemia (19), and the general conclusion is that 35% hematocrit represents the best combination of cardiac output and hematocrit. If all patients were in perfect health, a transfusion trigger could be simply defined as 35%.

The problem, of course, is that patients, by definition, are not in perfect health, and the ability to compensate for loss of hemoglobin by raising cardiac output, for example, may be quite variable. In addition, it is not always simple to deter-

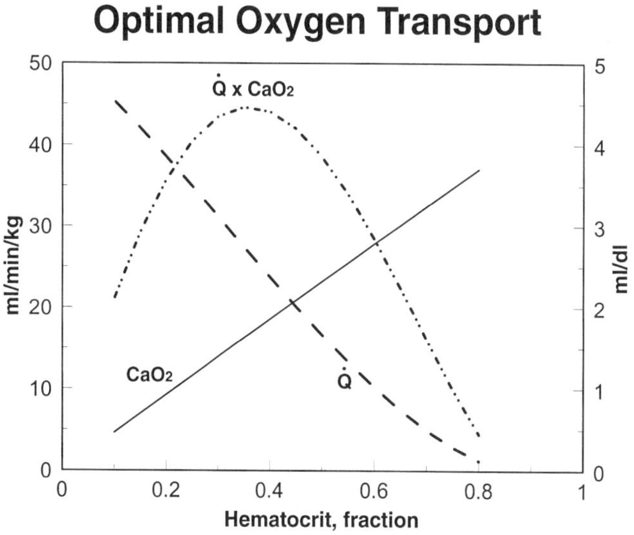

Figure 3.6. The relationship between blood viscosity, hematocrit, and cardiac output. (Reprinted with permission from Winslow RM. Hemoglobin-based red cell substitutes. Baltimore: John Hopkins University Press, 1992.)

mine which patients can use compensatory mechanisms and which cannot or which ones are in greater danger of localized tissue ischemia because of restrictions such as coronary stenosis.

Therefore, the "optimal" hematocrit is of limited value in determining a target hematocrit or transfusion trigger. To understand the basis of rational clinical decisions in this regard, we must examine first the different indications for blood transfusion and then some of the physiological and clinical transfusion triggers that are available.

PHYSIOLOGICAL TRANSFUSION TRIGGERS

Using this quantitative framework, is it possible to identify physiological markers that can be used as a transfusion trigger that might be more useful than hemoglobin or hematocrit? Obviously, a number would be more useful in clinical practice than subjective measurements and could lead to uniform criteria for the transfusion of red blood cells.

As our examples show, when the hemoglobin drops as the demand for O_2 rises, more of the arterial O_2 is used, venous O_2 is depleted, and $P\bar{v}O_2$ falls. Our calculations can be used to explore a range of O_2 delivery values ($Q \times CaO_2$ or DO_2) to predict what effect might be seen on $P\bar{v}O_2$ (Fig. 3.7). In this figure, DO_2 was reduced by reducing hematocrit at 5% intervals and calculating various potential physiological transfusion triggers.

$P\bar{v}O_2$ drops and the oxygen extraction ratio (OER) rises as continuous functions over the range of anemia down to a hematocrit of about 10%. Although we would agree that a transfusion would be desirable at some point in that interval, the data do not provide a clear-cut transfusion trigger. Cardiac output increases, $(a\text{-}v)O_2$ decreases, and the OER becomes greater, as shown in Figure 3.7, *lower left*. Calculation of the "critical O_2" (Fig. 3.7, *lower right*) appears to be the most useful, but it occurs at a hematocrit of 10%, clearly too low for clinical safety, and it is a derived calculation, often not readily available to the clinician. Thus, the goal of transfusion is to maintain an "O_2 reserve" such that the critical DO_2 is not reached.

Thus, although there is no clear-cut physiological transfusion trigger, many parameters have been proposed as indicative of the need for transfusion. The thoughtful clinician observes all possible signs of tissue ischemia and, based on experience, attempts to transfuse before the critical DO_2 is reached. In the following section, a brief discussion of some useful potential triggers is discussed briefly.

HEMATOCRIT/HEMOGLOBIN CONCENTRATION

The most commonly used parameter, the hematocrit (or hemoglobin concentration) is useful in some clinical situations but not in others, and it is important to be aware of its limitations. For example, in chronic anemia, an expanded plasma volume gives the impression that the red cell mass is smaller than it really is. In acute blood loss, some time is required for the fluid spaces to re-equilibrate and the hematocrit to once again reflect the red cell mass.

In one study of surgical patients, Spahn et al. (20) found that although hematocrit significantly correlated with red cell mass both intraoperatively and postoperatively, the ability of the hematocrit to predict red cell mass in individual patients was poor. In their study, hemodynamic parameters did not contribute to prediction of the red cell mass, plasma volume, or total blood volume at any time, and the authors believe that some patients, particularly those at risk for coronary ischemia, may be undertransfused if traditional hematocrit "triggers" are used. Similarly, Kim et al. (21) found no correlation with the level of hemoglobin at discharge, preoperative hemoglobin, or drop in hemoglobin during hospitalization with the number of inpatient days. They concluded that the use of blood transfusion as a means to shorten hospitalization is probably not justified. However, in another study of patients with postoperative myocardial ischemia (22), a postoperative hematocrit less than 28% was found to be associated with significantly more ischemic events than a hematocrit over 28%.

The hemoglobin concentration in Jehovah's Witness patients who undergo surgery with severe anemia is only a

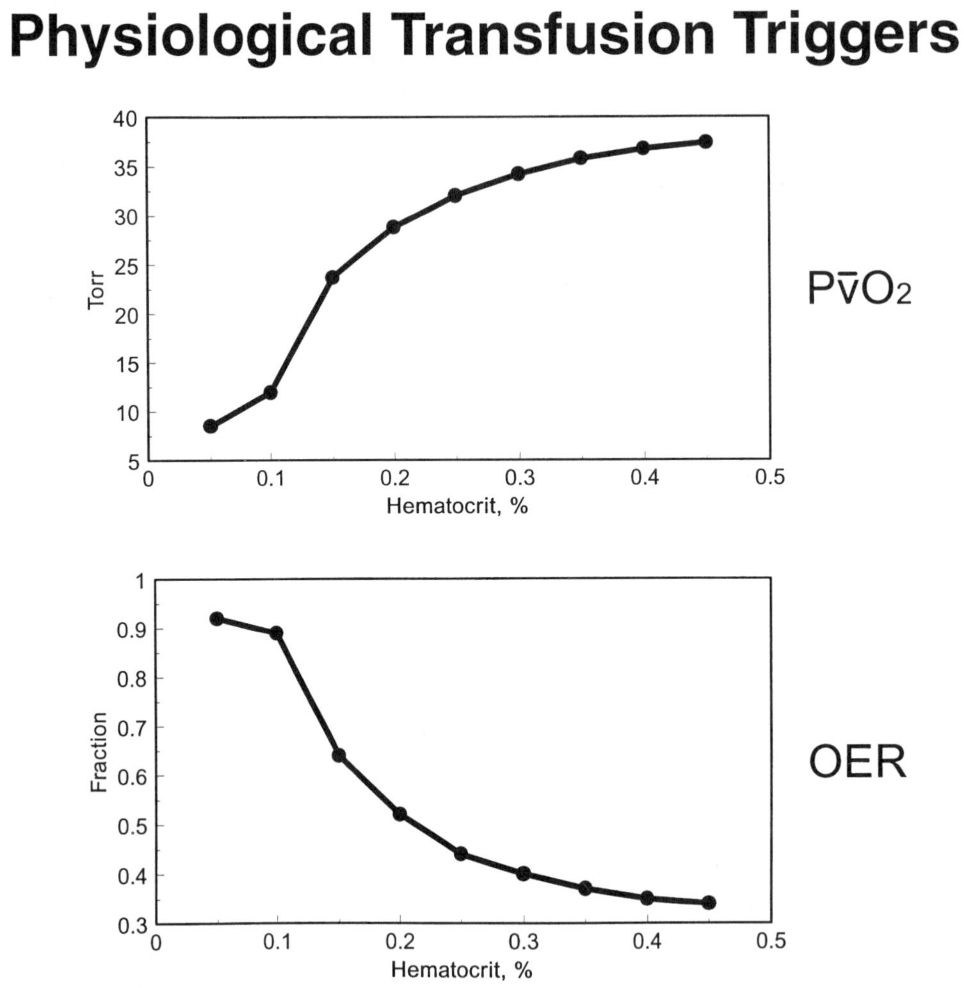

Figure 3.7. The effect of decreasing O_2 delivery (hematocrit) on two potential physiological transfusion triggers: $P\bar{v}O_2$ and the oxygen extraction ratio (OER). A rising cardiac output and falling $P\bar{v}O_2$ compensate over most of the range. The vertical line shows the hematocrit value at which tissues deteriorate (decreased VO_2) and is predicted from Figure 3.4. All parameters appear to be continuous functions and do not provide clear triggers.

predictor of overall outcome when less than 3 g/dL. Multiple independent factors influence outcome of these severely anemic surgical patients, the strongest being sepsis and active bleeding (23).

MIXED VENOUS PO_2

Mixed venous PO_2 ($P\bar{v}O_2$) would seem an obviously important parameter to assess adequacy of tissue oxygenation because, in theory, the mixed venous blood should be in equilibrium with tissue. Some clinical studies have shown that $P\bar{v}O_2$ decreases when VO_2 is supply dependent (Fig. 3.7) (24). However, as is now known, the tissue PO_2 is much lower than mixed venous values (25, 26) and $P\bar{v}O_2$ can be normal in severe anemia (27). The reason for this is complex but includes the fact that capillary blood can be shunted to different vascular beds in the face of hypovolemia, for example, so that $P\bar{v}O_2$ does not necessarily reflect the oxygenation state of *all* tissues. In addition, it is now understood that there is significant O_2 loss from arterioles and uptake in venules, so that the capillary PO_2 is much lower than mixed venous values (28, 29).

Nevertheless, a decreasing $P\bar{v}O_2$ has been used as a classic indicator of reduced tissue oxygenation, and perhaps a dropping value should be more meaningful to clinical evaluation of a given patient than an absolute value. Traditional textbooks of critical care medicine indicate that transfusions may be helpful when the $P\bar{v}O_2$ drops.

$S\bar{v}O_2$ may be a more useful indicator of severe O_2 extraction. Because of the steepness of the hemoglobin-O_2 dissociation curve, when mixed venous PO_2 falls below approximately 30 Torr, the hemoglobin saturation falls rapidly. As the hemoglobin reserve depletes, small drops in $P\bar{v}O_2$ will drop the $S\bar{v}O_2$ more rapidly. $S\bar{v}O_2$ falls dramatically at hematocrits less than approximately 20%. In one clinical study, Spiess et al. (30) showed that $S\bar{v}O_2$ is a sensitive indicator of overall O_2 consumption in liver transplant patients. In those patients, removal of the liver with attendant reduction in VO_2 produced a measurable rise in $S\bar{v}O_2$. When the new liver became functional, $S\bar{v}O_2$ fell back to normal values.

O_2 CONSUMPTION

Hemoglobin concentration may limit maximal VO_2 in some circumstances. However, the potential advantages of "blood doping" have not been fully realized, and, in general, the increased VO_2 associated with transfusion has been marginal and limited to well-trained athletes performing maximal work (31). Extending these observations to patients may be of little value, because patients never consume O_2 at or near their maximal rate.

Published literature suggests that reduced VO_2 in postoperative and trauma patients is associated with a poor prognosis and that increasing DO_2 by intervention (fluid boluses, administration of blood products, the use of inotropes) reduces mortality rate (32). In contrast, other evidence indicates that the *way* in which DO_2 is increased is critical; volume resuscitation more effectively raises VO_2 than transfusion, even though both raise DO_2.

In septic shock, VO_2 may be pathologically dependent on DO_2 (33–35). Patients whose cardiac output (and therefore DO_2) can be increased with dobutamine (36, 37) or adrenaline (38) can increase VO_2, possibly by improving specific organ perfusion (39). However, when DO_2 is raised by increasing hemoglobin concentration by transfusion, no effect is seen on VO_2 (38, 40, 41). In fact, when 23 critically ill patients with sepsis were transfused with stored blood, not only did the VO_2 (measured by calorimetry) fail to rise, but there was an inverse relationship between gastric mucosal pH and the age of the transfused blood (42), indicating poorer tissue oxygenation. In other studies, VO_2 failed to correlate with lactate levels in septic patients given either fluid therapy, transfusions, or dobutamine (43–45). These studies all indicate that pathological reduction of VO_2 in sepsis is due to reduced tissue perfusion, not reduced O_2 content of the perfusing blood.

Acute respiratory distress syndrome (ARDS) patients may represent another case in which O_2 uptake and utilization do not agree; they may not increase VO_2 after increasing DO_2 (46, 47). Hanique et al. (40) studied three groups of patients: septic, ARDS, and hepatic failure. They increased cardiac output by volume loading to increase DO_2 and measured VO_2 by calorimetry and calculated VO_2 by Fick (Equation 1). They found that the calculated VO_2 (Fick) increased, whereas the measured VO_2 (calorimetry) did not. By using an increase in VO_2 as a criterion for successful transfusion, as many as 58% of transfusions may be of questionable importance (48).

OXYGEN EXTRACTION RATIO

The OER is the fraction of arterial O_2 delivery extracted by tissue. In other words,

$$\text{OER} = \frac{CaO_2 - C\bar{v}O_2}{CaO_2} \tag{4}$$

In dogs with experimental stenotic lesions in the left anterior descending coronary arteries, hearts did not raise their output in response to bleeding, showed greater lactate production, and failed at a higher hematocrit (17%) than controls (10.6%) (49). The authors of this study concluded that in the normal heart, lactate production occurs when OER is greater than 50% and hematocrit less than 10%, but in the stenotic animals, an OER greater than 50% corresponded to a hematocrit less than 20%. Thus, an OER greater than 50% indicated a need for transfusion in these animals, and the findings indicate that the transfusion trigger, in terms of hematocrit or hemoglobin concentration, is higher in hearts with underlying coronary ischemia. Similar results have been reported for primates (50). These observations are consistent with experience in patients (51).

HEMODYNAMIC INSTABILITY

In shock, reduced O_2 capacity and blood volume contraction exist at the same time. Most resuscitations are carried out first with volume expanders and then with replacement of lost red cells. However, it is not clear whether volume or O_2 capacity reduction is more important. Thus, Deitrich et al. (52) studied patients with a variety of diagnoses who had undergone volume resuscitation in shock. They concluded that an increase of DO_2 by transfused red blood cells did increase O_2 capacity, but they could not demonstrate any benefit measured as increased VO_2, decreased lactate, or myocardial work.

BLOOD LOSS

Blood loss itself, apart from the attendant hemodynamic changes, is an important indicator of the need for transfusion. Carson et al. (53) carried out a careful study of 125 surgical patients who declined to be transfused on religious grounds and found that mortality was inversely related to hemoglobin concentration. Mortality rose from 7.1% for patients with hemoglobin concentrations over 10 g/dL to 61.5% for those with hemoglobin concentrations below 6 g/dL. Mortality was 8% for patients in whom 500 mL or less blood was lost but rose to 42.9% for those in whom loss was greater than 2000 mL.

SYMPTOMS

Although a quantitative index of the need for a red blood cell transfusion would be optimal, in many instances, especially in cases of chronic anemia, the decision to transfuse is based on subjective symptom evaluation. Some signs and symptoms that might indicate inadequate tissue oxygenation due to anemia are fatigue, dyspnea, angina, or claudication. None of these subjective symptoms is uniquely indicative of anemia per se, and so they must be evaluated in the context of the patient's total clinical presentation. However, these symptoms are of most benefit in patients in whom other more quantitative "triggers" do not provide the clinician with a clear decision as to whether or not to transfuse.

OTHER SIGNS OF ISCHEMIA

It would seem that demonstration of hemoglobin-dependent oxygenation of specific tissues should be possible using modern sophisticated techniques of measurement. In general, this has not been the case. For example, when ^{19}F magnetic resonance spectroscopy was used to examine the in vivo bioenergetics in forearm muscles, no effect of increasing the hemoglobin concentration from 8.9 to 12.9 g/dL could be shown (54). Although O_2 is needed for wound healing, deposition of new collagen requires very little of it. Jonsson et al. (55) were not able to demonstrate any correlation of hematocrit and collagen deposition in 33 postoperative surgical patients.

INDICATIONS FOR BLOOD TRANSFUSION

ACUTE BLOOD LOSS (SHOCK)

Acute blood loss can be considered at three levels: mild (up to 20% blood volume), moderate (20–40% blood volume), and severe (over 40% blood volume). Most patients do not survive hemorrhage of greater than 50% blood volume (56). Compensatory mechanisms come into play in all three, but the degree of compensation varies with the severity of blood loss.

Apparently, chemoreceptors play little or no role in the acute response to blood loss at sea level. For example, Meyers et al. (57) found in the fetal lamb that arterial PO_2 did not drop, even after loss of 40% estimated blood volume because of hyperventilation and mild alkalosis. In contrast, in environmental hypoxia, arterial PO_2 falls despite hyperventilation and alkalosis. In the latter instance, O_2 uptake in the lung is diffusion-limited and an increase in pulmonary red cell transit time will limit full oxygenation of red cells (58).

Thus, the initial response to blood loss is mediated by baroreceptor (pressure) reflexes. These include increased heart rate and hyperventilation. Both increase cardiac output, the former by increasing heart rate and the latter by increasing right heart filling. An additional consequence of hyperventilation is a fall in PCO_2 and rise in arterial pH, both of which increase arterial hemoglobin saturation via the Bohr effect.

The second part of the response to acute hemorrhage in restoration of blood pressure is mediated by the almost immediate secretion of vasoactive hormones, catecholamines, and angiotensin II. The degree of hormone response is proportional to the degree of blood loss (57). Both mechanisms, baroreflex and hormone secretion, increase blood pressure and peripheral vascular resistance selectively; that is, blood flow is redistributed in a predictable way, decreasing sharply to muscle, skin, gut, and kidney while preserved to heart and brain.

A third response to blood loss is a redistribution of water, from the extravascular to intravascular space. This redistribution is responsible for the falling hemoglobin concentration observed after hemorrhage and occurs with impressive rapidity. Meyers et al. (57) found in the fetal lamb that hemoglobin concentration was significantly lower after as little as 2 minutes after a 40% controlled hemorrhage.

Several mechanisms account for this rapid refilling of the vascular space. First, falling hydrostatic pressure results in a net flux of water from the interstitial to intravascular space. Second, albumin is mobilized from the interstitial matrix and increases the oncotic pressure of the plasma. Third, albumin synthesis is increased in the liver, as is production of glucose and amino acids, which further increase the plasma oncotic pressure. This increase in oncotic pressure contributes to further refilling of the vascular space. Acute reduction of circulating blood volume can impair liver function (59).

As the vascular volume refills, hematocrit falls; consequently, blood viscosity is lowered. Lowered blood viscosity reduces resistance to blood flow, increases venous return to the heart, and maintains or increases cardiac output.

If these compensatory mechanisms are inadequate to preserve tissue oxygen requirements, lactic acid may be produced, dropping arterial pH. Acidosis presents a further stimulus to hyperventilation and reduces hemoglobin oxygen affinity via the alkaline Bohr effect. This may actually augment tissue oxygen delivery, especially in regions of the circulation in which O_2 requirements are high, such as in cardiac muscle or brain (60).

Finally, erythropoiesis is stimulated. The precise mechanism of this stimulation is not yet completely understood, because, as mentioned above, arterial PO_2 is preserved or increased in hemorrhage. Thus, the renal sensors that signal increased erythropoietin secretion must be sensitive to O_2 flux rather than O_2 concentration (Po_2). In any case, erythropoietin concentration can be seen to rise within 2–3 days of hemorrhage, a reticulocyte response is present between 2 and 7 days, and, in humans, the hemoglobin concentration can be seen to rise at about 7 days posthemorrhage. Of course, in many surgical patients, this sequence of events may be delayed or prevented if there are other limitations to erythropoiesis such as chronic inflammation, iron deficiency, or other concomitant problems.

This brief discussion illustrates that although most healthy patients can tolerate loss of up to 40% of their blood volume, many surgical patients who are not healthy may be much less tolerant of blood loss. For example, elderly patients with ischemic heart disease may suffer tissue infarction as a result of decreased organ blood flow. Patients with borderline or inadequate pulmonary function may not be able to maintain arterial oxygenation when red cell capillary transit time decreases with increased cardiac output. Patients with liver disease may not be able to increase albumin synthesis to increase plasma oncotic pressure, and so on. These factors must be kept firmly in mind when considering the clinical indications for transfusion in an individual patient.

To some extent, restitution of blood volume by crystalloid and/or colloid resuscitation can in itself restore cardiac output. Thus, Mitzner et al. (61) found that administration of epinephrine increased cardiac output by 55% partly due to lowered right atrial pressure (caused by improved cardiac function) and increased pressure (caused by the volume shift to the systemic circulation). The choice of plasma expanders in the treatment of shock is still debated (62), but some workers believe that colloids such as urea-linked succinylated gelatin (Gelofusine) and 6% hetastarch (Hespan) or Pentastarch are more effective than crystalloid in restoring myocardial blood flow and O_2 after acute hemorrhage.

It should be emphasized, however, that blood and red blood cells are not recommended as the first plasma expanders administered to shock patients because of their high viscosity. If the plasma space needs to be expanded to restore hemodynamic stability, colloid or crystalloid should be given first, with blood or red blood cells being given after hemodynamic stability is achieved.

CHRONIC ANEMIA

Transfusion practices in chronic anemia are not well documented in the literature, but clinicians tend to use the same hemoglobin and hematocrit triggers as in other types of anemia. This may not be appropriate because chronically anemic patients develop significant adaptation to their anemia, including increased cardiac output, expanded plasma volume, and hyperventilation.

Transfusion in chronic anemia may be part of a more disturbing indifference in physicians' attitudes and practices. Saxena et al. (63) studied transfusions in 265 iron-deficient patients in a large metropolitan medical center and found that in most cases, transfusions were given to raise the hematocrit or hemoglobin to arbitrary values rather than using clinical signs or symptoms as a guide. Furthermore, iron was not prescribed for almost one third of the patients, including those in whom blood was not given when it was clearly indicated.

HEMODILUTION

Much of the literature concerned with the transfusion trigger does not distinguish between acute blood loss and the more controlled condition, surgical hemodilution. The important difference is that in the latter instance, blood volume is controlled. Thus, strategies for conservation of allogeneic blood in the surgical setting involve removal of blood before surgery and replacement with crystalloid or colloid (or both) so that during surgery, loss of the patient's red cells can be minimized (64–66). These techniques can be very effective in blood sparing and reducing a patient's transfusion exposure.

A separate, but similar, situation, however, is the patient who presents with (relatively) long-standing anemia that is well compensated. One example of such patients is Jehovah's Witnesses, who refuse transfusions on religious grounds (67, 68). Hemoglobins as low as 5 g/dL have been reported not to be associated with increased mortality (65). Similarly, the recommendation has been made that otherwise healthy African children with a hemoglobin of 5 g/dL or higher should not be transfused unless congestive heart failure is detected (69, 70). Some of these children can tolerate hemoglobin concentrations as low as 3 or 3.5 g/dL (70).

These examples from clinical practice illustrate the importance of understanding that if blood volume is restored, either in the hospital (hemodilution) or by physiological refilling of the intravascular space (long-standing anemia), rather low hemoglobin concentrations can be managed successfully in many patients. This concept is in agreement with the above argument that chemoreceptors are relatively less significant in adjusting to hemorrhage than are baroreceptors.

THE TRANSFUSION TRIGGER: CURRENT PRACTICE

It is almost impossible to summarize the state of current transfusion practice. In fact, data are very difficult to obtain.

Probably the best compilation comes from the European SANGUIS study (71), which found tremendous variation from hospital to hospital regarding the use of blood and blood products.

In the United States, Goodnough (5) examined hematocrit in respect to blood loss in a group of surgical patients and found 26% of women but 13% of men were transfused in excess of their estimated blood loss. In another study, Friedman et al. (72) found that the same trigger was used in both men and women, even though the normal hematocrit ranges for the two sexes is well known to be different, and questioned whether this is appropriate. Current experience suggests that otherwise healthy patients with hemoglobin values of 10 g/dL or greater rarely require perioperative transfusion, whereas those with hemoglobin values of less than 7 g/dL will frequently require transfusion (8).

THE RISK OF UNDERTRANSFUSION

In our enthusiasm to spare patients the risks of blood transfusions, there is a risk of undertransfusion. Although a National Institutes of Health (NIH) consensus conference (8) recommended that the lower safe limit of hemoglobin concentration could be below 10 g/dL, no definite lower limit guideline was provided. Experimental studies by Wilkerson et al. (73) in hemodiluted baboons suggested that a hematocrit of 10% could be reached before the OER rose or mortality increased. Cain showed that the Vo_2/Do_2 slope did not reach a critical Do_2 until the hematocrit was less than 10% in dogs (16). Levine et al. (6) found adaptive physiological changes during progressive hemodilution down to 15% hematocrit, and a number of studies in Jehovah's Witness patients who refuse blood transfusion show that extremely low hemoglobin and hematocrit levels can be tolerated (74).

Animal studies underscore the risks of undertransfusion. Spahn et al. (20) hemodiluted dogs in whom experimental stenoses had been placed on the left anterior descending coronary artery. They then measured regional function of the myocardium by sonomicrometry and found that the lowest hemoglobin concentration tolerated without compromised function was 7.5 g/dL and an increase of as little as 1.9 g/dL by transfusion restored function and O_2 consumption in the affected region. Other investigators have also found that coronary stenosis in dogs limits coronary O_2 supply reserve in progressive hemodilution (75).

Similar observations have been made in patients. A hematocrit lower than 29% was associated with significant cardiac ischemia (76) in a group of surgical patients with peripheral vascular disease. Significantly more coronary ischemia occurred in patients undergoing peripheral vascular reconstructive surgery in whom the hematocrit was less than 28% (77). A hematocrit value of 28% appears to be the lower limit that can be safely reached in patients with clear evidence of coronary ischemia (78).

These animal and clinical studies suggest that the current practice of tolerating hemoglobin concentrations of 8 g/dL is probably as low as is reasonable and that further lowering of the transfusion trigger, especially in patients at risk for coronary ischemia, could be very dangerous.

In patients in whom the hematocrit must fall below approximately 28%, the astute clinician must assess the patient's ability to compensate for the reduced O_2 capacity, and if there is evidence of ischemia, careful monitoring of ECG, blood pressure, oxygen saturation, and ST segment analysis is indispensable (79).

CLINICAL TRANSFUSION TRIGGERS

Although a physiological transfusion trigger is elusive, actual clinical situations are far more complicated. For example, not all patients can raise cardiac output in response to the challenge of anemia. In others, tissue ischemia, such as in coronary artery disease, can raise the local Do_2 requirement, reducing the O_2 reserve for that area. In other patients, pulmonary disease may impose a diffusion barrier (increased DMO_2) or restrict ventilation, which can restrict pulmonary O_2 uptake.

An enormous amount has been written about the transfusion trigger since the NIH clinical conference in 1988. In some ways, focusing attention on this issue has resulted in physicians' attitudes drifting away from using "clinical judgement" toward the search for hard quantitative triggers that relieve the clinician from the responsibility for making a decision (80). In reality, a decision to transfuse (or not to transfuse) is a clinical judgement, and the astute clinician distills many different data, objective and subjective, in coming to a final decision.

Figure 3.8 shows some factors that can influence the O_2 delivery as described by the Fick equation. As already mentioned, these are highly iterative. It is beyond the scope of this discussion to explore each of them, but the examples and calculations above should make plain that the transfusion trigger will vary from patient to patient, is not quantifiable given our current state of quantitation, and the use of good clinical judgement cannot be avoided.

How, then, should the responsible physician consider the decision to transfuse? Table 3.2 presents an attempt at a rational approach. It is difficult to imagine a situation in which a hemoglobin over 10 g/dL would be desired. The issue of the optimal hematocrit has been explored in the literature exten-

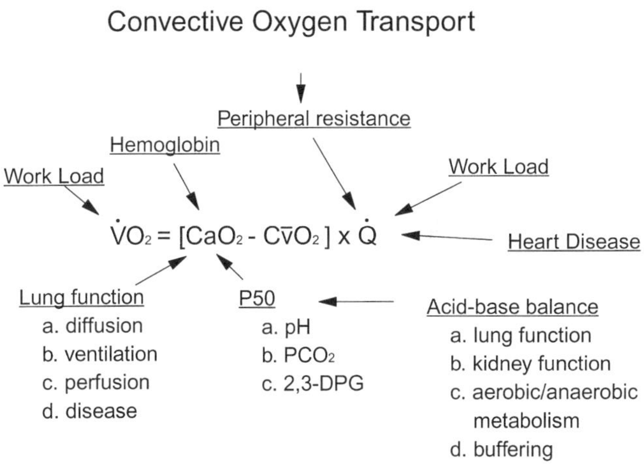

Figure 3.8. Interactions of the determinants of oxygen transport in health and disease. (Reprinted with permission from Winslow RM. Hemoglobin-based red cell substitutes. Baltimore: Johns Hopkins University Press, 1992.)

TABLE 3.2. CLINICAL TRANSFUSION TRIGGERS

Hemoglobin (g/dL)	Risk	Strategy
>10	Very low	Avoid
8–10	Low	Avoid; transfuse if demonstrably better after trial
6–8	Moderate	Try to avoid; decrease $\dot{V}O_2$ Clinical evaluation Volume status Pulmonary status Cardiac status (ischemia) Cerebrovascular status Duration of anemia Dyspnea on exertion Estimated blood loss during surgery Extent of surgery, risk of rebleed
<6	High	Usually requires transfusion

Modified from Swisher SN, Petz LD. Clinical practice of transfusion medicine. 2nd ed. New York: Churchill Livingstone, 1989: 531–548.

sively, and it appears that there is little justification for maintaining a hematocrit over 35% either at sea level or in high altitude natives (19). The reason for this is that as hematocrit rises, viscosity rises exponentially with increased resistance to flow and reduced cardiac output (18).

When the hemoglobin is between 8 and 10 g/dL, the risk to most patients is very low. Some patients, especially elderly ones, will report subjective improvement in symptoms of shortness of breath or dyspnea on exertion when their hematocrits are maintained over 8 g/dL. Transfusion in these patients would appear to be justified, but elevation to values over 10 g/dL would seem unnecessary.

A hemoglobin concentration between 6 and 8 g/dL requires a thoughtful approach to the clinical evaluation of the patient. One should try to avoid transfusion, and a number of alternatives are available, such as lowering V_{O_2} (e.g., rest, pharmacological agents, hypothermia) or treatments to modify the cause of anemia (e.g., stop the bleeding, treat underlying disease). But if neither can be done, then specific evaluation of a number of factors should be considered:

- Volume status: Is the patient hemodiluted or dehydrated? In other words, does the hemoglobin concentration reflect the true red cell mass?
- Pulmonary status: Is the patient able to oxygenate arterial blood? If not, why? Is the limitation diffusion or restricted ventilation? If the patient is a surgical candidate, will his or her ventilation be controlled?
- Cardiac status: Is there a history of myocardial ischemic disease or infarction? Such history would favor transfusion. Is the patient able to increase the cardiac output? The patient's age and symptoms are important factors here. The onset of coronary ischemic disease is most commonly seen one to two decades earlier in men than in women, and so sex can be an important consideration also. In general, one should assume coronary ischemia increases with age in both sexes.
- Cerebrovascular status: The considerations here are similar to those for cardiac status, except that the symptoms of ischemia may be more difficult to appreciate, particularly in the elderly. Is there a history of cerebrovascular accident? Are there neurological signs?
- Chronicity of anemia: An otherwise healthy person can adjust quite well to a hematocrit of 15% if the fall is slow; but if it is abrupt, it will usually cause severe symptoms.
- Symptoms: Does the patient complain of dyspnea on exertion, shortness of breath, or claudication?
- Estimated blood loss: If a patient is undergoing a procedure in which the extent of blood loss is expected to be high, the O_2 reserve should be maximized.
- Extent of surgery, risk of rebleeding: In such cases (e.g., coronary artery bypass graft procedures), rebleeding causes a significant risk of morbidity and mortality, especially in elderly high-risk patients. Included here should also be any patients with increased risk for bleeding, such as thrombocytopenic, or patients with liver disease.

When the hemoglobin is less than 6 g/dL, few would argue with the decision to transfuse except when the anemia is long-standing. Such cases would include, for example, some patients with pernicious anemia who are well adapted to a very low hematocrit. But the adaptation is due to, in part, chronically increased cardiac output and expanded blood volume, and a too vigorous transfusion can push the patient into overt congestive heart failure.

IMPACT OF BLOOD SUBSTITUTES ON THE TRANSFUSION TRIGGER

The use of cell-free hemoglobin, liposome-encapsulated hemoglobin, or perfluorocarbon emulsions as temporary red cell substitutes adds a new dimension to the transfusion trigger problem. They deliver O_2 in ways that are different from red cells (81, 82). For example, when animals are hemodiluted with cell-free hemoglobin, the cardiac output does not increase as expected from experience with conventional crystalloids or colloids. The reason for this is not clear, nor is it certain that all types of artificial O_2 carriers behave in the same way in this regard. Rosen et al. (83) showed that dextran hemodilution of animals that have already been hemodiluted with hemoglobin solution can raise their cardiac output in response to decreasing O_2 content, but for a given hemoglobin concentration the cardiac output is less than in animals with intact red cells. In contrast, Hess and coworkers (84) have claimed that failure of the cardiac output to rise in pigs after resuscitation with a cross-linked hemoglobin is a result of a specific hemoglobin-induced peripheral vasoconstriction. This matter may take some time to resolve. The physiological properties of cell-free O_2 carriers will have to be carefully studied. As an example, Stork et al. (85) found a complex interaction between blood viscosity (hematocrit) and blood flow distribution under hypoxic compared with normoxic conditions. Because cell-free O_2 carriers have Newtonian flow properties, these relationships can be expected to be quite different from those in whole blood.

In contrast to hemoglobin solutions, exchange transfusion with perfluorocarbon emulsions does not seem to limit cardiac output, but blood flow redistribution does occur and the pattern of redistribution might be unique to each product (86). In one study (87), the critical DO_2 was lowered in dogs given Fluosol DA, but the $P\bar{v}O_2$ was inexplicably high, calling into question the utility of this parameter as a measure of tissue PO_2. In other studies of perfluorocarbon emulsions, PO_2 measured with a Clark electrode has been increased, even though the O_2 increment is very small (88). Until results such as these can be rationalized, the use of PO_2 in patients who have been given perfluorocarbon emulsions must be viewed with skepticism.

If a red cell transfusion is given to prevent tissue hypoxia, how can a rational transfusion trigger be selected for clinical trials of red cell substitutes? When a transfusion is given to alleviate specific signs of ischemia (ECG changes, shortness of breath, angina, etc.), then one might see evidence of improvement after transfusion, and, conceivably, tests could be designed in which the goal would be to determine whether the indications are reversed.

Unfortunately, the optimal use of red cells is to prevent tissue hypoxia rather than to alleviate tissue ischemia, and so interpretation of clinical trials could be difficult if not impossible. It seems most likely that the best chance for a clear-cut demonstration of efficacy for a red cell substitute is in fully instrumented surgical patients whose detailed measurements of O_2 transport can be made. After efficacy is established in these patients, then the products could be used with more confidence in less intensively monitored patients.

SUMMARY AND CONCLUSIONS: INDIVIDUALIZED TRANSFUSION TRIGGERS

The transfusion trigger may not only be an elusive goal, it may not even be an appropriate one. Physiological studies cited in this chapter have shown animals can survive with hemoglobin concentrations lower than most clinicians would permit in patients. A recent NIH clinical conference (8) recommended that a 10-g/dL hemoglobin concentration might be too high for a transfusion trigger, and recent editorials (81) have recommended that when the hemoglobin is between 7 and 10 g/dL, many physiological and clinical data have to be considered before an intelligent decision can be made. Indeed, it might be time to abandon the concept of a transfusion trigger.

What effect should age, sex (42), heart disease (animal studies [42] suggest baboons can be lowered to a hematocrit of 15%, but failure occurs at a higher hematocrit in animals with experimental stenotic lesions), sickle cell (89), and sepsis (37, 90) (increased capillary permeability) have on the decision to transfuse? The decision to transfuse a patient should be based on his or her need for augmented O_2 delivery to tissue and the risk of *not* transfusing. Transfusion of blood or blood products is done for several reasons, and these should be carefully defined for each patient. The most important distinction that needs to be made is between the need for volume and the need for increased O_2 content of the arterial blood. The two do not necessarily go together; in acute hemorrhage, volume replacement may be more critical than it is in the chronically anemic patient in which O_2 content may be of primary concern.

There is no alternative to the exercise of good clinical judgement in the decision to transfuse a patient, but this requires an understanding of the fundamental determinants of

O_2 transport and the way these determinants interact and compensate for anemia in individual patients.

REFERENCES

1. Dodd RY. Viral contamination of blood components and approaches for reduction of infectivity. Immunol Invest 1995;24:25–48.
2. Tomasulo P. Transfusion alternatives: impact on blood banking worldwide. In: Winslow RM, Vandegriff KD, Intaglietta M, eds. Blood substitutes. Physiological basis ot efficacy. Boston: Birkhauser, 1995:1–19.
3. Tartter PI, Quintero S, Barron DM. Perioperative blood transfusion associated with infectious complications after colorectal cancer operations. Am J Surg 1986;152:479–482.
4. Stehling L, Simon TL. The red blood cell transfusion trigger. Physiology and clinical studies. Arch Pathol Lab Med 1994;118:429–434.
5. Goodnough LT, Verbrugge D, Vizmeg K, Riddell J IV. Identifying elective orthopedic surgical patients transfused with amounts of blood in excess of need: the transfusion trigger revisit [published erratum appears in Transfusion 1992;32:838]. Transfusion 1992;32:648–653.
6. Levine E, Rosen A, Sehgal L, Gould S, Sehgal H, Moss G. Physiologic effects of acute anemia: implications for a reduced transfusion trigger. Transfusion 1990;30:11–14.
7. Robertie PG, Gravlee GP. Safe limits of isovolemic hemodilution and recommendations for erythrocyte transfusion. Int Anesth Clin 1990;28: 197–204.
8. NIH Consensus Conference. Perioperative Red Cell Transfusion. JAMA 1988;260:2700–2703.
9. Mollison PL. Blood transfusion in clinical medicine. 7th ed. Philadelphia: F.A. Davis, 1983.
10. Roughton FJW, Forster RE. Relative importance of diffusion and chemical reaction rates in determining rate of exchange of gases in the human with special reference to true diffusing capacity of pulmonary. J Appl Physiol 1957;11:290–302.
11. Winslow RM. A model for red cell O_2 uptake. Int J Clin Monit Comput 1985;2:81–93.
12. Guyton AC, Jones CE, Coleman TG. Cardiac output and its regulation. 2nd ed. Philadelphia: WB Saunders, 1973.
13. Samaja M, Winslow RM. The separate effects of H+ and 2,3-DPG on the oxygen equilibrium curve of human blood. Br J Haematol 1979;41: 373–381.
14. Winslow RM, Samaja M, Winslow NJ, Rossi-Bernardi L, Shrager RI. Simulation of the continuous O_2 equilibrium curve over the physiologic range of pH, 2,3-diphosphoglycerate, and pCO_2. J Appl Physiol 1983;54:524–529.
15. Wagner PD. Diffusion and chemical reaction in pulmonary gas exchange. Physiol Rev 1977;57:257–312.
16. Cain SM. Oxygen delivery and uptake in dogs during anemic and hypoxichypoxia. J Appl Physiol 1977;42:228–234.
17. Crowell JW, Smith EE. Determination of the optimal hematocrit. J Appl Physiol 1967;22:501–504.
18. Guyton AC, Jones CE, Coleman TG. Cardiac output and its regulation. 2nd ed. Philadelphia: WB Saunders, 1973.
19. Winslow RM, Monge CC. Hypoxia, polycythemia, and chronic mountain sickness. Baltimore: Johns Hopkins University Press, 1987.
20. Spahn DR, Smith LR, Veronee CD, et al. Acute isovolemic hemodilution and blood transfusion. Effects on regional function and metabolism in myocardium with compromised coronary blood flow. J Thorac Cardiovasc Surg 1993;105:694–704.
21. Kim DA, Brecher ME, Estes TJ, Morrey BF. Relationship of hemoglobin and duration of hospitalization after total hip arthroplasty: implications for the transfusion target. Mayo Clin Proc 1993;68:37–41.
22. Nelson AH, Fleisher LA, Rosenbaum SH. Relationship between postoperative anemia and cardiac morbidity in high-risk vascular patients in the intensive care unit. Crit Care Med 1993;21:860–866.
23. Rice HE, Virmani R, Hart CL, Kolodgie FD, Farb A. Dose-dependent reduction of myocardial infarct size with the perfluorochemical Fluosol-DA. Am Heart J 1990;120:1039–1046.
24. Shibutani K, Komatsu T, Kubal K, Sanchala V, Kumar V, Bizzarri DV. Critical level of oxygen delivery in anesthetized man. Crit Care Med 1983;11:640–643.
25. Piiper J, Meyer M, Scheid P. Dual role of diffusion in tissue gas exchange: blood-tissue equilibration and diffusion shunt. Respir Physiol 1984;56:131–144.
26. Tenney SM. A theoretical analysis of the relationships between venous blood mean tissue oxygen pressures. Respir Physiol 1974;20:238–296.
27. Gould SA, Rosen AL, Sehgal LR, et al. O_2 extraction ratio: a physiologic indicator of transfusion need [abstract]. Transfusion 1983;23: 416.
28. Tenney SM. Oxygen diffusion from arterioles to capillaries. News Physiol Sci 1990;5:224–225.
29. Kerger H, Torres-Filho IP, Rivas M, Winslow RM, Intaglietta M. Systemic and subcutaneous microvascular oxygen tension in conscious Syrian golden hamsters. Am J Physiol 1995;268:H802-H810.
30. Spiess BD, Tuman KJ, McCarthy RJ, et al. Oxygen consumption and mixed venous oxygen saturation monitoring during orthotopic liver transplantation. J Clin Monit 1992;8:7–11.
31. Hoppeler YH, Noti C, Gurtner HP, et al. Limitations to Vo_2^{max} in humans after blood retransfusion. Respir Physiol 1993;92:329–341.
32. Yu M, Levy MM, Smith P, Takiguchi SA, Miyasaki A, Myers SA. Effect of maximizing oxygen delivery on morbidity and mortality in critically ill patients: a prospective, randomized, controlled study [comments]. Crit Care Med 1993;21:830–838.
33. Slanetz PJ, Lee R, Page R, Jacobs EE Jr, LaRaia PJ, Vlahakes GJ. Hemoglobin blood substitutes in extended preoperative autologous blood donation: an experimental study. Surgery 1994;115:246–254.
34. Cain SM, Curtis SE. Experimental models of pathological oxygen supply dependency. Crit Care Med 1991;19:603–612.
35. Cain SM. Assessment of tissue oxygenation. Crit Care Clin 1986;2: 537–550.
36. Mink RB, Pollack MM. Effect of blood transfusion on oxygen consumption in pediatric septic shock. Crit Care Med 1990;18:1087–1091.
37. Lorente JA, Landin L, De Pablo R, Renes E, Rodriguez-Diaz R, Liste D. Effects of blood transfusion on oxygen transport variables in severe sepsis. Crit Care Med 1993;21:1312–1318.
38. Seear M, Wensley D, MacNab A. Oxygen consumption-oxygen delivery relationship in children. J Pediatr 1993;123:208–214.
39. Silverman HJ, Tuma P. Gastric tonometry in patients with sepsis. Effects of dobutamine infusions and packed red blood cell transfusions. Chest 1992;102:184–188.
40. Hanique G, Dugernier T, Laterre PF, Dougnac A, Roeseler J, Reynaert MS. Significance of pathologic oxygen supply dependency in critically ill patients: comparison between measured and calculated methods. Intensive Care Med 1994;20:12–18.
41. Lucking SE, Williams TM, Chaten FC, Metz RI, Mickell JJ. Dependence of oxygen consumption on oxygen delivery in children with hyperdynamic septic shock and low oxygen extraction. Crit Care Med 1990;18:1316–1319.

42. Marik PE, Sibbald WJ. Effect of stored-blood transfusion on oxygen delivery in patients with sepsis. JAMA 1993;269:3024–3029.
43. Steffes CP, Bender JS, Levison MA. Blood transfusion and oxygen consumption in surgical sepsis. Crit Care Med 1991;19:512–517.
44. Silverman HJ. Lack of a relationship between induced changes in oxygen consumption and changes in lactate levels. Chest 1991;100:1012–1015.
45. Conrad SA, Dietrich KA, Hebert CA, Romero MD. Effect of red cell transfusion on oxygen consumption following fluid resuscitation in septic shock. Circ Shock 1990;31:419–429.
46. Ronco JJ, Phang PT, Walley KR, Wiggs B, Fenwick JC, Russell JA. Oxygen consumption is independent of changes in oxygen delivery in adult respiratory distress syndrome. Am Rev Respir Dis 1991;143: 1267–1273.
47. Ronco JJ, Montaner JS, Fenwick JC, Russell JA. Pathologic dependence of oxygen consumption on oxygen delivery in a respiratory failure secondary to AIDS-related *Pneumocystis carinii* pneumonia. Chest 1990;98:1463–1466.
48. Babineau TJ, Dzik WH, Borlase BC, Baxter JK, Bistrian BR, Benotti PN. Reevaluation of current transfusion practices in patients in surgical intensive care units. Am J Surg 1992;164:22–25.
49. Levy PS, Chavez RP, Crystal GJ, et al. Oxygen extraction ratio: a valid indicator of transfusion need in l coronary vascular reserve? J Trauma 1992;32:769–774.
50. Wilkerson DK, Rosen AL, Gould SA, Sehgal LR, Sehgal HL, Moss GS. Whole body oxygen extraction ratio as an indicator of cardiac status in anemia. Curr Surg 1988;45:214–217.
51. Mathru M, Kleinman B, Blakeman B, Sullivan H, Kumar P, Dries DJ. Myocardial metabolism and adaptation during extreme hemodilution in humans after coronary revascularization. Crit Care Med 1992;20: 1420–1425.
52. Dietrich KA, Conrad SA, Hebert CA, Levy GL, Romero MD. Cardiovascular and metabolic response to red blood cell transfusion in critically ill volume-resuscitated nonsurgical patients. Crit Care Med 1990;18:940–944.
53. Carson JL, Spence RK, Poses RM, Bonavita G. Severity of anaemia and operative mortality and morbidity. Lancet 1988;1:727–729.
54. Thompson CH, Kemp GJ, Taylor DJ, Ledingham JG, Radda GK, Rajagopalan B. No effect of blood transfusion on muscle metabolism. Q J Med 1992;85:897–899.
55. Jonsson K, Jensen JA, Goodson WH, et al. Tissue oxygenation, anemia, and perfusion in relation to wound healing in surgical patients. Ann Surg 1991;214:605–613.
56. Wisner DH, Holcroft JW. Surgical critical care. Curr Prob Surg 1990; 27:467–569.
57. Meyers RL, Paulick RP, Rudolph CD, Rudolph AM. Cardiovascular responses to acute, severe haemorrhage in fetal sheep. J Dev Physiol 1991;15:189–197.
58. Curtis SE, Cain SM. Systemic and regional O_2 delivery and uptake in bled dogs given hypertonic saline, whole blood, or dextran. Am J Physiol 1992;262:H778-H786.
59. Ping Wang ZF, Ba M-CL, Ayala A, Harkema JM, Chaudry IH. Measurement of circulating blood volume in vivo after trauma-hemorrhage and hemodilution. Am J Physiol 1994;266:R368-R374.
60. Wasserman K, Hansen JE, Sue DY. Facilitation of oxygen consumption by lactic acidosis during exercise. News Physiol Sci 1991;6:29–34.
61. Mitzner W, Goldberg HS, Lichenstein S. Effects of thoracic blood volume changes on steady state cardiac output. Circ Res 1976;38:255–261.
62. Gould SA, Sehgal LR, Sehgal HL, Moss GS. Hypovolemic shock. Crit Care Clin 1993;9:239–259.
63. Saxena S, Rabinowitz AP, Johnson C, Shulman IA. Iron-deficiency anemia: a medically treatable chronic anemia as a model for transfusion overuse. Am J Med 1993;94:120–124.
64. Stehling L, Zauder HL. Acute normovolemic hemodilution. Transfusion 1991;31:857–868.
65. Viele MK, Weiskopf RB. What can we learn about the need for transfusion from patients who refuse blood? The experience with Jehovah's Witnesses. Transfusion 1994;34:396–401.
66. Weiskopf RB. Mathematical analysis of isovolemic hemodilution indicates that it can reduce the need for allogeneic blood transfusion. Transfusion 1995;35:37–41.
67. Polley JW, Berkowitz RA, McDonald TB, Cohen M, Figueroa A, Penney DW. Craniomaxillofacial surgery in the Jehovah's Witness patient. Plastic Reconstruct Surg 1994;93:1258–1263.
68. Marelli TR. Use of a hemoglobin substitute in the anemic Jehovah's Witness patient. Crit Care Nurse 1994;February:31–38.
69. Lackritz EM, Campbell CC, Ruebush TK, et al. Effect of blood transfusion on survival among children in a Kenyan hospital. Lancet 1992;340:524–528.
70. Newton CR, Marsh K, Peshu N, Mwangi I. Blood transfusions for severe anemia in African children. Lancet 1992;340:916–917.
71. Baele PL, De Bruyere M, Deneys V, et al. The SANGUIS Study in Belgium: an overview. Acta Chir Belg 1994;94:69–74.
72. Friedman BA, Burns TL, Schork MA. An analysis of blood transfusion of surgical patients by sex: a question for the transfusion trigger. Transfusion 1980;20:179–188.
73. Wilkerson DK, Rosen AL, Sehgal LR, Gould SA, Sehgal HL, Moss GS. Limits of cardiac compensation in anemic baboons. Surgery 1988;103: 666–670.
74. Kitchens CS. Are transfusions overrated? Surgical outcome of Jehovah's Witnesses. Am J Med 1993;94:117–119.
75. Levy PS, Kim SJ, Eckel PK, et al. Limit to cardiac compensation during acute isovolemic hemodilution: influence of coronary stenosis. Am J Physiol 1993;265:H340-H349.
76. Christopherson R, Frank S, Norris E, Rock P, Gottlieb S, Beattie C. Low postoperative hematocrit is associated with cardiac ischemia in high-risk patients. Anesthesiology 1991;75:A99.
77. Nelson AH, Fleisher LA, Rosenbaum SH. Relationship between postoperative anemia and cardiac morbidity in high risk vascular patients in the intensive care unit. Crit Care Med 1993;21:860–866.
78. Johnson RG, Thurer RL, Kruskall MS, et al. Comparison of two transfusion strategies after elective operations for myocardial revascularization. J Thorac Cardiovasc Surg 1992;104:307–314.
79. Dick W, Baur C, Reiff K. Which factors determine the critical hematocrit as an indication of transfusion? (published erratum appears in Anaesthesist 1992;41:113). Anaesthesist 1992;41:1–14.
80. Faust RJ. Perioperative indications for red blood cell transfusion: has the pendulum swung too far? Mayo Clin Proc 1993;68:512–514.
81. Stehling L, Zauder HL. How low can we go? Is there a way to know? Transfusion 1990;30:1–3.
82. Homer LD, Weathersby PK, Kiesow LA. Oxygen gradients between red blood cells in the microcirculation. Microvasc Res 1981;22: 308–323.
83. Rosen AL, Gould S, Sehgal LR, et al. Cardiac output response to extreme hemodilution with hemoglobin solutions of various P_{50} values. Crit Care Med 1979;7:380–384.
84. Hess JR, MacDonald VW, Brinkley WW. Systemic and pulmonary hypertension after resuscitation with cell-free hemoglobin. J Appl Physiol 1993;74:1769–1778.

85. Stork RL, Bredle DL, Chapler CK, Cain SM. Regional hemodynamic responses to hypoxia in polycythemic dogs. J Appl Physiol 1988;65: 2069–2074.
86. Breuninger HG, Rubenstein SD, Wolfson MR, Shaffer TH. Effect of exchange transfusion with a red blood cell substitute on neonatal hemodynamics and organ blood flows. J Pediatr Surg 1993;28: 144–150.
87. Faithfull NS, Cain SM. Critical levels of O_2 extraction following hemodilution with dextran or Fluosol-DA. J Crit Care 1988;3:14–18.
88. Eastaugh SR. Valuation of the benefits of risk-free blood. Willingness to pay for hemoglobin solutions. Int J Technol Assess Health Care 1991;7:51–57.
89. Lester LA, Sodt PC, Hutcheon N, Arcilla RA. Cardiovascular effects of hypertransfusion therapy in children with sickle cell anemia. Pediatr Cardiol 1990;11:131–137.
90. Lucas CE, Ledgerwood AM, Rachwal WJ, Grabow D, Saxe JM. Colloid oncotic pressure and body water dynamics in septic and injured patients. J Trauma 1991;31:927–933.

Chapter 4

The Surgeon and the Transfusion Service: Essentials of Compatibility Testing, Surgical Blood Ordering, Emergency Blood Needs, and Adverse Reactions

LAWRENCE D. PETZ

INTRODUCTION

Appropriate blood ordering and smooth interaction between surgeons and the blood bank depends on an understanding by surgeons of a number of activities carried out by the hospital's transfusion service. This chapter describes those aspects of compatibility testing and blood ordering procedures that are critical for blood availability. The chapter also reviews the means of diagnosing and managing adverse reactions to transfusion.

WHAT SURGEONS NEED TO KNOW ABOUT BLOOD BANK PROCEDURES

PRINCIPLES OF COMPATIBILITY TESTING

The purpose of compatibility testing is to prevent hemolytic transfusion reactions that may be caused by red cell antibodies of the ABO blood group system ("expected" antibodies) or by antibodies to other blood group antigens ("unexpected" antibodies). If the patient has such antibodies, one must select red blood cells (RBCs) for transfusion that lack the antigens with which the antibodies react.

Compatibility testing includes a verification of the ABO-Rh of the donor blood and ABO and Rh typing, a screening test for unexpected antibodies, and a cross match between donor RBCs and recipient serum on the recipient's blood (1).

SIGNIFICANCE OF COMPONENTS OF COMPATIBILITY TESTING

ABO Typing

ABO typing is accomplished by testing the patient's RBCs with anti-A and anti-B antisera and by testing the patient's serum for anti-A and anti-B. The ABO system is unique in that a subject's serum has "naturally occurring" antibodies (i.e., not stimulated by exposure to foreign RBCs) to the ABO RBC antigens that are absent from his or her own RBCs.

Although ABO typing is the most critical test in determining the safety of transfused RBCs, it is quickly performed so that it plays little role in the time required to complete compatibility testing.

Rh Typing

The presence or absence of the D antigen in the Rh blood group system defines whether a person is Rh positive or Rh negative. As with ABO typing, testing for the D antigen can be accomplished quickly.

Cross-Match Tests

Previously, the cross-match test has played the dominant role in RBC compatibility testing, but in recent years the antibody screen has become the focal point and is particularly important in planning for blood for elective surgical procedures (see below). That blood cannot be available quickly unless it has been previously cross matched is a misconception. However, with the use of sensitive antibody screening tests, it is now recognized that the cross match can be abbreviated provided that an antibody screening test has been done in advance and is found to be negative.

A cross match consists of testing the patient's serum against a sample of RBCs from the actual unit that has been selected for transfusion. There are two types of cross matches. First, the immediate spin cross match is accomplished by mixing the patient's serum with a sample of RBCs from the unit selected for transfusion and observing immediate agglutination (as will be caused by ABO antibodies). The primary purpose of the immediate spin cross match is to confirm ABO compatibility; it does not reliably detect unexpected antibodies. The immediate spin cross match takes about 5 minutes to perform.

Second, a full cross match (or "Coombs' cross match") is done by incubating the patient's serum with the cells to be transfused for at least 15 minutes and then observing for agglutination and performing an antiglobulin (Coombs') test. The purpose of the full cross match is to detect all clinically significant RBC antibodies. The full cross match test takes about 30–45 minutes to perform.

The Antibody Screen

It is common policy for blood banks to perform an antibody screen in conjunction with cross-match tests, but the antibody screen may be ordered without the cross match as part of a "type and screen" order (see below).

The test that is most important regarding the complexity of compatibility testing in a given case and that provides the surgeon with an indication of the time required before compatible blood can be available is the antibody screen. This test is the focal point in developing preoperative compatibility test policies.

An antibody screen is performed by testing the patient's serum against the RBCs from several normal group O blood samples from persons who have been extensively typed. The test is performed under conditions that detect clinically significant RBC antibodies, that is, those that are known to have caused hemolytic transfusion reactions.

If the antibody screen is negative and blood bank records show no previous history of antibody, the interpretation is that the patient has no unexpected RBC antibodies and therefore may be transfused with any unit of the appropriate ABO/Rh type. All that is required before the release of blood from the blood bank is that ABO compatibility is confirmed, which is generally accomplished by an immediate spin cross match, which takes just a few minutes. Thus, blood should be available within 15 minutes after it is ordered, including the necessary clerical tasks. Although most blood transfusion services now perform only an abbreviated cross match in patients with negative antibody screening tests, some persist in performing a full cross match. The full cross match will rarely detect a clinically significant RBC antibody but will result in a delay in availability of blood and added expense (2–5).

If the antibody screen is positive, the transfusion service must determine the specificity of the antibody by testing the serum against a "panel" of 8–12 samples of RBCs of varying phenotypes. The pattern of positive and negative reactions with the cells on the panel identifies the antigen against which the antibody is directed. If a clinically significant antibody is found, the transfusion service must find RBCs that are negative for the relevant antigen. For example, if the antibody is anti-Kell, RBCs that are ABO and Rh compatible with the patient will be tested with Kell typing serum and only Kell-negative RBCs will be selected for transfusion. For added safety, a full cross-match test, including an antiglobulin test, is also performed.

Even if only a type and screen (and not a type and cross match) has been ordered, blood bank protocols should indicate that a positive antibody screen will result in the performance by the transfusion service of antibody identification tests and full cross-match tests on an appropriate number of units for the surgical procedure planned. Thus, even if the antibody screen is positive, blood will be available in a timely fashion before surgery.

From the above, it is evident that when the antibody screen is positive, additional time is required to identify the antibody(ies) and to select antigen-negative RBC units for transfusion. This time can range from about an hour, when the patient has an antibody for which antigen-negative blood is readily available, to many hours or even days if multiple antibodies or antibodies against high incidence antigens are present (see below). The surgeon should be informed if such a problem arises, because delays may be encountered if more blood than was ordered initially is needed.

Summary of Significance of the Antibody Screen

On the basis of the above, one may summarize the significance of the antibody screen as follows.

If the antibody screen has not been performed, it is impossible to predict how much time may be required to obtain compatible blood.

If an antibody screen is negative, compatible RBC units can be obtained quickly by relying on the results of an abbreviated cross-match test (providing there is an adequate inventory of blood of appropriate ABO type).

If an antibody screen is positive, at least an hour, frequently several hours, and possibly up to several days may be needed to obtain compatible blood.

If an antibody screen is positive but has been performed well in advance of surgery, the transfusion service will have adequate time to obtain compatible blood.

These facts are the basis for the strong recommendation that an antibody screen should be performed well in advance of surgery if there is a reasonable chance of requiring blood.

SURGICAL BLOOD ORDERING

SURGERY WITHOUT A BLOOD ORDER

For many surgeries, the likelihood of requiring a transfusion is so low that it is unnecessary to order even a type and screen.

THE "TYPE AND HOLD" OR "HOLD CLOT" ORDER

In some facilities, physicians are allowed to send a blood sample to the blood bank in advance of a defined request. The blood may be typed, but no antibody testing is performed. The specimen is logged in and stored should blood be needed within 3 days of sample collection. Physicians perhaps believe that blood can be made available more quickly if a specimen has already been sent to the blood bank. However, as explained above, the critical point in compatibility testing is the antibody screen. Having a sample available in the blood bank will not significantly shorten the length of time needed to complete compatibility tests unless an antibody screen has been performed. Therefore, if there is a reasonable likelihood that blood will be needed, a type and screen or type and cross match are more appropriate.

TYPE AND CROSS MATCH

If it is reasonable to assume a need for transfusion (at least 10% of patients for a given surgical procedure will require blood), it is justifiable to request a type and cross match of an appropriate number of units so that blood will be available at the time of surgery. The number of units cross matched should be sufficient to meet the anticipated total blood requirement of at least 90% of the patients who undergo the procedure.

If cross-matched blood is ordered, an antibody screen has been done so if more blood is needed than originally anticipated, it can be available expeditiously.

TYPE AND SCREEN

A type and screen procedure should be ordered when a surgical patient may require blood but the likelihood of transfusion is too low to justify setting aside cross-matched units. The extra expense of full cross matching and setting aside individual units is not justified when the probability of transfusion is low. Each institution should develop guidelines for which type and screen is appropriate rather than a full cross match (see below). Keep in mind that if only a type and screen is ordered but emergency blood needs arise, it should be possible to have blood available within 15 minutes in patients who have a negative screening test. For patients with a positive antibody screen, compatible blood should be identified well in advance of surgery. Accordingly, a type and screen is an appropriate preoperative order for a large percentage of elective surgical procedures.

The procedures for which type and screen are appropriate at a given institution will depend on the efficiency of the transfusion service in supplying blood quickly and the anxiety level of the surgeons. The latter is inversely proportional to the surgeon's confidence in the transfusion service's ability to supply blood quickly when a sudden need arises in cases in which only a type and screen has been ordered preoperatively.

MAXIMUM SURGICAL BLOOD ORDER SCHEDULE

A maximum surgical blood order schedule (MSBOS) is a listing of surgical procedures performed at a given institution, accompanied by an indication of the most appropriate preoperative blood order for each procedure (i.e., no blood order, type and screen, or type and cross match for a certain number of units) (6, 7). An override mechanism must be available so that if mitigating circumstances exist, these can be specified to the blood bank verbally or in writing to avoid having an inadequate number of cross-matched units available for a given patient's surgery.

An example of an MSBOS is presented in Table 4.1. An MSBOS should reflect local (institutional) blood use experience and should be prepared by a joint effort of the transfusion service and the surgical staff. Moreover, it should be revised every several years on the basis of current blood usage. Therefore, the example in Table 4.1 should not necessarily be used in another hospital but should merely serve as a model.

It is evident that a type and screen is the appropriate order for many surgical procedures. Also, because indications for transfusion are becoming increasingly more stringent, fewer units than indicated may need to be cross matched for a number of the procedures listed.

TABLE 4.1. TRANSFUSION SERVICE GUIDELINE FOR ELECTIVE SURGICAL PROCEDURES

Surgical Procedure	Transfusion Service	Surgical Procedure	Transfusion Service
General surgery		Ear, nose, and throat surgery	
Cholecystectomy	T&S[a]	Caldwell-Luc	T&S
Exploratory laparotomy (celiotomy)	T&S	Laryngectomy	T&S
Ileal bypass	T&S	Plastic surgery	
Hiatal hernia repair	T&S	Mammoplasty	T&S
Colectomy and hemicolectomy	2 units	Thoracoabdominal flap	T&S
Splenectomy	2 units	Oral surgery	
Breast biopsy	T&S	Osteotomy	T&S
Radical mastectomy	1 unit	Genioplasty	T&S
Modified radical mastectomy	1 unit	Bilateral subcondylar osteotomy	T&S
Simple mastectomy	1 unit	Vestibuloplasty	T&S
Gastrectomy	2 units	Le Forte I osteotomy	T&S
Antrectomy and vagotomy	2 units	Anterior maxillary osteotomy	T&S
Inguinal herniorrhaphy	T&S	Neurosurgery	
Liver biopsy	T&S	Craniotomy	2 units
Vein stripping	T&S	Herniated disk	T&S
Cardiovascular surgery		Ventriculoperitoneal shunt	T&S
Saphenous vein bypass	8 units	Transsphenoidal hypophysectomy	2 units
Congenital open heart surgery	8 units[b]	Orthopedics	
Valve replacement	8 units	Open reduction	2 units
Pleurodesis	T&S	Scoliosis fusion	3–4 units
Aortobifemoral bypass	8 units	Herniated disk	T&S
Thoracotomy	3 units	Arthroplasty	T&S
Closed mediastinal exploration	T&S	Shoulder reconstruction	T&S
Resection abdominal aortic aneurysm	8 units	Total hip replacement	2–3 units
Carotid endarterectomy	2 units	Total knee replacement	T&S
Obstetrical-gynecological surgery		Genitourinary surgery	
Total abdominal hysterectomy	T&S	Transurethral resection of prostate	T&S
Exploratory laparotomy	T&S	Radical nephrectomy	1 unit
Total vaginal hysterectomy	T&S	Renal transplantation	1 unit
Vaginal resuspension	T&S	Penile prosthesis insertion	T&S
Laparoscopy	T&S	Prostatectomy	2 units
Repeat cesarean section	T&S	Patch graft	T&S
Labor and delivery requests (oxytocin drips and cesarean sections)	T&S		

Reprinted with permission from Boral LI, Dannemiller FJ, Stanford W, et al. A guideline for anticipated blood usage during elective surgical procedures. Am J Clin Pathol 1979;71:680.

[a] Type and antibody screen (T&S) consists of an ABO-Rh typing and a screen for unexpected antibodies.

[b] Two heparinized.

Some guidelines suggest that if a surgical procedure requires transfusion in fewer than 10% of cases, a type and screen request rather than a type and cross match is appropriate (7). However, performing only a type and screen in a higher percentage of cases may be preferable with an efficiently operating transfusion service. Indeed, at some institutions, a type and screen is performed for all surgical procedures for which need for transfusion is anticipated and no blood is set up before surgery. A cross match is performed only when blood is actually required in the operating room (or in patients with a positive antibody screen).

CROSS MATCH-TO-TRANSFUSION RATIO

The success of an MSBOS may be measured by calculating a ratio known as the cross match-to-transfusion ratio (C:T). The C:T is well established as a useful indicator of the efficiency of physician blood-ordering practices. The more accurately physicians predict a patient's blood needs during the perioperative period, the closer the C:T will approach 1:1. Based on a study by the College of American Pathologists (8), over 50% of hospitals have a C:T of less than 2:1 and 75% have a C:T of less than 2.2:1.

Once an MSBOS is in place, it should be revised periodically if the overall C:T for surgical patients exceeds 2:1. However, even if the overall C:T is 2:1 or less, it may be appropriate to consult with the appropriate surgeons and consider revising the standard blood orders for a specific procedure if the C:T for that procedure exceeds 2:1.

EMERGENCY BLOOD ORDERS

Written SOPs (surgical order of products) should be in place before a patient requires an emergency blood transfusion. These SOPs should take into account emergency transfusion requirements of patients who suddenly need blood during an existing hospitalization and patients who are brought to the hospital in need of emergency treatment.

The physician requesting an emergency uncross-matched transfusion must document in the patient's medical record the urgent need for the blood. However, it is inappropriate for blood bank staff to demand that the physician "sign" for the blood before it can be released for transfusion, because such a requirement could delay blood availability (9).

BLOOD AVAILABILITY AND RELATIVE RISKS IN EMERGENCY BLOOD ORDERING

In the emergency room or, more rarely, for patients who develop unexpected bleeding during scheduled surgery, there may not be time to wait for type-specific cross-matched blood. The urgency of the surgical setting will dictate the appropriate blood order among the various options that are available as outlined in Table 4.2.

Surgeons should be familiar with the relative risks of transfusing each type of blood (i.e., group O negative versus type specific versus cross matched versus uncross matched, etc.) and the approximate times required for their availability.

If the actual turnaround times are longer than expected, a systems problem may be at fault, and this needs to be investigated. A careful analysis of each step in the process of emergency compatibility testing might reveal information that could shorten the turnaround time and improve patient care.

GROUP O, RH NEGATIVE, UNCROSS MATCHED

If blood is needed immediately and no blood specimen has previously been made available to the blood bank, the safest blood is group O, Rh negative, uncross matched. There

TABLE 4.2. RELATIVE RISKS OF VARIOUS BLOOD PRODUCTS AND APPROXIMATE TIME REQUIRED FOR THEIR AVAILABILITY

Type of Red Blood Cell	Time Required in a Blood Bank	Risks and Comments
O Negative, uncross matched	5 min	0.2–0.6% of population will have red cell antibody; serious hemolysis is rare. Wait for type specific only if a 10–15 min wait does not cause significant risk.
Type specific, uncross matched	15 min after specimen arrives in blood bank	Risk no less than group negative uncross-matched blood.
Type specific, cross matched	45 min after specimen arrives in blood blank	Cross-matched blood should be used if a 45-min wait does not cause significant risk.
Type specific, cross matched in a patient with red cell antibody	90 min to several hours; rarely even longer	If patient has red cell antibody, antibody identification may take 90 min to several hours. If blood is needed before compatibility testing is completed, hemolysis may occur but transfusion should not be withheld if absolutely necessary; life-threatening morbidity is rare.

is no risk of the transfused cells being hemolyzed by anti-A or anti-B. However, the patient may have RBC antibodies to other blood group systems (e.g., Rh, Kell, Kidd, Duffy) if previously transfused or pregnant so that the possibility of a hemolytic transfusion reaction is not completely avoided.

The response time to an emergency blood order should be short. At some institutions, particularly trauma centers, emergency blood orders can be honored at once because uncross-matched group O RBCs are routinely stored in the emergency room and operating rooms. Rough estimates of the number of units to be kept on hand can be obtained from periodic review of transfusion practices and discussion with the trauma staff. In well-administered transfusion services supporting trauma services and emergency rooms, type-specific blood can be made available quickly enough so that only a small number of group O, Rh-negative units are required. It may take several minutes or longer to provide uncross-matched blood in hospitals that store uncross-matched blood only in the blood bank.

GROUP O, RH POSITIVE, UNCROSS MATCHED

Because supplies of Rh-negative blood may be inadequate, it may be necessary to use Rh-positive blood when the need for transfusion is urgent.

The use of Rh-positive uncross-matched RBCs rather than Rh negative does engender a risk of a hemolytic transfusion reaction. However, this occurs only in that 15% of patients who are Rh negative and only if the patient has developed an anti-D as a result of pregnancy or prior transfusion of Rh-positive blood. About 0.27–0.56% of transfusion recipients will have anti-D.

TYPE SPECIFIC, UNCROSS MATCHED

Group O blood is often in short supply and must be reserved for patients who are group O because they can receive no other type. Therefore, type-specific uncross-matched blood is the most appropriate blood to transfuse as soon as the patient's blood type has been determined.

One should be aware that type-specific uncross-matched blood is no safer than group O uncross-matched blood; indeed, it is less safe. This is true because laboratory error, clerical error, or patient misidentification may result in ABO incompatible blood being transfused, whereas this is not a potential problem if only group O RBCs are used.

Because blood typing requires only a few minutes, only a short time is necessary to have type-specific blood available. Most of this time is caused by transportation of the blood specimen to the blood bank, administrative tasks, and transportation of the units of blood to the surgical suite. If the blood bank is in close proximity to the surgical suites and emergency room, type-specific blood should be available in minutes after the blood bank receives a specimen.

TYPE SPECIFIC, CROSS MATCHED

Type-specific cross-matched blood requires about 45 minutes after the specimen arrives in the blood bank, provided the patient has no RBC antibodies. Efficient transfusion services may reduce this time requirement, but transportation times and record keeping often make 45 minutes a realistic time.

If an RBC antibody is found, it must be identified, and antigen typing must be performed to select antigen-negative units. This may require 90 minutes to several hours or even longer depending on the number of antibodies and the ease of obtaining antigen-negative units.

TRANSFUSION POLICIES AT TIMES OF INADEQUATE INVENTORY

An institution must have SOPs to deal with occasional shortages in blood inventory. Such preplanning may minimize the impact of a shortage on an elective surgery schedule or on a specific patient. The inability of a hospital blood bank to meet the transfusion needs of its patients may result either from a shortage of blood within the national/regional system or from a local depletion of blood inventory, despite an adequate national/regional blood resource.

USE OF BLOOD NOT ABO/RH IDENTICAL TO THE PATIENT

During times of blood shortage, the surgeon should not feel constrained to only transfused blood that is ABO/Rh identical to that of the patient. The use of RBCs that are not ABO identical but are compatible ("minor incompatibility") is an effective means of increasing the number of available units during a shortage situation. Principles to be followed when switching blood groups and types due to shortages are outlined in Table 4.3 (10).

When nonidentical ABO groups are used, the transfused blood should always be in the form of RBCs rather than whole blood to avoid the transfusion of incompatible ABO alloantibodies.

Conversely for plasma, group O patients can receive non-group O fresh-frozen plasma (FFP). In cases of very extreme plasma use, it may be necessary to use ABO-incompatible plasma transfusions. For example, if a group AB patient needed quantities of AB plasma that were so large that the supply was threatened, the patient could be switched first to

TABLE 4.3. PRINCIPLES FOLLOWED WHEN SWITCHING BLOOD GROUPS AND TYPES DUE TO SHORTAGES

Patient's Group and Type	Principles to Follow
O negative	Use only O, Rh negative if patient is sensitized to D
	Use group O, D, and Du negative, C and/or E positive in preference to Rh(D) positive
	Avoid transfusing anything but O, Rh negative to patients (*especially females*) under age 45
	Restrict the use of O, Rh-positive blood for O, Rh negative patients to acute emergency situations and then use only if the patient either has a negative antibody screen or definitely lacks Rh antibodies
	If massive volumes of blood are required and switching to Rh positive is inevitable, avoid wasting O, Rh-negative blood by switching as early as possible
A negative or B negative	Use only Rh negative if patient is sensitized to D; i.e., group-specific Rh negative or O, Rh negative (as packed cells if possible)
	Use D and Du negative, C and/or E positive in preference to Rh(D) positive
	Avoid transfusing anything but Rh-negative blood to patients (*especially females*) under age 45
	Restrict use of Rh-positive blood to acute emergency situations and then use only if the patient has a negative antibody screen or definitely lacks Rh antibodies
	If massive volumes of blood are required and switching to Rh positive is inevitable, avoid wasting Rh-negative blood by switching as early as possible
	Conserve group O blood. Only group O can be given to a group O recipient
AB negative	Use only Rh negative if patient is sensitized to D
	Use D and Du negative, C and/or E positive in preference to Rh(D) positive
	Group A blood may be used (as packed cells if possible) unless the patient has anti-A_1. The patient initially should be switched to group A, then secondarily may be switched to O. *Always do this before switching Rh types* (see text)
	Avoid transfusing anything but Rh negative to patients (*especially females*) under age 45
	Restrict the use of Rh positive to acute emergency situations and then use only if the patient has a negative antibody screen or definitely lacks Rh antibodies
	If massive volumes of blood are required and switching to Rh positive is inevitable, avoid wasting Rh negative by switching as early as possible
	Conserve group O blood. Only group O can be given to a group O recipient
O positive	A group O patient may receive only group O blood
	Rh negative may be used, but this should be avoided due to supply problems
A positive or B positive	Group O blood may be given (as packed cells if possible)
	Rh negative may be used, but this should be avoided due to supply problems
AB positive	Group A blood may be used (as packed cells, if possible) unless the patient has anti-A_1. The patient initially should be switched to group A and then secondarily to group O
	Conserve group O blood. Only group O can be given to a group O recipient
	Rh negative may be used, but this should be avoided due to supply problems

Reprinted with permission from Shulman IA, Spence RK, Petz LD. Surgical blood ordering, blood shortage situations, and emergency transfusions. In*:* Petz LD, Swisher SN, Kleinman S, Spence RK, Strauss RG, eds. Clinical practice of transfusion medicine. 3rd ed. New York: Churchill-Livingstone, 1995.

group A RBCs and then after two or three blood volumes to group A FFP (even though it contains anti-B). At the end of surgery, the patient could be switched back in the reverse order, with AB FFP first and then to AB RBCs once cross matches showed compatibility due to a sufficient decline in titer of the passive anti-B.

USE OF RH-POSITIVE BLOOD FOR RH-NEGATIVE PATIENTS

When Rh-negative blood is in short supply, it may be necessary to transfuse Rh-positive blood to some Rh-negative patients. Transfusion of Rh-positive blood should be avoided in women with childbearing potential and in female children because of the risk of Rh alloimmunization and subsequent hemolytic disease of the fetus or newborn. Transfusion of Rh-positive blood should also be avoided in patients who have anti-D (regardless of gender), except for life-threatening situations. On the other hand, group O Rh-positive RBCs may be administered to Rh-negative male patients with very little risk of a reaction because they will not have developed anti-D unless they have been alloimmunized by a prior transfusion of Rh-positive blood.

During life-threatening emergency situations, most institutions have a policy of supplying group O Rh-negative blood, but some routinely provide group O Rh-negative RBCs for females and group O Rh-positive RBCs for males.

PATIENTS WITH MULTIPLE ALLOANTIBODIES OR ALLOANTIBODIES TO HIGH-INCIDENCE ANTIGENS

Some patients have multiple RBC alloantibodies. For example, when a patient has anti-Fy^a, anti-Jk^b, anti-E and anti-S, blood bank technologists need to test units of the appropriate ABO type until they find units that are negative for all four antigens and then they must perform a full cross match on each unit. In this example, the probability of a given unit of RBCs lacking all four antigens is less than 1:70. If a transfusion is required on an emergency basis or if large numbers of units are required urgently, it may be impossible to supply antigen-negative blood.

Patients with an alloantibody to an antigen that is on an extremely high percentage of allogeneic RBCs (i.e., a "high-incidence" antigen) may be incompatible with all RBCs available in the blood bank. Some of these antibodies are clinically insignificant, but others may cause shortened RBC survival. In the latter case, the blood bank may have to search for suitable donors among family members or rare donor files.

TEMPORARY USE OF INCOMPATIBLE BLOOD DURING MASSIVE TRANSFUSION

In certain circumstances, if only a limited number of compatible units can be located but massive bleeding is anticipated or is occurring, it might be prudent to divide up the compatible units that are available and use a portion of them for the patient's initial RBC transfusions. Once the patient's blood loss and fluid replacement therapy have diluted the serum alloantibodies, it may be safe to switch to incompatible RBC units under close observation. As soon as the patient's blood loss is under control and the supply of remaining compatible units is sufficient to meet the transfusion needs of the patient, the patient should be switched back to receive compatible RBC units. Such an approach could limit the volume of incompatible RBCs in the patient's circulation at the conclusion of surgery. This minimizes but may not completely prevent hemolytic transfusion reactions. Nevertheless, only rarely will an intraoperative hemolytic reaction be seen, and delayed hemolytic transfusion reactions have not been severe. This strategy has been used successfully on a number of occasions in liver transplant surgery (11, 12).

COMMUNICATION BETWEEN THE SURGEON AND THE BLOOD TRANSFUSION SERVICE

In the event a patient's serological problem cannot be resolved in time or in case a sufficient number of compatible units cannot be found, it becomes the responsibility of the blood bank/transfusion service medical director to apprise the surgeon of the clinical relevance of the particular incompatibility the patient is facing. Because the clinical relevance of an RBC antibody depends in part on the antibody specificity and in vitro reactivity, it should be possible for the blood bank physician to guide the surgeon and blood bank staff on the safest selection of incompatible blood. For example, if multiple antibodies are present and incompatible RBCs must be transfused, the donor RBCs should be selected so that they are incompatible with the antibody expected to be the least clinically significant.

CLINICAL SIGNIFICANCE OF RBC ALLOANTIBODIES

Unfortunately, as yet there is no recognized in vitro characteristic or group of characteristics that can be used to indicate the in vivo significance of all RBC antibodies. Serological characteristics of an antibody correlated empirically with past clinical experience have provided most of our present knowledge. In addition, RBC survival studies have contributed significantly. The two serological characteristics that have been found most helpful in predicting in vivo significance are an antibody's specificity and its ability to react in vitro at 37°C. The clinical significance of some RBC alloantibodies is reviewed.

CLINICALLY SIGNIFICANT ANTIBODIES`

Antibodies that react at 37°C and cause a significant majority of hemolytic transfusion reactions are antibodies of the ABO, Rh, Kell, Kidd, and Duffy blood group systems and S and s antibodies of the MNSs system (Table 4.4, group I).

When antibodies of group I are found or if the patient's record indicates that these antibodies have been present in the past, it should be assumed that incompatible blood will lead to a hemolytic transfusion reaction, and RBCs negative for

TABLE 4.4. CLINICAL SIGNIFICANCE OF SOME RED CELL ALLOANTIBODIES

Group I: clinically significant antibodies
ABO
Rh
Kell
Duffy
Kidd
Ss
Group II: benign antibodies
Chido/Rodgers (Ch^a/Rg^a)
Xg^a
Bg
"HTLA"
Cs^a
Kn^a
McC^a
JMH
Group III: clinically insignificant if not reactive at 37° C; possibly significant when reacting at 37° C
Lewis (Le^a/Le^b)
M, N
P_1
Lutheran (Lu^a/Lu^b)
A_1
Group IV: antibodies that are sometimes clinically significant
Yt^a
Vel
Ge
Gy^a
Hy
Sd^a
York (Yk^a)

the appropriate antigen should be transfused. Even here, it must be realized that serious hemolysis will not necessarily ensue if RBCs carrying these antigens are given. The severity of hemolysis caused by antibodies that are considered clinically significant varies strikingly. Anti-A and anti-B antibodies usually, but not always, cause immediate symptomatic transfusion reactions that in some cases may even be fatal. Some antibodies in the Rh, Kell, and Kidd blood group systems may cause serious degrees of hemolysis, whereas in other instances only modest shortening of RBC survival occurs and there are no important clinical sequelae.

Experience derived from transfusing such subjects out of absolute necessity in life-threatening situations, as in liver transplantation when supplies of compatible blood are exhausted, has indicated that the anticipated hemolysis may not occur or may be minimal and cause tolerable morbidity. Thus, every effort should be made to supply antigen-negative blood, but one must keep in mind that some extraordinary circumstances require transfusion of incompatible blood even to patients with antibodies of specificities in group I of Table 4.4.

BENIGN ANTIBODIES

Other alloantibodies are "benign" or cause only minimal RBC destruction even though they react at 37°C; some of these are listed in Table 4.4, group II. Hemolytic transfusion reactions caused by antibodies of group II have not been reported. It is an appropriate policy to transfuse RBCs having the pertinent antigen regardless of in vitro incompatibility when patients have antibodies of group II.

ANTIBODIES THAT ARE USUALLY BENIGN

The significance of some other antibodies previously thought capable of causing hemolytic transfusion reactions has been reassessed. Experience indicates that antibodies that are reactive in vitro only at temperatures below 37°C are clinically benign, and many examples of the antibodies in group III react only in the cold. Thus, cold-reactive antibodies such as anti-A_1, -P_1, -M, -N, and -Lu^a can safely be ignored (13). Even when antibodies of these specificities react at 37°C, their in vivo significance is uncertain, but they should be considered potentially clinically significant, and antigen-negative blood or cross match-compatible blood should be transfused.

ANTIBODIES THAT ARE SOMETIMES CLINICALLY SIGNIFICANT

Antibodies in group IV are inconsistent in regard to their in vivo significance. These are all rather unusual antibodies, and when an antibody of one of these specificities is detected, the surgeon and the transfusion service director should discuss the most appropriate course of action. This will depend on the urgency of the surgery and the probability of the antibody being of clinical significance.

SUMMARY OF CLINICAL DECISION-MAKING WHEN A PATIENT WHO HAS RBC ALLOANTIBODIES REQUIRES TRANSFUSION

When an RBC alloantibody is present that reacts at 37°C, the following approach is recommended. If the antibody is expected to be clinically significant (e.g., has a specificity listed in group I of Table 4.4), antigen-negative blood should be transfused except in an extreme emergency. If the antibody reacts at 37°C but is an antibody listed in group II of Table 4.4, antigen-positive blood may be transfused even though it is incompatible in vitro.

For antibodies of group III, cross match-negative blood may be issued without the necessity of ensuring that the blood is negative for the antigen in question. For antibodies in group IV, possible approaches include obtaining antigen-negative blood from rare donor files (through reference laboratories) and/or by typing of family members. Consideration should be given to autologous transfusion including the freezing of the patient's RBCs for long-term storage. If antigen-negative blood cannot be obtained, an in vivo survival study may be performed (see below).

TRANSFUSING PATIENTS WITH AUTOIMMUNE HEMOLYTIC ANEMIA

Table 4.5 summarizes the essential serological findings in patients with various kinds of autoimmune hemolytic anemia (AIHA). Of these, warm antibody AIHA is by far the most frequent and affords the biggest challenge to the blood transfusion service to provide an appropriate unit for transfusion. It must be emphasized that for most patients whose AIHA is serious enough to require transfusion, it will be impossible to find compatible blood because the antibody in the patient's serum is likely to react with essentially all RBCs. Nevertheless, transfusion may be indicated and should not be withheld until the patient's condition is critical. A common error is to withhold transfusion in the mistaken belief that it is impossible or improper to transfuse incompatible blood under any circumstance.

TABLE 4.5. CHARACTERISTIC SEROLOGICAL FINDINGS IN AUTOIMMUNE HEMOLYTIC ANEMIAS

Type of AIHA	Result of DAT	Tests for Serum Antibody	Antibody Specificity
Warm antibody	IgG or C3 or both	IAT positive (57%); enzyme-treated RBC (89%)	Usually within Rh system
Cold agglutinin	C3 alone	Agglutinating activity up to 30°C	Usually anti-I or anti-i
Paroxysmal cold hemoglobinuria	C3 alone	Biphasic hemolysin	Anti-P

AIHA, autoimmune hemolytic anemia; DAT, direct antibody test; IAT, indirect antiglobulin test; RBC, red blood cell.

There are unique risks associated with transfusion in patients with AIHA (14). The autoantibody often complicates the compatibility test and may make it difficult to exclude the presence of coexisting alloantibodies, thus increasing the risk of a hemolytic transfusion reaction. In addition, the autoantibody itself may cause marked shortening of the survival of donor RBCs. Despite these added risks, blood should never be denied in a patient with a justifiable need even though the compatibility test may be strongly incompatible. On the other hand, the course of lesser risk may be to withhold blood transfusion in some settings in which the initial clinical judgment would suggest their need; that is, it is appropriate to be somewhat more stringent with indications for RBC transfusion.

When warm autoantibodies complicate compatibility tests, the autoantibody may be absorbed from the patient's serum so that alloantibodies may be detected. When cold autoantibodies are present, compatibility testing is performed strictly at 37°C. Occasionally, the autoantibody itself has RBC specificity, and this is taken into account in selecting the optimal unit of blood for transfusion.

A critical aspect of transfusing patients with AIHA is to avoid overtransfusion (15–17). The kinetics of RBC destruction always describe an exponential curve of decay, indicating that the number of cells removed in a unit of time is a percentage of the number of cells present at the start of this time interval (15). Thus, raising the hemoglobin level abruptly is likely to increase the amount of hemolysis that is occurring and may precipitate disseminated intravascular coagulation (DIC) as a result of procoagulant substances present in RBC lysates. Indeed, the most common cause of posttransfusion hemoglobinemia and hemoglobinuria in AIHA may not be alloantibody-induced hemolysis but instead the quantitative effect of transfusion in increasing the RBC mass subjected to ongoing autoantibody-mediated destruction (16). Accordingly, transfusion of comparatively small volumes of blood may be the optimal means of minimizing the danger of transfusion-induced intravascular hemolysis (15–17). The patient's hemoglobin level should be maintained just at a tolerable level until more specific therapy of the AIHA becomes effective.

IN VIVO CROSS-MATCH TESTS

Because there is added risk of a hemolytic transfusion reaction, "in vivo compatibility testing" may be performed in which only a small volume (about 25 mL) of the selected unit is transfused initially (more precise studies using radiolabeled RBCs may also be performed but require a radioisotope laboratory experienced in RBC survival studies). Immediately after transfusion of this aliquot and before proceeding with the remainder of the unit, a blood sample is observed for visual evidence of plasma hemoglobin (and urine, if available, is observed for hemoglobinuria) to exclude the presence of acute intravascular hemolysis.

In vivo compatibility testing provides only limited information. The lack of hemoglobinemia and hemoglobinuria offers a degree of assurance that an acute hemolytic reaction will not occur with transfusion of the entire unit. However, if the patient is seriously ill, the survival of transfused RBCs is very unlikely to be normal.

Further, if the aliquot of RBCs does result in acute hemolysis, one may still find it necessary to transfuse the patient if the clinical findings so dictate. Before doing so, one should communicate with the blood bank to ensure that RBC absorption tests have been done to exclude alloantibodies.

SURGERY IN PATIENTS WITH RBC AUTOANTIBODIES AND AIHA

Occasionally, surgery patients will have RBC autoantibodies in their serum. Some such patients will have no anemia and either no evidence of hemolysis or only minimal signs of hemolysis, suggesting normal or essentially normal RBC survival. Because transfused RBCs are likely to survive as well as the patient's own RBCs, transfusion is unlikely to result in an adverse reaction.

Other patients with autoantibodies may have overt AIHA. It is, of course, preferable to delay elective surgery until the AIHA can be brought under control, but if this is not possible, the transfusion service will supply the optimal units for transfusion, even though they may be strongly incompatible. The risk of transfusion is likely related to the severity of the hemolysis that the patient is experiencing as can be judged by the degree of anemia and the compensatory responses (e.g., reticulocyte count).

If practical, begin with slow administration of a small volume of RBCs (15–20 mL of packed RBCs over 30 minutes), carefully monitor the patient for symptoms, and obtain a blood sample from the patient after 30 minutes to observe for hemoglobinemia. Continued clinical observation and follow-up blood samples for hemoglobinemia, perhaps after each unit, will allow repeat assessment of the results of the transfusion. Most patients with AIHA tolerate transfusions quite well unless they are overtransfused or have RBC alloantibodies that have not been identified in addition to their autoantibodies. It may be preferable to initiate transfusion before surgery (see above, In Vivo Cross-Match Tests) if this is feasible, because it is easier to judge the patient's symptoms before being anesthetized. It is the surgeon's responsibility to use blood judiciously to maintain a tolerable level of hemoglobin.

BLOOD TRANSFUSION IN MINOR ABO-MISMATCHED SOLID ORGAN TRANSPLANTATION

PASSENGER LYMPHOCYTE SYNDROME

A syndrome of immune hemolysis known as the "passenger lymphocyte syndrome" may occur in some patients after solid organ or bone marrow transplantation when there is a minor ABO blood group mismatch. The syndrome has been attributed to proliferation and antibody production by "passenger" lymphocytes that are infused with the transplanted organ or donor marrow product (18–24).

The syndrome occurs in only a minority of patients (perhaps 15%) who receive a minor ABO-mismatched transplant, and only rare cases have been associated with antibodies other than anti-A and anti-B. Patients generally (although not always) received cyclosporine for posttransplant immunosuppression.

Immune hemolysis generally has its onset near the end of the first week or during the second week posttransplant. Hemolysis is usually abrupt in onset and may be severe, with a rapidly dropping hemoglobin level, signs of intravascular hemolysis (hemoglobinemia and hemoglobinuria), and renal failure. Less-severe cases are characterized by a falling hemoglobin level, an increase in serum bilirubin and lactate dehydrogenase, and absent serum haptoglobin. In patients who have received a liver transplant, some signs of hemolysis are difficult to interpret, especially serum bilirubin and serum haptoglobin. Nevertheless, hemolysis is often quite evident as a result of a rapidly dropping hemoglobin without evident bleeding and a bilirubin and lactate dehydrogenase not in keeping with other laboratory findings of liver function.

Hemolysis usually persists for 5–10 days and then ceases as antibody production by the passenger lymphocytes ceases (or, in the case of bone marrow transplant, when the hemolyzed RBCs of the marrow recipient are replaced by transfused group O RBCs or by RBCs of donor origin). Transfusions of group O RBCs are indicated and are often necessary for 4–10 days as a result of the hemolysis. Rarely, hemolysis is so severe as to justify an emergency RBC exchange transfusion to replace the patient's RBCs with group O RBCs (25).

Serological Findings

Characteristic serological findings in patients with the passenger lymphocyte syndrome are a positive direct antiglobulin test and the presence of anti-A and/or anti-B in the patient's serum and in an eluate from RBCs. Pretransplant anti-A and anti-B titers in the donor do not appear to be helpful in predicting which patients will develop the passenger lymphocyte syndrome or the severity of the hemolysis. Of particular interest is that in some patients, overt signs of hemolysis may precede by 1–2 days one's ability to detect the expected antibody. It appears that small concentrations of anti-A or anti-B may cause hemolysis at a time in which they cannot be detected by routine serological tests.

Management

Appropriate management of patients who develop the passenger lymphocyte syndrome after solid organ transplantation generally requires only RBC transfusion. The patient should be transfused with group O RBCs to minimize the number of incompatible RBCs present in the circulation. In cases in which the hemolysis is unusually severe, exchange transfusion is indicated, but this is required only rarely. Either plasma exchange to remove the offending antibody or RBC exchange to replace incompatible RBCs with group O RBCs is effective.

ADVERSE REACTIONS TO TRANSFUSION AND THEIR MANAGEMENT

Adverse reactions to transfused blood products can occur, and physicians and nursing staff must be prepared to deal with them (26). Because the signs and symptoms of different types of adverse reactions overlap and their severity can vary considerably, all transfusions must be carefully monitored and stopped as soon as symptoms of a reaction are detected (with the exception of urticaria reactions; see below). Early recognition is the key to minimizing serious complications.

SIGNS AND SYMPTOMS OF TRANSFUSION REACTIONS

Table 4.6 lists the signs and symptoms that are indicative of a transfusion reaction. While a patient is under anesthesia, a number of these manifestations may not be evident. Hemoglobinuria is a sign that is particularly alarming because it is indicative of a serious hemolytic reaction that can be life-threatening or fatal.

When a transfusion reaction is suspected, the following immediate steps should be taken:

1. Always stop the transfusion and disconnect the entire infusion set from the needle/catheter unless hives are the only symptom (see step 7).
2. Using a new infusion set, keep the intravenous (IV) line open with a "keep open" drip of normal saline.
3. Check the blood bag label and paperwork against the patient's identification band to confirm that the patient received the correct unit.
4. If the manifestations of a transfusion reaction are noted by someone other than the attending physician, the patient's physician should be notified immediately.
5. Notify the blood bank and describe the signs and symptoms.
6. A posttransfusion blood sample (10 mL of clotted blood) should be sent to the blood bank with an order for a transfusion reaction workup. Accompanying the order should be the remainder of the unit and the attached administration set.
7. First voided urine should be sent to the blood bank for evaluation. If pink, red, or dark colored, a specimen should be sent to the laboratory for analysis of free hemoglobin.
8. Urticarial reactions are an exception to the above policies. An antihistamine may be prescribed, and if the patient's symptoms resolve and hospital policy permits, the blood transfusion may be restarted.

TABLE 4.6. SYMPTOMS INDICATIVE OF TRANSFUSION REACTIONS

Fever ($\geq$1°C rise without any other explanation)		
Chills	Headache	Itching
Chest/back pain	Nausea	Wheezing
Heat at infusion site	Facial flushing	Coughing
Hemoglobinuria	Uneasy feeling	Cyanosis
Hypotension	Myalgia	Dyspnea
Abnormal bleeding	Urticaria (hives)	Pulmonary edema
Oliguria/anuria	Rash	Jaundice

TYPES OF TRANSFUSION REACTIONS

Acute Hemolytic Transfusion Reaction

The most severe and life-threatening hemolytic reactions are almost always associated with ABO incompatibility between the donor and recipient because of a clerical or management error in identifying the patient or blood unit. These reactions are manifested by signs of intravascular hemolysis that consist of hemoglobinemia and hemoglobinuria. Fever is a prominent sign, and the clinical findings may progress to include DIC, multisystem organ failure, and death.

Occasionally, a non-ABO antibody may also trigger acute intravascular hemolysis. Usually, however, these antibodies (primarily of the IgG class and unrelated to ABO blood groups) are associated with extravascular hemolysis.

The most important aspect of management is to maintain adequate intravascular volume and blood pressure with adequate fluid intake. One should monitor the patient's electrocardiogram, blood pressure, cardiac output, urine output, and renal function. Although there is no good evidence that the use of diuretic agents can reverse acute renal failure once it has developed, it is reasonable to attempt a trial of furosemide, 80–400 mg i.v. in the early oliguric phase in the hope of inducing a diuresis. Medical consultation should be obtained as necessary for management of renal failure and/or DIC, if present.

It should be noted that most hemolytic reactions are the result of a clerical or management error and are eminently preventable. One should always carefully identify the patient, the blood product sent for transfusion, and all blood samples drawn for testing (27, 28).

Delayed Hemolytic Transfusion Reactions

Delayed hemolytic transfusion reactions (DHTRs) occur in patients who have been previously sensitized by transfusion or pregnancy but in whom the RBC antibodies have diminished to undetectable levels so that seemingly compatible antigen-positive units are transfused (29, 30). In response to a "secondary" antigen exposure, the patient's immune system increases antibody production, usually within several days, and these newly formed antibodies cause destruction of the RBCs transfused. The resultant anemia is frequently misdiagnosed as posttransfusion bleeding because the index of suspicion for DHTR is low. Often the blood bank is the first to recognize the reaction from subsequent antibody detection tests. If antibody is detected but there is no clinical hemolysis, the reaction is classified as a delayed serological transfusion reaction.

Usually, the only management required is transfusion with compatible blood as required. It is impossible to prevent all DHTRs because the patient may not have compatibility tests done after the transfusion or pregnancy that stimulated the original antibodies to develop. However, when RBC antibodies are identified by the blood bank, physicians should inform their patients and counsel them to provide this information when they are hospitalized elsewhere. Carrying a transfusion alert card is recommended.

Nonimmune Hemolytic Transfusion Reactions

When symptoms of hemolysis are observed and antibody detection tests are negative, nonimmune causes of hemolysis should be investigated. These include excessive heating of donor units, accidental freezing of donor units, contact with incompatible IV solutions in the donor bag or infusion line, older RBCs infused under pressure or with an IV pump, mechanical trauma from intraoperative blood collection devices or cardiopulmonary pump-oxygenators, large-volume infusions of hypotonic solutions, bacterial contamination, and rare RBC/hemoglobin defect in the donor.

Acute hemolysis not caused by an immune mechanism less often leads to serious sequelae. It is essential to correct the cause of hemolysis to minimize complications.

Febrile Nonhemolytic Transfusion Reactions

These are by far the most common type of transfusion reactions. Because they are relatively common and have no long-term effects, there is a tendency to minimize their significance. A major aspect of their importance lies in the fact that symptoms of fever and chills are also cardinal features of acute hemolytic reactions, the presence of which must be promptly excluded.

Febrile reactions are self-limiting and are usually seen in multitransfused or multiparous patients who have an antibody directed against donor leukocytes or platelets. Such antibody-antigen reactions can activate complement and stimulate cytokine production, which results in the release of endogenous pyrogens. Newer theories suggest that in some cases, cytokines accumulating in stored blood may directly activate endogenous pyrogens (31). Once acute hemolysis is ruled out, supportive care, including the use of antipyretics (aspirin or acetaminophen), will relieve symptoms.

Only 15% of patients experiencing a febrile nonhemolytic reaction will have another reaction at their next transfusion. If a second reaction does occur, leukocyte-reduced blood components should be requested. Routine use of prophylactic antipyretics is not recommended because they may mask symptoms from acute hemolysis.

Allergic Reactions

Simple allergic reactions are the second most common type of transfusion complication. These are attributed to soluble substances in donor plasma that react with IgE antibody in the patient attached to mast cells and basophils. The antibody-antigen reaction initiates histamine release, which causes hives, itching, and, rarely, laryngeal edema.

The patient should be monitored carefully because urticaria can be the first sign of a more serious allergic reaction. The patient should be treated with an antihistamine to ease discomfort: diphenhydramine HCl (Benadryl) 10–50 mg i.m. or i.v. depending on severity for adults and 1–1.5 mg/kg for children. If the only symptom is skin rash or hives, if the symptoms resolve within 30 minutes of treatment, and if hospital policy permits, the transfusion may be restarted.

Patients who have had two or more allergic reactions may benefit from oral or parenteral antihistamine prophylaxis 1 hour before transfusion and at the start of transfusion. Transfusing saline-washed RBCs may help patients with frequent severe allergic reactions. Corticosteroids are indicated only in severe repetitive cases.

Anaphylactic Reactions

Anaphylactic reactions result in a massive release of vasoactive and smooth muscle-reactive mediators after an antibody-antigen reaction. These increase vascular permeability and smooth muscle contraction to severe life-threatening proportions. In many cases, the implicated donor antigen is not identifiable. These reactions are rarely due to congenital IgA deficiency and concurrent high-titered IgG antibody to IgA (32).

Symptoms consist of a sudden onset of flushing and hypertension followed by hypotension, widespread edema, respiratory distress, and shock, and sometimes nausea, vomiting, and diarrhea can occur within minutes of starting the transfusion. The reactions are potentially fatal because of shock or respiratory failure; early recognition and treatment are critical.

Appropriate management consists of the immediate administration of subcutaneous epinephrine, 0.2–0.5 mL of 1:1000 epinephrine, and repeat as necessary. The patient's intravascular volume and blood pressure should be maintained with crystalloid infusions. If intractable hypotension develops, give 0.1 mL of 1:1000 epinephrine diluted to 10 mL with normal saline i.v. over 5 minutes. Consider using dopamine 1.0 μg/kg/min (contraindicated with volume depletion). If hypoxia develops, give oxygen by nasal catheter or mask. Endotracheal intubation may be necessary.

For those rare patients with a history of an anaphylactic reaction to blood who have congenital IgA deficiency and anti-IgA antibodies, blood components depleted of plasma should be used. For RBC transfusion, this can be accomplished by using saline-washed or frozen-thawed RBCs. If plasma is needed, it should be from a known IgA-deficient donor. Extra time is needed to order and prepare these special components.

Transfusion-related Acute Lung Injury

Also known as noncardiogenic pulmonary edema, this unusual life-threatening complication is associated with altered permeability of the pulmonary capillary bed from activation of complement, histamine-mediated events, or prostaglandins, which leads to fluid accumulation, inadequate oxygenation, and reduced cardiac return. The reaction is commonly attributed to leukocyte-agglutinating antibodies in donor plasma that react with recipient leukocytes in the pulmonary microvasculature (33). Other suggested causes include cytokines in the donor units (31), recipient antibody to donor cells or protein, and use of extracorporeal perfusion circuits.

Transfusion-related acute lung injury (TRALI) is manifested by an acute onset of respiratory distress, dyspnea, cyanosis, fever, and chills. An x-ray will show bilateral pulmonary infiltrates, but no other signs of left heart failure are seen. Potentially fatal hypoxia may occur and persist for 24–48 hours.

The cornerstone of therapy is effective supportive care for respiratory insufficiency. Intubation may be required. Corticosteroids are often used empirically, but their effectiveness has not been proven.

Patients who develop TRALI are unlikely to have another reaction because it is most often donor-specific. Donors who have been implicated in a case of TRALI and who possess potent leukoagglutinins can trigger reactions in other patients and should be deferred from donating.

Circulatory Overload

Circulatory overload may be the most underdiagnosed of the adverse reactions to transfusion. Patients who are very young or very old, who have underlying congestive heart failure, or who have chronic anemia and an expanded blood volume are at greatest risk from circulatory overload. When too much blood is transfused too quickly, these patients cannot handle the volume increase and consequently develop heart failure and acute pulmonary edema.

Patients at risk should be identified before a transfusion is started, and they should be transfused slowly. The blood bank can split blood units and issue only one-half at a time if very slow infusion rates are critical. One should avoid whole blood and extra priming saline. Patients should be monitored carefully during transfusion.

Bacterial Contamination

Bacterial contamination of blood is being recognized more frequently and is one of the most serious complications of transfusion (34). If bacteria are introduced into donor units during collection, processing, or pooling, they may cause sepsis or life-threatening endotoxic shock. Such reactions are unusual but frequently fatal. They are more commonly attributed to platelet transfusions, because platelet products are stored at room temperature for optimal platelet viability.

Bacterial contamination of blood products should be suspected when a patient develops high fever (often greater than 2°C rise) and shaking chills. Other manifestations may include severe hypotension, abdominal pain, vomiting, hemoglobinuria, DIC, renal failure, circulatory collapse, and a "warm" shock picture, which can occur within minutes of starting the transfusion. Because the reactions are potentially fatal, they must be recognized and treated at once. One should not wait for confirmatory laboratory data.

Patients should be managed with aggressive broad-spectrum antibiotic therapy and supportive care; corticosteroids are often given empirically. The patient's intravascular volume should be maintained with crystalloid solutions and possibly vasopressor drugs such as dopamine.

REFERENCES

1. Klein HG. Standards for blood banks and transfusion services. Bethesda, MD: American Association of Blood Banks, 1994.
2. Boral LI, Henry JB. The type and screen: a safe alternative and supplement in selected surgical procedures. Transfusion 1977;17:163–168.
3. Oberman HA, Barnes BA, Friedman BA. The risk of abbreviating the major crossmatch in urgent or massive transfusion. Transfusion 1978; 18:137–141.
4. Shulman IA, Nelson JM, Saxena S, et al. Experience with the routine use of an abbreviated crossmatch. Am J Clin Pathol 1984;82:178–181.
5. Heddle NM, OHoski P, Singer J, McBride JA, Ali MA, Kelton JG. A prospective study to determine the safety of omitting the antiglobulin crossmatch from pretransfusion testing. Br J Haematol 1992;81: 579–584.
6. Boral LI, Dannemiller FJ, Stanford W, Hill SS, Cornell TA. A guideline for anticipated blood usage during elective surgical procedures. Am J Clin Pathol 1979;71:680–684.
7. Mintz PD, Nordine RB, Henry JB, Webb WR. Expected hemotherapy in elective surgery. N Y J Med 1976;76:532–537.
8. Renner S. Q-probe 89–08A. Short-term studies of the laboratory's role in quality care. Blood utilization data analysis and critique. College of American Pathologists, 1990.
9. Shulman IA, Morales J, Nelson JM, Saxena S. Emergency transfusion protocols. Lab Med 1989;20:166–168.
10. Shulman IA, Spence RK, Petz LD. Surgical blood ordering, blood shortage situations, and emergency transfusions. In: Petz LD, Swisher SN, Kleinman S, Spence RK, Strauss RG, eds. Clinical practice of transfusion medicine. New York: Churchill-Livingstone, 1995.
11. Ramsey G, Cornell FW, Hahn LF, Fonzi F, Starzl TE. Incompatible blood transfusions in liver transplant patients with significant red cell alloantibodies. Transplant Proc 1989;21:3531.
12. Ramsey G, Cornell FW, Hahn L, et al. Red cell antibody problems in 1000 liver transplants [abstract]. Transfusion 1987;27:552.
13. Giblett ER. Blood group alloantibodies: an assessment of some laboratory practices. Transfusion 1977;17:299–308.
14. Petz LD. Transfusing the patient with autoimmune hemolytic anemia. Clin Lab Med 1982;2:193–210.
15. Rosenfield RE, Jagathambal K. Transfusioin therapy for autoimmune hemolytic anemia. Semin Hematol 1976;13:311–321.
16. Chaplin H Jr. Special problems in transfusion management of patients with autoimmune hemolytic anemia. In: Bell CA, ed. A seminar on laboratory management of hemolysis. Washington, D.C.: American Association of Blood Banks, 1979:135–150.
17. Bilgrami S, Cable R, Pisciotto P, Rowland F, Greenberg B. Fatal disseminated intravascular coagulation and pulmonary thrombosis following blood transfusion in a patient with severe autoimmune hemolytic anemia and human immunodeficiency virus infection. Transfusion 1994;34:248–252.
18. Hows J, Beddow K, Gordon Smith E, et al. Donor-derived red blood cell antibodies and immune hemolysis after allogeneic bone marrow transplantation. Blood 1986;67:177–181.
19. Ramsey G, Nusbacher J, Starzl TE, Lindsay GD. Isohemagglutinins of graft origin after ABO-unmatched liver transplantation. N Engl J Med 1984; 311:1167–1170.
20. Lundgren G, Asaba H, Bergstrom J, et al. Fulminating anti-A autoimmune hemolysis with anuria in a renal transplant recipient: a therapeutic role of plasma exchange. Clin Nephrol 1981;16:211–214.
21. Mangal AK, Growe GH, Sinclair M, Stillwell GF, Reeve CE, Naiman SC. Acquired hemolytic anemia due to "auto"-anti-A or "auto"-anti-B induced by group O homograft in renal transplant recipients. Transfusion 1984;24:201–205.
22. Nyberg G, Sandberg L, Rydberg L, et al. ABO-autoimmune hemolytic anemia in a renal transplant patient treated with cyclosporin. A case report. Transplantation 1984; 37:529–530.
23. Bird GW, Wingham J. Formation of blood group "autoantibodies" after transplantation [letter]. Transfusion 1995;22:400.
24. Salamon DJ, Ramsey G, Nusbacher J, Yang S, Starzl TE, Israel L. Anti-A production by a group O spleen transplanted to a group A recipient. Vox Sang 1985;48:309–312.
25. Gajewski JL, Petz LD, Calhoun L, et al. Hemolysis of transfused group O red blood cells in minor ABO-incompatible unrelated-donor bone marrow transplants in patients receiving cyclosporine without post-transplant methotrexate. Blood 1992;79:3076–3085.
26. Beauregard P, Blajchman MA. Hemolytic and pseudo-hemolytic transfusion reactions: an overview of the hemolytic transfusion reactions and the clinical conditions that mimic them [review]. Transf Med Rev 1994;8:184–199.
27. Linden JV, Kaplan HS. Transfusion errors: causes and effects [review]. Transf Med Rev 1994;8:169–183.
28. Sazama K. Reports of 355 transfusion-associated deaths: 1976 through 1985. Transfusion 1990;30:583–590.
29. Shirey RS, Ness PM. New concepts of delayed hemolytic transfusion reactions. In: Nance SJ, ed. Clinical and basic science: aspects of immunohematology. Arlington, VA: American Association of Blood Banks, 1991:179.
30. Vamvakas EC, Pineda AA, Reisner R, Santrach PJ, Moore SB. The differentiation of delayed hemolytic and delayed serologic transfusion reactions: incidence and predictors of hemolysis. Transfusion 1995;35: 26–32.
31. Davenport RD, Kunkel SL. Cytokine roles in hemolytic and non-hemolytic transfusion reactions [review]. Transf Med Rev 1994;8: 157–168.
32. Sandler SG, Mallory D, Malamut D, Eckrich R. IgA anaphylactic transfusion reactions. Transf Med Rev 1995;9:1–8.
33. Popovsky MA, Chaplin HC Jr, Moore SB. Transfusion-related acute lung injury: a neglected, serious complication of hemotherapy [see comments]. Transfusion 1992;32:589–592.
34. Wagner SJ, Friedman LI, Dodd RY. Transfusion-associated bacterial sepsis [review]. Clin Microbiol Rev 1994;7:290–302.

Chapter 5

Platelet Production, Physiology, Hemostasis, and Transfusion Therapy

SHERRILL J. SLICHTER

PLATELET PRODUCTION

Platelets are cytoplasmic fragments of bone marrow megakaryocytes that are released into circulation. Regulation of megakaryocytopoiesis is under hormonal control and proceeds as a two-step process. In the first phase, there are two types of proliferating progenitor cells that eventually produce identifiable megakaryocytes. These proliferating progenitors are designated burst-forming unit megakaryocyte and colony-forming unit megakaryocyte (CFU-Mk). At some point, cell mitosis ceases, and the second process of nuclear endoreduplication begins, resulting in polyploid megakaryocytes. Megakaryocytes divide synchronously, resulting in 2, 4, 8, 16, 32, and 64 nuclei. The median number is 8. For each nuclei formed, a finite amount of cytoplasm is generated. As the megakaryocyte increases in size, the number of platelets produced by each megakaryocyte also increases because platelets are derived from megakaryocyte cytoplasm (1). During or after polyploidization, the megakaryocyte cytoplasm matures, resulting in protein and granule synthesis (2).

Two hypotheses have been advanced to explain how platelets are formed from the megakaryocyte cytoplasm. The first is that demarcation membranes divide the megakaryocyte cytoplasm to form platelets. Alternatively, platelets are formed by a demarcation membrane system that envelopes cytoplasm, resulting in the formation of platelets. Cytoplasmic processes extend into the marrow sinuses through endothelial fenestration, giving rise to the platelets. Most investigators consider the marrow the major site of platelet production; however, some studies have suggested that platelet production may also occur in the lung, because pulmonary venous blood has lower numbers of platelets than the pulmonary arterial circulation. Megakaryocyte fragments and intact megakaryocytes may be released from the bone marrow into the venous blood and lodge in the pulmonary vasculature with release of platelets into the arterial circulation (3).

Evidence for a two-step regulatory process, with potentially one or more hormonal agents controlling platelet production, comes from the marrow's response to thrombocytopenia. With acute thrombocytopenia, megakaryocytes show increased nuclear polyploidization, resulting in larger mega-karyocytes that mature in a shorter time interval that results in the release of increased numbers of large, potentially hyperfunctional platelets into the circulation. Only when there is an actual reduction in the number of bone marrow megakaryocytes is there a proliferative response observed in the marrow with an increase in the number of CFU-Mk (3). In support of the hypothesis that at least two hormones regulate megakaryocytopoiesis is the generation of thrombopoietic stimulatory activity in the plasma of animals made acutely thrombocytopenic or in the plasma and urine of patients with peripheral thrombocytopenia. However, megakaryocyte colony-stimulating activity (CSA-Mk) is only increased in patients with bone marrow or selective megakaryocytic aplasia.

A variety of cytokines has demonstrated effects on induction of megakaryocyte colonies in vitro, on megakaryocyte maturation in vitro, or on thrombopoiesis in vivo (2, 3). The cytokines with effects on some aspect of megakaryocytopoiesis include granulocyte macrophage colony-stimulating factor, granulocyte colony-stimulating factor, interleukin (IL)-1, IL-3, IL-4, IL-6, CSA-Mk, and erythropoietin. Although these factors were found to have various types of stimulatory effects on megakaryocytopoiesis, they were not believed to represent a cell-specific thrombopoietin. However, recent reports from several laboratories have indicated that thrombopoietin has been isolated and cloned (4–7). If so, this factor could be administered both before and after elective surgeries known to commonly result in thrombocytopenia (e.g., cardiopulmonary bypass surgery) to avoid this side effect. However, because data suggest that platelets released under a thrombopoietic stimulus may be young and hyperfunctional, it will have to be determined in what clinical situations the benefits of increased platelet production may be outweighed by the potential hazards of thrombosis if, indeed, large numbers of hyperfunctional platelets enter the circulation.

PLATELET PHYSIOLOGY

As anucleated cytoplasmic fragments of megakaryocytes, platelets have only vestigial remnants of the cell machinery that regulates gene expression; however, they rely on proteins synthesized by their parent cell—the megakaryocyte—to perform complex metabolic tasks such as preserving vascular integrity and controlling hemorrhage after injury. Normally, platelets do not adhere to the endothelial lining of blood vessels but respond rapidly to the loss of endothelial cells by attaching themselves to exposed subendothelial structures. Platelets form an adherent layer on the surface of any thrombogenic surfacc (e.g., a nonendothelialized surface or an artificial surface introduced into the circulation). When the continuity of a normal blood vessel is interrupted, the initial response to the injury is defined as primary hemostasis (Fig. 5.1) (8). Platelets immediately adhere to collagen in the subendothelium that has been exposed by the injury. Collagen is a strong platelet agonist that induces platelet activation, leading to secretion of additional agonists. These include ADP, thromboxane A_2, and serotonin. Secretion leads

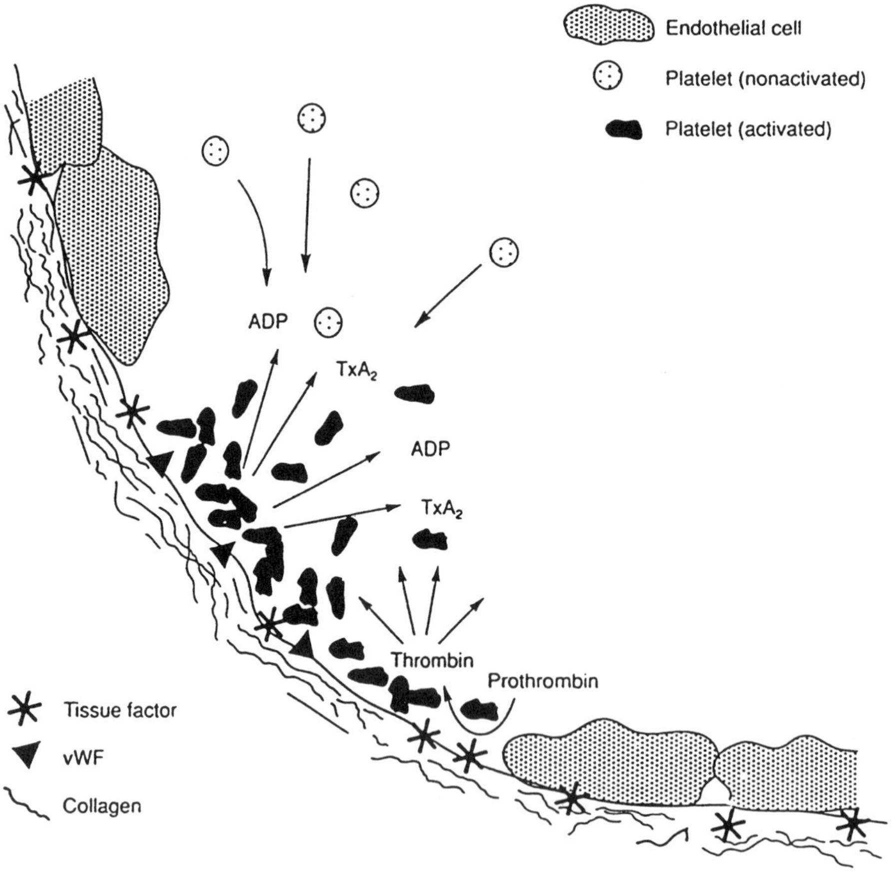

Figure 5.1. Platelet activation at the vessel wall. Platelet activation begins when vascular damage strips away endothelial cells, exposing collagen and tissue factor. Circulating platelets adhere to the exposed collagen, either directly or via von Willebrand factor (vWF). Others are activated by locally generated thrombin. These events are followed by a change in the platelet's shape, storage granule secretion, and the formation of multicellular aggregates as additional platelets are recruited into the growing platelet plug. The recruitment of nonadherent platelets is facilitated by the release of soluble factors from the platelets, such as ADP and thromboxane A_2. This phase of hemostasis is completed when the platelet plug is stabilized by a meshwork of fibrin. (Reprinted with permission from Brass LF. Molecular basis for platelet activation. In: Hoffman R, Benz EJ Jr, Shatill SJ, et al., eds. Hematology: basic principles and practice. 2nd ed. New York: Churchill-Livingstone, 1995:1536.)

to recruitment of other platelets that aggregate on the initial layer of adherent platelets, thereby forming the hemostatic plug. Activated platelets also undergo a change in shape from a disc to a spiny sphere. In the process, rearrangement of membrane phospholipoprotein components forms a potent catalytic procoagulant surface. Activated coagulation factor X is bound to the platelet surface in the presence of activated factor V. Factor VII of the extrinsic coagulation system is also platelet-surface activated. This series of events results in the formation of thrombin, which transforms fibrinogen into fibrin, stabilizing the platelet plug by providing individual fibrin links between the aggregated platelets. In addition, thrombin is also a strong platelet agonist. Secondary hemostasis results from thrombin-mediated reinduction of platelet activation and recruitment, along with coagulation. The hemostatic platelet plug is now consolidated and impermeable, preventing further hemorrhage (9).

The following detailed discussion of platelet physiology expands on this brief overview of hemostasis by dividing the platelet hemostatic process into endothelial cell structure and function, platelet adhesion, platelet activation, platelet aggregation, and platelet procoagulant activity. However, because formation of the hemostatic platelet plug is a dynamic sequential process, some overlap between these discussions occurs.

ENDOTHELIAL CELL STRUCTURE AND FUNCTION

Characteristically, endothelial cells form a single layer in vivo. Weibel-Palade bodies, unique rod-shaped secretory organelles, are associated with endothelial cells. von Willebrand factor (vWF) is contained within Weibel-Palade bodies and is secreted both constitutively and in response to a variety of agonists (10, 11). vWF synthesized by megakaryocytes is ultimately secreted by activated platelets. When the endothelium is disrupted under conditions of high shear stress, the primary adhesion protein for platelets is vWF (12). Platelet adhesive interactions in vessels in which shear stress is low (e.g., the venous circulation) are not well characterized (13). However, a number of vascular endothelial basement membrane and matrix proteins have the potential to serve as adhesive ligands for platelets in vivo. Vascular endothelial cells make several types of collagen (IV, V, and VIII) (14–16). Initial platelet adhesion to collagen does not appear to require platelet activation, and it results in platelet spreading. Other vascular basement membrane and matrix proteins that are candidate adhesion molecules for platelets are vitronectin and fibronectin. Platelets contain both vitronectin and fibronectin receptors. Platelets also adhere to thrombospondin through receptors that remain to be fully characterized. Thrombospondin is made by vascular endothelium and by megakaryocytes and is released from the platelet alpha granule during platelet secretion. Platelets also contain an integrin receptor for laminin that codistributes with type IV collagen (13).

Endothelial cells also act to regulate the size of the platelet thrombus because of several thromboresistant properties. Several substances and shear stress stimulate the release of a potent vasodilator, endothelium-derived relaxing factor (EDRF) (17). EDRF induces vasodilation by increasing cyclic 3′5′-guanosine monophosphate (cGMP) in vascular smooth muscle (18). EDRF also stimulates guanylyl cyclase in platelets, resulting in inhibition of platelet activation (19). Prostacyclin (PGI_2) is formed from arachidonic acid in response to thrombin, shear stress, fibrin, and a variety of other agents (13). PGI_2 is also a potent platelet activation inhibitor because it increases platelet cAMP (20). Platelet endoperoxides are also converted to PGI_2 by endothelial cells, suggesting a potential negative feedback regulatory mechanism inhibiting further platelet activation (21). In addition, the endothelial cell membrane ectonucleotidases are enzymes that metabolize released platelet ADP to AMP and adenosine, thereby limiting platelet recruitment (9). The endothelium also synthesizes glycosaminoglycans (heparin-like molecules), which enhance the activity of antithrombin III and heparin cofactor 2, thrombomodulin that inhibits thrombin and enhances the activation of protein C and tissue plasminogen activator. Thus, a delicate balance is maintained between the prothrombotic and antithrombotic properties of the endothelium.

PLATELET ADHESION

The first step in the response of platelets to vascular injury is their irreversible attachment to the altered surface. This stage requires that platelets recognize the site of vascular injury as different from the normal vessel wall. Two possible mechanisms may lead to site-specific platelet adhesion: circulating "resting" platelets react with adhesive substrates exposed when the vessel wall is damaged or agonists generated because of the injury act on neighboring platelets, "activating" them so they interact with the injured vessel wall. Some combination of both processes is likely to occur during the formation of platelet thrombi, with the most probable sequence being that adhesion always precedes, and is necessary for, platelet activation (22).

As previously mentioned, the adhesion of platelets to subendothelial structures after vascular injury depends on whether the lesion has occurred in the arterial or venous circulation. In the arterial circulation, with high flow rates, glycoprotein Ib (GPIb) receptors on the surface of platelets bind to vWF ligands on the vascular surface, resulting in platelet adhesion. In the venous circulation, fibrin forms in the presence of red cells, and platelet deposition is less prominent. The vWF factor/GPIb system is an "on" and "off" system. Soluble vWF in plasma will not bind to the GPIb receptor on platelets in the absence of shear forces. However, when shear forces are present, these two factors develop a specific affinity for one another, and the system switches on. Bound vWF on the subendothelial surface, as opposed to soluble circulating vWF, may be more reactive with platelet GPIb receptors.

Once the GPIb-vWF bond has been formed, the platelets are activated, and they spread to cover the surrounding subendothelial surface. Spreading on collagen also leads to platelet activation, possibly by multipoint attachment, inducing receptor clustering and transmission of activation signals (23). Activation of platelets, by either interaction with collagen or other mediators such as thrombin, leads to conformational changes in the integrin GPIIb/IIIa that allows it to mediate additional spreading on the matrix by binding to at least four adhesive ligands: fibrinogen, fibronectin, vWF, and vitronectin (Fig. 5.2) (24–26).

Using high-resolution scanning electron microscopy, circulating platelets have a very corrugated appearance that resembles the surface of the brain (Fig. 5.3*A*) (27). Once the platelet becomes activated, long filiform processes are formed. The wrinkled surface of the resting cell provides a significant amount of membrane to cover the elongations as discoid cells are converted to dendritic forms (Fig. 5.3*B*) (27). A major objective of the platelet in hemostasis is to cover as much of the damaged area as possible to restore vascular integrity. It accomplishes this by expanding its cytoplasm to fill spaces between the pseudopods. This process converts the dendritic platelet into a fully spread form (Fig. 5.3*C*) (27). The mechanism underlying pseudopod formation and spreading is the assembly of cytoplasmic actin. The actin filaments form into parallel bundles, pushing out pseudopods. During the conversion of discoid platelets to fully spread forms, the spread surface area increases by over 400%. Membranes to accomplish this spreading process come from the open canalicular system and from the convoluted surface of the platelet. Spreading is possible because the platelet surface receptors are a mo-

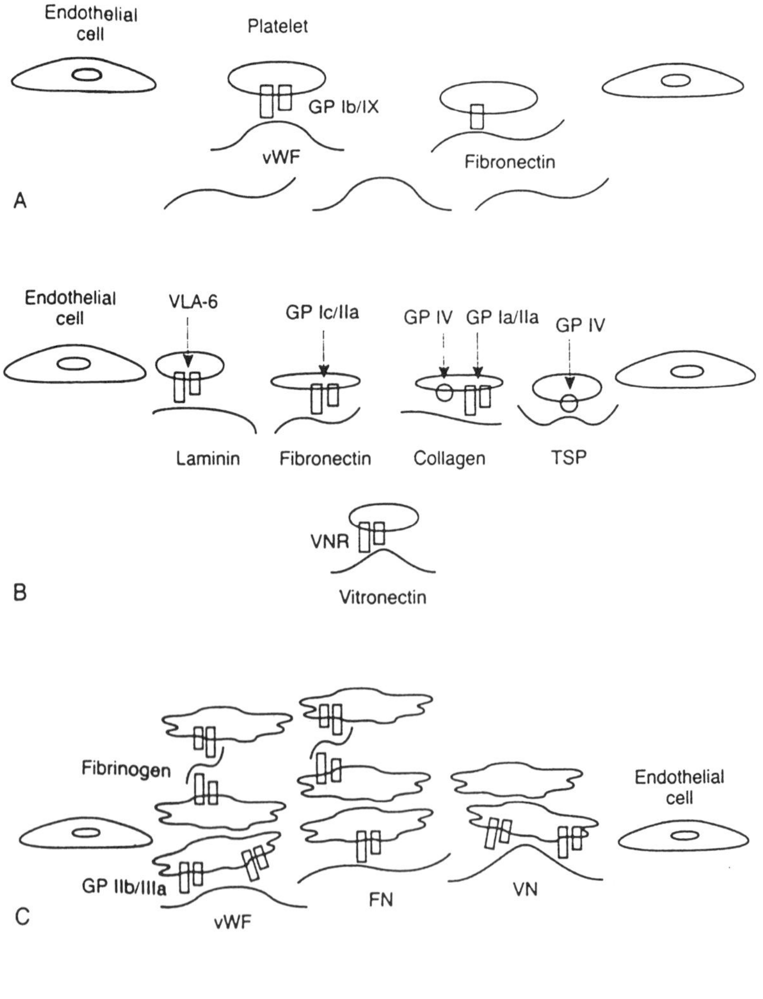

Figure 5.2. The role of membrane glycoproteins in mediating platelet adhesion and aggregation. **A.** When flowing blood encounters an exposed subendothelial surface, platelets initially adhere to vWF through the membrane GPIb-IX complex and to fibronectin through a receptor not yet identified. **B.** After these initial adherence events, platelets use several other membrane glycoprotein receptors to bind additional matrix macromolecules. The adherence of platelets to collagen and fibronectin also facilitates spreading of platelets on the subendothelial surface. **C.** The spreading of platelets on collagen and the release of procoagulant mediators, such as thrombin, lead to platelet activation. Cellular activation generates a conformational change in the platelet receptor GPIIb-IIIa that makes it competent to bind the adhesive ligands fibrinogen, fibronectin (FN), vWF, and vitronectin (VN). The binding of the former is particularly important in supporting platelet aggregation. The binding of the other ligands facilitates further platelet spreading on the damaged vessel wall. Not shown is the stabilization of platelet aggregates by interactions of GPIV with the adhesive macromolecule thrombospondin (TSP) that is released from the alpha granules of activated platelets. Also not shown are the multiple interactions of adhesive proteins with each other. (Reprinted with permission from McEver RP. The clinical significance of platelet membrane glycoproteins. Hematol Oncol Clin North Am 1990;4:87.)

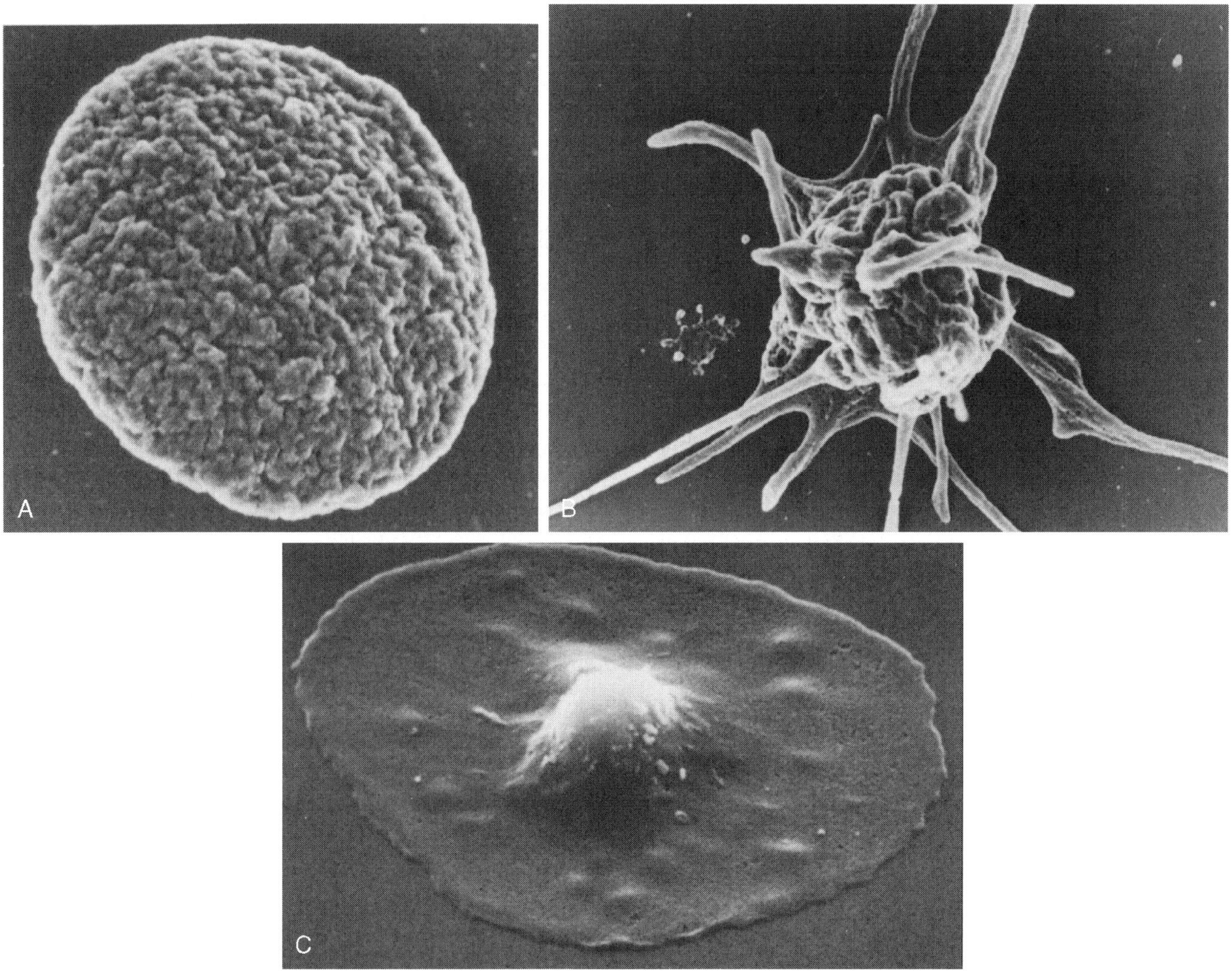

Figure 5.3. Platelet appearance during different phases of normal hemostasis. **A.** Circulating discoid platelet photographed in the low-voltage high-resolution scanning electron microscope (LVHR-SEM) demonstrating that the outside of the cell resembles the surface of the brain. Gyri and sulci alternate in a convoluted fashion, resulting in the wrinkled appearance. Magnification ×40,000. **B.** After platelet adhesion to an injured vessel wall, the platelet becomes activated, resulting in the formation of fine processes that extend in all directions as shown by LVHR-SEM. Surfaces of the pseudopods are smooth compared with the central body from which they extend. Convolutions similar to those on the discoid cell in **A** are present on the platelet body. Magnification ×16,000. **C.** To cover as much of the injured vessel wall as possible, the platelet expands its cytoplasm to fill the spaces between the pseudopods shown in **B.** The central body has almost disappeared on the spread cell, as shown with conventional SEM. The marked difference in surface area of the smooth spread cell and the convoluted discoid platelet is apparent. Magnification ×12,000. (Reprinted with permission from White JG, Escolar G. Current concepts of platelet membrane response to surface activation. Platelets 1993;4:175.)

bile facili-tating extension of the surface membrane over a wide surface area.

PLATELET ACTIVATION

Not only does platelet contact with subendothelial connective tissue (collagen) lead to platelet activation, but activation is also a result of platelet interaction with a variety of other agents such as plasma proteins (vWF, plasma proteases such as thrombin), circulating hormones (epinephrine and vasopressin), and products of platelet metabolism (ADP and thromboxane A_2) (28). Platelet agonists are commonly classified as strong or weak, but the distinctions between them are often blurred. By one definition, strong agonists are those that can trigger the secretion of factors that are normally stored in the platelet's cytoplasmic granules; that is, these agonists can cause a "release reaction" to occur even when aggregation is prevented. Thrombin and collagen are examples of strong agonists. By contrast, weak agonists, such as ADP and epinephrine, require aggregation for granule secretion to occur (8). Platelets have three types of storage granules—dense granules, alpha granules, and lysosomes—with different contents that may be secreted during a release reaction (Fig. 5.4) (29). Platelets are also partially activated when brought into close contact with foreign surfaces (e.g., plastics) or with each other (close cell contact). Although activation is caused by substances varying markedly in chemical structure, the platelets respond with the same series of identifiable responses: shape change, aggregation, three different secretory events, and liberation of arachidonic acid that is rapidly converted to prostaglandins, thromboxanes, and lipoxygenase products (30).

Even weak agonists will cause dense body and alpha granule secretion and arachidonic liberation when positive feedback is allowed to occur. There are three main mechanisms for positive feedback: secretion of the dense granule constituents ADP and serotonin, which are platelet agonists, either of which will act synergistically with another stimulus; formation of platelet-stimulating prostaglandins and thromboxanes from liberated arachidonic will also enhance the effect of the primary agonist; or close cell contact achieved through aggregation also provides a substantial increase in total stimulus, but the underlying mechanism is not known.

The two morphologically prominent platelet storage granules, alpha granules and dense bodies, have a limiting membrane and, thus, the final secretory event involves exocytosis (i.e., fusion of the secretory granule membrane with the plasma membrane) (31). The incorporation of an alpha granule membrane marker into the plasma membrane (P-selectin/GMP-140) directly establishes that exocytosis occurs during the secretion of alpha granule contents (32–34). However, in human platelets, most alpha granules are seen to move toward the center of the cell during secretion and are thus not in a locale that would permit fusion with the peripheral plasma membrane (35, 36). However, two hypotheses have been formulated to explain how exocytosis may occur. First, there may be deep invaginations of the plasma membrane into the center of the platelet, allowing alpha granule membranes to fuse with these invaginations. The secretory products then move to the outside of the cell through the open canalicular system (37, 38). Second, alpha granules may fuse with each other or with another cellular compartment to form a compound granule that then moves toward and fuses with the plasma membrane (39, 40).

PLATELET AGGREGATION

Once activation and spreading are underway, the adherent platelet becomes a nidus, or target, for other platelets, and by a

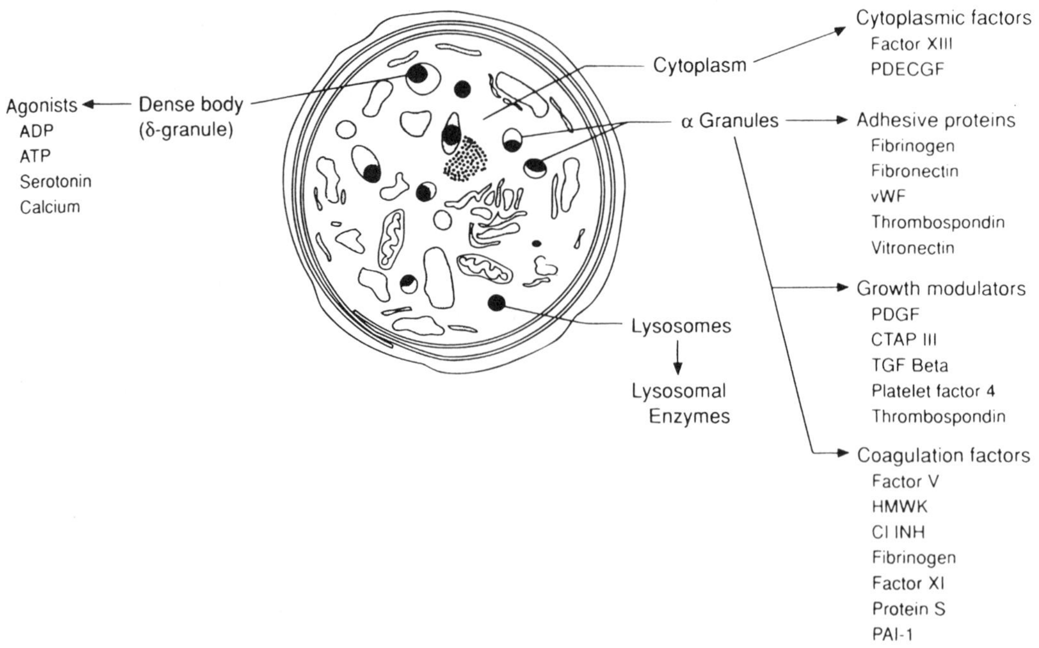

Figure 5.4. Substances released by platelets and their intraplatelet sources. Illustrated are some of the bioactive substances released from dense bodies, alpha granules, lysosomes, the cytoplasm, and the platelet membrane. PDECGF, platelet-derived endothelial cell growth factor; HMWK, high-molecular-weight kininogen; C1 INH, C1 inhibitor; PAI-1, plasminogen activator inhibitor-1; PDGF, platelet-derived growth factor; CTAP, connective tissue-activating peptide; and TGF, transforming growth factor. (Reprinted with permission from Plow EF, Ginsberg MH. Molecular basis of platelet function. In: Hoffman R, Benz EJ Jr, Shatill SJ, et al., eds. Hematology: basic principles and practice. 2nd ed. New York: Churchill Livingstone, 1995:1524.)

series of platelet-platelet interactions (aggregation events), a platelet mass (plug/thrombus) accumulates (41). Although the receptors involved in platelet adhesion appear to be functional on resting platelets (42), the major membrane receptor GPIIb/IIIa, which is involved in platelet aggregation through fibrinogen binding, is normally present in a nonfunctional state. This is indicated by the fact that little fibrinogen binds to nonstimulated platelets. However, when platelets become activated through the processes just discussed, conformational changes in the GPIIb/IIIa molecule occur, allowing it to bind fibrinogen in the presence of calcium. The resting platelet has 40,000–80,000 copies of GPIIb/IIIa on its surface, and platelet activation can increase this number by 0–100%. Each GPIIb/IIIa molecule is capable of binding one fibrinogen molecule (29). All major platelet agonists can initiate platelet aggregation through receptor induction, that is, the conversion of a latent cell surface receptor to a state in which it can bind fibrinogen. Receptor induction is very rapid, and the cell is fully competent to bind fibrinogen within seconds after its initial encounter with an appropriate agonist. The most likely and the simplest possibility to explain how fibrinogen binding to GPIIb/IIIa results in platelet aggregation is that a single fibrinogen molecule, by virtue of its dimeric structure, bridges two GPIIb/IIIa molecules symmetrically on adjacent platelets (29). Thrombospondin stored within the alpha granules of nonactivated platelets is released upon platelet activation and binds to unique receptors on the platelet surface (43). It is thought that thrombospondin may then play an auxiliary role in platelet aggregation by stabilizing the platelet aggregate (44).

Of additional interest in the aggregation process is the role played by red cells. Red cells have long been known to participate in hemostasis; for example, anemic patients have prolonged bleeding times that normalize upon correction of the erythrocyte deficit. Intact erythrocytes promote biochemical and functional responsiveness of activated platelets (45, 46). Furthermore, there is evidence that the presence of red cells in the bloodstream induces the localization of platelets to the periphery of the vessel next to the endothelium, thus promoting platelet adhesion to denuded endothelium with vascular injury. In addition, releasates obtained from mixtures of erythrocytes and platelets contain very high concentrations of secreted ADP (46). Erythrocytes are also capable of increasing platelet serotonin release (activation) despite aspirin treatment, enzymatic removal of released ADP, protease inhibition, or combinations of the above.

PLATELET PROCOAGULANT ACTIVITIES

Another consequence of platelet activation is the translocation of coagulant active phospholipids from the inner leaflet of the platelet membrane bilayer to the outer surface of the platelet where they can interact with other components of the tenase and prothrombinase activation complexes, thus accelerating thrombin generation (47, 48). Expression of receptors for the prothrombinase complex (i.e., factor Va, factor Xa, and calcium) catalyzes the conversion of prothrombin to thrombin. Platelets protect the serine proteases produced in these reactions from inactivation by antithrombin III. Further receptors are made available for proteins of the contact, fibrinolytic, and protein C/protein S systems. Platelets are, therefore, involved at all stages of hemostasis and are able to direct hemostatic reactions where they are required and also localize reactions so that the whole vascular compartment does not become involved (48).

Platelets also store a large number of plasma proteins involved in coagulation in their alpha granules. During thrombopoiesis, these plasma proteins are taken up by megakaryocytes (49, 50). Megakaryocytes also must synthesize factor V (51, 52); this conclusion is based on the fact that more factor V is present in platelet alpha granules than can be accounted for by their uptake from plasma (53). Platelets also contain protein S (54) and plasminogen activator inhibitor-1 (PAI-1) (55). Protein S is a cofactor for the action of activated protein C, and PAI-1 is an inhibitor of urokinase and tissue plasminogen activators. Thus, the concentration of these proteins in platelets suggests that platelets may be a favored site for the anticoagulant action of protein C. Similarly, the local release of PAI-1 from platelets may play a role in modulating the fibrinolytic events in the vicinity of thrombi (29).

Thus, in summary, the platelet performs a large number of complex metabolic processes that eventually result in the formation of a hemostatic plug at sites of vascular injury without simultaneously occluding the vessel because of unregulated growth of the thrombus.

PLATELET HEMOSTASIS IN PATIENTS WITH PRODUCTION-RELATED THROMBOCYTOPENIA

Patients with uncomplicated production-related thrombocytopenia and stable platelet counts provide an opportunity to determine how thrombocytopenia per se, independent of other disease factors, affects platelet hemostasis. Therefore, studies in these patients provide a baseline for identifying how other factors affect platelet hemostasis in patients who become thrombocytopenic by other mechanisms.

Platelet hemostasis represents the combined interaction of platelet number and function. Abnormalities in either of these two parameters may be associated with bleeding, and if there is both a decrease in platelet number as well as function, the bleeding risk is substantially increased.

PLATELET RECOVERY AND SURVIVAL MEASUREMENTS

Autologous radiochromium-labeled platelet recovery and survival measurements in 27 thrombocytopenic patients with platelet counts between 12 and 70 × 10^9/L demonstrated a direct relationship between platelet count and platelet survival (Fig. 5.5) (56). Platelet life span was only modestly reduced in patients having platelet counts in the range of 50–100 × 10^9/L (7.0 ± 1.5 days versus 9.6 ± 0.6 days in normal controls; $P < .01$) but was markedly reduced when the platelet count fell below 50 × 10^9/L (5.1 ± 1.9 days; $P < .001$). The recovery of autologous platelets was normal in thrombocytopenic patients when the platelet count exceeded 50 × 10^9/L (74 ± 15%) but was reduced in patients with low counts (50 ± 20%; $P < .01$). Autologous platelet recovery values in 16 normal controls averaged 66 ± 8%. Although the survival of homologous platelets in these thrombocytopenic patients was equivalent to their autologous survival and thus correlated directly with their posttransfusion platelet counts, the recovery of donor platelets in severely thrombocytopenic patients was 60 ± 15% and was equivalent to the control values ($P > .20$). Further analysis of these data indicated that platelets are removed from circulation by two mechanisms—a fixed number of platelets are removed daily, presumably in an endothelial supportive function, whereas the remainder are lost through senescent mechanisms. It is this fixed daily random loss of platelets from the circulation that accounts for the progressive decrease in platelet survival at low platelet counts. Although this fixed fraction represents only 18% of the daily platelet loss at normal platelet counts and therefore has little impact on platelet survival, at lower platelet counts, a progressively larger fraction of the circulating platelets is involved in this process, with a direct effect on platelet survival.

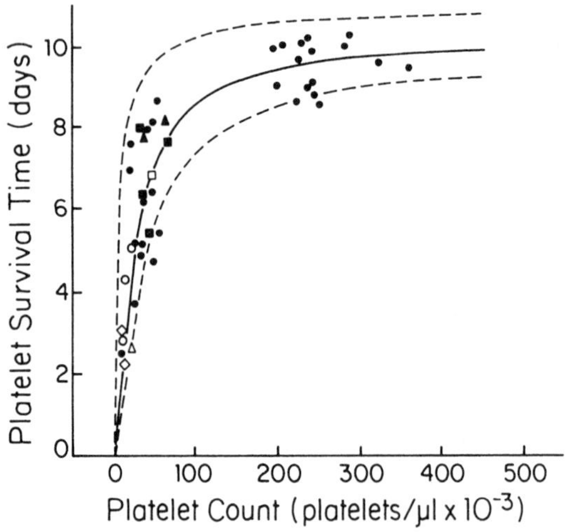

Figure 5.5. Relationship between platelet count and the survival of autologous or homologous platelets. The relationship between platelet count and the survival of autologous (closed symbols) or homologous (open symbols) ^{51}Cr-labeled platelets in normal and thrombocytopenic subjects with no evidence of hypersplenism (circles). Complications included splenectomy (squares), splenomegaly (triangles), and prior transfusions (diamonds). The data are well correlated (solid line) under the assumption of a finite platelet life span (T) of 10.5 days and a fixed rate of platelet destruction (k) averaging 4700 platelets/µL/day. The data are bounded by the region (between dashed lines). (Reprinted with permission from Hanson SR, Slichter SJ. Platelet kinetics in patients with bone marrow hypoplasia: evidence for a fixed platelet requirement. Blood 1985;66:1105.)

PLATELET FUNCTION

The usual in vitro technique of measuring platelet function involves adding a variety of platelet aggregating agents to platelets as they are stirred in an aggregometer. Changes in light transmission, as the stirred platelets agglutinate in response to the aggregating agents, are recorded as a measure of platelet function.

The only in vivo measure of platelet function is the bleeding time test. The relationship between bleeding time and platelet count was determined in 70 individuals with marrow failure and platelet counts of less than 150 × 10^9/L (57). As long as the platelet count remained at levels of greater than 100 × 10^9/L, the bleeding time was within the normal range of 4.5 ± 1.5 minutes. However, in patients with platelet counts between 10 and 100 × 10^9/L, there was a direct inverse relationship between bleeding time and platelet count that could be predicted by the following equation:

$$\text{Bleeding Time (minutes)} = 30.5 - \frac{\text{Platelet Count} \times 10^9/\text{L}}{3.85}.$$

At platelet counts of less than 10 × 10^9/L, the bleeding time is unmeasurable at greater than 30 minutes (Fig. 5.6). Similar observations were obtained when platelet transfusions were given to thrombocytopenic patients.

PLATELET TRANSFUSION THERAPY

Previous sections of this chapter provided a framework for understanding the role of platelets in hemostasis and the effects of thrombocytopenia on platelet hemostasis. This section discusses the indications for platelet replacement therapy, what are the expected responses to platelet therapy, and how these responses may be affected by the disease process causing the patient's thrombocytopenia.

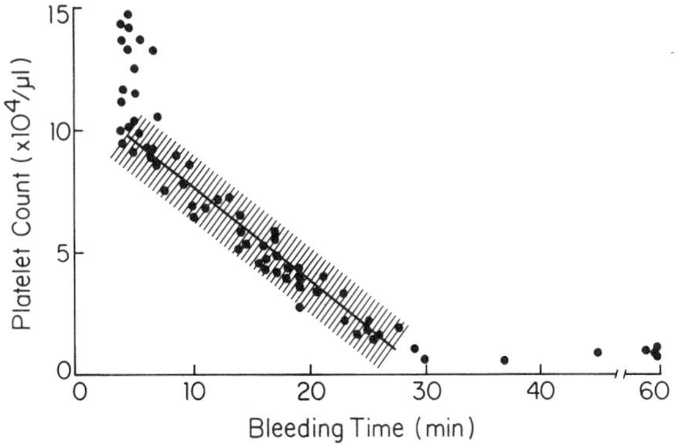

Figure 5.6. Relationship between bleeding time and platelet count. The relationship between bleeding time and platelet count was determined in 70 individuals with marrow failure and platelet counts of less than 150×10^9/L. As long as the platelet count remained at levels of 100×10^9/L or more, the bleeding time was within the normal range of 4.5 ± 1.5 minutes. However, in patients with platelet counts between 10 and 100×10^9/L, there was a direct inverse relationship between bleeding time and platelet count that could be predicted by the following equation: bleeding time (minutes) = 30.5 − platelet count $\times 10^9$/L ÷ 3.85. At platelet counts of less than 10×10^9/L, the bleeding time is unmeasurable at greater than 30 minutes. (Reprinted with permission from Harker LA, Slichter SJ. The bleeding time as a screening test for evaluating platelet function. N Engl J Med 1972;287:155, Massachusetts Medical Society.)

PLATELET PRODUCTS AVAILABLE FOR TRANSFUSION

Platelet concentrates can be prepared from routinely donated units of whole blood, or, alternatively, platelets can be obtained by apheresis procedures. To reduce the need for platelet transfusions, platelet products that have been appropriately collected and stored must be available for transfusion. Important variables are to optimize the yield of platelets in the product while ensuring that neither the preparation nor the storage procedure has compromised the viability and/or function of the platelets.

Random Donor Platelet Concentrates

The yield of platelets in a platelet concentrate varies with the time and force of centrifugation used to prepare the platelet-rich plasma (PRP) from whole blood and subsequently to sediment the platelets from the PRP into a concentrate. It is possible to consistently harvest 85–90% of the whole blood platelets into a platelet concentrate (58). Federal guidelines require at least 5.5×10^{10} platelets per concentrate; however, optimum techniques should produce an average yield of at least 7.0×10^{10}.

A substantial amount of work has been done to determine the variables that must be controlled to provide platelets with normal recovery, survival, and function after storage. Currently, platelets are licensed for up to 5 days of storage. In normal volunteers, autologous radiolabeled platelet viability studies demonstrate platelet recoveries in the range of only 38 ± 7% to 48 ± 6% and survivals of 5.1 ± 1.4 days to 6.3 ± 1.3 days after 5 days of storage, compared with fresh recoveries of 59 ± 4% and survivals of 8.1 ± 0.2 days (59–63).

In addition, some investigators have also performed stored platelet concentrate transfusion studies in thrombocytopenic patients (64–66). In every instance in which stored platelets were compared with fresh platelet transfusions, there was a statistically significant decrease in platelet increments at both 1 and 24 hours after transfusion. As a percentage of the expected or observed fresh platelet recovery values, only 11–76% of the stored platelets circulated in thrombocytopenic patients. Thus, these data raise the question of whether some thrombocytopenic patients are being appropriately supported by stored platelet concentrates. Indeed, there may be multiple types of "storage lesions" that need to be characterized and modified to improve patient responses to stored platelets.

In summary, the evidence suggests that the optimum methods of maintaining the viability and function of platelets during storage have yet to be identified. For some patients, platelets stored for a relatively short period of time (24–48 hours) may improve their transfusion response, and this may be worth trying in patients who become refractory to stored platelet transfusions (i.e., they demonstrate very poor post-transfusion platelet recoveries and survivals).

Apheresis Platelets

Platelet apheresis procedures are well established and have a long history of efficacy in collecting large numbers of platelets. After 5 days of storage, radiolabeled autologous platelet recoveries averaged 72 ± 10% and 67 ± 15%, and survivals averaged 6.7 ± 1.2 and 5.6 ± 1.1 days in normal volunteers, respectively (67, 68). Although these autologous apheresis stored platelet recoveries compare favorably with autologous fresh platelet apheresis recoveries in normal volunteers (58 ± 8%), the poststorage survivals are clearly shorter than the normal value of 9.6 ± 0.6 days (69).

INDICATIONS FOR PLATELET TRANSFUSIONS

Determining a patient's need for platelet transfusion requires an assessment of platelet count, platelet function, and the integrity of the vascular system. A patient's response to a platelet transfusion depends on the product provided and on the patient's underlying disease and associated aberrant physiology.

Platelet transfusions are indicated for any patient with active bleeding as a result of a documented severe deficiency in either platelet number (normal platelet count $250 \pm 50 \times 10^9$/L) or function (normal bleeding time 4.5 ± 1.5 minutes).

Active bleeding implies more than just the presence of petechiae or ecchymoses; these findings alone are not adequate to justify a platelet transfusion. Often, the bleeding is sufficient to require red cell transfusions and may be spontaneous from mucous membranes (gastrointestinal [GI], genitourinary, or oral-pharyngeal) or from one or more sites of vascular damage. The interaction of the relevant factors and how they affect a patient's bleeding risk are outlined in Table 5.1. The first important determination is whether the vascular system is intact or whether there is a pathological, traumatic, or surgically induced disruption of the vessel wall. The number and function of platelets needed to prevent oozing from intact vessels are much less than those required to form hemostatic platelet plugs and control blood loss when there is blood vessel damage.

Intact Vascular System

Platelet Count Less Than 5 × 10^9/L Prophylactic platelet transfusions should be given to any patient with thrombocytopenia and a platelet count of less than 5 × 10^9/L because the bleeding risk is substantial. Based on stool blood loss studies in patients with hypoproliferative thrombocytopenia, excessive bleeding does not occur spontaneously until the platelet count reaches this critical level (70). At this level, the bleeding time exceeds 30 minutes and cannot be used as an indicator of in vivo platelet function. These patients bleed not only from the GI tract, but also from other mucous membrane sites. They usually have prominent petechiae and ecchymoses, and bleeding into the urinary tract and central nervous system may occur.

Platelet Count Between 10 and 50 × 10^9/L When a patient has significant bleeding at a platelet count higher than 10 × 10^9/L, platelet dysfunction usually is present, as shown by a bleeding time longer than expected based on the inverse relationship between bleeding time and platelet count (Fig. 5.6) (57).

Platelet Count Greater Than 50 × 10^9/L When the platelet level is higher than 50 × 10^9/L, even with severe platelet dysfunction, significant bleeding is unlikely. In this category of patients, onset of substantial bleeding almost always signifies underlying vascular damage (e.g., erosion by an ulcer or incomplete surgical repair of a vessel). The bleeding is usually limited to a single site or organ system in contrast with the diffuse bleeding found in patients with extremely low counts or modestly low counts combined with severe platelet dysfunction. A workup aimed at identifying the vascular defect, followed by a direct approach to its repair, is needed. Platelet transfusions should only be used as adjunct therapy until the lesion can be identified and repaired.

Damaged Vascular System

Platelet Count Less Than 100 × 10^9/L As previously discussed, at platelet counts less than 100 × 10^9/L, the bleeding time becomes prolonged and varies inversely with the platelet count (Fig. 5.6) (57). Any such patient is at risk of bleeding with vascular injury, particularly if the lesion is arterial, where the intravascular pressure is greater than in the venous system.

Platelet Count Greater Than 100 × 10^9/L At platelet counts of 100 × 10^9/L or greater, bleeding times are normal. This combination of number and function is usually sufficient to control bleeding when the microvascular system is disrupted and does not make bleeding worse even with large vessel injury. However, marked prolongation of the bleeding time to more than 30 minutes, regardless of the platelet count, is usually accompanied by severe bleeding that is due wholly or in part to the platelet defect. If the platelet dysfunction is milder (bleeding time less than 20 minutes), any bleeding is probably not platelet related; thus, only repair of the vascular defect, rather than platelet transfusion, is needed.

One specific situation that may be associated with platelet dysfunction requiring platelet transfusions even with platelet counts of 100 × 10^9/L or more may occur after cardiopulmonary bypass procedures. When bleeding time measurements were followed serially throughout the preopertive, in-

TABLE 5.1. ASSESSMENT OF NEED FOR PLATELET TRANSFUSIONS

Vascular Integrity	Platelet Count (× 10^9/L)	Platelet Function (Bleeding Time)	Bleeding Risk
Intact	<5	Expected[a] (>30 min)	Increased
Intact	10–50	Dysfunctional (>30 min)	Increased
Intact	>50	Expected or dysfunctional	Unlikely
Damaged	<100	Expected or dysfunctional	Increased
Damaged	>100	Dysfunctional (>30 min)	Increased
Damaged	>100	Normal or dysfunctional but <20 min	Unlikely

[a]The bleeding time varies inversely with the platelet count at platelet levels of <100 × 10^9/L (Fig. 5.6).

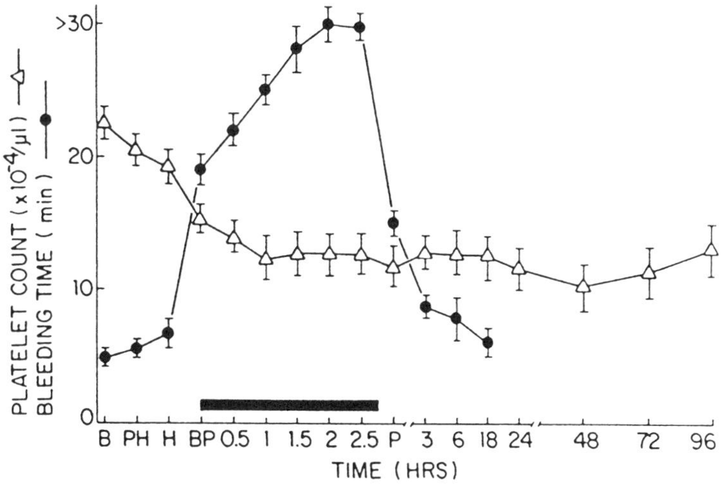

Figure 5.7. Changes in platelet behavior during cardiopulmonary bubble oxygenator bypass. Platelet count (△) falls progressively during the initial operative and bypass period in part due to dilution by nonblood priming solutions. Thereafter, the platelet count remains about half baseline, exceeding 100×10^9 platelets/L throughout the 4-day period of observation. The bleeding time (●) is unaffected by heparinization but increases abruptly after the initiation of bypass and lengthens progressively during the first 2 hours of bypass, at which time it is greater than 30 minutes. Bleeding time measurements fall quickly after termination of bypass. The horizontal solid bar identifies the period of bypass. Symbols on the horizontal axis areas follows: B, baseline; PH, preheparin; H, heparin; BP, bypass; time on bypass in hours; P, postprotamine; followed by hours postbypass. (Reprinted with permission from Harker LA, Malpass TW, Branson HE, et al. Mechanisms of abnormal bleeding in patients undergoing cardiopulmonary bypass: acquired transient platelet dysfunction associated with selected alpha granule release. Blood 1980;56:824.)

traoperative, and postoperative period, it was observed that the bleeding time increased immediately after initiation of bypass, although all patients had platelet counts greater than 100×10^9/L. Thereafter, the bleeding time progressively increased with the duration of bypass (Fig. 5.7) (71). Protamine administration after bypass produced an immediate improvement in the bleeding time, and further normalization occurred within the 3–6 hours after surgery in these prospectively studied patients. However, in a separate analysis of 10 patients who had excessive postbypass bleeding, a persistent bleeding time prolongation to values greater than 25 minutes was found in all patients. This bleeding time prolongation persisted for hours despite platelet counts of greater than 100×10^9/L. After a platelet transfusion was given, the bleeding time rapidly improved and bleeding ceased. In animal studies, the long bleeding time could be produced by either hypothermia or a bypass procedure (72).

EXPECTED RESPONSE TO PLATELET TRANSFUSIONS AND DOSE CONSIDERATIONS

The measurements that are used to determine the efficacy of transfused platelets are platelet increment and/or platelet recovery, platelet survival, platelet function, and clinical evaluation of hemostasis.

Platelet Increment

The increment is usually determined by subtracting the pretransfusion platelet count from the count measured at 1 hour after the transfusion; however, a similar result can be obtained using the 10-minute posttransfusion platelet count instead of the 1-hour count (73).

Platelet Recovery Normally, about 60 ± 15% of the transfused platelets circulate in thrombocytopenic patients (56), calculated by the formula

$$\text{Platelet Recovery (\%)} = \left[\frac{\text{(Platelet Increment)} \times \text{(Patient's Weight in kg)} \times \text{(Blood Volume Estimated at 75 mL/kg)}}{\text{(Platelet Count of Transfused Product)} \times \text{(Volume of Product in mL)}}\right] \times 100$$

Any noncirculating platelets are pooled in the spleen. Thus, in asplenic individuals, the posttransfusion platelet recovery approaches 100%, whereas in hypersplenism, the recovery is reduced proportionally to the size of the spleen (74). As each platelet concentrate is expected to contain a minimum of 5.5×10^{10} platelets per unit, a single platelet concentrate should increase the peripheral platelet count in a 75-kg recipient by approximately 6×10^9/L. However, if the average platelet yield is higher at 7.0×10^{10} (a reasonable expectation for most blood centers to achieve), the increment will be about 8×10^9/L. These estimates assume normal splenic pooling. Therefore, the usual pooled transfusion dose of 4–6 units of platelet concentrates or the transfusion of one apheresis platelet product (usually contains the equivalent number of platelets as in six platelet concentrates) should increase the platelet count enough to control bleeding in most patients.

Survival

As previously discussed, although normal autologous platelet survivals average 9.6 ± 0.6 days, there is a direct relationship between platelet count and survival at platelet counts of less than 100×10^9/L, giving an average of 5.2 ± 1.1 days in 23 patients with production-related thrombocytopenia and platelet counts of less than 70×10^9/L (56). The survival of transfused platelets in thrombocytopenic patients can be determined by following daily platelet counts, and this determines transfusion frequency. However, in addition to the fixed platelet-vessel wall loss and platelet senescence, as determinants of platelet life span, numerous clinical events may also adversely affect the survival of transfused platelets, for example, any condition associated with disseminated intravascular coagulation (DIC) (e.g., bacteremia, metastatic malignancies, leukemia, obstetrical catastrophes) (75, 76), viral infections (77), increased platelet utilization associated with wound healing (78), amphotericin therapy (77), fever (77), and, undoubtedly, other factors not yet identified. Tissue injury, whether by trauma or a surgical procedure, has profound effects on the hemostatic system. Radiochromium-labeled autologous platelet survival measurements in patients undergoing elective surgical procedures have demonstrated increased platelet utilization during and after surgery. Both the amount and duration of the associated platelet consumption were found to be directly related to the extent of the surgical injury (Fig. 5.8) (78). However, platelet counts were well maintained in these patients at greater than 193 × 10^9/L, even without platelet transfusions, because of an immediate compensatory shift in platelets from the splenic reservoir into the systemic circulation. This shift occurred in those patients with the shortest platelet survivals and therefore the most need for additional platelets (Fig. 5.9) (78). In addition, the fibrinogen survival in these patients was reduced in proportion to their platelet survival, and there was evidence for accumulation of the labeled clotting factors at the operative site. Thus, not unexpectedly, tissue injury activates the coagulation mechanism and uses clotting factors in the hemostatic response to injury and its subsequent repair.

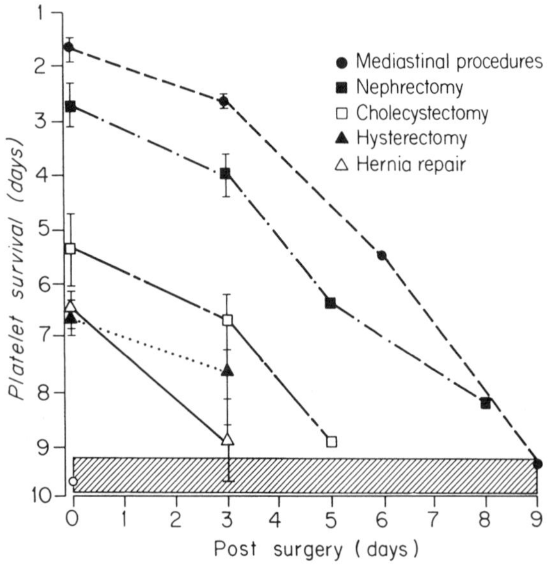

Figure 5.8. Platelet use as a consequence of surgery. As the amount of tissue injury increases, the shorter the survival of autologous platelets becomes and the longer it takes, postsurgery, for the platelet survival time to return to normal. Autologous platelets were labeled on the day before each operative procedure; in some cases, the labeling was repeated on the second, third, fourth, or eighth postoperative day. Mediastinal procedures (●) are shown nephrectomy (■), hysterectomy (▲), cholecystectomy (□), hernia repair (△), and lipectomy (○). The average normal survival + 1 SD is given in the hatched area. (Reprinted with permission from Slichter SJ, Funk DD, Leandoer LE, Harker LA. Kinetic evaluation of hemostasis during surgery and wound healing. Br J Haematol 1974;27:115.)

Function

Further documentation of the efficacy of transfused platelets is demonstrated by measuring the bleeding time and correlating it with the platelet count (Fig. 5.6) (57). As with autologous platelets, transfused donor platelets, if functioning normally, will show the expected inverse relationship between platelet count and bleeding time (57, 79). This permits the bleeding time to be used as a method of documenting whether transfused platelets demonstrate the expected relationship between platelet count and bleeding time or whether they are dysfunctional (bleeding time disproportionately prolonged for the platelet count) or hyperfunctional (bleeding time disproportionately reduced for the platelet count). Evidence of post-transfusion platelet dysfunction implies either some extrinsic factor (usually the patient's medications or disease processes) that alters the function of the transfused platelets or, alternatively, that the transfused platelets are defective. The most common causes of platelet dysfunction in thrombocytopenic patients are those related to drugs (aspirin or other anti-inflammatory drugs and semisynthetic penicillins) (80–82) or to specific disorders such as uremia (83), hyperfibrinolysis secondary to DIC (84), or to other aspects of the patient's underlying disease process. For example, dysfunctional platelets are often found in patients with leukemia (85), myeloproliferative disorders (86), or fever/infection (87). Aspirin or other anti-inflammatory drugs should be avoided in any thrombocytopenic patient. However, it has been documented that if a

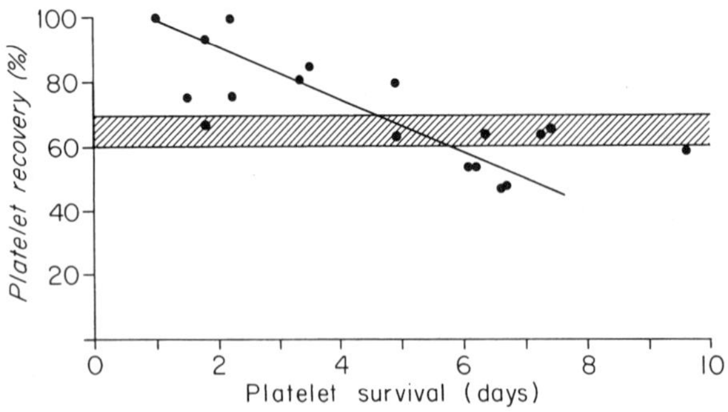

Figure 5.9. Platelet mobilization from the spleen. Relationship between platelet recovery and survival measured in the first 10 days after surgery. Increased platelet recoveries are correlated with survivals of less than 5 days (normal recovery ± 1 SD is shown by the hatched area). Correlation coefficient between platelet recovery and survival, as indicated by the line, is 0.74 ($P < .01$). (Reprinted with permission from Slichter SJ, Funk DD, Leandoer LE, Harker LA. Kinetic evaluation of hemostasis during surgery and wound healing. Br J Haematol 1974;27:115.)

platelet transfusion is given to a patient who has aspirin-induced platelet dysfunction, the bleeding time will improve as long as the transfused platelets constitute at least 10% of the circulating platelets (88). This observation may be particularly important for patients undergoing emergency open heart surgery who may be receiving aspirin as antithrombotic therapy. It has been documented that such patients have a larger red cell transfusion requirement than do patients not on aspirin; thus, aspirin-treated bleeding patients may benefit from platelet transfusions (89). However, the overall ability of platelet transfusions to correct the platelet dysfunction associated with other drugs or diseases has not been well documented. Lacking relevant data to guide therapy, it is probably reasonable to give platelet transfusions if bleeding is severe. Their efficacy can be documented by performing pretranfusion and posttransfusion bleeding times and by monitoring red cell transfusion requirements.

If there are no apparent patient factors to account for posttransfusion platelet dysfunction, then poor platelet collection techniques, inadequate platelet storage procedures, or the possibility that the platelet donor has taken aspirin within the preceding several days may account for posttransfusion platelet dysfunction. Surprisingly, aspirin-affected donor platelets show progressive improvement in function with time after a transfusion. Usually only 4–9 hours is required to achieve their expected function (90). The reversibility of the platelet dysfunction means that whole blood donors who are taking aspirin can be used as a source of platelet concentrates. Adequate recipient hemostasis is ensured by giving pooled platelet concentrates; by chance, at least half the donors will not be taking aspirin, and these nonaspirinized platelets will substantially reduce the initial impact of any dysfunctional aspirin-affected platelets. However, if apheresis platelets are to be used and the transfusion is being given for active bleeding rather than prophylaxis, platelets from a nonaspirinized donor should be used.

Hemostasis

The most important parameter reflecting the efficacy of a platelet transfusion is cessation of bleeding. Hemostasis can be evaluated directly by clinical observation and indirectly by noting a reduction in red cell transfusion requirements.

EFFECTS OF THE MECHANISM OF A PATIENT'S THROMBOCYTOPENIA ON RESPONSE TO PLATELET TRANSFUSIONS

Responses to platelet transfusions may also be directly affected by the patient's underlying pathophysiology that has produced the thrombocytopenia. The four major causes of thrombocytopenia are decreased platelet production, splenomegaly, increased platelet destruction, and dilutional thrombocytopenia. The effects of each of these on patient responses to platelet transfusions will be discussed separately.

Decreased Platelet Production

The effects of production-related thrombocytopenia on platelet hemostasis was previously discussed. This type of thrombocytopenia has little relevance to surgical hemostasis except to recognize that platelet transfusions to increase the platelet count to greater than 100×10^9/L may be required to provide adequate hemostasis during and after surgery. For the immediate postoperative period to maintain enough platelets to allow wound healing and prevent blood loss from damaged vessels, a platelet count of 50×10^9/L may be required. However, transfusions should be given at higher levels if bleeding occurs.

Hypersplenism

Normally, approximately one-third of the platelets produced by the bone marrow are pooled in the spleen, accounting for the normal platelet recovery value of $66 \pm 8\%$ (74). If the spleen becomes enlarged, more platelets are pooled in the spleen and thrombocytopenia may ensue. However, it is unusual for hypersplenism alone to cause a platelet count of less than 40×10^9/L. Thus, even though the patient may have a big spleen, if the platelet count is less than 40×10^9/L, an additional cause of thrombocytopenia should be pursued. If patients with hypersplenism—resulting in low platelet counts—require platelet transfusions because of disruption of their vascular system, just as there is increased pooling of autologous platelets, there will also be increased pooling of donor platelets requiring a higher dose of platelets to achieve the desired increment. However, platelet survival is not reduced by the hypersplenism so transfusion frequency will not need to be increased.

Increased Platelet Destruction

In these disorders, the frequency of platelet transfusions may have to be substantially increased to compensate for reduced platelet survival. In certain situations, survival may be so compromised that it is very difficult to maintain a constant platelet level.

Consumptive Thrombocytopenia In surgical patients, although the resultant tissue injury causes increased platelet and plasma coagulation factor use during wound healing and repair, as reflected in reduced platelet and fibrinogen survivals, compensatory mechanisms are usually sufficient to maintain platelet counts of greater than 100×10^9/L, as previously discussed. Thus, postsurgical thrombocytopenia suggests additional factors besides the surgical injury that must be contributing to the patient's thrombocytopenia. Postsurgical thrombocytopenia is most likely a result of other causes of platelet consumption added to the surgically induced platelet consumption and/or dilutional thrombocytopenia.

There are basically two types of platelet consumption. The first represents an exaggeration of the physiological hemostatic response in which not only platelets but other coagulation factors are removed from circulation at an accelerated rate. With more extensive injury than is seen during elective surgery (e.g., with trauma), platelet use may be so marked that thrombocytopenia may occur (91). Furthermore, injuries of a specific type (e.g., cerebral injury releases large amounts of tissue thromboplastin into the circulation with resultant depression of coagulation factors) may also produce thrombocytopenia (92). This type of consumption also occurs in a wide variety of other types of patients: those with venous thrombosis (75), widespread malignancy (75), obstetrical complications (75), bacteremia (75), shock (93), acidosis (93), or hypoxemia (94). These clinical conditions are associated with ongoing platelet consumption. However, whether the patient becomes thrombocytopenic depends on whether compensatory mechanisms of increased platelet production or release of platelets from the splenic pool are able to adequately compensate for the increased platelet removal rates. Management of patients who are consuming platelets calls for therapy directed at the underlying disease process that is causing the consumptive state, but for many of these patients, platelet transfusions are required until the disease process is resolved. These situations may be associated with not only reduced platelet survivals necessitating frequent transfusions, but also very poor platelet increments, making transfusion support extremely difficult.

The second consumptive process is characterized by isolated platelet destruction and appears to reflect platelet thrombus formation on abnormal surfaces in the arterial system, including prosthetic devices (artificial heart valves, prosthetic aortic grafts, plastic arteriovenous cannula, and intra-aortic assist devices) and arterial thrombosis, thrombotic thrombocytopenic purpura, hemolytic uremic syndrome, and other disorders associated with vasculitis (75). These processes can often be managed by providing platelet function inhibitors or other forms of therapy. However, if platelet transfusions are required, survival times less than expected can be anticipated.

Dilutional Thrombocytopenia

Mathematical models have been formulated to predict the disappearance rate of a substance confined to the intravascular volume when blood is periodically removed and replaced with a fluid not containing that substance (95). An exchange transfusion of one blood volume will reduce the concentration of any substance by approximately two-thirds. The next equivalent exchange will reduce the remaining one-third by two-thirds, and so on.

During massive blood loss and replacement with 4°C stored blood that contains no viable platelets, exchange of one blood volume (about 11 units of blood in a man weighing 75 kg) will decrease the platelet count from its normal value of $250 \pm 40 \times 10^9$/L to approximately 80×10^9/L. As it may require up to 100×10^9 platelets/L to maintain hemostasis with a disrupted vascular system (as would likely be the situation in a massively bleeding patient), even a one-volume exchange may increase the bleeding risk. Other factors beside dilution that might contribute to an even lower than calculated postexchange platelet count are a lower than normal preexchange platelet count and any complicating condition causing accelerated platelet destruction. For example, if massive bleeding occurs during the course of a major operative procedure such as open heart surgery or with severe traumatic injuries, then accelerated platelet consumption, due to the tissue injury, may result in a lower than expected postexchange platelet count (96).

One physiological factor that may mitigate the low platelet count expected from dilution or consumption may be increased platelet mobilization from the splenic storage pool. In young soldiers transfused for combat injuries, the postexchange platelet count was higher than predicted, particularly in those given more than 20 units of blood (Fig. 5.10) (97).

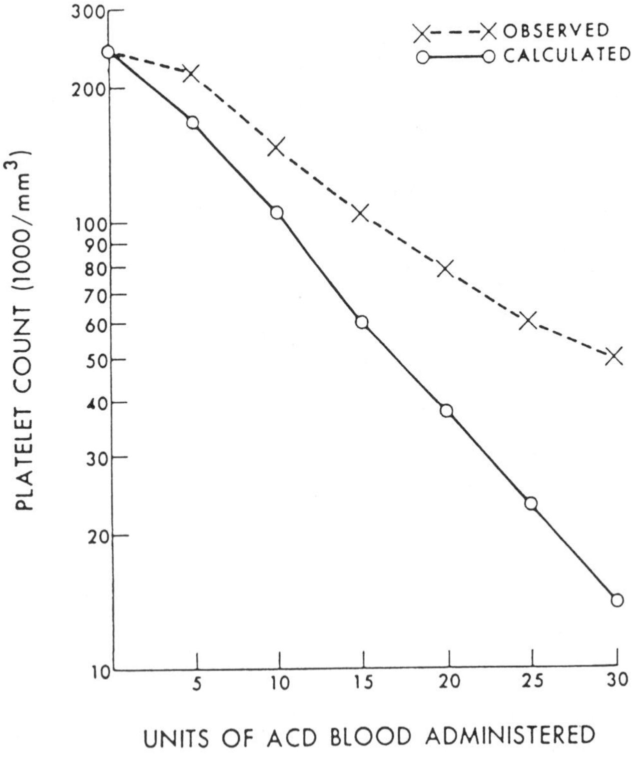

Figure 5.10. Platelet counts after massive transfusion. Comparison between mean observed platelet counts after multiple transfusions of acid-citrate-dextrose (ACD) stored blood and the predicted platelet count based on mathematical models. (Reprinted with permission from Miller RD, Robbins TO, Tong MJ, Barton SL. Coagulation defects associated with massive blood transfusion. Ann Surg 1971;174:794.)

This finding suggests that in a basically healthy population, platelet mobilization from the spleen and perhaps premature release of marrow platelets may prevent platelet counts from falling to predicted levels.

REFERENCES

1. Harker LA. Kinetics of thrombopoiesis. J Clin Invest 1968;47:458–465.
2. Burstein SA. Platelets and cytokines. Curr Opin Hematol 1994;1: 373–380.
3. Grossi A, Vannucchi AM, Rafanelli D, Ferrini PR. Regulation of platelet production. Platelets 1990;1:111–116.
4. Bartley TD, Bogenberger J, Hunt P, et al. Identification and cloning of a megakaryocyte growth and development factor that is a ligand for the cytokine receptor Mpl. Cell 1994;77:1117–1124.
5. Lok S, Kauchansky K, Holly RD, et al. Cloning and expression of murine thrombopoietin cDNA and stimulation of platelet production in vivo. Nature 1994;369:565–568.
6. Wendling F, Maraskovsky E, Debili N, et al. c-Mpl ligand is a humoral regulator of megakaryocytopoiesis. Nature 1994;369:571–574.
7. De Sauvage FJ, Hass PE, Spencer SD, et al. Stimulation of megakaryocytopoiesis and thrombopoiesis by the c-Mpl ligand. Nature 1994;369: 533–538.
8. Brass LF. Molecular basis for platelet activation. In: Hoffman R, Benz EJ Jr, Shattil SJ, Furie B, Cohen HJ, Silberstein LE, eds. Hematology: basic principles and practice. 2nd ed. New York: Churchill Livingstone, 1995:1536–1552.
9. Marcus AJ. Platelets and their disorders. In: Ratnoff OD, Forbes CD, eds. Disorders of hemostasis. 2nd ed. Philadelphia: WB Saunders, 1991:75–140.
10. Wagner DD, Olmsted JB, Marder VJ. Immunolocalization of von Willebrand protein in Weibel-Palade bodies of human endothelial cells. J Cell Biol 1982;95:355–360.
11. Sporn LA, Marder VJ, Wagner DD. Differing polarity of the constitutive and regulated secretory pathways of von Willebrand factor in endothelial cells. J Cell Biol 1989;108:1283–1289.
12. Turrito VT, Weiss HJ, Zimmerman TS, Sussman II. Factor VIII/von Willebrand factor in subendothelium mediates platelet adhesion. Blood 1985;65:823–831.
13. Shuman MA. Endothelial cell structure and function. In: Hoffman R, Benz EJ Jr, Shattil SJ, Furie B, Cohen HJ, Silberstein LE, eds. Hematology: basic principles and practice. 2nd ed. New York: Churchill Livingstone, 1995:1552–1565.
14. Laurie GW, Leblond CP, Martin GR. Localization of type IV collagen, laminin, heparin sulfate proteoglycan, and fibronectin to the basal lamina of basement membrane. J Cell Biol 1982;95:340–344.
15. Sage H, Trueb B, Bornstein P. Biosynthetic and structural properties of endothelial cell type VIII collagen. J Biol Chem 1983;258:13391–13401.
16. Kittelberger R, Davis PF, Greenhill NS. Immunolocalization of type VIII collagen in vascular tissue. Biochem Biophys Res Commun 1989; 159:414–419.
17. Brenner BM, Troy JL, Ballermann BJ. Endothelium-dependent vascular responses: mediators and mechanisms. J Clin Invest 1989;84:1373–1378.
18. Rapaport RM, Murad F. Agonist-induced endothelium-dependent relaxation in rat thoracic aorta may be mediated through cyclic cGMP. Circ Res 1983;52:352–357.
19. Busse R, Luckhoff A, Bassenge E. Endothelium-derived relaxant factor inhibits platelet activation. Naunyn Schmiedbergs Arch Pharmacol 1987;336:566–571.
20. Smith WL. The eicosanoids and their biochemical mechanism of action. Biochem J 1989;259:315–324.
21. Marcus AJ, Weksler BB, Jaffe EA, et al. Synthesis of prostacyclin from platelet-derived endoperoxides by cultured human endothelial cells. J Clin Invest 1980;66:979–986.
22. Ruggeri ZM. New insights into the mechanisms of platelet adhesion and aggregation. Semin Hematol 1994;31:229–239.
23. Barnes MS, Bailey A, Gordon JL, et al. Platelet aggregation by basement membrane-associated collagen. Thromb Res 1980;18:375–388.
24. McEver RP. The clinical significance of platelet membrane glycoproteins. Hematol Oncol Clin North Am 1990;4:87–105.
25. Pytela R, Peierschbacher MD, Ginsberg MH, et al. Platelet membrane glycoprotein IIb/IIIa: member of a family of arg-gly-asp-specific adhesion receptors. Science 1986;231:1559–1562.
26. Weiss HJ, Hawiger J, Ruggeri ZM, et al. Fibrinogen-independent platelet adhesion and thrombus formation on subendothelium mediated by glycoprotein IIb-IIIa complex at high shear rate. J Clin Invest 1989;83:288–297.
27. White JG, Escolar G. Current concepts of platelet membrane response to surface activation. Platelets 1993;4:175–183.
28. Rao AK. Congenital disorders of platelet function. Hematol Oncol Clin North Am 1990;4:65–86.
29. Plow EF, Ginsberg MH. Molecular basis of platelet function. In: Hoffman R, Benz EJ Jr, Shattil SJ, Furie B, Cohen HJ, Silberstein LE, eds. Hematology: basic principles and practice. 2nd ed. New York: Churchill Livingstone, 1995:1524–1535.
30. Holmsen H. Physiological functions of platelets. Ann Med 1989;21: 23–30.
31. Allen RD, Zacharski LR, Widirstky ST, et al. Transformation and motility of human platelets: details of the shape change and release reaction observed by optical and electron microscopy. J Cell Biol 1979; 83:126–142.
32. Wencel-Drake JD, Plow EF, Kunicki TJ, et al. Localization of internal pools of membrane glycoproteins involved in platelet adhesive responses. Am J Pathol 1986;124:324–334.
33. Berman CL, Yeo EL, Wencel-Drake JD, et al. A platelet alpha granule membrane protein that is associated with the plasma membrane after activation. Characterization and subcellular localization of PADGEM glycoprotein. J Clin Invest 1986;78:130–137.
34. Stenberg PE, McEver RP, Shuman MA, et al. A platelet alpha-granule membrane protein (GMP-140) is expressed on the plasma membrane after activation. J Cell Biol 1985;101:880–886.
35. White JG. Current concepts of platelet structure. Am J Clin Pathol 1979;71:363–378.
36. Stenberg PE, Shuman MA, Levine SP, Bainton DF. Redistribution of alpha-granules and their contents in thrombin-stimulated platelets. J Cell Biol 1984;98:748–760.
37. White JG. A search for the platelet secretory pathway using electron dense tracers. Am J Pathol 1970;58:31–49.
38. Behnke O. Electron microscopic observations on the membrane systems of the rat blood platelet. Anat Rec 1967;158:121–137.
39. Morgenstern E, Neumann K, Patscheke H. The exocytosis of human blood platelets. A fast freezing and freeze-substitution analysis. Eur J Cell Biol 1987;43:273–282.
40. Painter RG, Ginsberg MH. Centripetal myosin redistribution in thrombin-stimulated platelets. Relationship to platelet factor 4 secretion. Exp Cell Res 1984;155:198–212.
41. Roth GJ. Platelets and blood vessels: the adhesion event. Immunol Today 1992;13:100–105.

42. Coller BS. Platelets and thrombolytic therapy. N Engl J Med 1990;322:33–42.
43. Aiken ML, Ginsberg MH, Plow EF. Identification of a new class of inducible receptors on platelets. Thrombospondin interacts with platelets via GPIIb-IIIa-independent mechanism. J Clin Invest 1986;78: 1713–1716.
44. Kunicki TJ. Role of platelets in hemostasis. In: Rossi EC, Simon TL, Moss GS, eds. Principles of transfusion medicine. Baltimore, MD: Williams & Wilkins, 1991:181–192.
45. Santos MT, Valles J, Marcus AJ, et al. Enhancement of platelet reactivity and modulation of eicosanoid production by intact erythrocytes. J Clin Invest 1991;87:571–580.
46. Valles J, Santos MT, Aznar J, et al. Erythrocytes metabolically enhance collagen-induced platelet responsiveness via increased thromboxane production, ADP release, and recruitment. Blood 1991;78:154–162.
47. Zwaal RFA, Hemker HC. Blood cell membranes and haemostasis. Haemostasis 1982;11:12–39.
48. Mackie IJ, Bull HA. Normal haemostasis and its regulation. Blood Rev 1989;3:237–250.
49. Handagama PJ, George JN, Shuman MA, et al. Incorporation of a circulating protein into megakaryocyte and platelet granules (peroxidase/endocytosis/guinea pig). Proc Natl Acad Sci USA 1987;84:861–865.
50. Handagama PJ, Shuman MA, Bainton DF. Incorporation of intravenously injected albumin, immunoglobulin G, and fibrinogen in guinea pig megakaryocyte granules. J Clin Invest 1989;84:73–82.
51. Nichols WL, Gastineau DA, Solberg LA Jr, Mann KG. Identification of human megakaryocyte coagulation factor V. Blood 1985;65:1396–1406.
52. Chiu HC, Schick PK, Colman RW. Biosynthesis of factor V in isolated guinea pig megakaryocytes. J Clin Invest 1985;75:339–346.
53. Wencel-Drake JD, Dahlback B, Ginsberg MH. Ultrastructural localization of coagulation factor V in human platelets. Blood 1986;68:244–249.
54. Schwarz HP, Heeb MJ, Wencel-Drake JD, Griffin JH. Identification and quantitation of protein S in human platelets. Blood 1985;66:1452–1455.
55. Mann KG, Nesheim ME, Hibbard LS, Tracy PB. The role of factor V in the assembly of the prothrombinase complex. Ann NY Acad Sci 1981;370:378–388.
56. Hanson SR, Slichter SJ. Platelet kinetics in patients with bone marrow hypoplasia: evidence for a fixed platelet requirement. Blood 1985;66: 1105–1109.
57. Harker LA, Slichter SJ. The bleeding time as a screening test for evaluating platelet function. N Engl J Med 1972;287:155–159.
58. Slichter SJ, Harker LA. Preparation and storage of platelet concentrates. I. Factors influencing the harvest of viable platelets from whole blood. Br J Haematol 1976;34:393–402.
59. Rock G, Sherring VA, Tittley P. Five-day storage of platelet concentrates. Transfusion 1984;24:147–152.
60. Murphy S, Holme S, Nelson E, Carmen R. Paired comparison of the in vivo and in vitro results of storage of platelet concentrates in two containers. Transfusion 1984;24:31–34.
61. Simon TL, Nelson EJ, Murphy S. Extension of platelet concentrate storage to 7 days in second-generation bags. Transfusion 1987;27:6–9.
62. Holme S, Heaton A, Momoda G. Evaluation of a new, more oxygen-permeable, polyvinylchloride container. Transfusion 1989;29:159–164.
63. Snyder EL, Ezekowitz M, Aster R, et al. Extended storage of platelets in a new plastic container. II. In vivo response to infusion of platelets stored for 5 days. Transfusion 1985;25:209–214.
64. Hogge DE, Thompson BW, Schiffer CA. Platelet storage for 7 days in second-generation blood bags. Transfusion 1986;26:131–135.
65. Lazarus HM, Herzig RH, Warm SE, Fishman DJ. Transfusion experience with platelet concentrates stored for 24 to 72 hours at 22°C. Transfusion 1982;22:39–43.
66. Peter-Salonen K, Bucher U, Nydegger UE. Comparison of posttransfusion recoveries achieved with either fresh or stored platelet concentrates. Blut 1987;54:207–212.
67. Rock G, Tittley P, McCombie N. 5-Day storage of single-donor platelets obtained using a blood cell separator. Transfusion 1989; 29:288–291.
68. Shanwell A, Gulliksson H, Berg BK, et al. Evaluation of platelets prepared by apheresis and stored for 5 days. In vitro and in vivo studies. Transfusion 1989;29:783–788.
69. Slichter SJ. Efficacy of platelets collected by semi-continuous flow centrifugation (Haemonetics model 30). Br J Haematol 1978;38:131–140.
70. Slichter SJ, Harker LA. Thrombocytopenia: mechanisms and management of defects in platelet production. Clin Hematol 1978;7:523–539.
71. Harker LA, Malpass TW, Branson HE, et al. Mechanisms of abnormal bleeding in patients undergoing cardiopulmonary bypass: acquired transient platelet dysfunction associated with selected alpha granule release. Blood 1980;56:824–834.
72. Malpass TW, Hanson SR, Savage B, et al. Prevention of acquired transient defect in platelet plug formation by infused prostacyclin. Blood 1981;57:736–740.
73. O'Connell B, Lee EJ, Schiffer CA. The value of 10-minute posttransfusion platelet counts. Transfusion 1988;28:66–67.
74. Harker LA. The role of the spleen in thrombokinetics. J Lab Clin Med 1971;77:247–253.
75. Harker LA, Slichter SJ. Platelet and fibrinogen consumption in man. N Engl J Med 1972;287:999–1005.
76. McFarland JG, Anderson AJ, Slichter SJ. Factors influencing the response to HLA-selected apheresis platelets in patients refractory to random platelet concentrates. Br J Haematol 1989;73:380–386.
77. Bishop JF, McGrath K, Wolf MM, et al. Clinical factors influencing the efficacy of pooled platelet transfusions. Blood 1988;71:383–387.
78. Slichter SJ, Funk DD, Leandoer LE, Harker LA. Kinetic evaluation of hemostasis during surgery and wound healing. Br J Haematol 1974;27: 115–125.
79. Scott EP, Slichter SJ. Viability and function of platelet concentrates stored in CPD-adenine (CPDA-1). Transfusion 1980;20:489–497.
80. Weiss HJ, Aldeort LM, Kochwa S. The effect of salicylates on the hemostatic properties of platelets in man. J Clin Invest 1968;47: 2169–2180.
81. Brown CH, Natelson EA, Bradshaw MW, et al. The hemostatic defect produced by carbenicillin. N Engl J Med 1974;291:265–270.
82. Brown CH, Bradshaw MW, Natelson EA, et al. Effect on platelet function following the administration of penicillin compounds. Blood 1976;47:949–956.
83. Remuzzi G, Marchesi D, Livio M, et al. Altered platelet function and vascular prostaglandin-generation in patients with renal failure and prolonged bleeding time. Thromb Res 1978;13:1007–1015.
84. McKay DG. Disseminated intravascular coagulation: an intermediary mechanism of disease. New York: Harper & Row, 1965:493.
85. Van der Weyden MB, Clancy RL, Howard MA, Firkin BG. Qualitative platelet defects with reduced life-span in acute leukemia. Aust NZ J Med 1972;4:339–345.
86. Cardamon JM, Edson R, McArthur J, Jacob H. Abnormalities of platelet function in the myeloproliferative disorders. JAMA 1972;221:270–273.
87. Freeman G, Buckley ES. Serum polysaccharide and fever in thrombocytopenic bleeding in leukemia. Blood 1954;9:586–594.
88. Cerskus AL, Ali M, Davies BJ, McDonald JWD. Possible significance of small numbers of functional platelets in a population of aspirin-treated platelets in vitro and in vivo. Thromb Res 1980;18:389–397.

89. Torosian M, Michelson EL, Morganroth J, MacVaugh H. Aspirin- and coumadin-related bleeding after coronary artery bypass graft surgery. Ann Intern Med 1978;89:325–328.
90. Slichter SJ, Harker LA. Separation and storage of platelet concentrates. II. Storage variables influencing platelet viability and function. Br J Haematol 1976;34:403–419.
91. String T, Robinson AJ, Blaisdel FW. Massive trauma, effect of intravascular coagulation on prognosis. Arch Surg 1971;102: 407–411.
92. Attar S, Boyd D, Layne E, McLaughlin J, Mansberger AR, Cowley RA. Alterations in coagulation and fibrinolytic mechanisms in acute trauma. J Trauma 1969;9:939–965.
93. Broersma RJ, Bullemer GD, Mammen EF. Blood coagulation changes in hemorrhagic shock and acidosis. Thromb Diath Haem 1969;36 (Suppl):171–176.
94. Steele P, Ellis JH, Weily HS, Genton E. Platelet survival time in patients with hypoxemia and pulmonary hypertension. Circulation 1977; 55:660–661.
95. Marsaglia G, Thomas ED. Mathematical consideration of cross-circulation in exchange transfusion. Transfusion 1971;11:216–219.
96. Slichter SJ. Identification and management of defects in platelet hemostasis in massively transfused patients. In: Collins JA, Murawski K, Shafer AW, eds. Massive transfusion in surgery and trauma. New York: Alan R. Liss, Inc., 1982:225–258.
97. Miller RD, Robins TO, Tong MJ, Barton SL. Coagulation defects associated with massive blood transfusion. Ann Surg 1971;174:794–801.

Chapter 6

Physiology of Hemostasis

RICHARD B. COUNTS

INTRODUCTION

Because it is the business of the surgeon to cure or ameliorate diseases by cutting the tissues of the body, control of the resulting bleeding is essential to his or her success. Over the history of surgical technique, a great variety of ways to control bleeding have been tried, ranging from tourniquets and pressure to cautery and chemicals to magical potions applied to the wound. Only a few of these methods consistently control bleeding without injuring the tissue. Mastery and application of these methods are an essential part of the surgeon's training.

Many techniques control bleeding from larger blood vessels where the relatively high pressure and large volume of blood flow require temporary clamping, ligature, or some other mechanical occlusion to stop the flow of blood. At the other end of the size distribution of blood vessels, the microvasculature, individual arterioles and venules cannot be tied off, and one must depend on the body's intrinsic hemostatic systems to stop bleeding from wounds and to maintain hemostasis for the 10–14 days necessary for wound healing and restoration of the normal vascular integrity. Although hemostasis can be thought of as a simple process that begins with tissue injury and ends with the formation of a clot and the cessation of bleeding, it is, in fact, a redundant, tightly regulated process consisting of three separate but interrelated steps: platelet plug formation, fibrin clot formation, and fibrinolysis. The most important stimulus for both platelet and coagulation activation is exposure of subendothelial tissue as a result of vascular injury. An overview of the concerted mechanism can be gained by considering three critical questions: Why does the blood ordinarily not clot within the vasculature? How is the hemostatic plug formed after vascular injury? How is the process regulated so that circulation is reestablished after the injured blood vessels are healed?

WHY DOES BLOOD ORDINARILY NOT CLOT WITHIN THE VASCULATURE?

Normal vascular endothelium is nonthrombogenic. After more than 100 years of experimental study of the hemostatic system, we know more about how platelet and fibrin thrombi form than we do about why the blood circulating in the vessels does not clot. One reason is the difficulty of doing controlled in vivo experiments under physiological conditions. However, in the last 10 years, our knowledge of the physiological anticoagulant mechanisms has increased dramatically. In addition to aiding our understanding of thrombosis, the natural anticoagulant properties of endothelium give insight into the mechanisms of platelet plug formation and coagulation.

It has long been known that both platelets and blood clotting are activated by vascular damage that exposes blood to contact with the subendothelium. For this reason, one important way in which vascular endothelium is a barrier to blood activation is simply that it prevents blood from contacting proteins in subendothelial tissue, which would activate platelets or the coagulation system. Disorders that cause endothelial damage, such as certain viral or rickettsial infections or vasculitides, may be associated with local microthrombus formation. In addition to being a passive barrier, endothelium produces and releases inhibitors of both platelets and clotting. The main platelet inhibitors, prostacyclin (PGI_2) and nitric oxide radical ($NO^\bullet$), prevent the initial steps of thrombosis: adhesion and aggregation; the clotting inhibitors, thrombomodulin and heparin sulfates, are involved in limiting the extent of thrombin generation and clot formation.

PGI_2 and nitric oxide are synthesized by endothelial cells; both relax smooth muscle on the adventitial side of vessels and both are potent, although labile, inhibitors of platelet aggregation. The arachidonic acid pathway, by generating both activators and inhibitors of platelets, is a means of regulating platelet function (1). PGI_2 released from endothelial cells inhibits platelet aggregation by increasing cAMP. It is rapidly degraded in plasma and thus has mainly a local effect at the endothelial surface. Thromboxane A_2 (TXA_2), generated in platelets, induces platelet aggregation and vasoconstriction. Both PGI_2 and TXA_2 are formed from arachidonic acid released from membrane phospholipids by phospholipase A_2. The enzyme cyclooxygenase begins a sequence leading to the cyclic endoperoxide PGH_2 (prostaglandin H_2). From PGH_2, PGI_2 synthetase in endothelium makes PGI_2, and thromboxane synthetase in platelets makes TXA_2.

The secretion of PGI_2 by endothelial cells also accounts for aspirin's antiplatelet effects. Aspirin irreversibly acetylates cyclooxygenase that is present in both platelets and endothelium (2). However, the effects of aspirin on platelets differ from its effects on endothelial cells. The reason is that cyclooxygenase is made constitutively in endothelial cells, but circulating platelets do not make it. All cyclooxygenase in platelets is synthesized in the megakaryocytes before the platelets are released. After low-dose aspirin exposure, endothelial cells soon recover the ability to make PGI_2, but only newly released platelets make TXA_2 (1). Therefore, the net effect of low-dose aspirin is that endothelium continues to make the platelet inhibitor, PGI_2, but the thromboxane activation pathway in platelets is blocked.

The main function of $NO^•$ appears to be to regulate vascular tone. But $NO^•$ also inhibits platelet aggregation and adhesion by raising platelet cGMP. Synergism between subthreshold concentrations of $NO^•$ and PGI_2 has been demonstrated (3).

When thrombin is generated after vascular injury, two important inhibitory mechanisms limit the extent of thrombosis. Thrombin formed in situ at an injured area binds to the protein thrombomodulin on the surface of endothelial cells. The effects of this are twofold. First, thrombin is removed from circulation, minimizing the chance of generalized clotting of fibrinogen. Second, binding to thrombomodulin causes a conformational change in thrombin, resulting in both a loss of fibrinogen-clotting activity and the development of the ability to activate protein C, which then inactivates factors Va and VIIIa. Proteolytic inactivation of these two critical coagulation cofactors limits the factor X activation and prothrombin-converting steps.

HOW IS THE HEMOSTATIC PLUG FORMED AFTER VASCULAR INJURY?

The initial hemostatic plug is formed by platelets. The coagulation cascade is then triggered to produce a renewable fibrin clot. Whenever the vascular endothelium is disrupted or damaged, the exposure of subintimal proteins to the blood stimulates the formation, first of a platelet plug and then of a fibrin clot. The major steps leading to the platelet plug are adhesion to subendothelial tissue; activation of platelets, which leads to the release of messengers that amplify the activation of other platelets; and the aggregation of activated platelets (Fig. 6.1).

The first reaction to vascular injury, other than vasoconstriction, is formation of a platelet plug. Platelets in blood flowing past exposed subendothelial tissue adhere to the tissue and are activated to release intracellular messengers that stimulate other platelets to aggregate into a plug that occludes the area of injury. These reactions, adhesion, activation, and aggregation, are the prototypic sequence of all hemostatic mechanisms; amplifying reactions, triggered by a small external stimulus, are characteristic of hemostasis. In addition to forming the initial hemostatic plug, the activated, aggregated platelets stimulate two later series of reactions. By expression on their surface of high-affinity binding sites for factor X, they provide a catalytic surface that greatly promotes the rate of thrombin generation and clot formation, and by the release of growth factors, they play an important role in initiating angiogenesis and wound healing.

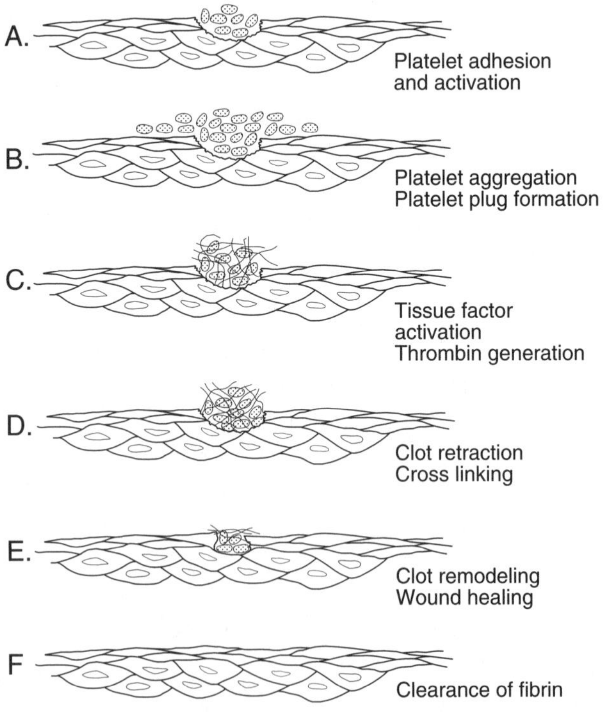

Figure 6.1. Sequence of major steps in hemostasis from platelet adhesion at an area of endothelial injury to restoration of blood flow after wound healing.

How do platelets adhere to subendothelial tissue and how are they activated? Of the proteins and polysaccharides in the subendothelial basement membrane, the most important ligands in platelet adhesion appear to be collagen and von Willebrand factor (vWF). In addition, a number of other subendothelial adhesive proteins can bind to platelet membrane receptor proteins: fibronectin, fibrinogen, laminin, vitronectin, and thrombospondin. Their role in platelet adhesion is not well understood.

Under the usual condition of flowing blood, the reaction between vWF and glycoprotein Ib/IX (GPIb/IX) on the platelet membrane seems by far to be the most important interaction (4). Under conditions of low shear rates, adhesion of platelets to subintimal tissue can be mediated through the binding of the membrane receptor GPIa/IIa to subendothelial collagen. However, the GPIb/IX-vWF interaction is required for adhesion at higher shear rates.

Adhesion of platelets to a wound results in a monolayer that anchors the platelet plug to tissue and stimulates the release from the adherent platelets of agonists that activate other platelets to aggregate with each other through fibrinogen receptors on their cell membranes (GPIIb/IIIA) (Table 6.1).

The substances that directly cause the activation of platelets that adhere to subendothelial tissue are not known. Most agonists that have been well studied in vitro are themselves released from activated platelets (ADP, ATP, serotonin, TXA_2) or are generated by clotting reactions (thrombin). Of the agonists that are not, fibrillar collagen seems a likely candidate to be the dominant initial activator in vivo. Platelets bind to collagen through the membrane receptor GPIa/IIa (5).

An important common path in platelet activation is the release of intracellular granule contents (Fig. 6.2). Most platelet membrane receptors studied are linked to G proteins (6). Binding of ligands leads to the activation of phospholipase C in the platelet membrane. Phospholipase C hydrolyzes phosphatidylinositol biphosphate to yield the intracellular messengers inositol 1,4,5-triphosphate (IP_3) and diacyl glycerol (DG). IP_3 stimulates the release of Ca^{++} from the dense tubular stores and an influx of extracellular Ca^{++}, rapidly raising the intracellular Ca^{++} concentration. DG activates protein kinase C, which leads to release of granule contents by mechanisms that are not yet known but which must involve phosphorylation of intracellular proteins.

Another direct effect of activation is the expression on the platelet surface of GPIIb/IIIa and conformational changes in the subunits of this protein that increases its affinity for fibrinogen (7). Fibrinogen molecules are the links that hold together the platelet aggregates and GPIIb/IIIa is the main platelet membrane receptor for fibrinogen. In addition to the initial wave of aggregation, activation of platelets produces a series of reactions that greatly amplify the initial activation. Phospholipase A_2 hydrolyzes membrane phospholipids to give arachidonic acid from which various icosanoids are derived, the most potent promoter of platelet aggregation being TXA_2. ADP and serotonin are released from dense granules and act synergistically with TXA_2, and with thrombin when it is generated, to produce maximal aggregation and a dense plug that occludes the damaged arteriole or venule.

Although it is the most important element in initial microvascular hemostasis, the platelet plug is a temporary hemostatic plug that appears to be dependent on platelet energy metabolism and disaggregates over 24–48 hours if a fibrin clot has not formed in and around it. Once it breaks down, it usually does not reform. An illustration of this is the well-known pattern of delayed bleeding in hemophiliacs or individuals with other coagulation protein deficiencies. In hemophilia, platelet function is essentially normal; small or moderately sized wounds usually stop bleeding in a few minutes, as they

TABLE 6.1. PLATELET PROTEINS AND ORGANELLE

Membrane Proteins	Function
GPIb-IX	vWF binding
GPIIb-IIIa	Fibrinogen binding
GPIV, Ia-IIa	Collagen binding
Alpha granules	Storage of intracellular protein PDGF, DF4, BTG, TGF-β ECGF, vWF, V fibrinogen
Dense bodies	Storage of ADP, serotonin, ATP, Ca^{++}
Open canalicular system	External delivery of secreted agonists
Dense tubular system	Ca^{++} storage; prostaglandin synthesis

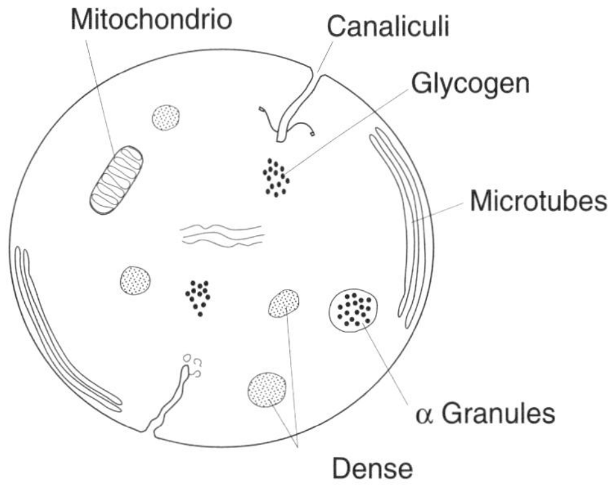

Figure 6.2. Simplified schematic diagram of a platelet in the quiescent discoid form.

would in someone without hemophilia. When the platelet plug disperses in 24–48 hours, however, the wound begins to bleed, and prolonged oozing is the rule, because the clotting factor deficiency blocks the formation of a renewable fibrin clot.

In addition to comprising the first hemostatic plug to form, activated platelets also contribute to the rapid activation of the coagulation cascade, which leads to the platelet thrombus being invested with a fibrin clot (Fig. 6.1). The clot, through a continuous process of fibrinolysis and regeneration, maintains hemostasis until healing of the damaged vessel is complete. It is then cleared away by plasmin and flow through the vessel is reestablished.

This two-stage mechanism, the temporary platelet plug and then the renewable longer term fibrin clot, is the key to understanding hemostasis as it applies to surgery. In the next section, parallels to this sequential process within the branches of the clotting cascade itself are shown. One can begin to see the outlines of steps by which the hemostatic system evolved from the earliest mechanism using only reactive cells analogous to platelets (8) to a series of reactions in mammals that combine rapidly acting, highly regulated steps with a more permanent clot that can be replenished as long as it is needed.

HOW IS THE PROCESS REGULATED SO THAT CIRCULATION IS REESTABLISHED AFTER THE INJURED BLOOD VESSELS ARE HEALED?

The coagulation-fibrinolytic system continually renews the clot until healing is complete and then rapidly clears it. The coagulation system has evolved to respond to vascular damage by generating an in situ fibrin clot, a strong plug consisting of red cells and platelets trapped in a net of fibrin strands while at the same time limiting the spread of the clotting process to the site of injury to avoid widespread thrombosis. The substrate for clots, fibrinogen, is, of course, omnipresent, being in the blood at a concentration of 2–3 mg/mL. The control of the clotting process comes through regulation of thrombin generation, limiting the dispersion of active clotting factors, and more or less continuous removal of fibrin by the fibrinolytic enzymes.

Coagulation pathways use a series of proteolytic enzymes as a biological amplification system that responds rapidly to small activating stimuli and generates locally high concentrations of thrombin, the fibrinogen-activating enzyme. Thrombin cleaves N-terminal activation peptides from fibrinogen, exposing polymerization sites, and long strands of fibrin then form, enveloping the platelet plug and trapping additional platelets, red cells, and white cells to form the clot. In addition to activating fibrinogen, thrombin has three additional activities, one of which reinforces the formation of thrombus, whereas the other two limit its extent. Thrombin is a potent activator of platelets and of factors V and VIII. These activities promote further accretion to the growing thrombus. But, on the other hand, thrombin also activates plasminogen activators that convert plasminogen, bound to the fibrin clot, into the active protease, plasmin, thus beginning the dissolution and remodeling of the thrombus. An ongoing process is established in which coagulation and fibrinolysis alternate, until the wound is healed and the last fibrin is cleared away. Throughout the process, excess thrombin, upon binding to thrombomodulin on endothelial cell membranes, loses its ability to cleave fibrinogen and acquires the ability to convert protein C from a zymogen to an active protease that then inactivates both factors V and VIII, thereby exerting feedback control to limit further thrombin generation.

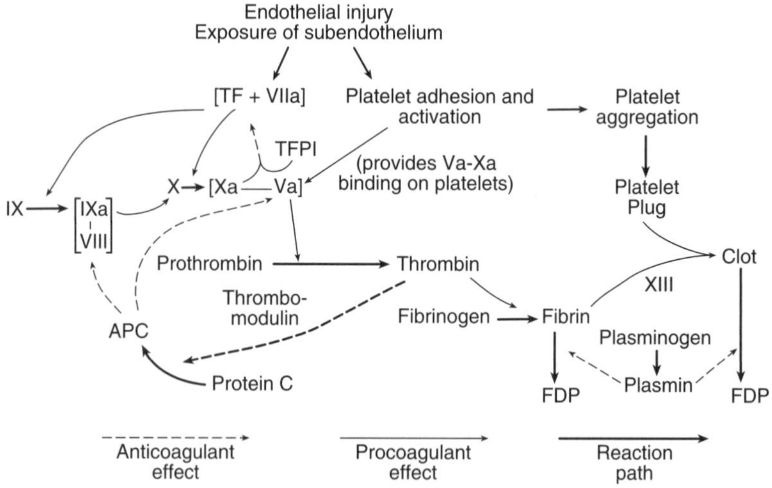

Figure 6.3. The main reaction steps leading to the generation and dissolution of the fibrin clot. Procoagulant enzyme complexes and feedback control steps are shown by solid and dashed arrows, respectively.

Plasma also contains various other protease inhibitors (e.g., antithrombin III [ATIII] and α-macroglobulin, which inactivate thrombin) that diffuse away from the site of clotting. An illustration of the main events in clot formation is given in Figure 6.3. The details of the important steps—initial activation, generation of thrombin, clotting of fibrinogen, regulation of the process, and dissolution and clearance of the fibrin clot—are given in the following sections.

FINGER IN THE DIKE: PLATELETS AND THE PLATELET PLUG

ORIGIN AND STRUCTURE OF PLATELETS

Platelets are small nonnucleated cells derived from megakaryocytes and released from the bone marrow by budding off fragments of megakaryocyte cytoplasm. Recently, production of platelets has been shown to be regulated by the growth factor thrombopoietin, which has been cloned (9–11). Other growth factors as well may also be involved in controlling platelet production. Platelets have a complex structure as might be expected from their multiple properties of adhesion to vascular surfaces, secretion, uptake of plasma constituents, aggregation with other platelets, and contraction. The structural features important in carrying out these functions include critical membrane proteins, intracellular storage granules, intracellular tubular and canalicular systems, and contractile and structural proteins. Figure 6.2 is a schematic diagram of a platelet.

Platelet membrane glycoproteins that mediate adhesion to subendothelial surfaces and platelet aggregation have been isolated; some important adhesion proteins are listed in Table 6.1. Adhesion to subendothelium involves binding of platelets to collagen and vWF. The most important receptor for vWF is GPIb-IX, a negatively charged protein by virtue of sialic acid residues. The average number of copies per platelet is 25,000. GPIb is a heterodimer consisting of a molecular weight of 145,000. GPIba subunit is disulfide-bonded to a smaller (molecular weight of 24,000) GPIbb subunit (12). These are noncovalently associated in the membrane with GPIX, which has a molecular weight of 17,000 (13). Under normal conditions of rapid blood flow, vWF-mediated adhesion is necessary for normal hemostasis. Patients with Bernard-Soulier syndrome, a moderate bleeding disorder characterized by a long bleeding time and a normal vWF level, lack one or several of the components of GPIb-IX (14). Their platelets do not adhere normally to exposed subendothelial tissue.

The major platelet receptor mediating aggregation is the GPIIb-IIIa complex. GPIIb has two disulfide-bonded chains, a heavy chain (M_r = 132,000) and a light chain (M_r = 23,000). GPIIIa is a single chain containing 762 amino acids. It has an apparent molecular weight (when reduced) of 114,000 and is extensively folded, the structure being maintained by a number of intrachain disulfide bonds. Around 50,000–70,000 copies of GPIIb-IIIa are present on each platelet; it is the most abundant platelet glycoprotein. A number of proteins, including fibrinogen, vitronectin, fibronectin, and vWF, bind to GPIIb-IIIa. The most important for platelet aggregation appears to be fibrinogen, which has six GPIIb-IIIa binding sites per fibrinogen molecule. Lack of GPIIb-IIIa causes the most severe congenital disease of platelet dysfunction, Glanzmann's thrombasthenia. People with thrombasthenia have normal platelet counts but a moderately severe bleeding disorder commonly manifested by prolonged life-threatening bleeding in childhood or early adolescence. The platelets in thrombasthenia have no ability to form a hemostatic plug. The bleeding time is infinite and platelet aggregation is zero (15, 16).

PLATELET PRODUCTION AND KINETICS

The normal platelet count in humans is 180,000–400,000, the mean being 250,000. There is little difference in the platelet count by age or sex. The average life span of platelets in the circulation is 9–10 days. The disappearance of platelets is normally age related; however, there appears to be a small fixed daily random loss on the order of about 10,000 platelets/μL/day or about 10% of the circulating mass (17, 18). This random disappearance is normally not noticeable; however, in severely thrombocytopenic individuals, it can be a large fraction of the total platelet mass and can make platelet transfusion support difficult. In rapid destruction states such as immune thrombocytopenia or disseminated intravascular coagulation (DIC), the kinetic pattern is quite different from normal, being dominated by random (first-order) disappearance in which the number of platelets disappearing per minute is a function of the platelet count.

About 30–50% of the platelets are in the spleen at any given time. This splenic pool is in equilibrium with blood platelets. However, in humans, unlike in the dog, the splenic pool cannot be rapidly mobilized to increase the platelet count because people do not have a contractile spleen. In cases of significant splenomegaly from any cause, splenic pooling of platelets is greatly increased, platelet counts in the 60,000–80,000 range being typical. The platelets may still equilibrate freely with the blood; such splenic pooling does not necessarily mean increased splenic destruction and is often not associated with increased bleeding. However, with increased splenic pooling, the increment in platelet count after platelet transfusions is much less than normal.

The formation of a platelet plug by aggregation of activated platelets depends on the platelet concentration. In vitro, dilution of platelet suspensions to a platelet count below 100,000/mL greatly decreases the aggregation reaction. However, the normal in vivo platelet count of 250,000/mL is far in excess of the minimum needed for hemostasis. In the absence of vascular injury, a platelet count of 5,000–10,000 usually suffices to prevent serious spontaneous bleeding, although patients with a platelet count this low often have petechiae and ecchymoses. Although the practice is widespread of trying to maintain the platelet count of patients on chemotherapy above 20,000/mL, there is little data to support a level that high for prophylactic transfusions (19). It is a different matter if a patient has vascular damage (e.g., trauma, surgery, or vasculitis). Higher platelet counts are then needed for platelet hemostasis. The level somewhat depends on the severity of the wound. In the case of infection or trauma, such as an uncomplicated fracture, which does not produce wide microvascular injury, a platelet count of 30,000–50,000 is often adequate. For extensive vascular damage, especially if coupled with some degree of dysfunction of platelets, as is commonly seen in cardiopulmonary bypass or major soft-tissue trauma, platelet counts in excess of 100,000/mL may be required, depending on the degree of dysfunction.

FUNCTION OF PLATELETS

The reactions of platelets are triggered by binding of various molecules to membrane receptor proteins. The sequence can be considered as three steps: adhesion of platelets to subendothelial tissue, activation of the adherent platelets, and aggregation of the activated platelets (Fig. 6.1). The activation step, on the one hand, causes the expression on the platelet membrane of adhesion molecule binding sites, resulting in aggregation, and on the other stimulates the secretion from the activated platelets of additional activating molecules (agonists) that recruit more platelets to the growing aggregate. Thus, the pattern of amplification of a small stimulus to form a large hemostatic plug, well known in the enzyme cascade of coagulation reactions, is also a property of platelets.

In vitro studies have characterized a variety of platelet agonist molecules. Some are proteins (e.g., collagen, vWF, and thrombin), whereas others are small molecules (e.g., ADP, serotonin, and epinephrine). Platelets encounter them in several ways. Some, such as collagen or thrombin, are external to platelets, whereas many of the others, such as ADP or serotonin, are stored in platelet granules and released upon activation.

Adhesion

Although there are likely several subendothelial proteins to which unstimulated platelets can adhere, the best characterized interactions are with vWF and collagen. Platelets, particularly at relatively high shear rates in flowing blood, adhere to exposed subendothelial vWF through GPIb-IX on the platelet surface (4). Although there is not much evidence that this plays a major role in platelet activation, it is critical for adhesion, as shown by the bleeding disorder in patients with Bernard-Soulier disease who have abnormalities in GPIb that interfere with vWF binding. The other important basement membrane protein involved in platelet adhesion is collagen. The major platelet receptor for collagen binding seems to be GPIa-IIa (5). In addition to mediating adhesion, collagen binding also activates platelets through a G-protein stimulation of phospholipase C. Experimental studies of platelets circulated past damaged vascular endothelium show that the first noticeable step is the formation of a monolayer of platelets adherent to the exposed subendothelial tissue. These platelets become activated, leading to changes in their shape and surface receptors and release of granule contents to recruit other platelets into large aggregates.

Activation

As in most reactive cells, the most prominent activation pathways involve membrane receptors linked to G proteins. It seems likely that the major in vivo activation stimuli are the binding of collagen and traces of thrombin. Collagen is, of course, present in subendothelial tissue. Thrombin is generated in small amounts by release of tissue factor soon after disruption of endothelium. Both thrombin and collagen are potent activators of platelets. Both have been shown to bind platelet receptors and activate phospholipase C via G-protein links. Of a large number of activators, the best characterized sequence to date involves inositol phosphatides and calcium ions as intracellular messengers. Binding of the agonist to the cell membrane receptor activates the related G protein, causing it to release the GDP bound to the Ga subunit in the quiescent state and to bind GTP instead. The subunit with GTP bound to it dissociates and activates phospholipase C on the inner surface of the cell membrane. Phospholipase C hydrolyzes membrane phosphatidylinositol-1,4-biphosphate, releasing the messengers IP_3 and DG. IP_3 causes the rapid release from endoplasmic reticulum of about half of the Ca^{++} stored there, producing a sudden rise in intracellular Ca^{++} concentration. As in muscle cells, the Ca^{++} ion concentration in platelets is normally maintained at a low (less than 0.2 mM) concentration. With release of Ca^{++} from dense granules and endoplasmic reticulum, the concentration is raised above 1 mM, sufficient to cause the release of adhesive proteins (fibrinogen, vWF,) stored in alpha granules and of additional platelet agonists (ATP, ADP, serotonin) stored in dense granules. In addition, conformational changes are initiated in the main adhesive protein receptor of the membrane, GPIIb-IIIa, which increases its affinity for fibrinogen and plasma vWF, thus setting in motion the events leading to the formation of aggregates. There are a number of intracellular activation pathways; for example, DG has been shown to activate protein kinase C in platelets. The reader is referred to more specialized reviews (20, 21) for details of recent work.

Aggregation

GPIIb-IIIa, which is present on platelet membranes in high concentration, is the most important receptor mediating aggregation. In inactivated platelets, GPIIb-IIIa does not bind fibrinogen. If they did, of course, the result would be constant intravascular aggregation, making it impossible for platelets to circulate. Indeed, some such mechanism may play a role in the platelet consumption associated with cardiopulmonary bypass surgery in which there is low-level but widespread activation of platelets, which can lead to formation of microaggregates that are then removed in the lungs or spleen. By mechanisms incompletely understood, activation causes conformational changes and rearrangement of GPIIb-IIIa, which greatly increases its affinity for fibrinogen and plasma vWF. These proteins then bind and form bridges between platelets generating platelet aggregates. As in the case with other integrins, GPIIb-IIIa appears to interact with fibrinogen and its other ligands through Arg-Glu-Asp-x sequences (RGD sequences) (22) and in fibrinogen through γ-chain sequences as well. Short RGD-containing peptides have been shown to block platelet aggregation, but binding of a carboxy-terminal sequence in γ-chains of fibrinogen has been shown recently to be essential to platelet aggregation, whereas the γ-chain RGD sequences are not essential (23).

In addition to alterations in the affinity of GPIIb-IIIa for fibrinogen, activation of platelets causes a change in their shape from small discs to elongated shapes having long protrusions, filopodia, which presumably increase the interaction with other platelets. The shape change and later contraction of platelets causing consolidation of platelet aggregates involve platelet actin polymerization, also triggered by the rise in intracellular Ca^{++}.

Platelets are metabolically very active cells. They have abundant glycogen stores. In storage of platelet concentrates, care must be taken to agitate the suspensions and provide for adequate O_2 and CO_2 exchange through the plastic bags. Upon stimulation by aggregating agents, such as collagen or thrombin, there is a burst of oxidative metabolic activity. ATP seems to be required both for contractility and maintenance of the platelet plug. A likely cause of the dissociation of the platelet plug after 1–2 days is depletion of ATP.

PLATELETS AND COAGULATION

Not only is the platelet plug the initial hemostatic plug, it also promotes thrombin generation and the formation of a fibrin clot that then invests the aggregated platelets and traps red cells as it grows in size. Another consequence of platelet activation is the expression on the surface of factor V released from alpha granules. The released factor V migrates to the platelet membrane where it becomes activated and serves as a high affinity factor X binding site. The surface-associated factor V-factor X complex permits very efficient assembly of the prothrombin-converting complex on platelets with an increase of several orders of magnitude in the rate of thrombin generation over that of the proteins in solution (24).

COAGULATION

The coagulation system, as it is now understood, consists of four interacting cascades, each containing sequentially activated serine proteases: two pathways of activation, the tissue factor pathway and the intrinsic, or blood, pathway; the common path of thrombin generation from prothrombin by activated factor X; and the activated protein C pathway for feedback regulation of thrombin generation. In addition, thrombin, through proteolytic cleavages, activates fibrinogen to fibrin monomer, activates plasminogen activators, and activates platelets.

CLOTTING PROTEINS

The coagulation proteins fall into several groups having such structural similarities that they must have evolved from common ancestral proteins. At our present understanding of their structures, the vitamin K-dependent serine proteases, prothrombin, factor VII, factor IX, and factor X, the enzymes involved in thrombin generation, have extensive homologies (25). In addition to the active serine protease domain, they share an N-terminal calcium-binding domain composed of from 9 to 12 γ-carboxyglutamic acid (Gla) residues that result from posttranslational carboxylation of the newly synthesized proteins. This is the step that requires vitamin K (26, 27). Historically, these four proteins have been grouped together because of the common requirement for vitamin K (and conversely, the production of inactive forms by the anticoagulant warfarin, a vitamin K antagonist). Also, because they are copurified by procedures that are based on the calcium-binding properties of the Gla residues, they have been referred to as the prothrombin complex factors.

But, because their full structures have been elucidated, it is clear that the vitamin K-dependent factors have more fundamental similarities than simply their hepatic synthesis and their calcium-binding properties. Factors VII, IX, and X share two epidermal growth factor-like domains of about 50 amino acids each, whereas in the same region of the molecule, prothrombin has two kringle domains, so-called because of the resemblance of the sequence diagrams to a Scandinavian cake, the kringle (28). Two regulatory proteins, protein S and protein C, show considerable structural similarity to the vitamin-K-dependent proteins. Both have N-terminal Gla domains and repeats of epidermal growth factor domains. However, protein S is not a serine protease, although protein C does have the serine protease domain.

The two high-molecular-weight cofactors involved in the assembly of activation complexes, factors VIII and V, also have many homologous regions. Both have three A domains that are homologous to the three A domains of ceruloplasmin and both have two carboxy-terminal C domains that, like the A domains, show about 40% sequence identity between the two proteins. Between the A2 and A3 domains, both have a large, heavily glycosylated, connecting region. But the connecting region of factor V is completely different from that of factor VIII. Both proteins circulate in an inactive form and can be converted to the active cofactor by minor proteolytic cleavage by either factor Xa or thrombin. Factor V is found in platelet alpha granules and on platelet membranes in addition to circulating in solution in plasma. Factor VIII is mostly bound to vWF, circulating as a very high-molecular-weight multimeric complex (29).

The two other plasma clotting factors, fibrinogen and factor XI, bear little resemblance to the proteins in the groups just discussed. Fibrinogen consists of three pairs of different polypeptide chains held together by disulfide bonds. Each fibrinogen molecule has three large globular regions separated by long, thin helical peptide strands, so that by electron microscopy, it resembles "three balls on a string" (30). Factor XI is a dimer of identical subunits disulfide bonded to each other. Although it is a serine protease, factor XI is not homologous with the vitamin K-dependent factors in its amino-terminal region. It shares with other serine proteases only the trypsin-like protease domain in the carboxy-terminal portion of the molecule (25).

COAGULATION CASCADE AND REGULATION OF THROMBIN GENERATION

A useful conceptual framework for understanding blood coagulation and for interpreting the results of clotting screening tests is provided by considering the series of clotting reactions as being comprised of three phases:

1. The early, or activation, phase, beginning with the initiation of clotting and ending with the generation of activated factor X (Xa), the prothrombin-converting enzyme.
2. The middle phase, which is the assembly of the prothrombinase complex and conversion of prothrombin to thrombin.
3. The last phase, which is the cleavage of the fibrinopeptides from fibrinogen and the polymerization of the resultant fibrin monomer to form the clot.

In addition to the basic reactions leading to clot formation, inhibitory reactions have been discovered that regulate each stage.

The Early Phase: Initiation of Coagulation

In 1904, Morawitz (31) propounded his celebrated theory that a substance, which he called thrombokinase, was generated in blood when it contacted tissues or foreign surfaces. He conceived of thrombokinase as activating prothrombin in plasma to thrombin, the factor that clots fibrinogen. In 1912, Howell (32) described an activity residing in a phospholipid fraction from tissue that did not activate prothrombin directly but accelerated thrombin generation. Over the next 80 years, biochemists sought to explain the mechanisms that these early observations suggested. It was readily agreed that thrombin caused fibrinogen to clot and that prothrombin was activated to thrombin. The puzzle, and years of confusion, lay in the initiation of clotting: What activated prothrombin? From the first decade of the century, there was evidence that clotting could be initiated in at least two ways: by contact of plasma either with tissue or tissue extracts or with glass. Thus, two ways of generating the prothrombin-converting enzyme "thrombokinase" came to be appreciated. In one, the blood contained all the necessary factors (the blood or intrinsic pathway); in the other, a factor or factors present in tissue were involved (the extrinsic or tissue pathway). By the early 1960s, these studies led to the recognition of the main pathways of coagulation reactions, the waterfall sequence or enzymatic cascade, in which a series of serine proteases in plasma is sequentially activated (33, 34). With the isolation and cloning of the main clotting proteins, and particularly with the recent characterization of the lipoprotein-associated coagulation inhibitor (now renamed the tissue factor pathway inhibitor [TFPI]) (35), the regulation and mechanisms of the initial phase of clotting are reasonably well understood.

The pattern that has emerged is a sort of fractal pattern; just as hemostasis is arranged with a rapid initial step, platelet plug formation, followed by generation of a longer lasting plug, the fibrin clot, so clotting itself begins with two steps that now appear to be not really redundant but sequential. The tissue factor pathway is the critical path in the initiation of clotting, but its action is short-lived because it is inhibited by TFPI when the prothrombin-converting enzyme, factor Xa, begins to form. Once small amounts of thrombin are formed, the intrinsic pathway begins to be activated (through activation of factor XI by thrombin). This pathway seems to be the physiologically important one in the long-term maintenance of the clot until the wound is healed. The evidence for this sequential activity of the two initial phase pathways is twofold. First, the mechanism of action of TFPI, which inhibits tissue factor activity in the presence of factor Xa but not in its absence, suggests a negative control process. Second, the observation that hemophilia, the most severe of the congenital bleeding disorders, is characterized by prolonged microvascular bleeding shows that the intrinsic activating pathway is essential to long-term clot maintenance. Within this framework of two different ways of activation factor X and a common path for prothrombin activation and fibrinogen clotting, we can now describe the sequence of enzymatic reactions and then their physiological regulation.

The activation of clotting begins with tissue factor. Damage to tissues and their microvasculature exposes blood to subendothelium-associated tissue factor. Tissue factor is a glycoprotein of a molecular weight of 29,600 that is present on the surface of fibroblasts and is also found in tissue stroma and other cells associated with blood vessels throughout the body (36, 37). Released tissue factor binds to factor VII in the plasma, changing the conformation of the factor VII peptide chain in such a way as to enhance its activation by traces of proteases. The enzyme primarily responsible for the cleavage and activation of factor VII-tissue factor is not yet known (38). It has been shown that factors Xa and IXa can activate the factor VII-tissue factor complex, but the source of traces of these activated factors in vivo has not been determined (39, 40). Although some authors have suggested the possibility of autoactivation of factor VII-tissue factor (41), there is also evidence that native factor VII-tissue factor complexes cannot autoactivate factor VII (42). Factor VII is activated by cleavage of a single peptide bond to yield a serine protease that is a very potent activator of both factor IX and factor X. Tissue factor appears to have two roles. First, it binds to factor VII, promoting the activation of factor VII. Phospholipid is required for this association, but it can be a neutral phospholipid. Second, it participates in the assembly of a catalytic complex of factor VIIa and either factor IX or factor X, Ca^{++} ions, and phospholipid, which results in the activation of the factor IX or factor X by factor VIIa (38). In this case, a negatively charged phospholipid is required. The reason for this is that the assembly of the catalytic complex proceeds by the binding of both factor VIIa and the substrate factor (the zymogen form of IX or X) to a phospholipid surface through the Gla domains in the clotting factors and the interpolation of positively charged Ca^{++} ions. In the absence of either phospholipid (or an equivalent surface, such as platelet membranes) or of Ca^{++}, the rate of the reaction is negligible. This is also one of the reactions blocked by the anticoagulant warfarin, which, by antagonizing the action of vitamin K, prevents the formation of the Gla residues in factors VII, IX, and X and prothrombin.

Factor Xa is the enzyme that converts prothrombin to thrombin. The thrombin generated, in turn, cleaves the negatively charged fibrinopeptides from the amino-terminal ends of the α and β chains of fibrinogen to give fibrin monomers that then spontaneously polymerize to form the fibrin clot. The main chain of clotting reactions, then, begins with factor VII binding to tissue factor and proceeds as follows:

$$\text{FVIIa/tissue factor} \rightarrow \text{FXa} \rightarrow \text{thrombin} \rightarrow \text{fibrin}$$

Each step represents a large biological amplification in which each enzyme acts on a substrate with a much higher plasma concentration than the one preceding it in the sequence.

Protein	Concentration (nmol/L)	$t_{1/2}$ (hr)
Factor VII	10	6
Factor X	170	45
Prothrombin	1400	72
Fibrinogen	7000	120

It is interesting that symptomatic factor VII deficiency is rare and that levels even as low as 5% of the normal level usually are not associated with severe bleeding. Why might this be? Probably, because only an exceedingly small amount of activation of factor X by factor VIIa-tissue factor is required to initiate thrombin generation, both because of the great amplification at each step and also, as we will soon see, because once any Xa is formed, it participates in a positive feedback loop involving factors IX and VIII to accelerate and continue factor X activation. Prothrombin deficiency is also not a severe bleeding risk unless the lack of the protein is nearly complete. The reason for this is different; it probably has to do with the large molar excess of prothrombin over the minimum needed and with the explosive generation of thrombin. Under physiological conditions, the conversion of only 10–15% of the prothrombin in plasma provides more than enough thrombin for normal fibrinogen clotting. Factor X deficiency does result in a bleeding disorder, clinically hardly distinguishable from the hemophilias, reflecting its central position in the sequence of reactions. But levels as low as 15–20% of normal may not be associated with abnormal bleeding. On the other hand, not only are the hemophilias, factor VIII deficiency, and factor IX deficiency the most common congenital bleeding disorders, they are the most severe. Levels of either of these factors must be above 25–30% of the normal level to avoid abnormal bleeding. What is the role of factors VIII and IX that there is an absolute requirement for them?

In 1935, Quick applied the prothrombin time, determined by adding a tissue extract (a source of tissue factor and phospholipid) and $CaCl_2$ to citrate plasma, to the study of patients with liver disease and hemophilia. He thus demonstrated that the prothrombin time was normal in hemophilia, indicating the abnormality lay outside the direct tissue factor pathway. In 1952, Biggs et al., making use of their newly developed thromboplastin generation test, showed that patients with hemophilia could be put into two groups: those who had an abnormality of a clotting factor present in plasma but not in serum and those who had an abnormality of a factor active in serum but not in adsorbed plasma (43, 44). The latter deficiency, named Christmas disease, after the surname of the first family in which it was detected, was subsequently named hemophilia B, which is a factor IX deficiency. The more common deficiency, accounting for 70% of cases of hemophilia (hence referred to as hemophilia A) is a deficiency of factor VIII, the factor activity present in normal plasma but missing in serum. For years, it was thought that factor VIII was consumed in clotting, but this is not strictly correct; it is inactivated by activated protein C after thrombin is generated, one of the main control steps of clotting.

Factors IX and VIII function together in one of the enzyme-cofactor-phospholipid-substrate complexes characteristic of clotting reactions to activate factor X. Factor IXa, the serine protease in the complex, cleaves factor X to generate the active protease Xa. Factor VIII is the nonenzymatic cofactor, although slight proteolytic modification by thrombin greatly increases its activity. The complex is illustrated in Figure 6.4, which shows the remarkable similarity to the VIIa-tissue factor and Xa-V complexes, the other proteolytic complexes assembled on a phospholipid surface: the recurring paradigm of clotting reactions.

The importance of factors VIII and IX in normal hemostasis appears to result from the regulation of clotting, namely, that the tissue factor pathway is restricted, by TFPI, to the initial activation of factor X and factor IX. Factor IX can also be activated by activated factor XI. This is a well-characterized reaction that for years was believed to be initiated mostly by the contact phase of activation, beginning with the activation of Hageman factor, factor XII, by negatively charged surfaces such as silica or kaolin. Although these minerals are clearly not normally present in the body, factor XIIa was for a long time the only known activator of factor XI, and it was presumed that some other physiological

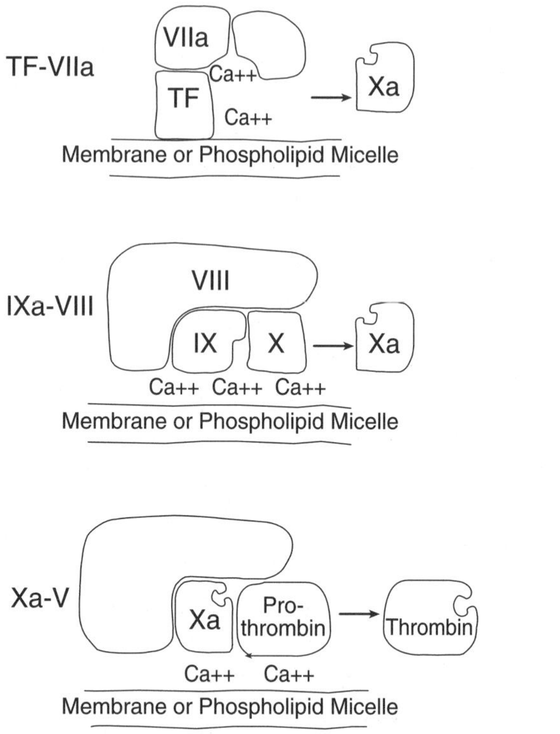

Figure 6.4. Schematic patterns of the main enzymatic complexes that generate the key active proteases, Xa and thrombin. The top two sketches show the two ways of activating factor X, one involving factor VIIa and the other, factor IXa. The lower sketch shows the conversion of prothrombin to thrombin.

activator of factor XII existed to start the contact phase of the intrinsic activation pathway of which the result was the generation of factor IXa. However, factor XII is not required for normal clotting, although contact activation is important in the in vitro assays based on the partial thromboplastin time and, possibly, in cardiopulmonary bypass or other situations in which blood contacts artificial vascular surfaces.

The recent demonstrations that factor XI can be activated by thrombin under physiological conditions provide a key to the in vivo function of the intrinsic pathway (45, 46). They suggest a model in which a small amount of thrombin formed through the initial activation of factor X by the tissue factor pathway in turn activates factor XI. The factor XIa then activates factor IX, which in a complex with factor VIII continues to generate factor Xa and hence additional thrombin generation even after the inactivation of the tissue factor pathway. Thus, the tissue pathway is a rapid, sensitive "trigger" initiating clotting, whereas the intrinsic pathway, driven by positive feedback by the thrombin it generates, is the main path by which additional thrombin is made for the purpose of extending a thrombus or remodeling clots after partial degradation by fibrinolysis. The great importance of continued thrombin generation during the entire 10- to 14-day period of wound healing is shown by the clinical observation that patients with hemophilia must be given factor VIII or factor IX, depending on their deficiency, for this length of time after surgery or they are likely to develop bleeding. In special cases, such as bleeding from tooth sockets, where a clot can be protected and stabilized by blocking fibrinolysis with EACA (ϵ-amino caproic acid) continual maintenance of the clotting factor level is not necessary. However, in the case of skin, muscle, or other soft tissue, where immobilization cannot be achieved, even inhibition of fibrinolysis does not usually suffice to prevent delayed bleeding.

The Middle Phase: Thrombin Generation

Factor Xa, once formed, binds into a complex with its substrate, prothrombin, through the mediation of factor V, another high-molecular-weight cofactor, having structural similarities, as we have seen, to factor VIII. It is likely that the cofactors function to aid assembly of the catalytic complex on the phospholipid surfaces and also to promote the specific binding of the proper substrate to the complex. Prothrombin is activated by Xa by cleavage of two peptide bonds, as mentioned above: Arg_{271}-Thr and Arg_{320}-Ile. Thrombin, the serine protease, is released from the complex (24). Under physiological conditions, the generation of thrombin is represented by an S-shaped curve. There is a lag phase representing the time required for earlier activation steps during which very little thrombin is formed. Then, after the formation of small amounts of thrombin, the positive feedback promoted by the increasing activation of factor XI by thrombin and therefore of factor X by the intrinsic pathway, a rapid burst of thrombin generation takes place so that high local concentrations of thrombin are formed in situ at a wound site. Later, feedback inhibition decreases new thrombin generation by inactivating factors V and VIII and protease inhibitors bind excess proteases; therefore, the reaction reaches a plateau (47).

The Last Phase: Formation of the Fibrin Clot

The final stage of clot formation is the activation of fibrinogen to fibrin monomer, which then polymerizes to form fibrin. The reaction differs from all earlier clotting reactions in four ways: (*a*) it takes place readily in solution and is not enhanced by membrane binding; (*b*) it does not require a high-molecular-weight cofactor; (*c*) although Ca^{++} ions do facilitate fibrin monomer polymerization, Ca^{++} is not required for the enzymatic step; and (*d*) the products of the reaction do not seem to regulate the reaction either positively or negatively. Thrombin cleaves four peptide bonds near the amino-terminal ends of the chains of fibrinogen, one in each of the two α chains (Arg_{18}-Gly) and one in each of the β chains (Arg_{16}-Gly) (48). The fibrinopeptides A and B are released, exposing polymerization sites that then allow the overlapping assembly of fibrin monomers as diagrammed in Figure 6.5 (48). Because of the high local concentrations of thrombin usually formed, the polymerization of fibrin monomer is ordinarily the rate-limiting reaction in vivo. Unless there is inhibition of thrombin (e.g. by heparin or hirudin), this is a function of the plasma concentration of fibrinogen. The normal fibrinogen, 2–2.5 mg/mL, is substantially in excess of the minimum needed for normal clot formation under most conditions. Usually, reasonably normal surgical hemostasis can be expected if the plasma fibrinogen is greater than 1.0–1.2 mg/mL. On the other hand, studies with fibrin glue preparations suggest that clot strength increases with increased Fg concentration even well above the normal range, and it is plausible that the increased Fg concentrations late in pregnancy help decrease bleeding at delivery.

Fibrin polymerization can be inhibited in a number of ways. Certain abnormal fibrinogens polymerize slowly, either because of delayed release of one or the other fibrinopeptide or because of an inherently slower rate of association of fibrin monomer. Probably the most common inhibitors of fibrin monomer polymerization are the high-molecular-weight fibrin degradation products (FDP) that result from partial cleavage of fibrin by the fibrinolytic protease, plasmin.

After fibrin polymers have formed by noncovalent association of fibrin monomers, amide bonds are formed between certain γ-glutamyl groups and ϵ-amino groups of lysines in adjacent chains. The enzyme that carries out this covalent cross-linking of fibrin chains is factor XIII (49). It circulates as a tetrameric protein comprised of two α chains each of 82,000 molecular weight (50) and two β chains, each of 76,000 mo-

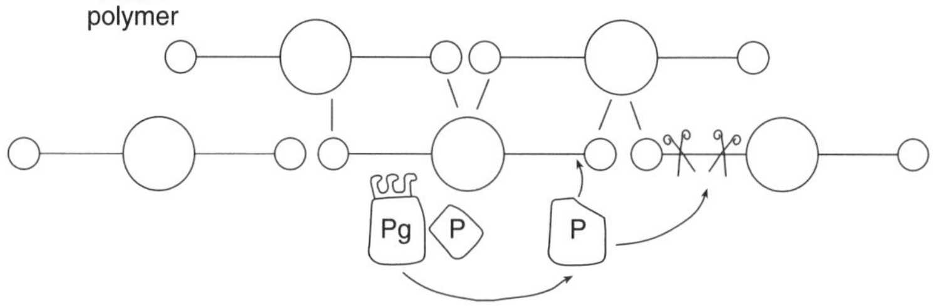

Figure 6.5. The structure of fibrin showing the manner of alignment of fibrin monomer units and indicating the attack by plasmin to cleave fibrin into FDP. Pg, plasminogen; PA, plasminogen activators; P, plasmin. (Redrawn and adapted with permission from Doolittle RF. Fibrinogen and fibrin. Sci Am 1981;45:126–135.)

lecular weight (51). Factor XIII is present in different forms in platelets, monocytes, and macrophages (52). The enzymatic active site for the transamination reaction catalyzed by factor XIII is in the α subunits that are cleaved by thrombin between Arg_{37} and Gly_{38} to give the active transamidase. A deficiency of factor XIII, although not affecting the formation of the fibrin clot, causes a bleeding disorder that can be moderately severe if the deficiency is nearly complete. The congenital deficiency in its symptomatic form is rare. Although early studies of factor XIII deficiency emphasized a pattern of delayed bleeding and poor wound healing, a similar initial cessation of bleeding, followed by delayed bleeding and poor wound healing, is seen in many coagulation factor deficiencies. So, although patients with factor XIII deficiency may have delayed bleeding, it is not pathognomonic of this disorder.

Bleeding from factor XIII deficiency is usually easy to manage. Low levels of the protein, 3–5% of normal, are usually sufficient, and the relatively long factor XIII in plasma of about 10 days (53) makes it possible to treat the deficiency with transfusions of 1–2 units of plasma in an adult.

The sites of cross-links are relatively few, fibrin having only 4–6 cross-links/mol (54). The cross-links give mechanical strength to the clot and provide some hindrance to fibrinolysis. However, plasmin associated with fibrin readily attacks the cross-linked clot.

As the clot is formed, plasmin is activated and begins its dissolution. The third of the physiological systems of hemostasis besides platelet plug formation and fibrin clot generation is fibrinolysis. Like clot formation, fibrinolysis is a finely balanced sequence of proteases regulated both by localization of reactions and by an abundance of inhibitors.

Plasminogen and Plasmin Plasminogen, the proenzyme form of plasmin, is synthesized as a single-chain protein of 92,000 molecular weight. It is present in plasma in a concentration of 2.4 mM and is activated by either of the two human plasminogen activators by cleavage Arg_{560}-Val to give a disulfide-linked two-chain molecule that has the active proteolytic site on the light chain. Lysine binding sites, by which plasmin associates with fibrin, are located in five kringle structures in the heavy chain between positions 83 and 560. The full-length plasminogen molecule has an NH_2-terminal glutamyl residue. Proteolysis at one of several sites removes a short peptide and exposes a new amino-terminal amino acid, methionine, lysine, or valine. These forms are generally all referred to as Lys-plasminogen. Lys-plasmin has both a higher affinity for fibrin and a higher enzymatic specific activity than Glu-plasmin. Activation of plasminogen can occur either directly from Glu-plasminogen or via one of the Lys-plasminogen intermediates.

Plasminogen Activators There are two physiological plasminogen activators: the tissue type (tPA), which is produced mostly by endothelial cells, and urokinase (uPA), originally isolated from urine but present in plasma also, although at about half the concentration of tPA. Of the two, tPA is the main physiological plasminogen activator in hemostasis (55). Although uPA can be activated in plasma and can cause widespread activation of plasminogen, its major locus of action appears to be extracellular, in tissues. uPA is readily bound to cell membranes by GPI-linked uPA receptors and can be active in this form as a cell-associated plasminogen activator, its function presumably being more to keep nonvascular cells free of immobilizing fibrin and to keep small vessels free of adherent clots than to lyse the bulk of a fibrin clot. Recent evidence suggests that specific uPA receptors are important in clearing fibrin from the liver but that uPA alone can keep most tissues clear of fibrin without significant contributions from uPA receptors or, for that matter, from tPA (56).

tPA is synthesized largely by endothelial cells, although also by other cells, notably monocytes/macrophages. It is continually released into plasma where it has a rapid transit, being removed by the liver with a $t_{1/2}$ for disappearance from plasma of about 4 minutes. The plasma concentration is about 5 mg/L (73 pM). Normally, tPA in plasma does not cause plasminogen activation. Not only is the molar concentration less than 10^{-5} that of plasminogen, but tPA also has little affinity for plasminogen in the absence of fibrin. Furthermore, tPA in plasma is rapidly bound to plasminogen activator inhibitor-1 (PAI-1), its major proteolytic inhibitor that is present in about a threefold molar excess over tPA (about 200 pM). Despite the low plasma concentration of tPA, the total daily amount synthesized is substantial, and if the high efficiency of normal hepatic clearance is interrupted, the levels rise rapidly (57). If appreciable fibrin is also present because of physiological hemostasis, the high tPA levels may induce excessive plasminogen activation (58). This appears to be one cause of the hypofibrinogenemia sometimes seen in liver transplantation.

There is diurnal variation in tPA. The level is lowest at night and in the early morning, with a threefold increase during the day to peak levels in the afternoon. PAI-1 shows a pattern that is the inverse of tPA, the lowest levels being in the afternoon and the highest in the early morning, suggesting less variation in its synthesis and that the changes in its plasma levels are related to variations in tPA. A number of factors are known to increase tPA levels significantly, including exercise, vasopressin and vasopressin congeners such as desmopressin (DDAVP), and physiological stress such as surgery, hypotension, hypoxia, and acidosis. Like the release of vWF from endothelial cells, the release of tPA seems to be mediated by β-adrenergic receptors; β-adrenergic drugs increase the levels and the effect is inhibited by β-blockers (59).

tPA has a marked affinity for fibrin. Not only does binding to fibrin give specificity to tPA, but also it enhances the rate at which it activates plasminogen (60). The increase in activation rate is largely the result of the locally high concentrations promoted by the common affinity of tPA and plasminogen for fibrin. As the kringle domains of plasminogen are the sites of its binding to fibrin, so the second kringle domain of tPA is the site of its fibrin binding. Curiously, the first kringle of tPA, although it has considerable homology with the kringles in plasminogen, does not contribute substantially to the binding. In addition to the kringles, tPA has a folded, disulfide-bonded domain from residues 4 to 50, which also participates in binding to fibrinogen.

In contrast to tPA, which is released into plasma by endothelial cells, uPA is prominently associated with cells, although not particularly with endothelial cells. It is made by fibroblasts and monocytes and is found in most tissues, associated with these cells and in interstitial spaces. uPA is synthesized as a single chain molecule (scuPA) having little or no plasminogen-activating activity. It is activated by kallikrein and plasmin (55), resulting in a two-chain form (tcuPA), with no affinity for fibrin but high plasminogen-activating activity. Although its prominent association with cell membranes and its low affinity for fibrin along with a low plasma concentration limit the physiological role of uPA in the normal clearance of small intravascular clots, in the presence of widespread activation of clotting (e.g., in DIC), it can be converted in significant quantities to active tcuPA and may contribute to generalized fibrinogenolysis. It has, however, been shown using transgenic mice that uPA does play a significant role in clearing fibrin from tissues independent of tPA and that the two activators have complementary functions (56).

Fibrinolytic Inhibitors There are two main serine protease inhibitors involved in the control of fibrinolysis: PAI- 1 and α_2-antiplasmin.

PAI-1 is a glycoprotein of 52,000 molecular weight with a plasma concentration estimated at 10–25 μg/L, three to five times the molar concentration of tPA. It inhibits both tPA and tcuPA, binding at the active site of the protease and forming an essentially irreversible stoichiometric complex in typical serine protease inhibitor fashion. It shows little binding to scuPA. tPA bound to PAI-1 is cleared from plasma by the liver as is free tPA. The binding to PAI-1 is limited to soluble tPA. Binding to fibrin protects tPA from inactivation by PAI-1. Thus, the PAI system is designed to limit activation of plasminogen by tPA to fibrin clots while protecting against random activation of plasminogen in solution.

α_2-Antiplasmin is the principal inhibitor of soluble plasmin in the circulation. It is a protein of 70,000 molecular weight having a concentration of 70 mg/L (1 μM). Although the molar concentration is high relative to the free plasmin concentrations to be found in plasma under most circumstances, it is about half the molar concentration of plasminogen. Thus, in the rare instances of generalized activation of plasminogen in severe DIC, it is possible that significant depletion of α_2-antiplasmin may occur. Like other serine protease inhibitors, it forms a 1:1 molar complex with the active protease, irreversibly blocking the active site serine. It has little inhibitory activity against plasmin associated with fibrin.

FIBRINOLYSIS IS ACTIVATED BY CLOTTING AND IS DIRECTED TOWARD CLEARING THROMBI FROM THE MICROVASCULATURE

Normally, in plasma one cannot detect any significant basal fibrinolytic activity. tPA, although possessed of an active proteolytic site, has little affinity for soluble plasminogen, and therefore because of the low plasma concentrations of both, it has virtually no plasminogen-activating effect in the absence of fibrin. scuPA is mostly extravascular in its distribution and associated with cell surfaces. Although it is present in plasma in low concentration, it is an inactive proenzyme until it is activated by kallikrein or plasmin. The major factor in the activation of plasmin seems to be the formation of fibrin polymers to which both plasminogen and tPA bind, causing the enzymatic activation of plasmin. In addition, if kallikrein is generated by the contact phase of clotting, uPA can be converted to the active tcuPA.

The plasmin, formed by whichever means, attacks fibrin in the relatively exposed α-helical regions to form first high-molecular-weight FDP and then, with continued attack, lower molecular weight forms (61). If fibrinogen and fibrin are degraded in the circulation, the higher molecular weight fragments X have one polymerizing site potentially exposed. Having one site, they can bind fibrin monomer, but lacking two, they cannot make polymers. Higher molecular weight FDP are thus inhibitors of clotting. Most FDP also have some affinity for platelets; on binding to platelet membranes, they can interfere with aggregation by interfering with the binding of intact fibrinogen to GPIIb/IIIa.

Hemostatic reactions are limited to areas of vascular injury by spatial localization, feedback control, and plasma inhibitors of activated proteases.

HEMOSTATIC REACTIONS ARE INHERENTLY LOCAL RESPONSES TO INJURY

Both activation of platelets and of coagulation are designed as localized processes. Both are initiated by endothelial injury; they are propagated either directly by cellular interactions (platelet aggregation) or by enzymatic complexes associated with cell surfaces (clotting activation). Probably only in the last stage of clotting—the activation of fibrinogen by thrombin—is a relatively stable serine protease released into solution in large amounts. Even then, it is likely that the diffusion of thrombin is constrained to some degree by its formation within a growing platelet plug. Several anatomical and structural features limit activation to areas of vascular damage:

- Tissue factor is associated with cell membranes;
- Platelet plugs form at the sites of exposure of subendothelial tissues;
- Factor Xa receptors on activated platelets are sites of assembly of prothrombin-activating complexes;
- Platelet activation is irreversible and platelets do not disaggregate and remain functional;
- Plasminogen and tPA bind to fibrin, localizing fibrinolysis.

FEEDBACK INHIBITION CONTROLS THE KEY STEPS OF COAGULATION

Both the main initiating step and the central step in clotting are subject to feedback controls (Table 6.2). The main control sequences involve TFPI, which switches the pathway of factor X activation from tissue factor to the plasma factor XI-IX-VIII system (the "intrinsic"pathway), and thrombomodulin, which binds from thrombin and, through proteins C and S, inactivates factors V and VIII (Fig. 6.3).

The first control step in coagulation is the switching of factor X activation from the tissue pathway to the intrinsic, or blood, pathway. It is unlikely that the effect of this feedback step is the overall limitation of thrombin generation. Rather, by limiting activity of the tissue factor-factor VII complex once some factor Xa is formed, it redirects the process of factor X activation. There must be an advantage of the intrinsic system in extension of clotting or a disadvantage of uncontrolled activation of the tissue factor pathway, perhaps excessive risk of thrombosis. Because individuals with TFPI deficiency have not been reported, the effects of a loss of this inhibitor are not known (35). This inactivation of the tissue factor pathway provides an explanation for the severe bleeding in individuals with hemophilia A or B as the step involving these two proteins becomes the predominant or only means of activating factor X. The ready supply of factors XI, IX, and VIII in plasma normally ensures the maintenance of a clot until the injury is healed. It is easy to see the advantage of this plasma system over the tissue factor system for clot maintenance. How the rapid feedback inhibition of tissue factor is important to the overall process is, as yet, not clear.

After some thrombin is formed, two scavenger systems, thrombomodulin and ATIII, limit its diffusion, preventing excessive activation of additional platelets and clotting of fibrinogen. Thrombomodulin is a membrane glycoprotein mainly associated with vascular endothelium. The molecule contains 575 amino acids. After thrombin binds to thrombomodulin, it is unavailable for clotting fibrinogen, activating platelets, or activating factors V, VIII, and XIII. Thrombomodulin has a further regulatory role; the thrombomodulin-thrombin complex is a potent activator of protein C, a plasma protein that, in its active form, is a major regulator of the extent of thrombin generation as it inactivates factors V and VIII, the essential high-molecular-weight cofactors, respectively, for the generation of activated factor X and thrombin. Protein C can be activated by thrombin alone in solution, but the thrombin-thrombomodulin complex activates protein C 20,000-fold faster (62). That the activated protein C pathway is an important control step is demonstrated by the discovery of a rather common mutation in the factor V gene that makes factor V resistant to the proteolytic effect of activated protein C and consequently increases the risk of deep-vein thrombosis (63–65). The G1691A substitution has a frequency of about 3% in North American and European populations studied and accounts for up to 40% of the patients with recurrent familial venous thrombosis. The frequency of heterozygotes is 6% of the population; even heterozygosity for the guanosine mutation increases the risk of deep vein thrombosis two- to threefold over that for individuals having adenosine at position 1691.

In addition to the feedback control mechanisms, plasma contains ATIII in relatively high concentration. This protein,

TABLE 6.2. REGULATORS AND INHIBITORS OF CLOTTING

Protein	Action
Tissue factor (TF) pathway inhibitor	Limits VIIa-TF to early activation by inactivating it once some Xa is formed
Thrombomodulin	Binds thrombin; inhibits its fibrinogen-clotting activity; converts it to a protein C activator
Protein C	Activated protein C (APC) inactivates V and VIII, resulting in feedback control of thrombin generation
Protein S	Acts as a cofactor with APC
Antithrombin III	Binds and inhibits proteases: thrombin, IXa, Xa, XIa; controls rate of thrombin generation; limits clotting to sites of vascular damage
Plasmin	Cleaves fibrin to FDP

the so-called heparin cofactor, binds and inactivates thrombin. In the absence of heparin or cell-associated heparin sulfates, the kinetics of the reaction are slow. Heparin greatly accelerates the binding by causing a conformational change in the ATIII molecule. But because the plasma concentration is high, ATIII plays a role in keeping stray thrombin out of the circulation. Normally, these control mechanisms are effective in localizing thrombus formation to an area of microvascular injury where a clot is required. Occasionally, however, the controls can be overwhelmed, either by rapid, widespread activation of clotting and excessive generation of thrombin or by excessive generation of plasminogen, perhaps by action of kallikrein on uPA or else simply as a secondary effect of thrombin formation.

WOUND HEALING

Disorders of hemostasis are characterized not only by prolonged bleeding, but also by slow wound healing. Although the formation of wound hematomas and the greater risk of infections that accompany hematomas play a role in poor wound healing, evidence is accumulating that the hemostatic mechanisms are also the primary initiators of wound healing.

Wound healing is generally considered under three broad stages: attraction and migration of monocytes and neutrophils to an injured area over the first 1–3 days; activation by cytokines of macrophages and fibroblasts leading to synthesis of collagen and other extracellular matrix materials and to proliferation of fibroblasts, a process of 14–21 days; and the longer term remodeling and consolidation of new collagen and other tissue constituents over a period of months. Hemostasis reactions, particularly platelet plug formation, play a primary role in initiating the first stage and perhaps the second (66).

Activated platelets initiate wound healing and angiogenesis by the release of growth factors and chemotactic factors from their alpha granules. Of the many alpha granule proteins, the following are so far known to exert significant effects. Platelet factor 4 is chemotactic for neutrophils and even more so for fibroblasts (67). It is a major component of the alpha granule protein pool that is released in large quantities immediately on activation and aggregation of platelets. Platelet-derived growth factor is a 30,000 molecular weight growth factor that has been the most-studied platelet cytokine. It has a number of functions critical to wound healing and seems to play the central role in initiating wound healing. It is strongly chemotactic for monocytes and neutrophils but also attracts fibroblasts and smooth muscle cells. It stimulates the proliferation of smooth muscle cells, activates neutrophils and monocytes, and also is an inducer of transcription of certain genes of the small inducible gene family that seem likely to further promote wound repair (66). Two other alpha granule proteins, β-thromboglobulin and transforming growth factor-β are chemoattractants for fibroblasts (67). Transforming growth factor-β also stimulates procollagen type I synthesis in fibroblasts (68).

So far the role of activated platelets has been the most studied, and it appears that the platelet plug initiates most of the early mobilization of both inflammatory cells and fibroblasts to begin wound repair. But there may be additional stimuli contributed by coagulation reactions. Thrombin, for example, is mitogenic in vitro for fibroblasts, macrophages, and smooth muscle cells, a reaction dependent on specific cell surface thrombin receptors. Urokinase bound to cell membranes has been shown to be mitogenic for epidermal cells (69). In addition to these preliminary findings that indicate important links between hemostasis and wound healing, there may be other mechanisms. For example, poor wound healing has often been mentioned in patients with factor XIII deficiency, a bleeding disorder resulting in failure of fibrin cross-linking in which platelet function, thrombin generation, and fibrinolysis are all normal.

CHANGES IN HEMOSTASIS IN SURGICAL PATIENTS

The surgeon should be aware of several common and predictable alterations in components of the hemostasis system that are seen in patients undergoing surgery. In patients suffering injuries or undergoing surgery, one finds significant increases in the release into plasma of factor VIII and vWF (70, 71). These proteins are noncovalently associated in plasma and presumably on endothelial cells, from which a pool approximately equal to the circulating pool can be released by β-adrenergic stimulation or, indirectly, by DDAVP. Thus, surgical patients usually have factor VIII and vWF levels about twice their preoperative level, and it is very rare that they develop significant deficiencies of either proteins unless they have a preexisting deficiency.

The levels of fibrinogen and various components of the fibrinolytic system also increase with injury, although consumption of fibrinogen by clotting with widespread trauma, or even DIC, can reduce the circulating level. Significantly low levels of fibrinogen are more often seen than low levels of factor VIII, and it is likely that the compensatory mechanisms are more effective for the latter.

Postoperatively, in uncomplicated cases, one may expect to see increased fibrinogen, factor VIII, vWF, and shortened clot lysis times indicative of increased fibrinolytic activity. These changes slowly return to preoperative levels over 1–3 weeks. They all have some physiological significance as seen by the high risk of venous thrombosis postoperatively in bedridden patients. The balance between increased procoagulant factors (to provide for control of bleeding until vascular healing is complete) and fibrinolysis (to clear fibrin from occluded vessels and protect against excessive thrombosis) is, even in normal individuals, a delicate one. In elderly patients or in patients in any way predisposed to venous thrombosis, the normally protective hemostatic mechanisms can become a threat.

REFERENCES

1. Vane JR, Anggard EE, Botting RM. Regulatory functions of the vascular endothelium. N Engl J Med 1990;323:27–36.
2. Roth GJ, Majerus PW. The mechanism of the effect of aspirin on human platelets. I. Acetylation of a particulate fraction protein. J Clin Invest 1975;56:624–632.
3. Radomski MW, Palmer RM, Moncada S. The anti-aggregating properties of vascular endothelium: interactions between prostacyclin and nitric oxide. Br J Pharmacol 1987;92:639–646.
4. Ruggeri ZM. The platelet glycoprotein Ib-IX complex. Prog Hemost Thromb 1991;10:35–68.
5. Saelman EUM, Nieuwenhuis HK, Hese KM, et al. Platelet adhesion to collagen types I through VIII under conditions of stasis and flow is mediated by GPIa/IIa (a2B1-Integrin). Blood 1994;83:1244–1250.
6. Clapham DE. The G-protein nanomachine. Nature 1996;379:297–299.
7. Philips DR, Charo IF, Scarborough RM. GPIIb-IIIa: the responsive integrin. Cell 1991;65:359–362.
8. Belamarich FA. Hemostasis in animals other than mammals: the role of cells. New York: Grune and Stratton, 1976:191–209.
9. Lok S, Kaushansky K, Holly RD, et al. Cloning and expression of murine thrombopoietin cDNA and stimulation of platelet production in vivo. Nature 1994;369:565–568.
10. Kaushansky K, Lok S, Holly RD, et al. Promotion of megakaryocyte progenitor expansion and differentiation by c-Mpl ligand thrombopoietin. Nature 1994;369:568–571.
11. Kaushansky K. Thrombopoietin: the primary regulator of platelet production. Blood 1995;86:419–431.
12. Lopez JA, Chung DW, Fujikawa K. The alpha and beta chains of human platelet glycoprotein Ib are both transmembrane proteins containing a leucine-rich amino acid sequence. Proc Natl Acad Sci USA 1988; 85:2135.
13. Hickey MJ, Williams SA, Roth GJ. Human platelet glycoprotein IX: an adhesive prototype of leucine-rich glycoproteins with flank-center-flank structures. Proc Natl Acad Sci USA 1989;86:6773.
14. Nurden AT, Caen JP. Specific roles for platelet surface glycoproteins in platelet function. Nature 1975;255:720.
15. Nurden AT, Caen JP. An abnormal glycoprotein pattern in three cases in Ganzmann's thrombasthenia. Br J Haemotol 1974;28:253–260.
16. Phillips DR, Agin PP. Platelet membrane defects in Glanzmann's thrombasthenia. Evidence for decreased amounts of two major glycoproteins. J Clin Invest 1977;60:535–545.
17. Shulman NR, Jordan JV. A fixed-loss component of platelet utilization accounting for short survival of transfused platelets. Clin Res 1981;29: 572A.
18. Hanson SR, Slichter SJ. Platelet kinetics in patients with bone marrow hypoplasia: evidence for a fixed platelet requirement. Blood 1985;66: 1105–1109.
19. Beutler E. Platelet transfusions: the 20,000/μL trigger. Blood 1993; 81:1411–1413.
20. Ware JA, Coller BS. Platelet morphology, biochemistry, and function. In: Beutler E, Lichtman MA, Coller BS, Kipps TJ, eds. Williams hematology. New York: McGraw-Hill, 1995:161–1201.
21. Brass LF, Manning DR, Shattil SJ. GTP-binding proteins and platelet activation. Philadelphia: WB Saunders, 1991:127–174.
22. Hawiger J, Kloczewiak M, Bednarek MA, Timmons S. Platelet receptor recognition domains on the alpha chain of human fibrinogen: structure-function analysis. Biochemistry 1989;28:2909–2914.
23. Farrell DA, Thiagarajan P, Chung DW, Davie EW. Role of fibrinogen alpha and gamma sites in platelet aggregation. Proc Natl Acad Sci USA 1992;89:10729–10732.
24. Mann KF, Neshiem ME, Church WR, Haley R, Krishnaswamy S. Surface-dependent reactions of the vitamin K-dependent enzyme complexes. Blood 1990;76:1–16.
25. Davie EW, Fujikawa K, Kisiel W. The coagulation cascade: initiation, maintenance, and regulation. Biochemistry 1991;30:10363–10370.
26. Stenflo J, Fernlund P, Egan W, Roepstorff P. Vitamin K dependent modification of glutamic acid residues in prothrombin. Proc Natl Acad Sci USA 1974;71:2730–2733.
27. Esmon CT, Suttie JW. Vitamin K-dependent carboxylase. Solubilization and properties. J Biol Chem 1976;251:6238–6243.
28. Magnusson S, Petersen TE, Sottrup-Jensen L, Claeys H. Complete primary structure of prothrombin: isolation, structure and reactivity of ten carboxylated glutamic acid residues and regulation of prothrombin activation by thrombin. In: Reich E, Rifkin DB, Shaw E, eds. Proteases and biological control. Cold Spring Harbor, NY: Cold Spring Harbor Laboratory, 1975:123–149.
29. Counts RB, Paskell SL, Elgee SK. Disulfide bonds and the quaternary structure of factor VIII/von Willebrand factor. J Clin Invest 1978;62: 702–709.
30. Hall CE, Slayter HS. The fibrinogen molecule: its size, shape, and mode of polymerization. J Biophys Biochem Cytol 1959;5:11–15.
31. Morawitz P. Beitraege zur Kenntnis der Blutgerinnung. Deutsch Arch Klin Med 1904;79:1–28.
32. Howell WH. The nature and action of the thromboplastic (zymoplastic) substance of the tissues. Am J Physiol 1912;31:1–31.
33. Davie EW, Ratnoff OD. Waterfall sequence for intrinsic blood clotting. Science [A]145:1310–1312, 1964.
34. Macfarlane RG. An enzyme cascade in the blood clotting mechanism, and its function as a biochemical amplifier. Nature 1964;202:498–499.
35. Broze GJ. Tissue factor pathway inhibitor and the revised theory of coagulation. Annu Rev Med 1995;46:103–112.
36. Nemerson Y. Tissue factor and hemostasis. Blood 1988;71:1–8.
37. Eddleston M, De La Torre JC, Oldstone MB, Loskutoff DJ, Edgington TS, Mackman N. Astrocytes are the primary source of tissue factor in the murine central nervous system. J Clin Invest 1993;92:349–358.
38. Rapaport SI, Rao LVM. The tissue factor pathway: how it has become a "prima ballerina." Thromb Haemost 1995;74:7–17.
39. Rao LVM, Rapaport SI. Activation of factor VII bound to tissue factor: a key early step in the tissue factor pathway of blood coagulation. Proc Natl Acad Sci USA 1988;85:6687–6691.
40. Eichinger S, Mannucci PM, Tradati F, Arbini AA, Rosenberg RD, Bauer KA. Determinants of plasma factor VIIa levels in humans. Blood 1995;86:3021–3025.

41. Nakagaki T, Foster DC, Berkner KL, Kisel W. Initiation of the extrinsic pathway of blood coagulation: evidence for the tissue factor dependent autoactivation of human coagulation factor VII. Biochemistry 1991;30:10819–10824.
42. Rao LVM, Rapaport SI, Bajaj SP. Activation of human factor VII in the initiation of tissue factor-dependent coagulation. Blood 1986;68:685–691.
43. Biggs R, Douglas AS. The thromboplastin generation test. J Clin Pathol 1953;6:23.
44. Biggs R, Douglas AS, Macfarlane RG, et al. Christmas disease: a condition previously mistaken for haemophilia. Br Med J 1952;2:1378.
45. Naito K, Fujikawa K. Activation of human blood coagulation factor XI independent of factor XII: factor XI is activated by thrombin and factor XIa in the presence of negatively charged surfaces. J Biol Chem 1991;266:7353–7358.
46. Gailane D, Broze GJ. Factor XI activation in a revised model of blood coagulation. Science 1991;253:909–912.
47. Beltrami E, Jesty J. Mathematical analysis of activation thresholds in enzyme-catalyzed positive feedbacks: application to the feedbacks of blood coagulation. Proc Natl Acad Sci USA 1995;92:8744–8748.
48. Doolittle RF. Fibrinogen and fibrin. Sci Am 1981;45:126–135.
49. Lorand L, Losowsky MS, Miloszewsky KJM. Human factor XIII: fibrin stabilizing factor. Prog Hemost Thromb 1980;5:245–290.
50. Ichinose A, Davie EW. Characterization of the gene for the α subunit of human factor XIII (plasma transglutaminase), a blood coagulation factor. Proc Natl Acad Sci USA 1988;85:5829–5833.
51. Bottenus RE, Ichinose A, Davie EW. Nucleotide sequence of the gene for the β subunit of human factor XIII. Biochemistry 1990;29:11195–11209.
52. Henriksson P, Backer S, Lynch G, McDonagh J. Identification of intracellular factor XIII in human monocytes and macrophages. J Clin Invest 1985;76:528–534.
53. Fear JD, Miloszewski KJM, Losowsky, MS. The half life of factor XIII in the management of inherited deficiency. Thromb Haemost 1983;49:102.
54. Chen R, Doolittle RF. Crosslinking sites in human and bovine fibrin. Biochemistry 1971;10:4486.
55. Vassalle JD, Sappino AP, Belin D. The plasminogen activator/plasmin system. J Clin Invest 1991;88:1067–1072.
56. Bugge TH, Flick MJ, Danton MJS, et al. Urokinase-type plasminogen activator is effective in fibrin clearance in the absence of its receptor or tissue-type plasminogen activator. Proc Natl Acad Sci USA 1996;93: 5899–5904.
57. Fuchs, HE, Berger H, Pizzo SV. Catabolism of human tissue plasminogen activator in mice. Blood 1985;65:539–544.
58. Dzik WH, Arkin CF, Jenkins RL, Stump DC. Fibrinolysis during liver transplantation in humans: role of tissue type plasminogen activator. Blood 1988;71:1090–1095.
59. Winther K. The effect of beta-blockade on platelet function and fibrinolytic activity. J Cardiovasc Pharmacol 1987;10:594.
60. Hoylaerts M, Rijken DC, Lijnen HR, Collen D. Kinetics of the activation of plasminogen by human tissue plasminogen activator. Role of fibrin. J Biol Chem 1982;257:2912.
61. Marder VJ, Shulman NR, Carroll WR. High molecular weight derivatives of human fibrinogen produced by plasmin. J Biol Chem 1969;244: 2111–2119.
62. Clouse LH, Comp PC. The regulation of hemostasis: the protein C system. N Engl J Med 1986;314:1298–1304.
63. Bertina RM, Koeleman BPC, Koster T, et al. Mutation in blood coagulation factor V associated with resistance to activated protein C. Nature 1994;369:64–67.
64. Voorberg J, Roelse J, Koopman R, et al. Association of idiopathic venous thromboembolism with single point mutation of Arg 506 of factor V. Lancet 1994;343:1535–1536.
65. De Stefano V, Finazzi G, Mannucci PM. Inherited thrombophilia: pathogenesis, clinical syndromes, and management. Blood 1996;87: 3531–3544.
66. Deuel TF, Kawahara RS, Mustoe TA, Pierce GF. Growth factors and wound healing: platelet-derived growth factor as a model cytokine. Annu Rev Med 1991;42:567–584.
67. Senior RM, Griffin GL, Huang JS, Walz DA, Deuel TF. Chemotactic activity of platelet alpha granule proteins for fibroblasts. J Cell Biol 1983;96:382–385.
68. Ignotz RA, Massague J. Transforming growth factor-beta stimulates the expression of fibronectin and collagen and their incorporation into the extracellular matrix. J Biol Chem 1986;261:4337–4345.
69. Altieri DC. Coagulation assembly on leukocytes in transmembrane signaling and cell adhesion. Blood 1993;81:569–579.
70. Counts RB, Haisch C, Simon TL, Maxwell NG, Heimbach DM, Carrico CJ. Hemostasis in massively transfused trauma patients. Ann Surg 1979;190:91–99.
71. Wall RT, Counts RB, Harker LA, Stryker GE. Binding and release of factor VIII/von Willebrand's factor by human endothelial cells. Br J Haematol 1980;46:287–298.

Chapter 7

Infectious Risks of Transfusion

MARK A. WARNER

INTRODUCTION

Few areas in clinical anesthesia and surgery have changed as much in the past 10 years as transfusion practices. For example, indications for the perioperative transfusion of blood and blood products are more restrictive now than a decade ago, preoperative autologous blood donation is common, and the use of perioperative red blood cell (RBC) salvage techniques continues to expand. Clearly, these changes have been prompted by constraints on the blood supply and widespread concerns of transfusion-induced disease.

The limit on the blood supply is generated simply by supply and demand. Despite restricted transfusion indications, the total number of persons with disease processes or undergoing procedures associated with an increased probability of transfusion is growing (1). Concomitantly, donations have decreased because of restrictions placed on donor eligibility and infectious screening processes that eliminate potentially contaminated blood units. The aging population of the United States is particularly important; the elderly donate less and receive more blood products than other adult segments of the population.

Although transfusion-induced disease was well known to the medical community five decades before 1983, the infectious and immunological risks of blood transfusions generated only low levels of interest there and in the general populace until the epidemiological link of the acquired immunodeficiency syndrome (AIDS) to transfused blood and blood products in that year. The transition was abrupt; physicians, provided with evidence of the infective risks of transfusion and swept by a wave of public concern for safety, responded rapidly by altering transfusion practices. Blood banking programs, supported by major advances in detection of infectious agents and the identification of associated markers, were soon able to provide and document a very safe supply of blood and blood products.

The recent changes in perioperative transfusion practices have been made to decrease demand and limit exposure of patients to blood and blood products. To guide these changes, multiple studies and national consensus conferences (e.g., the 1988 National Institutes of Health Consensus Conference on Perioperative Red Cell Transfusion [2]) have made recommendations for appropriate uses of blood and blood products. Are these recommendations uniformly accepted or applied? In 1990, Salem-Schatz et al. (1) surveyed 122 general surgeons, orthopedic surgeons, and anesthesiologists to evaluate the influence of several clinical and nonclinical factors on perioperative transfusion decision making. They found widespread deficiencies in physicians' knowledge of transfusion risks and indications. In particular, the more years of practice of the physician, the lower the knowledge score and the greater frequency of ordering blood products inappropriately. Two conclusions were drawn: there is a need to provide practicing physicians with updates of rapidly changing estimates of transfusion risks and involvement of respected colleagues plays an important role in encouraging older physicians to be receptive to new information and to consider modifying their transfusion practices. Unfortunately, no resurvey of this group has been performed to determine whether perioperative transfusion practices have changed. Because many transfusion decision-making processes are made in the perioperative period, surgeons and anesthesiologists must keep abreast of current practices and perspectives in this rapidly progressing field.

This chapter describes the infectious risks related to the transfusion of blood and blood products. The risk of infectious agent transmission of selected agents has been recently estimated by Etchason et al. (3) and is shown in Table 7.1. In addition, the infectious risks of autologous blood are considered.

TABLE 7.1. ESTIMATED RISK OF INFECTIOUS AGENT TRANSMISSION

Variable	Estimate
Probability of infection (per allogeneic unit)	
Hepatitis C virus	0.0003
Hepatitis B virus	0.000005
HIV	0.0000067
HTLV-I and HTLV-II	0.000017
Probability of disease[a]	
Hepatitis C virus	
Persistent hepatitis	0.28
Active hepatitis	0.12
Cirrhosis	0.10
Fulminant hepatitis	0.01
Hepatitis B virus	
Carrier status	0.04
Persistent hepatitis	0.02
Active hepatitis	0.01
Cirrhosis or cancer	0.01
HIV	
AIDS	1.0
HTLV-I and HTLV-II	
ATL or HAM	0.04
Quality adjustments for various health states	
Persistent hepatitis	0.99
Active hepatitis	0.90
Cirrhosis or cancer	0.90
Fulminant hepatitis	0
HIV infection	0.75
AIDS	0.50
ATL or HAM	0.90

Reprinted with permission from Etchason J, et al. The cost effectiveness of preoperative autologous blood donations. N Engl J Med 1995;332:19–724.
[a]Per unit of infected blood transfused.
ATL, adult T-cell lymphoma; HAM, HTLV-associated myelopathy.

DISEASE TRANSMISSION

The risk of infectious complications was recognized with the increasing use of homologous blood and blood products in the 1930s. Transfusion-associated hepatitis, marked by jaundice, was reported in 1943. Since then, many infective agents, including bacteria, spirochetes, parasites, and viruses, have been identified as being associated with transfusion-transmitted disease.

BACTERIA

Blood and blood products, homologous or autologous, may be contaminated with microorganisms. Various microorganisms, both pathogenic and nonpathogenic, can be cultured in up to 5% of collection systems and blood products. This number may be artificially inflated because of contamination occurring during the culturing process. A more likely estimate is 1–2%, a figure that corresponds to the rate of positive blood cultures obtained from healthy adults (4). In general, bacterial contamination of blood occurs from either a break in sterile technique during collection and processing of blood, bacteria in sweat glands, hair follicles, and other protected sites or unsuspected bacteremia in donors.

Avoidable sources for blood product contamination can include inadequate skin preparation, poor venipuncture technique, coring of a small piece of tissue by the needle, defects in the plastic collection bags, and inadequate sterilization of collection equipment. The first two account for most contaminated units and are the presumed source for many of the Gram-negative organisms associated with severe bacterial transfusion reactions (5, 6). The use of modern collection systems and strict standards for skin preparation, collection, and storage of blood products has reduced, but not eliminated, the risk of bacterial contamination.

Unsuspected transient bacteremia often occurs after normal activities or minor trauma to mucosal membranes in healthy adults (4, 7). In most cases, the bacteria are cleared from the blood within 30 minutes (7, 8). Because bacteremia may be a part of acute or subacute infections, the American Association of Blood Banks (AABB) recommends that persons with oral temperatures greater than 38°C should defer from donating.

Although 1–2% of donated blood units may contain bacteria, there is a very low risk of nonfatal or fatal transfusion reactions. In general, the number of bacteria present in donated blood is small. In 38 contaminated units, Braude et al. (9) found only 1 that contained greater than 14 bacteria/mL. Viable white blood cells, complement, opsonins and various plasma components in fresh donated blood can eliminate small loads of bacteria, particularly those that are Gram positive. Approximately 75% of culturable contaminants from freshly collected blood are Gram-positive organisms (e.g., *Staphylococci* and *Streptococci*). In addition, these organisms cannot survive refrigerator temperatures of 4°C for more than a few days (10).

Although Gram-negative bacteria contaminate donated blood units less frequently than Gram-positive organisms, their presence is more often associated with serious transfusion reactions. Many Gram-negative bacteria, particularly bacilli, produce potent endotoxins. In addition, some strains are psychrophilic and able to proliferate at refrigerator temperatures (10, 11). The growth rates of psychrophilic bacteria are slowed but not stopped by cold temperatures (Fig. 7.1). The longer the storage period, the greater the number of organisms and amount of endotoxin present (12).

Improvements in blood preservatives have extended the shelf-life of RBCs. Prolonged storage periods of RBCs contaminated with the enteric pathogen *Yersinia enterocolitica* have been associated recently with 15 cases of severe endotoxic shock, including persistent hypotension, renal failure, and disseminated intravascular coagulopathy (13). In all cases, blood contamination resulted from asymptomatic *Y. enterocolitica* bacteremia in the blood donors at the time of donation. *Y. enterocolitica* most often presents as a self-limited acute bacterial gastroenteritis. Most of these donors had symptoms of gastroenteritis within 2 months of donation. Potential measures to prevent endotoxic shock from Gram-negative psychrophilic bacteria include screening blood donors for a recent history of gastroenteritis, reducing the shelf-life of RBCs, and testing RBC units at least 25 days old for endotoxin or the presence of bacterial organisms. Screening asymptomatic donors would probably not be effective, because such a program could result in the exclusion of 1–13% of the current donor population (13). Reducing the shelf-life of RBCs to 25 days would decrease blood availability at many centers. Preliminary studies suggest that screening of blood units at least 25 days old with acridine-orange, Wright, or Wright-Giemsa stains may be effective in detecting units of blood with low levels of *Y. enterocolitica* (Centers for Disease Control and Prevention, unpublished data).

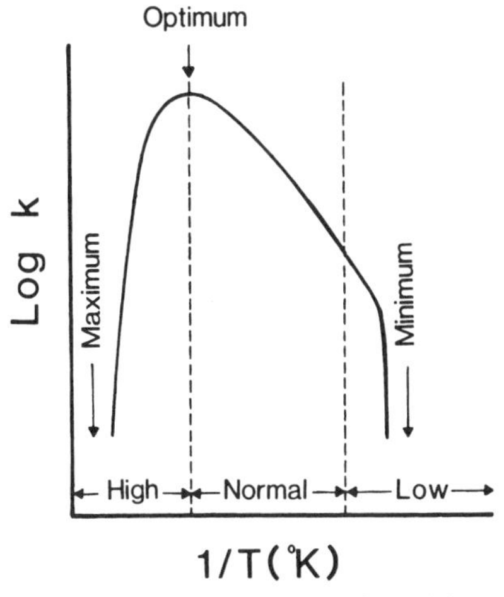

Figure 7.1. The influence of temperature on bacterial growth rate. The log of the bacterial growth rate (k) declines from its optimum peak as the temperature (in degrees Kelvin) decreases. The cardinal temperatures (maximum, optimum, and minimum for growth) and the growth temperature ranges (high, normal, and low) are shown. Although the growth rate of psychrophilic bacteria decreases at low-normal (e.g., refrigerator) temperatures, replication continues. (Reprinted with permission from Hamill TR. The 30-minute rule for reissuing blood: are we needlessly discarding units? Transfusion 1990;30:58–62, published by the American Association of Blood Banks.)

Since November 1975, the U.S. Food and Drug Administration (FDA) has required that all registered blood establishments report deaths associated with blood collection or transfusion and with plasmapheresis. Of 355 transfusion-associated deaths from 1976 through 1985, 26 (7.3%) were caused by transfusion of bacterially contaminated blood product units (14). The implicated blood products and bacterial contaminants were evenly distributed (Table 7.2).

Although there are many drawbacks to the FDA reporting system, patterns of unusual events that need immediate attention can be noted. For example, in 1981 new techniques and plastic bags made it possible to store platelets at room temperature for up to 5 days (15). This technique greatly increased the supply and availability of pooled platelets. Further refinement of platelet storage in 1984 extended the shelf-life of platelet storage at room temperature to 7 days. This improvement was not without risk; bacteria in contaminated platelet units can proliferate rapidly at room temperature. From 1980 to 1983, there were nine reported transfusion-associated deaths from sepsis in the United States (16). Six of these occurred in patients who received platelets stored at room temperature for greater than 3 days. *Salmonella* and *Staphylococcus* species were the contaminating organisms. The reporting mechanism led to an FDA bulletin that reduced the maximum platelet storage period to 5 days and alerted readers to this potentially fatal problem.

SPIROCHETES

Spirochetes, specifically *Treponema pallidum,* have a limited ability to survive at refrigerator temperatures (4°C) (17). Infectivity and survival time of treponemas stored at refrigerator temperatures is less than 120 hours. The only blood product not stored at refrigerator temperature is platelet concentrate (stored at room temperature, 20–25°C), and it is this blood product that has the greatest theoretical risk of treponemal transmission. Yet in the past 25 years, only two cases of posttransfusion syphilis have been reported (18, 19). Both occurred after transfusion of fresh platelet concentrate prepared from blood donors whose Venereal Disease Research Laboratories (VDRL) tests were negative. *T. pallidum* seropositivity usually occurs 4–6 weeks after the initial infection. Therefore, a "window" of seronegative infectivity is present, and susceptible blood product recipients may become infected. In recent years, the demand for fresh blood products, especially platelets, has increased, but this in-

TABLE 7.2. DEATHS FROM BACTERIAL OR PROTOZOAN CONTAMINATION OF BLOOD COMPONENTS: 1976–1985 (n = 26)

Red cells or Whole Blood		Platelets		Cryoprecipitate	
Gram-negative organisms					
Pseudomonas aeruginosa	2	*Klebsiella* sp.	3	*Pseudomonas cepacia*	1
Yersinia enterocolitica	2	*Salmonella* sp., type B	1		
Enterobacter cloacae	1	*Proteus mirabilis*	1		
		Serratia sp. + *Staphylococcus* sp.	1		
Gram-positive organisms					
Staphylococcus aureus	1	*Staphylococcus epidermidis*	3		
+ enterococci		*Bacillus* sp.	2		
Clostridium perfringens	1	*S. aureus*	1		
Proprionibacterium acnes	1	Gram-positive cocci	1		
Protozoa					
Plasmodium sp.	1				

Reprinted with permission from Sazama K. Reports of 355 transfusion-associated deaths: 1976 through 1985. Transfusion 1990;30:583–590, published by the American Association of blood banks.

creased use has not been paralleled by an increased number of posttransfusion syphilis cases. This lack of infectivity, despite the existing window of seronegativity and increasing prevalence of syphilis in general, may be associated with the near-universal use of antibiotics in patients who receive platelets and storage of platelets at room temperature in aerobic conditions. *T. pallidum* requires an anaerobic atmosphere, and its viability decreases quickly in the presence of oxygen (20).

For years, serological tests for syphilis have been routinely performed on donated blood. These screening tests include cardiolipin antigen (VDRL) and *T. pallidum* hemagglutination assay. After screening, the seropositivity of blood is confirmed with a fluorescent treponemal antibody-absorption test. Because syphilis is so rarely transmitted, the efficacy of routine testing in industrialized nations has been questioned (21). The FDA still requires this testing, however, because individuals with this venereal disease may also be at higher risk for concomitant human immunodeficiency virus (HIV) infection. Transmission by transfusion of other spirochetes, including the tropical treponemal diseases of yaws and pinta and also Lyme disease, has not been reported (22).

PARASITES

Parasites that infect humans often spend part of their life cycles in blood and may, therefore, be transmittable to the recipient of a donated blood product. Many parasites have been implicated in transfusion-associated infection, including malaria, Chagas' disease, babesiosis, toxoplasmosis, filariasis, and kala-azar. In general, major morbidity or mortality from transfusion-associated parasitic infection is rare. Most parasitic endemic areas are located in underdeveloped countries. In these countries, the prevalence of the parasitic disease is high, and many transfusion recipients already have immunity to the parasite.

There is concern, however, for the importation of these diseases to developed countries and its effect on transfusion practices. In endemic areas and worldwide, transmission of malaria is the most common infectious agent carried with blood transfusions. For example, the prevalence of malaria in Great Britain increased exponentially in the 1970s (23). As the prevalence increases, so does the risk of infection from homologous blood products. In the United States from 1972 to 1981, there were 26 blood product recipients who developed malaria; of these, 4 died (24). Because very few organisms are required to transmit malaria, most blood products have been implicated. Yet, because the number of cases in the United States is sufficiently small and predonation interview techniques eliminate almost all potential donors with previous infection or those who have traveled to endemic areas, there is no routine testing of donor blood for *Plasmodium* species.

Chagas' disease, caused by *Trypanosoma cruzi,* is transmissible by transfusion and is endemic in many areas in Central and South America. In some rural areas of Argentina and Brazil, nearly a quarter of blood donors are seropositive for *T. cruzi* (25). Transfusion of seropositive blood does not always result in transmission of infection, but serological screening of donated blood is worthwhile. In addition, gentian violet, which kills the organism within 24 hours, is routinely added to blood in some endemic areas. Chagas' disease is not an immediate threat to the blood supply of the United States, but an influx of immigrants from Central and South America may increase the risk of seropositive blood being donated. Screening procedures in areas with large immigrant populations from endemic areas may need to be reassessed periodically.

Babesiosis is worthy of mention because of its presence in the heavily populated areas of the northeast United States, particularly southeastern Massachusetts, its islands, and rural Long Island (26). It is a parasitic disease associated with fever, fatigue, and hemolytic anemia. The parasite is *Babesia microtia,* a protozoan that dwells in RBCs and is transmitted to humans from nymphal ticks carried by woodland rodents and white tail deer (27). Babesiosis has been transmitted by both platelet and RBC transfusions (28). Posttransfusion babesiosis is most likely to occur in elderly immunocompromised patients or asplenic blood recipients. The serious complications of babesiosis are those associated with hemolytic anemia. Fortunately, it is a rare problem, and routine donor screening is not warranted (29).

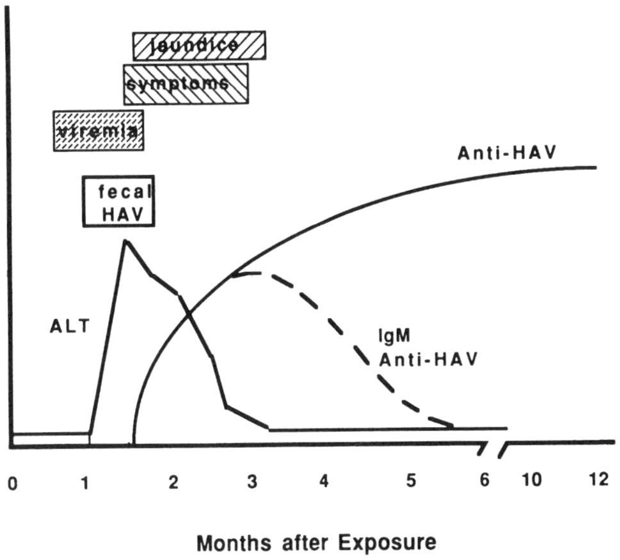

Figure 7.2. Time course of symptoms, viral presence, and serological markers with hepatitis A. Note that the onset of symptoms and serological markers follow the brief period of viremia, creating a "window" during which an asymptomatic person could donate blood. HAV, hepatitis A virus. Immunoglobulin M antibody to HAV (IgM anti-HAV) is present only during the acute infection. Immunoglobulins G and M antibodies to HAV (anti-HAV) indicate acute and past infection. (Reprinted with permission from Berry AJ. Viral hepatitis. Anesth Clin North Am 1989;7:771–794.)

VIRUSES

Hepatitis

The most frequent major morbidity in the United States attributable to transfusion of blood products is viral hepatitis. There are five major types of viral hepatitis: hepatitis A, hepatitis B, hepatitis C, delta hepatitis, and hepatitis E. In addition, cytomegalovirus (CMV), Epstein-Barr virus, and several rare viruses may be associated with transfusion-induced viral hepatitis. Although there has been much progress in identification of these hepatotropic viral agents and their specific clinical effects, our understanding of them is still evolving. The most common of the viral hepatitides, hepatitis A, B, and C, and CMV-associated hepatitis, are reviewed.

Hepatitis A is caused by a small RNA virus, hepatitis A virus (HAV), that is usually transmitted by oral-fecal contamination. The disease, formerly known as infectious hepatitis, is usually mild and self-limiting. In general, there is a brief period of low-titer viremia that precedes the onset of symptoms, and no carrier state develops (Fig. 7.2). Because the viremia is at very low levels and transient and anti-HAV is common in recipients and other blood units that may be transfused concomitantly, HAV is rarely transmitted by blood products (30–32). The most recent reports of posttransfusion hepatitis A have been limited to neonatal seroconversions and subsequent outbreaks of hepatitis A in family members and nursing personnel (33–34). The neonates received blood products from single-unit donors who subsequently became ill with hepatitis A, demonstrating the "window" during which asymptomatic persons may donate blood. In both instances, HAV was apparently transmitted to family members and nurses by fecal material and, in one case, ileostomy drainage.

Hepatitis B is caused by a DNA virus, hepatitis B virus (HBV), that is transmitted parenterally primarily through blood contamination (transfusion, needle stick, tattoo, etc.) but can also be transmitted perinatally and through sexual contact. HBV has distinct antigens and antibodies that allow its identification. In brief, there is a surface protein coat antigen (HBsAg—originally called the Australia antigen) and its antibody (anti-HBs), an antibody (anti-HBc) to an inner core antigen (HBcAg), a derivative of the core antigen called "e" antigen (HBeAg) and its antibody (anti-HBe), a specific DNA polymerase, and HBV DNA itself.

Routine donor screening for HBsAg has markedly decreased the occurrence of posttransfusion HBV in the United States. Much less than 1% of recipients of blood transfusions develop hepatitis B, and these cases account for approximately 10% of all posttransfusion hepatitis (35, 36). The efficacy of HBsAg testing depends on the prevalence of hepatitis B. As a worst case, in underdeveloped countries where HBV infection is endemic, identification of HBV infection with HBsAg may be falsely negative in up to 70% of donors carrying HBV (37). The test is much more reliable (at least 90%) in countries where HBV infection is not endemic (38).

The AABB recommends that all donated blood products be tested not only for HBsAg, but also for antibody to HBcAg (anti-HBc) and alanine aminotransferase (ALT) (Table 7.3). Anti-HBc (IgM) appears early in the serum of patients with acute hepatitis B, and higher levels of anti-HBc (IgG and IgM) are found in chronically infected individuals. ALT is a sensitive indicator of hepatocellular damage, but it cannot indicate the etiological cause of the damage. Before the discovery of a specific test for the hepatitis C virus (HCV), routine screening of all donors for the presence of anti-HBc and/or an elevated ALT level in donated blood was associated with a 40–60% decrease in posttransfusion non-A, non-B (NANB) hepatitis (now known to be predominantly hepatitis C) (39–42).

The addition of anti-HBc and ALT testing in the mid-1980s as surrogate tests for NANB hepatitis infection has been associated with a decrease in the incidence of transfusion-associated hepatitis (Table 7.4) (43). Also playing roles in decreasing the incidence of transfusion-associated hepatitis are the self-deferral and exclusion questionnaire programs of the blood banks. Although these programs were originated to limit donations from persons in groups at risk for HIV infection, similar epidemiological risks exist for HIV, HBV, and HCV infections.

Despite routine screening, posttransfusion hepatitis B

TABLE 7.3. ROUTINE TESTS ON DONATED BLOOD

ABO and Rh type
Screen for antibodies to red blood cell antigens
Infectious diseases
Serology for syphilis (VDRL)
Hepatitis B surface antigen (HBsAg)
Antibody to hepatitis B core antigen (anti-HBc)
Antibody to hepatitis C virus
Antibody to HIV-1
Antibody to HTLV-I/II
Serum ALT

Reprinted with permission from Warner MA, Faust RJ. Risks of transfusion. Anesth Clin North Am 1990;8:503.

TABLE 7.4. INCIDENCE OF POSTTRANSFUSION HEPATITIS B AFTER TRANSFUSION OF BLOOD WITH OR WITHOUT DETECTABLE ANTI-HBc

Reference	Number of Recipients of Blood	Rate of HBV Infection After Receipt of Blood Tested for Anti-HBc: Anti-HBc-Positive (%)	Anti-HBc-Negative (%)
Cossart et al. (39)	842	8.6 (3/35)	0 (0/807)
Koziol et al. (40)	481	3.6 (7/193)	1.7 (5/288)
Katchaki et al. (43)	282	2.1 (3/141)	0 (0/141)

Reprinted with permission from Hoofnagle JH. Posttransfusion hepatitis B. Transfusion 1990;30:385, published by the American Association of Blood Banks.

Values in parentheses are number of recipients estimated from data on number of units.

continues to occur. Hoofnagle (35) suggests that the simplest explanation is that the disease occurs after but not because of transfusion. In one study, an HBsAg-positive gynecologist apparently transmitted HBV to four patients who underwent surgical procedures and received HBsAg-negative blood products (44). Nevertheless, this type of occurrence must be very rare. Other explanations for continued posttransfusion hepatitis B are mistakes made in the testing of blood, infectious donors who are in the incubation (seronegative "window") period of acute hepatitis B, and infectious donors who are chronic carriers of low undetectable levels of HBV. Of these, the most plausible is the presence of low undetectable levels of HBV in donors. In studies of individuals who developed posttransfusion hepatitis B after receiving HBsAg-negative blood, the implicated blood units had high titers of anti-HBc, suggesting the presence of low levels of infective HBV (45, 46).

Before the routine testing of donated blood for HBsAg, approximately 30% of posttransfusion hepatitis patients were found to be positive for HBsAg in random tests (47). With the introduction of routine donor blood testing for HBsAg, this rate dropped to less than 10%. It became clear that an agent or agents other than HAV and HBV were responsible for most posttransfusion hepatitis cases. With no specific agent identified, the agent was referred to as the NANB hepatitis virus. In 1989, Choo et al. (48) reported the identification of an NANB hepatitis agent, designated it as the HCV, and cloned it. Kuo et al. (49) from the same investigative group then developed and used an assay to detect HCV antibody (anti-HCV).

In late April 1990, the FDA approved commercial distribution and use of tests for anti-HCV. Using this test retrospectively and prospectively, approximately 90% of what was formerly NANB hepatitis has proven to be caused by HCV (50–53). Even before the routine use of anti-HCV testing, the incidence of transfusion-associated NANB hepatitis caused by HCV had decreased by half in the preceding 4 years (Fig. 7.3) (54–56). This decrease was associated with the implementation of surrogate testing with anti-HBc and ALT for NANB hepatitis and increased deferral and testing of individuals at risk for HIV infection (57).

The posttransfusion hepatitis of HCV differs clinically from that of HBV. In general, HBV is associated with an acute icteric illness, with an incubation period of less than 24 weeks. Approximately 10% of patients progress to chronic carrier states, and one quarter of these develop histological evidence of chronic active hepatitis or cirrhosis. In contrast, hepatitis C is usually mild; patients are usually asymptomatic and anicteric. It occurs after a mean incubation period of 7–8 weeks, with 80% of cases occurring between 5 and 12 weeks after transfusion. There is no correlation between time to seroconversion and the degree of illness (56, 57). Greater than half of hepatitis C cases progress to chronic disease states and 20% of those to cirrhosis (58). Some patients with these posttransfusion chronic liver diseases will develop hepatocellular carcinoma. In a longitudinal study, Kiyosawa et al. (59) evaluated the long-term effects of chronic liver disease. Twenty-one of their 54 patients with hepatocellular carcinoma had previous transfusions, and all were seropositive for HCV.

If greater than 90% of patients with NANB hepatitis have been shown to have hepatitis C, what is the etiology of the remaining cases? Some may have HCV, but the blood sample was taken early before a titer sufficient for detection is present, given the insensitivity of the first-generation test. Following precedent, these cases may be categorized as non-A, non-B, non-C hepatitis. In this unending alphabetic progression, there are a number of likely etiologic candidates. For example, a variety of distinct subsets of HCV have been identified (60, 61).

CMV, a member of the herpes virus family, is ubiquitous. Seroprevalence is directly related to population density. In the United States, nearly 100% of the population is seropositive for anti-CMV by age 70, with Californians having the highest rates (62). In some nonindustrialized countries, 100% of the population may be affected as early as 2 years of age.

CMV infects mononuclear white blood cells, including monocytes, helper and suppressor lymphocytes, B lymphocytes, and natural killer cells (62). Although polymorphonuclear leukocytes may be infected in rare instances, mononuclear cells are primarily responsible for transfusion-transmitted CMV infection. CMV may be present, therefore, in any blood products that have white blood cells. Unfortunately, any RBC products, even those that have been frozen and deglycerolized or washed to be leukocyte-poor, and platelet concentrates may transmit CMV infection (63). Although anti-CMV is present in most donated blood products in the United States, CMV is rarely pathogenic after transfusion (64–66). Most transfusion recipients are already immune to CMV, and many donors have neutralizing antibodies that provide passive protection. Because most donated blood has anti-CMV, it is not practical to screen all donated blood for CMV.

CMV can, however, cause serious morbidity in immunosuppressed recipients or low-birthweight infants, and CMV-negative blood products should be used for these patients. In

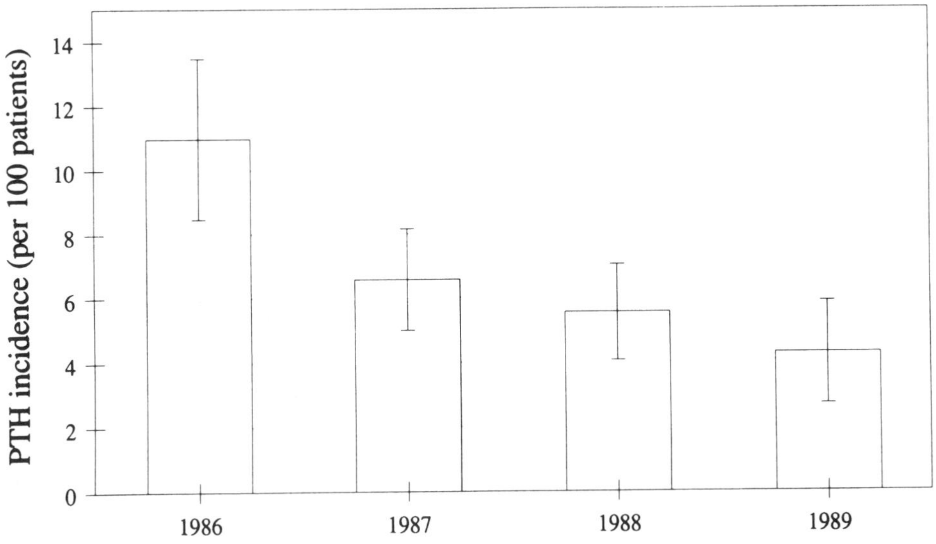

Figure 7.3. Declining incidence of posttransfusion hepatitis (PTH) (columns, ±SEM), 1986 through 1989. Ninety-six percent of these cases were NANB hepatitis. Preliminary data gathered since the routine use of anti-HCV began suggests that most of these NANB cases were caused by HCV. (Reprinted with permission from Sirchia G, Giovanetti AM, Parravicini A, et al. Prospective evaluation of posttransfusion hepatitis. Transfusion 1991;31:299–302, published by the American Association of Blood Banks.

immunosuppressed adults, CMV infection may cause pneumonia, hepatitis, or symptoms of graft rejection. This infection can be primary when the donor has an active or latent infection or secondary from reactivation of a recipient's own latent infection (Table 7.5) (67). Seronegative blood products can eliminate the risk of transfusion-transmitted CMV if both the donor and recipient are seronegative (62). In transplant patients, if a seropositive organ or bone marrow is transplanted, seronegative blood products are probably not necessary. In neonates, CMV infection may be associated with atypical lymphocytosis, hepatosplenomegaly, and pneumonia (68, 69). In general, CMV seronegative blood is used in neonates who are born to CMV-negative mothers and who weigh less than 1200 g at birth.

Retroviruses

Retroviruses differ from most organisms and viruses because their replication depends on the flow of genetic material from RNA to DNA. This passage of material is the reverse of the usual transfer of genetic information and is made possible by reverse transcriptase, a special viral DNA polymerase. Retroviruses had been postulated since early in this century, but their reproductive biology was unknown until the discovery of reverse transcriptase in 1970 (70, 71). Although retroviral infection of humans was first noted in 1978 (72), the study of retroviruses was not well supported until the association of AIDS with human T-cell lymphotropic virus-type III (HTLV-III; now known as HIV type 1, the causative factor in AIDS). At least six retroviruses infect humans, and five are pathogenic (73, 74). All are cytotropic for T4 lymphocytes, monocytes, and macrophages (75).

TABLE 7.5. TYPE OF CMV INFECTION IN TRANSPLANT RECIPIENTS BY SEROLOGICAL STATUS OF RECIPIENT AND TRANSFUSED PRODUCTS

	Blood Products	
Recipients	**Seronegative**	**Seropositive**
Seronegative	No risk of transfusion-transmitted infection	Risk of transfusion-transmitted primary infection
Seropositive	Reactivation of latent infection	Risk of transfusion-transmitted secondary infection or reactivation of latent infection (theoretical)

Reprinted with permission from Hillyer CD, Snydman DR, Berkman EM. The risk of cytomegalovirus infection in solid organ and bone marrow transplant recipients: transfusion of blood products. Transfusion 1990;30: 660, published by the American Association of Blood Banks.

Within a year of the first report in 1981 of opportunistic infection and Karposi's sarcoma in homosexual men (76), *Pneumocystis carinii* pneumonia was reported in three hemophilic patients who had no risk factors other than their use of factor VIII concentrates (77). Shortly thereafter, Ammann et al. (78) reported an infant who received multiple transfusions and developed pneumocystis pneumonia. One donor of blood to this child later developed signs and symptoms of the same infectious process. Subsequently, the association of blood transfusions and transmission of the causative agent of AIDS became evident.

Although the etiological agent of AIDS was unknown at the time, the AABB called for self-deferral from donating by members of high-risk groups in March 1983 (79–81). The controversial identifications of the presumptive etiologic agent, HIV-1, by Barre-Sinoussi et al. (82) and Gallo et al. (83) in 1983 and 1984, respectively, and the development of serological tests for antibody to HIV-1 led to evaluation of effective heat treatment techniques of pooled blood products in November 1984 (84) and donor screening of all blood products in April 1985 (85). These key events effectively improved the safety of the U.S. blood supply. When donor screening was implemented in the United States in 1985, 0.04% of blood donations were positive for HIV-1 (86). Over the next 2 years, donor education, confidential self-exclusion, and selective recruitment of donors contributed to decrease HIV seropositive donors by 50% (87).

The safety of the blood supply from HIV-1 contamination improved further by asking donors very explicit and direct questions regarding their risk status. The Centers for Disease Control and Prevention's HIV Blood Donor Study Group reviewed 2,153,600 blood donations from May 1988 to April 1989 from 19 transfusion centers (88). They found that 68% of the 462 donors who had seropositive blood also had easily identifiable risk factors for HIV-1 infection, and only 5% used the confidential exclusion option. A similar study confirmed their findings that most HIV-1-infected donors could be excluded by using simple language and more explicit questions when interviewing potential blood donors (89).

Currently, 1 in 5000 to 1 in 10,000 donors test positive for HIV-1 antibody by enzyme-linked immunosorbent assay (ELISA) and Western blot assay (American Red Cross, unpublished data). There is another small group who have positive ELISA but indeterminate Western blot test results. Most of these indeterminate cases are believed to be related to HLA cross-reactivities. A prospective study evaluated donors with indeterminate screening tests over several years and did not document any donors who converted to both ELISA and Western-blot positive or who developed any symptoms of HIV-1 infection (90). In contrast, Perrin et al. (91) used DNA amplification to identify a blood donor with indeterminate Western blot who later seroconverted to positive. Because the results are controversial and only a minor part of the total blood supply has an indeterminate screen, the AABB has recommended that the blood products of these donors not be used.

The risks of transfusion-acquired HIV infection are very low but not absent despite screening tests that approach 100% sensitivity and specificity. Estimates of risk of transmission of HIV from transfusions of screened seronegative blood range from 1 in 38,000 (92) to 1 in 300,000 (3, 93) per unit of blood. These estimates are based on either epidemiological models or the demonstration of seroconversion in recipients. Busch et al. (94) used sensitive cultures and polymerase chain reactions on seronegative blood pools made from blood donations in San Francisco and estimated the probability that a screened donor unit would be positive for HIV-1 as 1 in 61,171.

There are two major reasons for the continuing occurrence of HIV-1 infections after transfusion. First, there is a variable period after initial acquisition of HIV-1 infection when infectious HIV-1 is present but antibody titers are insufficient to be detected by the screening tests (Fig. 7.4). During this period or "window" of silent infection, infectious blood may test seronegative. Ward et al. (92) reported 13 recipients of seronegative blood (from seven donors) who later developed detectable antibodies to HIV-1. Second, clerical errors can lead to transfusion of seropositive blood. In 1985, 13 units of blood products known to be seropositive were mistakenly transfused because of clerical errors (93). As more tests are conducted on each donated unit of blood, the risk of clerical error rises. Many blood banks are evaluating or using computerized tracking systems to decrease the risk of clerical errors.

If HIV-1 seropositive blood is transfused, there is a 90% chance of seroconversion for a seronegative recipient. The Transfusion Safety Group retrospectively tested 200,000 donor blood component specimens stored in late 1984 and early 1985 before routine testing of donated blood for antibody to HIV-1 (95). The group contacted recipients of a seropositive blood product and found 90% had seroconverted. The rate of progression to AIDS within 3 years was similar to that reported for homosexual men.

Improvements in laboratory identification of HIV-1-seropositive blood will make an already very safe blood supply in the United States even safer. The use of immunoassays made with recombinant technology, particularly those with low cost, rapid analyses, and high sensitivity and specificity, will further strengthen the safety of the U.S. blood supply and have marked benefits in the blood supply of less developed countries (96). Health care systems in many less developed countries do not have the resources or personnel to evaluate donated blood using the ELISA and Western blot tests common to more developed countries. In addition, in countries where refrigeration is scarce and whole blood fresh within 4 hours of donation is the most commonly

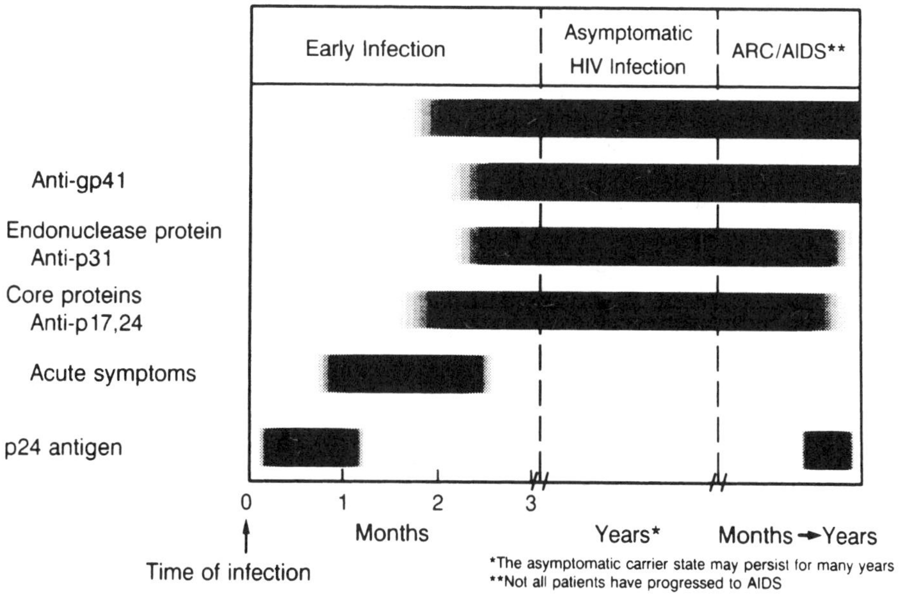

Figure 7.4. Usual time course of HIV-1 serologic responses. Infectious HIV-1 is present from initial exposure. Within 1–2 weeks of initial exposure, p24 antigen may be detected, but the sensitivity of the p24 antigen screening test is poor, and its use is no longer recommended. There is a period of 2–3 months before antibodies common to the screening ELISA have developed in sufficiently high titers to cause a positive finding. (Reprinted with permission from Warner MA, Kunkel SE. Human immunodeficiency virus infection. Anesth Clin North Am 1989;7: 795–811.)

transfused blood, identification techniques that take minutes instead of hours may greatly diminish the risk of HIV-1-seropositive transfusions (97).

In 1986, a West African with symptoms of AIDS was found to have a retroviral infection that was immunologically distinct from HIV-1 (98). The retrovirus was identified as HIV type 2 (HIV-2, formerly HTLV-IV) (99). Since that initial case report, there have been other well-documented cases of HIV-2 infection, including several in the United States (100). In mid-1989, the Retrovirus Study Group of the French Society of Blood Transfusion reported on 18 asymptomatic blood donors who were found to have HIV-2 antibodies that initially cross-reacted with HIV-1 ELISA (101). By studying patients who were HIV-2 seropositive and also symptomatic with AIDS, they found that most persons with HIV-2 were identifiable because their HIV-2 antibodies cross-reacted with HIV-1 ELISA tests. As these persons became overtly symptomatic, the cross-reactivity was less pronounced. In the United States, HIV-2-specific tests on sera from 22,699 asymptomatic persons, including 8503 randomly selected blood donors, failed to reveal an HIV-2 infection (100).

If potential donors who are symptomatic for AIDS are excluded as well as donors from West Africa, it appears at this time that HIV-1 screening tests are sufficient to identify HIV-2 seropositive blood. As the prevalence of HIV-2 infection increases in various populations, it may be necessary to test donated blood specifically for the presence of HIV-2 or its antibodies.

In 1978, HTLV-I became the first retrovirus identified in humans (72). It is associated with a rare, highly malignant adult T-cell leukemia and also a myelopathy known as tropical spastic paraparesis (102). An immunologically similar human T-cell lymphotropic virus, HTLV-II, may be associated with a type of leukemia known as hairy cell leukemia (102, 103). Because these viruses are similar immunologically, passive agglutination or indirect immunofluorescence for HTLV-I is indistinguishable from HTLV-II. As a result, epidemiological data based on available screening and confirmatory assays without further detailed laboratory evaluation do not discern HTLV-I from HTLV-II.

The epidemiology of HTLV-I/II is not as well documented as that of HIV. HTLV-I is endemic in southern Japan, where 1 in 15 potential blood donors is seropositive (104), and also in areas of the Caribbean, South America, and equatorial Africa. In contrast, estimates suggest that less than 1 in 4000 of U.S. donors are HTLV-I/II seropositive (105), and most of these donors are intravenous drug users. Although the most common routes for the spread of HTLV-I/II infection in endemic areas are mother-to-child and sexual transmission, transfusion of infected cellular blood components can introduce the virus(es) into nonendemic populations.

The efficacy of screening donated blood for HTLV-I/II in nonendemic areas is controversial. There is no doubt that HTLV-I/II is readily transmitted by transfusion. Up to 10% of the HTLV-I/II-infected Japanese population may have been infected by transfusion (102). In the United States, the Red Cross has estimated that approximately 2800 transfusion recipients could contract HTLV-I/II infection if the blood supply was not screened for these viruses (105). Cardiac surgical patients who were multiply transfused with HIV-screened but HTLV-I/II-unscreened blood products were found to have an estimated risk of HTLV-I/II transmission of 0.028% for each unit of cellular blood component they received (106). This risk is low but almost 10 times greater than the risk of HIV transmission of 0.003% per cellular component. The implementation of a screening program for HTLV-I/II in blood banks in Japan resulted in a dramatic decline in recipient seroconversion rate from 53.6% to 0.9% (107). Based on this information, the U.S. Public Health Service and the American Red Cross have recommended, and blood banks have implemented, screening of the U.S. blood supply for HTLV-I/II (108).

Other countries with low prevalence of HTLV-I/II have chosen to forego screening in favor of allocating resources to other public health issues. Because most HTLV-I/II-seropositive blood donors in the United States are intravenous drug users who are also at risk for HIV infection (109, 110), screening blood donors for HIV, plus self-deferral programs and stringent donor exclusion criteria, may eliminate many donors at risk of transmitting HTLV-I/II.

What is the risk to the recipient of a unit of blood infected with HTLV-I/II? The seroconversion rate after exposure to HTLV-I/II-infected cellular blood products ranges from 35 to 60% (111, 112). The time to seroconversion has been reported from 20 to 90 days, with a mean time of 40 days (111). Seropositivity to HTLV-I/II after transfusion has been linked to the development of tropical spastic paraparesis (sometimes referred to as HTLV-I-associated myelopathy) (112). This paraparesis may develop with 3 months of transfusion. Because there is a latent period estimated at between 20 and 30 years between time of infection and actual development of adult T-cell leukemias or lymphomas (113), transfusion-acquired HTLV-I/II infection has not yet been linked to their development.

INFECTION AND AUTOLOGOUS DONATIONS

Preoperative collection and storage of autologous blood is the most popular mechanism to provide patients with "safe" blood. In 1990, an estimated 5% of all blood collected for transfusion was intended for use by the patient-donor from whom it was collected (114). Although there is no disagreement that autologous blood is the safest blood, there are infectious risks associated with its collection, processing, and transfusion (115). The basic risks are those associated with homologous blood, including contamination of collecting systems, proliferation of psychrophilic bacteria, and testing and clerical errors. There are, however, few national guidelines or standards for the testing of autologous blood for infectious disease processes, and blood bank medical directors make their independent decisions based on patient demographics and the experience of their institution. If autologous blood is donated and processed at a hospital-based blood-drawing facility and used in that same institution, neither the FDA nor AABB requires any infectious disease testing. On the other hand, if the blood is donated and processed in a community blood center for possible transfusion in another facility, the FDA requires all autologous units to be tested for HBSAg, syphilis, and anti-HIV-1. The standards of the AABB differ from those of the FDA only by not requiring testing for syphilis.

Testing of autologous blood for infectious processes is controversial, with compelling arguments for both routine testing and no testing of autologous blood. Complete infectious disease testing makes "crossover" of unused autologous blood products into the homologous community blood supply possible. In terms of safety, it is unclear if crossover autologous blood is as safe as homologous blood. The overall safety of the homologous blood supply depends on donor screening and testing for infectious processes. For autologous blood, donor screening may be partially eliminated, and legitimate concerns can be raised regarding the donor's understanding of the nature of his or her illness (116–118). Complete testing also enables large blood collection centers to avoid breaks in their standard operating procedures, a critical step for the success or failure of testing procedures (14, 119). In contrast, no testing results in cost savings, simplified bookkeeping, and avoidance of falsely positive tests. A strong case can be made for no testing in institutions that have tight control over blood collection, processing, and release processes and that do not practice crossover.

What should be done with autologous units that test positive for an infectious disease marker? Again, there are no firm guidelines, and the practice differs between institutions. Some release all units, without regard to test results, to autologous donors. Others do not release units that test positive for HIV-1, HBsAg, anti-HCV, or HTLV-I/II. This conservative release policy protects health care workers who handle the infected blood and also prevents transmission of disease should the unit be given to the wrong patient.

SUMMARY

At present, there are few alternatives to blood transfusion in clinical practice. Autologous blood transfusion is available and increasing in popularity, primarily because of patient fear of contracting HIV-1 infection. Although many infectious risks of transfusion may be avoided by the use of autologous blood, autologous transfusion is susceptible to the clerical and bacterial contamination problems associated with use of homologous blood. For patients with refractory anemia or those undergoing emergency or extensive surgical procedures, there is no practical alternative currently to the transfusion of homologous blood products. Because many transfusions may be unnecessary, modification of improper transfusion practices is a logical first step to the reduction of transfusion risks.

The blood supply in the United States is remarkably free of infectious diseases. In the past decade, transmission of HIV-1 by transfusion has been virtually eliminated and the incidence of posttransfusion hepatitis has been reduced dramatically. As these improvements continue, other infectious problems, including transfusion-induced immunosuppression and the recent evolution of psychrophilic bacteria, become increasingly important. As public health concerns call for more testing of blood for markers of infectious disease to attain a "zero-risk" blood supply, physicians in transfusion medicine will be progressively confronted by the medicolegal problems associated with false-positive and false-negative markers of infectious diseases in donated and transfused blood.

Future directions in research to decrease the risk of infectious processes associated with blood transfusion include the development of blood substitutes, increased utilization of autologous blood, generation of cellular blood components from omnipotent stem cell lines, and improvements in blood testing and transfusion practices based on epidemiological studies. Because many transfusion decision-making processes are made in the perioperative period, surgeons and anesthesiologists must keep abreast of current practices and perspectives in this rapidly progressing field.

REFERENCES

1. Salem-Schatz SR, Avorn J, Soumerai SB. Influence of clinical knowledge, organizational context, and practice style on transfusion decision making. JAMA 1990;264:476–483.
2. Office of Medical Applications and Research. National Institutes of Health. Perioperative red cell transfusion. JAMA 1988;260:2700–2703.
3. Etchason J, Petz L, Keeler E, et al. The cost effectiveness of preoperative autologous blood donations. N Engl J Med 1995;332:719–724.
4. Wilson WR, Van Scoy RE, Washington JA. Incidence of bacteremia in adults without infection. J Clin Microbiol 1975;2:94–95.

5. Myrhe BA. Fatalities from blood transfusion. JAMA 1980;244: 1333–1335.
6. Honig CL, Bove JR. Transfusion associated fatalities: review of Bureau of Biologics reports 1976–1978. Transfusion 1980;20:653–661.
7. Ness PM, Perkins HA. Transient bacteremia after dental procedures and other minor manipulations. Transfusion 1980;20:82–85.
8. LeFrock IL, Ellis CA, Turchik JB, Weinstein L. Transient bacteremia associated with sigmoidoscopy. N Engl J Med 1973;289:467–469.
9. Braude AI, Sanford JP, Bartlett JE, Mallery OT. Effects and clinical significance of bacterial contaminants in transfused blood. J Lab Clin Med 1952;39:902–916.
10. Braude AI, Carey FJ, Siemienski J. Studies of bacterial transfusion reactions from refrigerated blood: the properties of cold-growing bacteria. J Clin Invest 1955;34:311–325.
11. Aber RC. Transfusion-associated *Yersinia enterocolitica.* Transfusion 1990;30:193–195.
12. Ratkowsky DA, Olley J, McMeekin TA, Ball A. Relationship between temperature and growth rate of bacterial cultures. J Bacteriol 1982;149:1–5.
13. Tipple MA, Bland LA, Murphy JJ, et al. Sepsis associated with transfusion of red cells contaminated with *Yersinia enterocolitica.* Transfusion 1990;30:207–213.
14. Sazama K. Reports of 355 transfusion-associated deaths: 1976 through 1985. Transfusion 1990;30:583–590.
15. Heal JM, Singal S, Sardisco E, Mayer T. Bacterial proliferation in platelet concentrates. Transfusion 1986;26:388–390.
16. Braine HG, Kickler TS, Charache P, et al. Bacterial sepsis secondary to platelet transfusion: an adverse effect on extended storage at room temperature. Transfusion 1986;26:391–393.
17. Seidl S. Syphilis screening in the 1990s. Transfusion 1990;30:773–774.
18. Risseeuw-Appel IM, Kothe FC. Transfusion syphilis: a case report. Sex Transm Dis 1983;10:200–201.
19. Chambers RW, Foley HT, Schmidt PJ. Transmission of syphilis by fresh blood components. Transfusion 1969;9:32–34.
20. Van der Sluis JJ, Onvlee PC, Kothe FCHA, Vezevski VD, Aelbers GMN, Menke HE. Transfusion syphilis, survival of *Treponema pallidum* in donor blood. (I). Report of an orientating study. Vox Sang 1984;47:297–304.
21. International Forum. Does it make sense for blood transfusion services to continue the time-honored syphilis screening with cardiolipin antigen? Vox Sang 1981;41:183–192.
22. Seidl S, Kuhnl P. Transmission of diseases by blood transfusion. World J Surg 1987;11:30–35.
23. Bruce-Chwatt LJ. Imported malaria. An uninvited guest. Br Med Bull 1982;38:179–185.
24. Guerrero IC, Weniger BC, Schultz MG. Transfusion malaria in the United States 1972–1981. Ann Intern Med 1983;99:221–226.
25. Schumis GA. Chagas' disease and blood transfusion. Prog Clin Biol Res 1985;182:127–145.
26. Popovsky MA. Transfusion-transmitted babesiosis. Transfusion 1991;31:296–298.
27. Gombert ME, Goldstein EJC, Benach JL, et al. Human babesiosis: clinical and therapeutic considerations. JAMA 1982;248:3005–3007.
28. Jacoby GA, Hunt JV, Kosinski KS, et al. Treatment of transfusion-transmitted babesiosis by exchange transfusion. N Engl J Med 1980;303:1098–1100.
29. Popovsky MA, Lindberg LE, Syrek AL, Page PL. Prevalence of *Babesia* antibody in a selected blood donor population. Transfusion 1988;28:59–61.
30. Hollinger FB, Khan NC, Oefinger PE, et al. Posttransfusion hepatitis type A. JAMA 1983;250:2313.
31. Sherertz RJ, Russell BA, Reuman PD. Transmission of hepatitis A by transfusion of blood products. Arch Intern Med 1984;144:1579–1580.
32. Giusti G, Galanti B, Gaeta GB, Gallo C. Etiological, clinical and laboratory data of post-transfusion hepatitis: a retrospective study of 379 cases from 53 Italian hospitals. Infection 1987;15:111–114.
33. Azimi PH, Roberto RR, Guralnik J, et al. Transfusion-acquired hepatitis A in a premature infant with secondary nosocomial spread in an intensive care nursery. Am J Dis Child 1986;140:23–27.
34. Giacoia GP, Kasprisin DO. Transfusion-acquired hepatitis A. South Med J 1989;82:1357–1360.
35. Hoofnagle JH. Posttransfusion hepatitis B. Transfusion 1990;30: 384–386.
36. Dienstag JL, Alter HJ. Non-A, non-B hepatitis: evolving epidemiologic and clinical perspective. Semin Liver Dis 1986;6:67–81.
37. Lai ME, Farci P, Figus A, Balestrieri A, Arnone M, Vyas GN. Hepatitis B virus DNA in the serum of Sardinian blood donors negative for the hepatitis B surface antigen. Blood 1989;73:17–19.
38. Ferec C, Verlingue C, Saleum JP. HBV DNA in blood donors [letter]. Transfusion 1988;28:84–85.
39. Cossart YE, Kirsch S, Ismay SL. Post-transfusion hepatitis in Australia. Report of the Australian Red Cross Study. Lancet 1982;1:208–213.
40. Koziol DE, Holland PV, Alling DW, et al. Antibody to hepatitis B core antigen as a paradoxical marker for non-A, non-B hepatitis agents in donated blood. Ann Intern Med 1986;104:488–495.
41. Alter HJ, Purcell RH, Holland PV, Alling DW, Koziol DE. Donor transaminase and recipient hepatitis. Impact on blood transfusion services. JAMA 1981;246:630–634.
42. Aach RD, Szmuness W, Mosley JW, et al. Serum alanine aminotransferase of donors in relation to the risk of non-A, non-B hepatitis in recipients: the transfusion-transmitted viruses study. N Engl J Med 1981;304:989–994.
43. Katchaki JN, Siem TIY, Brouwer R, Brandt KH, van der Waart M. Detection and significance of anti-HBc in the blood bank: preliminary results of a controlled prospective study. J Virol Methods 1980;2: 119–125.
44. Carl M, Blakely DL, Francis DP, Maynard JE. Interruption of hepatitis B transmission by modification of a gynaecologist's surgical technique. Lancet 1982;1:731–733.
45. Hoofnagle JH, Seeff LB, Bales ZB, Zimmerman HJ, the Veterans Administration Hepatitis Cooperative Study Group. Type B hepatitis after transfusion with blood containing antibody to hepatitis B core antigen. N Engl J Med 1978;298:1379–1383.
46. Larsen J, Hetland G, Skaug K. Posttransfusion hepatitis B transmitted by blood from a hepatitis B surface antigen-negative hepatitis B virus carrier. Transfusion 1990;30:431–432.
47. Aach RD, Kahn R. Posttransfusion hepatitis. Current perspectives. Ann Intern Med 1980;92:539–546.
48. Choo Q-L, Kuo G, Weiner AJ, Overby LR, Bradley DW, Houghton M. Isolation of a cDNA clone derived from a blood-borne non-A, non-B viral hepatitis genome. Science 1989;244:359–362.
49. Kuo G, Choo QL, Alter HJ, et al. An assay for circulating antibodies to a major etiologic virus of human non-A, non-B hepatitis. Science 1989;244:362.
50. Alter HJ, Purcell RH, Shih JW, et al. Detection of antibody to hepatitis C virus in prospectively followed transfusion recipients with acute and chronic non-A, non-B hepatitis. N Engl J Med 1989;321:1494–1500.
51. Alter MJ, Hadler SC, Judson FN, et al. Risk factors for acute non-A,

non-B hepatitis in the United States and association with hepatitis C virus infection. JAMA 1990;264:2231–2235.
52. Esteban JI, Gonzalez A, Hernandez JM, et al. Evaluation of antibodies to hepatitis C virus in a study of transfusion-associated hepatitis. N Engl J Med 1990;323:1107–1112.
53. Cuthbert JA. Hepatitis C. Am J Med Sci 1990;299:346–355.
54. Sirchia G, Giovanetti AM, Parravicini A, et al. Prospective evaluation of posttransfusion hepatitis. Transfusion 1991;31:299–302.
55. Zuck TF, Rose GA, Dumaswala UJ, Geer NJ. Experience with a transfusion recipient education program about hepatitis C. Transfusion 1990;30:759–761.
56. Alter MJ, Hadler SC, Judson FN, et al. Risk factors for acute non-A, non-B hepatitis in the United States and association with hepatitis C virus infection. JAMA 1990;264:2231–2235.
57. Richards C, Holland P, Kuramoto K, Douville C, Randell R. Prevalence of antibody to hepatitis C virus in a blood donor population. Transfusion 1991;31:109–113.
58. Zuck TF, Sherwood WC, Bove JR. A review of recent events related to surrogate testing of blood to prevent non-A, non-B post-transfusion hepatitis. Transfusion 1987;27:203–206.
59. Kiyosawa K, Sodeyama T, Tanaka E, et al. Interrelationship of blood transfusion, non-A, non-B hepatitis and hepatocellular carcinoma: analysis by detection of antibody to hepatitis C virus. Hepatology 1990;12:671–675.
60. Arima T, Mori C, Takamizawa A, Nakajima T, Kanai K. Cloning of serum RNA associated with hepatitis C infection suggesting heterogeneity of the agent(s) responsible for the infection. Gastroenterol Jpn 1989;24:685–691.
61. Takeuchi K, Boonmar S, Kubo Y. Hepatitis C viral cDNA clones isolated from a healthy carrier donor implicated in post-transfusion non-A, non-B hepatitis. Gene 1990;91:287–291.
62. Hillyer CD, Snydman DR, Berkman EM. The risk of cytomegalovirus infection in solid organ and bone marrow transplant recipients: transfusion of blood products. Transfusion 1990;30:659–666.
63. Tegtmeier GE. The use of cytomegalovirus-screened blood in neonates. Transfusion 1988;28:201–203.
64. Adler SP, Baggett J, McVoy M. Transfusion-associated cytomegalovirus infections in seropositive cardiac surgery patients. Lancet 1985;2:743–745.
65. Preiksaitis JK, Grumet FC, Smith WK, Merigan TC. Transfusion-acquired cytomegalovirus infection in cardiac surgery patients. J Med Virol 1985;15:283–290.
66. Wilhelm JA, Matter L, Schopfer K. The risk of transmitting cytomegalovirus to patients receiving blood transfusion. J Infect Dis 1986;154:169–171.
67. Tegtmeier GE. Posttransfusion cytomegalovirus infections. Arch Pathol Lab Med 1989;113:236–245.
68. Adler SP, Chandrika T, Lawrence L, Baggett J. Cytomegalovirus infections in neonates acquired by blood transfusions. Pediatr Infect Dis 1983;2:114–118.
69. Benson JWT, Bodden SJ, Tobin JOH. Cytomegalovirus and blood transfusion in neonates. Arch Dis Child 1979;54:538–541.
70. Baltimore D. RNA dependent DNA polymerase in virions of RNA tumor viruses. Nature 1970;226:1209–1211.
71. Temin NM, Mizutani NS. RNA-directed DNA polymerase in the virions of Rous sarcoma virus. Nature 1970;226:1211–1213.
72. Poiesz BJ, Ruscetti FW, Ritz MS, Kalyanaraman VS, Gallo RC. Isolation of a new type C retrovirus, HTLV, in primary cultural cells of a patient with Sezary T cell leukemia. Nature 1981;294:268–271.
73. Broder S. Pathogenic human retroviruses. N Engl J Med 1988;318: 243–245.
74. Streicher H, Schlar L. Human retroviruses and their associated diseases: biology, pathophysiology, and clinical consequences of human retroviral infection. Clin Chest Med 1988;9:363–376.
75. Gallo RC, Montagnier L. AIDS in 1988. Sci Am 1988;259:41–48.
76. Centers for Disease Control. Pneumocystis pneumonia. Los Angeles. MMWR 1981;30:250–252.
77. Centers for Disease Control. Pneumocystis carinii pneumonia among persons with hemophilia A. MMWR 1982;31:365–367.
78. Ammann AJ, Cowan MJ, Wara DW, et al. Acquired immunodeficiency in an infant: possible transmission by means of blood products. Lancet 1983;1:956–958.
79. Centers for Disease Control. Prevention of acquired immune deficiency syndrome (AIDS): report of inter-agency recommendations. MMWR 1983;32:101–103.
80. Joint statement on acquired immune deficiency syndrome (AIDS) related to transfusion. Transfusion 1983;23:87–88.
81. Busch MP, Young MJ, Samson SM, et al. Risk of human immunodeficiency virus (HIV) transmission by blood transfusions before the implementation of HIV-1 antibody screening. Transfusion 1991;31:4–11.
82. Barre-Sinoussi F, Chermann JC, Rey F, et al. Isolation of a T-lymphotropic retrovirus from a patient at risk for acquired immune deficiency syndrome (AIDS). Science 1983;220:868–871.
83. Gallo RC, Salahuddin SZ, Popovic M, et al. Frequent detection and isolation of cytopathic retroviruses (HTLV-III) from patients with AIDS and at risk for AIDS. Science 1984;224:500–503.
84. Centers for Disease Control. Acquired immunodeficiency syndrome (AIDS) in persons with hemophilia. JAMA 1984;252:2679–2680.
85. Centers for Disease Control. Provisional public health service inter-agency recommendations for screening donated blood and plasma for antibody to the virus causing acquired immunodeficiency syndrome. MMWR 1985;34:5–7.
86. Schorr JB, Berkowitz A, Cumming PD, Katz AJ, Sandler SG. Prevalence of HTLV-III antibody in American blood donors. N Engl J Med 1985;313:384–385.
87. Cumming PD, Wallage EL, Schorr JB, Dodd RY. Exposure of patients to human immunodeficiency virus through the transfusion of blood components that test antibody-negative. N Engl J Med 1989;321:941–946.
88. Petersen L, CDC. Surveillance and epidemiology of blood donors positive for HIV antibody. Transfusion 1989;29:S200.
89. Rutter P, Arnold E, Rykaczewski C, Sherwood W. HTLV-I antibody testing and counseling experience. Transfusion 1989;29:27S.
90. Nushbacher J, Naiman R. Longitudinal follow-up of blood donors found to be reactive for antibody to human immunodeficiency virus (anti-HIV) by enzyme linked immunoassay (EIA+) but negative by Western blot (WB−). Transfusion 1989;29:365–367.
91. Perrin LH, Yerly S, Adami N, et al. Human immunodeficiency virus DNA amplification and serology in blood donors. Blood 1990;76: 641–645.
92. Ward JW, Holmberg SD, Allen JR, et al. Transmission of human immunodeficiency virus (HIV) by blood transfusions screened as negative for HIV antibody. N Engl J Med 1988;318:473.
93. Zuck TF. Greetings—a final look back with comments about a policy of a zero-risk blood supply. Transfusion 1987;27:447–448.
94. Busch MP, Eble BE, Khayam-Bashi H, et al. Evaluation of screened blood donations for human immunodeficiency virus type 1 infection by culture and DNA amplification of pooled cells. N Engl J Med 1991;325:1–5.

95. Donegan E, Stuart M, Niland JC, et al. Infection with human immunodeficiency virus-positive blood donations. Ann Intern Med 1990;113: 733–739.
96. Quinn TC, Riggin CH, Kline RL, et al. Rapid latex agglutination assay using recombinant envelope polypeptide for the detection of antibody to the HIV. JAMA 1988;260:510–513.
97. Heyward WL, Curan JW. Rapid screening tests for HIV infection. JAMA 1988;260:542.
98. Clavel F, Guetard D, Brun-Vezinet F, et al. Isolation of a new human retrovirus from West African patients with AIDS. Science 1986;233: 343–346.
99. Essex M, Kanki PJ. The origins of the AIDS virus. Sci Am 1988;259: 64–71.
100. Centers for Disease Control. AIDS due to HIV-2 infection—New Jersey. JAMA 1988;259:969–972.
101. Courouce AM, Barin F, Baudelot J, et al. HIV 2 infection among blood donors and other subjects in France. The "retrovirus" study group of the French Society of Blood Transfusion. Transfusion 1989;29:368–370.
102. Manns A, Blattner WA. The epidemiology of the human T-cell lymphotrophic virus type I and type II: etiologic role in human disease. Transfusion 1991;31:67–75.
103. Rosenblatt JD, Golde DW, Wachsman W, et al. A second isolate of HTLV-II associated with atypical hairy cell leukemia. N Engl J Med 1986;315:372–377.
104. Bove JR, Sandler SG. HTLV-1 and blood transfusion. Transfusion 1988;28:93–94.
105. Williams AE, Fang CT, Slamon DJ, et al. Seroprevalence and epidemiological correlates of HTLV-I infection in U.S. blood donors. Science 1988;240:643–646.
106. Cohen ND, Munoz A, Reitz BA, et al. Transmission of retroviruses by transfusion of screened blood in patients undergoing cardiac surgery. N Engl J Med 1989;320:1172–1176.
107. Kamihira S, Nakasima S, Oyakawa Y, et al. Transmission of human T cell lymphotropic virus type I by blood transfusion before and after mass screening of sera from seropositive donors. Vox Sang 1987;52: 43–44.
108. Larson CJ, Taswell HF. Human T-cell leukemia virus type I (HTLV-I) and blood transfusion. Mayo Clin Proc 1988;63:869–875.
109. Perez G, Ortiz-Interian C, Lee H, et al. Human immunodeficiency virus and human T-cell leukemia virus type I in patients undergoing maintenance hemodialysis in Miami. Am J Kidney Dis 1989;14: 39–43.
110. Williams AE, Fang CT, Slamon DJ. Seroprevalence and epidemiological correlates of HTLV-I infection in U.S. blood donors. Science 1988;240:643–646.
111. Okochi K, Sato H, Hinuma Y. A retrospective study on transmission of adult T cell leukemia virus by blood transfusion: seroconversion in recipients. Vox Sang 1984;46:245–253.
112. Osame M, Izumo S, Igata A, et al. Blood transfusion and HTLV-I associated myelopathy. Lancet 1986;2:104–105.
113. Blattner WA, Nomura A, Clark JW, et al. Modes of transmission and evidence for viral latency from studies of human T-cell lymphotropic virus type I in Japanese migrant populations in Hawaii. Proc Natl Acad Sci USA 1986;83:4895–4898.
114. Surgenor DM, Wallace EL, Hao SHS, Chapman RH. Collection and transfusion of blood in the United States, 1982–1988. N Engl J Med 1990;322:1646–1651.
115. Silvergleid AJ. Preoperative autologous donation: what have we learned? Transfusion 1991;31:99–101.
116. Starkey JM, MacPherson JL, Bolgiano DC, Simon ER, Zuck TF, Sayers MH. Markers for transfusion-transmitted disease in different groups of blood donors. JAMA 1989;262:3452–3454.
117. AuBuchon JP, Dodd RY. Analysis of the relative safety of autologous blood units available for transfusion to homologous recipients. Transfusion 1988;28:403–405.
118. Kruskall MS, Popovsky MA, Pacini DG, Donovan LM, Ransil BJ. Autologous versus homologous donors: evaluation of markers for infectious disease. Transfusion 1988;28:286–288.
119. Sherwood WC. To err is human. Transfusion 1990;30:579–580.

Chapter 8

Preoperative Autologous Blood Donation

MARK A. POPOVSKY
ROBERT L. THURER
ANDA KUO

INTRODUCTION AND HISTORY

Preoperative autologous donation (PAD) is the collection and anticoagulation of whole blood from a patient or donor for anticipated perioperative transfusion. Autologous transfusion is one of the oldest known transfusion techniques, with its first recorded use dating to the 19th century (1). In the first half of this century, PAD use was infrequent and limited primarily to situations involving patients with rare red cell phenotypes or serological problems complicating the identification of compatible allogeneic blood (2). In these situations, the patient served as the ideal compatible blood donor. However, the anticoagulant and preservative solutions available limited liquid storage to a maximum of 21 days and therefore often limited the number of units that could be collected before an anticipated transfusion need.

Autologous transfusion continued to be infrequently practiced into the early 1980s, when it evolved into an important mode of hemotherapy. Although some transfusion medicine specialists and other clinicians had espoused the use of autologous blood, the real impetus for its acceptance was the recognition that the acquired immune deficiency syndrome (AIDS) was a transfusion-transmitted disease (3). Appreciation of other complications of transfusion only hastened this process. By the mid-to-late 1980s, autologous transfusion was embraced as the standard of practice by major medical organizations (4–6). Interest in autologous blood has not been limited or defined solely by the medical community. A public confused and made anxious by AIDS has often been the standard bearer for this therapy, serving as the catalyst for increased use (3).

Based on data available from the member institutions of the American Association of Blood Banks, PAD increased more than 17-fold during the 1980s, from less than 0.41% of blood collections to almost 7% in 1991 (7). This is deceptive, however, because autologous donations may not be used by the intended recipient. In many cases, the blood is discarded (3, 8). Wallace et al. (8) showed that 286,000 (44%) of 655,000 autologous units were never used.

A survey of more than 600 North American hospitals showed that autologous units represent only a median of 2.5% of transfused red cells. A 10% rate of autologous transfusion was reached in slightly more than 8% of the hospitals surveyed (9). Many experts believe that the potential for use is closer to 10–15% (10, 11), depending on the particular patient population at a given hospital. Clearly, many physicians and hospitals have yet to incorporate this technique into routine practice.

BENEFITS OF AUTOLOGOUS TRANSFUSION

Before 1980 and the introduction of human immunodeficiency virus (HIV) into the United States, the primary advantage of autologous over allogeneic blood was the avoidance of the viruses that cause hepatitis B and non-A, non-B. Clearly, the risk of acquiring any bloodborne infection is significantly, if not completely, eliminated by autologous transfusion. Although the list of potential infectious agents is long, the most important ones, in addition to hepatitis, are HIV and cytomegalovirus. Fortunately, the introduction of more extensive medical history questions as part of the blood donation process and the use of sensitive assays for the detection of HIV, hepatitis B, and, more recently, hepatitis C has decreased the risk of transmission of viral hepatitis to approximately 1:3,000 (12) and the risk of HIV to about 1:225,000 (13).

However, as the risks of transfusion-transmitted disease became less foreboding, another complication, immune modulation, has caused increasing concern. Several studies have described an association between transfusion (either at surgery or before a surgical event) and an increased risk for perioperative bacterial infection in patients having major orthopedic procedures (14, 15). These infections are not limited to the operative wound; they have been observed in distant sites involving the lung, bowel, and blood. Triulzi et al. (14), Murphy et al. (15), and Jensen et al. (16) have shown that exposure to allogeneic blood components increases a patient's perioperative infectious risk by as much as five- to sixfold. The mechanism or mechanisms for this phenomenon are not well understood, but it appears that the immunosuppressive and immunomodulatory properties of allogeneic plasma and/or leukocytes play a significant role. It is well known that allogeneic blood impairs numerous aspects of the immune effector system, including natural killer cell activity (16), but how such in vitro observations are connected to perioperative infection is not known.

Other hazards of transfusion that are eliminated by the use of autologous blood include hemolytic reactions; alloimmunization to red cell, platelet, and white cell antigens; anaphylactic and allergic reactions; transfusion-related acute lung injury; and graft-versus-host disease (GVHD) (17, 18). GVHD has long been recognized as a serious transfusion threat in the immunocompromised host, but only recently has it been reported in apparently immune-competent blood recipients (19). Because of its high mortality rate, avoidance of this complication is desirable.

When autologous blood is used in lieu of blood components from the community blood supply, more units become available from the latter to meet community needs. Unfortunately, blood shortages are not a thing of the past, particularly during the major holiday periods and summer months. Although autologous transfusion could never completely replace the need for volunteer blood donors, if used in significant numbers, it could act as a buffer for a sometimes fragile system.

Stimulation of erythropoiesis is one of the overlooked benefits of PAD. For the patient with adequate bone marrow and iron reserves and/or iron repletion, blood donation can increase red cell production by two- to threefold before surgery (20). In adult male baboons, an aggressive program of twice weekly autologous donations led to intense reticulocytosis during the first 4 postoperative days and significantly steeper hematocrit increases than in controls (21). In many cases, however, patients are iron deficient, and, as a result, red cell regenerative capabilities are limited.

INDICATIONS AND ELIGIBILITY

The selection of patients appropriate for PAD is difficult because of both the lack of clear data and the financial implications of this practice. Compared with the costs of allogeneic collections, PAD is an expensive and time-consuming process. Therefore, PAD is generally reserved for patients having surgical procedures in which there is a reasonable likelihood of a blood transfusion. At the very minimum, PAD should be considered only if blood is normally reserved for patients having a particular procedure and more than 10% of similar patients are, in fact, transfused (22).

One approach that clarifies the boundaries between judicious and inappropriate requests for PAD was developed by Axelrod et al. (23). This group integrated a maximum surgical blood-ordering system into their hospital's autologous transfusion practices. By evaluating actual transfusion rates of allogeneic and autologous blood for their hospital's surgical procedures, the authors developed recommendations for the "optimal" number of PAD units that should be collected per procedure. The investigators used as their standard for maximum autologous collections the number of units that would prevent exposure to allogeneic blood in at least 90% of patients having a given procedure. For example, the collection of 5 units of autologous blood would be recommended for sanguineous procedures such as coronary artery bypass grafting and heart valve replacement, 1 unit for transurethral resection of the prostate, and none for dilatation and curettage or nasal sinus repair (Table 8.1).

One impediment to the early growth of PAD was concern over patient and donor safety. Numerous studies and significant empirical evidence support the view that PAD is a very safe procedure in a wide variety of circumstances.

Although a limited number of studies examine the use of PAD for young patients, several demonstrate that the preoperative collection of blood from children and young adults who are scheduled for elective surgery is safe and effective in reducing their exposure to allogeneic blood sources (24–26). An increase in the rate of donation reactions, however, is associated with decreasing age and weight (27). At present, most pediatric patients selected for PAD are scheduled for orthopedic or cosmetic surgery and are more than 7 years old.

The amount of blood collected during a single donation is typically limited to 10% of the total blood volume. The size of the units collected from pediatric patients and the amount

TABLE 8.1. SCHEDULE OF OPTIMAL PREOPERATIVE COLLECTION OF AUTOLOGOUS BLOOD

Surgical Procedure	Suggested Collection (units of blood)
Coronary artery bypass graft	5
Heart valve replacement	5
Total hip replacement	3
Prostatectomy	3
Laminectomy	3
Hysterectomy	2
Transurethral resection of the prostate	1
Knee arthroscopy	0
Burch repair	0
Dilation and curettage	0
Nasal sinus repair	0

Reprinted with permission from Axelrod FB, Pepkowitz SH, Goldfinger D. Establishment of a schedule of optimal preoperative collection of autologous blood. Transfusion 1989;29:677–680, published by the American Association of Blood Banks.

of anticoagulant used are determined by the patient's weight. Although the bone marrow of healthy pediatric patients eligible for donation may be able to withstand a more intense phlebotomy schedule than that of adults (25), a weight minimum for donors is established by most autologous programs. Of three university hospitals examined by McVay et al. (28), one of the most frequent reasons autologous blood was not donated by pediatric patients undergoing surgery for which blood was ordered was concern about limited venous access. Patients at Boston's Children's Hospital who weigh less than 75 pounds are not accepted for autologous donation, and PAD at the American Red Cross is limited to patients weighing more than 85 pounds. A 1974 study (24), however, reported blood collection from patients weighing as little as 25 kg and did not find an adverse outcome.

Although lower weight patients are less likely to participate in PAD, they also have a decreased risk of homologous blood exposure because fewer units are usually administered. In addition to low weight and poor venous access, the contraindications used for all patients considering PAD should also apply to the pediatric population. Other factors to be considered for pediatric blood donors are the need to obtain informed consent from the patient and the parents and the extra time and attention from staff that younger donors and patients may require (25). In general, however, once the unit size is adjusted to reflect the weight of the patient, autologous blood donation by pediatric patients is analogous to that of adults. A pediatric autologous blood program may be most effective if other autologous blood sources, such as intraoperative blood collection, hemodilution, and postoperative blood collection, are incorporated (26, 29).

At the other extreme is the older donor. It is clear that age alone is not a barrier to PAD. Haugen and Hill (30) found that patients 80 years and older were comparable with donors less than 50 years of age in the incidence of adverse reactions. In an analysis of more than 2000 autologous donations, elderly donors were found least likely to have reactions (31). These data complement findings among allogeneic blood donors over 60 years old, reported by Simon et al. (32). These investigators found that of 900 donations, there were no severe reactions, 10 (1.1%) moderate reactions, and 73 slight reactions. In another study of allogeneic donors, older donors were found to have fewer adverse reactions than younger donors (33).

PAD may, however, be more complicated for elderly patients because they have a greater rate of deferrals (30, 33). One group froze most of the blood collected from elderly patients because unexpected medical or surgical complications often arose during the donation period, causing an increase in the time necessary to collect the desired units or delays in the scheduled surgery (30). However, frozen storage is expensive and may not be a cost-effective solution to making PAD more available to the elderly. Donation reactions may be reduced in some elderly patients with fluid replacement (34). In general, an analysis of the eligibility of elderly patients for PAD should emphasize the physical health or biological age of the patient rather than his or her chronological age.

The criteria for PAD are intended to be more liberal than those for allogeneic blood donation. There is no age limit. The requirements of the donor for PAD are relatively few: the cardiovascular system must be able to withstand an acute decrease in volume of approximately 10% (450 mL ± 10%), there should be no ongoing bacterial infections, and the hematocrit should be at least 0.33 (33%) or hemoglobin greater than 11 g/dL before each donation (35). The last point is perhaps the most arbitrary but is intended to protect the patient from reaching a level of anemia that might precipitate a decision to transfuse before there is significant intraoperative blood loss, thereby defeating the purpose of the autologous procedure. There must also be adequate venous access. For donors weighing less than 50 kg, proportionately less blood than the standard 450- to 500-mL unit should be collected.

DONATION SCHEDULE

Although it is desirable to establish a schedule of donations, there are no inviolable "rules" that apply. At many centers, it has become customary to collect a unit of blood on a weekly basis. This approach works well because it allows adequate volume repletion between donations and some regenerative erythropoiesis. However, current operative scheduling often provides only a narrow window between the time a procedure is scheduled and the actual surgical date. This means that patients may need to donate at more frequent intervals. If there are adequate iron reserves, patients may donate on a more aggressive schedule, but because many eligible candidates are older, the procedure may fatigue the individual and venous access can become problematic. To allow for intravascular equilibration, there should be at least 72 hours between the last donation and surgery (35).

ELEMENTS OF A SUCCESSFUL AUTOLOGOUS BLOOD DONATION PROGRAM

Although phlebotomy for purposes of autologous transfusion is itself a relatively simple procedure (exceptions include patients with difficult venous access or physically disabled persons), successful PAD programs require good communication and coordination between multiple parties both within and outside the hospital. The key groups include physicians, hospital (and possibly community) blood banks, and patients. Model programs usually have an individual who champions autologous practice and is responsible for coordination of the process. To be successful, programs must meet the needs of both patients and surgeons. They should provide convenience for the patient and donor and a minimum of administrative burden for the requesting physician. A tracking system is needed to ensure blood availability and reduce the risk of transfusion errors.

As of 1989, slightly more than half of autologous blood donations were made through blood centers that manage the collection process for an entire community (8). The remainder were collected in hospitals. For the blood center-managed programs, phlebotomies may occur in blood center donor rooms or blood mobiles. In the early to mid-1980s, there was some reluctance to collect autologous blood outside the hospital, because of concern that the lack of immediate access to emergency care facilities placed a patient or donor at increased risk in the event of a severe reaction. However, studies by AuBuchon and Popovsky (36) and McVay et al. (37) demonstrated the relative safety of PAD in the out-of-hospital setting. Both groups showed that the overall frequency of severe reactions in autologous donors is low, 0.45% and 0.039%, respectively. In the analysis by AuBuchon and Popovsky, many patients had a history of cardiovascular disease. Because of adverse hemodynamic changes (e.g., systolic and diastolic hypotension, premature ventricular contractions) during donation in individuals characterized as high risk (38), it is unclear whether some patients should not donate outside of the hospital setting.

Whether PAD is performed by the blood center or the hospital, there are several important steps that are critical to a program's success.

IDENTIFICATION OF POTENTIAL CANDIDATES FOR DONATION

In the first national multicenter study of its kind, Toy et al. (39) found that only 5% of eligible candidates made PADs. Obviously, the more systematic the process used to identify patients, the greater the likelihood of having appropriate individuals donate blood for themselves. Procedures that automatically notify a patient's surgeon of a likely candidate when specific surgical procedures (e.g., when the surgical blood order for that procedure is for 2 or more units) are scheduled have been described (40). The important point is that notification of physicians and screening of patients must occur far enough in advance of surgery so that phlebotomies can be arranged if the patient is a good candidate for PAD.

SCREENING OF POTENTIAL PATIENTS

In either the blood center or hospital blood bank model, patients need to be assessed as to their suitability as donors. As discussed elsewhere, the patient may have an underlying condition that would preclude PAD or require in-hospital collection. If the patient is not an acceptable PAD candidate or the method is likely to provide only partial transfusion needs, other techniques such as intraoperative blood salvage or perioperative isovolemic hemodilution should be considered. In one medical center model, 269 patients scheduled for elective orthopedic surgery were automatically referred to the department of transfusion medicine for evaluation of autologous blood needs. The assessment considered the appropriateness of either PAD or intraoperative blood salvage (41). Compared with controls, automatic referral increased the percentage of elective orthopedic surgical patients who received only autologous blood from 26% to 86%.

OBTAINING INFORMED CONSENT FOR TRANSFUSION

This has become a more complicated issue because of AIDS and legislative initiatives in certain states. It is important that patients understand the small, but finite, risks to allogeneic transfusion and that even with the use of autologous techniques, there can be no guarantees that allogeneic blood will be avoided entirely. Obviously, it is less than desirable to initiate a discussion of a patient's transfusion options the night before or day of surgery.

Consent for PAD should be obtained before the initial donation. The document should note the same risks that can complicate allogeneic blood donation (e.g., fainting, hematoma) and should also mention other problems, including the possibility that autologous units may not be available at the time of surgery because of difficulties with collection, storage, or testing (42). It is advisable to inform the donor that abnormal test results (e.g., presence of hepatitis B surface antigen) will be reported to the ordering surgeon and the patient. This provides the opportunity for appropriate medical care and counseling.

Iron Supplementation

A single unit of blood contains approximately 450 mg of iron. The donation of 1 unit generally lowers the hemoglobin approximately 1 g/dL and the hematocrit 3%. Because the rate of erythropoiesis after phlebotomy depends primarily on the availability of iron, oral iron supplementation is considered an important adjunct during the donation period. The patient should be instructed to take at least 320 mg of iron three times a day (with meals). Although enteric-coated tablets may cause less gastrointestinal side effects, these are not as well absorbed as those that lack the enteric coating (43). The tablets should be taken as close as possible to the time of the first phlebotomy and continued until the red cell mass has been restored.

In a study of oral iron supplementation in autologous donors, Biesma et al. (44) came to a different conclusion. They found that in 34 subjects who had donated 4 units of blood preoperatively, those who received 287 mg of ferrous sulfate per day starting 1 week before the first blood donation showed no change in hemoglobin or erythropoietin levels, compared with control patients who did not receive iron supplementation. They concluded that supplemental iron does not affect erythropoiesis and is insufficient to maintain iron stores in autologous blood donors. It should be noted that these data are subject to question because the dose of iron these patients were prescribed is only one-third the typical dose in autologous donors, thereby reducing the amount of elemental iron that the patients received (45).

Serological Testing

The American Association of Blood Banks requires that the ABO group and Rh type be determined by the collecting facility on every unit (35). Transfusing facilities must retest units drawn at other facilities (46). The U.S. Food and Drug Administration (FDA) recommends that registered blood establishments perform all FDA-required tests (at the time of this writing, this includes anti-HIV-1, anti-HIV-2, anti-HBc, syphilis, HBsAG, and anti-HCV) (47). The FDA provides exceptions to these testing requirements provided that the establishment collects and uses autologous blood products only for the autologous donor, these products are used at the site of collection, and all products not used by the donor are destroyed.

Production of Blood Components

Most autologous blood is made into packed red blood cells suspended in a protein-poor anticoagulant-preservative solution with a storage life of 42 days. The plasma is usually discarded, provided for research, or sent to fractionation facilities for the manufacture of plasma derivatives. However, in some programs, liquid plasma remains attached to the red cell container. Special requests for frozen plasma are also accommodated by many collecting facilities. Although most surgical cases do not require plasma transfusions, the availability of this option for selected cases (such as cardiac reoperations) is attractive.

Although a 6-week storage period of liquid red cells can accommodate most patient needs, autologous blood can be frozen. Frozen red cells can be stored for 10 years from the date of phlebotomy (35). This may be helpful in circumstances in which a large number of units are needed for surgery. The freezing procedure adds considerable cost and exposes the unit to a higher probability of breakage. Frozen units must be deglycerolized and require more preoperative preparation time.

COST-EFFECTIVENESS OF AUTOLOGOUS BLOOD

As discussed previously, the risk of the infectious complications of allogeneic transfusion has been dramatically reduced. This has occurred as the costs of administering autologous programs have increased because of greater patient participation, difficulties in reimbursement, and the burden of disposal of blood collected but not transfused. Is autologous transfusion cost-effective? Do the benefits of a safer product justify these costs? Given the public's fear of AIDS, some patients might justify any cost associated with PAD. However, many of these patients do not directly bear the costs of PAD, whereas hospitals do.

Because of the additional procedures used to identify autologous patients and collect and track their blood, PAD is more costly than the provision of allogeneic transfusions. The patient-specific nature of autologous services eliminates the advantages of economies of scale seen with allogeneic blood collection. Birkmeyer et al. (48) examined the cost-effectiveness of PAD by patients undergoing total hip and knee replacement and estimated the cost per quality-adjusted year of life saved to range from $40,000 to $1,467,000, depending on the center and the procedure. For example, bilateral or revision joint replacement was most cost-effective, whereas primary unilateral knee replacement was least cost-effective. Using the same method of analysis, the cost-effectiveness of autologous blood use is significantly less than that for other common procedures such as bypass surgery for patients with left main disease and angina, which has a $6000 cost per year of life saved when compared with medical therapy. Although the cost of autologous blood is relatively low, the cost-effectiveness is poor because of the minimal estimated gains (i.e., 0.03–0.18 days increased life expectancy for each patient/donor).

A study by Elawad et al. (49), however, suggests that autologous blood use in elective orthopedic operations is cost-effective when the costs of health care and loss of productivity for patients who contract chronic non-A, non-B hepatitis (NANBH) from transfused homologous blood are considered. The cost savings for PAD were estimated at $753–$8172. For example, the cost of collecting 1.5 units from a 40-year-old patient were estimated at $1800, whereas the total expenses associated with NANBH (taking into account the risk per transfused unit of allogeneic blood) are $5386. The transfusion of more autologous blood units to younger patients was associated with greater cost-effectiveness.

The discrepancy between the two studies and the general difficulty in analyzing the cost-to-benefit ratio of autologous blood are due, in part, to variations in the estimated risks of allogeneic blood transfusions. Birkmeyer et al. calculated the cost-effectiveness of autologous blood by estimating the risk of hepatitis C infection as 0.03% per unit (a higher estimate of 0.1% per unit was also used). The risk per unit of HIV infection was estimated as 0.001%. Elawad et al. estimated the risk of NANBH resulting in health care costs as 0.5% per unit of allogeneic blood and the risk of production loss as 0.1%; the risk of HIV infection was not examined. Neither study included risks associated with autologous blood donation that would decrease the cost-effectiveness. On the other hand, the potential risk of immunosuppression due to allogeneic blood transfusions was also not included by either study. These studies must be considered preliminary and more work in this area is clearly needed.

CONTRAINDICATIONS AND RISKS

When considering patients for PAD, the risks related to both the delay of surgery required for donation and the possibility of adverse reactions should be weighed against the benefits of autologous transfusion.

RISK OF DELAY

Generally, a PAD program involves the collection of 1 unit of blood from the donor/patient each week for 2–4 weeks before surgery, leaving at least 72 hours between the last donation and operation. During the collection period, the patient's condition may worsen, and this risk must be considered when weighing the benefits gained by the patient in using autologous blood. The time necessary for PAD may be of particular consequence for patients with cardiac conditions, vascular disease, and/or cancer.

Adverse outcomes caused by a delay in elective cardiac surgery are difficult to measure. Although several studies have demonstrated the successful donation of autologous blood by patients having elective cardiac surgery (50–55), the presence of significant heart disease (usually atherosclerotic coronary artery disease) carries with it a small but definite risk of clinical deterioration and even death during the donation period. In addition, deferral of donations due to anemia or vasovagal reaction will either prolong the time required for donation or make preoperative donation a less-effective source of blood. Autologous blood donors may have an increased rate of deferrals because they are more likely to have poorer baseline health than allogeneic blood donors. One study examining 180 patients eligible for autologous blood donation found that 25.5% of all scheduled donations were deferred (40). Although the incidence of at least one deferral was 47.8% for all patients, 63.8% of the cardiac patients experienced deferral. Two cardiac patients in the program died before their scheduled surgery; and although the cause of deaths could not be directly related to donation, they likely would have been avoided by early operation.

Another study examining the use of autologous blood in 104 patients scheduled for elective cardiac surgery also had two preoperative deaths occur among the autologous donors and one among the 111 patients in the control group (52). The report concluded that "patients with severe coronary artery disease risk experiencing increasing symptoms during preoperative delay required for donation." An estimate of the risk of donation in light of the extent of delay necessary for PAD might preclude the referral of patients with cardiac conditions. In particular, patients scheduled for cardiac surgery who have unstable syndromes, severe left main coronary disease, or aortic stenosis may be less able to tolerate a delay in surgery and may not be appropriate autologous donors. Although a recent study reports that 79 patients with serious aortic valve disease donated 1–3 units of blood before elective aortic valve surgery without negative outcome (53), severe aortic stenosis, unstable coronary artery disease, and refractory congestive heart failure are typically considered contraindications for preoperative donation before cardiac surgery not only because of the risk of donation but also because of the risk of delay of surgery.

Patients in a PAD program with abdominal aortic aneurysms (AAA) risk sustaining a rupture during the donation period. At what size an aneurysm's risk of rupture becomes significant is controversial. Larger aneurysms (greater than 6–7 cm) are associated with an increased risk of rupture when compared with small aneurysms (less than 6 cm) (56–59). However, the data also demonstrate a significant risk of rupture of small aneurysms (57–59). Small AAAs have been measured to grow on an average of 0.4 cm per year, but sporadic periods of latency and rapid enlargement are also noted (60, 61). In addition to the size of the aneurysm and perhaps more relevant in determining the risk of delaying surgery is the presence of a symptomatic aneurysm. Thirty percent of the patients in a study of untreated aneurysms of the abdominal aorta and its branches died within 1 month of the onset of symptoms and 74% died within less than 6 months (58).

Some investigators have found that intraoperative salvage, which eliminates the risk of delay, is a more practical autologous blood source than PAD blood for patients undergoing AAA repair. Of the autologous units used for elective AAA repair in 100 patients, 91% of the units were salvaged intraoperatively, whereas 9% were donated preoperatively (62). Recently, however, other studies have demonstrated the successful use of PAD in AAA surgery (63, 64). Generally, donation should be reserved for elective asymptomatic patients. A combination of PAD and intraoperative salvage may minimize surgical delay while also diminishing the use of allogeneic blood.

The risk of delay for patients undergoing elective surgery for cancer is probably small but is difficult to accurately determine. Metastases are more likely to occur before detection of the primary tumor than in the much shorter interval between detection and operation. However, the delay of surgery required by PAD may have negative psychological effects on patients who are anxious about their condition. On the other hand, autologous blood may be preferable to allogeneic blood for patients with cancer because several studies report an increased rate of recurrence in patients with cancer using allogeneic blood transfusions (65–67).

Although the coordination of preoperative therapy (e.g., radiation therapy) with PAD has been shown to have no adverse effects on the radiosensitivity of tumors (68), such scheduling may not actually minimize the delay of surgery. An examination of autologous blood donation by 25 patients with bladder cancer undergoing preoperative irradiation followed by radical cystectomy reported that 10 patients avoided allogeneic blood completely without adverse effects related to donation (69). However, the preoperative period was 11 weeks, involving 5 weeks of treatment and withdrawal followed by a 6-week recuperative delay before surgery; each donated unit was centrifuged into components and then frozen for later transfusion. Because it involves a substantial delay of surgery and the expense of frozen storage, the coordination of preoperative therapy with PAD may not be an effective option for patients with cancer. In addition, surgery for cancer is often associated with minimal blood loss, which obviates the need for PAD. On the other hand, patients with cancer who have a high probability of requiring transfusions, such as patients having radical prostatectomy, and who can tolerate a 1-month delay of surgery are ideal candidates for PAD.

RISK OF DONATION

In light of the potential benefits the patient/donor gains by using autologous blood, the standards for blood donation are altered from those established for volunteer blood donors and should be determined by the medical director of the blood bank. Adverse reactions may be mild, such as diaphoresis, nausea, and lightheadedness, or severe, such as loss of consciousness accompanied by convulsions. When considering all blood donors, mild vasovagal donation reactions are sustained in approximately 1–3% (70). Of particular concern are serious cardiovascular reactions in "high-risk" donors.

Several studies (27, 37, 40, 50, 51) report no significant difference in the overall reaction rate of autologous donors compared with that of allogeneic donors, although one study (36) reports a 2.7% reaction rate for donors meeting allogeneic donation requirements versus a 4.3% reaction rate for donors missing at least one requirement. An examination of donation reactions among 2091 autologous donors and 4737 allogeneic donors also found an increased rate of reaction for repeat autologous donors (5.8%) versus that for repeat allogeneic donors (2.6%) (27). The higher frequency of donation for PAD may increase the risk of sustaining a donation reaction.

Independent factors such as first-time donors, age less than 17 years, low weight (less than 110–120 lbs), and female gender also correlate with a higher reaction rate among all donors (27, 36), although one report examining these factors did not find that they increased the risk of donation (71). An analysis of the risk of PAD should consider that allogeneic blood donors are more likely than allogeneic donors to be first-time donors and to have a condition (e.g., coronary artery disease) that may reduce their ability to recover from a reaction.

The effect of the donor's medical condition on reaction rate is unclear. One study reports significant adverse hemodynamic changes (e.g., systolic hypotension) in high-risk autologous donors with blood donation (38). Yet, predisposition to a donation reaction and to a diminished capacity to recover from a reaction is difficult to predict. Lin et al. (72) examined phlebotomy and convulsive syncope in random donors at a community center and did not find a significant change in pulse rate, blood pressure, and mean arterial pressure between donors with syncope and those with convulsive syncope. Similarly, 40 candidates for heart or lung transplants did not demonstrate significant differences in physiological parameters when compared with the control group (73). Most patients scheduled for various elective surgical procedures (40, 74–76), including cardiac and high-risk cases (40, 50–55), have donated blood without adverse outcome. Even patients taking antihypertensive medication, including beta-blockers, which may precipitate severe postural hypotension, have given blood without notable event (74, 77).

Serious donation reaction and death during or after phlebotomy, however, have been reported (36, 52, 54, 74, 78). Although increased reaction rates in patients with various conditions such as neurological disorders are of theoretical concern, reaction rates in cardiac patients remain the center of attention. In particular, there are cases reporting a correlation between donation and an increase of angina and myocardial infarction in some patients with cardiac conditions (36, 40, 52, 54, 74, 78).

Precautions with high-risk patients may include precluding donation by patients with unstable angina or a recent history of myocardial infarction and enhanced monitoring of the patient. In addition, volume replacement with crystalloid solutions may reduce the risk of donation because changes in heart rate, blood pressure, and oxygen uptake after blood loss are associated with volume depletion rather than loss of red blood cell (RBC) mass (34). A study of fluid replacement after blood donation by the elderly and by patients with compromising cardiovascular conditions reports that the maintenance of blood volume using crystalloid solutions hemodynamically stabilized the patients and avoided adverse effects of donation (34). It should be noted that most patients with cardiac disease donate without incident and without fluid replacement.

CONTRAINDICATIONS

Given the potential benefits the patient/donor gains by using autologous blood, most contraindications for allogeneic donation are not applied to autologous donors. Guidelines for autologous donation are established by the blood collection facility medical director. Patients considered for autologous donation who have one or more of the following conditions should be selected carefully: suspected or potential bacteremia, angina, myocardial infarction in the past 3 months, congestive heart failure, aortic stenosis, transient ischemic attacks, arrhythmias, and hypertension. Generally, if an evaluation of a patient's anesthetic risk allows elective surgery, the patient should also be able to safely donate autologous blood units.

Another factor to consider when determining the eligibility of a patient for autologous blood is the potential psychological effect PAD may have on the patient/donor. Autologous blood donation can have positive psychological effects on patient/donors by reducing anxiety associated with allogeneic blood transfusion and by involving patients in their own treatment. However, PAD may also have deleterious effects on patients who are distressed about their weakened condition and about the postponement of surgery.

SPECIAL PATIENTS

CARDIAC SURGERY

Although the presence of cardiovascular disease is not in itself a contraindication to preoperative donation, unstable coronary artery disease, aortic stenosis (moderate to severe), and congestive heart failure are conditions that generally exclude patients from PAD. Despite advances in blood conservation, many patients having elective cardiac surgery still require transfusions. Because PAD can reduce the need for allogeneic transfusions, several groups have explored the use of preoperative donation for patients having elective cardiac surgery. The donation of autologous blood by patients undergoing cardiac surgery has been documented by several studies to be safe and effective (50–55) in reducing the exposure of patients to allogeneic blood. Nonetheless, the routine donation of autologous blood by patients scheduled for cardiac surgery remains controversial because of lingering concerns about the safety of donation and the risk of delaying operations.

That most patients with cardiac conditions donate without adverse outcome and without an increase in overall reaction rate does not preclude a need for precaution when including them in an autologous donation program. One study found significant changes in the hemodynamics of patients with major cardiovascular or multiple-organ disease during phlebotomy even though an increase in reaction rate was not demonstrated (38). Also of concern is that a patient with cardiovascular disease may be less able to recover from a donation reaction. A study of the safety of autologous blood donation in a nonhospital setting reported the occurrence of four severe reactions in 5660 donations (36). Although this figure is extremely low, of interest is that all four patients had cardiovascular disease. Given the uncertainty of the effect of donation on patients with compromising cardiovascular conditions, the risks of donation must be weighed against the risks associated with allogeneic blood transfusions. One study estimated that the risk of donating autologous blood must be less than 1 in 100,000 to offset the risk of allogeneic blood exposure (48).

Even if autologous blood donation is considered safe for patients undergoing cardiac surgery, its effectiveness in reducing the exposure of patients to allogeneic blood is limited by the number of patients with cardiac conditions who can donate. Cardiac surgery often occurs soon after diagnosis, and this does not provide adequate time for autologous blood collection (BD Spiess, MD, unpublished data). In one study, 57% of 674 patients underwent open heart surgery during the diagnostic admission and were unable to donate; only 36.8% of the remaining 291 patients participated in the autologous blood program (54). Current trends to shorten lengths of stay and waiting lists will exacerbate this problem. In addition, of those who donate, the high incidence of deferrals among patients with coronary artery disease may limit the number of units collected for later transfusion (40).

Excessively liberal use of transfusions also minimizes the effectiveness of autologous blood. The use of autologous blood does not address the root cause of allogeneic blood exposure if transfusions are not given appropriately. The practice of transfusion medicine in coronary artery bypass surgery varies significantly among institutions, in part as a result of the administration of unnecessary transfusions (79). The availability of autologous blood for cardiac surgery may only aggravate the overuse of transfusions by providing a source of "risk-free" blood. In fact, although the exposure to allogeneic blood was reduced for autologous donors having cardiac surgery, data from several studies also demonstrated that significantly fewer autologous donors avoided any transfusion when compared with nondonors (51–55). Coupled with the availability of "safe" blood, this trend may be a result of a reduced preoperative hematocrit associated with multiple phlebotomies. An autologous blood program in cardiac surgery, and in other types of surgery, is effective only if all transfusions are indicated.

A careful analysis of the potential blood needs and of the physical condition of patients scheduled for cardiac surgery should precede recommendation for preoperative donation. In general, stable patients likely to require transfusions are acceptable candidates.

AAA AND CARDIOVASCULAR DISEASE

The risk analysis of a patient with AAA should include a careful examination of the medical condition of the patient, particularly because many patients with AAA also have coronary artery disease (57, 58, 80). Of 90 patients with AAA that did not undergo surgical repair and died, 41.1% died of coronary atherosclerosis and 27.8% died of a ruptured AAA (57). In another study, myocardial infarction was responsible for 37% of the early postoperative deaths after AAA resection (80). Cardiac stress tests and careful monitoring of the aneurysm may provide an indication of a patient's capacity to undergo elective AAA repair and PAD. In some patients, coronary angioplasty or bypass surgery may be recommended before AAA repair (81). Because the blood loss associated with the two procedures (whether performed separately or concurrently) is substantial, PAD should be considered.

ORTHOPEDIC SURGERY

As elective procedures associated with significant blood loss, some orthopedic operations present ideal opportunities for patients to donate autologous blood. Successful donations by patients undergoing elective orthopedic surgery is well documented and includes donation by elderly patients (76, 82–86). Because of the nature of the pathology being treated, there is little risk in delaying operation. Although two studies demonstrate a significantly lower preoperative hematocrit among allogeneic donors compared with allogeneic recipients (a potential concern given the high volume of blood loss that often accompanies orthopedic surgery), ensuing complications have not been reported (76, 85). In fact, stimulation of erythropoiesis by preoperative donation may hasten postoperative recovery of red cell mass (76).

Preoperatively donated blood eliminates the need for allogeneic transfusion in most patients undergoing elective orthopedic surgery. However, the number of donor/patients who receive allogeneic transfusions ranges from 2% to 90% (76, 82–86). Some patients are unable to donate the requested amount of blood because of deferrals or a patient may have an unexpectedly high volume of blood loss during surgery. Without resorting to the expensive option of frozen storage, an autologous blood program may increase the number of collected units with erythropoietin (EPO) therapy (87). Patients scheduled for hip replacement surgery, in general, can have their transfusion needs met by the donation of approximately 3 units (85). In a 1991 study of preoperative donation in elderly patients undergoing hip arthroplasty, 40 of 45 patients received less than 2 units of donated blood, and a total of 40 autologous units were discarded (76).

In the absence of contraindications for donation (e.g., osteomyelitis, which may be associated with bacteremia [70]), patients undergoing elective orthopedic operation associated with transfusion should be encouraged to donate. The number of units collected should be estimated according to the amount of blood typically ordered. The reduction of allogeneic blood use may be improved by using other autologous blood sources such as hemodilution and salvage.

PREGNANT WOMEN

Transfusions are administered to 1–2% of all patients giving birth, with a slightly lower transfusion rate for women having vaginal deliveries than for those having cesarean sections. Kruskall et al. (88) reported a 1.6% transfusion frequency for all deliveries at the Beth Israel Hospital, with a 1.2% transfusion rate after vaginal deliveries and a 2.2% rate after cesarean sections. In another study, 0.57% of 2265 patients received transfusions (0.28% of vaginal deliveries, 1.9% of primary cesareans, and 0.66% of repeat cesarean sections) (89). Given the small number of patients receiving transfusions, autologous donation may be most effective if targeted toward those patients with conditions that predispose them to blood loss. Some risk factors associated with postpartum transfusion are placenta previa, multiple gestation, cesarean sections, preeclampsia, a history of postpartum hemorrhage, and third-trimester bleeding. Although some studies report a greater rate of transfusion for pregnant women with complications, many demonstrate that the rate of postpartum transfusion for patients with risk factors remains relatively low and unpredictable (89–94). Andres et al. (89) report that less than 2% of patients predicted to require transfusions actually received them (89). In another report, only 1 donor/patient of 37 obstetrical patients (32 with risk factors) received the unit of blood that had been donated preoperatively (93). Of the risk factors reported, placenta previa is more consistently associated with transfusions (95).

Physicians caring for pregnant women should also consider that many pregnant patients (approximately 44%) can donate only 1 unit of autologous blood because of a low hematocrit (less than 34%) (88, 90). Yet, only 8% and 11.2% of pregnant women requiring transfusions in two studies had their needs met by only 1 unit of blood (89, 91). Another study reports that 27% of patients with placenta previa require allogeneic units in addition to autologous blood (95). Thus, although PAD is most effective for pregnant women with a high risk for transfusions, this represents a small and unpredictable group of patients.

The donation of blood antepartum was originally recommended for pregnant patients in their second trimester due to the potential risks of abortion during the first trimester and premature delivery in the third trimester. Several studies, however, report the safety of PAD by pregnant women in their third trimester (88, 90, 93, 95, 96). This avoids the costly storage of frozen blood required by second-trimester donation. One argument for third-trimester donation is that an occurrence of fetal distress or premature labor resulting in delivery may have better outcomes with increased length of gestation (93).

Although female gender has been associated with a higher risk of sustaining a donation reaction (27, 36), the rate of reaction due to donation by pregnant donors is consistent with that for all donors (88, 90). A comparison of the hemodynamic responses in uncomplicated pregnant donors and nonpregnant donors did not find a significant difference between the two groups (although the pregnant group experienced a reduced heart rate response to orthostasis compared with the nonpregnant group) (96). However, in addition to the potential risk of reaction faced by all donors, pregnant donors must consider the donation effect on the fetus. Risks of particular import to pregnant donors are induced delivery, hypovolemia/hypotension, and anemia. Unfortunately, at present the effect of a maternal donation reaction on the fetus is unclear, and an obstetrician recommending autologous blood donation should obtain informed consent from the patient/donor (97).

Studies that examined the effect of donation on the fetus by using various monitoring devices reported no significant changes in fetal conditions during donation (88, 90, 93, 96). Two reports, however, noted early delivery in several donor/patients, although these patients had underlying complications with pregnancy (90, 93). Six donor/patients in one study underwent cesarean section for fetal distress; one patient delivered 6 hours after an uneventful phlebotomy when fetal bradycardia occurred during active labor (93). Another patient with a twin pregnancy went into spontaneous labor the day after donation (90).

In addition to the potential for donation-related fetal distress and induced labor, PAD may affect fetal circulation if the mother/donor experiences hypovolemia or hypotension (88, 92). Two studies each reported two patients who sustained hypotension, one of which was severe, although the fetal heart rate remained normal throughout the incidents (90, 93). Because these incidents occur infrequently, the effect of hypovolemia and hypotension on the fetus is not known.

Another concern involving pregnant donors is donation-induced anemia despite the use of iron supplementation (98). In addition to having a potentially adverse effect on the fetus, a reduced maternal hematocrit may limit the units of blood collected (as discussed above) and increase the risk for postpartum transfusion. McVay et al. (95) suggested that donations within 1 week of delivery may decrease the predelivery hematocrit and increase the need for postpartum transfusion. The study found that women who donate blood during the week before delivery have a greater rate of transfusion than those who donate 1 week or more before delivery (21% versus 9.4%). Yet, an increase in the time between donation and delivery also increases the risk of the blood expiring and the need for frozen blood, which raises the cost of PAD.

Blood transfusion in women giving birth, including those

with complications, is infrequent. Donated units are often wasted, particularly in the absence of a crossover program for allogeneic use (94). Autologous blood donation by pregnant women may not be cost-effective unless applied to a selected population of patients (i.e., third-trimester patients in stable condition with a high risk for blood loss). Donor/patients may benefit most if there is at least 1 week between the last donation and delivery. A determination of the benefits of autologous blood use in deliveries associated with substantial blood loss should also consider the low number of units generally donated by pregnant patients.

CANCER SURGERY

The presence of cancer does not contraindicate autologous blood donation. In fact, autologous blood may be preferable to allogeneic blood for patients with malignant disease because an increased rate of recurrence in patients with cancer is associated with the transfusion of allogeneic blood (66–68). This correlation may be related to an immunosuppressive effect of allogeneic blood on the recipient. However, increased recurrence of cancer (99, 100) and decreased survival of patients with cancer may be associated with all blood transfusions—autologous and allogeneic alike. Several studies found no significant difference in recurrence rates between patients with cancer who received autologous blood and those transfused with allogeneic blood (99, 100). In addition, patients transfused with any blood had increased recurrence rates when compared with patients who did not require blood products. The effect of blood transfusions on tumor recurrence remains controversial. A recent study comparing tumor growth in animal models reports a significant increase of metastases in mice receiving allogeneic blood compared with mice transfused with syngeneic blood (101). The study also found that leukodepletion of allogeneic blood significantly mitigated the deleterious effects of allogeneic transfusions, suggesting the presence of a tumor growth-promoting factor in allogeneic blood.

Autologous blood donation may not be recommended in cancer surgery if the delay of surgery required is deemed unacceptable by the surgeon or the patient. In addition, PAD is not recommended for cancer surgery that is associated with low blood loss. One study examining the effectiveness of donation in 129 patients with left-sided colonic or rectal cancer found that of the 60 units withdrawn from 28 donors, only 52% of the blood was transfused; 48% of the units were discarded (68). The time and expense of using autologous blood in elective cancer surgery should be weighed against the low blood loss associated with such surgery. Few patients undergoing procedures like colectomies, mastectomies, or pulmonary lobectomies require blood transfusion. Of 48 consecutive patients having colon resection for cancer at Boston's Beth Israel Hospital, 75% did not receive any blood; 2 patients donated 1 unit of which only one was transfused along with allogeneic blood. Of 39 patients having mastectomies, 38 did not require any transfusions (the patient who required allogeneic blood had a hemorrhagic complication). Two patients gave a total of 3 units that were discarded. For patients having pulmonary lobectomy, less than 15% require transfusion.

Patients undergoing radical prostatectomies, however, may be ideal autologous donors given the likelihood for substantial blood loss during these operations. Ninety-three percent of 60 consecutive patients undergoing radical prostatectomy for cancer at Boston's Beth Israel Hospital were transfused. An average of 3 units was given by 56 patients, fulfilling the blood needs of all but 4 of these donor/patients. A total of 44 units of autologous blood were discarded. A study by Toy et al. (102) demonstrated that PAD reduced the rate of allogeneic transfusion for this procedure from 66% to 20%. In light of this information, PAD is generally recommended for patients having cancer surgery only when perioperative transfusion is likely.

CONTROVERSIES

CROSSOVER OF AUTOLOGOUS BLOOD

In the United States, more than 40% of autologous units are never used (8). In some hospitals, the proportion of discarded PADs is much higher. Why is this happening? Why is there an excess of autologous units and, when available, why are these units not being integrated into the blood bank's allogeneic supply?

The explanation for the excess of available units is clear. Physicians are requesting patients to make PADs for surgical procedures for which there is little, if any, likelihood of transfusion (3). Examples of such procedures include routine cholecystectomy, abdominal laparoscopy, or tubal ligation. Although the rate of transfusion after uncomplicated vaginal delivery is only 1–2% (103), it is common for women with normal pregnancies to donate 1–2 units of autologous blood. The overzealous use of PAD can be accounted for partly by the fear of litigation related to transfusion-associated complications. In such cases, the physician may be responding to pressure from the patient who wants to eliminate any risk of an allogeneic transfusion. Another contributing factor may be the overestimation of both the need for blood and risks associated with transfusion (104).

The transfusion of "unused" autologous blood for allogeneic recipients, termed "crossover," is a controversial topic often fought on emotional rather than scientific grounds. The proponents of crossover argue that if an autologous unit is fully tested for the same infectious disease markers as allogeneic blood and the tests are negative, then such units should be considered as safe as any unit collected from community volunteer donors. Are autologous units as safe? The evidence is contradictory. Several studies point to increased rates of abnormalities in the two nonspecific hepatitis markers, alanine aminotransferase and anti-HBc, in autologous compared with volunteer donors (105, 106). These data must be interpreted cautiously in that they lack proper controls and consist of small cohorts. Using much larger populations of autologous and allogeneic donors, Kruskall et al. (107) found that a comparison of marker rates yielded no biologically significant differences between these populations. Other investigators have also found no significant differences in antibody to hepatitis C virus (108). Because the published data have methodological flaws, it is difficult to make strong conclusions about the relative safety of autologous blood compared with blood from volunteer blood donors. The consequence of the controversy, however, has been a reluctance to make autologous units available for the general blood supply.

As a practical matter, many autologous donations cannot be used for other recipients because the original donor does not meet either U.S. Food and Drug Administration or American Association of Blood Banks standards for blood donation. The most frequent reason is a low predonation hemoglobin. Other reasons may include the underlying disease process (e.g., malignancy) or medications that would disqualify the individual as an allogeneic donor. Finally, some blood banks do not perform all donor screening tests on autologous units, usually as a cost-saving measure. Unless subjected to the same testing as allogeneic units, autologous units cannot be transfused for others.

ERYTHROPOIETIN

A major limitation to PAD is the inadequate erythropoietic response to mild anemia (109). In studies performed at University Hospitals of Cleveland, 30 of 175 patients overall and 23 of 58 patients asked to store 4 or more units were unable to do so because of progressive anemia (109). Not surprisingly, McVay et al. (110) found that women were less likely (42% versus 86%; $P = .001$) than men to make four donations, and the difference was more striking at the 5-unit level. Patients not able to meet the requested number of autologous units are more likely to be transfused with allogeneic blood (109). Another manifestation of inadequate erythropoietic response in autologous blood donors is the finding that RBC mass decreases with successive PADs. In one study, mean RBC mass of 188 consecutively collected autologous units was, on average, 13% less than that of 300 consecutively collected allogeneic units (111). (It is this difference in RBC mass that is used as one of the arguments against crossover of autologous units; such units would provide less therapeutic benefit per unit dose compared with allogeneic red cells.)

To maximize the erythropoietic response, two approaches have been evaluated: increasing the aggressiveness of the donation schedule and the use of recombinant human EPO. The rationale for decreasing the donation interval is based on the observation of peak concentration in endogenous EPO levels within 1 day of phlebotomy followed by a plateau at lower, although still elevated, levels after each subsequent donation (donations were scheduled on days 1, 3, 7, 14, and 21) (112). In adult baboons, increased donation frequency alone (donation occurred when the hematocrit was greater than 30%) yielded 10 units of blood over a 5-week period, whereas the addition of intravenous EPO further increased the yield 35% (113). In a controlled trial involving 47 adults scheduled for elective orthopedic procedures, the mean red cell volume donated by the patients receiving EPO was 41% greater than that donated by patients receiving placebo (87). In humans, a twice-weekly (for 3 weeks) blood donation schedule yielded a 27% and 47% increase in red cell mass for 23 placebo and 21 EPO-treated patients, respectively (114). The authors concluded that in patients unsuited for aggressive autologous phlebotomy (such as some cardiac surgery patients), EPO may be a preferable approach.

Although the use of EPO to increase the yield of PAD might, at first glance, look attractive, it is premature to embrace this as routine practice. First, most patients are able to successfully donate the number of requested PADs. As transfusion practices become more conservative and fewer transfusions are needed, the number of procedures that necessitate 4 or more units should also diminish. Second, optimum methods for drug delivery and dosage schedule have yet to be determined. The initial studies of EPO used the intravenous route, usually administered at least three times weekly. Because PAD is an outpatient procedure, often performed outside the hospital, most patients would find this method and schedule of delivery to be impractical.

Several groups have investigated the subcutaneous use of EPO as an alternative delivery route. Preliminary results in relatively small cohorts of patients awaiting heart surgery and hip replacement surgery are promising (115, 116). Watanabe et al. (115) found that subcutaneous EPO (administered on preoperative days 14 and 7 and oral iron for 14 days) was as effective as intravenous EPO in stimulating erythropoiesis in 14 patients undergoing coronary artery bypass procedures.

Finally, the cost of EPO must be viewed as a barrier to use in the autologous setting. At current prices, a single course of the drug may cost $1000–3000, depending on the dosage.

INDICATIONS FOR TRANSFUSION OF AUTOLOGOUS BLOOD

The efficacy of autologous blood donation in reducing patient exposure to allogeneic blood products is well documented (9, 24, 25, 30, 40, 51–55, 75, 76, 84, 85). However, the extent to which autologous blood collected preoperatively should be transfused remains controversial. The benefits of increasing oxygen delivery, the usual reason for administering blood, must be weighed against the risks of transfusion. Some believe that a more liberal transfusion practice should be followed for autologous blood than allogeneic blood (RD Miller, unpublished data). However, others support the use of universal indications for autologous and allogeneic transfusions alike because autologous blood is not entirely risk-free and the extent to which the risk-to-benefit ratio is altered by autologous blood is difficult to measure (SA Gould, unpublished data).

An analysis of the benefits gained by receiving blood units and the risks associated with autologous blood transfusion is necessary to determine when and how much PAD blood to transfuse. One study reported that erythrocyte reinfusion in healthy individuals absent of anemia correlates with an increase in hemoglobin concentration and an improved exercise performance (117). However, another report comparing the "conservative" transfusion (hematocrit 25%) and "liberal" transfusion (hematocrit 32%) of autologous donors after elective operations for myocardial revascularization found no direct correlation between hematocrit level and exercise capacity (118). Other parameters of postoperative recovery were also unaffected.

Although the benefits of a liberal transfusion practice are somewhat ambiguous, the potential adverse outcomes of autologous blood transfusions, although few, pose substantial risks that require consideration. Administrative errors, fluid overload, and sepsis due to bacterial infection during phlebotomy or storage are risks of particular concern. Physicians may also have an increased tendency to transfuse autologous blood because of its mere availability, pressure to fulfill patients' expectations, and concern for blood wastage (especially in light of the decline of crossing over unused units for allogeneic transfusion). Indeed, several studies (39, 51, 53–55, 95, 119) reported an increased rate of transfusion in autologous donors than in nondonors. Autologous blood programs may be most effective if combined with efforts to reduce inappropriate transfusions. Similarly, iron replacement, accelerated wound healing, and the normalization of hemoglobin levels are not considered indications to administer autologous blood (120).

When a need for autologous blood transfusion is determined, intraoperatively salvaged blood, because of its short storage period, should be transfused before preoperatively donated blood. PAD blood ideally should be transfused after blood loss, and the fresher units should be administered first. A system should be established to prevent the transfusion of allogeneic blood when autologous blood is available and to inform the ordering physician of the blood available for transfusion. In addition, because autologous blood collection and storage provides ample opportunity for administration error, blood unit should always be double-checked for identity.

In addition to the potential to reduce allogeneic blood use and mitigate the concerns associated with allogeneic blood transfusions, the hemodilution associated with autologous blood may also decrease operative blood loss and enhance circulation (75, 76). However, the availability and utilization of autologous blood may also conceal, and perhaps reinforce, inappropriate transfusion practices. Although one study found that physicians in autologous blood programs accepted lower admission and discharge hematocrits in autologous donors than in nondonors (119), various reports suggested that autologous blood use may aggravate misperceptions of transfusion risks by the physicians and patients (3, 9, 120). Such distortions may result in the overordering of PADs and the inappropriate application of autologous blood donation to patients having procedures associated with minimal blood loss and/or high donation risks (3, 9, 121).

The appropriate application of autologous blood requires a delicate balance between overordering and underordering, excessive transfusion and blood wastage, and risk and benefit of transfusion. Careful analysis and commitment by the surgeon and anesthesiologist are necessary. However, given a request for a necessary transfusion and the appropriate coordination between the blood bank and the surgical team, autologous blood provides a safer and more readily available alternative than banked blood and reduces the potential for transfusion-related complications during and after surgery.

PLATELETPHERESIS

The collection of autologous platelet-rich plasma during the early stages of a cardiac procedure for reinfusion after cardiopulmonary bypass has been suggested as a potential means of decreasing postoperative bleeding. This is based on the fact that postoperative bleeding by such patients may be the result of platelet dysfunction. Thus, plateletpheresis could potentially minimize the number of blood products transfused. Several studies demonstrate that the transfusion of autologous platelet-rich plasma to patients undergoing cardiac surgery reduces the amount of RBC, platelets, and plasma administered and increases the percentage of patients who avoid allogeneic products (122–124). In contrast, a "blind" study of the effectiveness of autologous platelet-rich plasma in 31 patients having repeat vascular surgery and a prospective study in cardiac patients reported no significant difference in the administration of allogeneic products to patients who did and did not receive autologous plasma (125, 126). Postoperative bleeding is often associated with aspirin-induced platelet dysfunction, a problem not solved by plateletpheresis because the salvaged platelets will also be impaired by this drug.

The routine use of platelet transfusions in cardiac surgery is not appropriate. Despite known platelet defects after cardiopulmonary bypass, most patients do not have substantial bleeding, and platelet therapy is not required. According to a National Institutes of Health Consensus Conference, there is a lack of evidence correlating platelet counts and bleeding after coronary artery bypass graft, and prophylactic platelet administration is unjustified (127). An examination of the variability of transfusion practice in coronary artery bypass surgery found that of 540 patients at 18 institutions, 22% received platelets, with an institutional range of 0–80% (79). The variation, in part, could be attributed to the disparate distribution of patients with platelet-associated bleeding risk factors and the increased likelihood of transfusion in such patients; however, there was no difference in blood loss between patients with and without risk factors, suggesting that platelet transfusions were often administered unnecessarily.

Benefits from plateletpheresis in cardiac surgery may not be the result of the postoperative reinfusion of healthy platelets but the enhanced tissue perfusion and reduced blood loss of the hemodiluted patient. One report found that patients who had plateletpheresis had a significant reduction in operative loss of red cell mass (124). This observation is unrelated to the postoperative reinfusion of platelet-rich plasma and weakens the premise that plateletpheresis can reduce postoperative bleeding. In the same study, the postoperative blood loss did not differ significantly between patients who did and did not receive autologous platelets.

COMPREHENSIVE BLOOD PROGRAMS

Throughout this chapter, we have emphasized the importance of PAD as part of a comprehensive effort to minimize the allogeneic exposures received by patients having surgery. Clearly, the benefits of a PAD program will be diminished if unnecessary units of allogeneic products are given. An effective approach requires the commitment of the entire care team to reducing blood exposure throughout the patient's hospital stay.

Preoperatively, in addition to PAD, any associated bleeding diatheses should be corrected and anticoagulant medications (including aspirin and warfarin) discontinued, if possible. Hematinics should be administered when indicated.

During operation, surgical hemostasis must be meticulous and obligate blood loss should be salvaged when feasible. When anticoagulation is indicated (such as in cardiac or vascular surgery), it should be carefully controlled and properly reversed. After operation, postoperative drainage should be salvaged and infused when appropriate (after cardiac and perhaps after orthopedic surgery).

Throughout the perioperative period, blood and blood components should be transfused only when clearly indicated. Prophylactic therapy of red cells and other components is inappropriate. Transfusion decisions should be made on an individual basis rather than by protocol. Blood loss through laboratory testing should be minimized. If these comprehensive principles are followed, the effectiveness of PAD will be enhanced and the full benefit of the PAD program achieved.

REFERENCES

1. Blundell J. Experiments on the transfusion of blood by the syringe. Med Chirg Trans 1818;9:56–92.
2. Grant FC. Autotransfusion. Ann Surg 1921;74:253–254.
3. Popovsky MA. Autologous blood transfusion in the 1990s. Where is it heading? Am J Clin Pathol 1992;97:297–300.
4. Surgenor DM. The patient's blood is the safest blood. N Engl J Med 1987;316:542–544.
5. Council on Scientific Affairs. Autologous blood transfusions. JAMA 1986;256:2378–2380.
6. The National Blood Resource Education Program Expert Panel. The use of autologous blood. JAMA 1990;263:414–417.
7. American Association of Blood Banks. Annual Report, Bethesda, MD, 1992.
8. Wallace EL, Surgenor DM, Hao HS, et al. Collection and transfusion of blood and blood components in the United States, 1989. Transfusion 1993;33:139–144.
9. Renner SW, Howanitz PJ, Bachner P, et al. Preoperative autologous blood donation in 612 hospitals. Arch Pathol Lab Med 1992;116:613–619.
10. Yomtovian R. Increasing the use of predeposited autologous blood for transfusion [letter]. N Engl J Med 1987;317:569.
11. Columbo M, Rebulla P, Zanieso F, et al. Increasing the use of predeposited autologous blood for transfusion [letter]. N Engl J Med 1987;317:570.
12. Donahue JG, Munoz A, Ness PM, et al. The declining risk of post-transfusion hepatitis C virus infection. N Engl J Med 1992;327:419–421.
13. Dodd RY. The risk of transfusion-transmitted infection. N Engl J Med 1992;327:369–373.
14. Triulzi DJ, Vanek K, Ryank DH, et al. A clinical and immunologic

study of blood transfusion and postoperative bacterial infection in spinal surgery. Transfusion 1992;32:517–524.
15. Murphy P, Heal JM, Blumberg N. Infection or suspected infection after hip replacement surgery with autologous or homologous blood transfusions. Transfusion 1991;31:212–217.
16. Jensen LS, Andersen AJ, Christiansen PM, et al. Postoperative infection and natural killer cell function following blood transfusion in patients undergoing elective colorectal surgery. Br J Surg 1992;79:513–516.
17. Popovsky MA, Moore SM. Diagnostic and pathogenetic considerations in transfusion-related acute lung injury. Transfusion 1985;25:573–577.
18. Shivdasani RA, Haluska FG, Dock NL, et al. Brief report: graft-versus-host disease associated with transfusion of blood from unrelated HLA-homozygous donors. N Engl J Med 1993;328:766–770.
19. Otsuka S, Kuneida K, Kitamura F, et al. The critical role of blood from HLA-homozygous donors in fatal transfusion-associated graft-versus-host disease in immunocompetent patients. Transfusion 1991;31: 260–264.
20. Coleman DH, Stevens AR, Dodge HT, et al. Rate of blood regeneration after blood loss. Arch Intern Med 1953;92:341–349.
21. Levine E, Rosen A, Sehgal L, et al. Accelerated erythropoiesis: the hidden benefit of autologous donation. Transfusion 1990;30:295–297.
22. Simon TL, Smith KJ. The issues in autologous transfusion. Hum Pathol 1989;20:3–6.
23. Axelrod FB, Pepkowitz SH, Goldfinger D. Establishment of a schedule of optimal preoperative collection of autologous blood. Transfusion 1989;29:677–680.
24. Cowell HR, Swickard JW. Autotransfusion in children's orthopedics. J Bone Joint Surg [A] 1974;56:908–912.
25. Silvergleid AJ. Safety and effectiveness of predeposit autologous transfusions in preteen and adolescent children. JAMA 1987;257: 3403–3404.
26. Novak RW. Autologous blood transfusion in a pediatric population. Clin Pediatr 1988;27:184–187.
27. McVay PA, Andrews A, Kaplan EB, et al. Donation reactions among autologous donors. Transfusion 1990;30:249–252.
28. McVay PA, Strauss RG, Stehling LC, Toy PTCY. Probable reasons that autologous blood was not donated by patients having surgery for which crossmatched blood was ordered. Transfusion 1991;31:810–813.
29. DePalma L, Luban NLC. Autologous blood transfusion in pediatrics. Pediatrics 1990;85:125–128.
30. Haugen RK, Hill GE. A large-scale autologous blood program in a community hospital. A contribution to the community's blood supply. JAMA 1987;257:1211–1214.
31. McVay PA, Andrews A, Kaplan EB, et al. Donation reactions among autologous donors. Transfusion 1990;30:249–252.
32. Simon TL, Rhyne RL, Wayne SJ, Garry PJ. Characteristics of elderly blood donors. Transfusion 1991;31:693–697.
33. Pindyck J, Avorn J, Kuriyan M, et al. Blood donation by the elderly. Clinical and policy considerations. JAMA 1987;257:1186–1188.
34. Daneshvar A. Fluid replacement after blood donation: implications for elderly and autologous blood donors. Md Med J 1988;37:787–791.
35. Standards for blood banks and transfusion services. 15th ed. Bethesda, MD: American Association of Blood Banks, 1993.
36. AuBuchon JP, Popovsky MA. The safety of preoperative autologous blood donation in the non-hospital setting. Transfusion 1991;31:513–517.
37. McVay PA, Andrews A, Hoag MS, et al. Moderate and severe reactions during autologous blood donations are no more frequent than during homologous blood donations. Vox Sang 1990;59:70–72.
38. Spiess BD, Sassetti R, McCarthy RJ, et al. Autologous blood donation: hemodynamics in a high-risk patient population. Transfusion 1992;32:17–22.
39. Toy PTCY, Strauss RG, Stehling LC, et al. Predeposited autologous blood for elective surgery. N Engl J Med 1987;316:517–520.
40. Kruskall MS, Glazer EE, Leonard SS, et al. Utilization and effectiveness of a hospital autologous preoperative blood donor program. Transfusion 1986;26:335–340.
41. Moore SB, Swenke PK, Foss ML, et al. Simplified enrollment for autologous transfusion: automatic referral of presurgical patients for assessment for autologous blood collections. Mayo Clin Proc 1992;67:323–327.
42. Kruskall MS. Autologous blood collection and transfusion in a tertiary-care center. In: Taswell HF, Pineda AA, eds. Autologous transfusion and hemotherapy. Boston: Blackwell Scientific Publications, 1991:53–77.
43. Fairbanks VF, Beutler E. Iron deficiency. In: Williams WJ, Beutler E, Erslev AJ, Lichtman MA, eds. Hematology. 3rd ed. New York: McGraw-Hill, 1983:466–489.
44. Biesma DH, Kraaijenhagen RJ, Poortman J, et al. The effect of oral iron supplementation on erythropoiesis in autologous blood donors. Transfusion 1992;32:162–165.
45. Strauss RG. Iron for autologous blood donors needs more work [letter]. Transfusion 1992;32:788–789.
46. Autologous transfusion. In: American Association of Blood Banks technical manual. 11th ed. Bethesda, MD: American Association of Blood Banks, 1993:491–506.
47. Autologous blood collection and processing procedures: January 1990. Addendum to FDA guidance for autologous blood and blood components memorandum of March 15, 1989.
48. Birkmeyer JD, Goodnough LT, AuBuchon JP, et al. The cost-effectiveness of preoperative autologous blood donation for total hip and knee replacement. Transfusion 1993;33:544–551.
49. Elawad A, Benoni G, Montgomery F, et al. Cost effectiveness of blood substitution in elective orthopedic operations. Acta Orthop Scand 1991;62:435–439.
50. Mann M, Sacks HJ, Goldfinger D. Safety of autologous blood donation prior to elective surgery for a variety of "high-risk" patients. Transfusion 1983;23:229–232.
51. Love TR, Hendren WG, O'Keefe DD, Daggett WM. Transfusion of predonated autologous blood in elective cardiac surgery. Ann Thorac Surg 1987;43:508–512.
52. Britton LW, Eastlund DT, Dziuban SW, et al. Predonated autologous blood use in elective cardiac surgery. Ann Thorac Surg 1989;47: 529–532.
53. Dzik WH, Fleisher AG, Ciavarella D, et al. Safety and efficacy of autologous blood donation before elective aortic valve operation. Ann Thorac Surg 1992;54:1177–1181.
54. Owings DV, Kruskall MS, Thurer RL, Donovan LM. Autologous blood donations prior to elective cardiac surgery. JAMA 1989;262: 1963–1968.
55. Zussa C, Polesel E, Salvador L, et al. Efficacy and safety of predeposit autodonation in 500 cases of myocardial revascularization. Scand J Thorac Cardiovasc Surg 1990;24:171–175.
56. Hollier LH, Rutherford RB. Infrarenal aortic aneurysms. In: Rutherford RB, ed. Vascular surgery. 3rd ed. Vol. 2. Philadelphia: WB Saunders, 1989.
57. Szilagyi DE, Elliott JP, Smith RF. Clinical fate of the patient with asymptomatic abdominal aortic aneurysm and unfit for surgical treatment. Arch Surg 1972;104:600–606.
58. Gleidman ML, Ayers WB, Vestal BL. Aneurysms of the abdominal aorta and its branches: a study of untreated patients. Ann Surg

1957;146:214.
59. Darling RC, Brewster DC. Elective treatment of abdominal aortic aneurysms. World J Surg 1980;4:661–667.
60. Bernstein EF, Dilley RB, Goldberger LE, et al. Growth rate of small abdominal aortic aneurysms. Surgery 1976;80:765–773.
61. Ernst CB. Current concepts. Abdominal aortic aneurysm. N Engl J Med 1993;328:1167–1172.
62. Pittman RD, Inahara T. Eliminating homologous blood transfusion during abdominal aortic aneurysm repair. Am J Surg 1990;159:522–524.
63. Tulloh BR, Brakespear CP, Bates SC, et al. Autologous predonation, haemodilution and intraoperative blood salvage in elective abdominal aortic aneurysm repair. Br J Surg 1993;80:313–315.
64. Nicholls MD, Janu MR, Davies VJ, Wedderburn CE. Autologous blood transfusion for elective surgery. Med J Aust 1986;144:395–399.
65. Blumberg N, Agarwal MM, Chuang C. Relation between recurrence of cancer of the colon and blood transfusion. Br Med J 1985;290: 1037–1039.
66. Heal JM, Chuang C, Blumberg N. Perioperative blood transfusions and prostate cancer recurrence and survival. Am J Surg 1988;156:374–379.
67. Burrows L, Tartter P, Aufses A. Increased recurrence rates in perioperatively transfused colorectal malignancy patients. Cancer Detect Prevent 1987;10:361–369.
68. Harrison S, Steele RJC, Johnston AK, et al. Transfusion in patients with colorectal cancer: a feasibility study. Br J Surg 1992;79:355–357.
69. Swanson DA, Lo RK, Lichtiger B. Predeposit autologous blood transfusion in patients undergoing irradiation and radical cystectomy. J Urol 1983;130:892–894.
70. The National Blood Resource Education Program Expert Panel. The use of autologous blood. JAMA 1990;263:414–417.
71. Mazzei C, Imberciadori G, Saccone F, et al. Risks of donation reactions among autologous and homologous donors [letter]. Transfusion 1991;31:285.
72. Lin JT-Y, Ziegler DK, Lai C-W, Bayer W. Convulsive syncope in blood donors. Ann Neurol 1982;11:525–528.
73. Klapper E, Inducil C, Pepkowitz SH, et al. Objective hemodynamic measurements support the safety of autologous blood donations by patients awaiting heart and lung transplantations. Transfusion 1992;32 (suppl):S255.
74. Howard MR, Chapman CE, Dunstan JA, et al. Regional transfusion centre preoperative autologous blood donation programme: the first two years. Br Med J 1992;305:1470–1473.
75. Rebulla P, Giovanetti AM, Petrini G, et al. Autologous blood predeposit for elective surgery: a program for better use and conservation of blood. Surgery 1985;97:463–466.
76. Elawad AAR, Jonsson S, Laurell M, Fredin H. Predonation autologous blood in hip arthroplasty. Acta Ortho Scand 1991;62:218–222.
77. Pisciotto P, Sataro P, Blumberg N. Incidence of adverse reactions in blood donors taking antihypertensive medications. Transfusion 1982; 22:530–531.
78. Kiraly JF III, Feldmann JE, Wheby MS. Hazards of phlebotomy in polycythemic patients with cardiovascular disease. JAMA 1976;236: 2080–2081.
79. Goodnough LT, Johnston MFM, Toy PTCY. The variability of transfusion practice in coronary artery bypass surgery. JAMA 1991;265: 86–90.
80. Hertzer NR. Fatal myocardial infarction following abdominal aortic aneurysm resection. Ann Surg 1980;192:667–673.
81. Hertzer NR, Young JR, Kramer JR, et al. Routine coronary angiography prior to elective aortic reconstruction. Arch Surg 1979;114: 1136–1144.
82. Mallory TH, Kennedy M. The use of banked autologous blood in total hip replacement surgery. Clin Orthop 1976;117:254–257.
83. Thomson JD, Callaghan J J, Savory CG, et al. Prior deposition of autologous blood in elective orthopaedic surgery. J Bone Joint Surg [A] 1987;69:320–324.
84. Bailey TE, Mahoney OM. The use of banked autologous blood in patients undergoing surgery for spinal deformity. J Bone Joint Surg [A] 1987;69:329–331.
85. Woolson ST, Marsh JS, Tanner JB. Transfusion of previously deposited autologous blood for patients undergoing hip-replacement surgery. J Bone Joint Surg [A] 1987;69:325–328.
86. James SE. Autologous blood transfusion in elective orthopaedic surgery. J R Soc Med 1987;80:284–285.
87. Goodnough LT, Rudnick S, Price TH, et al. Increased preoperative collection of autologous blood with recombinant human erythropoietin therapy. N Engl J Med 1989;321:1163–1168.
88. Kruskall MS, Leonard SL, Klapholz H. Autologous blood donation during pregnancy: analysis of safety and blood use. Obstet Gynecol 1987;70:938–941.
89. Andres RL, Piacquadio KM, Resnik R. A reappraisal of the need for autologous blood donation in the obstetric patient. Am J Obstet Gynecol 1990;163:1551–1553.
90. Herbert WNP, Owen HG, Collins ML. Autologous blood storage in obstetrics. Obstet Gynecol 1988;72:166–170.
91. Klapholz H. Blood transfusion in contemporary obstetric practice. Obstet Gynecol 1990;75:940–943.
92. Combs CA, Murphy EL, Laros RK. Cost-benefit analysis of autologous donation in obstetrics. Obstet Gynecol 1992;80:621–625.
93. Druzin ML, Wolf CFW, Edersheim TG, et al. Donation of blood by the pregnant patient for autologous transfusion. Am J Obstet Gynecol 1988;159:1023–1027.
94. Kruskall MS. Are autologous donations necessary for pregnant women? In: Maffei LM, Thurer RL, eds. Autologous blood transfusion: current issues. Arlington, VA: American Association of Blood Banks, 1988.
95. McVay PA, Hoag RW, Hoag MS, Toy PTCY. Safety and use of autologous blood donation during third trimester of pregnancy. Am J Obstet Gynecol 1989;160:1479–1488.
96. Droste S, Sorensen T, Price T, et al. Maternal and fetal hemodynamic effects of autologous blood donation during pregnancy. Am J Obstet Gynecol 1992;167:89–93.
97. Goldfinger D. Strategies for reducing the risk of transfusion in pregnancy: unanswered questions regarding safety and effectiveness. In: Maffei LM, Thurer RL, ed. Autologous blood transfusion: current issues. Arlington, VA: American Association of Blood Banks, 1988.
98. Sayers MH. Controversies in transfusion medicine. Autologous blood donation in pregnancy: con. Transfusion 1990;30:172–174.
99. Ness PM, Walsh PC, Zahurak M, et al. Prostate cancer recurrence in radical surgery patients receiving autologous or homologous blood. Transfusion 1992;32:31–36.
100. Busch ORC, Hop WCJ, van Papendrecht H, et al. Blood transfusions and prognosis in colorectal cancer. N Engl J Med 1993;328:1372–1376.
101. Blajchman MA, Bardossy L, Carmen R, et al. Allogeneic blood transfusion-induced enhancement of tumor growth: two animal models showing amelioration by leukodepletion and passive transfer using spleen cells. Blood 1993;81:1880–1882.
102. Toy PTCY, Menozzi D, Strauss RG, et al. Efficacy of preoperative do-

nation of blood for autologous use in radical prostatectomy. Transfusion 1993;33:721–724.
103. Kamani AA, McMorland GH, Wadsworth LD. Utilization of red blood cell transfusion in an obstetric setting. Am J Obstet Gynecol 1988;159: 1177–1181.
104. Salem-Schatz SR, Avorn J, Soumerai SB. Influence of clinical knowledge, organizational context, and practice style on transfusion decision making. Implications for practice change strategies. JAMA 1990; 264:471–475.
105. Grossman BJ, Steward NC, Grindon AJ. Increased risk of a positive test for antibody to hepatitis B core antigen (anti-HBc) in autologous blood donors. Transfusion 1988;28:283–285.
106. Niceley I, Lugo J, Glacken K, et al. Infectious disease markers in autologous donors compared to the random population [abstract]. Transfusion 1987;27:517.
107. Kruskall MS, Popovsky MA, Pacini DG, et al. Autologous versus homologous donors. Evaluation of markers for infectious disease. Transfusion 1988;28:286–288.
108. Conover PT, Fang CT, Lam E, et al. Antibodies to hepatitis C virus in autologous blood donors. Transfusion 1991;31:616–619.
109. Goodnough LT. Toward bloodless surgery: erythropoietin therapy in the surgical setting. Semin Oncol 1992;19:19–24.
110. McVay PA, Hog MS, Lee SJ, et al. Factors associated with successful blood donation for elective surgery. Am J Clin Pathol 1992;97: 304–308.
111. Goodnough LT, Bravo JR, Hsueh Y, et al. Red blood cell mass in autologous and homologous blood units. Implications for risk/benefit assessment of autologous blood crossover and directed blood transfusion. Transfusion 1989;29:821–822.
112. Lorentz A, Eckardt KU, Osswald PM, et al. Erythropoietin levels in patients depositing autologous blood in short intervals. Hematology 1993;64:281–285.
113. Levine EA, Rosen AL, Gould SA, et al. Recombinant human erythropoietin and autologous blood donation. Surgery 1988;104:365–369.
114. Goodnough LT, Price TH, Rudnick S. Preoperative red cell production in patients undergoing aggressive autologous blood phlebotomy with and without erythropoietin therapy. Transfusion 1992;32:441–445.
115. Watanabe Y, Fuse K, Naruse Y. Subcutaneous use of erythropoietin in heart surgery. Ann Thorac Surg 1992;54:479–484.
116. Graf H, Watzinger U, Ludvik B, et al. Recombinant human erythropoietin as adjuvant treatment for autologous blood donation. Br Med J 1990;300:1627–1628.
117. Sawka MN, Young AJ, Muza SR, et al. Erythrocyte reinfusion and maximal aerobic power. An examination of modifying factors. JAMA 1987;257:1496–1499.
118. Johnson RG, Thurer RL, Kruskall MD, et al. Comparison of two transfusion strategies after elective operations for myocardial revascularization. J Thorac Cardiovasc Surg 1992;104:307–314.
119. Wasman J, Goodnough LT. Autologous blood donation for elective surgery. Effect on physician transfusion behavior. JAMA 1987;258: 3135–3137.
120. Silvergleid AJ. Preoperative autologous donation: what have we learned [editorial]? Transfusion 1991;31:99–101.
121. Jaffray B, King PM, Gillon J, Basheer MM. Efficiency of blood use and prospects for autologous transfusion in general surgery. Ann R Coll Surg Eng 1991;73:235–238.
122. Giordanao GF, Rivers SL, Chung GKT, et al. Autologous platelet-rich plasma in cardiac surgery: effect on intraoperative and postoperative transfusion requirements. Ann Thorac Surg 1988;46:416–419.
123. Giordanao GF Sr, Giordanao GF Jr, Rivers SL, et al. Determinants of homologous blood usage utilizing autologous platelet-rich plasma in cardiac operations. Ann Thorac Surg 1989;47:897–902.
124. Jones JW, McCoy TA, Rawitscher RE, Lindsley DA. Effects of intraoperative plasmapheresis on blood loss in cardiac surgery. Ann Thorac Surg 1990;49:585–590.
125. Ereth MH, Oliver WC Jr, Beynen FM. Autologous platelet-rich plasma does not reduce transfusion of homologous blood products in patients undergoing repeat vascular surgery. Anesthesiology 1993;79:540–547.
126. Tobe CE, Vocelka C, Sepulvada R, et al. Infusion of autologous platelet rich plasma does not reduce blood loss and product use after coronary artery bypass. J Thorac Cardiovasc Surg 1993;105: 1007–1014.
127. Platelet Transfusion Therapy. National Institutes of Health Consensus Conference. JAMA 1987;257:1777–1780.

Chapter 9

Role of Recombinant Human Erythropoietin as a Perioperative Adjuvant

MICHAEL N. D'AMBRA
EDWARD CHEN
DOUGLAS HANSELL

INTRODUCTION

Erythropoietin (EPO), a glycoprotein hormone, is the primary regulator of erythropoiesis. The humoral regulation of red blood cell (RBC) production was first suggested in 1906 by Carnot and Deflandre (1) and later confirmed by a large number of subsequent studies (2, 3). EPO is produced primarily in the kidney in the adult, with a small amount produced in the liver. Under normal physiological conditions, there is an inverse correlation between tissue oxygenation and circulating EPO levels, with kidney hypoxia being the main stimulus to EPO production. EPO acts on committed erythroid progenitor cells to stimulate their proliferation and differentiation into mature RBCs.

The process of Miyake et al. (4) of purification and amino acid sequencing of human urinary EPO has permitted the production of large quantities of EPO in mammalian expression vectors through the use of recombinant DNA technology (5, 6). The recombinant human EPO produced in mammalian cells is biologically active and biologically indistinguishable from human urinary EPO and is referred to generically as epoetin alfa.

Based on the known biological activity of EPO, epoetin alfa is considered an important pharmacological agent for the treatment of anemia. Numerous clinical trials have established epoetin alfa as a clinically effective treatment for anemia of various etiologies, including anemia associated with chronic renal failure (7, 8), human immunodeficiency virus (HIV) infection (9, 10), and cancer (11).

Recent clinical trials have demonstrated the safety and efficacy of perioperative epoetin alfa for increasing erythropoiesis, and thus RBC mass, and in reducing exposure to allogeneic blood transfusions in patients undergoing major elective surgical procedures (12–15). This chapter reviews the use of epoetin alfa as a perioperative adjuvant with concomitant iron supplementation in surgical blood management.

CLINICAL PHARMACOLOGY AND PHYSIOLOGY OF EPO

Human EPO produced by recombinant DNA technology in mammalian expression vectors (i.e., epoetin alfa) and human EPO purified from human urine have indistinguishable biological activity. Furthermore, epoetin alfa and human urinary EPO are similar in structure, with an identical amino acid sequence and similar, but not identical, oligosaccharide chains. EPO is a glycoprotein with a molecular mass of approximately 30,400 Da, consisting of approximately 30% carbohydrate (16) linked to a polypeptide backbone (17). As seen in Figure 9.1, this single-chain polypeptide backbone has a sequence of 165 amino acids with a molecular mass of 18,400 Da and two intrachain disulfide bonds that are important for the conformation and biological activity of the molecule (18, 19).

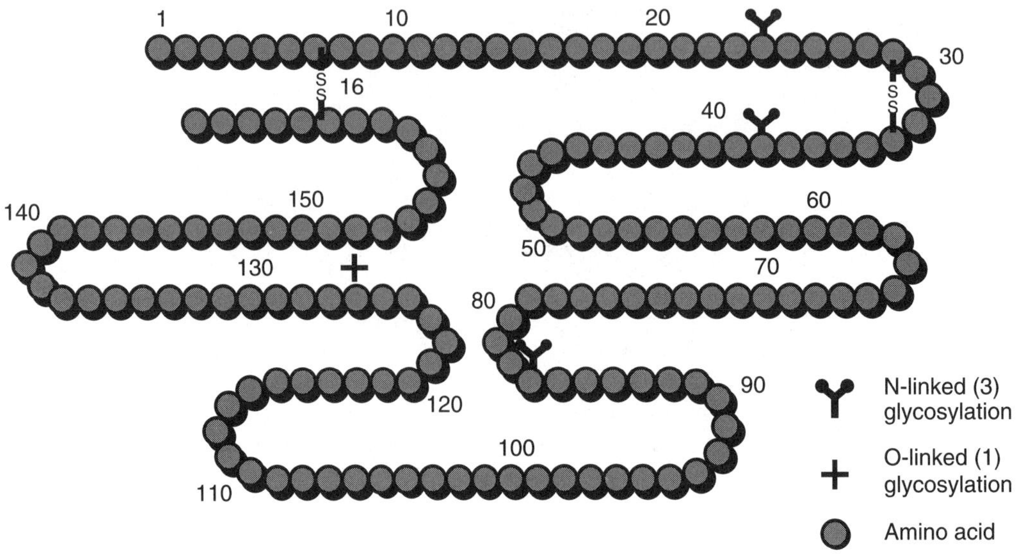

Figure 9.1. Erythropoietin amino acid sequence.

The major functions of EPO are to recruit, maintain, and induce the differentiation of erythroid progenitor cells. EPO is primarily, but not completely, restricted in its target cell specificity to cells in the erythroid differentiation pathway. EPO dependence develops in parallel with expression of the soluble EPO receptor. The burst-forming unit erythroid (BFU-E) and the colony-forming unit erythroid (CFU-E) are the earliest erythroid progenitor cells that demonstrate EPO dependence and peak EPO receptor expression (20). The BFU-E are the most primitive erythroid progenitor cells that respond to EPO and require the synergistic action of EPO with interleukin-3 and/or granulocyte–macrophage colony-stimulating factor to differentiate into a colony of recognizable RBC precursors (21). The CFU-E, progeny of the BFU-E, are committed erythroid cells that differentiate into morphologically recognizable erythroblasts (22). The CFU-E are completely dependent on EPO for proliferation, viability, and differentiation. As differentiation of the erythroid cell line proceeds through the late CFU-E stage, EPO receptors and dependence on EPO decline in parallel. The proerythroblast, the progeny of the CFU-E, is the earliest morphologically recognizable RBC precursor in the bone marrow and does not appear to require EPO for maturation into the reticulocyte (Fig. 9.2).

In adults, the primary site of EPO production is the kidney (24–26). However, the identity of the EPO-producing cell within the kidney remains controversial. In situ hybridization techniques using EPO cDNA suggest a peritubular, interstitial cell in the inner cortex and outer medulla (27). Although the kidney is the major site of EPO production in the adult, the liver is the principal EPO-producing organ in the fetus (28). Small quantities of EPO are produced in the liver in the adult, usually under conditions of renal dysfunction or absence (29).

The regulation of EPO production involves a classic feedback loop (Fig. 9.3). Under normal physiological conditions, there is an inverse correlation between tissue oxygenation and circulating EPO levels, with kidney hypoxia the main stimulus to EPO production (31). Hypoxia induces increased EPO gene transcription and increased EPO messenger RNA levels, leading to increased production and secretion of biologically active EPO (31–33).

The increased RBC mass produced in response to increased EPO levels results in an increase in the oxygen-carrying capacity of the blood. This decreases the hypoxic stimulus to the kidney, thereby decreasing EPO production. The linkage between the production and action of EPO in this negative feedback loop maintains the RBC mass at a volume that is optimal for oxygen transport.

The expected inverse correlation between the serum EPO level and RBC mass has been extensively observed in the clinical setting. Serum EPO levels have been demonstrated to be inversely proportional to hematocrit (Hct) and hemoglobin (Hgb) in anemic patients with normal renal function (34–36). In individuals with Hgb levels within the normal range, endogenous serum EPO levels range from 5 to 30 mU/mL of plasma (21, 37). EPO levels increase exponentially in the presence of anemia, and with an Hct less than 20%, 100-fold or greater increases in plasma EPO levels have been observed (Fig. 9.4) (36).

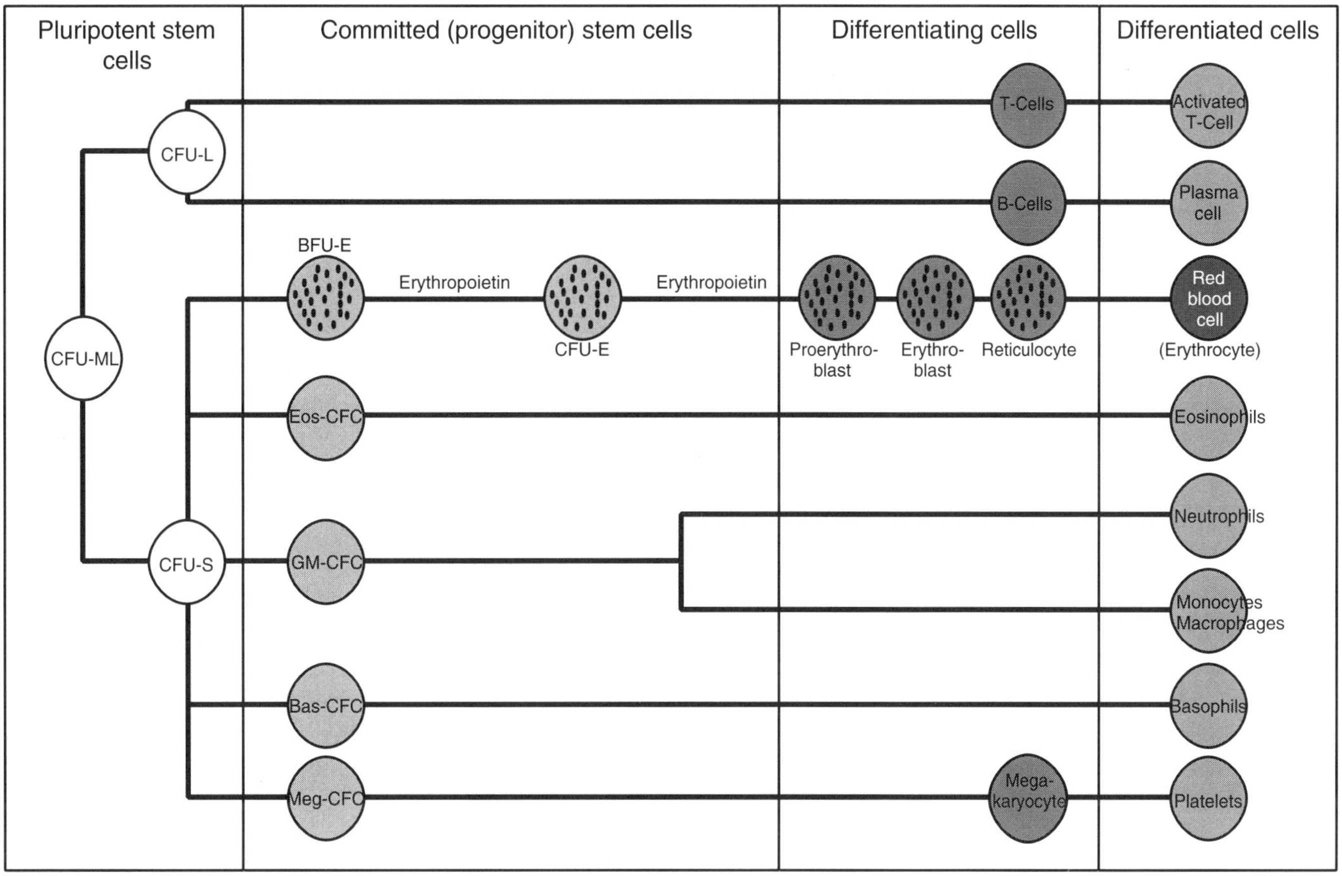

Figure 9.2. Site of erythrocyte differentiation. (Adapted with permission from Gilbert SF. Developmental biology. 3rd ed. Sunderland, MA: Sinauer Associates, 1991:891.)

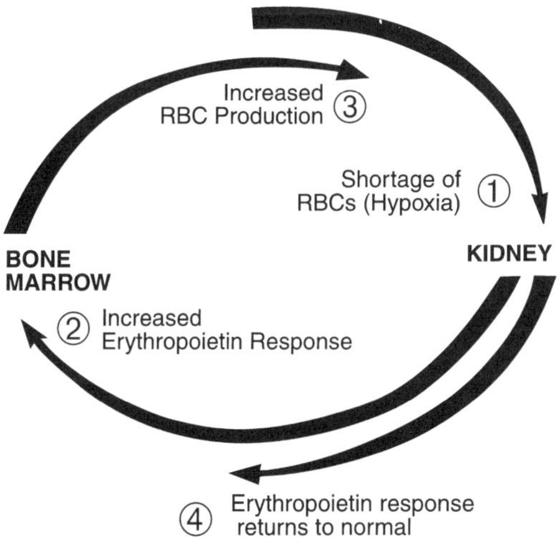

Figure 9.3. Red blood cell (RBC) production and oxygen demand feedback loop. (Reprinted with permission from Rieger PT. Anemia—the forgotten problem. In: Fighting fatigue: resolving issues for the cancer patient. Beachwood, OH: Pro Ed Communications, 1994:2–12. Monograph.)

ERYTHROPOIESIS IN THE ANEMIC PATIENT

Anemia is a powerful stimulus to EPO production in patients with normal renal function and Hgb-oxygen affinity. However, the anemia that is a consequence of various clinical disorders, such as chronic renal failure, chronic inflammatory disorders, and infectious disorders, does not stimulate production of EPO in quantities sufficient to restore the RBC mass. In patients with chronic renal failure (34), cancer (38), HIV (39), and rheumatoid arthritis (40), the expected exponential relationship between serum EPO levels and degree of anemia has been observed. However, in these patients, the EPO response is blunted in comparison with that of iron-deficient patients with a comparable degree of anemia. This results in EPO levels insufficient to overcome the degree of anemia found in these disorders.

Anemia of Iron Deficiency

Iron Metabolism and Regulation Body iron stores are conserved, with no physiological pathway for iron removal from the body. The small amounts of iron that are lost,

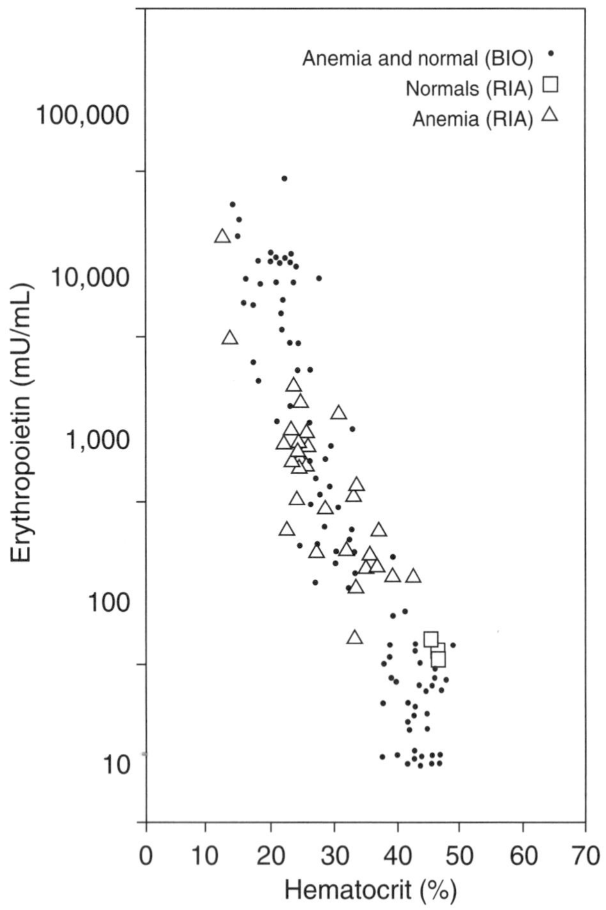

Figure 9.4. Correlation between Hct and serum EPO levels. (Reprinted with permission from Erslev A, Caro J. Physiologic and molecular biology of erythropoietin. Med Oncol Tumor Pharm 1986;3:159–164.)

approximately 1 mg/day in males and 1.5–2 mg/day in females, are usually balanced by the daily absorption of approximately 1 mg iron/day, which represents absorption of about 10% of the 10–20 mg of dietary iron ingested daily (41). Under normal conditions, iron homeostasis is strictly maintained, but a heightened demand for iron due to accelerated erythropoiesis can increase iron absorption and alter iron kinetics.

Effective erythropoiesis results in the incorporation of 80–90% of iron into Hgb in circulating erythrocytes. As a consequence, iron availability has been identified as a major rate-limiting factor for erythropoiesis. Iron kinetics are closely coupled with the rate of erythropoiesis. A correlation exists between the serum ferritin concentration and body iron stores, with serum ferritin levels providing an indirect measure of the level of tissue iron stores. Serum ferritin levels range from 30 to 250 ng/mL of blood in normal individuals. Normal values for transferrin saturation range between 20% and 45% and are much lower in patients with iron deficiency. A serum ferritin level of less than 30 ng/mL or a transferrin saturation level of less than 20% indicates iron deficiency (42).

Stages of Iron Deficiency Iron deficiency develops when the rate of iron loss exceeds the rate of iron intake. The development of iron deficiency progresses in three stages. The first stage is depletion of stored iron, during which iron reserves are lost without compromising the iron supply necessary for erythropoiesis. At this stage, the serum ferritin level is decreased. Iron-deficient erythropoiesis occurs when the erythroid iron supply is reduced yet anemia is not present. This second stage of iron deficiency is characterized by a rise in the serum total iron-binding capacity (TIBC), followed by a decrease in serum iron levels. As a result, transferrin saturation falls to less than the 15% of that required to support erythropoiesis. The final stage is the development of iron-deficiency anemia (42).

Anemia of Perioperative Blood Donation

A clinical situation of particular relevance to surgical blood management is the development of mild, asymptomatic anemia in patients participating in a perioperative autologous blood donation (PAD) program. A standard PAD program usually involves the donation of 450 mL ± 10% of RBCs every third day, provided that the patient maintains an Hct level greater than 34% (Hgb greater than 11 g/dL) (43). Many donors, however, fail to maintain an adequate Hct during the course of repeated phlebotomy and thus fail to donate sufficient blood to meet operative needs (44–46). Anemia develops in these patients, which is accompanied by an increase in serum EPO level, but not to a magnitude necessary to maintain adequate erythropoiesis and RBC mass (44).

PHARMACOLOGY AND PHARMACOKINETICS OF EPOETIN ALFA

Epoetin alfa has been shown to produce a dose-dependent stimulation of RBC production in healthy patients and in patients with anemia of various etiologies. The efficacy of the route of administration of epoetin alfa has been extensively investigated both in healthy patients and in patients with chronic renal failure and end-stage renal disease.

Epoetin alfa administered intravenously to patients with chronic renal failure is eliminated at a rate consistent with first-order kinetics, with a half-life circulation range of approximately 4–13 hours. The peak serum EPO level is reached within 1 hour. Within the therapeutic dose range, detectable levels of plasma EPO are maintained for at least 24 hours (47). In healthy volunteers, the half-life of intravenously administered epoetin alfa is approximately 20% shorter than that found in chronic renal failure patients (Fig. 9.5).

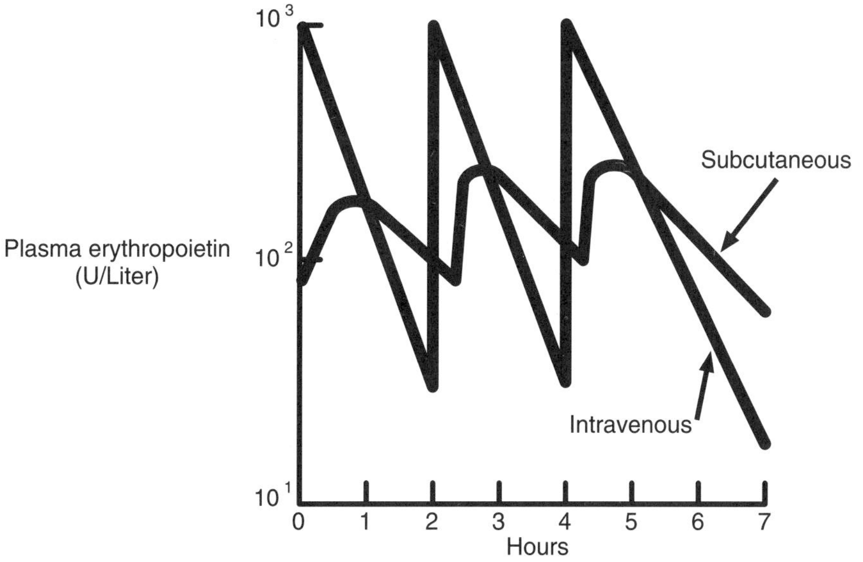

Figure 9.5. Pharmacokinetics of epoetin alfa. (Adapted with permission from Erslev AJ. Erythropoietin. N Engl J Med 1991;324:1339–1344.)

Subcutaneous administration of epoetin alfa to patients with chronic renal failure yields a volume of distribution and elimination half-life identical to that obtained through intravenous administration. However, the time required to reach peak serum EPO levels is substantially longer in subcutaneous than in intravenous administration, ranging from 5 to 24 hours (47, 49) and declines slowly thereafter, with a half-life of more than 24 hours (49). Peak serum EPO levels reached with subcutaneous administration are significantly lower than those after comparable intravenous doses (47, 49).

In adult hemodialysis patients, the intravenous and subcutaneous routes of administration are equally effective in *raising* Hct levels. However, the subcutaneous route of administration has been found to be more effective in *maintaining* desired Hct levels (50). More important, a 30% lower dose of epoetin alfa administered subcutaneously has been shown to provide erythropoietic stimulation comparable with a higher intravenous dose (51). In addition, subcutaneous administration of epoetin alfa to ambulatory patients is more convenient than intravenous administration. Thus, subcutaneous administration of epoetin alfa is safe and cost-effective for patients scheduled for major elective surgery.

IRON SUPPLEMENTATION

Normal iron stores, although adequate for basal erythropoiesis, may not be sufficient for the accelerated erythropoiesis associated with epoetin alfa therapy, even with oral iron supplementation (52, 53). In a randomized trial, Rutherford et al. (52) evaluated the effect of accelerated erythropoiesis on iron indices and RBC hemoglobinization in 24 healthy, iron-replete men. Patients were administered epoetin alfa subcutaneously in one of three dosing schedules, with a total dose of 1200 IU/kg over 10 days. All received 300 mg of elemental iron orally each day for 10 days. The patients showed statistically significant increases in Hct level, Hgb concentration, and absolute reticulocyte counts during the 24-day study period. Increases in Hct level positively correlated with log baseline serum ferritin ($P<.001$). Subcutaneous administration of epoetin alfa was associated with a 74% ($P = .0005$) decrease in serum ferritin and a marked decrease in percent saturation of TIBC, from 39% ± 14% to 14% ± 4% ($P = .0005$) (52). The maximum increase in Hct was higher in patients with serum ferritin levels greater than 100 ng/mL (8.1 ± 1.7% versus 5.4 ± 1.9%, $P = .005$). Patients with relatively low iron stores, as estimated by baseline serum ferritin, produced reticulocytes with decreased Hgb content, thus confirming observations in other studies (54). Further clinical observations have indicated that epoetin alfa treatment causes significant mobilization of iron stores and that iron is a rate-limiting factor for erythropoiesis (42). This is due to the accelerated erythropoiesis induced by epoetin alfa.

Supplemental oral iron is generally poorly absorbed in the gastrointestinal tract. Various preparations have been devised to improve the absorption rate, but at present the maximum reliable absorption rate is approximately 20 mg of elemental iron per day. Using the simplified formula that equates 1 g of Hgb with 150 mg of elemental iron in an average-sized adult man, a 2-g/dL increase in Hgb would require 300 mg of elemental iron. To attain this, patients would require 15 days of oral iron supplementation therapy, assuming continual optimum absorption, which is seldom attained.

IRON SUPPLEMENTATION DURING SURGERY

Parenteral iron therapy in the perioperative period has been suggested as an effective strategy for augmentation of endogenous iron stores and facilitation of the increased rate of erythropoiesis associated with epoetin alfa therapy. The effects of epoetin alfa therapy on iron metabolism in patients participating in autologous blood donation has been recently studied. Before elective surgery, 62 autologous blood donors were randomly assigned to two study groups: 32 patients received 500 IU/kg epoetin alfa subcutaneously twice weekly during a 3-week period and 30 patients received no treatment (control group). Epoetin alfa treatment was associated with restoration of the prephlebotomy Hgb concentration and a fourfold increase in erythropoietic activity. However, reticulocyte counts declined despite continuous epoetin alfa treatment and oral iron supplementation, reflecting a failure to prevent depletion of iron stores (55).

Intravenous iron supplementation has also been investigated and has been demonstrated to be clinically effective in supporting erythropoiesis. A placebo-controlled trial of 50 women who had Hct levels below 40% and who were undergoing PAD before elective orthopedic surgery were randomized to either a placebo group or one of two epoetin alfa dosage groups. The efficacy of 125–270 mg/day oral iron supplementation alone was then compared at the time of blood donation with oral iron supplementation combined with 100 mg iron saccharate intravenously every third or fourth day. No difference was observed between the effects of the two epoetin alfa dosages studied. However, patients receiving intravenous iron saccharate therapy achieved the highest sustained reticulocyte response, the greatest volume of PAD blood, and the least exposure to allogeneic blood. In contrast, patients treated with oral iron alone did not maintain their reticulocyte response (56).

Intravenous iron supplementation has been suggested for patients with presurgery serum ferritin less than 100 ng/mL undergoing epoetin alfa therapy (49). However, rapid administration of high doses of intravenous iron may saturate the available iron-binding capacity and result in free plasma iron. Because free plasma iron is toxic and can lead to hemodynamic instability, small test doses should be administered (41). Further, allergic reactions have been associated with certain intravenous iron preparations. Saccharated iron preparations not associated with allergic reactions are currently available in Europe for intravenous administration in increments of 150 mg.

Adequate iron supplementation is required to achieve the maximum erythropoietic response to epoetin alfa treatment. The observations made in these clinical trials indicate that intravenous saccharated iron preparations, rather than oral iron supplements, are significantly more effective in supporting erythropoiesis.

PERIOPERATIVE EPOETIN ALFA THERAPY

The enhanced erythropoietic activity of epoetin alfa therapy has been studied in multiple surgical settings in which blood loss is extensive, including urological, orthopedic, gynecological, and coronary artery bypass graft (CABG) surgeries. Three clinical strategies for the perioperative use of epoetin alfa have been studied. These strategies include the use of epoetin alfa as an adjunctive therapy that enhances the patient's ability to undergo PAD, enhances perioperative Hgb levels and erythropoiesis without PAD, and increases erythropoiesis in preparation for hemodilution.

ENHANCEMENT OF PAD FOR ELECTIVE SURGERY

Patients undergoing major elective surgical procedures in which significant blood loss is expected often participate in a PAD program. In such programs, the patient predonates 1 unit of blood per visit, usually once each week for 2–3 weeks. The 2–3 units of blood collected are then returned to the patient during or after surgery. Autologous blood donations are usually scheduled at least 3 days apart. This allows the collection of several units of blood if Hct level of at least 33% is maintained (43). However, it has been estimated that 15–25% of potential autologous donors are unable to start or complete a PAD program due to an Hct of no more than 33%.

Analysis of orthopedic patients enrolled in a PAD program demonstrated that approximately 32% of the patients, most of them women, were unable to donate the requested number of autologous blood units and that almost 33% of these patients subsequently received allogeneic blood. For these patients, the primary determinants for risk of receiving allogeneic blood were the number of requested units and the presence of anemia at first blood donation, especially in patients asked to predonate 4 or more autologous units (57). Additionally, sequential donation of autologous blood units was found to correlate with a linear decrease in mean RBC volume, thereby demonstrating an absence of compensatory erythropoiesis under normal blood donation conditions (58).

Clinical trials evaluating the EPO response to serial phlebotomy have confirmed that the most likely cause for the development of anemia in PAD donors is the inadequate stimulation of endogenous serum EPO production. The anemia does not appear to be due to iron deficiency in most cases. As shown in a clinical trial documenting the result of repeated phlebotomy on serum EPO levels, most iron-supplemented patients in whom anemia developed did not demonstrate increased RBC-free protoporphyrin levels (44). A study involving 69 autologous blood donors, of whom 11 men and 2 women were anemic at the time of initial donation, showed that during the course of repeated donation, anemia developed in an additional 17 men and 14 women. As a consequence, the anemic condition precluded donation of the required units of autologous blood to meet operative needs. The anemia in these patients was accompanied by an increase in endogenous serum EPO level. However, this increase in endogenous serum EPO level, although statistically significant, was not above the upper normal limit and was clearly insufficient to maintain adequate erythropoiesis (44).

Consistent with this observation are the analyses of the inverse relationship between Hgb concentration and endogenous serum EPO level. Studies demonstrated that an Hgb of no more than 11 g/dL is required for significant stimulation of endogenous serum EPO production (35, 59). It has been observed that a major blood loss, greater than 1500 to 2000 mL, is required for a substantial increase in endogenous serum EPO production and rate of erythropoiesis in healthy subjects (49).

The conclusion that the anemia induced by PAD does not stimulate sufficient production of endogenous EPO to stimulate erythroid regeneration, and thus compensate for RBC loss, provides a rationale for administration of perioperative epoetin alfa to augment RBC production in PAD patients scheduled for major elective surgery. This rationale has been confirmed in a large number of randomized, controlled studies showing that perioperative epoetin alfa therapy diminishes or prevents the development of anemia in patients undergoing PAD and increases the volume of autologous blood donated by anemic and nonanemic patients before undergoing elective surgery. Several clinical trials evaluating the efficacy of epoetin alfa in PAD patients undergoing elective surgical procedures, including orthopedic and cardiac procedures, are summarized in Table 9.1.

Several studies reported that epoetin alfa administered two times per week in doses of 150–600 IU/kg per dose over a 3-week preoperative period was effective in increasing erythropoiesis in patients with both low (65, 66) and normal (45, 46, 56, 60, 61, 67) baseline Hct levels. Patients receiving 600 IU/kg epoetin alfa twice weekly donated 41% greater blood volume than did placebo-treated patients (46). These studies demonstrate that epoetin alfa-treated patients were able to donate a significantly greater number of units of blood, with a greater RBC volume, than placebo-treated patients. A direct correlation between preoperative RBC volume and epoetin alfa dose was observed.

Epoetin alfa is most efficacious in the subset of patients who are anemic at first blood donation. Subsequent allogeneic blood needs in a group of anemic (i.e., Hct no more than 40%) orthopedic surgery patients asked to predonate 4 or more autologous units were reduced with epoetin alfa treatment (in conjunction with intravenous iron supplementation) compared with placebo treatment (56). A recent trial studied orthopedic patients participating in a PAD program. The study found that for patients with an Hct no more than 37% at first donation, six doses of 600 IU/kg epoetin alfa intravenously over a 3-week period reduced allogeneic blood exposure to 28% of epoetin alfa-treated patients compared with 49% of placebo-treated control patients (68).

Several studies have reported the benefits of epoetin alfa with PAD before cardiac surgery (62, 69, 70). Hayashi et al. (62) found that the subcutaneous administration of epoetin alfa at 24,000 IU/week for 3 weeks, in combination with an oral iron preparation, permitted the safe donation of 800 mL of autologous blood before cardiac surgery (Table 9.1). In a subsequent study, 40 patients donated 800 mL of blood before undergoing coronary bypass procedures in a randomized, controlled trial. Reticulocyte counts increased significantly in patients receiving epoetin alfa therapy ($P < .01$), but little increase was observed in the control group. The Hgb levels immediately before surgery were higher in the epoetin alfa-treated patients, none of whom required allogeneic blood transfusions (71).

In summary, perioperative epoetin alfa therapy in patients undergoing major elective surgery has been shown to significantly increase the volume of autologous blood donated before surgery through expansion of the RBC mass. Finally, clinical observations demonstrate that administration of epoetin alfa in combination with a PAD program bolsters pre-PAD Hgb levels in both nonanemic and anemic patients, allowing their entry into a PAD program, prevents PAD-induced anemia, allowing completion of scheduled PAD, and thereby reduces the exposure to allogeneic transfusion.

EPOETIN ALFA REDUCES OR ELIMINATES EXPOSURE TO ALLOGENEIC BLOOD AND ENHANCES ERYTHROPOIESIS WITHOUT PAD

Perioperative epoetin alfa therapy has demonstrated significant efficacy in reducing allogeneic transfusion in surgical patients who were unable to participate in a PAD program. Recent clinical trials have demonstrated that treatment with perioperative epoetin alfa alone, without concomitant PAD, reduces the need for allogeneic transfusion in patients undergoing major elective orthopedic surgery. Epoetin alfa has been found to produce a dose-dependent increase in RBC volume before elective surgery in patients who might otherwise

TABLE 9.1. EFFICACY OF ERYTHROPOIETIN ON PREOPERATIVE AUTOLOGOUS BLOOD DONATION BY ELECTIVE SURGERY

Reference	Patients/Procedures	Study Design	Preoperative EPO Dosing	Results
45	EPO = 49 C = 52 Orthopedic, cardiac, other	R, C, MC	150–180 IU/kg, 3×/wk, Weeks 4 and 2	Controls had significantly greater decrease in Hgb (P<.001). Reticulocyte count increased earlier and to higher levels in EPO patients. Trend to increased transfusion requirement in controls.
60	EPO = 50 C = 45 Primary unilateral hip replacement	R, C, MC	500 IU/kg, 2×/wk for 3 wk	RBC volume increased to predonation values in EPO group but not in controls. Absolute reticulocyte count increased more than twofold in control group and almost sixfold in EPO group. 100% of EPO patients and 84% of controls donated 2 units. Autologous transfusions required in 89% of controls and 46% of EPO patients (P<.001). Allogeneic transfusions required in 36% of controls and 10% of EPO patients (P<.01). Blood loss and blood volume predicted allogeneic transfusion requirement.
55	EPO = 32 C = 30 Primary total hip replacement	R, C, MC	500 IU/kg, 2×/wk for 3 wk	Hgb, EPO, and serum transferrin receptor concentrations and absolute reticulocyte counts were significantly higher in EPO group (P<.05). Hgb concentration returned to predonation values in EPO group but decreased in controls after 2 units donated.
61	600 IU/kg = 28 300 IU/kg = 30 150 IU/kg = 29 Placebo = 29 Orthopedic	R, DB, PC, MC parallel, dose-ranging	600 IU/kg 300 IU/kg 150 IU/kg, 2×/wk for 3 wk	Significantly more units and volume of RBCs donated by EPO groups (P<.05). Direct correlation between preoperative RBC volume expansion and EPO dose (P= .024). Placebo patients had the largest mean decrease in Hct compared with 600 U/kg EPO group. No significant difference observed among groups in blood transfusions required.
46	EPO = 23 Placebo = 24 Orthopedic	R, DB, PC, MC	600 IU/kg, 2×/wk for 3 wk	EPO group donated significantly more units, 41% greater RBC volume (P<.05). Significantly (P<.05) more EPO patients donated ≥ 4 units. The EPO group had significantly greater Hct and reticulocyte increase (P<.05). The number of patients with low Hct unable to donate was significantly greater in placebo group (P<.05).
62	12,000 IU = 28 2400 IU = 30 Placebo = 28 Cardiac	R, DB, PC, MC, dose-ranging	12, 000 IU 24,000 IU, 1×/wk for 3 wk	Two units were donated by 100% in 24,000 IU EPO group, 92.9% in 12,000 IU EPO group, and 78.5% in placebo group (P = .018). Allogeneic blood transfusion was avoided in 62% of placebo group, 89% of 12,000 U EPO group, and 90% of 24,000 EPO group (P = .013).

TABLE 9.1. EFFICACY OF ERYTHROPOIETIN ON PREOPERATIVE AUTOLOGOUS BLOOD DONATION BY ELECTIVE SURGERY *(continued)*

References	Patients/Procedures	Study Design	Preoperative EPO Dosing	Results
63	EPO IV = 2 EPO SC = 8 Hb < 10 g/dL Cardiac	Open	100 IU/kg/day i.v., 2–3 wk 600 IU/kg/wk s.c., 2–12 wk	Hgb levels increased in all patients until day of operation. Blood donated by the 8 EPO s.c. patients but not by the 2 EPO i.v. patients. Allogeneic blood required in 1 EPO i.v. patient with blood loss of 1530 mL.
64	PAD group: 3000 IU = 31 6000 IU = 40 9000 IU = 26 C = 13 Cardiac	R, C, MC, dose-ranging	3000 IU 6000 IU 9000 IU per dose, 2 or 3×/wk, for 3 wk before surgery (and 2 wk after surgery)	Preoperative Hgb decrease with PAD was alleviated by 6000 IU and 9000 IU EPO 3×/wk. Hgb significantly increased in all EPO groups given EPO 3×/wk ($P<.05$) and demonstrated a dose-dependent increase. The allogeneic transfusion rate in patients with moderate perioperative blood loss (15–50 mL/kg) was 40% in controls, 20% with 3000 IU, 26.9% with 6000 IU, and 12.5% with 9000 IU. The allogeneic blood transfusion rate significantly reduced by combination of preoperative EPO 3×/wk and PAD ($P<.0001$).
65	EPO = 11 C = 12 Hct < 34% Rheumatoid arthritis Primary total hip or total knee replacement	Open, pilot	300 IU/kg, 2×/wk for 3 wk	EPO patients had increased Hct values and reticulocyte counts. Control patients could not participate in PAD; 10/11 EPO patients donated ≥ 2 units (mean 2.6 ± 0.6, range 2–4) ($P<.001$). The control group received more allogeneic blood (2.6 ± 1.6 vs 0.8 ± 0.8) ($P=.009$). 50% of EPO patients and 8% of controls did not receive allogeneic transfusion.
66	300 IU/kg = 19 600 IU/kg = 20 Placebo = 9 Total hip replacement	R, PC	300 IU/kg 600 IU/kg, 2×/wk for 3 wk	The study demonstrated a significant increase of reticulocytes in EPO patients ($P<0.5$). EPO patients donated significantly more blood units and greater RBC volume than did placebo patients ($P<.05$). The total number of units transfused/patient similar with placebo and EPO. The number of allogeneic units transfused significantly higher ($P<.05$) in placebo than in EPO patients. 75% of EPO patients and 50% of placebo patients did not receive allogeneic blood.

EPO, epoetin alfa; C, control; R, randomized; MC, multicenter; DB, double-blind; PC, placebo controlled.

have required up to 3 units of allogeneic blood. The rationale for epoetin alfa therapy is that if RBC mass can be increased preoperatively and the rate of erythropoietic recovery can be increased postoperatively, the RBCs remaining after surgical blood loss should be sufficient to avoid allogeneic blood exposure.

Three major studies have evaluated the use of epoetin alfa as a perioperative adjuvant in 724 patients undergoing major elective surgery (12–14). These studies indicate that compared with placebo, epoetin alfa therapy results in a significantly lower incidence of exposure to allogeneic blood transfusion (Table 9.2). Specifically, 300 IU/kg epoetin alfa administered subcutaneously for 10 days before, on the day of, and for 4 days after surgery results in a significantly lower

TABLE 9.2. SUMMARY DESIGN OF PERIOPERATIVE ORTHOPEDIC STUDIES

			No. Subjects					
Reference	**Study Type**	**Dose Regimen[a]**	**600 IU/kg qw**	**300 IU/kg qd**	**150 IU/kg qd**	**100 IU/kg qd**	**Placebo**	**Total**
12	Orthopedic surgery (hip), randomized double-blind placebo-controlled multicenter	Stratification by type of hip surgery (primary or revision). Subjects randomly assigned to receive 300 IU/kg epoetin alfa or placebo s.c. daily, given 10 days before surgery, on the day of surgery, and for 3 days after surgery (total, 14 doses). Additional group: placebo given 5 days followed by epoetin alfa given 5 days before surgery, on the day of surgery, and for 3 days after surgery (total, 14 doses; or nine doses epoetin alfa). Surveillance for DVTs by venography or ultrasound.	—	77 (14-day)	—	—	78	155
				53 (9-day)				53
				130			78	208
13	Orthopedic surgery (hip, knee, back, shoulder, leg, arm, elbow), randomized double-blind, placebo-controlled, multicenter	Subjects randomly assigned to receive 300 or 100 IU/kg epoetin alfa or placebo s.c. daily, given 10 days before surgery, on the day of surgery, and for 4 days after surgery (total, 15 doses).	—	60	—	71	69	200
14	Orthopedic surgery (hip or knee), randomized, double-blind, placebo-controlled, multicenter	Stratification by baseline Hgb level (≤10, > 10 to ≤13, and >13 g/dL). Subjects randomly assigned to receive 300 or 100 IU/kg epoetin alfa or placebo s.c. daily, given 10 days before surgery, on the day of surgery, and for 4 days after surgery (total, 15 doses). Surveillance for DVTs by ultrasonography.	—	112	—	101	103	316
15[b]	Orthopedic surgery (hip or knee), randomized open-labeled, multicenter	Subjects randomly assigned to receive 600 IU/kg epoetin alfa once a week for 3 weeks before surgery and on the day of surgery (total, 4 doses) or 300 IU/kg epoetin alfa given 10 days before surgery, on the day of surgery, and for 4 days after surgery (total, 15 doses).	73	72	—	—	—	145

Data on file from the R.W. Johnson Pharmaceutical Research Institute; 1996.

qw, once a week; qd, once a day.

[a]Subjects also received iron supplements (300 or 325 mg ferrous sulfate tablets [12–14] or polysaccharide-iron complex containing 200 mg elemental iron [15]) throughout the treatment period, starting either on or before the first day of study medication (14,15) or 3 weeks (12) and at least 10 days (13) before surgery.

[b]Included only patients with a baseline Hgb level of ≥10 to ≤13 g/dL.

incidence of exposure to allogeneic blood transfusion compared with placebo in patients with baseline Hgb more than 10 to no more than 13 g/dL. Epoetin alfa was also well tolerated in this patient population, with a safety profile similar to that seen with placebo treatment.

A randomized, multicenter study was recently completed that compared the safety and efficacy of two epoetin alfa dosing regimens in increasing Hgb and Hct levels before surgery in patients who were undergoing elective hip or knee replacement and who were at risk for receiving allogeneic blood transfusions (i.e., baseline Hgb more than 10 to no more than 13 g/dL). One group of patients received 600 IU/kg epoetin alfa subcutaneously once per week for 3 weeks before surgery and on the day of surgery (total dose, 2400 IU/kg); the second group received 300 IU/kg epoetin alfa subcutaneously once per day for 10 days preoperatively, on the day of surgery, and for 4 days postoperatively (total dose, 4500 IU/kg) (69).

Both regimens were well tolerated. The increase in Hgb from prestudy to presurgery was greater in the weekly regimen group (1.44 ± 1.029) than in the daily regimen group (0.73 ± 0.867). There was no significant difference between the groups with regard to transfusion requirements (16% in the weekly group and 20% in the daily group).

These data suggest that 600 IU/kg epoetin alfa weekly was at least as effective as 300 IU/kg epoetin alfa daily. The once-weekly dosing of epoetin alfa is obviously more convenient. Therefore, if the period before surgery is at least 3 weeks, 600 IU/kg epoetin alfa may be administered as an alternative dosing regimen once weekly for 3 weeks (e.g., days - 21, - 14, - 7) before surgery and on the day of surgery. In addition to being more convenient for patients and physicians, the amount of total drug for the weekly dosing regimen would be reduced by almost half.

The efficacy of epoetin alfa therapy has also been studied in cardiovascular surgery (63, 64, 70, 71). Recent advances in perioperative blood management using epoetin alfa therapy have reduced and in some cases eliminated the need for allogeneic RBC transfusions in cardiac surgery patients (72, 73).

In a randomized, controlled study, 205 patients undergoing open-heart surgery were randomized to either treatment with epoetin alfa or control. One hundred ten patients in this study also participated in a PAD program and are reported in Table 9.1. In the 95 non-PAD patients, 3000 IU/kg intravenous epoetin alfa was administered two or three times a week for 2 weeks before surgery and for 2 weeks after surgery with concomitant iron supplementation. Patients with moderate perioperative blood loss (15–50 mL/kg) treated with epoetin alfa without PAD had a lower rate of allogeneic transfusions than did control subjects (64).

A recent double-blind, placebo-controlled study (74) found that perioperative epoetin alfa decreased allogeneic blood transfusions in routine CABG patients. The study evaluated 182 cardiac patients in three groups: epoetin alfa 300 IU/kg (n = 63), epoetin alfa 150 IU/kg (n = 63), and placebo (n = 56). Study medication was administered subcutaneously for 8 consecutive days, starting 5 days preoperatively. All patients received oral ferrous sulfate for 5 days preoperatively. Although only 5 days of preoperative epoetin alfa therapy were administered, attenuating the erythropoietic response, epoetin alfa therapy did reduce allogeneic transfusion exposure in a number of these patients (300 IU/kg, 33.3%; 150 IU/kg, 27.9%; placebo, 48.1%; P = .054). When patients who experienced surgical complications were retrospectively excluded from the analysis (n = 22), epoetin alfa therapy significantly (P = .001) reduced the percentage of patients requiring allogeneic blood transfusion (300 IU/kg, 21.6%; 150 IU/kg, 13.7%; placebo, 44.9%). Epoetin alfa therapy increased the postoperative Hct in both epoetin alfa groups compared with placebo. Adverse events, including thrombotic and vascular events, were equally distributed among the three treatment groups (300 IU/kg, n = 5; 150 IU/kg, n = 4; placebo, n = 0; P = .098); patient deaths were not related to the study medication. Further work is warranted to evaluate the dose, route, and frequency of administration of epoetin alfa and the safety profile in CABG patients.

These studies demonstrate that epoetin alfa is effective as an alternative to PAD in eliminating or reducing the risk of transfusion in elective surgery patients. In addition, the cost-effectiveness of epoetin alfa without PAD may provide a distinct advantage.

PREDICTIVE POWER OF HEMOGLOBIN FOR TRANSFUSION RISK

Retrospective analysis of data from two recent studies (12, 13) indicated that presurgery baseline Hgb is an important prognostic variable for the risk of transfusion in patients undergoing major elective orthopedic surgery. In patients with a presurgery Hgb greater than 10 to no more than 13 g/dL, the risk of transfusion was much greater than in those with a presurgery Hgb greater than 13 g/dL. In high-risk patients (e.g., presurgery Hgb greater than 10 to no more than 13 g/dL), the reduction in risk of transfusion provided by a 14- to 15-day regimen of 300 IU/kg PROCRIT was substantial and superior to that of the 9-day or 100 IU/kg regimens. In lower risk patients (e.g., presurgery Hgb greater than 13 g/dL), both regimens showed similar levels of efficacy. Because of the small number of patients with presurgery Hgb no more than 10 g/dL, no conclusions could be drawn about this subset of patients.

A retrospective logistic regression analysis from these studies (12, 13) was conducted to examine the value of seven baseline variables as predictors of the need for transfusion in surgical patients: Hgb, age, endogenous EPO level, ferritin, serum iron, TIBC, and predicted normal blood volume (PBV). Among these, Hgb and PBV were found to be the most important as predictive variables. Although PBV can improve on the prediction available from using only Hgb, it was shown that Hgb alone is nevertheless a consistent and reliable predictive variable, especially in the orthopedic surgery setting (12, 13).

Because Hgb is a more readily ascertainable value than PBV and because by itself it is highly predictive of transfusion risk, further statistical analysis considered the predictiveness of Hgb alone. The upper cutoff point for which baseline Hgb defined a responsive subpopulation varied across analyses from approximately 13–16 g/dL. Although the choice of the exact cutoff point is arbitrary, depending on the desired degree of relative assurance of avoidance of transfusion, the upper cutoff point chosen for further evaluation was 13 g/dL. This patient subpopulation, defined by a baseline Hgb of greater than 10 to no more than 13 g/dL, was believed to essentially define a clinically relevant patient population with mild anemia.

Additional logistic regression analysis revealed a consistent relationship between baseline Hgb and avoidance of transfusion and a consistent effect of 300 IU/kg epoetin alfa daily treatment for 14 or 15 days preoperatively (12–14). Thus, perioperative epoetin alfa has proven efficacious both in elevating the Hgb levels of high-risk orthopedic patients (e.g., Hgb greater than 10 to no more than 13 g/dL) and in decreasing the risk of transfusion in these patients.

PERIOPERATIVE EPOETIN ALFA AS AN ADJUNCT TO HEMODILUTION

Acute normovolemic hemodilution (ANH) involves removing and temporarily storing 2–4 units of a patient's blood just before major elective surgery in which major blood loss is anticipated. The blood that has been withdrawn is then reinfused into the patient during or after surgery. During the period of ANH, normal circulatory volume is maintained by infusing the patient with acellular fluid. Simultaneous infusions of crystalloid (3 mL crystalloids per 1 mL blood withdrawn) or colloid (1 mL hydroxyethyl starch per 1 mL blood withdrawn) have been recommended. Hemodilution is also being used in clinical trials of synthetic oxygen carriers and Hgb solutions. In such trials, blood (removed by hemodilution in an oxygen-carrying solution) greatly enhances the safety and benefit of ANH.

The rationale for the use of hemodilution is that if intraoperative blood loss is relatively constant with or without preoperative normovolemic hemodilution, then it is better to lose blood at a lower rather than at a higher level of Hct. This procedure lowers the patient's preoperative Hct to 28%. If the perioperative Hct level falls to 24%, the ANH blood units are reinfused in reverse order of their collection (i.e., last unit collected is the first unit transfused). The first unit of blood collected, and therefore the last unit reinfused, has the highest Hct, contains the most platelets, and has the highest concentration of clotting factors (75).

Clinical observations show that ANH reduces allogeneic blood use in 20–90% of patients with no difference in postoperative outcomes (76, 77). Furthermore, ANH is substantially more cost-effective than transfusion. Total transfusion costs are significantly lower for patients who are treated with ANH, and a unit of autologous blood obtained by hemodilution is more cost-effective than allogeneic blood preoperatively donated (76).

Hemodilution is enhanced with the effects of epoetin alfa on RBC mass. A recent prospective, randomized trial evaluated perioperative anemic patients undergoing radical prostatectomy with PAD (3 units) compared with ANH (up to 4 units), with or without epoetin alfa therapy (600 IU/kg subcutaneously at 3 weeks and 2 weeks before surgery and 300 IU/kg subcutaneously on the day of surgery). This study found that preoperative epoetin alfa was effective in minimizing perioperative anemia, despite hemodilution and surgical blood loss. In these patients, the mean nadir Hct levels exceeded 30% throughout surgical hospitalization (78). This preservation of RBC volume was accompanied by the transfusion of only 1 unit of allogeneic blood to 1 of 24 patients in the epoetin alfa-treated group. This represents a substantial improvement over hemodilution alone—wherein 6 of 26 patients were transfused with a total of 16 allogeneic units—or PAD alone—wherein 4 of 26 patients were transfused with a total of 5 allogeneic units. In summary, epoetin alfa therapy in conjunction with PAD and ANH increases preoperative Hct levels and reduces the need for allogeneic blood (78).

ADVERSE EVENTS ASSOCIATED WITH PERIOPERATIVE EPOETIN ALFA THERAPY

Epoetin alfa treatment before major elective surgery increases the rate of erythropoiesis in patients with normal renal function. In addition, perioperative epoetin alfa is safe and generally well tolerated. In randomized, placebo-controlled clinical trials in patients scheduled for major elective surgery, the frequency of adverse events, including thrombotic vascular events and hypertension, was comparable in epoetin alfa-treated and placebo-treated patients (13, 45, 46, 65, 66).

Epoetin alfa does not have direct pressor effects; therefore, increases in blood pressure in epoetin alfa-treated patients may be related to the effects of drug administration on blood viscosity and changes in vascular resistance (79).

Thrombotic and vascular events, including myocardial infarction, angina, deep vein thrombosis (DVT), superficial phlebitis, and peripheral arterial thrombosis, are adverse events that have been found to be associated with rapid increases in Hgb and Hct levels. Furthermore, patients undergoing joint replacement surgery are at high risk of DVT. The frequency of thrombotic and vascular events was analyzed in three large, randomized, placebo-controlled trials in patients undergoing epoetin alfa therapy before major elective orthopedic surgery. Thrombotic and vascular events were reported in less than 15% of patients in these three studies. The overall prevalence of these adverse events in the groups of patients who received epoetin alfa (100 IU/kg and 300 IU/kg per dose) did not differ significantly from the rate in the placebo-treated patients (12–14).

EFFECTS OF EPOETIN ALFA ON COAGULATION

Some investigators have suggested that hypertensive and thrombotic complications are the result of the rapidly rising Hct induced by epoetin alfa therapy, whereas others contend that induction of abnormally high RBC aggregation at a low shear rate is of concern (80–82). Further, it has been suggested that epoetin alfa improves platelet adhesion and aggregation independent of its effect on Hct (83–88). Moreover, a number of hemostatic and fibrinolytic changes that might predispose patients to a thrombotic tendency have been described in patients with end-stage renal disease (89–93).

These data are, however, of limited value in the perioperative patient. Perioperative patients receive higher dosages of epoetin alfa during a relatively short period of time and have no uremic bleeding disorder as do patients with end-stage renal disease. Biesma et al. (93) studied alterations in blood rheology or hemostatic function and fibrinolysis in autologous donors treated with 500 IU/kg epoetin alfa. The study parameters were not influenced by epoetin alfa; only activated patient thromboplastin time (APTT) and protein C antigen decreased significantly, whereas levels of protein C and S did not reach those associated with a thrombotic tendency. Although decreased, both APTT and protein C levels remained within normal ranges and were unlikely to have any important clinical impact (93). In the same study, therapy with epoetin alfa led to a modest increase in platelets. The absence of evident prothrombotic changes in this study confirms the safety of perioperative epoetin alfa in patients scheduled for major elective surgery.

Increased platelet production has been reported in other studies (94–97). However, a comparable increase in platelets has been observed in autologous blood donors with a pronounced decrease in iron stores who received no epoetin alfa (93). It is therefore more likely that the increase in platelets observed by Biesma et al. was related to the development of iron deficiency rather than to a direct effect of epoetin alfa.

Despite conflicting data from studies in patients undergoing dialysis, the use of epoetin alfa in at-risk patients may predispose them to a slightly higher incidence of thrombotic complications. DVT is a serious and frequent complication of total joint replacement and cardiovascular surgery. It is therefore important to determine whether treatment with epoetin alfa contributes to the risk of thrombotic events in patients undergoing major elective surgery. An increase of thrombotic tendency can be provoked by alteration in hemostatic and fibrinolytic function and by changes in blood rheology that are dependent on whole blood and plasma viscosity, erythrocyte deformability, and erythrocyte aggregation.

In studies of a daily epoetin alfa dosing regimen in the orthopedic surgery setting (12–15), the rates of thrombotic and vascular events or of DVTs alone were similar across treatment groups. Hypertension also occurred at similar rates in epoetin alfa-treated and placebo-treated patients (12–14). The differences in whole blood viscosity before and after epoetin alfa therapy resembled changes in Hct. When corrected for Hct, whole blood viscosity had only small alterations. Most patients even showed a slight decrease in corrected whole blood viscosity at low and high shear rates (12, 13).

Whole blood viscosity can be influenced by many factors, including Hct, RBC deformability and aggregation, and plasma composition. The changes in whole blood volume are highly correlated with the epoetin alfa-induced rise in Hct. However, RBC deformability did not change at low and high shear rates throughout these studies (12–14). Reticulocytes and young erythrocytes, having large cell sizes, might accelerate erythrocyte aggregation, but this effect was apparently too small to induce any changes in RBC deformability. The increase in plasma viscosity is typically due to large molecular weight plasma proteins, but no alteration in fibrinogen was observed in autologous donors treated with epoetin alfa. No explanation for the small increase in plasma viscosity was found, and the investigators reported no rheological consequences.

PERIOPERATIVE EPOETIN ALFA IN JEHOVAH'S WITNESSES

Patients who refuse blood transfusions for religious reasons may benefit from epoetin alfa therapy. Jehovah's Witness patients generally refuse allogeneic blood products and any autologous blood that has been removed from the body for any length of time. Most Jehovah's Witnesses will accept epoetin alfa, however, because the amount of human albumin it contains is minimal and not intended to be used as a blood product (98).

Epoetin alfa therapy has been shown to be beneficial to available blood conservation programs by expanding available options to transfusion for Jehovah's Witness patients undergoing elective cardiovascular surgery (99). In one study, epoetin alfa was administered subcutaneously to two Jehovah's Witness patients with Hct levels of 34% and 36%, respectively, before cardiac surgery at a total dose of 900 IU/kg (100 IU/kg three times weekly for 3 weeks), in conjunction with oral iron supplementation (100). The two patients entered surgery with Hct levels of 45% and 41%, respectively, and underwent successful surgery. Similar doses of epoetin alfa have been administered to Jehovah's Witness patients undergoing major urological surgical procedures. A total dose of 600 IU/kg (50 IU/kg subcutaneously three times weekly for 4 weeks), along with oral iron supplementation, increased the preoperative Hct level in a Jehovah's Witness with cervical carcinoma from 34% to 37%.

SUMMARY

In recent years, the transmission of infectious diseases and other complications associated with allogeneic blood transfusion have made it a less attractive therapeutic intervention in perioperative blood loss. Attention has therefore been focused on the need to reassess current medical practices, with the goal of establishing effective surgical blood management strategies that reduce the use of allogeneic blood transfusions. Epoetin alfa offers a safe and effective means of reducing the need for allogeneic blood products in patients undergoing major elective surgery.

The accelerated erythropoiesis associated with epoetin alfa not only increases preoperative Hgb and RBC mass but also accelerates depletion of serum iron stores that may contribute to the development of iron-deficiency anemia. Further, iron availability has been identified as a rate-limiting factor for the response to epoetin alfa (12, 52, 55, 101). Thus, perioperative iron supplementation should be considered for iron-deficient patients and as an adjunct to epoetin alfa therapy. Close monitoring of serum iron levels throughout epoetin alfa therapy is also indicated, both for avoiding iron overload and for ensuring adequate levels of serum iron to meet the accelerated erythropoietic need.

Epoetin alfa is a valuable therapeutic tool in surgical blood management of patients undergoing major elective surgical procedures with anticipated major blood loss, patients with a preoperative Hgb greater than 10 and no more than 13 g/dL, patients who require elective surgery, and patients with inadequate time for PAD or who are unable to participate in a PAD program due to concomitant medical conditions (e.g., cardiac disease). In addition, epoetin alfa has proven invaluable for patients in whom use of blood or blood products is contraindicated.

The future prospects for epoetin alfa in surgical blood management are based on its efficacy in increasing erythropoiesis to reduce or eliminate allogeneic transfusion. Epoetin alfa can be used alone; as an adjunct to autologous blood use via PAD, normovolemic hemodilution, or perioperative cell salvage; or simultaneously with blood substitutes. Studies are underway to determine the lowest dose and most convenient dosing regimen of epoetin alfa that would provide the greatest cost-to-benefit ratio.

REFERENCES

1. Carnot P, Deflandre C. Sur l'activite hemopoietique du serum. Comp Rend Acad Sci 1906;143:384.
2. Erslev A. Humoral regulation of red cell production. Blood 1953;8: 349–357.
3. Krantz SB, Jacobson LO. Erythropoietin and the regulation of erythropoiesis. Chicago, IL: University of Chicago Press, 1970.
4. Miyake T, Kung CK, Goldwasser E. Purification of human erythropoietin. J Biol Chem 1977;252:5558–5564.
5. Jacobs K, Shoemaker C, Rudersdorf R, et al. Isolation and characterization of genomic and cDNA clones of human erythropoietin. Nature 1985;313:806–810.
6. Lin FK, Suggs S, Lin CH, et al. Cloning and expression of the human erythropoietin gene. Proc Natl Acad Sci USA 1985;82:7580–7584.
7. Winearls CG, Oliver DO, Pippard MJ, Reid C, Downing MR, Cotes PM. Effect of human erythropoietin derived from recombinant DNA on the anemia of patients maintained by chronic hemodialysis. Lancet 1986;2:1175–1178.
8. Eschbach JW, Abdulhadi MH, Browne JK, et al. Recombinant human erythropoietin in anemic patients with end-stage renal disease: results of a phase III multicenter clinical trial. Ann Intern Med 1989;111:992–1000.
9. Fischl M, Galpin JE, Levine JD, et al. Recombinant human erythropoietin for patients with AIDS treated with zidovudine. N Engl J Med 1990;322:1488–1493.
10. Phair JP, Abels RI, McNeill MV, Sullivan DJ. Recombinant human erythropoietin treatment: investigational new drug protocol for the anemia of the acquired immunodeficiency syndrome. Arch Intern Med 1993;153:2669–2675.
11. Abels R. Use of recombinant human erythropoietin in the treatment of anemia in patients who have cancer. Semin Oncol 1992;19(suppl 8):29–35.
12. Canadian Orthopedic Perioperative Erythropoietin Study Group. Effectiveness of perioperative recombinant human erythropoietin in elective hip replacement. Lancet 1993;341:1227–1232.
13. Faris PM, Ritter MA, Abels RI, the Erythropoietin Study Group. The effects of recombinant human erythropoietin on perioperative transfusion requirements in patients having a major orthopaedic operation. J Bone Joint Surg 1996;78A(suppl):62–72.

14. de Andrade JR, Jove M, Landon G, Frei D, Guilfoyle M, Young D. Baseline hemoglobin as predictor of risk of transfusion and response to epoetin alfa in orthopedic surgery patients. Am J Orthop 1996;25: 533–542.
15. Goldberg MA, McCutchen JW, Jove M, et al. A safety and efficacy comparison study of two dosing regimens of epoetin alfa in patients undergoing major orthopedic surgery. Am J Orthop 1996;25:544–552.
16. Dordal MS, Wang FF, Goldwasser E. The role of carbohydrate in erythropoietin action. Endocrinology 1985;116:2293–2299.
17. Goldwasser E, Beru N, Smith D. Erythropoietin: the primary regulator of red cell formation. In: Sporn MB, Roberts AB, eds. Handbook of experimental pharmacology. Berlin: Springer-Verlag, 1990:747–770.
18. Boissel JP, Bunn HF. Erythropoietin structure-function relationships. Prog Clin Biol Res 1990;352:227–232.
19. Wang FF, Kung CKH, Goldwasser E. Some chemical properties of human erythropoietin. Endocrinology 1985;116:2286–2292.
20. Krantz SB. Erythropoietin. Blood 1991;77:419–434.
21. Goldberg MA, Bunn HF. Molecular and cellular hematopoiesis. In: Isselbacher KJ, Braunwald E, Wilson JD, eds. Harrison's principles of internal medicine. 13th ed. New York: Mc Graw-Hill, 1994:1714–1717.
22. Stephenson JR, Axelrod AA, McLeod DL, Shreeve MM. Induction of colonies of hemoglobin-synthesizing cells by erythropoietin in vitro. Proc Natl Acad Sci USA 1971;68:1542–1546.
23. Gilbert SF. Developmental biology. 3rd ed. Sunderland, MA: Sinauer Associates, 1991:891.
24. Jacobson LO, Goldwasser E, Fried W, Plzak L. Role of the kidney in erythropoiesis. Nature 1957;179:633–634.
25. Erslev AJ. Renal biogenesis of erythropoietin. Am J Med 1975;58: 25–30.
26. Beru N, McDonald J, Lacombe C, Goldwasser E. Expression of the erythropoietin gene. Mol Cell Biol 1986;7:2571–2575.
27. Koury ST, Bondurant MC, Koury MJ. Localization of erythropoietin synthesizing cells in murine kidneys by in situ hybridization. Blood 1988;71:524–527.
28. Zanjani ED, Poster J, Burlington H, Mann LI, Wasserman LR. Liver as the primary site of erythropoietin formation in the fetus. J Lab Clin Med 1977;89:640–644.
29. Fried W. The liver as a source of extrarenal erythropoietin production. Blood 1972;40:671–677.
30. Rieger PT. Anemia—the forgotten problem. In: Fighting fatigue: resolving issues for the cancer patient. Beachwood, OH: Pro Ed Communications, Inc., 1994:2–12. Monograph.
31. Krantz SB, Goldwasser E. On the mechanism of erythropoietin-induced differentiation. II. The effect on RNA synthesis. Biochim Biophys Acta 1965;103:325–332.
32. Costa-Giomi P, Caro J, Weinmann R. Enhancement by hypoxia of human erythropoietin gene transcription in vitro. J Biol Chem 1990;265: 10185–10189.
33. Schuster SJ, Wilson JH, Erslev AJ, Caro J. Physiologic regulation and tissue localization of renal erythropoietin messenger RNA. Blood 1987;70:316–318.
34. Erslev AJ, Caro J, Kansu E, Miller O, Cobbs E, Silver R. Plasma erythropoietin in health and disease. Ann Clin Lab Sci 1980;10: 250–257.
35. Sherwood JB, Goldwasser E, Chilcote R, Carmichael LD, Nagel RL. Sickle cell anemia patients have low EPO levels for their degree of anemia. Blood 1986;67:46–49.
36. Erslev A, Caro J. Physiologic and molecular biology of erythropoietin. Med Oncol Tumor Pharm 1986;3:159–164.
37. Goldwasser E, Sherwood JB. Radioimmunoassay of erythropoietin. Br J Haematol 1981;48:359–363.
38. Miller CB, Jones RJ, Piantadosi S, Abeloff MD, Spivak JL. Decreased erythropoietin response in patients with the anemia of cancer. N Engl J Med 1990;322:1689–1692.
39. Spivak JL, Barnes DC, Fuchs E, Quinn TC. Serum immunoreactive erythropoietin in HIV-infected patients. JAMA 1989;261:3104–3107.
40. Baer AN, Dessypris EN, Goldwasser E, Krantz SB. Blunted erythropoietin response to anaemia in rheumatoid arthritis. Br J Haematol 1987;66:559–564.
41. Bridges KR, Bunn HF. Anemias with disturbed iron metabolism. In: Isselbacher KJ, Braunwald E, Wilson JD, eds. Harrison's principles of internal medicine. 13th ed. New York: McGraw-Hill, 1994:1721–1726.
42. VanWyck DB. Iron management during recombinant human erythropoietin therapy. Am J Kidney Dis 1989;14(suppl 1):9–13.
43. Holland PV, Schmidt PJ, eds. Standards for blood banks and transfusion services. Arlington, VA: American Association of Blood Banks, 1987:39.
44. Kickler TS, Spivak JL. Effect of repeated whole blood donations on serum immunoreactive erythropoietin levels in autologous donors. JAMA 1988;260:65–67.
45. Beris P, Mermillod B, Levy G, et al. Recombinant human erythropoietin as adjuvant treatment for autologous blood donation: a prospective study. Vox Sang 1993;65:212–218.
46. Goodnough LT, Rudnick S, Price TH, et al. Increased preoperative collection of autologous blood with recombinant human erythropoietin therapy. N Engl J Med 1989;321:1163–1168.
47. Egrie JC, Eschbach JW, McGuire T, Adamson JW. Pharmacokinetics of recombinant human erythropoietin (r-HuEPO) administered to hemodialysis (HD) patients. Kidney Int 1988;33:262.
48. Erslev AJ. Erythropoietin. N Engl J Med 1991;342:1339–1343.
49. Goldberg MA. Erythropoiesis, erythropoietin, and iron metabolism in elective surgery: preoperative strategies for avoiding allogeneic blood exposure. Am J Surg 1995;170 (suppl):37S–43S.
50. Bommer J, Ritz E, Weinreich T, Bommer G, Zeigler T. Subcutaneous erythropoietin. Lancet 1988;2:406.
51. McMahon FG, Vargas R, Ryan M, et al. Pharmacokinetics and effects of recombinant human erythropoietin after intravenous and subcutaneous injections in healthy volunteers. Blood 1990;76:1718–1722.
52. Rutherford CJ, Schneider TJ, Dempsey H, Kirn DH, Brugnara C, Goldberg MA. Efficacy of different dosing regimens for recombinant human erythropoietin in a simulated perisurgical setting: the importance of iron availability in optimizing response. Am J Med 1994;96:139–145.
53. Goodnough LT, Price TH, Rudnick S. Iron restricted erythropoiesis as a limitation to autologous blood donation in the erythropoietin-stimulated bone marrow. J Lab Clin Med 1991;118:289–296.
54. Brugnara C, Colella GM, Cremins J, et al. Effects of subcutaneous recombinant human erythropoietin in normal subjects: development of decreased reticulocyte hemoglobin content and iron-deficient erythropoiesis. J Lab Clin Med 1994;123:660–667.
55. Biesma DH, van de Weil A, Beguin Y, Kraaijenhagen RJ, Marx JJ. Erythropoietic activity and iron metabolism in autologous blood donors during recombinant human erythropoietin therapy. Eur J Clin Invest 1994; 24:426–432.
56. Mercuriali F, Zanella A, Barosi G, et al. Use of epoetin alfa to increase the volume of autologous blood donated by orthopaedic patients. Transfusion 1993;33:55–60.
57. Goodnough LT. Clinical application of recombinant erythropoietin in the perioperative period. Hematol/Oncol Clin North Am 1994;8: 1011–1020.

58. Goodnough LT, Bravo J, Hsueh Y, Keating L, Brittenham GM. Red blood cell mass in autologous and homologous blood units: implications for risk/benefit assessment of autologous blood crossover and directed blood transfusion. Transfusion 1989;29:821–822.
59. Spivak JL, Hogans BB. Clinical evaluation of a radioimmunoassay (RIA) for serum erythropoietin (EPO) using reagents derived from recombinant erythropoietin (rEPO). Blood 1987;70(suppl 1):143.
60. Biesma DH, Marx JJ, Kraaijenhagen RJ, Franke W, Messinger D, van de Wiel A. Lower homologous blood requirement in autologous blood donors after treatment with recombinant human erythropoietin. Lancet 1994;344:367–370.
61. Goodnough LT, Price TH, the Erythropoietin Study Group. A phase III trial of recombinant human eyrthropoietin therapy in nonanemic orthopedic patients subjected to aggressive removal of blood for autologous use: dose, response, toxicity, and efficacy. Transfusion 1994;34: 66–71.
62. Hayashi J, Kumon K, Takanashi S, et al. Subcutaneous administration of recombinant human erythropoietin before cardiac surgery: a double-blind, multicenter trial in Japan. Transfusion 1994;34:142–146.
63. Konishi T, Ohbayashi T, Kaneko T, Ohki T, Saitou Y, Yamato Y. Preoperative use of erythropoietin for cardiovascular operations in anemia. Ann Thorac Surg 1993;56:101–103.
64. Kyo S, Omoto R, Hirashima K, Eguchi S, Fujita T. Effect of human recombinant erythropoietin on reduction of homologous blood transfusion in open-heart surgery: a Japanese multicenter study. Circulation 1992;86(suppl 5):413–418.
65. Mercuriali F, Gualtieri G, Singaglia L, et al. Use of recombinant human erythropoietin to assist autologous blood donation by anemic rheumatoid arthritis patients undergoing major orthopedic surgery. Transfusion 1994;34:501–506.
66. Mercuriali F, Inghilleri G, Biffi E, et al. Erythropoietin treatment to increase autologous blood donation in patients with low basal hematocrit undergoing elective orthopedic surgery. Clin Invest 1994;72:S16-S18.
67. Goodnough LT, Verbrugge D, Marcus RE, Goldberg V. The effect of patient size and dose of recombinant human erythropoietin therapy on red blood cell volume expansion in autologous blood donors for elective orthopedic operation. J Am Coll Surg 1994;179:171–176.
68. Price TH, Goodnough LT, Vogler W, et al. The impact of recombinant erythropoietin administration on the efficacy of autologous blood strategies in patients with low hematocrits [abstract]. Blood 1992;80:219a.
69. The R.W. Johnson Pharmaceutical Research Institute. Data on File, 1996.
70. D'Ambra MN, Lynch KE, Boccagno J, et al. The effect of perioperative administration of recombinant human erythropoietin (r-HuEPO) in CABG patients: a double blind, placebo-controlled trail [abstract]. Anesthesiology 1992;77:A159.
71. Watanabe Y, Fuse K, Naruse Y, et al. Subcutaneous use of erythropoietin in heart surgery. Ann Thorac Surg 1992;54:479–483.
72. Cooley DA. Conservation of blood during cardiovascular surgery. Am J Surg 1995;170(suppl 6):53S-59S.
73. D'Ambra MN, Lynch KE, Boccagno J, et al. The effect of perioperative administration of recombinant human erythropoietin (epoetin alfa) in CABG patients [abstract]. Br J Anaesth 1995;74(suppl 1):64.
74. D'Ambra MN, Finlayson DC, Gray R, et al. The effect of recombinant human erythropoietin on transfusion risk in coronary bypass patients. Ann Thorac Surg (in press).
75. Goodnough LT. Erythropoietin in the surgical setting. In: Garnik M, ed. Erythropoietin in clinical applications. Cambridge, MA: Marcel Dekker; 1990:287–300.
76. Monk TG, Goodnough LT, Birkmeyer JD, Brecher ME, Catalona WJ. Acute normovolemic hemodilution is a cost-effective alternative to preoperative autologous blood donation by patients undergoing radical retropubic prostatectomy. Transfusion 1995;35:559–565.
77. Spence RK, Cernaianu AC, Carson J, DelRossi AJ. Transfusion and surgery. Curr Probl Surg 1993;30:1103–1180.
78. Monk TG, Goodnough LT, Andriole GL, et al. Preoperative recombinant human erythropoietin therapy enhances the efficacy of acute normovolemic hemodilution. Anesth Analg 1995;80:S320.
79. Goodnough LT. Erythropoietin. In: Anderson K, Ness P, eds. Scientific basis of transfusion medicine. Philadelphia, PA: WB Saunders, 1994: 830–842.
80. Maeda N, Kon K, Tateishi N, et al. Rheological properties of erythrocytes in recombinant human erythropoietin-administered normal rat. Br J Haematol 1989;73:105–111.
81. Macdougall IC, Davies ME, Hutton RD, Coles GA, Williams JD. Rheological studies during treatment of renal anaemia with recombinant human erythropoietin. Br J Haematol 1991;77:550–558.
82. Koppensteiner R, Stockenhuber F, Jahn C, Balcke P, Minar E, Ehringer H. Changes in determinants of blood rheology during treatment with haemodialysis and recombinant human erythropoietin. Br Med J 1990; 300:1626–1627.
83. Moia M, Mannucci PM, Vizzotto L, et al. Improvement in the haemostatic defect of uraemia after treatment with recombinant human erythropoietin. Lancet 1987;2:1227–1229.
84. Van Geet C, Hauglustaine D, Verresen L, Vanrusselt M, Vermylen J. Haemostatic effects of recombinant human erythropoietin in chronic haemodialysis patients. Thromb Haemost 1989;61:117–121.
85. Van Geet C, Van Damme-Lombaerts R, Vanrusselt M, et al. Recombinant human erythropoietin increases blood pressure, platelet aggregability and platelet free calcium mobilisation in uraemic children: a possible link? Thromb Haemost 1990;64:7–10.
86. Akizawa T, Kinugasa E, Kitaoka T, Koshikawa S. Effects of recombinant human erythropoietin and correction of anemia on platelet function in hemodialysis patients. Nephron 1991;58:400–406.
87. Taylor JE, Henderson IS, Stewart WK, Belch JJ. Erythropoietin and spontaneous platelet aggregation in haemodialysis patients. Lancet 1991;338:1361–1362.
88. Zwaginga JJ, Ijsseldijk MJW, de Groot PG, et al. Treatment of uremic anemia with recombinant erythropoietin also reduces defects in platelet adhesion and aggregation caused by uremic plasma. Thromb Haemost 1991;66:638–647.
89. Canavese C, Stratta P, Pacitti A, et al. Impaired fibrinolysis in uremia: partial and variable correction by four different dialysis regimes. Clin Nephrol 1982;17:82–89.
90. Panicucci F, Sagripanti A, Pinori E, et al. Comprehensive study of haemostasis in chronic uraemia. Nephron 1983;33:5–8.
91. Huraib S, Al-Momen AK, Gader AMA, et al. Effect of recombinant human erythropoietin (r-HuEPO) on the hemostatic system in chronic hemodialysis patients. Clin Nephrol 1991;36:252–257.
92. Wirtz JJ, van Esser JW, Hamulyak K, Leunissen KM, van Hooff JP. The effects of recombinant erythropoietin on hemostasis and fibrinolysis in hemodialysis patients. Clin Nephrol 1992;38:277–282.
93. Biesma DH, Bronkhorst PJH, de Groot PG, van de Wiel A, Kraaijenhagen RJ, Marx JJM. The effect of recombinant human erythropoietin on hemostasis, fibrinolysis, and blood rheology in autologous blood donors. J Lab Clin Med 1994;124:42–47.
94. Ishibashi T, Koziol JA, Burstein SA. Human recombinant erythropoietin promotes differentiation of murine megakaryocytes in vitro. J Clin Invest 1987;79:286–289.

95. Burstein SA, Ishibashi T. Erythropoietin and megakaryocytopoiesis. Blood Cells 1989;15:193–201.
96. Tsukada J, Misago M, Kikuchi M, et al. The effect of high doses of recombinant human erythropoietin on megakaryocytopoiesis and platelet production in splenectomized mice. Br J Haematol 1990;76: 260–268.
97. Ishida Y, Yano S, Yoshida T, et al. Biological effects of recombinant erythropoietin, granulocyte-macrophage colony-stimulating factor, interleukin 3, and interleukin 6 on purified rat megakaryocytes. Exp Hematol 1991;19:608–612.
98. Spence RK. Surgical red blood cell transfusion practice policies. Am J Surg 1995;170(suppl 6):3S-15S.
99. Rosengart TK, Helm RE, Klemperer J, Krieger KH, Isom OW. Combined aprotinin and erythropoietin use for blood conservation: results with Jehovah's Witnesses. Ann Thorac Surg 1994;58:1397–1403.
100. Gaudiani VA, Mason HD. Preoperative erythropoietin in Jehovah's Witnesses who require cardiac procedures. Ann Thorac Surg 1991;51: 823–824.
101. Stivelman JC. Resistance to recombinant human erythropoietin therapy: a real clinical entity? Semin Nephrol 1989;(suppl 2):8–11.

Chapter 10

Red Cell Substitutes

Part A: Clinical Development of Human Polymerized Hemoglobin

STEVEN A. GOULD
LAKSHMAN R. SEHGAL
HANSA L. SEHGAL
GERALD S. MOSS

INTRODUCTION

There continues to be great interest in developing a clinically useful O_2 carrier to serve as a red blood cell (RBC) substitute. The goal is to develop a safe and effective alternative to human blood. Although the current blood supply is safer than ever because of improved donor screening and testing, it is likely that disease transmission will always occur (1). This is due to the inevitable occurrence of new viruses and to the small but real incidence of false-negative screening tests, often due to the window period of infectivity before conversion of the markers used for screening. In addition, the use of allogeneic blood will always involve the need for compatibility testing and will include a limited shelf-life.

The potential benefits of an RBC substitute include universal compatibility and the accompanying immediate availability, freedom from disease transmission, and long-term storage. The two potential candidates to serve as clinically useful RBC substitutes include hemoglobin solutions and perfluorochemical emulsions (2). We have had considerable experience with the perfluorochemicals, including a clinical trial in patients with a first-generation 20% (weight/volume or 10% volume/volume) perfluorochemical emulsion (3–5). The results of that trial showed that particular preparation was not effective as an O_2 carrier (see Chapter 7). This chapter deals with the history and development of hemoglobin solutions.

BACKGROUND

The basic concept of developing a hemoglobin solution can be illustrated by examining the red blood cell (Fig. 10.1). The "active ingredient" in the red blood cell is the four-part hemoglobin molecule, the tetramer, that chemically binds and actually carries the oxygen. The hemoglobin molecule has several important characteristics. For example, 1 g of hemoglobin binds 1.39 mL of oxygen and is almost fully saturated with oxygen at ambient pressure. Few, if any, biologically acceptable substances have a greater oxygen-binding capacity. Oxygen is normally unloaded from hemoglobin in the capillaries at a PO_2 of approximately 40 Torr, allowing oxygen molecules to diffuse from hemoglobin to the intracellular mitochondria without producing interstitial hypoxia. The physiological capability of the hemoglobin molecule is clear.

The surrounding cell membrane accounts for the need for compatibility testing and the limited shelf-life. It has long been known that although the cell has a finite life span, the hemoglobin protein itself is rather durable and will survive and function outside of the cell. The history of the development of hemoglobin solutions is the tale of the efforts to harvest the hemoglobin protein and prepare it in a form that would be safe and useful in the clinical setting (6).

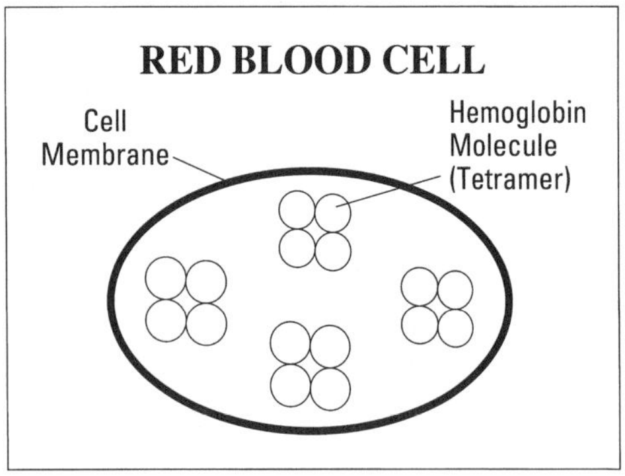

Figure 10.1. A schematic representation of the red blood cell containing the hemoglobin tetramer. (Reprinted with permission from Gould SA, Sehgal L, Sehgal H, Moss GS. The development of hemoglobin solutions as red cell substitutes. Transfusion Sci 1995;16:5–17.)

TABLE 10.1. HEMOGLOBIN SOURCE

- Human
- Bovine
- Recombinant
- Transgenic

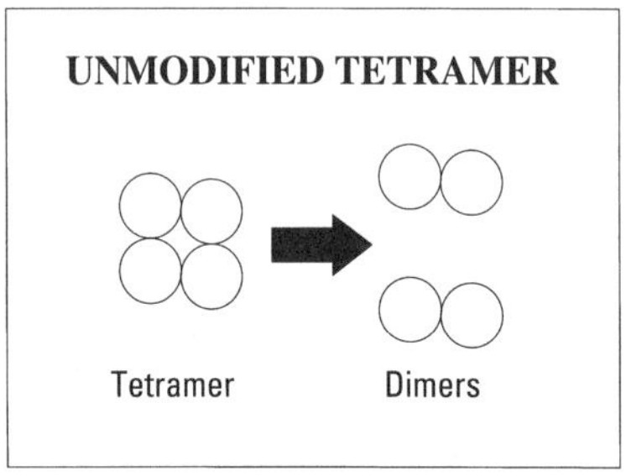

Figure 10.2. Representation of unmodified tetramer as it dissociates into dimers. (Reprinted with permission from Gould SA, Sehgal L, Sehgal H, Moss GS. The development of hemoglobin solutions as red cell substitutes. Transfusion Sci 1995;16:5–17.)

CONSIDERATIONS FOR A HEMOGLOBIN SOLUTION

There are several properties that must be considered when describing the nature of a hemoglobin solution. The first is the source of the hemoglobin to be used as the starting material (Table 10.1). We have always believed that the human source is the best known and readily available, making it the preferred choice. The bovine source has been proposed as a way of providing easier access to an unlimited supply. The recombinant and transgenic approaches have received considerable interest because of their use of the modern molecular biology approaches. However, there is no evidence to suggest any physiological or functional benefit of using any source other than human hemoglobin. In fact, the choice of source has not yet been a crucial issue in the development of an RBC substitute. Cost and availability of supply may yet modify which sources are most greatly used.

The limiting factor in this field has been the safety of the hemoglobin solution. It is now evident that unmodified tetrameric hemoglobin is unsafe because of the associated toxicities of renal dysfunction, gastrointestinal distress, and vasoconstriction (6). Therefore, the most important property of a hemoglobin solution is the nature of the hemoglobin preparation itself. Unmodified tetramer dissociates into dimers when removed from the RBC (Fig. 10.2). It is now believed that the observed toxicities are in large part due to this dissociation and the presence of free tetramer in the circulation. Efforts to eliminate these toxicities have consisted of a variety of attempts to stabilize the simple unmodified tetramer. Table 10.2 lists the various preparations. Each effort involves the use of a different approach to try to stabilize the tetramer and thereby avoid toxicity. A conjugated tetramer (Fig. 10.3) involves the binding of a macromolecule such as polyethylene glycol to form a larger molecule. Other agents have been used, such as diasporin, but to date, no comparison between cross-linking technologies has occurred. A cross-linked tetramer (Fig. 10.4) is an intramolecular chemical or genetic link to stabilize the native hemoglobin molecule. Polymerization involves intermolecular cross-linking of tetramers as shown in Figure 10.5. The polymerization results in a variety of molecular weight sizes. Finally, encapsulation, as shown in Figure 10.6, involves the "packaging" of the hemoglobin molecule within a lipid membrane or liposome to form a "synthetic" red blood cell. Only testing in humans will eventually resolve the issue of safety with these various preparations. However, it is clear that the nature of the actual hemoglobin preparation itself is far more important than the choice of source material.

The third characteristic of any hemoglobin solution is the intended clinical use. Table 10.3 lists some of the various potential applications for a safe and effective hemoglobin solution. Although they represent a diverse set of circumstances, it is likely that the major role of a hemoglobin solution will be as an RBC substitute for use in acute blood loss. The surgical implications are obvious and once again not fully appreciated because these solutions are not yet approved by the U.S. Food and Drug Administration.

There are numerous clinical trials underway in both volunteers and patients using a variety of these approaches. Ultimately, each effort involves a selection of hemoglobin source, preparation, and intended clinical use. Table 10.4

TABLE 10.2. HEMOGLOBIN PREPARATION

- Unmodified tetramer
- Conjugated tetramer
- Cross-linked tetramer
- Polymer
- Encapsulation

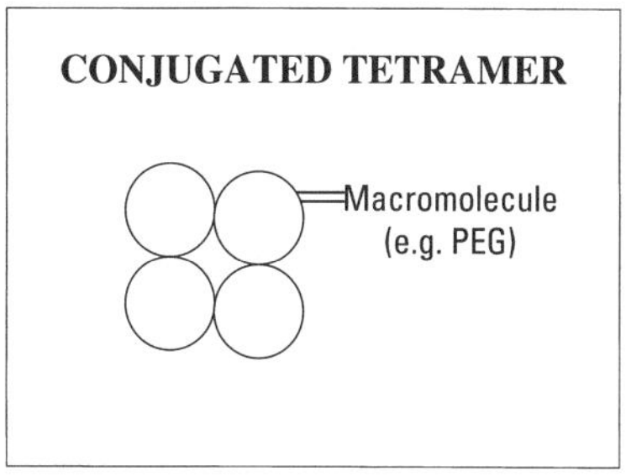

Figure 10.3. Conjugated tetramer. (Reprinted with permission from Gould SA, Sehgal L, Sehgal H, Moss GS. The development of hemoglobin solutions as red cell substitutes. Transfusion Sci 1995;16:5–17.)

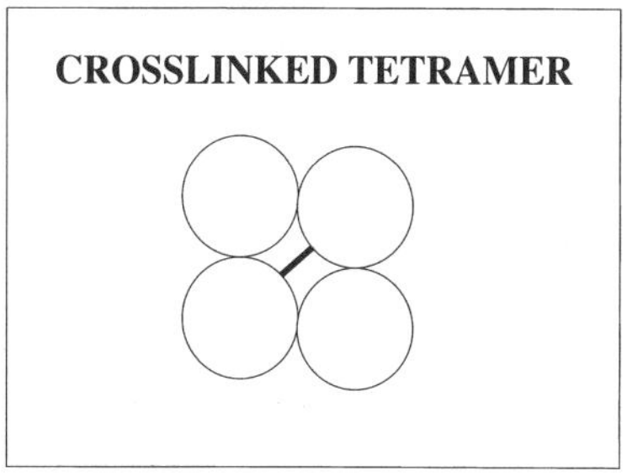

Figure 10.4. Cross-linked tetramer. (Reprinted with permission from Gould SA, Sehgal L, Sehgal H, Moss GS. The development of hemoglobin solutions as red cell substitutes. Transfusion Sci 1995;16:5–17.)

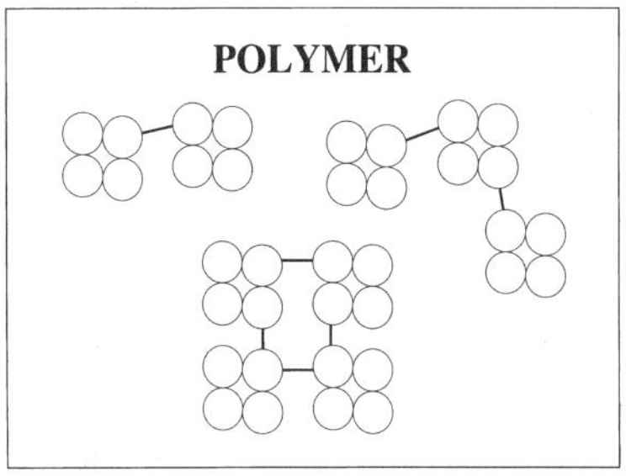

Figure 10.5. Polymers composed of two, three, and four tetramers linked together. (Reprinted with permission from Gould SA, Sehgal L, Sehgal H, Moss GS. The development of hemoglobin solutions as red cell substitutes. Transfusion Sci 1995;16:5–17.)

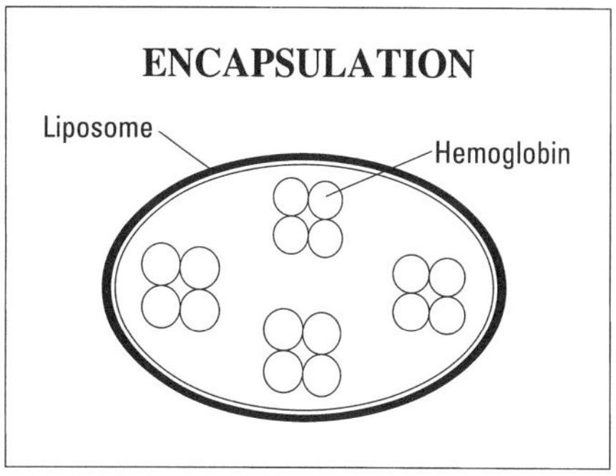

Figure 10.6. Liposome encapsulated hemoglobin. (Reprinted with permission from Gould SA, Sehgal L, Sehgal H, Moss GS. The development of hemoglobin solutions as red cell substitutes. Transfusion Sci 1995;16:5–17.)

TABLE 10.3. HEMOGLOBIN CLINICAL USE

- Acute blood loss
- Hemodilution
- Ischemia
- Cardioplegia
- Organ preservation
- Cancer therapy
- Sepsis

TABLE 10.4. CURRENT APPROACHES

- Human polymer, tetramer-free
- Human polymer, tetramer present
- Bovine polymer, tetramer present
- Human crossed-linked tetramer
- Recombinant cross-linked tetramer

shows a list of the source and preparation for each of the current approaches in clinical trials.

DEMONSTRATION OF EFFICACY

The concept of using a hemoglobin solution as an oxygen carrier was first fully tested by Amberson et al. in 1934 (7). Amberson et al. prepared a crude RBC lysate, which was an unmodified tetrameric form of the hemoglobin solution. In a rather remarkable experiment, they gradually removed all blood from cats and replaced it with this primitive hemoglobin solution. The results demonstrated the proof of concept and paved the way for all future efforts. The cats survived on a short-term basis and were able to walk normally. In an absolutely elegant maneuver, Amberson et al. evaluated neurological function by holding the cats on their backs and dropping them. The cats were able to land upright, demonstrating the fully intact nervous system required to perform this complicated neurological event. The potential utility of hemoglobin solutions was firmly established.

PROBLEM OF TOXICITY

Based on this early demonstration by Amberson et al., the efficacy of a hemoglobin solution was uncontestable. However, 60 years later there is still no hemoglobin solution in clinical use. The reason for this relates to the results in clinical trials (8–11). All prior clinical trials through 1978 had been done with unmodified tetrameric forms of hemoglobin solution. These trials consistently demonstrated major toxicities consisting of renal dysfunction, gastrointestinal distress, and systemic vasoconstriction characterized by a rise in blood pressure and a fall in heart rate (12). The Savitsky et al. study in 1978 (11) clearly established the futility of further efforts to develop a safe tetrameric form of hemoglobin solution.

MECHANISMS OF TOXICITY

The mechanisms of toxicity of the tetramer now seem to be better understood. In general, these toxicities are related to the presence of the tetramer outside of the RBC and the dissociation into dimers. The renal dysfunction is thought to be related to filtration and excretion of the hemoglobin molecule, primarily in the form of dimers, although vasoconstriction is also likely to play a role. Dimers are filtered and concentrated in renal tubules, and with pH changes, they can precipitate, leading to renal tubular plugging. The effect of vasoconstriction on renal blood flow may also have been a cause of renal impairment. The vasoconstriction and other adverse effects are currently thought to be related to extravasation of the tetrameric hemoglobin molecule (13).

Our understanding of the control of vasoconstriction of blood vessels has been improved with the identification of endothelium-derived relaxing factor, also known as nitric oxide (14, 15). It is known that nitric oxide avidly binds to hemoglobin. Figure 10.7 is a graphic representation of the control of vasoconstriction. It is a cross-section of a blood vessel representing the lumen, the endothelial cell layer, and the interstitial space within which reside the vascular smooth muscle cells. Nitric oxide is produced by the endothelial cells and is released on both the luminal and the abluminal sides. The physiological activity of nitric oxide occurs on the vascular smooth muscle cells in the interstitial space. The nitric oxide released into the lumen is rapidly bound by the hemoglobin within the circulating RBCs and does not act on the smooth muscle cells. It is also evident that RBCs do not normally move beyond the endothelial cell lining into the interstitial space, leaving the nitric oxide available to exert its vasorelaxant effect.

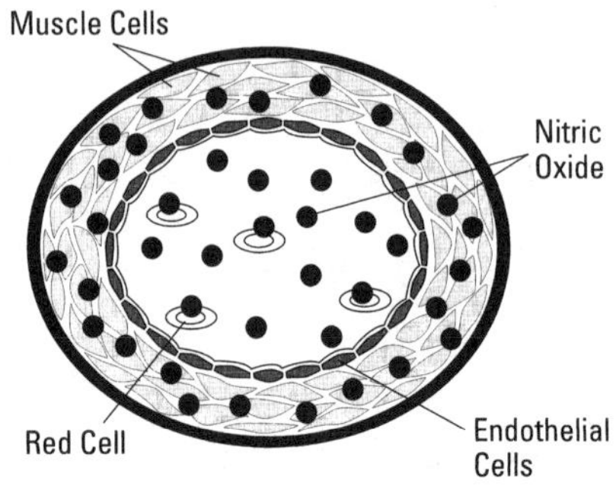

Figure 10.7. Control of vasoconstriction. (Reprinted with permission from Gould SA, Sehgal L, Sehgal H, Moss GS. The development of hemoglobin solutions as red cell substitutes. Transfusion Sci 1995;16:5–17.)

The vasoconstriction that occurs with the tetrameric form of the hemoglobin is considered to be due to extravasation of the hemoglobin beyond the endothelial cell barrier and the immediate binding of the nitric oxide to the hemoglobin, leading to unopposed vasoconstriction. This is illustrated in Figure 10.8. The presence of the tetramer in the interstitial space where nitric oxide normally acts thereby disrupts the normal control of vascular relaxation. Our working hypothesis has been that prevention of extravasation will prevent vasoconstriction, because nitric oxide would function normally. It has also been our contention that all forms of tetramer will extravasate and produce both vasoconstriction and the other toxicities historically associated with hemoglobin solutions (13, 16, 17). The only forms of hemoglobin that would appear to prevent extravasation include the polymer and encapsulation. The cross-linked tetramers have indeed been shown to extravasate (13, 17). Because the encapsulation approach is still in the developmental stage, only the polymer has been able to be evaluated in the clinical setting. Figure 10.9 illustrates the likely scenario when the polymer is infused. As with the RBC, the polymer will exist only in the lumen, leaving the nitric oxide to exert its normal physiological vasorelaxant role on the vascular smooth muscle cell in the interstitial space.

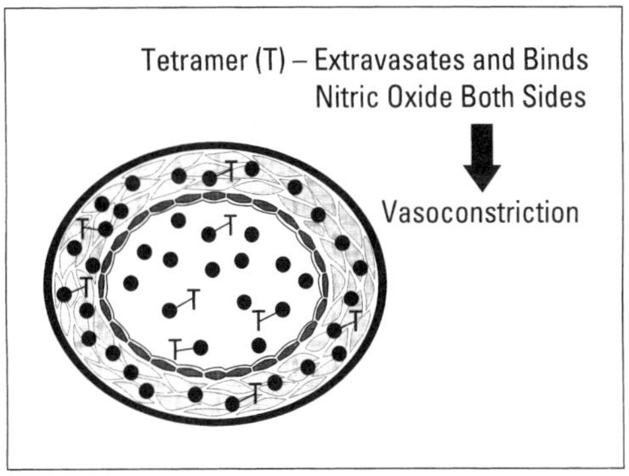

Figure 10.8. The effect of tetramer on extravasation and binding of nitric oxide. (Reprinted with permission from Gould SA, Sehgal L, Sehgal H, Moss GS. The development of hemoglobin solutions as red cell substitutes. Transfusion Sci 1995;16:5–17.)

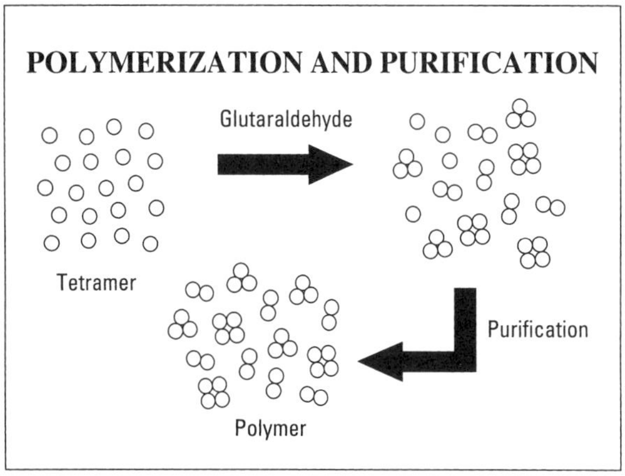

Figure 10.10. Preparation of Poly SFH-P, including polymerization and removal of unreacted tetramer. (Reprinted with permission from Gould SA, Sehgal L, Sehgal H, Moss GS. The development of hemoglobin solutions as red cell substitutes. Transfusion Sci 1995;16:5–17.)

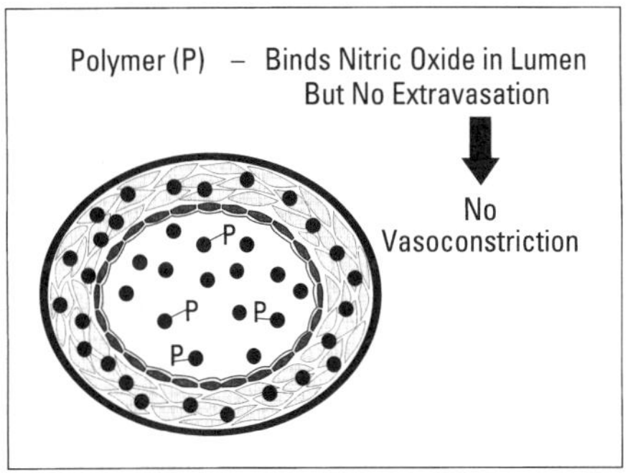

Figure 10.9. Representation of polymer and absence of extravasation. (Reprinted with permission from Gould SA, Sehgal L, Sehgal H, Moss GS. The development of hemoglobin solutions as red cell substitutes. Transfusion Sci 1995;16:5–17.)

Our approach, therefore, has been to specifically design a hemoglobin solution using a two-step process to create a tetramer-free form of polymerized hemoglobin (18–21). The first step is the polymerization, which results in an array of different size polymers. The second step, which is just as important, is the removal of all unreacted tetramer. Figure 10.10 is a representation of this process. Glutaraldehyde is used as the cross-linking (polymerizing) agent. The second step is to remove virtually all unreacted tetramer, leading to a pure polymeric solution. The remainder of this part of the chapter deals with the historical development of our human polymerized hemoglobin solution, including the physiological observations that led to the characteristics of our current preparation.

UNMODIFIED HEMOGLOBIN

The basic unmodified hemoglobin solution is currently prepared from outdated blood, beginning with the washing and lysis of the RBCs with pyrogen-free water. A series of filtration steps permits the complete separation of the RBC membrane debris (stroma) from the hemoglobin molecules. The resultant solution is referred to as stroma-free hemoglobin (SFH). Because the RBC antigens are located on the cell membrane, SFH is universally compatible and can be infused without regard to specific blood type. The properties of this unmodified, tetrameric, or "stripped" hemoglobin solution are given in Table 10.5.

TABLE 10.5. PROPERTIES AND PARAMETERS OF STROMA-FREE HEMOGLOBIN AND WHOLE BLOOD

Properties and Parameters	Stroma-Free Hemoglobin	Whole Blood
Hemoglobin content (g/dL)	6–8	12–14
Oxygen-carrying capacity (vol%)	8.0–11.0	16–19
Binding coefficient (mL O_2/g hemoglobin)	1.30	1.30
P_{50} (Torr) (P_{CO}=40 Torr; pH=7.40)	12–14	26–28
Methemoglobin (%)	<2	<1
Colloid osmotic pressure (Torr)	18–25	18–25
Osmolarity (mOsm)	290–310	290–310

Although SFH can be prepared with a hemoglobin concentration of 14 g/dL, this solution has a colloid osmotic pressure (COP) greater than 60 mm Hg, which renders it unacceptable for clinical use (22). The hemoglobin concentration of 7 g/dL is iso-oncotic. The low P_{50} is due to the loss of the organic ligand, 2,3-diphosphoglycerate (2,3-DPG), during preparation. The $[O_2]$ curve of SFH is thus both anemic (↓ hemoglobin content) and leftward shifted (↓ P_{50}).

Despite these limitations, SFH supports life in primates in the absence of RBCs (22). Animals survive a total exchange transfusion with SFH to zero hematocrit with maintenance of normal O_2 consumption ($\dot{V}O_2$), cardiac output, and arteriovenous oxygen content difference ($CaO_2 - CvO_2$), although a decline from baseline values occurs in some of these measures. In addition, a considerable decrease occurs in the $P\bar{v}O_2$ from roughly 50 to 20 Torr. The $P\bar{v}O_2$ is the partial pressure at which oxygen unloads from the hemoglobin molecule and is in equilibrium with the tissue PO_2. This decline indicates a marked increase in oxygen extraction and is the mechanism used to compensate for the fall in hemoglobin content and P_{50}. This low $P\bar{v}O_2$ is of some concern and led us to attempt to restore a more normal value (23).

PYRIDOXYLATED HEMOGLOBIN

A leftward shift in the $[O_2]$ curve, with no change in $\dot{V}O_2$, cardiac output, or $CaO_2 - CvO_2$, produces a decrease in the $P\bar{v}O_2$ (Fig. 10.11). Attempts to establish a normal P_{50} by the simple addition of 2,3-DPG to the hemoglobin solution were unsuccessful because the ligand disappears rapidly from the circulation after infusion. However, a modification of the hemoglobin molecule by the addition of pyridoxal phosphate results in a pyridoxylated hemoglobin (SFH-P) with a P_{50} of 20–22 Torr, which is considerably higher than the P_{50} of unmodified SFH (24–26).

We evaluated SFH-P in eight baboons (27). Four received SFH and four received SFH-P, with a final hemoglobin content of 7 g/dL and zero hematocrit. The $P\bar{v}O_2$ levels were significantly higher at the end of the exchange in the animals receiving SFH-P. Although hemodynamic parameters were normal, a decline from the baseline values occurred in both groups.

These results illustrate three points. First, a rightward shift in the dissociation curve (↑ P_{50}) results in an increased $P\bar{v}O_2$ because all else remained constant. This observation is of physiological importance because oxygen unloading can occur at a higher tissue PO_2. Second, although it was increased, the $P\bar{v}O_2$ level in the animals treated with SFH-P was still substantially lower than the normal value of 40–50 Torr found in control animals. Third, hemodynamic function still showed a reduction from the baseline values. It became apparent that a nonanemic hemoglobin solution was required (23).

NONANEMIC ISO-ONCOTIC HEMOGLOBIN SOLUTION

The advantages of a nonanemic hemoglobin solution are self-evident. Such a solution would have the same oxygen capacity as whole blood. In addition, according to our data, the infusion of a nonanemic solution should be associated with normal $P\bar{v}O_2$ levels, even at zero hematocrit (23). The principal obstacle to normalization of hemoglobin concentration is the effect of an elevation in protein concentration on oncotic pressure.

The relationship between hemoglobin concentration and oncotic pressure is shown in Figure 10.12. At hemoglobin concentrations of 7 g/dL, the oncotic pressure is similar to

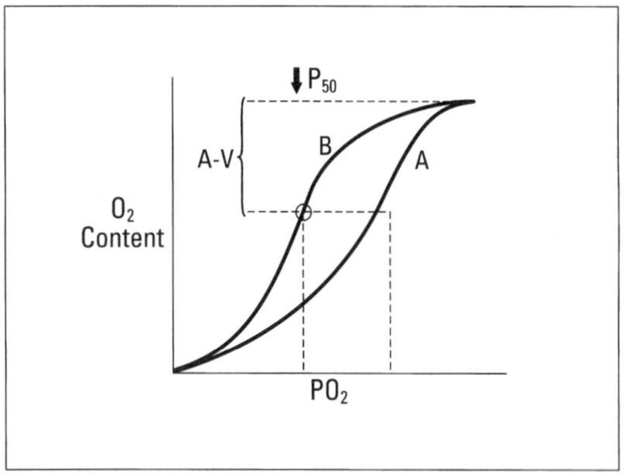

Figure 10.11. $[O_2]$ curves showing a leftward shift in P_{50} with a constant $CaO_2 - CvO_2$ leads to a lower $P\bar{v}O_2$. Curve B is shifted to the left compared with curve A. (Reprinted with permission from Moss GS, Sehgal LR, Gould SA, et al. Alternatives to transfusion therapy. Anesthesiol Clin North Am 1990;8:569.)

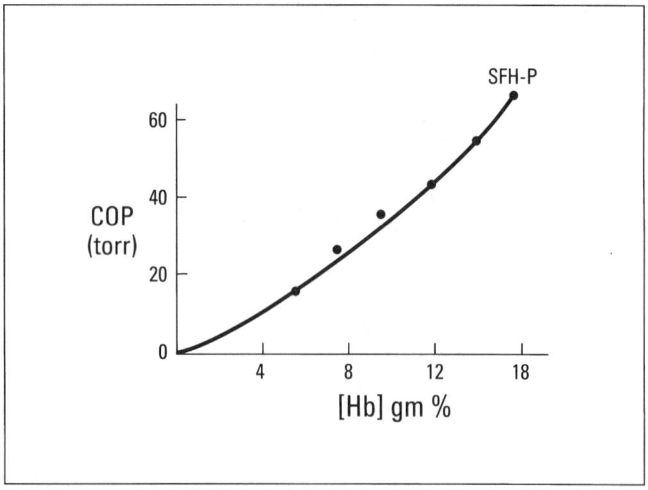

Figure 10.12. Relationship between COP and hemoglobin concentration for SFH-P. (Reprinted with permission from Moss GS, Sehgal LR, Gould SA, et al. Alternatives to transfusion therapy. Anesthesiol Clin North Am 1990;8:569.)

that of plasma (20 Torr). In contrast, at hemoglobin levels of 15 g/dL, oncotic pressure increases by more than 300%. The infusion of such a solution would theoretically produce large shifts of fluid from the extravascular space into the intravascular space. These changes are likely to be harmful.

One approach to producing a nonanemic hemoglobin solution with normal COP values is polymerization of the hemoglobin. The COP of any solution is proportional to the number of colloidal particles. If a 15-g/dL solution of hemoglobin could be polymerized, the result would be a reduction in COP, whereas no change would occur in hemoglobin concentration (Fig. 10.13). This idea was tested in our laboratories (18). The hemoglobin solution obtained was pyridoxylated by modification of previously described techniques. The characteristics of the final product are listed in Table 10.6.

TABLE 10.6. PROPERTIES OF POLYMERIZED PYRIDOXYLATED HEMOGLOBIN

Property	Parameter Range
Hemoglobin (g/dL)	12–14
Oxygen-carrying capacity (vol%)	16–19
Methemoglobin (%)	<5
Molecular weight range	64,000–400,000
Number average molecular weight	150,000
P_{50} (Torr)	18–22
Binding coefficient (mL O_2/g hemoglobin)	1.30
COP (Torr)	20–25

EFFICACY OF POLY SFH-P

Seven adult baboons were anesthetized, paralyzed, intubated, and mechanically ventilated with room air (28, 29). The respiratory rate and tidal volume were adjusted to maintain a $Paco_2$ between 35 and 45 Torr before the start of the study and were not changed during the study. The animals were surgically prepared with arterial and central venous catheters for infusion, blood sampling, and monitoring. A thermal dilution balloon-tipped catheter was floated into the pulmonary artery. A Foley catheter was inserted into the urinary bladder. Standard hemodynamic monitoring was performed for electrocardiogram, arterial pressures, pulmonary capillary wedge pressure, and central venous pressure. Cardiac output was determined by the thermal dilution method.

The study was conducted with the use of ketamine anesthesia. After stabilization of the animals, a set of baseline measurements was obtained. An isovolemic exchange transfusion with the Poly SFH-P was then performed. Whole blood was removed in 50-mL aliquots and was replaced with approximately equal volumes of the infusate. Additional volume adjustments were made as required to maintain the pulmonary capillary wedge pressure at baseline values. The exchange was stopped at hematocrits of 20, 10, and 5% to obtain additional sets of measurements. The exchange transfusion was then carried out to obtain a complete washout of the RBCs. A hematocrit of less than 1% was achieved.

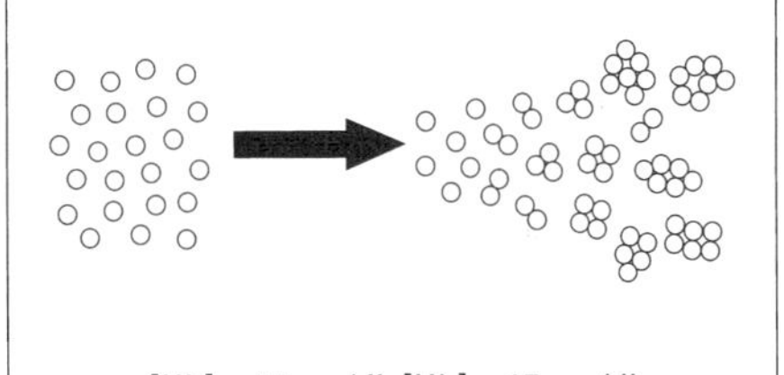

Figure 10.13. Polymerization. (Reprinted with permission from Moss GS, Sehgal LR, Gould SA, et al. Alternatives to transfusion therapy. Anesthesiol Clin North Am 1990;8:569.)

These animals, at zero hematocrit, had a Poly SFH-P concentration of approximately 10 g/dL. They were then exchanged-transfused with dextran 70 to a hemoglobin concentration of 1 g/dL (30). The data from the second half of the study were compared with a control group (n = 6) that underwent an exchange transfusion with dextran 70 to a hemoglobin concentration of 1 g/dL.

The efficacy of the Poly SFH-P was calculated as we have previously described (31). At each hematocrit level, the arterial $[O_2]([O_2]_a)$ was determined for each compartment by direct measurement or calculation. Total Vo_2 was calculated as the product of the cardiac output and $Cao_2 - Cvo_2$. The contribution of Poly SFH-P to oxygen delivery was calculated as the ratio of the Poly SFH-P to total arterial $[O_2]$:

$$\text{Poly SFH-P } O_2 \text{ delivery} = \frac{[O_2], \text{ Poly SFH-P}}{[O_2]_a, \text{ total}}$$

The contribution of Poly SFH-P to Vo_2 was calculated as the ratio of Poly SFH-P to total $Cao_2 - Cvo_2$:

$$\text{Poly SFH-P } Vo_2 = \frac{\text{Poly SFH-P } (Cao_2 - Cvo_2}{\text{Total } (Cao_2 - Cvo_2}$$

All contributions were expressed as their percent values.

All animals receiving Poly SFH-P survived the exchange transfusion, as did the previous animals receiving SFH-P.

The final hematocrit was 0.8 ± 0.4% (mean ± SEM). The difference in the initial bag P_{50} values of the two infusates was statistically significant ($P < .05$). However, the mean in vivo plasma P_{50} for the Poly SFH-P was 17.0 ± 0.5 Torr, which was not significantly different from the mean value of 17.6 ± 0.8 Torr for the SFH-P. Both plasma P_{50} values are significantly below the mean baboon RBC P_{50} of 31.3 ± 0.8 Torr. The Poly SFH-P $[O_2]_a$ is significantly greater than the SFH-P value at all hematocrits ($P < .001$). At a hematocrit of 5%, the $[O_2]_a$ was 9.5 ± 0.2 vol% for Poly SFH-P and 5.0 ± 0.4 vol% for SFH-P. The percent contributions of Poly SFH-P to total oxygen delivery and total Vo_2 were compared with those of SFH-P. Poly SFH-P makes a significantly greater contribution to total oxygen delivery than SFH-P at all hematocrit. The contribution to total Vo_2 is greater by Poly SFH-P at all hematocrit, with the difference significant ($P < .005$) at a hematocrit of 20%. These results document that Poly SFH-P is an effective O_2 carrier and provides benefit over the tetrameric form of SFH-P.

The in vivo P_{50} in the Poly SFH-P animals undergoing the second exchange transfusion with dextran 70 ranged from 18 to 11 Torr. In contrast, the in vivo P_{50} of the control group ranged from 31.5 to 25.5 Torr. The $P\dot{v}o_2$ was significantly lower in the Poly SFH-P group compared with the control group. Both groups of animals raised their cardiac output in an identical manner in response to their anemia. The critical oxygen delivery in the control group was 6.6 mL/min/kg of body weight compared with 5.7 mL/min/kg in the test group. These results indicate that the infusion of Poly SFH-P does not alter the normal physiological response to progressive anemia and therefore provides evidence of lack of vasoconstriction.

CLINICAL TRIALS

VOLUNTEER EXPERIENCE

Based on these preclinical observations, we began clinical trials in both healthy volunteers and patients to assess the safety and efficacy of Poly SFH-P. For these trials, a decision was made to prepare the Poly SFH-P in a fashion that would allow one unit of Poly SFH-P to deliver the equivalent amount of hemoglobin contained in a one-unit blood transfusion. Therefore, each unit contains 500 mL at a 10-g/dL concentration, thereby delivering 50 g of hemoglobin. In addition, continued improvement in the process enabled the P_{50} to be increased to 28–30 Torr. The characteristics of one unit of Poly SFH-P used for clinical trials is shown in Table 10.7. To date, the clinical trials have included both healthy volunteers (32), stable patients, and patients being resuscitated from hemorrhagic shock after major trauma (33, 34). Poly SFH-P was successfully infused in doses up to the equivalent of a one-unit transfusion of blood (50 g) in healthy volunteers without the undesirable effects historically associated with hemoglobin solutions, including vasoconstriction, kidney dysfunction, or gastrointestinal distress (Table 10.8). This experience provided sufficient evidence to begin therapeutic trials with Poly SFH-P in bleeding patients. A brief summary of these data are provided.

TABLE 10.7. CHARACTERISTICS OF POLY SFH-P FOR CLINICAL TRIALS

- Hemoglobin = 10 g/dL
- P_{50} = 28–30 Torr
- Methemoglobin <3%
- Tetramer <1%
- T ½ = 1 day
- 1 unit = 500 mL (50 g)

FIRST PATIENT TRIAL

The protocol was a dose-escalation, open-label investigation of the clinical utility of Poly SFH-P in the perioperative management of patients who have experienced acute blood loss after trauma, surgery, or both. Initially, one unit (50 g) of Poly SFH-P was infused in 10 patients. The dosage was increased to a maximum of three units (150 g) in the next 20 patients and finally to an allowable maximum dosage of six units (300 g) as needed in the last 9 recipients. Of 39 recipients, 8 received the maximum dose of six units of Poly SFH-P.

The protocol was rather straightforward. Patients were eligible after hemorrhage from trauma or surgery. The transfusion decision was based on clinical judgement. When the treating physician determined a blood transfusion was indicated, the infusion of Poly SFH-P was initiated in place of allogeneic blood. Infusions were given during resuscitation, intraoperatively and postoperatively, to both awake and anesthetized patients. Men and women of all racial and ethnic

TABLE 10.8. CLINICAL EXPERIENCE WITH 30 HEALTHY VOLUNTEERS

	Preinfusion	Postinfusion
Heart rate (bpm)	63 ± 8	60.0 ± 9.0
MAP	95 ± 12	100 ± 13
Inulin clearance (mL/min/m²)	52 ± 13	51 ± 12

groups ranging in age from 19 to 83 years of age received Poly SFH-P infusions.

No adverse effects attributed to the infusion of Poly SFH-P have been observed in any of these patients. Accordingly, no treatment with any drug before, during, or after the infusion of Poly SFH-P was necessary to prevent or eliminate any such effect in this group of patients experiencing acute blood loss. There was no evidence of fever in any recipient. There were no abnormal changes in heart rate or blood pressure attributed to Poly SFH-P, indicating no evidence of vasoconstriction. Kidney function was measured using creatinine clearance and serum creatinine determinations. There was no evidence of gastrointestinal distress, and serum amylase levels remained normal during and after the infusion of Poly SFH-P. In addition, there was no evidence of organ dysfunction in any recipient. These data indicate that Poly SFH-P is well tolerated when infused up to and including the equivalent of a six-unit transfusion of blood.

These clinical results also indicate the potential clinical utility of Poly SFH-P. The data illustrate that each unit of Poly SFH-P raises hemoglobin concentration and carries as much oxygen as one unit of transfused blood and that Poly SFH-P loads and unloads oxygen in the same manner as transfused blood (Tables 10.9–10.11) (33). None of these actively bleeding patients received transfusions of donated blood during the infusion of Poly SFH-P. Furthermore, 18 of 39 patients, or 46%, received only Poly SFH-P and did not receive any donated blood during the critical 24-hour period after their blood loss.

CURRENT PATIENT PROTOCOL

Based on this evidence, we recently began a randomized, controlled trial comparing the use of up to six units of Poly SFH-P to allogeneic blood in the treatment of acute blood loss. The protocol differs in several ways from the earlier study. Eligibility is limited to those patients experiencing moderate to severe hemorrhage for which urgent hemoglobin replacement is indicated. Elective surgical patients are not being enrolled. The decision to transfuse is made before a sealed envelope is opened to assign the patient to either the experimental (Poly SFH-P) or control (allogeneic blood) group. Furthermore, unlike the earlier study, Poly SFH-P is only infused during the period of active bleeding. Once the operation has ended, any further transfusions are given in the form of allogeneic blood, even if the maximum dose of six units of Poly SFH-P has not been infused.

The goal of this study is to assess the safety, physiological activity, and efficacy of Poly SFH-P in the treatment of acute blood loss. Although the trial is still in progress, more than 40 patients have been enrolled to date. The results continue to demonstrate Poly SFH-P is physiologically active in the presence of RBCs and so far does not produce any safety concerns to date. The primary focus on efficacy will be the ability to reduce the use of allogeneic blood. This trial is the first direct comparison of a hemoglobin-based blood substitute to donated blood in the treatment of bleeding patients. At present, the data suggest a virtual 1:1 replacement of Poly SFH-P for allogeneic blood. These findings are encouraging. Ultimately, the results of continued trials will fully assess the likely clinical utility of Poly SFH-P. Continued clinical trials

TABLE 10.9. THE [HB] DATA (G/DL) PREINFUSION AND AFTER EACH UNIT OF POLY SFH-P ARE SHOWN (MEAN ± SD)

	Plasma [Hb]	Red Cell [Hb]	Total [Hb]
Preinfusion	—	9.7 ± 2.6	9.7 ± 2.6
After 1 unit	1.3 ± 0.5	8.3 ± 1.9	9.3 ± 1.7
After 2 units	2.5 ± 0.7	6.4 ± 1.3	8.5 ± 1.2
After 3 units	3.4 ± 0.9	5.6 ± 1.1	8.5 ± 0.6
After 6 units	4.8 ± 0.8	2.9 ±1.2	7.5 ± 1.2

Poly SFH-P maintained total [Hb], despite the marked fall in red cell [Hb] due to blood loss.
[Hb], hemoglobin concentration.

TABLE 10.10. OXYGEN LOADING

	RBC	Poly SFH-P
[Hb] (g/dL)	7.7 ± 2.4	2.2 ± 1.2
$[O_2]_a$ (vol%)	10.3 ± 3.2	2.9 ± 1.7

[Hb], hemoglobin concentration.

TABLE 10.11. OXYGEN UNLOADING

	RBC	Poly SFH-P
$[O_2]_v$ (vol%)	7.3 ± 2.9	1.8 ± 1.1
$AVDO_2$ (vol%)	3.0 ± 2.2	1.1 ± 0.7
O_2 (%)	28 ± 16	37 ± 13

$AVDO_2$, arterovenous, difference in oxygen (volume %)

are necessary before any hemoglobin preparation is available for widescale perioperative use, but the time appears to be drawing closer when the dream of a true "blood substitute" will be a therapeutic option.

REFERENCES

1. Dodd RY. The risk of transfusion-transmitted infection. N Engl J Med 1992;327:419–421.
2. Gould SA, Rosen AL, Sehgal LR, et al. Red cell substitutes: hemoglobin solution or fluorocarbon? J Trauma 1982;22:736–740.
3. Gould SA, Rosen AL, Sehgal LR, et al. How good are fluorocarbon emulsions as O_2 carriers? Surg Forum 1981;32:299–303.
4. Gould SA, Sehgal LR, Rosen AL, et al. Assessment of 35% fluorocarbon emulsion. J Trauma 1983;23:72–24.
5. Gould SA, Rosen AL, Sehgal LR, et al. Fluosol-DA as a red cell substitute in acute anemia. N Engl J Med 1986;315:1653–1656.
6. Winslow RM. Hemoglobin-based red cell substitutes. Baltimore: Johns Hopkins University Press, 1992.
7. Amberson WR, Flexner J, Steggerda FR, et al. On the use of Ringer-Locke solution containing hemoglobin as a substitute for normal blood in mammals. J Cell Comp Physiol 1934;5:59–82.
8. Amberson WR, Jennings JJ, Rhode CM. Clinical experience with hemoglobin-saline solutions. J Appl Physiol 1949;1:469–49.
9. Brandt JL, Frank R, Lichtman HC. The effect of hemoglobin solutions on renal functions in man. Blood 1951;6:1152–1158.
10. Miller JH, McDonald RK. The effect of hemoglobin on renal function in the human. J Clin Invest 1951;30:1033–1040.
11. Savitsky JP, Doczi J, Black J, Arnold JD. A clinical safety trial of stroma-free hemoglobin. Clin Pharmacol Ther 1978;23:73–80.
12. Center for Biologics Evaluation and Research. Points to consider in the safety of hemoglobin-based oxygen carriers. Transfusion 1991;31: 369–371.
13. Keipert PE, Gonzales A, Gomez CL, MacDonald VW, Hess JR, Winslow RM. Acute changes in systemic blood pressure and urine output of conscious rats following exchange transfusion with diaspirin-crosslinked hemoglobin solution. Transfusion 1993;33:701–708.
14. Martin W, Villani GM, Jothianandan D, Furchgott RF. Selective blockade of endothelium-dependent and glycerol trinitrate-induced relaxation by hemoglobin and by methylene blue in the rabbit aorta. J Pharmacol Exp Ther 1985;232:708–716.
15. Moncada S, Palmer RMJ, Higgs EA. Nitric oxide: physiology, pathophysiology, and pharmacology. Pharmacol Rev 1991;40:109–142.
16. Hess JR, MacDonald VW, Brinkley WW. Systemic and pulmonary hypertension after resuscitation with cell-free hemoglobin. J Appl Physiol 1993;74:1769–1778.
17. Keipert PE, Gomez CL, Gonzales A, MacDonald VW, Hess JR, Winslow RM. Diaspirin-crosslinked hemoglobin: tissue distribution and long term excretion following exchange transfusion. J Lab Clin Med 1994;123:701–711.
18. Sehgal LR, Rosen AL, Gould SA, et al. Preparation and in vitro characteristics of polymerized pyridoxylated hemoglobin. Transfusion 1983; 23:158–162.
19. Sehgal LR, Gould SA, Rosen AL, Sehgal HL, Moss GS. Polymerized pyridoxylated hemoglobin: a red cell substitute with normal O_2 capacity. Surgery 1984;95:433–438.
20. Gould SA, Sehgal LR, Sehgal HL, Moss GS. Artificial blood. In: Carlson RW, Geheb MA, eds. Principles & practice of medical intensive care. Philadelphia: WB Saunders, 1993:151–160.
21. Moss GS, Gould SA, Sehgal LR, et al. Hemoglobin solution: from tetramer to polymer. Surgery 1984;95:249–255.
22. Moss GS, DeWoskin R, Rosen AL, et al. Transport of oxygen and carbon dioxide by hemoglobin-saline solution in the red cell-free primate. Surg Gynecol Obstet 1976;142:357–362.
23. Gould SA, Sehgal LR, Rosen AL, et al. Hemoglobin solution: is a normal [Hb] or P_{50} more important? J Surg Res 1982;33:189–193.
24. Benesch RE, Benesch R, Renthal RD, et al. Affinity labeling of the polyphosphate binding site of hemoglobin. Biochemistry 1972;11: 3576–3582.
25. Greenberg AG, Hayashi R, Siefert I, et al. Intravascular persistence and oxygen delivery of pyridoxylated, stroma-free hemoglobin during gradations of hypotension. Surgery 1979;86:13–16.
26. Sehgal LR, Rosen AL, Noud G, et al. Large volume preparation of pyridoxylated hemoglobin with high in vivo P_{50}. J Surg Res 1981;30:14–20.
27. Gould SA, Rosen AL, Sehgal LR, et al. The effect of altered hemoglobin-oxygen affinity on oxygen transport by hemoglobin solution. J Surg Res 1980;28:246–251.
28. Gould SA, Sehgal LR, Rosen AL, Sehgal HL, Moss GS. Polyhemoglobin: an improved red cell substitute. Surg Forum 1985;36:30–32.
29. Gould SA, Sehgal LR, Rosen AL, Sehgal HL, Moss GS. The efficacy of polymerized pyridoxylated hemoglobin solution as an O_2 carrier. Ann Surg 1990;211:394–398.
30. Rosen AL, Gould SA, Sehgal LR, et al. Effect of hemoglobin solution on compensation to anemia in erythrocyte-free primate. J Appl Physiol 1990;68:938–943.
31. Rosen AL, Gould SA, Sehgal LR, et al. Evaluation of efficacy of stroma-free hemoglobin solutions. In: Bolin RB, Geyer RP, eds. Blood substitutes. New York: Alan Liss, 1983:79–88.
32. Gould SA, Sehgal LR, Sehgal HL, Toyooka E, Moss GS. Clinical experience with human polymerized hemoglobin [abstract]. Transfusion 1993;33(suppl 9S):60S.
33. Gould S, Moore E, Moore F, et al. The clinical utility of human polymerized hemoglobin as a blood substitute following trauma and emergent surgery. J Trauma 1995;39:157.
34. Gould S. Human polymerized hemoglobin first therapeutic use as a blood substitute in trauma and surgery. American College of Surgeons, 81st Clinical Congress, New Orleans, LA, October 22–27, 1995.

Chapter 10

Red Cell Substitutes

Part B: Perfluorocarbon Emulsions: Artificial Gas Transport Media

BRUCE D. SPIESS

INTRODUCTION

Perfluorocarbon (PFC) emulsions are one of two main technologies in development to function as oxygen-carrying media. Hemoglobin preparations and PFC emulsions are sometimes referred to as "artificial blood" or "blood substitutes." Neither one is a true blood substitute or artificial blood. At best, these represent pharmacological approaches to intravenous gas transport. Blood functions in coagulation, inflammation, protein transport, humoral transport, and a multitude of other functions. Both PFCs and hemoglobin preparations will only partially fulfill the one function of moving respiratory gases through the circulation. There has long been a wish for a stable, nontoxic, effective intravenous solution that could be stored for long periods of time on a shelf, rapidly prepared, or simply infused and immediately function in the transport of oxygen. At best, these agents may be able to partially fulfill this role. However, they will have an entirely different pharmacological and physiological profile from human blood. Therefore, the misconception that a health care worker will simply turn to these instead of a unit of packed red cells is naive. There may be future indications for these gas transport solutions instead of human blood transfusion but with their own toxicity and intolerance issues, and it is hoped they will have their own unique indications that conceivably could go far beyond merely replacing a blood transfusion. This chapter discusses the state of the science as it exists today in PFC emulsions. One, Fluosol DA 20%, is U.S. Food and Drug Administration (FDA) approved for usage in coronary angioplasty, and other second-generation formulations are undergoing FDA testing. Some areas of very promising research are touched on. Almost certainly in 5–10 years, this chapter will be outdated as indications, contraindications, and perhaps formulations not now even conceived of will come to the forefront.

HISTORY

Carbon fluoride chemistry was a product of the second World War and was extremely active in the 1950s. Early observations that liquid fully fluoridated hydrocarbons could dissolve oxygen were very important. The carbon fluoride bond is extremely stable and of very high energy (504 kJ/mol) (1). To understand the effect of fluoridating hydrocarbons, one can examine what happens with a simple benzene ring (2). If one fluorine is added to each carbon atom of the ring, then hexafluorobenzene is created. Hexafluorobenzene is interesting in that it has potent anesthetic properties but is also quite toxic. It demonstrates almost no increase in respiratory gas solubilities. Hexafluorobenzene if then fully fluoridated becomes perfluorocyclohexane, and that molecule has no anesthetic properties. It can now solubilize twice the oxygen carried by benzene.

In 1966 Clark and Gollan (3) produced a fury of scientific and lay interest when they published photographs of mice and rats immersed in liquid PFC and breathing the oxygenated liquid. Persons speculated upon this liquid as a new method of breathing for undersea exploration and for submarine escape. Also, other researchers thought that if the compounds were effective enough to transport oxygen to the lungs, then they should be useful as intravenous oxygen transporters as well (4, 5). Perfusion of various isolated organs was demonstrated, and, indeed, mammal brain could be maintained electrically active with a warm PFC containing perfusate (5). It kept cellular activity going as long as a red cell-based perfusate. An isolated rat heart preparation could also be kept beating with either a perfluorobutyltetrahydrofuran (FX80) solution or red cell perfusion (4).

Infusion of these early PFC solutions caused gaseous microemboli and macroemboli, leading to disastrous pulmonary complications (6). The native PFC was largely immiscible with water, and therefore plasma and PFC would separate, much like olive oil and vinegar in salad dressing. However, if the mixture was sonicated before infusion, these complications could be decreased and partial transfusions of amphibians and total exchange transfusion of rats were possible (6–8).

One problem leading to gas embolism was not only the lack of ability of the PFC to mix with plasma, but also the vapor pressure of the PFC. Multiple different carbon skeletons were tested and fluoridated (9). Those with low vapor pressures will create intravascular gas bubbles at normal body temperatures (2, 6).

Clark (2) recognized these problems and made some early attempts to create an emulsion using the industrial surfactant pluronic F68 to stabilize it. A combination of perfluorodecalin and perfluorotributylamine was created and called FC-43. This was very stable and could be used to replace red cells in a number of animal species (2, 7, 9, 10). This was tried in Japan in 1978 as a treatment for anemia, and although initial results from Japan were encouraging, the trials in the United States could not support its usefulness (11–13). Also, FC-43 appeared to have a very long half-life (years) because perfluorotributylamine has a very high vapor pressure. Another formulation, Fluosol DA 20%, manufactured by the Green Cross Corporation of Osaka, Japan, used perfluorodecalin and perfluorotripropalamine with pluronic F68 and egg yolk phospholipids (10, 14). This preparation underwent considerable testing in animals and humans and will be extensively reviewed. In the United States, it did garner FDA approval for use not as a "blood substitute" but as a perfusion solution for infusion distal to coronary artery angioplasty catheters. Its use remains inconsequential because of the way it is supplied and the steps required for its preparation. Fluosol is supplied in frozen form and must be thawed, mixed with emulsifiers, and then sonicated before infusion. Also, before infusion in angioplasty, it must be oxygenated. These steps are time-consuming and cumbersome in an active cardiac catheterization laboratory where the decision to undergo angioplasty may be made in one moment and undertaken a few minutes later. There simply is not enough time to prepare Fluosol even if clinicians did want to use it.

These early preparations of PFC contained only 10% by volume of active PFC and 90% water, electrolyte, and emulsifying agents (10). Although most PFC compounds can carry 40–60 vol% of oxygen at 1 atmosphere (760 Torr), with the emulsions being only 10% PFC, the oxygen-carrying capacity is already limited. That limitation has led to the development of second-generation compounds that are now 40% by volume PFC (15, 16). These second-generation emulsions use emulsifiers other than pluronic F68 and therefore may have fewer side effects. At the present time, the second-generation compounds are undergoing FDA testing.

CHEMISTRY AND GAS-CARRYING CAPABILITIES

PFCs possess a unique ability for enhanced gas solubility. All nonpolar gases, including oxygen, nitrogen, and carbon dioxide, are solubilized within the liquid PFC. One way to conceive of this is that gas molecules are dissolved between PFC molecules. The concentration of any given gas within the PFC is dependent only on Henry's law and is therefore proportional to the partial pressure of a particular gas. One gas does not interfere with the transport potential for another gas. Therefore, if a patient is breathing a high oxygen content but has dissolved nitrogen within tissue, that nitrogen will be soluble within the PFC dependent only on the innate solubility and the partial pressure of each gas independently. Each gas is freely movable to another adjacent solution or tissue, again based only on partial pressure gradients. Therefore, oxygen carried in PFC is completely available for metabolic processes (Fig. 10.14). Because gas-carrying capacity is dependent only on Henry's law, a straight-line dissociation curve for oxygen is created with PFC.

The gas dissociation curve of PFC contrasts sharply with the sinusoidal curve of hemoglobin oxygen dissociation. Of course, oxygen is carried by hemoglobin chemically bound to its various heme moieties. Occupation of each of the four heme moieties in turn changes the stability of oxygen binding to the next one. A wide range of physiological conditions affect the oxyhemoglobin dissociation curve, including temperature, 2,3-diphosphoglycerate (2,3-DPG) concentration, and pH. PFC is completely unaffected by enzyme degrada-

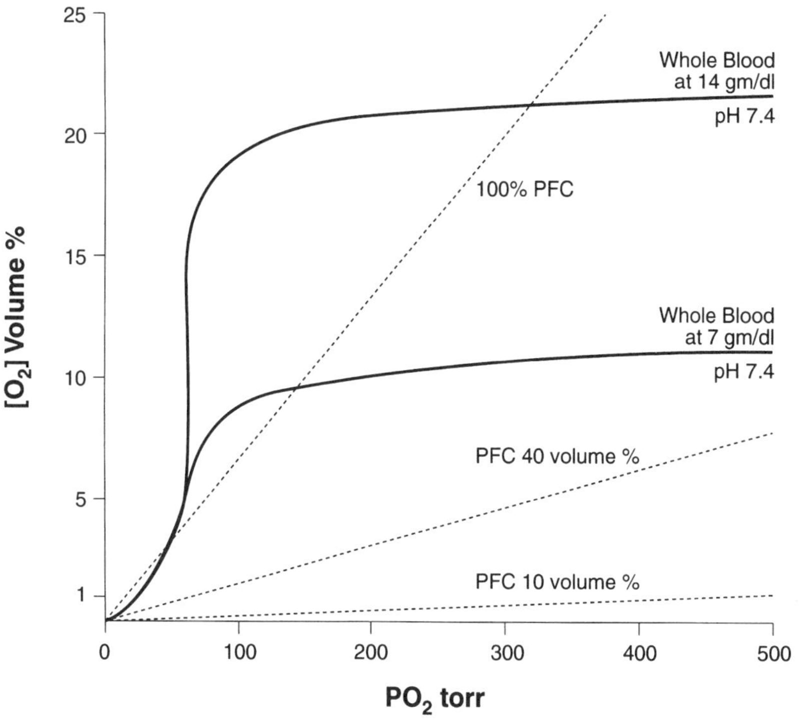

Figure 10.14. Oxygen content of whole blood at two different hemoglobin concentrations. Note the sinusoidal curve of the oxyhemoglobin dissociation curve. Changes in pH, body temperature, and 2,3-diphosphoglycerate shift the curves to the right or left. Note that the three PFC lines are not sinusoidal in relation to Po_2. Rather, a straight-line relationship exists between perfluorocarbon concentration and dissolved oxygen. In 100% pure PFC, as much as 40–60 vol% of oxygen can be carried. However, in stable emulsions administered intravenously, the total oxygen-carrying capacity is approximately 1 vol% for first-generation (Fluosol DA-20%) compounds and 4–8% for second-generation (40% v/v) emulsions. All dissolved oxygen in PFC is metabolically available.

tion, and pH changes have no effect on the gas solubilities. Furthermore, 2,3-DPG has no effect on oxygen release from PFC. Temperature does not cause the same effects as it does in hemoglobin oxygen binding. But, hypothermia does increase oxygen solubility in PFC just as hypothermia increases gas solubility in plasma.

Physiologically, the PFC gas transport therefore becomes quite unique and is dependent on the partial pressure of a gas (oxygen or nitrogen) and the available concentration of PFC within the bloodstream. As noted before, PFCs are organic compounds substituted with fluorides and therefore are quite immiscible with water. Stable emulsions must be formed using some sort of emulsifying agent. First- and second-generation PFC emulsions have created particles of 0.01–0.3 μm (17–19). Of note, these are considerably smaller than erythrocytes and therefore come close to acting as part of the plasma phase of the blood. Oxygen is very insoluble in plasma, and therefore the plasma acts as a barrier that oxygen must transit from erythrocytes to the tissues. PFC emulsions increase oxygen diffusion by as much as 17-fold when added to plasma (20). Much is yet unknown about what can change oxygen delivery characteristics from red cells. The very small particle size of the emulsions leads to a massive increase in surface area available from gas exchange. Once again, it is unclear how much this factor can assist in oxygen transport.

Hemoglobin can be affected by other factors than the oxyhemoglobin dissociation curve and also it may have a number of roles that clearly PFC does not possess. Hemoglobin has a buffering capacity as it binds carbon dioxide. A number of compounds can cause the formation of reduced hemoglobin or methoxyhemoglobin that cannot take part in oxygen transport at all. These compounds have no effect on the oxygen transport of PFC. Carbon monoxide irreversibly binds to hemoglobin, thereby occupying sites that could chemically bind and release oxygen. PFC is unaffected by carbon monoxide; however, PFC would carry it in equilibrium with the partial pressure. Hemoglobin is a profound nitric oxide binder (21–23). Free hemoglobin and some of the new polymerized hemoglobin compounds being investigated as blood substitutes create profound hypertension on infusion because of the preferential flow of nitric oxide to these molecules and away from their physiological target organ, the vascular smooth muscle. Once again, there is no suggestion that PFC would have any role in nitric oxide flow other than that dictated by Henry's law.

Because PFC must be emulsified for use as an intravenous infusion, the concentration of PFC in the emulsion is one determinant of total available gas-carrying capacity. Concentration of PFC in the emulsion can be reported as either weight to volume or volume to volume (v/v). The early emulsions, FC-43 and Fluosol DA 20%, were 10–11% v/v emulsions; however, Fluosol was designated 20% because it was 20% w/v. Most PFC pure compounds can carry between 40–60 vol% oxygen when equilibrated with 100% oxygen at

1 atmosphere pressure. With these early emulsions being only 10% PFC and 90% emulsifying agent and water, the effectiveness of the PFC was severely limited by the low PFC concentration. Even under the circumstances of the normal emulsion being equilibrated with room air, the available oxygen would have been 0.8–1.0 vol%. The total PFC emulsion volume able to be infused to a patient is limited by toxicity issues. In first-generation PFCs, that issue severely limited the amount that could be infused; therefore, although pure PFC has the ability to carry 40–60 vol% oxygen, the contribution in patients was quite low. Second-generation emulsions seem to have less toxicity and also have a higher concentration of PFC in the emulsion (40% v/v) so their ability to contribute to physiological oxygen requirements should be much better.

TOLERABILITY

PFCs in their pure form are biologically inert. No known enzyme system changes these compounds in any way, and there is no measurable fluoride release from them as well (24). The concerns regarding tolerability of the emulsions within biological systems can be separated into two problems. One is that these emulsions are taken up by the reticuloendothelial system and harbored there for some time (25–27). They do have effects on that organ group function. Second, the emulsion chemistry has inherent effects that have in the past created their own toxicity (28–33).

PFC particles when infused have a variable circulating half-life dependent on the dose and the type of PFC administered. Fluosol has been estimated to have a circulating half-life of between 13 and 24 hours (34–36). The second-generation PFCs (perfluoro-octylbromide and perfluorodichloro-octane) appear to have shorter half-lives of 5–9 hours. In animal models, these half-lives can be considerably extended if high dosages are administered.

After administration, the PFC is equally distributed throughout the circulation and is thought to stay confined to the vascular compartment. Macrophages ingest the PFC, and it is deposited in the liver and spleen (25, 32, 36). Dependent on the dosage, these organs can actually increase in size and weight within the first 24 hours after a PFC infusion, as the emulsion is deposited there. The emulsion itself is broken down within the reticuloendothelial system, and it appears that the free PFC is slowly carried (by partial pressure solubility) to the lungs and skin (37, 38). Most is volatilized and exhaled through the lungs; however, some may transpire through the skin itself. There may be some excretion through the biliary system and thus the fecal route; however, this has not been noted with the second-generation group of emulsions.

The effect that the PFC has on the reticuloendothelial system is a matter of some investigation and potential concern. Once again, the effects of early, first-generation compounds such as Fluosol may be different from those of the second-generation compounds. Both appear to cause some swelling of the liver, and there may be some element of dysfunction in some circumstances simply because of mechanical size changes. In Fluosol, there were well-documented increases in liver function enzymes (39–42). Presumably, this would signal that some cell damage or leakage had occurred. For this reason, it was always cautioned not to give Fluosol to patients with liver disease or impending liver failure. However, there was never any indication of these changes persisting beyond several days, and nowhere did patients go on to have liver damage or cirrhosis. In animal studies with the second-generation compounds, although liver swelling and hepatocellular sequestration of PFC can be demonstrated, there is no demonstrable organ damage. Perhaps the elevations of liver function enzymes from the Fluosol were in some way related to the presence of the emulsifying agent pluronic F68 and not just from the mechanical swelling of hepatocytes. Indeed, in animals, as opposed to human work with Fluosol, there is evidence for reduced drug metabolism by the liver, changes in hepatic blood flow, and decreases in microsomal enzyme activity (41, 42). In Fluosol-treated animals, hepatic Kupffer cells show reduced phagocytosis and engorgement with PFC (43).

The fact that some of these same effects are seen in second-generation PFC emulsions (perfluoro-octylbromide and perfluorodichlorooctane) but not to the same severity, even though the second-generation emulsions contain four times the PFC, would suggest that the emulsifying agents in Fluosol somehow contributed to the toxicity. Pluronic F68 is an industrial surfactant with a wide variety of uses. There is evidence that it is not toxic itself but that trace impurities in the actual formulation may be causing the effects. Neutrophil activation and complement activation occur with Fluosol and have been attributed to pluronic F68 (30, 31). Platelet aggregation is reduced, but complement itself is a platelet inhibitor and may be the cause of that effect (27). The neutrophil activation causes degranulation and suppression of inflammatory responsiveness for a number of hours (32, 33, 44). It is unclear whether that has any clinical relevance. However, the neutrophil inhibition may be partially responsible for animal findings of decreased reperfusion injury after Fluosol infusion (44). Again, are all these due to pluronic F68? If pluronic F68 is added to neutrophils and incubated, a degranulation situation will occur (32). In the second-generation PFC emulsions, platelet aggregation suppression may still occur with perfluoro-octylbromide but to a lesser degree than seen in Fluosol. Perfluorodichloro-octane appears to have less complement activation than does Fluosol, and in one in vitro study, adding perfluorodichloro-octane to a closed-loop cardiopulmonary bypass circuit actually seemed to inhibit complement formation (45). Both second-generation emulsions do not use pluronic F68 at all but rely on another as yet nondisclosed emulsification processes. They are thought to be quite similar to the egg yolk phospholipid-based emulsifiers used in intralipid preparations (46).

Once the PFC is broken free from its emulsion in the liver and spleen, elimination is dependent only on the volatility of the PFC. Those with high vapor pressures may be in tissues for a considerable length of time. FC-43, which has perfluorotributylamine, has a tissue half-life measured in years. That long half-life is why (along with its relatively low PFC concentration) it has not gained use in humans in the United States. Fluosol, a blend of perfluorodecalin and perfluorotripropalamine, has a tissue half-life of 6 days and 63 days, respectively, for the component PFC compounds (47). What is acceptable? We do not have an answer to that question because there are no data regarding any long-term effects of trace PFC within tissues. Second-generation PFCs appear to have considerably shorter tissue half-lives, probably much less than 7 days. However, again it does depend on the dosage administered.

With these organ effects, it is worthy to note that the effects of infusion are met with relatively few side effects. Fluosol has been given to a large number of patients and volunteers both in Japan and in the United States (12, 13, 27, 32, 48, 49). A flu-like syndrome of mild diffuse muscle aches was noted; however, in some Fluosol patients, chest pains and transient hypotension resulted (50). Facial flushing was also seen. The thought was that these side effects may have been due to macrophage activation and some complement formation (51). The second-generation compounds to date show no evidence of hypotension, although some flu-like symptoms may yet be encountered in persons not given any preventative measures (15, 16). The second-generation compounds are just now entering the part of FDA testing in which larger numbers of patients will be receiving them and therefore the potential for safety assurance or reporting of adverse events will increase.

POTENTIAL APPLICATIONS: OXYGEN TRANSPORT

The creation of a nontoxic, shelf-ready, small particle, stable oxygen-carrying intravascular infusion media has incredible wide-ranging applicability. Considerable animal and human testing has been done primarily with the 10% v/v compounds such as Fluosol but also with second-generation compounds. A great deal of hope and enthusiasm has been generated, particularly by animal research, yet today PFC emulsions are not part of the everyday pharmacological interventions used.

USE AS A BLOOD TRANSFUSION SPARING AGENT

The efficacy of a single red cell transfusion is very difficult to prove (52–56). This probably results from the fact that clinicians do not transfuse red cell products when the limits of physiology have been reached (i.e., organ ischemia) but rather do it as a preventative measure. Because efficacy of a given therapy cannot be proven, it is therefore considerably more difficult to show that a replacement for that therapy is also efficacious or even more efficacious. The use of PFC emulsions as a treatment for anemia or prevention of oxygen delivery debt is therefore rather hard to prove as effective. A number of physiological measurements may be helpful, but these are only surrogate markers of efficacy. This one problem alone plagues the entire blood substitute technology as it struggles to gain approval from government agencies.

The first use of PFC emulsions was to treat a gastrointestinal bleed in 1980 with Fluosol DA 20% (57). Shortly thereafter in 1982, a large series of patients (n = 186) was published from Japan (49). Most patients were experiencing surgical blood loss and had refused blood products for one reason or another. No major cardiovascular, biochemical, or anatomical abnormalities occurred in the series of patients. There was a slight leukocytosis and increase in their bleeding time. Some patients had changes in their liver enzymes that were transient. It was thought that the contribution to oxygen-carrying capacity was 1.2–1.3 vol%, although this was calculated and not measured. Also, although this series represents an initial enthusiastic endorsement for PFC emulsions as an alternative to blood, there was no randomized control group with which to compare either outcome or laboratory findings.

A report of another series, this time from China, of war casualties listed 140 patients given PFC (58). Once again, there was no control group that received colloid, crystalloid, or blood with which to compare. These authors did note some side effects, including flushing, chest tightness, a decrease in platelet count, and some changes in liver functions. Were those products of the PFC infusion or the natural course of injuries incurred in wartime?

In the United States and Canada, some small series were reported. One listed seven patients who received up to 3% fluorocrit when undergoing surgical blood loss (59). The contribution to measured oxygen delivery was 0.7–0.8 vol%, which the authors thought was not significant enough to warrant further pursuit. Also, patients had to breathe 100% oxygen, and the half-life of only 24 hours was believed by the authors to be insufficient for adequate erythropoiesis to replace the oxygen-carrying function of the Fluosol DA 20%. However, one should point out that if these patients derived some benefit from the added 0.7–0.8 vol%, then very little erythropoiesis would be needed to replace the effect of the PFC.

A Canadian study was attempted using Fluosol DA 20%, and only three patients were undertaken, as one had a severe reaction after a test dose (60). Here the authors noted that mixed venous oxygen saturation increased after PFC infusion and concluded that oxygen was being preferentially delivered from the PFC. Once again, no control group or randomization was done with either of the United States or Canadian early experiences. A case report notes the success of a pancreatoduodenectomy in a patient who entered the operating room with a hemoglobin of only 5 g/dL (61).

In two randomized studies of, respectively, 46 and 52 patients, there were higher oxygen concentrations measured in the group who received Fluosol DA 20% compared with control subjects who received only crystalloid resuscitation (13, 62). The survival and hemodynamics were no different between groups and, like the earlier work in the United States, it was concluded that the contribution to total oxygen content by the PFC, although statistically significant, was not worth the effort clinically.

Second-generation PFC formulations are presently undergoing some testing as oxygen-carrying media in lieu of blood transfusion. In one small study using volunteers undergoing surgery expected to have only small blood losses, perfluorooctylbromide appeared to be well tolerated (16). Unfortunately, one cannot judge the effectiveness of oxygen transport. In another abstract where a small series of patients were expected to lose more than 100 mL of blood during surgery, the patients were given perfluoro-octylbromide before blood loss (15) with mixed venous oxygen saturation pulmonary artery catheters and arterial lines. As the blood loss occurred, mixed venous oxygen saturation was stable or increased over the period of time before PFC infusion, yet actual oxygen-carrying capacity of the PFC was not reported.

Much work is yet to be done with randomized trials of second-generation PFC infusions during a number of blood loss situations. Massive hemorrhage seems to be one potential clinical indicator for PFC use, yet researching such events is fraught with a wide range of problems (62). If motor vehicle accident victims are to be studied, there may be questions about consent because most of these victims are incapable of communicating. Persons could not be randomized to receive either blood or PFC because withholding blood may be deemed inappropriate. The population is diverse, and the ability to control any hemodynamic or biochemical variable alone may be nearly impossible. Therefore, proving that PFC, even the more potent second-generation emulsions, is effective instead of or in addition to blood transfusion may be left for the surgical suite. Once again, the questions remain: which cases should one investigate, how should they be randomized, and what product, blood or crystalloid/colloid, should they receive? These questions and hopefully some meaningful outcome data will be forthcoming in the not-too-distant future. One thing is agreed upon and that is that Fluosol DA 20% is far too dilute to be of great use as a blood substitute alone in the face of acute hemorrhage. Therefore, it has not reached FDA approval for that indication.

OXYGEN TRANSPORT FOR ANGIOPLASTY

Coronary angioplasty is now used in as many patients annually as those having coronary artery bypass graft surgery. During coronary angioplasty, a balloon is inflated in a coronary artery at the site of an atherosclerotic plaque, thus fracturing, stretching, or otherwise dilating the plaque. Historically, this technique used catheters that obstructed flow of blood distal to the inflated balloon for some period of time. This obstruction of blood flow would either cause distal ischemia or hopefully be avoided by sufficient flow from collaterals. Short balloon inflations could thus avoid permanent myocardial damage but the effectiveness of the therapy might be less efficient. Today, there are angioplasty catheters with balloons that allow for some distal flow of blood. However, the inflation of even one of these causes significant flow reduction and can result in ischemia. PFC emulsions might therefore have a unique application if infused distal to such catheters. Fluosol DA 20% has gained its FDA approval for that indication alone. The evidence of its effectiveness is based on the following research.

In dog studies of coronary angioplasty, oxygenated Fluosol DA 20% showed in several studies that it could provide protection from angioplasty ischemia (63–65). Hemodynamic and electrocardiographic indices of ischemia were decreased in the first reported study (63). This was translated into histological evidence of better cellular preservation with Fluosol distal perfusion as compared with no infusion or crystalloid infusion. Interestingly, if autologous blood was infused distal to the catheter rather than Fluosol or no infusion, then subendocardial blood flow was better. There is no clear reason for this, but Fluosol is a profound histamine releaser in dogs and therefore the regional flow differences could be species-specific. Fluosol alone should have a lower viscosity than whole blood, and therefore one might have expected that it would create better subendocardial perfusion (65).

Human studies of distal perfusion during angioplasty began in 1985 with the report of a series of 34 patients (66). These patients could tolerate longer balloon inflations with Fluosol infusion than other patients historically not receiving PFC. Other reports noted less echocardiographic evidence of wall dysfunction, and lower lactate production if Fluosol DA 20% was oxygenated and infused at rates up to 60 mL/min distal to the balloon inflation site (66–69). Also, when compared with groups that received a lactated Ringer solution through the catheter, cardiac output was much better preserved with Fluosol (69). In a multicentered trial for the FDA, 245 patients had either Fluosol DA 20% or no fluid infused through the distal part of the catheter (70). Those who received the PFC had less chest pain during inflation, had fewer electrocardiograph indications of ischemia, and had better systolic function by echocardiography. There was no difference in long-term outcome, yet the FDA believed that these advantages were enough to grant an indication. To date, there are no published articles showing it in clinical use to be of great benefit for coronary angioplasty. One wonders whether those outcome statistics might not be forthcoming if used in conjunction with flowthrough catheters and particularly in the second-generation group of compounds. This is especially worthy of investigation in view of some evidence regarding PFC and reperfusion injury.

REPERFUSION INJURY AND INFLAMMATORY EFFECTS

Reperfusion injury is a complex series of events that occurs when tissues are made hypoxic for some period of time and then high-energy phosphate metabolism is shifted toward the breakdown of purines. When these purines are then exposed to oxygen upon reperfusion, that leads to the production of high-energy free radicals that can cause further cellular damage by destroying intracellular proteins (71–76). The production of high-energy intermediates is both a result of and a stimulus for white cell attraction and upregulation of neutrophil activity. Today, a great deal of work is ongoing with neutrophil activation, attachment molecules, and regulators of white cell activity. It is far beyond the scope of this chapter to attempt to explain the complex process of reperfusion injury, but there has been a significant amount of research suggesting that PFC emulsions may have effects on reperfusion injury (77–83). Once again, much of this research has focused on myocardial injury.

Dog and pig models of myocardial ischemia showed that the amount of tissue made ischemic can be reduced if PFC is added and the animals made to breathe 100% oxygen (82, 83). If left anterior coronary ligation is performed, infarct size in dogs is decreased when hemodiluted to 25% hematocrit and PFC is added, compared with those with only hemodilution alone (84). In the pig models, myocardial oxygen content was better with PFC and hemodilution as compared with hemodilution alone with colloid or no hemodilution at all (85). The onset of myocardial ischemia was delayed if Fluosol was infused before a coronary artery snare was placed. If reperfusion of an ischemic bed occurred with Fluosol and blood, that may not necessarily have shown improvement over blood reperfusion alone. However, if prolonged and preexisting PFC perfusion was present, then reperfusion ischemia was reduced. The thoughts were that myocardial ischemia could be reduced by oxygen delivery to tissues that it would not otherwise reach due to the small particle size of PFCs and its ability to enhance diffusion in slow or poorly moving plasma. Perhaps if tissues were never truly made ischemic, then reperfusion injury might be less.

Other studies in which dogs were subjected to 90 minutes of proximal left anterior descending coronary artery ischemia did show effects of Fluosol upon reperfusion. Animals that had PFC added just after reperfusion had better myocardial function, blood flow, and less neutrophil adhesion to their coronary arteries than nontreated animals (83). In another dog study in which Fluosol was infused just before reperfusion, a series of neutrophil function studies were performed (86). Chemotaxis and lysosome release were reduced in animals that received PFC, and it was concluded that the PFC caused a reduction in reperfusion injury that was independent of myocardial oxygen delivery alone during the ischemic period.

Studies of neutrophils in isolated preparations or in cell culture have shown that the PFC may have independent effects (32, 44). Neutrophil adherence, cytotoxicity, and lysosome release upon stimulation in vitro was decreased by PFC but not by the emulsifying agent alone (44). Electron microscopic inspection of neutrophils incubated with Fluosol showed that they had ingested the Fluosol because of vacuoles containing PFC (32). It was believed that the neutrophils had phagocytized the PFC particles and therefore were somehow unable to further react to normal stimuli. There still exists some controversy over whether some of the same effects can be created with the emulsion agents. In vitro incubation with pluronic F68 decreased neutrophil adhesion and reaction to stimulation. Also, in a rabbit model in which 30 minutes of myocardial ischemia was followed by reperfusion with either Fluosol added to systemic circulation or the detergent part of the emulsion, both Fluosol and the emulsifier alone did decrease the size of myocardial infarction as compared with the placebo control (87). It should be noted that only when the rabbits were given 100% oxygen did the effects of the Fluosol and the emulsifier become effective. Also, the infarct size was related to the dose of PFC with the higher dosages having a smaller infarct.

Human studies were undertaken in the late 1980s and early 1990s to test the effect of acute intervention with added infused Fluosol DA 20%. A small study using 26 patients used angioplasty within 4 hours of the onset of acute myocardial infarction and randomly assigned them to either intracoronary Fluosol (40 cc/min) or nothing with their angioplasty (88). The group that received the oxygenated PFC showed better improvement of their left ventricular function than those not receiving the Fluosol. Also, myocardial infarction size was reduced in the Fluosol group. Results from this study prompted a much larger study at multiple centers (89). Four hundred thirty patients in the Thrombosis and Angioplasty in Myocardial Infarction 9 Trial were studied with new-onset (less than 6 hours) symptoms of infarction. All patients received aspirin, heparin, tissue plasminogen activator, and angioplasty as quickly as possible. Two hundred thirteen of the 430 were randomized to also receive oxygenated Fluosol as an intravenous dose. It should be noted that the maximum dose received was 15 mL/kg, and a great number of patients received far less than that. Also, the Fluosol was not delivered peripherally through the angioplasty catheter at the time of inflation. At 5 and 14 days after infusion and angioplasty, multiple measurements of ventricular function were made, including stress thallium testing. There were no differences in stroke, death, or bleeding, but there were some small but significant decreases in infarct size in the Fluosol group. The PFC patients had less recurrent angina in the immediate postangioplasty period, but this group also suffered more pulmonary edema. This study is not conclusive and can be criticized for not intervening at an early time period (e.g., 1–4 hours) with intravenous infusion. Also, the dose of PFC might not be maximal. One certainly wonders how effective it might be to use a second-generation emulsion that is four times as concentrated. Unfortunately, no studies of neutrophil activation were done to assess the effect of the PFC on reperfusion injury, so the question still remains as to the effect of PFC on inflammatory responses.

In a second-generation PFC, perfluorodichloro-octane, unpublished data from our laboratories does show that the effects of PFC seen with Fluosol in inhibiting some inflammatory processes may translate into the second-generation compounds as well. In a closed-loop model of cardiopulmonary bypass, using fresh human whole blood and the standard bypass system but without any patient, complement levels were studied (45). It is well known that complement levels rise progressively during bypass, presumably as a response to white cell activation (90). Two groups were studied, those with routine crystalloid prime and those who had PFC emulsion added. The group with the PFC added had no rise in complement during the bypass run. Unfortunately, the reason for this was not given, and much work remains to be done to understand the effects of these newer PFCs on neutrophil activation.

ORGAN PROTECTION: CARDIOPLEGIA AND TRANSPLANTATION

During cardiopulmonary bypass, usually the aorta is cross-clamped and blood flow to the heart is stopped for an extended period of time. If some attempt to preserve cellular integrity is not undertaken, then myocardial infarction will result. It is impossible to discuss the various recipes and methods for delivering cardioplegia solutions because the types and applications of these solutions are quite variable from one institution to another. Preservation of organs for transport ex vivo and transplantation has had fantastic growth and development in the recent past. Once again, there has been widespread use of newer preservative solutions that have extended the time wherein solid organs can be outside the body and ischemic. Both techniques, cardioplegia and organ preservation for transplantation, are undertaken because there is no present way to continuously supply oxygen and metabolic substrates during the period of time in question. PFC emulsions, with their potential oxygen-carrying capacity, would seem to be perfect for fitting the role of organ preservation.

Heart transplantation has a limiting ischemic time of approximately 6 hours, and the organs are usually preserved with cold crystalloid infusion. Ideally, a system of continuous perfusion with a solution capable of transporting oxygen and containing metabolic requirements would be created. In heart transplantation, a trial of perfusion with Fluosol DA 20% had earlier heart failure, more lactate production, and an increased creatinine phosphokinase than those given colloid alone (91). The mechanism behind this potential failure is unknown, but if PFC is added to albumin, then some of these problems can be reduced (91). Multiple studies have shown in isolated animal organs that kidney, liver, pancreas, intestine, and some other heart protocols can preserve tissue with continuous or intermittent flushes of PFC (92–99). To date, however, there are no series using PFC as their primary solution for transport in human transplantation and no series using the newer second-generation PFCs in either animal organ preservation or in humans.

AIR EMBOLISM

Venous air embolism occurs during sitting craniotomy in probably upward of 40% of cases and is also common in total hip arthroplasty (100–102). Other surgeries have been noted as significant as well, including spine surgery, pelvic surgery, hepatectomy, and neck dissection. The effects of air embolism are dependent on the size of embolus entrained, the speed and site of entrainment and the eventual distribution of the air. A significant number of patients have a probe patent foramen ovale that, under the right circumstances, can lead to movement of the air from the right side of the heart to the arterial side (103). Hypotension, adult respiratory distress syndrome (ARDS), coagulopathy, stroke, and death are all possible consequences of venous air embolism. To date, there is no adequate treatment modality other than physical maneuvers to move the blockage to the circulation caused by the embolism (104).

Arterial air embolism can be caused by venous air embolism and migration through a patent foramen ovale. In cardiopulmonary bypass, massive air embolism is a rare but almost universally fatal complication caused by air entering the arterial side of the circuit (105). Smaller amounts of air embolism, including microair embolism, are much more commonly seen (106, 107). During cannulation of the aorta and decannulation, air is entrained. Open cardiac procedures such as valve replacement, congenital repair, or thoracic aneurysm repair, by necessity of opening the vasculature, have a large chance of distributing air emboli. Even coronary artery bypass graft surgery has a large number of microemboli associated with it. The cardiopulmonary bypass machine, because of its mechanism with pressure changes, causes the formation of microbubbles. These microbubbles have often been implicated as a possible primary cause of neuropsychological dysfunctions (106, 107, 108, 109, 110). Forty to eighty percent of patients 7 days after cardiopulmonary artery bypass have one or more abnormalities on very exacting tests of cognitive abilities, learning, and complex higher cortical function (111). These abnormalities persist in 20–40% of patients. Similar types of microair emboli occur during decompression sickness, and indeed the same types of neuropsychiatric changes can be seen in divers who have experienced "the bends" (112).

PFC emulsions have a unique ability not only to solubilize oxygen but also to carry nitrogen and other gases that would not be soluble in plasma. Indeed, nitrogen is 10,000 to 100,000 times as soluble in PFC as in plasma (17). A number of studies have shown promise that PFC emulsions may be useful in both venous and arterial air embolism (113–122).

In decompression sickness, a number of rodent models have been tested in which animals have been compressed to six or more atmospheres in room air and rapidly decompressed, with resultant air embolism (115, 118). Immediate treatment with a PFC (FC-43) and 100% oxygen has shown PFC to be very effective in preventing death (115). In dogs, a xenon solubility study has demonstrated that PFC can greatly speed the removal of xenon, a very insoluble gas, from muscle tissue (120). It was estimated that the removal of xenon in animals treated with PFC was at least 17 times as quick as that seen without PFC. It was also estimated that the removal of nitrogen from such tissues, because of physical chemical properties of the PFC, could cause the removal at least four times as fast as that of xenon. These studies were performed with first-generation PFC and one wonders if the efficacy would be even greater if a second-generation emulsion were used. To date, no human trials of prevention or treatment of decompression sickness have been performed with second-generation PFC.

Venous air embolism has been studied in several animal models with first-generation PFC (FC-43). A rabbit study looked at survival in animals pretreated with PFC or hetastarch and ventilated with either room air or 100% oxygen (113). Venous air embolism was delivered via the femoral vein continuously until death and the time until death noted. Animals who received PFC and were mechanically ventilated with 100% oxygen lived five times as long as all other groups of animals. In a larger animal study, cardiac and pulmonary hemodynamics were monitored in dogs pretreated with PFC (114). Again with femoral venous air embolism there were fewer hemodynamic complications in the dogs pretreated with PFC. The pulmonary artery pressures and cardiac outputs suggested that the air embolism in the PFC group was smaller or caused less mechanical obstruction than the one in the control group.

Arterial air embolism has been examined in cerebral and coronary artery air embolism. In rats given either a continuous air infusion in their internal carotid artery or a large bolus of air, those pretreated with PFC (FC-43) lived longer, had earlier return of their electroencephalograms, and had fewer ataxic events than animals pretreated with hetastarch (116). In a dog study with the left anterior descending coronary artery isolated and cannulated, 0.1 mL/kg of air was injected (117). Those animals that had again received a first-generation PFC before air embolism had fewer ventricular arrhythmias and quicker return of dP/dT than animals preloaded with colloid. In a recent work using swine and a second-generation PFC as an additive to the cardiopulmonary artery bypass machine, a model of massive air embolism was performed (123). Animals given Oxygent (Homage Inc., St. Louis, MO) as compared with colloid had better cerebral blood flow and higher electroencephalograms in the first few minutes after going onto bypass. The mechanism for these differences still is not completely understood, but others have suggested that the PFC actually will increase cerebral blood flow. One recent study using a hemoglobin blood substitute did not show the same increases in cerebral blood flow. The swine model previously described used a massive air insult of 5 mL/kg injected directly into the common carotid artery 10 minutes after bypass. End points were cerebral blood flow by calorimetric microspheres, electroencephalography, and infarction by triphenyl tetrazolium chloride stain 6 hours after insult. The cerebral blood flow was significantly better in the PFC group and the electroencephalogram did not fall as low in the PFC group and had a more rapid return to baseline. The infarct data showed that four of six animals in the colloid group had diffuse infarctions and no PFC animals showed any infarcts. In a treatment protocol, treatment of massive air embolism is clearly far less effective than priming the bypass machine with PFC.

Microembolism to the brain and systemic circulation can be assessed by viewing the retinal microcirculation (124, 125). Retinal fluorescein angiography has demonstrated that 3–5% of the capillaries are not perfused at the end of bypass and that by 1 day later, these are reperfused. In a dog study using the same retinal angiographic technique, if the cardiopulmonary bypass machine is primed with a second-generation PFC, the amount of capillary obstruction is decreased by 90% or more (K. Taylor, personal communication). In the swine model of massive air embolism, another set of studies using retinal angiography has shown about a 50% reduction in capillaries blocked if PFC is used in the prime and furthermore correlations by histology staining showed better preservation of capillary blood flow and less endothelial damage (unpublished results from our laboratory).

LIQUID VENTILATION

The initial work showing rodents breathing oxygenated liquid PFC led to speculation that such technology could be used in deep sea escape. Today, application of liquid PFC breathing shows promise in infant respiratory distress and ARDS (126–129). Both syndromes have severe problems with systemic oxygenation. There is a tremendous loss of alveolar activity with either loss of surfactant or diffuse inflammatory infiltrates that fill the alveolar spaces. Clearly, not all ARDS or respiratory distress syndromes are the same, and there is not only a continuum of severity but also a multitude of causes in the ARDS situation. Today, two methods are being investigated to assist in these syndromes. Liquid PFC ventilation involves filling the entire respiratory tree with PFC and then using some piston-driven ventilator device to move the liquid. Without a unique ventilator, the work of breathing would be so great as to make it impossible for these otherwise severely ill patients to respire. Animal studies have shown some promise with liquid PFC ventilation, and one early report showed some transient improvement in infants who had failed every other therapy (126). As yet unpublished ongoing trials of this technique are underway.

PFC associated gas exchange may be useful in ARDS more so than infant respiratory distress. The technique uses just enough PFC to fill the functional residual capacity. It thereby is thought to coat the alveolar spaces, perhaps working as a surfactant and also improving gas exchange across the alveoli. Animal models have shown good hemodynamic tolerance and improvement in compliance and gas exchange (127, 128). Once again, large-scale clinical data are not yet available.

RADIOLOGY APPLICATIONS

The PFCs may have some advantages because they can produce vascular contrast in a number of imaging techniques (130–132). If bromine or iodine is part of the PFC molecule as in perfluoro-octylbromide, then some amount of x-ray contrast is conferred. In rabbits with abdominal tumors who were infused with perfluoro-octylbromide, the tumors could be imaged more easily. Magnetic resonance imaging (MRI) has a number of advantages that routine x-ray does not have (132). There are presently no adequate MRI dyes, and PFCs may fill that role. The MRI can be tuned to a frequency that interrogates fluorine molecules, and also the PFC does not contain any hydrogen ion. MRI usually is tuned to hydrogens, and therefore the PFC can act as a negative contrast. Once again, future work is needed to see whether this can be developed as an advantage or whether it will be a potential problem. If PFC is infused as a blood substitute and a patient needs an emergency MRI or computed tomography, one can conceive of a scenario in which present technology has difficulty with the PFC in the vascular tree.

TUMOR THERAPY

Chemotherapy may be more effective in some tumors if oxygen is delivered effectively to that tumor (133). Tumors may have areas of poor capillary distribution that makes chemotherapy less effective. Also, radiotherapy is most effective in well-oxygenated tumors. PFCs with their ability to deliver oxygen to areas that may have poor perfusion otherwise theoretically would lend themselves to assisting tumor therapy. In animal models using both first- and second-generation PFC emulsions, there is considerable benefit to combining the chemotherapy and PFC. Although human trials are just now underway, this idea does seem encouraging. Also, there are considerations of housing the actual chemotherapeutic agents within the emulsion particle itself, thereby combining the delivery of oxygen and adjuvant therapy at the same time. Certainly, much work needs to be done before PFC is routinely seen as part of cancer therapy.

SUMMARY

The quest for a safe, economic, and effective blood substitute continues. The PFC emulsions have shown some promise, but initially their effectiveness was limited by the imperfect emulsion chemistry. Early 10% v/v emulsions could not supply enough tissue oxygen delivery to warrant their approval for use as whole-body oxygen delivery media. However, second-generation compounds have a four times greater concentration of active compound and therefore are quite effective. Also, second-generation compounds appear to have a better side-effect profile. These and PFC emulsions are now in extensive human testing.

Perhaps the most exciting applications of second-generation compounds go beyond merely enhancing oxygen delivery. Insoluble gases will become considerably more soluble if PFC is added to human blood. Problems that used to plague us, such a air embolism or decompression sickness, may become treatable or preventable. Also, use of radiology dyes and cancer adjuvant therapies will develop in the next few years. No matter what the eventual development of PFC infusions will be, they will be considerably different from infusing a unit of packed red blood cells or even a polymerized hemoglobin preparation. Indications, contraindication advantages, and limitations will become evident. This is a very exciting and potentially revolutionary group of compounds.

REFERENCES

1. Spiess BD, Cochran RP. Perfluorocarbon emulsions and cardiopulmonary bypass: a technique for the future. J Cardiothorac Vasc Anesth 1996;10:1–9.
2. Clark LC. Emulsion of perfluoronated solvents for intravenous gas transport. Federation Proc 1981;34:1468–1477.
3. Clark LC, Gollan F. Survival of mammals breathing organic liquids equilibrated with oxygen at atmospheric pressure. Science 1966;152: 1755–1756.
4. Gollan F, Clark LC. Organ perfusion with fluorocarbon fluid. Physiologist 1966;9:191.
5. Sloviter HA, Kamimoto T. Erythrocyte substitute for perfusion of brain. Nature 1967;216:458–460.
6. Sloviter HA, Petkovic M, Ogoshi S, Yamada H. Dispersed fluorochemicals as substitutes for erythrocytes in intact animals. J Appl Physiol 1969;27:666–668.
7. Geyer RP, Taylor K, Duffett EB, Eccles R. Successful complete replacement of the blood of living rats with artificial substitutes. Federation Proc 1973;32:927.
8. Geyer RP. Fluorocarbon—polyol artificial blood substitutes. N Engl J Med 1973;289:1077–1082.
9. Geyer RP. Substitutes for blood and its components. Prog Clin Biol Res 1978;19:1–26.
10. Geyer RP. “Bloodless” rats through the use of artificial blood substitutes. Federation Proc 1975;34:1499–1505.
11. Ohyanagi H, Sekita M, Yokoyama K, et al. Fourth International Symposium on Perfluorochemical Blood Substitutes, Kyoto, Japan. Amsterdam: Excerpta Medica, 1978:373–389.
12. Gould SA, Rosen AL, Sehgal LR, et al. Fluosol-DA as a red cell substitute in acute anemia. N Engl J Med 1986;314:1653–1656.
13. Spence RK, McCoy S, Constabile J, et al. Fluosol DA-20 in the treatment of severe anemia: randomized, controlled study of 46 patients. Crit Care Med 1990;18:1227–1230.
14. Marchbank A. Fluorocarbon emulsions. Perfusion 1995;10:67–88.
15. Wahr JA, Trowborst A, Spence RK. A pilot study of the efficacy of an oxygen carrying emulsion, Oxygent, in patients undergoing surgical blood loss [abstract]. Anesthesiology 1994;8:A313.
16. Cernaianu AC, Spence RK, Vassilidze TV, et al. A safety study of a perfluorochemical emulsion, Oxygent, in anesthetized surgical patients [abstract]. Anesthesiology 1994;81:A397.
17. Faithfull NS. Second generation fluorocarbons. In: Erdmann W, Bruley DF, eds. Oxygen transport to tissue XIV. Advances in experimental medicine and biology. Vol. 317. New York: Plenum Press, 1992:441–452.
18. Riess JG. Fluorocarbon-based oxygen carriers: new orientations. Artif Organs 1991;15:408–413.
19. Lowe KC. Synthetic oxygen transport fluids based on perfluorochemicals: applications in medicine and biology. Vox Sang 1991;60: 129–140.
20. O'Brien RN, Langlois AJ, Deufert WD. Diffusion coefficients of respiratory gases in a perfluorocarbon liquid. Science 1982;217:153–155.
21. Rimar S, Gillis CN. Selective pulmonary vasodilation by inhaled nitric oxide is due to hemoglobin inactivation. Circulation 1993;88: 2884–2887.
22. Kinsella JP, Abman SH. Methaemoglobin during nitric oxide therapy with high frequency ventilation. Lancet 1993;342:615.
23. Jacob TD, Nakagama DK, Seki I, et al. Hemodynamic effects and metabolic fate of inhaled nitric oxide in hypoxic piglets. J Appl Physiol 1994;76:1794–1801.
24. Faithfull NS. Fluorocarbons. Current status and future applications. Anaesthesia 1987;42:234–242.
25. Lutz J, Metzenauer P. Effects of potential blood substitutes (perfluorochemicals) on rat liver and spleen. Pflügers Arch 1980;387:175–181.
26. Kaufman RJ. Medical oxygen transport using perfluorochemicals. Biotechnology 1991;19:127–162.
27. Fujta J, Suzuki C, Ogana R. Effect of Fluosol-DA on the reticuloendothelial system function in surgical patients. In: Bolin RB, Geyer RP, Nemo GJ, eds. Advances in blood substitute research. Progress in clinical and biological research. Vol. 122. New York: Alan R Liss Inc, 1983:265.
28. Ingram DA, Forman MB, Murray JJ. Activation of complement by Fluosol attributable to the pluronic detergent micelle structure. J Cardiovasc Pharmacol 1993;22:456–461.
29. Mattrey RF, Hilpert PL, Long CD, Long DM, Mitten RM, Peterson T. Hemodynamic effects of intravenous lecithin-based perfluorocarbon emulsions in dogs. Crit Care Med 1989;17:652–656.
30. Mahe AM, Manoux J, Valla A, et al. Perfluoroalkylated surfactants: relationships between structure and acute toxicity in mice. Biomater Artif Cells Immobil Biotechnol 1992;20:1025–1027.
31. Bentley PK, Davis SS, Johnson OL, Lowe KC, Washington C. Purification of pluronic F-68 for perfluorochemical emulsification. J Pharm Pharmacol 1989;41:61–63.

32. Ingram DA, Forman MB, Murray JJ. Phagocytic activation of human neutrophils by the detergent component of Fluosol. Am J Pathol 1992;140:1081–1087.
33. Forman MB, Pitarys CJ II, Vidibill HD, et al. Pharmacological perturbation of neutrophils by Fluosol results in a sustained reduction in infarct size in the canine model of reperfusion. J Am Coll Cardiol 1992;19:205–216.
34. Mattrey RF. Perfluorooctylbromide: a new contrast agent for CT, sonography and MR imaging. Am J Roentgenol 1989;152:247–252.
35. Waxman K, Tremper KK, Cullen BF, Mason GR. Perfluorocarbon infusion in bleeding patients refusing blood transfusions. Arch Surg 1984;119:721–724.
36. Bentley PK, Johnson OL, Washington C, Lowe KC. Uptake of concentrated perfluorocarbon emulsions into rat lymphoid tissues. J Pharm Pharmacol 1993;45:182–185.
37. Yokoyama K, Yamanouchi K, Murashima R. Excretion of perfluorochemicals after intravenous injection of their emulsion. Chem Pharmacol Bull 1975;23:1368–1373.
38. Riess JG. Reassessment of criteria for the selection of perfluorochemicals for second-generation blood substitutes: analysis of structure/property relationships. Artif Organs 1984;8:44–56.
39. Smith DJ, Lane TA. Effect of a high concentration perfluorocarbon emulsion on platelet function. Biomater Artif Cells Immobil Biotechnol 1992;20:1045–1049.
40. Mattrey RF, Strich G, Shelton RE, et al. Perfluorochemicals as US contrast agents for tumor imaging and hepatosplenography: preliminary clinical results. Radiology 1987;163:339–343.
41. Shrewsbury RP. Effect of Fluosol-DA hemodilution on the kinetics of hepatically eliminated drugs. Res Commun Chem Path Pharmacol 1987;55:375–396.
42. Ravis WR, Ramakanth S, Brzozowski DM, Hamrick ME. Effect of perfluorochemical emulsion on rat hepatic mixed function oxidase system. J Pharm Pharmacol 1992;44:219–223.
43. Bottalico LA, Betensky HT, Min YB, Weinstock SB. Perfluorochemical emulsions decrease Kupffer cell phagocytosis. Hepatology 1991;14: 169–174.
44. Babbitt DG, Forman MB, Jones R, Bajaj AK, Hoover RL. Prevention of neutrophil-mediated injury to endothelial cells by perfluorochemical. Am J Pathol 1990;136:451–459.
45. Rosoff JD, Soltow LO, Vocelka CR, et al. Second generation perfluorocarbon (perfluorodichlorooctane) does not increase complement activation in ex-vivo extracorporeal bypass experiments [abstract]. Anesth Analg 1996;82:SCA-123.
46. Hammerschmidt DE, Vercelloti GM. Limitation of complement activation by perfluorocarbon emulsions: superiority of lecithin-emulsified preparations. In: Chang TMS, Geyer RP, eds. Blood substitutes. New York: Marcel Dekker, 1989:431–438.
47. Riess JG. Fluorocarbon-based in vivo oxygen transport and delivery systems. Vox Sang 1991;61:225–239.
48. Tremper KK, Friedman AE, Levine EM, et al. The preoperative treatment of severely anemic patients with perfluorochemical oxygen-transport fluid, Fluosol-DA. N Engl J Med 1982;307:277–283.
49. Suyama T, Yokoyama K, Naito R. Development of a perfluorochemical whole blood substitute Fluosol-DA (20%): an overview of clinical studies with 185 patients. Prog Clin Biol Res 1981;55:609–628.
50. Tremper KK, Vercelotti GM, Hammerschmidt DE. Hemodynamic profile of adverse clinical reactions to Fluosol-DA 20%. Crit Care Med 1984;12:428–431.
51. Hong F, Shastri KA, Logue GL, Spaulding MB. Complement activation by artificial blood substitute Fluosol: in vitro and in vivo studies. Transfusion 1991;31:642–647.
52. Weiskopf RB. More on the changing indications for transfusions of blood and blood components during anesthesia. Anesthesiology 1996; 84:498–501.
53. Vichinsky EP, Haberkern CM, Neumayr L, et al. A comparison of conservative and aggressive transfusion regimens in the perioperative management of sickle cell disease: the preoperative transfusion in sickle cell disease study group. N Engl J Med 1995;333:206–213.
54. Spiess BD, Kapitan S, Body S, et al. ICU entry hematocrit does influence the risk for perioperative myocardial infarction (MI) in coronary artery bypass graft surgery [abstract]. Anesth Analg 1995;80 (suppl. 1):47.
55. Task Force on Blood Component Therapy Practice Guidelines for Blood Component Therapy. A report by the American Society of Anesthesiologists Task Force on blood component therapy. Anesthesiology 1996;84:732–747.
56. Makuuchi M, Takayama T, Gunven P, et al. Restrictive versus liberal blood transfusion policy for hepatectomies in cirrhotic patients. World J Surg 1989;13:644–648.
57. Honda K, Hoshino S, Shoji M, et al. Clinical use of a blood substitute. N Engl J Med 1980;303:391–392.
58. Chen HS, Yang ZH, et al. Perfluorocarbon as blood substitute in clinical applications and in war casualties. In: Chang TMS, ed. Blood substitutes. New York: Marcel Dekker, 1989:403–409.
59. Tremper KK, Friedman AE, Levine EM, Lapin R, Camarillo D. The preoperative treatment of severely anemic patients with a perfluorochemical oxygen-transport fluid, Fluosol-DA. N Engl J Med 1982;307: 277–283.
60. Stefaniszyn HJ, Wynands JE, Salerno TA. Initial Canadian experience with artificial blood (Fluosol-DA 20%) in severely anemic patients. J Cardiovasc Surg 1985;26:337–342.
61. Atabek U, Spence RK, Pello M, Alexander J, Camishion R. Pancreatoduodenectomy without homologous blood transfusion in an anemic Jehovah's Witness. Arch Surg 1992;127:349–351.
62. Spence RK, McCoy S, Costabile J, et al. Fluosol-DA 20% in prehospital resuscitation. Crit Care Med 1989;17:166–172.
63. Spears JR, Serur J, Baim DS, Grossman W, Paulin S. Myocardial protection with Fluosol-DA during prolonged coronary balloon occlusion in the dog. Circulation 1983;68:317.
64. Roberts CS, Anderson HV, Carboni AAJ, et al. Usefulness of intracoronary infusion of fluorocarbon distal to prolonged coronary occlusion by angioplasty balloon in dogs. Am J Cardiol 1986;57:1202–1205.
65. Christensen CW, Reeves WC, Lassar TA, Schmidt DH. Inadequate subendocardial oxygen delivery during perfluorocarbon perfusion in a canine model of ischemia. Am Heart J 1988;115:30–37.
66. Lincoff AM, Popma JJ, Ellis SG, Vogel RA, Topol EJ. Percutaneous support devices for high risk or complicated coronary angioplasty. J Am Coll Cardiol 1991;17:770–780.
67. Cleman M, Jaffee CC, Wohlgelernter D. Prevention of ischemia during percutaneous transluminal coronary angioplasty by transcatheter infusion of oxygenated Fluosol-DA 20%. Circulation 1986;74:555–562.
68. Cowley MJ, Snow FR, DiSciascio G, Kelly K, Guard C, Nixon JV. Perfluorochemical perfusion during coronary angioplasty in unstable and high-risk patients. Circulation 1990;81:27–34.
69. Jaffe CC, Wohlgelernter D, Cabin H, et al. Preservation of left ventricular ejection fraction during percutaneous transluminal coronary angioplasty by distal transcatheter coronary perfusion of oxygenated Fluosol DA 20%. Am Heart J 1988;115:1156–1164.

70. Kent KM, Cleman MW, Cowley MJ, et al. Reduction of myocardial ischemia during percutaneous transluminal coronary angioplasty with oxygenated Fluosol. Am J Cardiol 1990;66:279–284.
71. Sellke FW, Shafique T, Ely DL, Weintraub RM. Coronary endothelial injury after cardiopulmonary bypass and ischemic cardioplegia is mediated by oxygen-derived free radicals. Circulation 1993;88:395–400.
72. Kalfin RE, Engelman RM, Rousou JA, et al. Induction of interleukin-8 expression during cardiopulmonary bypass. Circulation 1993;88:401–406.
73. Evora PR, Pearson PJ, Schaff HV. Crystalloid cardioplegia and hypothermia do not impair endothelium-dependent relaxation or damage vascular smooth muscle of epicardial coronary arteries. J Thorac Cardiovasc Surg 1992;104:1365–1374.
74. Wilson I, Gillinov AM, Curtis WE, et al. Inhibition of neutrophil adherence improves postischemic ventricular performance of the neonatal heart. Circulation 1993;88:372–379.
75. Maulik N, Engelman RM, Wei Z, Lu D, Rousou JA, Das DK. Interleukin-1α preconditioning reduces myocardial ischemia reperfusion injury. Circulation 1993;88:387–394.
76. Kubes P, Suzuki M, Granger DN. Nitric oxide: an endogenous modulator of leukocyte adhesion. Proc Natl Acad Sci USA 1991;88:4651–4655.
77. Jaffin JH, Magovern GJ, Kanter KR, Flaherty JT, Gardner TJ, Jacobus WE. Improved myocardial metabolism with oxygenated perfluorocarbon cardioplegia. Surg Forum 1981;13:290–293.
78. Magovern GJ, Flaherty JT, Gott VL, Bulkley BH, Gardner TJ. Optimal myocardial protection with Fluosol cardioplegia. Ann Thorac Surg 1982;34:249–257.
79. Flaherty JT, Jaffin JH, Magovern GJ, et al. Maintenance of aerobic metabolism during global ischemia with perfluorocarbon cardioplegia improves myocardial preservation. Circulation 1984;69:585–592.
80. Novick RJ, Stefaniszyn HJ, Michel RP, Burdon FD, Salerno TA. Protection of the hypertrophied pig myocardium. A comparison of crystalloid, blood, and Fluosol-DA cardioplegia during prolonged aortic clamping. J Thorac Cardiovasc Surg 1985;89:547–566.
81. Cusimano RJ, Asho KA, Chin ID, et al. Myocardial projection in the hypertrophied right ventricle. Ann Thorac Surg 1991;52:934–938.
82. Forman MB, Bingham S, Kopelman HA, et al. Reduction of infarct size with intracoronary perfluorochemical in canine preparation of reperfusion. Circulation 1985;71:1060–1068.
83. Forman MB, Puett DW, Bingham SE, et al. Preservation of endothelial cell structure and function by intracoronary perfluorochemical in a canine preparation of reperfusion. Circulation 1987;76:469–479.
84. Nunn GR, Dunn G, Peters J, Cohn LH. Effect of fluorocarbon exchange transfusion on myocardial infarct size in dogs. Am J Cardiol 1983;52:203–205.
85. Faithfull NS, Erdmann W, Fennema M, Kok A. Effects of haemodilution with fluorocarbons or dextran on oxygen tensions in the acutely ischaemic myocardium. Br J Anaesth 1986;58:1031–1040.
86. Bajaj AK, Cobb MA, Virmani R, Gay JC, Light RT, Forman MB. Limitation of myocardial reperfusion injury by intavenous perfluorochemicals. Circulation 1989;79:645–656.
87. Kolodgie FD, Farb A, Carlson GC, Wilson PS, Virmani R. Hyperoxic reperfusion is required to reduce infarct size after intravenous therapy with perfluorochemical (Fluosol-DA 20%) or its detergent component (Poloxamer 188) in a poorly collateralized animal model. J Am Coll Cardiol 1994;24:1098–1108.
88. Forman MB, Perry JM, Wilson BH, et al. Demonstration of myocardial reperfusion injury in humans: results of a pilot study utilizing acute coronary angioplasty with perfluorochemical in anterior myocardial infarction. J Am Coll Cardiol 1991;18:911–918.
89. Wall TC, Califf RM, Blankenship J, et al. Intravenous Fluosol in the treatment of acute myocardial infarction. Results of the Thrombolysis and Angioplasty in Myocardial Infarction 9 Trial. Circulation 1994;90:114–120.
90. Levy JH. The human inflammatory response. J Cardiovasc Pharmacol 1996;27:531–537.
91. Segel LD, Ensunsa JL, Boyle WAI. Prolonged support of working rabbit hearts with a perfluorochemical emulsion. In: Chang TMS, ed. Blood substitutes. New York: Marcel Dekker, 1989:619–621.
92. Silber R, Sauer B, Eigel P, Henrich HA, Elert O. Electron microscopic changes and edema after nine hours' perfusion of isolated canine hearts. Heart Vessels 1991;6:203–210.
93. Baba S, Nakai KK. Ex-vivo perfusion of surgically removed organs. In: Chang TMS, ed. Blood substitutes. New York: Marcel Dekker, 1989:623–624.
94. Berkowitz HD, McCombs P, Sheety S, Miller LD, Sloviter H. Fluorochemical perfusates for renal preservation. J Surg Res 1976;20:595–600.
95. Voiglio EJ, Cloix P, Zarif L, Gorry F, Riess J, Dubernard JM. Ex vivo normothermic preservation of rat multiple organ blocks using a perfluorooctyl bromide emulsion as oxygen carrier. Transplant Proc 1993;25:2558–2560.
96. Bando K, Teramoto S, Tago M, Teraoka H, Senoo S, Senoo Y. Successful extended hypothermic cardiopulmonary preservation for heart-lung transplantation. J Thorac Cardiovasc Surg 1988;95:465–473.
97. Gohra H, Mori F, Esato K. The effect of fluorocarbon emulsion on 24-hour canine heart preservation by coronary perfusion. Ann Thorac Surg 1989;48:96–103.
98. Segel LD, Ensunsa JL. Albumin improves stability and longevity of perfluorochemical-perfused hearts. Am J Physiol 1988;254:H1105–1112.
99. Segel LD, Minten JMO, Schweighardt FK. Fluorochemical emulsion APE-LM substantially improves cardiac preservation. Am J Physiol 1992;263:H730–739.
100. Spiess BD, Sloan MS, McCarthy RJ, et al. The incidence of venous air embolism during total hip arthroplasty. J Clin Anesth 1988;1:25–30.
101. Anderson K. Air aspirated from the venous system during total hip replacement. JAMA 1984;251:2720.
102. Michenfelder J, Martini J, Altenberg B, Reholer K. Air embolism during neurosurgery. JAMA 1969;208:1353–1358.
103. Gronert GA, Messick JM, Cuchiara RF, Michenfelder JD. Paradoxical air embolism from a probe patent foramen ovale. Anesthesiology 1979;50:548.
104. Artru A, Colley PS. Bunegin-Albin CVP catheter improves resuscitation from lethal venous air embolism in dogs. Anesth Analg 1986;65:57.
105. Mills NL, Ochsner JL. Massive air embolism during cardiopulmonary bypass: causes, prevention and management. J Thorac Cardiovasc Surg 1980;80:208–215.
106. Dahme B, Meffert HJ, Rodewald P, et al. Extracorporeal circulation and neuropsychological deficits. In: Smith P, Taylor K, eds. Cardiac surgery and the brain. London: Edward Arnold, 1993:34–55.
107. Slogoff S, Girgis KZ, Keatz AZ. Etiologic factors in neuropsychiatric complications associated with cardiopulmonary bypass. Anesth Analg 1982;61:903–911.
108. Smith PL, Treasure T, Newman SP, et al. Cerebral consequences of cardiopulmonary bypass. Lancet 1986;1:823–825.
109. Nussmeier NA. Neuropsychiatric complications of cardiac surgery. J Cardiothorac Vasc Anesth 1994;8:13–18.

110. Nussmeier NA, Frish KJ. Neuropsychological dysfunction after cardiopulmonary bypass: a comparison of two institutions. J Cardiothorac Vasc Anesth 1991;5:584–588.
111. Shaw PJ, Bates D, Cartlidge NE, et al. Early intellectual dysfunction following coronary bypass surgery. Q J Med 1986;58:59–68.
112. Francis TJR, Dutka AJ, Hallenbeck JM. Pathophysiology of decompression sickness. In: Bove AA, Davis JC, eds. Diving medicine. Philadelphia: WB Saunders, 1990:170–187.
113. Spiess BD, McCarthy R, Piotrowski D, Ivankovich AD. Protection from venous air embolism with fluorocarbon emulsion FC-43. J Surg Res 1986;41:439–444.
114. Tuman K, Spiess BD, McCarthy R, Ivankovich AD. Cardiorespiratory effects of venous air embolism in dogs receiving a perfluorocarbon emulsion. J Neurosurg 1986;65:238–244.
115. Spiess BD, McCarthy RJ, Tuman K, Tool K, Woronowicz A, Ivankovich AD. Treatment of decompression sickness with a perfluorocarbon emulsion. Undersea Biomed Res 1988;15:31–37.
116. Spiess BD, Braverman B, Woronowicz A, Ivankovich AD. Protection from cerebral air emboli with perfluorocarbons in rabbits. Stroke 1986;17:1146–1149.
117. Spiess BD, McCarthy RJ, Tuman KJ, Ivankovich AD. Protection from coronary air embolism by a perfluorocarbon emulsion (FC-43). J Cardiothorac Anesth 1987;1:210–215.
118. Menasché P, Pinard E, Desroches AM, et al. Fluorocarbons: a potential treatment of cerebral air embolism in open heart surgery. Ann Thorac Surg 1985;40:494–497.
119. Lynch PR, Krasner LJ, Vinciquerra T, et al. Effects of intravenous perfluorocarbon and oxygen breathing on acute decompression sickness in the hamster. Undersea Biomed Res 1989;16:275–281.
120. Novotny JA, Bridgewater PM, Him JF, et al. Quantifying the effect of intravascular perfluorocarbon on xenon elimination from canine muscle. J Appl Physiol 1993;74:1356–1360.
121. Cassuto Y, Nunneley SA, Farhi LE. Inert gas washout in rats: enhancement by fluorocarbon infusion. Aerosp Med 1974;45:12–14.
122. Kennann RP, Pollack GL. Solubility of xenon in perfluorocarbons: temperature, dependence, and thermodynamics. J Chem Phys 1988; 89:517–521.
123. Spiess BD, Cochran RP, Kunzelman K, et al. Cerebral protection from massive air embolism with a perfluorocarbon emulsion prime addition for cardiopulmonary bypass [abstract]. Anesthesiology 1994;81:A692.
124. Blauth C, Smith P, Newman S, et al. Retinal microembolism and neuropsychological deficit following clinical cardiopulmonary bypass. Comparison of a membrane and bubble oxygenator. Eur J Cardiothorac Surg 1989;3:135–138.
125. Arnold JV, Blauth CI, Smith PL, et al. Demonstration of cerebral microemboli occurring during coronary artery bypass graft surgery using fluorescein angiography. J Audiov Media Med 1990;13:87–90.
126. Greenspan JS, Wolfson MR, Rubenstein SD, Shaffer TH. Liquid ventilation of human preterm neonates. J Pediatr 1990;117:106–111.
127. Lachmann B, Tutuncu AS, Bos JAH, Faithfull NS, Erdmann W. Perflubron (perfluorooctylbromide) instillation combined with mechanical ventilation: an alternative treatment of acute respiratory failure in adult animals. In: Erdmann W, Bruley DF, eds. Oxygen transport to tissue XIV. Advances in experimental medicine and biology. Vol. 317. New York: Plenum Press, 1992:409–412.
128. Tutuncu AS, Akpir K, Mulder P, Erdmann W, Lachmann B. Intratracheal perfluorocarbon administration as an aid in the ventilatory management of respiratory distress syndrome. Anesthesiology 1993;79: 1083–1093.
129. Leach CL, Fuhrman BP, Morin FC III, Rath MG. Perfluorocarbon-associated gas exchange (partial liquid ventilation) in respiratory distress syndrome: a prospective, randomized, controlled study. Crit Care Med 1993;21:1270–1278.
130. Andre MP, Steinbach G, Mattrey RF. Enhancement of the echogenicity of flowing blood by the contrast agent perflubron. Invest Radiol 1993;28:502–506.
131. Mattrey RF, Brown JJ, Shelton RE, Ogino MT, Johnson KK, Mitten RM. Use of perfluorooctylbromide (PFOB) to detect liver abscesses with CT: safety and efficacy. Invest Radiol 1991;26:792–798.
132. Mattrey RF, Hajek PC, Gylys-Morin VM, et al. Perfluorochemicals as gastrointestinal contrast agents for MR imaging: preliminary studies in rats and humans. Am J Roentgenol 1987;148:1259–1263.
133. Teicher BA. Use of perfluorochemical emulsions in cancer therapy. Biomater Artif Cells Immobil Biotechnol 1992;20:875–882.

Chapter 11

Surgery in the Patient Who Refuses Transfusion

RICHARD K. SPENCE
RONALD J. ALVAREZ

INTRODUCTION

On occasion, the surgeon and anesthesiologist will deal with a patient who is a candidate for transfusion but either cannot or will not accept blood. Those who cannot represent a small group who are victims of logistics and include patients with antibody incompatibilities and those unfortunate enough to develop active bleeding at a time of acute blood shortage. The second group is represented by the Jehovah's Witness, who refuses blood transfusion because of religious beliefs. This chapter focuses on the latter group by offering an understanding of the beliefs and position of Jehovah's Witnesses on blood products. Alternatives to allogeneic blood transfusion acceptable to Jehovah's Witnesses are discussed as well as general guidelines for both elective and emergency surgery in these patients. The reader is referred to other chapters for a more in-depth presentation of specific transfusion alternatives. We believe that the proposed guidelines are as applicable to the general population as they are to the Jehovah's Witness patient.

BACKGROUND

The Jehovah's Witness religion started in the early 1800s, growing out of a Bible study group known as Millenniasts who believed in the imminent second coming of Christ and His rule over the earth for the ensuing 1000 years. The group was further organized by Charles Taze Russell in the 1870s. Russell expanded the role of Bible study and promoted the group's beliefs through the publication of religious tracts and books. In 1884, the group became known as the Zion's Watch Tower Tract Society. In 1916, upon Russell's death, the religious group's leadership was assumed by Joseph Franklin Russell. He used his talents as an attorney and organizer to restructure the group into a centrally run religion that became known as the Jehovah's Witnesses in 1931. Under his tutelage, the Jehovah's Witnesses further developed their goals of Bible study and community missionary work. The religion is currently run by a governing body based in Brooklyn, New York.

Of primary concern to surgeons is the Jehovah's Witnesses refusal to accept blood transfusion (1–5). This belief is based on a strict interpretation of passages from the Bible (6):

> *Every moving thing that liveth shall be meat for you; even as the green herb have I given you all things. But the flesh of the life thereof, ye shall not eat.* (Genesis 9:3–4) *For it [blood] is the life of all flesh; the blood of it is for the life thereof: therefore I say unto the children of Israel, ye shall eat the blood of no manner of flesh: for the life of all flesh is the blood thereof. Whosoever eateth it shall be cut off.* (Leviticus 17:14)

One can argue interminably that these passages should not be interpreted to include blood transfusion or that such dietary prohibitions have no place in the modern world. However, the true Jehovah's Witness cannot be dissuaded and frequently counters any philosophical or religious arguments with sound scientific reasons why blood transfusion is inherently dangerous (7–11).

Physicians tend to underestimate the importance of the Jehovah's Witness' prohibition against blood transfusion. This refusal to accept transfusion is not a minor infraction to be forgiven lightly. The consequences of transfusion for the Jehovah's Witness include excommunication from the church, forfeiture of a chance for eternal life, and severance of the individual's relationship with God. To die while upholding one's religious beliefs, in this case, refusing transfusion, is an ancient and accepted practice in the world's religions. Although the physician may not agree with this position, especially regarding transfusion, one must understand that the potential for life everlasting is an enormous incentive, especially when the alternative is so negative. The Jehovah's Witness whose life is saved by an unwanted transfusion may believe that he or she is eternally damned—a great price to pay for temporal salvation.

Physicians often have a difficult time with this issue, because their training is directed toward saving lives. To withhold blood transfusion, a relatively low-risk treatment with great life-saving potential, seems to violate the Hippocratic Oath. However, regardless of how "medically" correct transfusion may be to the physician, it can never be correct to the Jehovah's Witness. Moreover, it should never be "morally or ethically" correct for a physician to force an unwanted treatment on an unwilling patient (12–16). Each surgeon must make a personal decision as to whether or not this prohibition against transfusion is acceptable. If not, Jehovah's Witness patients should be referred or transferred to physicians who are willing to accept them. Approximately 40 Centers for Bloodless Surgery, hospitals with experienced personnel that have agreed to honor the wishes of the Jehovah's Witness, now exist throughout the United States. Following the doctrine of "If you can't transfuse, transfer" has saved many lives. Time should not be wasted in misguided attempts to convince the Witness by argument and logic or in waiting for the situation to worsen in hopes that the patient will convert at the operating room door (17–19). Unfortunately, we have seen just such actions rob actively bleeding patients of a chance for survival.

ACCEPTABLE TRANSFUSION ALTERNATIVES FOR THE JEHOVAH'S WITNESS

What do Jehovah's Witness patients accept? There is a common misconception that they refuse any type of medical care. To the contrary, Jehovah's Witnesses actively seek the best in medical treatment. As a group, they are the best-educated consumers the surgeon will ever encounter and are very knowledgeable, especially in areas of alternatives to transfusion. Their church has established local Liaison Committees, consisting of church members whose goals are to act as a link between the physician and the patient and to provide the physician with a clear understanding of the Witnesses' position, use of alternatives, and so on (20). Guidelines for the use of alternatives to blood transfusion have been published by the Watchtower society. These serve as information for the Jehovah's Witness with the caveat that the decision to use a specific alternative is a matter of individual conscience.

In general, the Jehovah's Witness refuses any and all allogeneic blood products and any autologous blood that has been separated from the body for any length of time. These prohibitions do not prevent most Witnesses from accepting the use of cardiopulmonary bypass, dialysis, and intraoperative blood salvage and reinfusion (4). Although the difference may seem small to the casual observer, the Jehovah's Witness distinguishes acceptable therapy from the unacceptable by deciding whether or not the diverted blood is still part of the circulatory system (21). Such is the case with dialysis and the heart-lung machine, because in both blood remains part of the circulation. Autotransfusion devices can be revised very simply to meet this test by dedicating an intravenous line from the collection device to the patient to maintain a closed circuit. This modification has been used successfully by our group and by others (22–28). Hemodilution can also be used in a similar fashion (29–32).

Most drugs, such as iron dextran, aprotinin, and desmopressin, and synthetic "blood substitutes" are readily accepted by the Jehovah's Witness because these contain no human blood products (33, 34). Perfluorocarbons, specifically Fluosol DA-20% (Green Cross, Osaka, Japan), were studied extensively as blood substitutes in the Jehovah's Witness (35–40). Fluosol had little beneficial effect in terms of improving survival in the anemic patient despite its ability to increase dissolved oxygen. In our experience, its main value was as a temporary adjunct in the severely anemic Jehovah's Witness. Unfortunately, this product is no longer available. Second-generation products such as Oygent (Alliance Pharmaceutical, San Diego, CA) have improved characteristics as oxygen carriers and may play a future role in the treatment of the Jehovah's Witness. Hemoglobin-based blood substitutes are unacceptable to the Jehovah's Witness if they are made of either human or animal blood. The acceptability of a blood substitute made from recombinant hemoglobin (Somatogen, Boulder, CO) remains to be determined.

Some products that contain portions of blood or blood products (e.g., immune globulin) may be accepted by the Jehovah's Witness. Such is the case with recombinant erythropoietin (Amgen, Thousand Oaks, CA), which contains a small amount of human albumin. This hormone has been used in its recombinant form in many Jehovah's Witnesses (22, 41–50). Albumin, when used as a volume expander, is considered an unacceptable blood product. Because the amount contained in erythropoietin is so small and it is not intended to be used as a blood product, the albumin is acceptable. In our experience, only a very small percentage of Jehovah's Witnesses have refused erythropoietin use. Erythropoietin has become a mainstay in our treatment of the anemic Jehovah's Witness, particularly in the postoperative period. We analyzed the use of erythropoietin in 20 such patients with severe anemia (hemoglobin less than 7.0 g/dL) and compared them with 20 others who were treated with iron dextran injections and nutritional support alone (unpublished data). The former group demonstrated a 3–4% rise in hematocrit within 1 week, whereas the latter group did not change. Although this amount of change may seem small, the reader should remember that it is the equivalent of the transfusion of 1 unit of packed red blood cells.

SURGERY, SURVIVAL, AND ANEMIA—LESSONS LEARNED FROM THE JEHOVAH'S WITNESS

The surgical world owes a debt of gratitude in a sense to the Jehovah's Witness population. Their refusal to accept blood transfusion has given us the opportunity to evaluate and assess the effect of anemia on outcome in surgery in the clinical setting. One could never design a randomized study that would allow avoidance of transfusion to the levels that have been reported in the Jehovah's Witness. Much has been published about individual experiences in treating Jehovah's Witness patients. Rather than list over 200 references dealing with this subject, we refer the reader to several articles dealing with either large groups of patients or summaries of smaller anecdotal experiences.

We reported several studies of anemia and the risk of postoperative morbidity and mortality in Jehovah's Witnesses (51–53). In the first, 125 patients undergoing either emergency or elective surgery were studied (51). The mean preoperative hemoglobin level in those who died was 7.6 g/dL and was significantly lower than that in the survivors (11.8 g/dL, $P < .002$). The percentage of patients who died with preoperative hemoglobin levels between 0 and 6 g/dL was 61.5%, between 6.1 and 8 g/dL was 33.3%, between 8.1 and 10 g/dL was 0%, and greater than 10 g/dL was 7.1%. None of the patients with preoperative hemoglobin levels greater than 8 g/dL and operative blood loss less than 500 mL died (upper 95% confidence interval, 5%). However, the study was too small to precisely describe the risk of death in patients in relation to hemoglobin levels, and it did not distinguish between elective and emergency surgery.

Our subsequent analysis of 113 elective operations in 107 Jehovah's Witness patients showed that mortality was 0 with hemoglobin levels as low as 6 g/dL as long as blood loss was kept below 500 mL (52). To date, we have accumulated data on over 1500 Jehovah's Witness patients who underwent elective surgery without transfusion. A subgroup of 238 patients who had operations that would have required transfusion based on traditional maximum surgical blood-ordering schedules were analyzed to determine the relationship between surgical blood loss, preoperative hemoglobin, and survival. Preoperative hemoglobin ranged between 6.0 and 16.4 g/dL, with a mean of 11.4 g/dL. Overall mortality was 5 of 238 patients, or 2.1%. All deaths occurred in those patients with blood loss greater than 500 mL. No deaths occurred with less than 500-mL blood loss regardless of the preoperative hemoglobin level. Outcome was based more on the amount of blood lost during surgery than the starting hemoglobin level.

Ott and Cooley's (54) classic study of cardiac surgery in Jehovah's Witness children demonstrated that such high-risk surgery was possible (mortality 9.4%) and also defined the standards for open heart surgery in this group. Similar reports of large series of patients showing that surgery can be performed safely have appeared for gynecological surgery (55), abdominal surgery (24), and orthopedic surgery (56). Viele and Weiskopf (57) reviewed 61 reports dealing with 4722 Jehovah's Witness patients. Fifty-four articles representing 134 patients with moderate to severe anemia, defined as hemoglobin below 8 g/dL, met their criteria for further analysis. They concluded from this study that major surgery with an acceptable mortality rate was feasible in the Jehovah's Witness.

These reports should not be dismissed only as proof that we can "get away with" performing surgery without transfusion even when confronted with severe anemia. They are of much greater value in providing the basis for much of what we know about the safety of performing "bloodless surgery" in all patients, not just the Jehovah's Witness. This body of work represents an essential part of the clinical support for lowering of the transfusion trigger below 10 g/dL.

ELECTIVE SURGERY IN THE JEHOVAH'S WITNESS

Elective surgery of all types and magnitudes, from pancreaticoduodenectomy (22) to major cardiovascular procedures (53), can be performed safely in the Jehovah's Witness patient. Because most surgical procedures do not result in significant blood loss, these types of cases (e.g., laparoscopic cholecystectomy) can be performed without major concern about transfusion needs in the nonanemic patient. It is our policy to delay elective surgery in the anemic Jehovah's Witness until such time as red cell mass can be restored to normal levels with the use of oral iron supplements, folic acid, attention to nutrition, and erythropoietin (Fig. 11.1). In some resistant patients, a

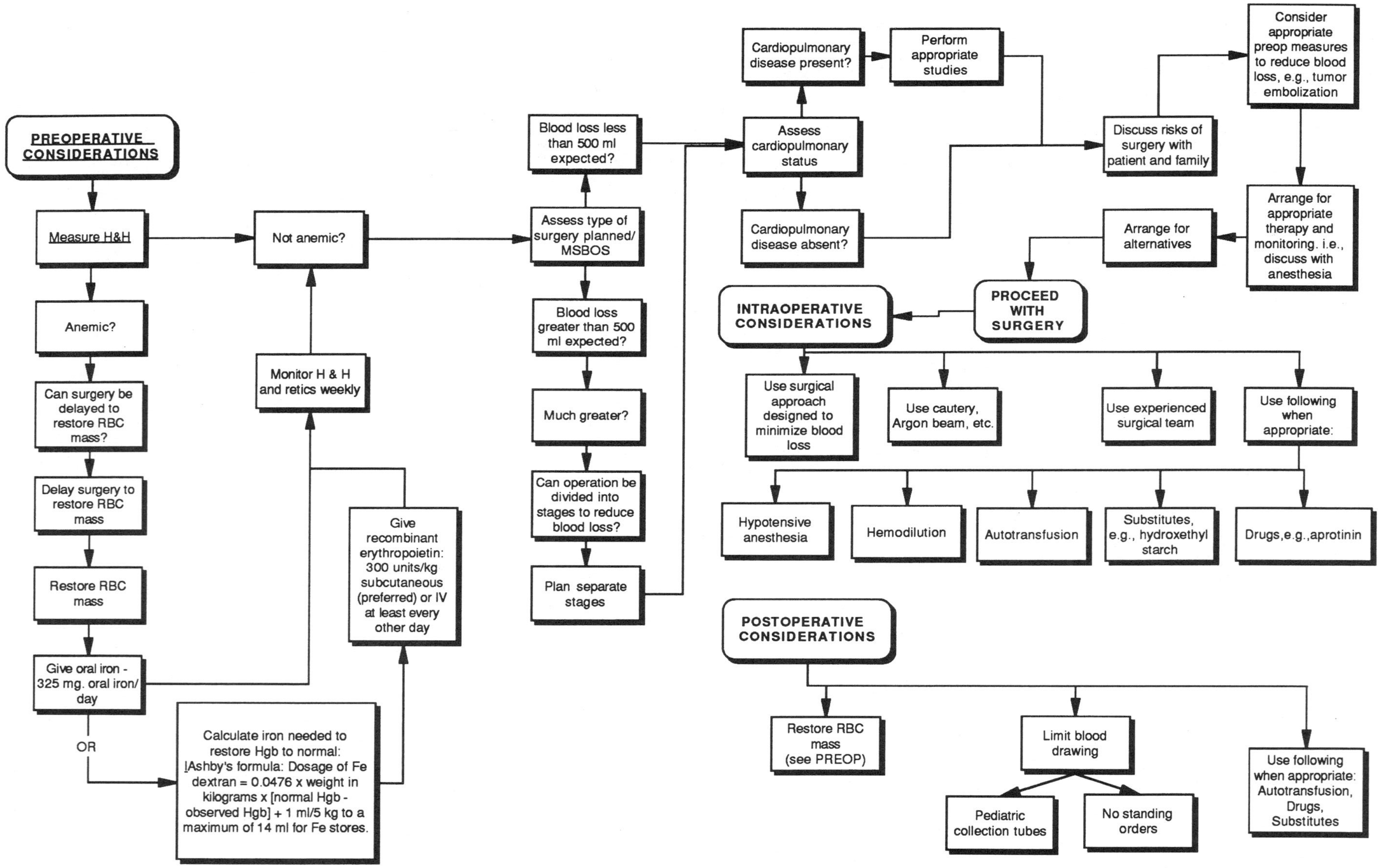

Figure 11.1. Elective surgery in the Jehovah's Witness.

complete hematological workup may be needed to diagnose and treat anemia.

Successful major surgery (i.e., surgery in which blood loss is great enough to require transfusion) requires limiting blood loss as much as possible, especially in the Jehovah's Witness. The importance of the latter is demonstrated by our analysis of mortality, preoperative hemoglobin level, and blood loss described above. The sine qua non of minimizing blood loss during surgery is careful, skillful operative technique. Dissection along anatomic, avascular planes is essential and requires a thorough knowledge of anatomy. "Rip and tear" surgical techniques only lead to avulsion of vessels and increased bleeding. All potentially vascular structures should be clamped and tied before being cut. Any vessel inadvertently cut or any unexpected bleeding, no matter how minor, must be controlled. Attention to what may seem to be insignificant detail at the time can lead to diminished blood loss. Bleeding from many small vessels can accumulate quickly. In our experience, as much as 100–200 mL of blood can be lost from unattended skin and subcutaneous vessels during the course of an operation, especially in the hypertensive patient.

A variety of cutting devices that decrease operative blood loss is available to the surgeon. The use of electrocautery has been shown to reduce blood loss without significant complications in many procedures, including tonsillectomy, gynecological excisions, laparoscopic cholecystectomy, and abdominal surgeries (58–68). The combination of electrocautery and ultrasonic capability has produced an efficient instrument for dissecting while maintaining a bloodless field (69). Similarly, both laser and argon beam devices reduce blood loss when used in either open or laparoscopic surgery (70–72). In an experimental model of splenic injury in swine, Dowling et al. (73) showed that hemostatic control was achieved faster and with less blood loss using argon beam coagulation compared with electrocautery, direct pressure, topical hemostatic agents, or suture ligation. Two reports from China have demonstrated the transfusion-sparing effect of microwave hepatic surgery. Microwave current transmitted through a monopolar needle electrode produced coagulation, reduced blood loss when compared with conventional hepatectomy (average, 244 versus 746 mL), and decreased transfusion need (74). However, this device may produce more septic complications from the coagulum of tissues left behind (75). In our experience, reduced blood loss is a function more of the surgeon's skill than of the device itself. The individual surgeon should gain experience with these tools to develop optimal surgical technique.

Multiple surgical techniques have been modified from existing techniques or developed anew to minimize blood loss in general, vascular, and orthopedic surgery. All are useful in the Jehovah's Witness patient. Some techniques are generic; others are procedure specific. The former group includes preoperative tumor embolization, the temporary use of clotting aids such as collagen pads, and laparoscopic surgery. Angiographic embolization with either clot, metal coils, or synthetic material can reduce blood loss at the time of surgery (76, 77). Laparoscopic surgical techniques have been shown to reduce blood loss in a wide range of procedures from cholecystectomy to adrenalectomy (78–82). However, the surgeon must understand that successful bloodless laparoscopic surgery is not inherent in the approach but comes only with practice. The inexperienced surgeon is capable of producing massive bleeding during laparoscopy if correct technique is not used.

Surgical procedures that entail little or no blood loss (e.g., hernia repair or breast biopsy) do not routinely lead to transfusion. Such operations can be done in the Jehovah's Witness without the need for extraordinary precautions. However, procedures that involve large vessels (e.g., abdominal aortic aneurysm repair), include extensive dissection (e.g., pancreaticoduodenectomy), or require resection of a portion of a well-vascularized organ (e.g., partial hepatectomy) have routinely led to transfusion of red cells in the past. Fortunately, these types of operations can be performed in a bloodless manner without resorting to allogeneic blood transfusion by using a combination of alternatives and modified techniques.

Hepatic surgery frequently leads to bleeding and the need for transfusion. Technique has been shown to be one of the most important determinants of the need for transfusion in both cancer resection and liver transplantation (83, 84). Intraoperative ultrasound and/or waterjet dissection, needle localization, and microwave cautery reduce blood loss (85, 86, 87). Several authors have reported great success using vascular isolation before parenchymal division, or VIP approach to liver resection (88–94). This includes parenchymal compression, the temporary cross-clamping of the portal triad (Pringle maneuver), a hepatic venous tourniquet, hilar division, hepatic vein division, and the use of temporary occlusion of the infrahepatic and suprahepatic vena cava (Heaney maneuver). As the name of the approach implies, bleeding is prevented before it occurs. Only 2 VIP patients in Ryan and Faulkner's series of 34 (6%) needed allogeneic transfusion compared with 18 of 24 patients (75%) done without this approach (94). Makuuchi et al. (88) discharged 87% of their hepatectomy patients without the need for whole blood transfusion. Kim et al. (90) reduced blood loss by approximately one-half with this approach. Experienced surgeons working as a team are essential for successful reduction of blood loss during liver surgery (91, 95). Terblanche et al. (91) performed operations with a two-person team of experienced surgeons using 4.5× magnification and completed the resection with occlusion times averaging 73 minutes. Although these reports do not deal directly with the Jehovah's Witness patient, they point out that successful bloodless hepatic surgery can be performed in most patients.

Modification of operative approaches may minimize blood loss in vascular surgery. Both the retroperitoneal approach to the abdominal aorta and the exclusion-bypass technique have been reported as superior to traditional surgical approaches and handling of the aorta in terms of blood loss, although some controversy exists in this area. In their study of a standard transperitoneal approach, Leather et al. (96) estimated that blood loss averaged 1700 mL. By switching to a retroperitoneal approach and excluding the aneurysm, blood loss was decreased to 900 mL, a reduction of almost one-half. Carrel et al. (97) found a similar decrease from 1300 to 630 mL in 42 retroperitoneal operations compared with 121 transperitoneal cases. In contrast, Cambria et al. (98) found no significant transfusion advantage to using one approach over the other in a series of 69 patients randomized to either a retroperitoneal or transperitoneal operation.

Woven Dacron grafts with minimal porosity, gelatin or collagen-sealed grafts, and polytetrafluoroethylene (PTFE) essentially eliminate blood loss from extravasation during aortic bypass and replacement, but their effect on reducing transfusion need is questionable. Reid and Pollock (99) reported that gelatin-sealed grafts had "no measurable blood loss at implantation." However, 47 patients still required transfusion for blood loss of greater than 750 mL or on clinical grounds. Fisher et al. (100) performed a comparative analysis of double velour woven Dacron grafts to PTFE using sophisticated blood loss measurement techniques and concluded that neither graft had an advantage over the other in decreasing blood loss or preventing transfusion. Their results may have been skewed by a significantly lower preoperative erythrocyte volume in the Dacron group, which may have accounted for increased transfusion need. In the lower extremity, Hans et al. (101) noted a greater blood loss with in situ femoral popliteal bypass versus reversed saphenous vein. They attribute this to an increased operative time and more release of blood in testing the vein.

We approach the abdominal aorta through a transperitoneal incision in most cases, because the midline is avascular and leads to less bleeding in our hands than an incision through muscle. All patients have blood salvaged, washed, and returned using autotransfusion, and we use low-porosity Dacron grafts for bypass. With this approach, we have results of total blood loss less than 500 mL in most patients, which results in an average postoperative hemoglobin level of 8–10 g/dL. By careful attention to detail and limiting bleeding from the anastomosed vein during in situ surgery, we have reduced blood loss in a small number of lower extremity bypass cases to approximately 150 mL, a level below the need for transfusion (53). Other groups have reported the performance of successful major vascular surgery in the Jehovah's Witness using many of these techniques (102, 103).

Advances have also been made in the performance of bloodless orthopedic surgery. Blood loss during lumbar fusion surgery is greater with a posterior versus an anterior approach, three-level versus two-level fusion, and the use of internal fixation (104). Two studies of hip surgery have shown that an anterior approach to total hip repair creates less blood loss than a transtrochanteric or posterior approach (105, 106). Blood loss is also greater for exchange arthroplasty when compared with internal fixation for hip fractures. Nelson et al. (107) attribute their success in performing total hip replacement in Jehovah's Witness patients to a variety of factors, including careful operative planning, meticulous technique, and hypotensive anesthesia. Lotke et al.'s (108) detailed analysis of tourniquet use in total knee replacement concluded that intraoperative release coupled with immediate, continuous, postoperative passive motion led to increased blood loss when compared with postoperative tourniquet release. Burkart et al. (109) studied this in 100 consecutive knee replacements, demonstrating that tourniquet release had no bearing on overall blood loss. Cemented prostheses and femoral intramedullary plugs offer an advantage in terms of reduced blood loss in knee replacement surgery (110, 111). Delayed hip fracture repair using traction as a temporary measure until red cell mass can be restored may be useful in the severely anemic patient who refuses or cannot be transfused (e.g., the Jehovah's Witness). Several reports of a variety of orthopedic procedures in the Jehovah's Witness demonstrate the ability to perform this type of surgery successfully (107, 112, 113).

Both the choice of anesthetic technique and operation can influence the amount of blood lost during surgery. Regional anesthetic techniques have been associated with decreased blood loss in orthopedic surgery. Bridenbaugh (114) showed less blood loss in patients who underwent total hip replacement under continuous epidural than in those who received a general anesthetic. Nelson and Bowen (56) saw similar results with hypotensive anesthesia. Oxygen consumption is reduced 15–20% under general anesthesia in most patients (115). Narcotic anesthesia may also reduce oxygen consumption by an additional 5–10%, providing a greater margin of safety. Our anesthesiologists favor narcotic anesthesia, usually with fentanyl, in anemic patients. If inhalational anesthetics are used, isoflurane is usually chosen because it has less inhibitory effect on the heart's conductivity. These anesthetic agents do not directly minimize blood loss, but they provide a somewhat safer environment for the stressed, anemic patient who may need increased cardiac reserves. For example, the use of propofol, an intravenously administered nonbarbiturate hypnotic agent, was associated with a reduction in blood loss compared with standard inhalational agents in a study of endoscopic sinus surgery (116).

Our approach to elective surgery in the Jehovah's Witness is summarized in Figure 11.1. This algorithm is useful in non-Jehovah's Witness patients as well, if one wishes to reduce or eliminate exposure to allogeneic blood. The only major addition to the outline would be the use of autologous predonation of blood, a process unacceptable to the Jehovah's Witness. Table 11.1 covers general guidelines for dealing with Jehovah's Witnesses in both elective and emergency situations.

TABLE 11.1. GUIDELINES FOR DEALING WITH THE JEHOVAH'S WITNESS

1. Discuss issues with patient, including the possibility of life-threatening hemorrhage and possible death if not transfused.
2. Document discussions in the record or as part of a refusal of treatment form.
3. If unable or unwilling to treat, stabilize and transfer to a sympathetic institution such as a Center for Bloodless Surgery.
4. Contact the local Jehovah's Witness liaison committee for information and help.
5. In an emergency or with an unconscious patient, look for an advance directive (e.g., card) and discuss with third party.
6. Seek legal assistance for minor or unconscious/incompetent adult.
7. Learn about and use alternatives.

TRAUMA, BLEEDING, AND THE JEHOVAH'S WITNESS

The key to successful, elective, bloodless surgery lies in following basic Halstedian principles of careful dissection and attention to detail. The actively bleeding patient or the trauma patient who needs emergency surgery presents a different challenge to the surgeon, especially if the patient is a Jehovah's Witness. Rapid control of bleeding from trauma is essential if the patient is to be saved.

In the bleeding patient, our first priority traditionally has been to correct volume losses and reverse hypotension with infusions of colloid and/or crystalloid solutions. The goal is to stabilize the patient and improve oxygen delivery by increasing cardiac output as quickly as possible. Once the patient is stabilized and is no longer hypovolemic, decisions are made concerning bleeding activity and the need for surgical intervention. This approach has been questioned recently because of the perception that fluid resuscitation designed to correct hypovolemia may prolong or reinitiate hemorrhage. Several investigators have demonstrated in animal models of uncontrolled hemorrhage that attempts to stabilize the animal with intravenous fluid infusions led to continued blood loss and increased mortality (117, 118). This issue was addressed clinically in a prospective study of the effect of fluid resuscitation in hypotensive patients who had sustained penetrating truncal injuries (119). No significant difference was noted in mortality between two groups of patients assigned to either initial or delayed resuscitation, although the trend was toward a higher death rate in the former group. These results can be viewed as supporting the traditional approach to early resuscitation as doing no harm; however, they do not show its benefit. Delaying fluid resuscitation until hemorrhage is controlled appears to be as safe as this traditional approach and may have the added benefit of reducing transfusion need, particularly for the Jehovah's Witness.

Two major resuscitation fluid alternatives to allogeneic blood transfusion exist—crystalloids and colloids. Both are capable of restoring blood pressure—at least temporarily—in the patient in shock after acute blood loss. Colloids have a longer intravascular half-life, but they do not differ significantly from crystalloids in their resuscitative properties. We have used hydroxyethyl starch extensively in our Jehovah's Witness population. This synthetic colloid is an acceptable substitute for albumin and can be infused in volumes of up to 2 L/day without producing clinical evidence of coagulopathy. A new addition to the family of crystalloids, hypertonic saline (HTS), has been studied extensively in both animals and humans, with mixed results (120–123). HTS infusions in animal studies have improved hemodynamics after hemorrhage, but they have also increased bleeding, decreased blood pressure, and increased mortality (120, 121). Younes et al. (122) randomized 105 patients with hypovolemia treated in the emergency room to either 7.5% NaCl HTS, a combination of HTS with Dextran 70, or saline. Initial mean arterial pressure was higher in HTS groups, and both fluid and blood required for overall resuscitation were less. However, there was no effect on mortality (122). A prospective, randomized, double-blind trial of an HTS/Dextran combination versus lactated Ringer's solution in 166 trauma patients conducted by Vassar et al. (123) showed no significant difference in either bleeding or amount of blood transfused. Outcome was improved only in patients with head injuries. Further studies are needed to assess if HTS with or without colloid will have a beneficial effect on blood loss and transfusion requirements and whether or not use of this agent will benefit the Jehovah's Witness.

Major vascular injuries are often fatal, not only in the Jehovah's Witness (124, 125). The traditional teaching regarding a retroperitoneal or pelvic hematoma in a blunt trauma patient is to leave it alone for fear of unleashing uncontrollable venous bleeding. In the patient with a suspected large vessel injury, this hands-off approach may lead to continued hemorrhage and deterioration. If transfusion is not an option, as in the Jehovah's Witness, death is inevitable. Brathwaite and Rodriguez (126) recommended an alternative approach of opening all central and lateral hematomas in blunt trauma victims after proximal and distal aortic control has been established. This philosophy, based on sound vascular surgical principles, permits expeditious repair of major injuries while minimizing blood loss.

Angiography remains the standard not only in identifying pelvic vascular injury but also in controlling bleeding by embolization or coil occlusion. Intraoperative ultrasound offers an alternative to preoperative angiography and may avoid dangerous delays (127). Occlusion, by either catheter or direct ligation, is appropriate in smaller vessels and in areas where collateral circulation is sufficient to maintain perfusion of the affected distal tissues or in life-threatening situations. However, occlusion of a proximal iliac vessel can be disastrous, leading to high amputation. Performance of a cross-femoral bypass graft in conjunction with iliac artery ligation can be both a life-saving and limb-saving procedure in the Jehovah's Witness (128).

Vascular injuries of the extremities are usually not exsanguinating. Ongoing bleeding can be controlled via direct compression and exploration to attain proximal control followed by either direct repair or bypass (129). The use of a stent-graft combination to treat a traumatic femoral arteriovenous fistula has been described by Marin et al. (130). These grafts, which can be placed through minimal incisions using angiographic techniques, may lead to dramatic reductions in operative blood loss and patient survival in ruptured aneurysms or similar vascular injuries. The endovascular approach to the ruptured aneurysm in the Jehovah's Witness may be the only way this type of patient can be saved.

In contrast to the trauma patient in which early surgical intervention to stop bleeding is the norm, it is common practice in the patient with gastrointestinal bleeding to determine the need for surgery based on the number of units of blood lost (read: transfused) within a 12- to 24-hour period. This approach is clearly unacceptable in the Jehovah's Witness. Early surgical intervention is essential when transfusion is not an option. Early intervention requires early diagnosis. Endoscopy will determine the cause of bleeding in the upper gastrointestinal tract in most patients and can provide a means of therapy. Failure to stop hemorrhage from an ulcer with electrocoagulation should prompt surgical intervention. Our own experience with bleeding Jehovah's Witness patients in whom blood transfusion is not an option points out the need for early, decisive intervention to control hemorrhage. In five such patients bleeding from peptic ulcer disease, we followed the traditional approach of volume resuscitation and monitoring to assess the rapidity of bleeding and need for surgery. Mortality was 75%. Dissatisfied with these results, we modified our approach to one of immediate endoscopy to identify the bleeding source, performed simultaneously with volume replacement. If bleeding could be stopped by coagulation with cautery or heater probe, this was done, followed by close monitoring. Specific indications for immediate surgery included active uncontrolled bleeding, the presence of a visible vessel in the ulcer crater, or ongoing shock despite active resuscitation. Surgery was performed while resuscitation was ongoing, usually within 6 hours of arrival in the hospital. By combining early endoscopy and surgery with simultaneous fluid resuscitation, we decreased mortality in a subsequent seven consecutive patients to 25%.

Most variceal bleeding can be controlled using a stepwise treatment plan that includes endoscopy, vasopressin infusion, balloon tamponade, and sclerotherapy followed by selective decompression with a shunt for persistent or recurrent bleeding (131). After confirmation by endoscopy of varices as the bleeding source, vasopressin may be infused at a rate of 0.4 U/min, increasing to a maximum of 1 U/min as needed. Nitroglycerin may be infused concomitantly to minimize coronary vasoconstriction. If bleeding does not stop with this approach, insertion of a Sengstaken-Blakemore tube provides rapid, temporary control. Although the balloon provides only temporary control and rebleeding rates are high after removal, one must remember that the primary goal here is to stop the continued bleeding quickly. Once control is achieved, endoscopic sclerotherapy provides further control.

Rebleeding with increased transfusion requirements and mortality rates as high as 45% after endoscopic sclerotherapy have led others to evaluate alternative methods of controlling variceal bleeding, including endoscopic ligation, esophageal interruption, and emergency shunting, the latter performed either surgically or through an endovascular approach. Stiegmann et al. (132) reduced allogeneic blood usage and decreased mortality from 44% with sclerotherapy to 28% using endoscopic ligation in a randomized trial of 129 patients. Burroughs et al. (133) reported decreased rebleeding using staple transection of the esophagus when compared with sclerotherapy. However, morbidity, mortality, and blood usage were similar for the two groups compared. Berard (134) stated in his report of 108 patients who underwent clip interruption of the esophagus via thoracotomy that this procedure can be done in less than 1 hour without transfusion and a mortality of 20%. Nagasue et al. (135) reduced blood loss from approximately 1400 to 800 mL using PTFE to construct a modified distal splenorenal shunt. Mortality was 11.1% using this technique in eight of nine emergency shunts.

Use of the transvenous intrahepatic portosystemic shunt (TIPS) follows catheter-directed vasopressin infusions as the next step in angiographically driven therapy for bleeding varices. This expandable metal shunt can be placed either angiographically between a branch of the hepatic vein and the right or left branch of the portal vein or directly into a small bowel mesenteric vein via a midline laparotomy incision (136). In Ring et al.'s (137) initial series of 13 patients, creation of a TIPS acutely stopped variceal bleeding by decreasing portal pressure approximately 10 cm H_2O. Four patients had previous portosystemic shunts; others were sclerotherapy failures. Bleeding recurred in only one patient after 3 months. Moreover, seven patients derived considerable long-term benefit by going on to successful liver transplantation. This group has subsequently reported similar results in over 100 patients, as have others in smaller series (138, 139).

We prefer definitive therapy (i.e., portacaval shunting) in the Jehovah's Witness after an initial episode of variceal bleeding because rebleeding must be avoided. We have used an end-to-side shunt because of its simplicity and minimal blood loss in four such patients. All survived their initial operation, but one died 8 days postoperatively after occluding the shunt and exsanguinating from his esophageal varices. The other three were discharged from the hospital in good condition. All shunts were done during the hospitalization for the initial bleeding episode. Definitive treatment (i.e., surgery) was not performed until hepatic function had improved. This was facilitated by initial volume replacement, nutritional support, and iron replacement. We believe that this approach, which works well with Jehovah's Witnesses, can be used with other patients to limit the need for allogeneic transfusion.

LEGAL ASPECTS

Legal decisions concerning medical practice are based on either constitutional law or precedent (i.e., case law) (140). Included in the former are three basic concepts: the right to freedom of religion, the right to privacy, and the right to accept or refuse basic medical care. Freedom of religion is guaranteed by the U.S. Constitution and applies here most directly to situations involving patients who refuse transfusion on religious grounds (i.e., Jehovah's Witnesses). Although the right to privacy is not part of the Constitution per se, it has been recognized and accepted by the Supreme Court as a basic right of U.S. citizens. The right to accept or to refuse medical care is based on an interpretation of these other rights found in a decision given by Justice Benjamin Cardozo in 1914: "Every human being of adult years and sound mind has a right to determine what shall be done with his own body. . . . " (141). This decision is the basis for the informed consent doctrine and its application to transfusion practices.

These basic rights have been balanced in the courts against the interests and powers of the State designed to regulate and protect the citizenry. The basic goals of the State are to preserve human life and to ensure that one individual's rights do not infringe on another's. These interests have come into play in transfusion issues primarily in attempts to define standards of care and informed consent and to preserve the lives of minor children of Jehovah's Witness parents.

Legal actions regarding Jehovah's Witnesses have defined treatment approaches for the surgeon. Controversial areas include transfusion of the minor, the use of emergency transfusion, and determinations of competency. Transfusion questions concerning minors usually arise only with children of Jehovah's Witnesses. Traditionally, the courts have ruled in favor of the physician in a decision to transfuse a minor, based on the doctrine of parens patriae, or the power of the State to preserve the lives of minors (142). However, times are changing. Courts are beginning to distinguish between life-threatening and nonlife-threatening situations (143). More and more, physicians are being required to document the life-threatening nature of an illness and to justify the benefits of transfusion, that is, to prove to the court that a transfusion will indeed be needed to save a child's life. In our experience, judges have required the physician to limit transfusion to the circumstances presented at the time of a court hearing and to report back to the court the success or failure of the transfusion. In other words, blanket orders "to transfuse as needed" are becoming rare. Similarly, if a surgical procedure is not needed to save a child's life and can safely be postponed until the child reaches adulthood, such a procedure may be denied by the court if it involves transfusion (144).

The teenage patient, or mature minor, presents other problems to the surgeon. If a child has married, joined the armed forces, or has been legally emancipated, he or she is considered to be a competent adult with all rights and privileges. Even without these factors, if the teenager is capable of understanding the nature and consequences of his or her actions, the courts may oppose transfusion. The Illinois Supreme Court recently found in favor of a 17-year-old girl with leukemia who opposed a transfusion because of her religious beliefs (145).

Luban and Leikin (143) suggest early, open discussion with the parents of the Jehovah's Witness child and involvement of the patient when appropriate. The surgeon should consider how essential transfusion is to the patient's outcome and whether or not alternatives are available. A wide variety of surgical procedures, including those with unavoidable attendant blood loss, have been performed safely in Jehovah's Witness children using combinations of hemodilution, hypothermic anesthesia, and intraoperative salvage (30, 54, 146–149).

In the emergency or when the patient is unconscious, the traditional approach is to stabilize the patient first, which may include the use of blood transfusion, and to seek consent later. Most states will permit transfusion in this setting, provided there is no advance directive known to the physician prohibiting transfusion and the transfusion is needed to save the patient's life. One may need to prove the latter after the fact. Most Jehovah's Witnesses carry a card proclaiming them as such and describing their refusal of blood and blood products. One must consider this card to be valid and binding, because it carries the weight of an advance directive. Some states have recognized the card's validity by law (20). In Malette *v*. Shulman, the Court of Ontario established this precedent by awarding damages to a Jehovah's Witness who was transfused despite the fact that she had such a card (16).

Informed consent with the Jehovah's Witness, or for that matter, any other patient, should include a discussion of the potential of life-threatening hemorrhage and its consequences. This need to include such discussions has been made clear in two recent decisions regarding Jehovah's Witnesses. In a case similar to Malette *v*. Shulman discussed above, the Michigan Court of Appeals ruled in favor of a surgeon who transfused his patient during a routine dilation and curettage when bleeding became life-threatening (150). The decision to uphold the surgeon's actions was based in large part on the fact that the patient did not fully comprehend that she might die during the operation if a transfusion became necessary and was not given. In a similar case in New Jersey in which a patient bled during a hysterectomy, the surgeon sought a court order to transfuse on the basis of the inability to inform the unconscious patient contemporaneously of the change in circumstances (i.e., bleeding that now threatened her life). Given the life-threatening circumstances, the court allowed the husband to act as a surrogate and grant permission to transfuse, even though the patient was a known Jehovah's Witness. However, in their decision, the court recognized that by failing to discuss the potential for life-threatening hemorrhage with the patient, the surgeon had not fulfilled his obligation to provide adequate informed consent. The appellate court subsequently upheld the decision while reaffirming the right of a Jehovah's Witness to refuse a blood transfusion while he or she is competent, or when incompetent, through an advance directive or Living Will. It is prudent, therefore, that the surgeon discuss the possibility of life-threatening hemorrhage, the possible need for additional surgery to stop bleeding (e.g., hysterectomy), and the possible need for transfusion with all Jehovah's Witness patients before surgery. Remember that the patient's refusal to accept such a transfusion does not protect the surgeon from liability for any negligent actions that may necessitate transfusion. Table 11.1 contains our general recommendations for dealing with the Jehovah's Witness patient. These can be used in conjunction with the algorithm presented in Figure 11.1 as an aid in dealing with the Jehovah's Witness patient.

This review has dealt with the major issues surgeons face in treating patients who refuse blood transfusion. The reader is referred to other chapters in the text for a more thorough discussion of the transfusion decision and the use of alternatives to allogeneic transfusion.

REFERENCES

1. Thurkauf GE. Understanding the beliefs of Jehovah's Witnesses. Focus Crit Care 1989;16:199–204.
2. Studdard PA, Greene JY. Jehovah's Witnesses and blood transfusion. Toward the resolution of a conflict of conscience. Ala J Med Sci 1986;23:454–459.
3. Singlenberg R. The blood transfusion taboo of Jehovah's Witnesses: origin, development and function of a controversial doctrine. Soc Sci Med 1990;31:515–523.
4. Ridley DT. Accommodating Jehovah's Witnesses' choice of nonblood management. Perspect Healthcare Risk Manage 1990;10:17–21.
5. Nielsen W. The Biblical laws against transfusions reexamined—a Christian physician's viewpoint. Transfus Med Rev 1991;5: 271–273.
6. Green M. Biblical laws relating to blood transfusion: the Judaic laws and principles. Transfus Med Rev 1991;5:247–252.
7. Jehovah's Witnesses and the question of blood. New York: Watchtower Bible and Tract Society, 1977:38–49.
8. Clarke JM. Surgery in Jehovah's Witnesses. Br J Hosp Med 1982;27: 497–500.
9. Dixon JL. Blood: whose choice and whose conscience? N Y State J Med 1988;88:463–464.
10. Findley LJ, Fletcher JC. Jehovah's Witnesses and the right to refuse blood. N Y State J Med 1988;88:464–465.
11. Trent B. Jehovah's Witnesses and the transfusion debate: we are not asking for the right to die [see comments]. Can Med Assoc J 1991; 144:770–776.
12. Macklin R. The inner workings of an ethics committee: latest battle over Jehovah's Witnesses. Hastings Cent Rep 1988;18:15–20.
13. Layon AJ, D'Amico R, Caton D, Mollet CJ. And the patient chose: medical ethics and the case of the Jehovah's Witness. Anesthesiology 1990;73:1258–1262.
14. Kleinman I. Written advance directives refusing blood transfusion: ethical and legal considerations. Am J Med 1994;96:563–567.
15. Grant AB. Exploring an ethical dilemma. Nursing 1992;22:52–54.

16. Fontanarosa PB, Giorgio GT. Managing Jehovah's Witnesses: medical, legal, and ethical challenges [editorial]. Ann Emerg Med 1991;20: 1148–1149.
17. Burrows R, Fabian J, Barker EM. Emergency treatment of Jehovah's Witnesses [see comments]. S Afr Med J 1991;80:218.
18. Vincent JL. Transfusion in the exsanguinating Jehovah's Witness patient—the attitude of intensive-care doctors. Eur J Anaesthesiol 1991;8: 297–300.
19. Vinicky JK, Smith ML, Connors RB Jr, Kozachuk WE. The Jehovah's Witness and blood: new perspectives on an old dilemma. J Clin Ethics 1990;1:65–71; discussion 71–74.
20. Jehovah's Witness cases raise critical issues for RMs [editorial]. Hosp Risk Manage 1990;12:101–104.
21. Letter to the editor. The Watchtower 1989;110:31–32.
22. Atabek U, Spence RK, Pello M, Alexander J, Camishion R. Pancreaticoduodenectomy without homologous blood transfusion in an anemic Jehovah's Witness. Arch Surg 1992;127:349–351.
23. Bengtsson A, Johansson S, Hahlin M, Crona N. Autotransfusion of blood cells made surgery of a Jehovah's Witness possible. Lakartidningen 1992;89:2955–2957.
24. Kambouris AA. Major abdominal operations on Jehovah's Witnesses. Am Surg 1987;53:350–356.
25. Kelley JL, Burke TW, Lichtiger B, Dupuis JF. Extracorporeal circulation as a blood conservation technique for extensive pelvic operations. J Am Coll Surg 1994;178:397–400.
26. Malan TP Jr, Whitmore J, Maddi R. Reoperative cardiac surgery in a Jehovah's Witness: role of continuous cell salvage and in-line reinfusion. J Cardiothorac Anesth 1989;3:211–214.
27. Ottesen S, Frysaker T. Use of Haemonetics Cell Saver for autotransfusion in cardiovascular surgery. Scand J Thorac Cardiovasc Surg 1982; 16:263–268.
28. Popovsky MA, Moore SB. Autologous transfusion in Jehovah's Witnesses [letter]. Transfusion 1985;25:444.
29. Grubbs PE Jr, Marini CP, Fleischer A. Acute hemodilution in an anemic Jehovah's Witness during extensive abdominal wall resection and reconstruction. Ann Plast Surg 1989;22:448–452.
30. Kraft M, Dedrick D, Goudsouzian N. Haemodilution in an eight-month-old infant. Anaesthesia 1981;36:402–404.
31. Chaney MA, Aasen MK. Severe acute normovolemic hemodilution and survival [letter; comment]. Anesth Analg 1993;76:1371–1372.
32. Trouwborst A, van Woerkens EC, van Daele M, Tenbrinck R. Acute hypervolaemic haemodilution to avoid blood transfusion during major surgery [see comments]. Lancet 1990;336:1295–1297.
33. Spence RK, Cernaianu AC, Carson J, DelRossi AJ. Transfusion and surgery. Curr Probl Surg 1993;30:1101–1180.
34. Dudrick SJ, O'Donnell JJ, Raleigh DP, et al. Rapid restoration of red blood cell mass in severely anemic surgical patients who refuse transfusion. Arch Surg 1985;120:721–722.
35. Brown AS, Reichman JH, Spence RK. Fluosol-DA, a perfluorochemical oxygen-transport fluid for the management of a trochanteric pressure sore in a Jehovah's Witness. Ann Plast Surg 1984;12:449–453.
36. Frackiewicz EJ, Lee R. Use of a blood substitute in a patient who refuses to accept a transfusion. Am J Hosp Pharm 1991;48:2176–2180.
37. Gonzalez ER. Fluosol—a special boon to Jehovah's Witnesses . . . [news]. JAMA 1980;243:720–724.
38. Karn KE, Ogburn PL Jr, Julian T, Cerra FB, Hammerschmidt DE, Vercellotti G. Use of a whole blood substitute, Fluosol-DA 20%, after massive postpartum hemorrhage. Obstet Gynecol 1985;65:127–130.
39. Waxman K, Tremper KK, Cullen BF, Mason GR. Perfluorocarbon infusion in bleeding patients refusing blood transfusions. Arch Surg 1984;119:721–724.
40. Spence RK, McCoy S, Costabile J, et al. Fluosol DA-20 in the treatment of severe anemia: randomized controlled study of 46 patients. Crit Care Med 1990;18:1227–1230.
41. Boshkov LK, Tredget EE, Janowska-Wieczorek A. Recombinant human erythropoietin for a Jehovah's Witness with anemia of thermal injury. Am J Hematol 1991;37:53–54.
42. DeMeester SR, Marsh EE, Gerkin TM, Rodriguez JL. Immediate use of recombinant erythropoietin in a Jehovah's Witness following major blunt trauma. Contemp Surg 1994;45:228–232.
43. Fletcher JL Jr, Perez JC, Jones DH. Successful use of subcutaneous recombinant human erythropoietin before cholecystectomy in an anemic patient with religious objections to transfusion therapy. Am Surg 1991;57:697–700.
44. Heinz R, Reisner R, Pittermann E. Erythropoietin for chemotherapy patient refusing blood transfusion [letter] [see comments]. Lancet 1990; 335:542–543.
45. Jim RT. Use of erythropoietin in Jehovah's Witness patients. Hawaii Med J 1990;49:209.
46. Johnson PW, King R, Slevin ML, White H. The use of erythropoietin in a Jehovah's Witness undergoing major surgery and chemotherapy [letter]. Br J Cancer 1991;63:476.
47. Kantrowitz AB, Spallone A, Taylor W, Chi TL, Strack M, Feghali JG. Erythropoietin-augmented isovolemic hemodilution in skull-base surgery. Case report. J Neurosurg 1994;80:740–744.
48. Koestner JA, Nelson LD, Morris JA Jr, Safcsak K. Use of recombinant human erythropoietin (r-HuEPO) in a Jehovah's Witness refusing transfusion of blood products: case report [see comments]. J Trauma 1990;30:1406–1408.
49. Larson B, Clyne N. A case report. Erythropoietin replaced blood transfusion. Lakartidningen 1993;90:1662.
50. Schiff SJ, Weinstein SL. Use of recombinant human erythropoietin to avoid blood transfusion in a Jehovah's Witness requiring hemispherectomy. Case report. J Neurosurg 1993;79:600–602.
51. Carson JL, Spence RK, Poses RM, Bonavita G. Severity of anemia and operative mortality and morbidity. Lancet 1988;2:727–729.
52. Spence RK, Carson JA, Poses R, et al. Elective surgery without transfusion: influence of preoperative hemoglobin level and blood loss on mortality. Am J Surg 1990;159:320–324.
53. Spence RK, Alexander JB, DelRossi AJ, et al. Transfusion guidelines for cardiovascular surgery: lessons learned from operations in Jehovah's Witnesses. J Vasc Surg 1992;16:825–831.
54. Ott DA, Cooley DA. Cardiovascular surgery in Jehovah's Witnesses. JAMA 1977;238:1256–1258.
55. Bonakdar MI, Eckhous AW, Bacher BJ, Tabbilos RH, Peisner DB. Major gynecologic and obstetric surgery in Jehovah's Witnesses. Obstet Gynecol 1982;60:587–590.
56. Nelson CL, Bowen WS. Total hip arthroplasty in Jehovah's Witnesses without blood transfusion. J Bone Joint Surg [A] 1986;68: 350–353.
57. Viele M, Weiskopf R. What can we learn about the need for transfusion from patients who refuse blood? The experience with Jehovah's Witnesses. Transfusion 1994;34:396–401.
58. Miller E, Paull D, Morrissey K, et al. Scalpel versus electrocautery in modified radical mastectomy. Am Surg 1988;54:284–286.
59. Pearlman NW, Stiegmann GV, Vance V, et al. A prospective study of incisional time, blood loss, pain, and healing with carbon dioxide laser, scalpel, and electrosurgery [see comments]. Arch Surg 1991;126: 1018–1020.

60. Ward P, Castro D, Ward S. A significant new contribution to radical head and neck surgery. The argon beam coagulator as an effective means of limiting blood loss. Arch Otolaryngol Head Neck Surg 1989;115:921–923.
61. Trent CS. Electrocautery versus epinephrine-injection tonsillectomy [see comments]. Ear Nose Throat J 1993;72:520–525.
62. Tan AK, Rothstein J, Tewfik TL. Ambulatory tonsillectomy and adenoidectomy: complications and associated factors. J Otolaryngol 1993;22:442–446.
63. Leach J, Manning S, Schaefer S. Comparison of two methods of tonsillectomy. Laryngoscope 1993;103:619–622.
64. Tchabo JG, Thomure MF, Tomai TP. A comparison of laser and cold knife conization. Int Surg 1993;78:131–133.
65. Bhatta N, Isaacson K, Flotte T, Schiff I, Anderson RR. Injury and adhesion formation following ovarian wedge resection with different thermal surgical modalities. Lasers Surg Med 1993;13:344–352.
66. Bordelon BM, Hobday KA, Hunter JG. Laser vs electrosurgery in laparoscopic cholecystectomy. A prospective randomized trial. Arch Surg 1993;128:233–236.
67. Shaha AR. Minimizing the blood loss during flap raising in thyroidectomy. J Surg Oncol 1993;52:153–154.
68. Andrews BT, Layer GT, Jackson BT, Nicholls RJ. Randomized trial comparing diathermy hemorrhoidectomy with the scissor dissection Milligan-Morgan operation. Dis Colon Rectum 1993;36:580–583.
69. Muraki J, Addonizio JC, Lastarria E, Eshghi M, Choudhury MS. New Cavitron system (CUSA/CEM): its application for kidney surgery. Urology 1993;41:195–198.
70. Wyman A, Rogers K. Randomized trial of laser scalpel for modified radical mastectomy [see comments]. Br J Surg 1993;80:871–873.
71. Neven P, Shepherd JH, Wilkinson DJ. Radical vulvectomy using the argon enhanced electro-surgical pencil. Br J Obstet Gynaecol 1993;100: 789–790.
72. Helkjaer PE, Eriksen PS, Thomsen CF, Skovdal J. Outpatient CO_2 laser excisional conization for cervical intraepithelial neoplasia under local anesthesia. Acta Obstet Gynecol Scand 1993;72:302–306.
73. Dowling RD, Ochoa J, Yousem SA, Peitzman A, Udekwu AO. Argon beam coagulation is superior to conventional techniques in repair of experimental splenic injury. J Trauma 1991;31:717–721.
74. Zhou XD, Tang ZY, Yu YQ, et al. Microwave surgery in the treatment of hepatocellular carcinoma. Semin Surg Oncol 1993;9:318–322.
75. Lau WY, Arnold M, Guo SK, Li AK. Microwave tissue coagulator in liver resection for cirrhotic patients. Aust N Z J Surg 1992;62:576–581.
76. Siniluoto TM, Luotonen JP, Tikkakoski TA, Leinonen AS, Jokinen KE. Value of pre-operative embolization in surgery for nasopharyngeal angiofibroma. J Laryngol Otol 1993;107:514–521.
77. Wakhloo AK, Juengling FD, Van Velthoven V, Schumacher M, Hennig J, Schwechheimer K. Extended preoperative polyvinyl alcohol microembolization of intracranial meningiomas: assessment of two embolization techniques [see comments]. AJNR Am J Neuroradiol 1993; 14:571–582.
78. Go H, Takeda M, Takahashi H, et al. Laparoscopic adrenalectomy for primary aldosteronism: a new operative method. J Laparoendosc Surg 1993;3:455–459.
79. Suzuki K, Kageyama S, Ueda D, et al. Laparoscopic adrenalectomy: clinical experience with 12 cases [see comments]. J Urol 1993;150: 1099–1102.
80. Pier A, Gotz F, Bacher C. Laparoscopic appendectomy in 625 cases: from innovation to routine. Surg Laparosc Endosc 1991;1:8–13.
81. Corbitt JD Jr. Laparoscopic cholecystectomy: laser versus electrosurgery [see comments]. Surg Laparosc Endosc 1991;1:85–88.
82. Senagore AJ, Luchtefeld MA, Mackeigan JM, Mazier WP. Open colectomy versus laparoscopic colectomy: are there differences? Am Surg 1993;59:549–554.
83. Jamieson GG, Corbel L, Campion JP, Launois B. Major liver resection without a blood transfusion: is it a realistic objective? Surgery 1992;112:32–36.
84. Deakin M, Gunson BK, Dunn JA, et al. Factors influencing blood transfusion during adult liver transplantation. Ann R Coll Surg Engl 1993;75:339–344.
85. Wu CC, Yang MD, Liu TJ. Improvements in hepatocellular carcinoma resection by intraoperative ultrasonography and intermittent hepatic inflow blood occlusion. Jpn J Clin Oncol 1992;22:107–112.
86. Baer HU, Stain SC, Guastella T, Maddern GJ, Blumgart LH. Hepatic resection using a water jet dissector. HPB Surg 1993;6:189–198.
87. Izumi R, Shimizu K, Kiriyama M, et al. Hepatic resection guided by needles inserted under ultrasonographic guidance. Surgery 1993;114: 497–501.
88. Makuuchi M, Kosuge T, Takayama T, et al. Surgery for small liver cancers. Semin Surg Oncol 1993;9:298–304.
89. Hannoun L, Borie D, Delva E, et al. Liver resection with normothermic ischaemia exceeding 1 h. Br J Surg 1993;80:1161–1165.
90. Kim YI, Nakashima K, Tada I, Kawano K, Kobayashi M. Prolonged normothermic ischaemia of human cirrhotic liver during hepatectomy: a preliminary report. Br J Surg 1993;80:1566–1570.
91. Terblanche J, Krige JE, Bornman PC. Simplified hepatic resection with the use of prolonged vascular inflow occlusion. Arch Surg 1991;126: 298–301.
92. Yamaoka Y, Ozawa K, Kumada K, et al. Total vascular exclusion for hepatic resection in cirrhotic patients. Application of venovenous bypass. Arch Surg 1992;127:276–280.
93. Elias D, Lasser P, Hoang JM, et al. Repeat hepatectomy for cancer. Br J Surg 1993;80:1557–1562.
94. Ryan JJ, Faulkner D II. Liver resection without blood transfusion. Am J Surg 1989;157:472–475.
95. Nagasue N, Kohno H, Chang YC, et al. Liver resection for hepatocellular carcinoma. Results of 229 consecutive patients during 11 years. Ann Surg 1993;217:375–384.
96. Leather RP, Shah DM, Kaufman JL, et al. Comparative analysis of retroperitoneal and transperitoneal aortic replacement for aneurysm. Surg Gynecol Obstet 1989;168:387–393.
97. Carrel T, Pasic M, Turina M, et al. The retroperitoneal approach: an excellent alternative to the transperitoneal route in elective aortic surgery. Int J Angio Winter 1992:1–5.
98. Cambria R, Brewster D, Abbott W, et al. Transperitoneal versus retroperitoneal approach for aortic reconstruction: a randomized prospective study. J Vasc Surg 1990;11:314–325.
99. Reid D, Pollock J. A prospective study of 100 gelatin-sealed aortic grafts. Ann Vasc Surg 1991;5:320–324.
100. Fisher JB, Dennis RC, Valeri CR, et al. Effect of graft material on loss of erythrocytes after aortic operations. Surg Gynecol Obstet 1991;173: 131–136.
101. Hans S, Masi J, Goyal V, et al. Increased blood loss with in situ bypass. Am Surg 1990;56:540–542.
102. Dorsey JS, Stone RM. Emergency portacaval shunting in Jehovah's Witnesses. Can J Surg 1980;23:197–198.
103. Simmons CW Jr, Messmer BJ, Hallman GL, Cooley DA. Vascular surgery in Jehovah's Witnesses. JAMA 1970;213:1032–1034.
104. Johnson RG, Murphy JM. The role of desmopressin in reducing blood loss during lumbar fusions. Surg Gynecol Obstet 1990;171: 223–226.
105. Keene GS, Parker MJ. Hemiarthroplasty of the hip—the anterior or

posterior approach? A comparison of surgical approaches. Injury 1993;24:611–613.
106. Grzeskiewicz J, Hall R, Anderson G, et al. Preoperative crossmatch guidelines for total hip arthroplasty. Orthopedics 1989;12:549–553.
107. Nelson IW, Sivamurugan S, Latham PD, Matthews J, Bulstrode CJ. Total hip arthroplasty for hemophilic arthropathy. Clin Orthop 1992;276:210–213.
108. Lotke PA, Faralli VJ, Orenstein EM, Ecker ML. Blood loss after total knee replacement. Effects of tourniquet release and continuous passive motion. J Bone Joint Surg [A] 1991;73:1037–1040.
109. Burkart BC, Bourne RB, Rorabeck CH, Kirk PG, Nott L. The efficacy of tourniquet release in blood conservation after total knee arthroplasty. Clin Orthop 1994;299:147–152.
110. Raut VV, Stone MH, Wroblewski BM. Reduction of postoperative blood loss after press-fit condylar knee arthroplasty with use of a femoral intramedullary plug. J Bone Joint Surg [A] 1993;75:1356–1357.
111. Heddle N, Brox W, Klama L, et al. A randomized trial on the efficacy of an autologous blood drainage and transfusion device in patients undergoing elective knee arthroplasty. Transfusion 1992;32:742–746.
112. Bowen JR, Angus PD, Huxster RR, MacEwen GD. Posterior spinal fusion without blood replacement in Jehovah's Witnesses. Clin Orthop 1985;198:284–288.
113. Brodsky JW, Dickson JH, Erwin WD, Rossi CD. Hypotensive anesthesia for scoliosis surgery in Jehovah's Witnesses. Spine 1991;16: 304–306.
114. Bridenbaugh LD. Regional anesthesia for outpatient surgery—a summary of 12 years' experience. Can Anaesth Soc J 1983;30:548–552.
115. Bjoraker D. Blood transfusion. What is a safe hematocrit? Prob Crit Care 1991;5:386–399.
116. Blackwell K, Ross D, Kapur P, et al. Propofol for maintenance of general anesthesia: a technique to limit blood loss during endoscopic sinus surgery. Am J Otolaryngol 1993;14:262–266.
117. Krausz M, Meital B, Rabinovici R, et al. "Scoop and run" or "stabilize" hemorrhagic shock by normal saline or small-volume hypertonic saline. J Trauma 1992;33:6–9.
118. Bickell W, Bruttig S, Millnamoro G, et al. The deterimental effects of intravenous crystalloid after experimental aortotomy in swine. Surgery 1991;110:529–534.
119. Martin R, Bickell W, Pepe P, et al. Prospective evaluation of preoperative fluid resuscitation in hypotensive patients with penetrating truncal injury: A preliminary report. J Trauma 1992;33:354–362.
120. Lilly M, Gala G, Carlson D, et al. Saline resuscitation after fixed-volume hemorrhage. Role of resuscitation volume and rate of infusion. Ann Surg 1992;216:161–171.
121. Rabinovici R, Krausz MGF. Control of bleeding is essential for successful treatment of hemorrhagic shock with 7.5 percent sodium chloride solution. SGO 1991;173:98–106.
122. Younes R, Aun F, Accioly C, et al. Hypertonic solutions in the treatment of hypovolemic shock: a prospective, randomized study in patients admitted to the emergency room. Surgery 1992;111:380–385.
123. Vassar M, Perry C, Gannaway W, et al. 7.5% sodium chloride/dextran for resuscitation of trauma patients undergoing helicopter transport. Arch Surg 1991;126:1065–1072.
124. Jackson M, Olson D, Beckett WJ, et al. Abdominal vascular trauma: a review of 106 injuries. Am Surg 1992;58:622–626.
125. Lopez-Viego M, Snyder WD, Valentine R, et al. Penetrating abdominal aortic trauma: a report of 129 cases. J Vasc Surg 1992;16:332–335.
126. Brathwaite C, Rodriguez A. Injuries of the abdominal aorta from blunt trauma. Am Surg 1992;58:350–352.
127. Williams D, Dake M, Bolling S, et al. The role of intravascular ultrasound in acute traumatic aortic rupture. Semin Ultrasound CT MR 1993;14:85–90.
128. Samuels L, Gross C, DiGiovanni R, et al. External iliac artery occlusion due to pelvic fracture: management with a cross-femoral bypass graft. South Med J 1993;86:572–574.
129. van Wijngaarden M, Omert L, Rodriguez, et al. Management of blunt vascular trauma to the extremities. Surg Gynecol Obstet 1993;177: 41–48.
130. Marin M, Veith F, Panetta T, et al. Percutaneous transfemoral insertion of a stented graft to repair a traumatic femoral arteriovenous fistula. J Vasc Surg 1993;18:299–302.
131. Gliedman M, Langer B, Rikkers L, et al. Management of variceal bleeding. Contemp Surg 1992;41:49–62.
132. Stiegmann G, Goff J, Michaletz-Onody P, et al. Endoscopic sclerotherapy as compared with endoscopic ligation for bleeding esophageal varices. N Engl J Med 1992;326:1527–1532.
133. Burroughs A, Hamilton G, Phillips A, et al. A comparison of sclerotherapy with staple transection of the esophagus for the emergency control of bleeding from esophageal varices. N Engl J Med 1989;321:857–862.
134. Berard P. Surgical treatment of hemorrhage from ruptured esophageal varices by an orally introduced clip to provoke sclerosis of the lower esophagus and ligation of the peri-esophageal veins through a thoracic approach. Results in 108 cases treated over a period of 5 years. J Chir (Paris) 1984;121:389–393.
135. Nagasue N, Kohno H, Ogawa Y, et al. Appraisal of distal spinal renal shunt in the treatment of esophageal varices: an analysis of prophylactic emergency and elective shunts. World J Surg 1989;13:92–99.
136. Harville L, Rivera F, Palmaz J, et al. Variceal hemorrhage associated with portal vein thrombosis: treatment with a unique portal venous stent. Surgery 1992;111:585–590.
137. Ring EJ, Lake JR, Roberts JP, et al. Using transjugular intrahepatic portosystemic shunts to control variceal bleeding before liver transplantation [see comments]. Ann Intern Med 1992;116:304–309.
138. LaBerge J, Ring E, Gordon R, et al. Creation of transjugular intrahepatic portosystemic shunts with the wallstent endoprosthesis: results in 100 patients. Radiology 1992;187:413–420.
139. Martin M, Zajko A, Orons P, et al. Transjugular intrahepatic portosystemic shunt in the management of variceal bleeding: indications and clinical results. Surgery 1993;114:719–726.
140. Goldman EB, Oberman HA. Legal aspects of transfusion of Jehovah's Witnesses. Transfus Med Rev 1991;5:263–270.
141. Schloendorff *v* Society of New York Hospital. 211 NY 1914:125.
142. Goldman E. Legal issues in blood transfusion. Alternatives to homologous blood use. Denver, CO: Education Design, 1992:16–20.
143. Luban NL, Leikin SL. Jehovah's Witnesses and transfusion: the pediatric perspective. Transfus Med Rev 1991;5:253–258.
144. In re Green. 292 A 2d 1971:387.
145. In re EG. No. 66089 Illinois Supreme Court 1989.
146. Ackerman TF. The limits of beneficence: Jehovah's Witnesses & childhood cancer. Hastings Cent Rep 1980;10:13–18.
147. Bausch LC. Blood transfusions and the Jehovah's Witness—neonatal perspectives. Nebr Med J 1991;76:283–284.
148. Henling C, Carmichael M, Keats A, Cooley DA. Cardiac operation for congenital heart disease in children of Jehovah's Witnesses. J Thorac Cardiovasc Surg 1985;89:914–920.
149. Kawaguchi A, Bergsland J, Subramanian S. Total bloodless open heart surgery in the pediatric age group. Circulation 1984;70(3 Pt 2):I30–37.
150. Battery claim of Jehovah's Witness rejected by Michigan Court [editorial]. Hospital Law Newsletter 1992;9:4–7.

Chapter 12

Quality Control of Hospital Transfusion Practices

LINDA S. BARNES
CYNTHIA M. MURRAY
THOMAS H. PRICE

INTRODUCTION

It is widely recognized that the blood supply has never been safer (1). The strides achieved in improved safety are in large part due to constant surveillance by blood banks and clinicians along with increased scrutiny by consumer groups and government bodies such as the U.S. Food and Drug Administration (FDA). Blood centers and transfusion services, as with other health care providers, have struggled mightily under the influence of competing interests that demand the ultimate in safety while forcing cost reductions.

Recent attention to blood safety has been directed almost exclusively toward reducing the risk of infectious disease transmission, yielding more intrusive donor health screening, expansion of rigorous donor selection criteria, and broadened infectious disease marker testing. The burgeoning battery of laboratory tests to which the volunteer blood donor is subjected signals a singular obsession with reducing the potential for viral or parasitic infection through blood. Rarely, if ever, does public examination of transfusion quality extend beyond infectious risk.

In the future, extensive DNA- and RNA-based tests will likely be regarded as seminal advances in blood safety. Yet the prominent admonition in the Circular of Information, "WARNING: The risk of transmitting infectious agents is present. Careful donor selection and available laboratory tests do not eliminate the hazard," will likely remain a permanent clause notwithstanding extraordinary efforts to surmount the risk (2). Despite the exhaustive scrutiny for infectious agents at exponential cost, the safety of blood transfusion cannot be reduced to the potential for disease transmission alone.

Far beyond the donor interview room and the laboratory bench, substantial possibilities for improving transfusion safety remain outside civic survey. Herein lie the hidden opportunities to further improve the quality of transfusion medicine. Ensuring the overall quality of blood transfusion necessitates evaluation of the entire system under which a transfusion is administered: materials, methods, people, and environment. This realm is within the purview of the physicians, clinical professionals, and health care institutions. Within this domain, the surgeon operates.

Rather than focusing narrowly on examination of the potential for disease transmission, the charge for those practicing transfusion medicine must broadly encompass the propriety of transfusion and the context in which the transfusion is administered. The quality of transfusion practice depends on appropriate controls in the systems supporting blood administration: procedures and policies, personnel training and competency, record-keeping and audit trails, and the establishment of oversight systems such as transfusion committees dedicated to monitoring efficacy.

Quality control in transfusion medicine requires a comprehensive understanding of the associated hazards, definition of mechanisms that ensure process control, and monitoring systems to assess appropriate practice. Complex interdependencies support clinical blood transfusion, requiring the establishment of rigid procedures to prevent error and delineate lines of communication between those on the floor and the transfusion service. Those ordering blood should be fully aware of the role of the transfusion committee and the standard formulas used by institutions to ensure the quality of transfusion practices. And if despite every effort to prevent it, a disease transmission occurs, it is the role of the transfusing physician to be aware of what follow-up is indicated.

The surgeon must be familiar with hospital transfusion policy, the systems that ensure safety and efficacy, and assert proper protocol. This chapter explores each of these areas in three sections.

GENERAL ASPECTS OF QUALITY CONTROL AND QUALITY ASSURANCE

AVOIDABLE RISK

In quantitative terms, blood transfusion remains one of the safest invasive medical procedures (3). The major adverse effects are the result of infection or immunological incompatibility. These adverse effects may be considered either avoidable or unavoidable. Examples of unavoidable risk may include window-period infections or rare incompatibilities. Avoidable risk, or that which can be prevented, may include use of the wrong unit for transfusion or the otherwise avoidable risks associated with administration of blood components when not indicated. Deaths attributed to such preventable cause as a mismatched transfusion may occur at least as frequently as deaths from transfusion-transmitted human immunodeficiency virus (HIV) (3). Despite the small hazard of death that blood transfusion presents—estimated at less than 1 in 100,000 patients transfused—this risk assumes new significance in the era of transfusion-transmitted HIV, which is calculated to occur with a similar, yet decreasing, frequency (4).

Excluding transfusion-transmitted disease, the most common cause of death secondary to transfusion is acute intravascular hemolysis (4). A recent FDA review of approximately 150 transfusion-related fatalities from 1990 to 1992 revealed that almost one-third of the deaths may have been prevented had appropriate controls been present or practiced at the time of transfusion (5). Such controls range from adequacy of procedures and properly trained personnel to appropriate use of equipment. It is estimated that between 800 and 900 misdirected transfusions occur each year in the United States, 10–20 of which lead to death (4). In a study of transfusion errors in New York State, the mortality rate was established to be 1 in 600,000 red blood cell transfusions. By virtue of the fact that most mismatched transfusions would not lead to incompatibility, the estimated incidence of transfusion error was determined to be 1 in 12,000 red blood cells transfused (6).

SOURCES OF ERROR

In examining the source of error in transfusion practice, clerical mistakes are by far the most commonly implicated cause (4, 6–8). A clerical error may be broadly defined as a failure to properly observe and record information (e.g., transcription errors) or recording the right test result on the wrong record (4). Closer examination reveals that wherever errors can be made, errors occur (Table 12.1). No aspect of transfusion is without the potential for omission, misinterpretation, or simple human error. Although it may seem inexcusable to fail to properly identify the intended patient, such omissions occur much too frequently to disregard the root causes. It may be tempting to blame the individual who made the mistake, but evaluation must extend beyond the particulars of the error into examination of the systems supporting transfusion.

System failures bear the brunt of responsibility for the continuing and increasing percentage of fatalities due to ABO incompatibility. Approximately two-thirds of ABO incompatibilities relate to misidentification. In examining where errors or omissions led to the wrong unit being administered, the following systems failed (9):

1. Pretransfusion sample was drawn from the wrong patient;
2. Pretransfusion sample was drawn from the right patient but labeled with the wrong name—usually when labeling occurred subsequent to the collection of the sample;
3. Mislabeling supplementary tubes aliquoted from the original sample;
4. Storing blood in an unmonitored operating room refrigerator from which the wrong unit of blood is all too easily removed;
5. Issuing the wrong unit from the blood bank;
6. Failing to adequately check patient identification to ensure that the unit is transfused to the correct patient.

TABLE 12.1. EXAMPLES OF PROCESS FAILURES LEADING TO TRANSFUSION ERROR

1. Failure to properly identify the patient at the time of phlebotomy;
2. Incorrectly labeled phlebotomy sample;
3. Improperly identified sample aliquot for serological assay;
4. Wrong sample tested;
5. Result recorded on the wrong record;
6. Wrong unit selected;
7. Wrong patient transfused because of inadequate identification or checking.

Reprinted with permission from Sazema K. Reports of 355 transfusion-related fatality reports—a summary. Nurs Mngmnt 1994;25:80I, 80L, 80O.

Each of these errors should have been prevented or at least identified through proper quality control mechanisms. If the system is robust, errors that do occur should be detected and corrected. All too often, subsequent omissions in protocol allow the error to result in significant patient risk. Although it may be easy to establish that the source of an error or omission occurred elsewhere in the process, the bedside is the last opportunity for a potentially fatal mistake to be detected. To err is human; appropriate safeguards must prevent harm.

A hospital that fails to manage the entire process of transfusion of blood components, including systems of administering blood to the correct recipient, puts itself at unnecessary liability (4). For this reason, efforts to eliminate transfusion error must be cooperative and hospital-wide. Facilities that lack established blood administration protocols and mechanisms dedicated to monitoring compliance are the ones most often implicated in transfusion-related fatalities (5).

It is through quality management initiatives that processes are standardized, controlled, and monitored. Although many institutions may ascribe to various theories of quality, including Total Quality Management, Total Process Control, and Continuous Quality Improvement, the approach is the same. Systems are subdivided into defined processes, the interdependencies examined, monitors established, and targeted improvements instituted.

QUALITY CONTROL AND ASSURANCE

Theoretically speaking, the practice of quality control encompasses establishing specifications for each quality characteristic of a process, assessing the procedures used to determine conformance to specifications, and instituting corrective actions necessary to achieve conformance. Quality control is the method by which actual performance is measured against quality goals. The difference is rectified through corrective action. Thus, quality control is largely directed toward meeting objectives and preventing adverse events (10). The emphasis is on controlling processes verified by inspection.

Built on the premise of quality control is that of quality assurance. Although quality control provides information on the performance of a given process and requires corrective action, quality assurance relies on analyzing quality control data to determine the source and magnitude of variation. This evaluation includes ongoing monitoring of activities that may or may not be directly related to the process being examined. For example, quality assurance in transfusion medicine may include broad considerations of financial impacts, competency assessment, and patient outcomes. Feedback from these considerations is used to error-proof the process rather than solely correct failures. The focus of quality assurance is in proactively reducing opportunities for error, thus preventing failures in the system (11).

Beyond quality assurance lies the realm of quality improvement where, in addition to evaluation of quality indicators and performance measures, information is proactively solicited to create beneficial change (10). Examples may include customer surveys, benchmarking against other peer institutions, and detailed methods analysis. Often, teams of professionals with profound knowledge of the process being examined are assigned to reengineer or significantly modify the system to reduce waste, prevent errors, or improve service to clients (12).

REGULATORY CONSIDERATIONS

Historically, regulatory bodies, accrediting agencies, and peer-review groups focused almost exclusively on quality control. The FDA through the Center for Biologics, Evaluation and Research gained oversight for the manufacture and transfusion of blood components via the U.S. Public Health Service Act and the Federal Food, Drug, and Cosmetic Act (13). The FDA's current Good Manufacturing Practices, amended for blood products in 1974, required procedure definitions and process controls for all blood establishments and transfusion services (14). The American Association of Blood Banks (AABB) and Joint Commission for the Accreditation of Health Care Organizations (JCAHO) relied heavily on strict standards of practice and subsequent evaluation of correction action for accreditation (15).

Even now, compliance with each of the above is assessed by external auditors who search for weakness and problems through inspection. If any are found, the facility is given a strict time frame to remedy the problem or face ostracism at the least. On the next inspection, evidence of remedies to prior citations is verified, and then the search for new deficiencies begins anew. In this manner, quality is retrospectively and artificially shaped by external review of operations and quality control (12). Performance on inspections is viewed as the gold standard.

In recent years, the transit from this classical perspective is plainly illustrated by increased emphasis on establishing internal evaluation mechanisms to reduce, if not prevent, system failures. In 1995, the FDA released the *Guidelines for Quality Assurance for Blood Establishments,* which stressed preventing errors rather than simply detecting them retrospectively (16). AABB requires institutional members to establish a quality control program complete with identification of systems, critical control points, key elements, and system checks. In 1994, AABB published a thorough compendium constituting the basic elements of a quality program inclusive of stipulations for transfusion services and blood administration (17). By 1995, JCAHO concluded the principal transition of the *Accreditation Manual for Hospitals* from a source that articulated requirements for structures and processes as ends in themselves to one that relates performance of essential processes to patient outcomes (18).

Although such paradigm shifts in the external climate may facilitate quality improvements, the mere ascription to philosophy merits little until practices are modified. Although increased attention to quality assurance activities in the blood bank over the past few years has been quite effective in reducing errors, more attention must be paid to transfusion-related activities on the hospital floor (3, 7). How these principles translate into day-to-day practice by transfusionists will be the true measure of success.

PROCESS CONTROLS

In examining the processes that must function without fail in transfusion practice, it is difficult to relegate the primary responsibility solely to phlebotomists, blood banking technologists, admissions staff, ordering physicians, nursing personnel, the surgeon, or the transfusionist. Each must realize the interconnected nature of the role played in ensuring transfusion quality. Critical control points constitute junctures in the process that must be performed correctly to ensure the quality of transfusion. AABB has defined multiple processes that must proceed without error during compatibility testing, blood administration, and investigation of adverse effects. A selection of these systems and related critical control points is shown in Table 12.2.

Each critical control point consists of key elements that must function correctly for the transfusion to proceed without additional risk. For example, when administering blood, a critical control point relies on the appropriate unit being dispensed from the transfusion service. There must be a mechanism in place to ensure that autologous and designated/directed donations are issued in the correct order, that there is a verification step that the right unit was selected, and that the transfusion tag is completed with the required information. If any of these key elements is lacking, it is likely that the system will fail at this critical control point and that an incorrect unit may be dispensed for transfusion (17).

TABLE 12.2. SELECTED SYSTEMS AND CORRESPONDING CRITICAL CONTROL POINTS THAT MAY AFFECT TRANSFUSION QUALITY

System: compatibility testing
Critical control point
Blood order request form
Recipient identification
Specimen collection
Component ABO/Rh verification
Patient pretransfusion compatibility testing
System: blood administration
Critical control points
Dispensing the blood component
Pretransfusion recipient identification
Blood component administration
Appropriate use of blood components
System: investigation of adverse effects
Critical control points
Recognition of adverse effects
Investigation of adverse effects
Investigation of delayed (immunological) effect
Investigation of suspected transfusion-transmitted disease
Lookback

Reprinted with permission from Quality program: self-assessment manual. Vol II. Bethesda, MD: American Association of Blood Banks, 1994:I.2–K.2

STANDARD OPERATING PROCEDURES

A rudimentary yet often overlooked method of ensuring process control is through the written word. Often referred to as standard operating procedures (SOPs), written procedures clearly delineate roles, responsibilities, and appropriate methods for transfusion. A process cannot be controlled without benefit of definition. Lack of written policies and procedures to serve as the definitive description of practice begs error. Failure to establish written mechanisms significantly compromises the efficacy of transfusion.

Certain process controls are critical in ensuring that the correct unit is transfused to the proper patient (Table 12.3). Although by no means all inclusive, each of these transactions necessitates definition through SOP. To some it may seem burdensome or overly didactic to inscribe every step in the process, yet the benefits are indisputable. Not only does the SOP satisfy the requirement for basic instructions, it also serves as an interdisciplinary communication tool, audit template, and training guide.

TRAINING

Unfortunately, the existence of detailed SOPs does not guarantee that errors will not occur. One institution reported 1 in 6000 patients undergoing transfusion received an ABO-incompatible component; over half of the variances resulted from improper blood administration practice (8). Although

TABLE 12.3. PROCESS CONTROLS TO BE DEFINED BY WRITTEN POLICY AND PROCEDURE

Dispensing the blood component
Mechanisms to ensure that autologous and designated/directed donations are dispensed before allogeneic
Verification that the correct unit was selected
Transfusion tag completed with required information
Pretransfusion recipient identification
Mechanism for verification of MD order before transfusion
Informed consent
Comparison of the unit label with the patient identification band and requisition
Identification of the transfusionist on the transfusion record
Blood component administration
Directions for documentation of pretransfusion vital signs
Instructions for how to use filters, infusion devices, and ancillary equipment
Periodic documentation of patient vital signs
Signs and symptoms of adverse reactions
Instructions for documentation in the patient record
Disposal of hazardous waste
Appropriate use of blood components
Peer-review process
Directions for establishing and reviewing ordering and use of blood components
Communications mechanisms
Directions for tallying blood use
Directions for tallying blood waste
Directions for establishing and reviewing preoperative blood order schedules for allogeneic and autologous transfusion

Reprinted with permission from Quality program: self assessment manual. Vol II. Bethesda, MD: American Association of Blood Banks, 1994:J.1–J.10.

phlebotomy and transfusion service errors are responsible for some ABO-incompatible transfusions, the greatest number continues to result from the failure of the transfusionist to properly identify the patient or the blood component that the patient receives (5, 8). A 1994 CAP Q Probe study of 497 institutions found 60% of participating hospitals failed to compare the patient's name on the wrist band to the name on the compatibility tag, despite the requirement to do so (6).

Interestingly, a contributing factor to many transfusion-related fatalities correlates to recognizing the signs and symptoms of a transfusion reaction. Thus, not only did the primary error occur, but systems were inadequate to promote rapid treatment (5). Although most facilities have documented policies and procedures that describe apparent signs or symptoms of transfusion reactions and measures for prompt intervention, they may not be routinely communicated to the appropriate personnel.

Such fundamental flaws definitively illustrate the need for appropriate training of personnel. Personnel must be knowledgeable and competent to administer and monitor transfusions according to written policy. Such training should be periodic and ongoing rather than confined to the initial orientation period. Although an emphasis on training requires time and resources, the elimination of variance due to insufficient knowledge or simply stressing the importance of system checks significantly reinforces process integrity and enhances staff awareness.

PHYSICIAN'S ROLE IN THE QUALITY OF TRANSFUSION PRACTICE

The systems that support clinical blood transfusion are designed to prevent errors by building quality into the outcome of all processes. This is done by establishing control over each significant step in each process. These systems are designed to operate continuously and invisibly in the background of the daily practice of medicine. The physician can and should assume that these systems are in place and function optimally unless there are signs to the contrary. When things go wrong, it is important to think of root causes while inquiring or investigating why processes fail.

Generally speaking, the transfusion service bears the responsibility for dispensing the blood component and must have mechanisms in place to ensure that the correct unit is selected and released in the appropriate order. Once blood components have been issued from the transfusion service, the responsibility for safe transfusion extends to the ordering physician and the nursing team who will administer the component. The transfusion service is directed by a qualified physician, most commonly a hematologist or clinical pathologist, who is available for consultation on all issues concerning transfusion.

If a transfusion practice process has slipped out of control, the physician requesting the blood transfusion will be notified whenever the well-being of the patient may have been compromised. Specific areas of transfusing physician involvement will include

- Patient identification issues;
- Need to transfuse incompatible or uncross-matched blood;
- Inadvertent transfusion of incompatible blood;
- Transfusion of a blood component that was not processed as specified by the ordering physician;
- A transfusion reaction;
- Need for patient notification after transfusion;
- Transfusion-transmitted disease.

The role that the physician should assume in these situations may not be apparent because most of the process operates largely outside of the physician's control. Nonetheless, understanding the critical points in the process that may require intervention will help the physician determine the best course of action to follow.

PATIENT IDENTIFICATION ISSUES

Controversy will always surround the transfusion service department's adherence to rigid rules regarding patient identification and the suitability of the blood sample used for pretransfusion testing. Blood samples are difficult to obtain from hospitalized patients, especially children. For outpatients, returning to the laboratory for a redraw is a major inconvenience. The physician is often drawn into disputes about the suitability of a blood sample for pretransfusion testing.

Problems that may occur often involve incorrect or incomplete labeling of the patient sample (19). Patient identification may be illegible or may not agree with records on file in the transfusion service, raising a healthy level of suspicion about the reliability of the identification process. The serum provided for pretransfusion testing may be hemolyzed, compromising in vitro compatibility testing that must be performed before transfusion. Any of these reasons may cause the transfusion service to "reject" the sample and request a redraw.

Although these policies may be regarded by those outside of the transfusion service as overly paranoid, study after study has shown that a large fraction of the errors that result in negative patient outcome can be attributed to failures in proper patient identification (4). Of the 800–900 cases involving the erroneous transfusion of ABO-incompatible blood that occur annually in the United States, 43% could be directly traced to the improper identification of the recipient or the unit at the time of transfusion (6). Because the integrity of the patient identification process is so central to patient safety, hospitals have adopted such policies as

- Requirement for a written release with patient name and identification number before the issue of a unit from the transfusion service to avoid confusion over the identity of the intended recipient;
- Use of a second blood bank wristband identification system to force a second method of identification (the second system is often only numerical);
- Use of a "blood lock" identification system that adds a physical barrier to misidentification by placing a preprogrammed disposable combination lock on a plastic bag containing the unit to be transfused;
- Limitation of the authorized storage locations for blood components within the hospital;
- Requirement for careful segregation of units for a given patient within the operating room.

Adherence to patient identification procedures can be particularly difficult in the operating room because identification bands may be cut off to allow venous access or covered by surgical drapes. Alternative policies may need to be developed to ensure positive identification of the surgical patient before transfusion (8). These procedures may include cross-checking the identification band with another document or item bearing the patient's name and identification number before covering or removing the wristband. The item to which the wristband was cross-checked then acts as the primary identification for the purpose of blood transfusion.

TRANSFUSION OF INCOMPATIBLE OR UNCROSS-MATCHED BLOOD

Clinical situations will occur where the only choice for transfusion will be blood that is, despite the laboratory's best efforts, serologically incompatible (20). The patient's physician must participate in the decision to transfuse incompatible blood and should understand the nature of the incompatibility, the likelihood that an adverse reaction will occur, and the measures to be taken to detect and manage such reactions. Consultation with the laboratory and/or transfusion service physician is usually required. Only after full consideration of the issues should the transfusion proceed.

In difficult cases, additional investigation by an advanced level Immunohematology Reference Laboratory may be indicated. These services should be available from the local blood supplier on a 24-hour basis if it is not available within the hospital itself. Advanced investigations may take time and may require the postponement of transfusion. If the cause for the incompatibility is identified as a red cell alloantibody to a high incidence antigen and if the alloantibody is known to be associated with clinically significant red cell destruction, it is reasonable to expect the hospital, with the assistance of the local blood supplier, to request compatible blood through a national registry of rare blood donors. It may be possible to locate red blood cells that have been frozen to allow extended storage and availability (21). If, after all options are exhausted, the best decision is still to transfuse serologically incompatible blood, the patient should be carefully monitored for signs and symptoms of immediate or delayed red cell destruction. Similarly, if a patient's serum appears to contain a red cell antibody but there is not sufficient time to allow laboratory confirmation or identification of its specificity, any blood made available is considered to be uncross matched. Although transfusion in this situation is undesirable, it may be preferable to waiting for pretransfusion testing in the face of a life-threatening hemorrhagic emergency.

FDA regulations specifically addressing pretransfusion testing are few in number but do include the requirement that certain conditions be met if an emergency situation requires the transfusion of uncross-matched blood (22). The decision that a patient's condition requires transfusion before cross-matched blood is available must be documented and that statement must be signed by the responsible physician.

INADVERTENT TRANSFUSION OF INCOMPATIBLE BLOOD

Occasionally, the physician may be notified by the transfusion service that a patient has received blood that, in retrospect, was found to be incompatible. There are four scenarios under which this may occur. First, a patient is transfused with uncross-matched blood under emergency conditions and subsequent compatibility testing reveals a red cell antibody directed toward antigens that have been transfused. Second, a subsequent cross match may reveal an emerging antibody that was not previously detected, and nonroutine test methods that enhance the antibody's reactivity may show the antibody to have been present in the original sample. Third, it may be learned after the transfusion that the patient has a prior history of a clinically significant red cell antibody not currently demonstrable. There would have been no attempt to select blood based on the antibody's specificity, and the patient may have received blood positive for the relevant antigen. Finally, a testing error could have been made that was not detected before transfusion. In all of these cases, the patient must be closely monitored for the signs and symptoms of immediate or delayed hemolytic transfusion reactions, the latter typically characterized by an otherwise unexplained drop in hemoglobin concentration often coupled with a positive direct antiglobulin test (23).

TRANSFUSION OF A BLOOD COMPONENT NOT PROCESSED AS SPECIFIED BY THE ORDERING PHYSICIAN

In modern transfusion practice, there are widely accepted indications for processing blood components differently for different patients, as described in Chapter 2. These processes typically include gamma irradiation, leukoreduction by filtration, or saline washing of cellular components. The physician order may specify the processing that is necessary for proper care of the patient or hospital policy may dictate that all patients with a specific diagnosis receive blood components that have been processed in a certain manner (24, 25). System deficiencies at any point between ordering and administration can result in the transfusion of a compatible unit that was not processed as specified. Depending on the patient's disease process, the transfusion of cellular components that have not been irradiated or leukoreduced may have significant effect on patient outcome. If this occurs, the ordering physician must be notified to initiate appropriate interventions.

TRANSFUSION REACTIONS

Immediate adverse reactions to transfusion can range from urticaria to acute hemolysis. In most cases, transfusion reactions are benign, but the nursing and laboratory investigation must assume that the patient's symptoms other than urticaria are indicative of a potentially life-threatening reaction until proven otherwise (26). The physician must be informed that the patient has experienced an adverse reaction and should direct the management of the patient in consultation with the laboratory or transfusion service physician. In the rare case of an error in pretransfusion testing or administration, the physician should expect thorough investigation of all contributing factors and corresponding corrective action. Each step in the process must be examined for weaknesses that might have allowed the event to occur. Although many situations may appear to be "close calls" (i.e., a group O unit inadvertently given to a group A patient), these incidents serve as important signals that a critical control point has failed. Concern should also be given to the possibility of a reciprocal error that may involve yet another patient (i.e., 2 units of red blood cells may have been mutually mislabeled and transfused to the wrong patients).

PATIENT NOTIFICATION AFTER TRANSFUSION

A basic tenet of transfusion medicine is that a continuous audit trail of blood components from donor to recipient should be maintained (27). This is critical to facilitate the investigation of transfusion-transmitted disease such as hepatitis and HIV. The transfusion service department maintains a record of all components issued to patients within the institution. The patient chart should mirror this record and corroborate that those units issued were actually transfused unless otherwise noted. Records of blood component disposition are essential in the event recipient tracing is required.

Information about a blood donor's medical history may be learned *after* the donation and transfusion of a blood component. In fact, postdonation reports are received with surprising frequency and account for 35% of all error and accident reports to the FDA (28). If this information could affect the health of the recipient, the patient's physician will be advised of the situation to counsel or treat the patient accordingly.

This practice is commonly referred to as "lookback" and may involve transfusions that occurred many years earlier. The donor information is typically received by the blood supplier and transmitted to the director of the transfusion service at the transfusing institution. The director determines the identity of the recipient of the blood components(s) involved, contacts the patient's physician, and advises the physician as to current notification practices for the situation at hand. The patient's physician must decide whether to contact the patient, what to tell the patient, and what to suggest to the patient with regard to follow-up testing.

Factors affecting this decision will necessarily include an estimate of risk to the patient, the patient's clinical situation, psyche, social considerations (is there a sexual contact), and applicable hospital policy. If the physician decides not to inform the patient, the decision should be documented in the patient chart. If the patient is informed, there should be clear record of the information conveyed and the subsequent actions.

Donor information stimulating a lookback may be gained in one of three ways. After the donation, the donor may volunteer information that was not mentioned at the time of the donation. This information may call into question not only the most recent donation, but many donations in the past. The donor may have neglected, for instance, to mention a history of past intravenous drug use.

The donor may seroconvert for an infectious disease marker between donations, raising the concern that a unit may have been collected during an infectious window period. Typically, the recipients of any blood components donated within a year of a donor's seroconversion for markers of hepatitis and HIV are notified and are encouraged to seek follow-up testing.

As new tests are added to the cadre of screening tests performed on blood donors, a long-time donor may suddenly become ineligible to donate. Those units donated before the implementation of the new test may have been infectious for the agent and it may be appropriate to test prior recipients for the transmissible disease marker as well.

TRANSFUSION-TRANSMITTED DISEASE

Clinical or laboratory evidence that an infectious disease such as hepatitis or acquired immunodeficiency syndrome has been transmitted to a patient by transfusion should be reported to the director of the transfusion service (29). Records of the blood donor may provide further information to determine whether the transfusion was implicated. Although donation centers may take different approaches to prevention, the permanent exclusion of donors whose blood has been clearly implicated in the transmission of disease is an important step in protecting the safety of the blood supply.

ROLE OF THE TRANSFUSION COMMITTEE

The transfusion committee plays a crucial role in ensuring the quality of the hospital's transfusion policies and practices (30–32). Originally formed to simply monitor the ordering and use of blood and blood components, over the last 10–15 years, these committees have assumed a much wider role, becoming instrumental in the development of hospital transfusion policy, education of the hospital staff, and continuous process improvement activities. Many of these activities have been undertaken in response to regulatory requirements. JCAHO requires that the medical staff evaluate and monitor the appropriateness of transfusion of all blood components. Continuous process improvement activities are required for all aspects of transfusion and include ordering; distribution, handling, and dispensing; administration; and the effects of transfusion on the recipient. In addition, all confirmed transfusion reactions must be assessed (18). AABB standards require that a peer-review mechanism be in place to monitor transfusion practice for all blood components (33). Finally, the FDA requires that every transfusion service have procedures for investigation and management of adverse reactions to transfusion (14).

Within the above requirements, the committee may choose to focus on a wide variety of transfusion-related issues, the most common of which are discussed in more detail below. For each area chosen, the committee should identify processes for improvement, implement changes, monitor and document the effect of the changes, and maintain those processes that are successful. Reports of committee activities should be prepared regularly for the hospital administration. The transfusion committee often deals with sensitive issues that may have medicolegal implications for the hospital; thus, it is important to be aware of applicable laws regarding discoverability concerning the minutes and the communications of the committee.

STRUCTURE OF THE TRANSFUSION COMMITTEE

The transfusion committee is ideally a council devoted entirely to transfusion issues, although there is no regulatory requirement that this should be the case. In some institutions, these activities are included in the duties of committees devoted to broader issues such as laboratory affairs or quality assurance. In either case, the committee reports to hospital administration. It is important that the composition of the committee is broadly based and includes individuals from all departments that deal regularly with transfusion. Thus, members routinely include representatives from surgery, medicine, pediatrics, anesthesia, obstetrics, nursing, laboratory, quality assurance, the transfusion service, and the regional blood center. It is probably wise for the chair of the committee to be a physician other than the director of the transfusion service because the success of the committee requires the broad-based support of the entire hospital medical staff.

UTILIZATION REVIEW

Historically, the primary role of the transfusion committee has been to monitor the appropriateness of transfusion therapy, to identify situations in which therapy is not appropriate, and to take action to correct the situation. To accomplish this, objective guidelines must be established, and adherence to these guidelines must be monitored for all blood components and for all hospital departments. Ideally, these activities are carried out in cooperation with the medical staff, the overall goal being to ensure optimal patient care rather than to punish physicians who appear to be ordering blood components inappropriately.

Audit Criteria

The first step in utilization review is to establish audit criteria so that instances of inappropriate practice can be detected. These criteria should be based on relevant literature, guidelines, and expert panels and developed in collaboration with the medical staff (32, 34–38). At a minimum, they should include criteria for all standard blood components (whole blood, red blood cells, platelets, fresh frozen plasma, and cryoprecipitate), but guidelines for additional components such as leukoreduced products, irradiated products, and autologous blood collection and transfusion should also be considered. In addition, the committee may want to develop criteria to assess underutilization of blood components, the use of therapeutic hemapheresis, or the appropriateness of the quantity of blood transfused. The JCAHO requirement is that areas for improvement must be identified by this process, so it is important that the criteria are not set so liberally that all transfusions are considered appropriate. The criteria should be widely publicized and should be regularly reviewed and modified when appropriate. It is important to realize that these criteria are not to be interpreted as indications for transfusion, rather they are criteria used for flagging charts for auditing. In the audit process, the appropriateness of the transfusion must be determined by the information available to the clinician at the time of transfusion and not by information that becomes known at a subsequent time.

Extent of Review

From 1985 until 1991, JCAHO required that all transfusions be reviewed until the results consistently supported the conclusion that transfusion practice was appropriate. After that, selective review was permitted. The 1995 guidelines still require utilization review but allow selective review depending on the local circumstances and the number of the various components transfused. Thus, reasonable leeway is allowed and the committee may elect to target the reviews to those areas in which opportunities for improvement are believed to be most likely.

Timing of Review

Review of transfusion orders may take place prospectively, "concurrently," or retrospectively, the latter being the method most often associated with the functions of the transfusion committee. With prospective review, the order is reviewed by the transfusion service before the blood component is sent to the patient. This approach is the optimal one from the patient's point of view in that it is most effective in ensuring that each transfusion is appropriate. However, it is time-consuming, it may not work well in emergent situations, and it may cause friction between the transfusion service and the ordering physician. As a variant of prospective review, some hospitals have designed transfusion order forms on which the accepted indications for transfusion are listed; the ordering physician is required to mark which indication applies. The form has an educational function, serves as a self-administered prospective review of the order, and may be easily audited at a later time. Experience with this method has shown it to be effective and that the information provided by the physicians on the form has been accurate (31).

A concurrent review is actually retrospective but takes place within 1–2 days of the transfusion. If the transfusion appears to have been inappropriate, the transfusion service physician discusses the case with the ordering physician while the details of the case are still fresh, providing education where needed. This approach is also time-consuming, but the interaction between the transfusion service and the ordering physician often occurs under calmer circumstances than with prospective review.

The more traditional retrospective review occurs several weeks or months after the fact, the episode having been identified by chart review long after the patient has left the hospital. Although less time-consuming than either prospective or concurrent review, retrospective review is the least effective in terms of either physician education or prevention of inappropriate transfusion. Chart documentation is often inadequate to determine whether the transfusion was really indicated, and time may have dimmed the memories of the event to such an extent that the interaction is not very useful.

ROLE OF THE COMMITTEE IN THE REVIEW

Once the transfusion committee has determined that a transfusion appears to have been inappropriate, the ordering physician is usually contacted for clarification. It should be clear at this stage that the committee is seeking information on the reasons for the transfusion and that no accusations are being made. If, after receiving the information from the ordering physician, the committee concludes that the transfusion was not indicated, further communication of an educational rather than punitive nature is sent to the physician and to his or her department chair. The committee should then monitor the effect of this action on transfusion practice. Several studies have shown that transfusion practice can be affected by well-designed and executed review and educational procedures. With the most successful programs, the reviews are performed before or shortly after the planned transfusion, and the educational efforts involve personal interactions between the transfusion medicine physician and the ordering physician (39–44).

MONITORING TRANSFUSION REACTIONS

One charge of the transfusion committee is to evaluate all confirmed transfusion reactions. Ideally, this would include febrile and allergic reactions as well as hemolytic reactions, the purpose being not only to detect errors that may have contributed to the occurrence of the reactions, but also to evaluate the management of the reactions. It is the duty of the committee to establish the procedures for reporting and monitoring the occurrence and management of transfusion reactions. Reporting forms may be developed that provide guidelines on proper workup and management and, when completed by the nursing and medical staff, include all pertinent information about the reaction and how it was handled. The difficulty is that minor febrile and allergic reactions are very common, particularly on a busy oncology service, and it may be hard to convince the nursing staff that filling out paperwork for each of these reactions is a productive use of their time. It will be up to the committee to decide whether these minor reactions need the same attention afforded to suspected hemolytic transfusion reactions.

PERFORMANCE OF BLOOD CENTER

An adequate and timely supply of properly labeled and tested blood is essential to the proper care of patients and is thus a concern of the transfusion committee. The performance of the hospital's supplier of blood should be routinely evaluated so that any problems are identified early. Situations in which patient care might be compromised, such as need to cancel or delay surgery, excessive delay in delivery of blood and blood components, or inaccurately labeled or processed components, should be carefully monitored. If problems are identified, the blood supplier should be notified.

ORDERING, HANDLING, AND DISPENSING PRACTICES

The ordering and handling of blood and blood components are an integral part of a hospital's transfusion service and, as indicated above, have been identified by the JCAHO as an area for attention by the transfusion committee. Inappropriate ordering of blood by physicians is usually excessive ordering. As such, there is no direct adverse effect on the patient's care, but the cost is excessive and blood is removed from central inventory where it may be needed by other patients. The appropriateness of ordering is usually assessed by the cross match-to-transfusion (C/T) ratio. The appropriate C/T ratio depends on the kind of patient being transfused; it is usually less than 1.5 for patients with highly predictable transfusion needs but larger with trauma patients, for example, where the needs are much less predictable. The overall C/T ratio for most hospitals is less than 2.0. Many hospitals have found that the C/T ratio can be improved by the establishment of ordering guidelines for surgical procedures (maximum surgical blood ordering schedules). These guidelines specify the routine appropriate blood order for each procedure (e.g., no blood, type and screen only, number of units to cross match) and are developed by the surgical staff in concert with the transfusion committee based on the local transfusion experience with the various surgical procedures (45).

The transfusion committee should ensure that there are proper procedures for handling and dispensing blood. Relevant issues include maintenance of proper storage temperatures for blood components; minimizing waste of components due to improper handling or improper ordering; and separation of autologous, directed, and allogeneic units intended for the same patient.

EDUCATION OF CLINICAL STAFF

As indicated above, one charge of the transfusion committee is to identify areas for improvement in transfusion practice. Once these areas are identified, the education of the medical and/or nursing staff is likely to be an important feature of the corrective action. The committee has an important role to play in these educational activities, whether they are in the form of communication with individual practitioners, the design and implementation of educational instruments such as order forms or transfusion reaction forms, or the scheduling of conferences or inservices.

DEVELOPMENT OF HOSPITAL TRANSFUSION POLICIES

The transfusion committee can play an important role in the development of various transfusion-related hospital policies and procedures, although the final approval of such policies usually rests with the hospital administration. With the development of these policies, mechanisms should be put in place to allow monitoring of compliance with the policy and evaluation of the policy by the committee. The list of possibilities is endless, but the more commonly addressed issues are listed below.

Informed Consent

To the extent possible, all patients receiving transfusions should be informed of the benefits and risks associated with the therapy. This is not only sound medical practice but also important from a risk management point of view, because lawsuits resulting from adverse effects of transfusion often hinge on the patient's claim that he or she was not adequately informed. There must be documentation that the informed consent process has occurred. There are many ways to do this. Sections of the hospital general consent form or the surgical consent forms may deal with transfusion, or separate consent forms may be developed for transfusion. A physician note in the patient's chart indicating that the risks and benefits of transfusion have been discussed with the patient and that he or she consents to the transfusion is probably the ideal approach, but it is usually difficult to get physicians to do this.

Documentation Requirements

Adequate documentation of the ordering and administration of blood and blood components and the effects of the transfusion on the patient are important for proper patient care, for medicolegal reasons, and for compliance with JCAHO requirements. The transfusion committee should set the standards for the required documentation and have mechanisms in place to monitor compliance.

Patient Identification Procedures

Proper patient identification is a critical step in safe transfusion practice, and mistakes in patient identification are one of the most frequent causes of fatal transfusion reactions. Nursing and laboratory procedures for patient identification should be in place and enforced. Errors in identification should be routinely reviewed by the committee and flaws in the process quickly identified and corrected.

Transfusion Devices

Policies and procedures related to the use of devices such as blood warmers, intraoperative cell savers, postoperative cell salvage equipment, and apheresis machines should be approved by the transfusion committee, and methods for monitoring the use of these devices should be in place.

Autologous and Directed Donation Blood Policy

Hospital policy regarding the collection, handling, and transfusion of autologous blood should be established and approved by the transfusion committee. The need for improved management of the transfusion of autologous units has been identified as this form of transfusion therapy grows in popularity (46). The most serious error, giving autologous units to an unintended recipient, raises great concern because blood banking requirements do not mandate the testing of autologous units for infectious disease markers nor is compatibility testing required. Procedures should be in place to guarantee that patients receive autologous blood before receiving allogeneic blood, and indications for collection and transfusion of autologous blood may be different from those of allogeneic blood. In particular, the committee may want to set up mechanisms to monitor underuse of autologous blood. Similar considerations apply for the use of directed donor blood. Autologous blood should always be given before directed donor blood. It is probably important from a risk management perspective to guarantee that directed donor blood is given before community allogeneic blood, although there is no medical reason to do so.

Lookback Procedures

Occasionally, the hospital may be notified that certain patients have received blood from donors who subsequently reported high-risk behavior or who have been found on a subsequent donation to be positive for an infectious disease marker (e.g., anti-HIV or anti-HCV). Hospitals should have policies and procedures for how to handle this; for example, under what circumstances should the patients be notified, who should notify them, and what follow-up is indicated.

SUMMARY

The physician is one of many professionals responsible for quality control of transfusion medicine. Given the complex nature of clinical transfusion, multiple safeguards secure the propriety of blood use and the systems within which blood components are administered. Fundamental support structures such as process controls, SOPs, and training are necessary to provide definition and ensure consistency. When unusual circumstances arise, the physician plays a critical role in the quality of transfusion practice, particularly in situations requiring immediate clinical intervention or decisive action. As an oversight body, the hospital transfusion committee broadly supervises the quality of transfusion medicine, assessing blood utilization, establishing policies, and reviewing practices. Although not always apparent to the casual observer, these elements ensure the overall quality control of transfusion practice.

REFERENCES

1. Wenz B, Burns ER. Improvement in transfusion safety using a new blood unit and patient identification system as part of safe transfusion practice. Transfusion 1991;31:401–403.
2. Circular of information: for the use of human blood and blood components. American Association of Blood Banks, American Red Cross, the Community Council of Blood Centers, March 1994:1.
3. Dodd RY. Adverse consequences of blood transfusion: quantitative risk estimates. In: Nance TS, ed. Blood supply: risks, perceptions and prospects for the future. Bethesda, MD: American Association of Blood Banks, 1994:1–19.
4. Sazama K. Reports of 355 transfusion-associated deaths 1976 through 1985. Transfusion 1990;30:583–590.
5. Mummert TB, Tourault MA. Transfusion-related fatality reports—a summary. Nurs Manage 1994;25:80I, 80L, 80O.
6. Linden JV, Paul B, Dressler KP. A report of 104 transfusion errors in New York State. Transfusion 1992;32:601–606.
7. Ringel M. Getting to the root of transfusion errors. CAP Today 1995;9: 12–16.
8. Shulman IA, Lohr K, Derdiarian AK, Picukaric JM. Monitoring transfusionist practices: a strategy for improving transfusion safety. Transfusion 1994;34:11–15.
9. Myrhe BA, Bove JR, Schmidt PJ. Wrong blood—a needless cause of surgical deaths [editorial]. Anesth Analg 1981;60:777–778.
10. Juran JM. Companywide planning for quality. In: Juran JM, Gryna FM, eds. Juran's quality control handbook. 4th ed. San Francisco: McGraw-Hill, 1988:6.31–6.32.
11. Cembrowski GS, Carey RN. Laboratory quality management: QC/QA. Chicago: American Society of Clinical Pathologists Press, 1989:5–6.
12. Berte LM. Managing quality in hospital transfusion medicine. Lab Med 1994:25;118–123.
13. Solomon JM. The evolution of the current blood banking regulatory climate. Transfusion 1994:31;272–277.
14. Code of Federal Regulations, 21 CFR 600–640.
15. Mintz PD. Quality assessment and improvement of transfusion practices. In: Rossi EC, Simon TL, Moss GS, Gould SA, eds. Principles of transfusion medicine. Baltimore: Williams & Wilkins, 1996:907–915.
16. FDA Guidelines: guidelines for quality assurance in blood establishments. Washington, DC: Food and Drug Administration, 1995.
17. Quality program: self assessment manual. Bethesda, MD: American Association of Blood Banks, 1994:I, J, K.
18. Accreditation manual for hospitals, 1995. Vol. 1. Oakbrook Terrace, IL: Joint Commission for the Accreditation of HealthCare Organizations, 1994.
19. Technical manual. 11th ed. Bethesda, MD: American Association of Blood Banks, 1993:310.
20. Habibi B. Pretransfusion compatibility assurance: past and present in quality assurance in transfusion medicine. Boca Raton, FL: CRC Press, 1992:267–292.
21. Mollison PL, Engelfriet CP, Contreras M. Blood transfusion in clinical medicine. 9th ed. London: Blackwell Scientific Publications, 1993:419.
22. Code of Federal Regulations, 21 CFR 606.151 (e).
23. Technical manual. 11th ed. Bethesda, MD: American Association of Blood Banks, 1993:484.
24. Anderson K. Clinical implications for blood component irradiation. Bethesda, MD: American Association of Blood Banks, 1992:31–49.
25. Wenz B. Clinical and laboratory precautions that reduce the adverse reactions, alloimmunization, infectivity and possibly immunomodulation associated with homologous transfusions. Transf Med Rev 1990;4:3–7.
26. Standards for blood banks and transfusion services. 16th ed. Bethesda, MD: American Association of Blood Banks, 1994:35.
27. Code of Federal Regulations, 21 CFR 606.160 (c).
28. FDA Center for Biologics, Evaluation and Research: Summary of error and accident reports, Fourth quarter FY-95, 1995.
29. Standards for blood banks and transfusion services. 16th ed. Bethesda, MD: American Association of Blood Banks, 1994:36.
30. Grindon AJ, Tomasulo PS, Bergin JJ, et al. The hospital transfusion committee. JAMA 1985;253:540–543.
31. Mintz PD. Quality assessment and improvement of transfusion practices. Hematol Oncol Clin North Am 1995;9:219–232.
32. Stehling L, Luban NLC, Anderson KC, et al. Guidelines for blood utilization review. Transfusion 1994;34:438–448.
33. Standards for blood banks and transfusion services. 16th ed. Bethesda, MD: American Association of Blood Banks, 1994:2.
34. Blanchette VS, Hume HA, Levy GJ, Luban NLC, Strauss RG. Guidelines for auditing pediatric blood transfusion practices. Am J Dis Child 1991;145:787–796.
35. Silberstein LE, Kruskall MS, Stehling LC, et al. Strategies for the review of transfusion practices. JAMA 1989;262:1993–1997.
36. Perioperative red cell transfusion. JAMA 1988;260:2700–2703.
37. Platelet transfusion therapy. JAMA 1987;257:1777–1780.
38. Fresh frozen plasma. Indications and risks. JAMA 1985;253:551–553.
39. Clark JA, Ayoub MM. Blood and component wastage report: a quality assurance function of the hospital transfusion committee. Transfusion 1989;29:139–142.
40. Despotis GJ, Grishaber JE, Goodnough LT. The effect of an intraoperative treatment algorithm on physicians' transfusion practice in cardiac surgery. Transfusion 1994;34:290- 296.
41. Rosen NR, Bates LH, Herod G. Transfusion therapy: improved patient care and resource utilization. Transfusion 1993;33:341–347.
42. Simpson MB. Prospective-concurrent audits and medical consultation for platelet transfusions. Transfusion 1987;27:192–195.
43. Soumerai SB, Salem-Schatz S, Avorn J, et al. A controlled trial of educational outreach to improve blood transfusion practice. JAMA 1993; 270:961–966.
44. Toy PTCY. Effectiveness of transfusion audits and practice guidelines. Arch Pathol Lab Med 1994;118:435–437.
45. Friedman BA. An analysis of surgical blood use in United States hospitals with application to the maximal surgical blood order schedule. Transfusion 1979;19:268.
46. AABB position on testing of autologous units. Bethesda, MD: American Association of Blood Banks, 1995.

Chapter 13

Legal Duties to Patients and Dispute Resolution

JIM MACPHERSON
STEVEN LABENSKY

INTRODUCTION

No physician today, including and especially the surgeon, treats his or her patient unaware of the legal responsibilities and potential consequences should an adverse outcome occur. The tragedy of transfusion-related acquired immunodeficiency syndrome (AIDS) has given rise to new approaches for determining whether a transfusion is necessary, whether additional options are available to the patient, or whether special informed consent is required for the transfusion. A large number of AIDS-related lawsuits have been instituted against attending physicians, the physicians who ordered the blood (if different), the hospitals where the transfusions took place, and the blood centers or hospitals collecting the blood. These and other cases have helped redefine responsibilities to patients, threatened to redefine what and who determines the appropriate standard of care, and spawned new and sometimes novel procedures for avoiding and managing transfusion-related medical malpractice claims. This chapter briefly reviews those developments.

TRANSFUSIONS AND MEDICAL MALPRACTICE CLAIMS

Transfusions have always contained risks. The widespread use of transfusions since the late 1960s, which made many highly complex surgeries and aggressive chemotherapies possible, coincided with improvements in transfusion safety and the sophistication of blood component therapy. Before near-universal reliance on volunteer donors and tests for hepatitis B introduced during the early 1970s, an estimated 20% of patients suffered an adverse and usually unavoidable consequence from a transfusion. By 1980, the safety of the blood supply was largely, and with justification, taken for granted. Unfortunately, we were unaware that viruses like human immunodeficiency virus (HIV) and human T-cell lymphotropic virus existed, much less that they had already entered the blood supply. We were also unaware of the extensive transfusion-associated infection with non-A, non-B hepatitis and the disease's long-term sequelae for many patients.

Transfusion-related HIV infection has indelibly changed the medical community and the public perception of transfusions. HIV has also shaken modern society's perception of invulnerability to infectious diseases. Where once a blood transfusion was viewed as an adjunct to improving the quality of life, it is now viewed as a dangerous and contaminated drug that should be largely reserved for life-threatening situations. Ironically, this has occurred at a time when all agree that the blood supply has never been safer. Yet this public perception, coupled with an ever-increasingly litigious society, has created a climate where physicians who prescribe blood, health care professionals who transfuse blood, hospitals where the blood is transfused, and blood centers which collect, test, and distribute it are subject to lawsuits for adverse results, some of which are known and unavoidable.

OVERVIEW

In a legal sense, a legal claim is a demand for compensation. A medical malpractice claim arises from the negligent provision of medical services. Usually, such claims are accompanied by a lawsuit, although as indicated below, increasingly claims are being resolved outside of the courts. A lawsuit is brought by a plaintiff, that is, the injured patient or, if the patient has died, the estate. Sometimes other plaintiffs, for example, the spouse or minor children, may bring derivative claims such as loss of consortium or loss of support as well as claims for personal injuries, such as the secondary transmission of bloodborne infections. To recover, however, in our fault-based system of justice, a plaintiff must still prove the underlying medical malpractice claim. The physician, hospital, and/or others involved in the delivery of the medical services are, obviously, the defendants.

Understanding when and why a plaintiff can prevail in a malpractice lawsuit can help a physician better know what actions should be taken before and during the delivery of a medical service. Our justice system, unfortunately, uses the terms winners and losers, although victims are often winners and losers can become victims. For the plaintiff to win, he or she must prove each of the following elements:

1. The defendant owed the plaintiff a duty to use reasonable care (also known as due care);
2. The defendant breached this duty;
3. The plaintiff was injured;
4. The defendant's breach caused the plaintiff's injury.

The plaintiff must prove each of these elements by a preponderance of the evidence. This means that the fact finder (usually the jury) must consider it is more likely than not that the proposition advanced by the plaintiff is true. Each of these elements is discussed below.

THE DEFENDANT'S DUTY AND THE PROFESSIONAL'S STANDARD OF CARE

The principal difference between an ordinary negligence action and a medical malpractice action is the nature and scope of the defendant's duty. In an ordinary negligence action, the defendant's duty is measured by what a reasonably prudent person would do under the circumstances of the case. The jury is presumed to have sufficient knowledge and experience to determine how this hypothetical reasonably prudent person would behave and to judge the defendant's conduct against this standard. For example, the law imposes on a driver the duty to use reasonable care when operating a car. The law presumes that a jury would know how a reasonably prudent driver would act under the circumstances of the case and whether the defendant driver has met this standard.

The physician-patient relationship creates a special duty on the part of the physician to exercise reasonable care when treating the patient. In a typical medical malpractice action, the jury is presumed not to possess the knowledge necessary to determine how a reasonably prudent professional such as a physician would act under the circumstances. Rather, courts have long afforded the medical (and other) professions a certain deference. Under most circumstances, the profession itself defines the appropriate conduct and the jury decides whether the defendant professional met this standard. This measure or level of appropriate behavior or conduct is the *standard of care*. It is often articulated as that degree of skill and knowledge possessed and exercised by members of the defendant's profession at or about the same time and under the same or similar circumstances. It is against this professional standard of care that the defendant professional is judged.

Traditionally, courts have afforded physicians four additional deferences with regard to the standard of care:

1. *The Locality Rule:* Until recently, most jurisdictions applied the locality rule providing that the standard of care was measured by the knowledge and skill of reasonably prudent physicians who practiced in the same locality as the defendant. Thus, a physician working in a rural area was not judged by what physicians were doing in urban medical centers but rather was judged by the conduct of other physicians practicing in rural communities. However, with the advent of nationwide standards, standardization of treatments, rapid and widespread dissemination of medical information, and uniform education and training, the locality rule has been, for the most part, abandoned. Now, a physician's acts or omissions are judged against a nationwide standard. The locality rule still exists to the extent that courts recognize that differences in available facilities, equipment, assistance, and logistics may dictate different but still appropriate behavior if, for example, the patient was in a rural or urban area.
2. *The Specialty Rule:* Although there may be a nationwide standard of care, one standard does not apply across the board to all professionals, regardless of their specialties. Instead, each physician is judged by the knowledge and skill of a reasonably prudent physician practicing in his or her specialty. Thus, a family practitioner in a rural community is not judged against the standards of an internist practicing in an urban area; his or her acts or omissions are measured against the knowledge and skill of reasonably prudent family practitioners. Courts, however, recognize that specialties may overlap. For example, although an orthopedic surgeon may not be qualified to describe the prevailing standard of care for a neurosurgeon performing the evacuation of a subdural hematoma, he or she may be qualified to opine on the neurosurgeon's performance of a cervical fusion at C5-C6, as both an orthopedic surgeon and a neurosurgeon perform that procedure.

3. *The Schools of Thought Doctrine:* An issue arises when there are two or more accepted practices or procedures; that is, there is no one standard of care. Under the schools of thought doctrine, a defendant's conduct will be judged against the measure of accepted practices of the school of thought to which he or she belongs. For this doctrine to apply, the defendant must establish two or more schools of thought on the medical practice or procedure at issue and that the adherence to one school of thought (normally, not the one espoused by the plaintiff) is reasonable.
4. *The Temporal Rule:* The prevailing standard of care is based on contemporaneous knowledge. Even though the lawsuit may come to trial years after the event at issue, the defendant should be judged by the standard prevailing at the time of the event. Subsequent developments and hindsight opinions are generally not allowed.

EXPERT WITNESSES

Because a jury is presumed not to know enough to set the standard of care for health care professionals, courts (as well as the parties and their attorneys) look to expert witnesses to assist with this task. Expert witnesses are those individuals who, based on their knowledge, training, education, skills, and experience, are familiar with the prevailing practices in their professions. They tell the jury how reasonably prudent physicians would act under the circumstances. They are also often allowed to tell the jury whether the defendant met or fell below this standard of care. Both the plaintiff and defendant are entitled to call one or more expert witnesses to define the standard of care, and the jury is then allowed to weigh competing expert testimony to reach its decision. The court instructs the jury that it cannot and should not substitute its own judgment for that of the experts when determining the standard of care. For all intents and purposes then, the typical medical malpractice action becomes a battle of the experts. Whose expert will the jury believe: the plaintiff's or the defendant's? This is often a matter of credentials, theatrics, and knowledge. An experienced expert witness with jury appeal and the right opinions (such a person is often known, politely, as a hired gun) could win a lawsuit.

Many legislatures and courts are attempting to set minimum standards for the qualifications of experts to prohibit testimony from marginally qualified or fringe professionals who proffer opinions that are out of the mainstream (so-called "junk science") but are presented to the jury with equal validity as those of contradictory but mainstream experts.

Expert testimony is not necessary, however, where the issue is one that a lay (i.e., nonprofessional) juror could presumably understand. For example, a jury has sufficient knowledge to understand that a reasonably prudent physician would not leave a scalpel in a surgical patient's gut; expert testimony to set the standard of care (i.e., a reasonably prudent surgeon does not leave a scalpel in a patient's gut) is not necessary.

COMMUNITY STANDARDS AND PUBLISHED GUIDELINES

In addition to expert testimony, the standard of care is often established by authoritative medical literature and clinical guidelines, standards, regulations, policies, and protocols. This is not to say, however, that published guidelines alone define standard of care. Rather, expert testimony establishing that reasonably prudent physicians would rely on these standards and that these standards are, in turn, reasonable is still needed.

Under most circumstances, the standard of care evolves over time and emerges from consensus. But reliance on such a standard of care may be inappropriate if the allegation of malpractice rests on the decision to develop or adopt state-of-the-art procedures. Sometimes a deviation from the accepted norm may be appropriate and the practice of cookbook medicine may not be. Given the increasing regimentation of health care and the adoption of specialty protocols, standards, and guidelines, rigidity may not always be desirable.

Reliance on community standards or published guidelines is not an absolute defense. Under certain circumstances, courts have found that although a defendant may have acted in accordance with the prevailing standard of care, the standard of care itself was unreasonable. Courts will not allow the defendant to excuse failure to exercise reasonable care simply because the entire professional community failed to exercise reasonable care. Of interest here, for example, is the manner in which courts have approached this issue in transfusion-transmitted HIV lawsuits. By way of background, these cases are generally limited to the period of late 1982, when medical literature first began to report that the then unknown causative agent of AIDS may be bloodborne, and the middle of 1985, when blood centers implemented the then recently licensed ELISA test to detect HIV antibodies in donated blood. From January 1983 on, the American Association of Blood Banks (AABB), the American Red Cross (ARC), and Council of Community Blood Centers (CCBC) published joint statements containing certain suggested guidelines regarding donor screening and blood testing procedures then believed to be possibly effective in decreasing the risk of transfusion-transmitted HIV infections. During the same time, the U.S. Food and Drug Administration (FDA) published similar guidelines. Many blood centers followed the AABB, ARC, and CCBC joint statements and FDA guidelines. Nevertheless, blood containing HIV was donated and transfused. The Centers for Disease Control and Prevention estimated that approximately 12,000 of these recipients survived whatever illness or trauma necessitated the transfusion. Attorneys who track lawsuits against blood centers believe that between 5 and 10% of these recipients (or their estates) have since sued blood centers and others they deem responsible for the recipient's HIV infection.

Defendant blood centers have often defended their donor screening and blood testing policies and procedures by noting their reliance on the AABB, ARC, and CCBC joint statements and FDA guidelines. Some courts have found that these joint statements and guidelines established the standard of care and that a defendant blood center that met this standard is not liable. A few courts have created an anomaly in the theory that a practitioner will be judged against the prevailing standard of care and have allowed plaintiffs in transfusion-related AIDS (and a few other) cases to attack the standard of care itself. In *Quintana v. Blood Systems, Inc.* (827 P.2d 509 [Colo. 1992]), for example, the Colorado Supreme Court recognized a national standard of care for blood collection and transfusion practices but said that the adequacy of such a professional community standard was subject to review by a jury. The Colorado Supreme Court did not limit its ruling to just blood practices but suggested that such review may be applied to all professional standards. For practical purposes, the *Quintana* ruling remains a minority view, but it serves as an additional warning that a professional practitioner cannot necessarily and completely rely on what others did or did not do as an absolute defense.

Several states are taking the standard of care defense to its absolute application, that is, by prescribing in law what the standard should be for judging a physician's conduct. In Maine and New Mexico, for instance, practice parameters are being developed that, in theory, will provide a physician with immunity from liability should he or she follow the parameters. In reality, the ability of such practice parameters to accurately reflect the standard of care will likely be subject to endless challenge except for all but the most well-established medical practices.

Increasingly, in cases of transfusion-related disease, claims are being filed against the patient's attending physician and/or the physician who ordered the transfusion questioning whether the transfusion was appropriate, whether proper consent was given, and whether the patient was given options, if feasible. This may even be true for autologous transfusion, which also carries risks, including misidentification of the patient. For example, although a surgeon may have a tendency to use available autologous blood in circumstances where he or she might not use homologous transfusions, an adverse outcome would call into question the transfusion's necessity.

THE DEFENDANT'S BREACH OF DUTY

Breach of duty means that the physician's malfeasance (bad act) or nonfeasance (failure to act or omission) deviated from the prevailing standard of care. Like the standard of care, this is often an area of expert testimony.

An error in judgment is not necessarily a breach of the prevailing standard of care if the erroneous judgment was reasonable. The data used to formulate the alleged erroneous judgment may, however, be challenged as unreasonable, and a good plaintiff's expert will argue that the error in judgment was unreasonable. If the plaintiff challenges the physician's judgment, then the defendant shoulders the burden of proving that the given medical decision was reasonable. As discussed above, an act or omission that the plaintiff may characterize as a bad medical judgment may actually be a reasonable medical judgment among physicians following a specific school of thought.

THE PLAINTIFF'S INJURY AND DAMAGES

The plaintiff must prove that he or she was injured. The plaintiff may ask for money to compensate for physical, financial, or emotional injuries. Lost wages, lost of income-earning potential, medical expenses, and the like are often recoverable as economic (also know as actual) damages; these damages are expenses and losses that can be mathematically computed or readily proven. Noneconomic damages are those that are most often attributed to pain and suffering or, in the case of death, the survivor's grief. Their computation is often subject to the jury's sympathy or antipathy. Some states have attempted by statutes to limit the amount of noneconomic damages.

Punitive damages are available if the plaintiff proves that more than mere negligence occurred. Although the rubric may differ from state to state, for a plaintiff to recover punitive damages, the plaintiff must show—in many states by clear and convincing evidence, a more onerous burden than a preponderance of the evidence—that the defendant's actions were willful and wanton, exhibited a conscious disregard for the plaintiff's safety, or exhibited an evil hand guided by an evil heart. Where awarded, punitive damages often bear no relationship to the plaintiff's economic damages. Rather, they are intended to punish the defendant and can be a portion of the defendant's earnings and net worth.

Punitive damages, once rare, are becoming more common as plaintiffs seek to truly punish bad players, because such damages are rarely covered by insurance.

CAUSATION

The plaintiff must show a causal connection, known as proximate cause, between the defendant's breach of the standard of care and the plaintiff's injury. Several legal standards for determining causation exist. Typically, the question asked of the jury is "but for" the defendant's conduct, would the plaintiff have been injured? A more expansive test is whether the defendant's conduct caused or contributed to the plaintiff's injury.

Sometimes causation is difficult to prove, especially when the plaintiff's preexisting condition deteriorates and it is unclear whether the defendant's acts or omissions caused or contributed to the deterioration. This is especially true for transfusion-associated diseases that are also commonly found in the general population and/or have a high incidence of nosocomial transmission, such as non-A, non-B hepatitis (hepatitis C). In a practical sense, juries are not practical. They will often look for an excuse to compensate an injured party even when negligence is not obvious.

INFORMED CONSENT

The medical community's thoughts about an informed consent for transfusion has evolved during the past several years, in part because of lawsuits brought by transfusion recipients who claim an injury as the result of the physician's failure to seek and receive a truly informed consent. A special informed consent for transfusion is now routinely recommended and in several states, such as California and New Jersey, is required by statute. Because the logistics of autologous transfusion, if feasible, require weeks and often months of preparation, a review with the patient of transfusion needs and options is recommended when a surgery is first contemplated.

GENERAL PRINCIPLES OF INFORMED CONSENT

Good communication is at the heart of the modern physician-patient relationship. The physician must communicate to the patient how he or she intends to treat a condition and the likely results of that treatment. The patient must communicate to the physician any concerns and questions he or she may have as well as his or her consent to the proposed treatment. This particular communication—the informed consent—allows the physician to treat the patient. Consents may be given by the patients or by others who have the legal right to act for the patient under the specific circumstances. Consents may be oral or written, express or implied. It is best, however, that they be express and memorialized in a document signed by the patient and then witnessed.

For a valid express informed consent

1. The physician must explain to the patient what is to be done, including the significant benefits, risks, and reasonable alternatives;
2. The patient must understand the physician's explanation at the time the consent is being given;
3. The patient or legally authorized representative must give consent to the proposed treatment.

The physician must decide what information to provide and then actually provide that information. Without an informed consent, a patient's fundamental right to decide what happens to his or her body will be violated. This unconsented interference with someone's body or the failure to receive consent can be the basis for a medical malpractice claim.

Except in an emergency, any injection, penetration of the skin, use of radiation for treatment, or comparable invasive procedure involving some interference of body tissues requires a patient's consent. In an emergency, consent generally is implied by law. (An emergency is typically defined as a situation where the patient requires immediate care, there is danger to health or life if care is delayed, and an attempt to secure a written or oral consent would delay treatment.) An implied consent exists only during the immediate emergency and is limited to the treatment necessary to resolve the emergency. An express consent is necessary for any further treatment.

CONSENT FOR TRANSFUSION

Time permitting, a physician should get an express, written informed consent for all transfusions. Thus, a surgeon who needs an informed consent for surgery should also get a separate informed consent for any transfusions anticipated during the course of the surgery or postoperative care (Fig. 13.1). An informed consent form for transfusions is preferable even if a general form (i.e., Conditions of Admission) has been signed.

A Conditions of Admission is the basic agreement routinely signed by the patient on admission; it is a broad consent designed to cover routine and customary hospital practices such as general duty nursing, release of information, statements about personal valuables, financial agreements, and a general consent for medical and surgical procedures. Although it often contains a provision regarding transfusions, patient sensitivity

CONSENT FOR TRANSFUSION OF BLOOD OR BLOOD PRODUCTS

Patient ____________________________ Date________Time_____a.m./p.m.
Chart or Social Security Number ___________________

1. I authorize the transfusion to me of whole blood or blood products as may be deemed advisable and recommended by Dr. ___________________, his associates, or assistants.

2. My physician has explained to me the nature, purpose and possible consequences of the procedures relating to transfusion, as well as significant risks involved, possible complications of and alternatives to transfusion, and options of obtaining blood and blood products. I understand that transfusion involves some risk to the patient even though precautions are taken. I also understand that despite the exercise of due care, the transfusion of blood and blood products may transmit infectious diseases such as hepatitis or HIV (AIDS) and may result in an allergic reaction. I have been advised of these risks and complications.

3. I have been advised that I may ask questions or receive further explanation if I so desire. I do not wish to receive any further information.

4. I have received no guarantees from anyone of the results that may be obtained by transfusion. I understand that there is no warranty, including warranties of merchantability and fitness, applicable to blood or blood products.

____
Patient's Signature

If patient is unable to consent, state reasons:

____
____
____

____
Signature of Legally Authorized Representative

____
Relationship to Patient

Witness:______________________

Witness:______________________

Figure 13.1. Example of a consent for transfusion. Note these are not widely used in hospitals.

to transfusions and possible adverse outcomes dictate that a patient's consent for a transfusion is treated no differently than informed consent for the specific surgery. Moreover, the physician should obtain a separate consent for each transfusion (unless multiple units are given within a short time period) and each separate consent should be accompanied by the appropriate informed consent discussion.

Generally, the physician intending to prescribe the blood should discuss with the patient the risks and benefits associated with the transfusion. Risks that should be noted include, but are not necessarily limited to,

1. Transmission of infectious agents such as HIV or hepatitis C (although blood is tested for these infectious agents, it is still possible, albeit remote, that such viruses can be transmitted through blood) and infectious agents for which blood cannot be tested and which pose a serious risk;
2. An allergic reaction.

Physicians should be familiar with risks and uses of blood, as outlined in the generic package insert for blood components jointly published by the AABB, ARC, and CCBC (1). The National Institutes of Health also publishes guidelines on the use of blood components (2).

The physician should also advise the patient of any reasonable alternatives to the transfusion. A rule of thumb is that the greater the risk or the lesser chance of benefit, the more information the physician should provide the patient. Also, the greater the severity of the risk, even if the odds of the risk occurring are minimal, and the greater the number of units to be transfused, the more information the physician should provide. For example, the chances of receiving blood from a donor infected with HIV are minimal, but if an HIV infection does occur, the outcome is very serious. There is often a direct relationship between the number of transfusions required and the overall benefit that may be derived from hemotherapy, as well as the decreasing ability for a patient to avail him or herself of alternatives. (Alternatives to perioperative homologous transfusions are outlined elsewhere in this book but may include presurgical autologous deposit, intraoperative cell salvage, and hemodilution.) There are many guides on the use of autologous transfusions, including one published by the National Institutes of Health (3).

The informed consent document for transfusion should generally include

1. Identifying information such as the patient's name and chart number, the date and time the informed consent discussion was held and the patient's consent was given, and the physician's name;
2. A statement that the physician has explained to the patient the nature, purpose, and possible consequences of the procedures relating to transfusion; the significant risks and possible complications involved; alternatives to the transfusion and possible options for obtaining blood;
3. A statement that a transfusion involves some risk to the patient even though precautions are taken and that despite the exercise of due care, the transfused blood may transmit infectious diseases such as hepatitis or HIV or result in an allergic reaction to the patient;
4. A statement that the patient was specifically warned of these risks and complications and that the patient understands this information;
5. A statement that the patient has been advised that he or she may ask questions or receive further explanations if he or she so desires but does not do so at the time;
6. A statement that the patient has received no guarantees from anyone of the results that may be obtained by transfusion and that no warranty, including warranties of merchantability and fitness for a particular purpose, apply to the provision of blood;
7. A statement that the patient authorizes the transfusion as deemed advisable and recommended by the doctor or his or her associates or assistants.

If an informed consent is not given or implied by the emergency situation and an untold or negative result occurs, the patient could argue that had he or she been informed of the risks associated with the transfusion, and specifically the risk that actually occurred, he or she would have refused the transfusion and the physician's failure to conduct an informed consent discussion injured the patient. The patient may also argue that even if he or she had not refused the transfusion, that had the physician disclosed the risks, the patient would have—assuming there was sufficient time—insisted on a directed donation or even an autologous transfusion.

Consent must be given by the patient unless someone else (often a guardian, spouse, or family member) is legally authorized to act for the patient. Any mentally competent adult may consent to the performance of a medical or surgical procedure on his or her body. The law assumes that an individual is mentally competent unless there is evidence to the contrary. Physicians should make the same assumption. Where it is apparent that the patient is not able to make a rational decision about treatment or does not understand the requested consent, however, a consent, in nonemergencies, needs to be supplied by a legally authorized representative. Such authority must be verified and recorded in the patient's medical records or hospital records.

For minors, the general rule is that the parent's or guardian's consent is required. Generally recognized exceptions include an emancipated minor (the minor lives away from his or her parents and is self-supporting or otherwise free of parental care, custody, and control), a married minor, a homeless minor, a minor suffering from a venereal disease and the purpose of the medical treatment relates to its diagnosis or treatment, and a minor 12 years of age or older under the influence of a dangerous drug or suffering withdrawal symptoms.

A competent patient has a right to refuse proposed medical treatment; this is an important aspect of the patient's right to privacy and self-determination. The physician must honor this right of refusal whether it is given at the time consent is sought or by advance directive. However necessary the proposed treatment is to the patient's health or however specious the reason for the refusal, a competent rational patient may refuse consent and forego all treatment. The worsened condition of a patient who earlier refused treatment is not an emergency giving rise to an implied consent for that treatment.

Nevertheless, courts regularly impose some limits on the rights of patients and legally authorized representatives to refuse consent. Courts are especially responsive in two situations. The first involves the refusal of a parent or guardian to consent to a minor's treatment. Under those circumstances, the state, physician, or hospital can ask a court to order the treatment. If the minor's life is in danger, a court order permitting necessary treatment may be issued even when the basis for the refusal is religious. This is especially true with regard to Jehovah's Witnesses who, for religious reasons, will sometimes refuse transfusions. The second situation in which courts may overrule an otherwise valid refusal is when a competent pregnant woman refuses to give consent. If the health of the fetus may be impaired, the state's interest may result in judicial intervention.

A valid, well-documented refusal should be a complete defense to a claim that a physician was negligent in not administering treatment, including a transfusion. When a competent patient refuses a suggested treatment, the physician should make an additional effort to apprise the patient of the nature of the treatment, the reasons it is urged, and the consequences of continued refusal. If the patient persists in refusing a transfusion, the patient should be asked to sign a form (Fig. 13.2). In addition to appropriate identifying information, the form should include

1. A statement that the patient releases the hospital, its personnel, the attending physician, and all others participating in the patient's care from any responsibility whatsoever for unfavorable reactions or untold results because of the patient's refusal to permit the transfusion;
2. A statement that the physician has explained the possible consequences of such refusal to the patient and the patient understands these possible consequences.

Like the informed consent document, the refusal should be placed in the patient's medical records or hospital records. Also, like most other medical records, informed consents and refusals should be retained for an appropriate period of time (10 years is often recommended for adults; longer for minors).

RISK MANAGEMENT APPROACHES TO ADVERSE OUTCOMES

In 1990, the New York State Department of Health published its landmark study on medical injuries conducted by Harvard's School for Public Health (4). In a review of over 30,000 patient charts, New York found that 3.7% of the patients suffered an injury that either prolonged their hospitalization or otherwise impeded recovery. In 28% of these patients (1% of the total), the injury was a result of negligence. Although most injuries were minor, 14% resulted in the death of the patient and nearly half were perioperative.

Many medical specialty groups have seized the New York findings to argue that injuries are low and medical care is overall very good. Critics say, however, that such an injury rate in any other service or business setting would be intoler-

REFUSAL TO PERMIT BLOOD TRANSFUSION

Patient________________ Date ______ Time ______ a.m./p.m.

Chart or Social Security Number ________________

I request that no blood or blood derivatives be administered to ________________(Patient) during this hospitalization.

I release the hospital, its personnel, the attending physician, and all others participating in my care from any responsibility whatsoever for unfavorable reactions or untoward results due to my refusal to permit the use of blood or its derivatives. The attending physician has explained to me, and I fully understand, the possible consequences of my refusal.

____
Patient's Signature

If patient is unable to consent by reason of age or some other factor, state reasons: ________________________________.

____
Signature of legally authorized representative

____
Relationship to patient

Witness:________________

Witness:________________

Figure 13.2. Example of a permit for refusal of blood transfusion. More hospitals have these forms available than they do consent for transfusion forms.

able. A one-in-four chance that a serious injury was the result of negligence understandably fuels lawsuits and patient mistrust, although the New York study found that only 1 in 10 patients negligently injured filed a malpractice claim. Although another study found that 80% of malpractice claims had no evidence of a negligently caused injury (5), suspicion or a desire "to assure that all that could be done to prevent future similar injuries" drives many claims.

The literature on why patients sue their physicians is surprisingly sparse but emerging. Several studies indicate that patients sue not to get money or prevent similar occurrences in the future, as is commonly believed, but to find out what really happened (6). Many injured patients also say they would not have sued if their physician had just apologized. Such findings are spawning a whole new approach by medical practitioners to patients with adverse outcomes. Whereas in the past physicians were counseled by legal advisers to avoid discussing the causes of an adverse outcome for fear of admitting negligence and increasing liability, physicians are now being counseled by risk managers at some hospitals and insurance companies to factually convey what happened and to generally and genuinely express sorrow for errors of omission or commission. The physician should also, along with the risk manager and patient, help determine whether the patient's needs can best be met by an early agreement or whether some formal dispute resolution mechanism may be necessary to settle a claim or potential claim of malpractice (7, 8). Although the strategy appears to be to keep the patient away from the lawyers, it is more fundamentally rooted in an attempt to continue to resolve problems within the physician-patient relationship.

These approaches, although new and controversial, have their origins in common sense and decency, but appear contradictory to the adversarial tort system and legal instincts commonly applied in the United States for resolving malpractice claims during the last 30 years.

Applying their ability to identify and correct sources of malpractice, risk management programs, whether conducted by health care institutions or insurance companies, have proven enormously successful in improving the standard of care, thereby reducing malpractice, so much so that, at least initially, as part of its comprehensive health care reform proposal, the Clinton Administration sought to force all providers to work for institutions that would use risk management techniques to reduce malpractice. This proposal for "enterprise liability" was withdrawn, however, after hospitals strongly objected to such risk-shifting and physicians expressed a fear of a loss of independence by being forced to affiliate with and have their practices governed by institutional overseers.

RESOLVING DISPUTES

As implied above, there are a number of methods for resolving medical malpractice disputes. The most common is the civil (tort) lawsuit. (Because most physicians are familiar with the course of lawsuits, we will not outline the usual steps.) For most physicians, the tort system often is an expensive, humiliating, time-consuming, and frustrating meat-grinder, especially for the physician who believes he or she did no wrong or, at least, performed at his or her best possible level. Although it is often selective in its truth finding, our civil justice system does cure many of society's ills. And although it may be inequitable in metering out compensation, several studies show that the system usually compensates the deserved individuals if not the right amounts (9).

The explosion of lawsuits, especially in the health care arena, has inspired doctors, hospitals, and others in the health care system to seek reforms by limiting patient options within the judicial system and/or the level of compensation. Such tort reforms vary by state. For example, California has medical malpractice limits ($250,000) on the amount of noneconomic damages a plaintiff can recover for losses such as pain and suffering, loss of consortium, or wrongful death. Such caps are believed to force early settlement of cases, although others believe that caps are unfair to the severely and egregiously injured patient. California and many other states also require that any awards for economic damages are reduced by compensation from other (collateral) sources, such as health, disability, or accident insurance.

Other states, like Indiana and Louisiana, have fault-based compensation patient programs under which a special board reviews malpractice claims and can award up to several hundreds of thousands of dollars if any negligence is suspected. Patients must reject any awards from the patient compensation board before they can sue for higher damages. Such systems do eliminate most lawsuits. Indiana physicians have among the lowest professional liability insurance premiums in the United States, although the required and separate contribution to the patient compensation fund brings the total payment near the average premiums seen in other states.

Most states have a standard of care defense with which negligence can be found only if it has been shown that a physician or other health care provider did not follow the generally recognized standard of care for patients with similar illnesses. As noted above, in practice, a standard of care defense often fails if the plaintiff can produce credible experts to show that the physician should have followed a higher or different course of care. Yet no matter how strong a case may be presented by a defending physician, as noted above, juries are sometimes swayed to compensate a grossly or fatally injured patient regardless of whether negligence was actually found.

Dissatisfaction with the tort system has spawned a near cottage industry in alternative dispute resolution methods. In the health care arena, many Health Maintenance Organizations, especially in California, are using preservice contracts to require binding arbitration to resolve disputes. Other forms of mediation and screening panels have been applied (10).

Recently, the AABB, ARC, and CCBC reported on the successful completion of a pilot study to apply "early neutral evaluation" (ENE) to cases of transfusion injury (11). ENE is essentially a minitrial with no witnesses except the plaintiff and defendant and very limited discovery. The process is often characterized as a "reality check" for the plaintiff and defendant to understand the validity of their respective positions early on in the process before much time, effort, and emotion have been invested in the case. Although most lawsuits, including medical malpractice cases, settle on or before the courthouse steps, this is, unfortunately, usually after both defense and plaintiff attorneys have spent considerable amounts of time, money, and energy in preparing for a trial that never happens. Settlement at such a late point raises not only the defense expenses but also the expectations of the plaintiff and his or her attorney. In blood cases, ENE cuts costs by nearly 50% by resolving the cases early, before much has been spent in discovery (e.g., interrogatories, requests for production of documents and depositions) and defense of the lawsuit.

The New York/Harvard study noted above questioned the premise of our fault-based malpractice system and proposed a no-fault-based system that would allow those injured, whether by negligence or not, to seek financial aid in coping with their injuries. The New York study estimates that although such a system would result in a dramatic increase in the number of claims filed, compensation based only on economic losses, coupled with a savings of legal process fees, would be no more expensive than our current tort system. Many have pointed out that if we are injured on the job, workers' compensation covers much of our losses and addresses most of our needs. Similarly, automobile-related injuries are covered by insurance. However, if we are injured most any place else, including a hospital, we need to sue to recover damages. Both Colorado and Utah plan extensive experimentation with no-fault medical injury compensation programs within the next few years.

The practical effect of these alternatives for most surgeons depends on where they live and who insures them. Physicians in states with progressive tort reform or judicially required settlement mechanisms may have less stressful experiences with malpractice claims than others who feel like victims of an unjust system. On the other hand, enlightened risk management approaches to resolving disputes or potential disputes require more will than legislation.

In the final analysis, a surgeon must determine where professional judgement and trust are placed. In the end, the surgeon who does not address the needs of a patient who suffered an adverse outcome may be forced to meet the patient's demands.

SUMMARY

Ironically, at a time when transfusion has never been safer, especially for the remote risk of HIV, the public's fear of blood transfusion has never been higher. Hence, the patient's need for disclosure and choices about transfusions is very acute. Good, well-documented informed consent will help a physician in his or her defense should a remote but very possible adverse outcome arise. Additionally, the surgeon should keep abreast of the standard of care and practice parameters involving the use of blood products and alternatives. When in doubt, consult the hospital's specialist in transfusion medicine. If an adverse outcome occurs, follow the hospital's risk management guidelines or your insurance carrier's advice regarding an in-depth discussion of the incident with the patient or patient's family. Although some good alternatives to litigation are emerging, the surgeon is largely a captive of his or her insurance carrier and state statutes in trying to resolve disputes.

SCENARIOS FOR A MEDICAL MALPRACTICE ACTION ARISING FROM BLOOD USAGE

The following scenarios are intended to provide a range of situations where a physician may or may not be concerned about liability for a transfusion-related incident and therefore whether the physician should inform his or her professional insurance carrier of the incident. Obviously, these are hypothetical examples, and carriers may have their own criteria for incident reporting. Also, even though a physician may not obviously be liable in an adverse transfusion-related incident, the prevailing practice in lawsuits arising from such cases is to name the attending physician in any claim to question whether the transfusion was really necessary, consent was proper, and/or options were provided. Often the best defense in these cases—and most other medical malpractice lawsuits—is based, in part, on *detailed* medical records identifying the bases for the physician's decision to prescribe blood and the information provided during the informed consent discussion.

Scenario 1: A surgeon determines that his patient needs to undergo a lobectomy and schedules surgery for 2 weeks later. The surgeon informs the patient of the scheduled date and advises her that the operation is "routine" and there are "normally no complications." No other discussion of risks, benefits, or alternatives occurs. The patient signs a general consent allowing the surgery. Blood transfusions are not discussed nor are they referred to in the surgical consent.

Before surgery and as part of his routine practice, the surgeon asks the hospital's transfusion service to "type and screen" 2 units of packed red blood cells. The transfusion service correctly types and cross matches the blood. During the surgery, unanticipated bleeding occurs and the surgeon administers the 2 units. The patient develops a severe allergic reaction to 1 unit and becomes critically ill, requiring several weeks of additional hospitalization.

Should the surgeon inform his carrier?

Answer: Yes. The patient was not informed of the specific risks and benefits associated with the surgeon's anticipated possible use of blood. Therefore, a very good argument could be made that the informed consent was neither informed nor a consent. Although a transfusion was not likely, it was sufficiently within the realm of possibility such that standby blood was ordered. Consequently, the surgeon should have discussed this possibility with the patient and disclosed the attendant risks and benefits. One risk that should have been discussed was a possible allergic reaction and such a reaction occurred. The surgeon, however, could argue that even if he fell below the standard of care by failing to receive an informed consent, his omission did not cause the patient's injury; rather, the patient's reaction is a known unavoidable complication. But the patient can argue that if she had known of the risk of an allergic reaction, she would have either declined the transfusion or insisted on an autologous transfusion, which may have decreased the risk of an allergic reaction. Thus, but for the surgeon's omission, the patient's reaction may not have occurred.

Scenario 2: A surgeon determines that his patient needs to undergo a colectomy and schedules surgery for the following week. The surgeon informs the patient of the scheduled date and advises her that the operation is "routine" and there are "normally no complications." No other discussion of risks, benefits, or alternatives occurs. The patient signs a general consent allowing the surgery. Blood transfusions are not discussed nor are they referred to in the surgical consent. The patient has no religious or other concerns about transfusions.

During the surgery, some abnormal bleeding occurs so the surgeon administers 2 units of packed red blood cells. The transfusion and surgery are completed with a good result.

Should the surgeon inform his carrier?

Answer: Probably no. Although the physician may have breached the prevailing standard of care, the plaintiff can show no injury.

Scenario 3: A physician decides to administer 2 units of whole blood to a patient suffering from pernicious anemia. Before the transfusion, the physician explains the risks, benefits, and alternatives of the transfusion and the patient asks detailed questions. An informed consent for a blood transfusion is executed. The blood is then administered; the patient develops an allergic reaction and becomes critically ill, requiring several weeks of additional hospitalization.

Should the physician inform his carrier?

Answer: Yes. A good argument can be made that the standard of care does not endorse the use of whole blood for a patient suffering from pernicious anemia. By prescribing the units, the physician may have breached the standard of care. Even though the injury was a naturally occurring one and may not be related to the use of whole blood as opposed to packed red cells, the physician set in force the sequence of events that gave rise to the injury.

Scenario 4: A blood center's laboratory technician fails to perform a test to detect the hepatitis B surface antigen; the blood is nevertheless processed and shipped to a hospital's transfusion service.

A physician decides to administer packed red blood cells to a patient suffering from postpartum hemorrhage. The hospital's transfusion service types and cross matches the blood and the transfusion service's technologist selects the untested unit, unaware that it was not tested for hepatitis B.

Before the transfusion, the physician explains the risks, benefits, and alternatives and the patient asks detailed questions about the procedure. An informed consent for a blood transfusion is executed. The blood is then administered and the patient develops hepatitis B.

Should the physician inform his carrier?

Answer: Probably no. Assuming that the physician did not know of the error or did not have a reasonably well-founded suspicion that the blood center was not reliable, the physician should not be liable. The blood center, however, may be liable for its employee's negligence.

Scenario 5: A surgeon decides to administer whole blood to a postoperative cardiac surgery patient. Before the transfusion, the physician explains the risks, benefits, and alternatives and the patient asks detailed questions about the procedure. An informed consent for a blood transfusion is executed. The blood is then administered and the patient develops a Yersinia infection. There is no licensed technology to screen blood for the presence of Yersinia.

Should the surgeon inform his carrier?

Answer: Probably no. The risk of a transfusion-transmitted Yersinia infection is exceedingly remote and blood centers cannot test blood for its presence. Provided the informed consent included a discussion of bloodborne antigens, the surgeon should not be liable.

REFERENCES

1. Circular of information for the use of human blood and blood components. Washington, DC: American Association of Blood Banks, American Red Cross, and Council of Community Blood Centers, February 1994.
2. National Blood Resource Education Program. Indications for the use of red blood cells, platelets, and fresh frozen plasma (NIH Publication no. 89–2974). Rockville, MD: National Institutes of Health, 1989.
3. National Blood Resource Education Program. Transfusion alert: use of autologous blood (NIH Publication no. 91–3038). Rockville, MD: National Institutes of Health, 1991.
4. Medical practice study: executive summary. New York: New York State Department of Health, February 1990.
5. Hiatt HH, BA Barnes, TA Brennan, et al. A study of medical injury and malpractice: an overview. N Engl J Med 1989;321:480–484.
6. Dauer EA. Three Goldbergs: Arthur, Molly and Rube and the irrelevance of legal rights. The Quinn Jordan Memorial Lecture. Washington, DC: American Association of Blood Banks, November 1994.
7. Applegate WB. Physician management of patients with adverse outcomes. Arch Intern Med 1986;146:2249–2251.
8. Holzer JF. Current concepts in risk management. Int Anesthesiol Clin 1984;22:91–116.
9. Jacobson PD. Medical malpractice and the tort system. JAMA 1989; 262:3320–3327.
10. Report of the task force on medical liability and malpractice. Washington, DC: Department of Health and Human Services, August 1987.
11. Alternative methods for managing transfusion injury claims. Report of a pilot program: mediation and early neutral evaluation. Washington, DC: American Association of Blood Banks, American Red Cross, and Council of Community Blood Centers, September 1994.

SELECTED DECISIONS RELATING TO BLOOD USAGE

Snyder v. American Association of Blood Banks, 282 N.J. Super. 23, 659 A.2d 482 (N.J. 1995).

During the course of an August 1984 coronary bypass surgery, the plaintiff received a blood contaminated with HIV. The plaintiff sued the AABB, alleging that AABB was negligent in failing to recommend that member blood centers and others using the AABB's *Standard for Blood Banks and Transfusion Services* adopt surrogate testing for AIDS. The lower court first determined that the AABB, a trade association that inspects and accredits blood centers, owed a duty of care to the recipients of blood whose health and lives depended on the reasonableness of the AABB's actions. The jury rendered a verdict for the plaintiffs, finding that the AABB's failure to recommend surrogate testing constituted negligence and that such negligence resulted in substantially enhancing the plaintiff's risk of contracting AIDS. The appellate court affirmed the jury's verdict against AABB, noting that the record contained adequate evidence to support the jury's findings.

Hoemke v. New York Blood Center, 912 F.2d 550 (2d Cir. 1990), *aff'g* 1989 WL 147642 (S.D. N.Y. Nov. 28, 1989).

As a result of a blood transfusion during a November 1981 kidney operation, Ms. Hoemke contracted an HIV infection. She sued the hospital for negligence, alleging that it failed to institute procedures for autologous or directed donations and to educate its medical staff to avoid ordering transfusions when blood loss is slight.

The lower court agreed with the hospital that it had not violated the standard of care because no other hospital in 1981 had instituted such procedures. The appellate court affirmed the lower court's decision but noted that the standard of care is not necessarily defined by an industry standard: "If a given industry lags behind in adopting procedures that reasonable prudence would dictate be instituted, then we are free to hold a given defendant to a higher standard of care than that adopted by the industry."

Spann v. Irwin Memorial Blood Centers, 40 Cal. Rptr.2d 360 (Cal. Ct. App. 1995).

In October 1984, Ms. Spann received more than 130 units of plasma and platelets to treat thrombotic thrombocytopenic purpura. One or more of the units contained HIV. Ms. Spann eventually died. Her husband sued the blood center for professional negligence, alleging that the blood center's failure to have a donor reduction plan (i.e., a plan to reduce the number of donors to which a plasmapheresis patient is exposed) fell below the standard of care and the blood center failed to obtain an adequate informed consent (it did not mention the risk of an HIV infection).

On the donor reduction issue, the trial court granted summary judgment in the blood center's favor because no other blood center in the United States offered a donor reduction plan in 1984 and therefore the blood center met the industry standard of care. It also granted summary judgment on the informed consent issue. It noted that the purpose of an informed consent is to inform the patient of a potential peril if it would be material to the patient's decision. The court determined that in this case, the element of causation had not been established because the decedent's husband failed to prove that the nondisclosure of the HIV risk caused his wife's injury.

Osborn v. Irwin Memorial Blood Bank, 7 Cal. Rptr.2d 101 (Cal. Ct. App. 1992).

Parents of a child who contracted an HIV infection from a February 1983 blood transfusion sued the blood center and hospital for negligent misrepresentation and negligence, among other claims. The parents based their negligent misrepresentation claim on the blood center's receptionist's statement that they could not give directed donations for their child. At the time, the blood center's actual policy was to discourage directed donations, not forbid them.

Although the jury found in the plaintiffs' favor on the negligent misrepresentation claim, the appellate court ordered a new trial. The appellate court noted that the child's rare blood type had been omitted from the evidence. It reasoned that because the child had a rare blood type, directed donations may not have been feasible and thus the blood center's failure to accurately inform the parents about this alternative may not have caused their child's injury; in other words, a jury needed to answer the question: But for the blood center's failure, would the child have received an HIV-contaminated unit?

For their negligence claim, the plaintiffs argued that the blood center and hospital should have implemented anti-HBc testing as a surrogate test for HIV. The defendants offered evidence that no other blood center or hospital was conducting such tests in February 1983. Therefore, the court concluded that the blood center's and hospital's actions met the professional standard of care.

McKnight v. American National Red Cross, 1994 U.S. Dist. LEXIS 9046 (July 6, 1994).

During a triple bypass operation in July 1984, physicians ordered fresh frozen plasma as part of the "usual" procedure after open heart surgery. Subsequently, the Red Cross discovered that the plasma came from an HIV-positive donor and the plaintiff eventually developed AIDS. Before surgery, the plaintiff had signed a consent form that neither mentioned blood transfusions nor the risks associated with such transfusions. The plaintiff sued the hospital and his physicians, alleging that they had breached their respective duties to obtain informed consent for the blood transfusions. The lower court granted summary judgment for the hospital, stating that the treating physician is solely responsible for obtaining informed consents and a hospital has no comparable duty. Although the appellate court affirmed the lower court's ruling, it recognized that plaintiffs may have cause of action against the hospital if the hospital's informed consent form provides misleading information on which the patient relied.

Gibson v. Methodist Hospital, 822 S.W.2d 95 (Tex. App. 1991), *rev'd in part,* 1992 Tex. LEXIS 78, 35 Tex. Supp. J. 974 (1972).

After a February 1983 surgery for colon cancer, Ms. Gibson's physician ordered 2 units of blood that were transfused in early March 1983. One unit contained HIV, and Ms. Gibson eventually died of AIDS. Her estate sued the hospital, blood center, and physicians for professional negligence. Specifically, they alleged that the hospital deviated from the standard of care when it unilaterally changed the physician's order for whole blood and administered packed red blood cells instead. The hospital moved for summary judgment relying on expert affidavits that there would be no material difference to a patient's health whether a unit of whole blood or packed cells were administered. Indeed, the expert opined that the administration of packed red cells was a "good, safe and improved way of filling an order for whole blood." This evidence went unchallenged, and the hospital was granted summary judgment. The blood center argued that it met the prevailing standard of care by following the recommendations for donor screening set forth in the "Joint Statement On Acquired Immune Deficiency Syndrome Related To Transfusions." Plaintiffs' expert opined that these standards were inadequate and that surrogate testing should have been adopted. Although the trial court granted summary judgment to the blood center, the court of appeals reversed, concluding that the jury must determine which expert is correct.

Doe v. Johnston, 476 N.W.2d 28 (Iowa 1991).

In February 1985, an orthopedic surgeon performed hip replacement surgery and ordered a blood transfusion as part of the postoperative care. Two years later, the patient learned that the blood he had received contained HIV and sued the physician, alleging that he had violated the standard of care by failing to advise the patient about the risk HIV posed to the blood supply and of the possibility of an autologous donation. Although the physician did not dispute the fact that he failed to advise the patient of the risk of HIV, he did testify that he had assessed the risk as 1 in 250,000 and this was too remote a concern to bother providing—and alarming—his patient. The jury rendered a verdict for the physician; it was upheld on appeal.

Hoffman v. Brandywine Hospital, 661 A.2d 397 (Pa. 1995).

During the course of preoperative, operative, and postoperative procedures for a radical mastectomy in December 1984, the patient's surgeon ordered several blood transfusions, one of which turned out to contain HIV. The deceased patient's estate sued the physician, alleging he had ordered unnecessary blood and failed to obtain informed consent for the transfusions. The lower court granted summary judgment in the physician's favor on the issue of unnecessary blood transfusions.

The appellate court decided, however, that a genuine issue of material fact existed because the plaintiff's expert opined that the physician breached the standard of medical care. Accordingly, the court reversed the summary judgment and remanded the issue to the lower court for further proceedings. On the informed consent issue, the appellate court first determined that the doctrine of informed consent should be limited to surgical procedures rather than the administration of drugs. Because the medical records revealed that the blood transfusion at issue occurred nearly 7 hours after the surgery, the appellate court held that the physician was not required to disclose the risks or alternatives to the transfusion. Accordingly, the court affirmed the grant of summary judgment in the physician's favor on the informed consent issue.

J.V. v. State of Florida, 516 So.2d 1133 (Fla. Ct. App. 1987).

Because J.V.'s parents, who were Jehovah's Witnesses, refused to consent to a blood transfusion for their child based on religious reasons, the court ruled that the parents had neglected their child and authorized Florida's Department of Health and Rehabilitative Services to approve any transfusion necessary to sustain the child's life. The court of appeals concluded that the lower court did not abuse its discretion based on a state statute allowing a court to order medical treatment for a minor if the parent does not furnish medically necessary services based on religious beliefs. The appellate court, however, reversed the trial court's finding of parental neglect, noting that the parents' refusal was motivated by sincere religious beliefs.

In the Interest of E.G., 161 Ill. App.3d 765, 515 N.E.2d 286 (Ill. Ct. App. 1987), *aff'd in part, rev'd in part,* 133 Ill.2d 98, 549 N.E.2d 322 (1989).

E.G., a 17-year old Jehovah's Witness, was diagnosed with acute leukemia. When asked to consent to blood transfusions, both E.G. and her parents refused based on religious beliefs. Her condition deteriorated, and the hospital petitioned the court for a finding that the patient was medically neglected. The court found probable cause of medical neglect; it authorized a hospital official to consent to necessary medical treatments and ordered the hospital to administer the recommended transfusions. Later, the court reconsidered its ruling and concluded that E.G. was a mature individual and she had arrived at the decision to refuse the blood transfusions independent of her parents' beliefs. Nonetheless, the court decided that the urgency of her condition justified a finding of medical neglect. The appellate court vacated the order, stating that once the lower court made a determination of E.G.'s maturity and independent decision to refuse the transfusion, the lower court violated her First Amendment right to freedom of religion. The Illinois Supreme Court affirmed the appellate court's decision to allow appellant to refuse consent.

Fosmire v. Nicoleau, 75, N.Y.2d 218, 551 N.E.2d 77, 551 N.Y.2d 876 (N.Y. 1990), *rev'd on other grounds,* 581 N.Y.S.2d 382 (N.Y. App. Div. 1992).

Before the delivery of her baby, an adult Jehovah's Witness refused to consent to any blood transfusions and continued to refuse consent even after losing a substantial amount of blood during her cesarean section. Her physicians submitted affidavits to the court indicating that the blood transfusions were necessary to save the patient's life and a lower court authorized the hospital to proceed with the transfusions despite the patient's objections. After receiving two transfusions, the patient appealed the order. The appellate court vacated the order, holding that the lower court erred in ordering the transfusions without providing the patient and her family notice and opportunity to oppose the order. The state's highest court of appeals affirmed the intermediary appellate court's decision because as a competent adult, the patient had a right to determine her own treatment.

Section III
Preoperative Preparation

Chapter 14

Practical Aspects of Resuscitation to the Hemorrhaging Patient

A. GERSON GREENBURG

INTRODUCTION

Hemorrhagic events can be life threatening to patients. It has long been recognized that acute and rapid loss of blood volume in the absence of an adequate and appropriate resuscitation is associated with poor outcome; definitive measures to control bleeding are, of course, required. It is also recognized that control of the hemorrhaging site may not, by itself, be sufficient to effect a desirable, beneficial outcome. The detrimental physiological consequences on many organs initiated by an acute decrease in blood volume, especially if left uncorrected for a period of time, may be of sufficient magnitude to create an irreversible situation at the cellular level.

This chapter presents an overview of acute vascular volume resuscitation as applied to the acutely hemorrhaging patient. Starting with an overview of the concept and a statement of the working definition and specific goals of resuscitation, there follows a discussion of the underlying pathophysiology of hemorrhagic hypovolemia, a physiological basis to support the interventions. This places in context the cellular-organ-organism derangements that result from acute hypovolemia, providing a specific rationale for the therapeutic interventions. Against this background, different resuscitation concepts are discussed and considered. Specific emphasis is given to describing the fluid attributes in general and the unique properties of each class of resuscitation solution and each individual solution. Because no therapeutic intervention is without the potential for adverse effects, this issue will be explored in the context of resuscitation decisions. The important issues and factors to consider in resuscitation are volume, composition, and timing of the resuscitation. These are the critical decision elements that could compound the resuscitation effort or confound the evaluation of endpoints. It is important to recognize that unexpected intraoperative hemorrhage in a monitored, anesthetized patient is quite different in its consequences from hemorrhage resulting from penetrating trauma. The "resuscitation" may be different because the timing issue may be moot. A synthesized plan for resuscitation based on the known macro- and microphysiological phenomena matched to fluid properties and patient status is offered.

PHYSIOLOGICAL CONSEQUENCES OF HEMORRHAGE

To appreciate the utility of therapeutic specificity, an understanding of the pathophysiological consequences of the hemorrhagic hypovolemia, the inciting event, is required. This subject has been extensively studied and investigated for well over a century; it is not the intent of this chapter to review this area of literature. It must be recognized that the experimental models of hemorrhagic hypovolemia have evolved with time since the era of Wiggers and his predecessors. More importantly, these models now more closely mimic the clinical situation, including elements of uncontrolled hemorrhage and dehydration and tissue damage in their design. With an increasing sophistication in the models has come a better appreciation of the assets and liabilities of various resuscitation schemes. When applied to clinical situations, improved outcomes are apparent, making the clinical situation a true reflection of the experimental animal models.

This exposition discusses only acute hypovolemic hypotension and the resuscitation model; it will exclude other forms of hypotension (e.g., septic shock, cardiogenic shock) to focus the discussion. Although these forms of shock all share at least "a functional component of hypovolemia," altered tissue perfusion, the associated perturbations create a complexity that confounds rather than clarifies the situation. A number of references and reviews take the broader perspective of shock and resuscitation based on an appreciation of the overall shock of pathophysiology (1–5).

An underlying assumption in the management of acute hemorrhagic hypovolemia is the rapid and appropriate restoration of intravascular volume to achieve hemodynamic stability *and* adequate tissue perfusion, the primary resuscitation goals. Generally accepted as sound concepts, the implementation of methods and techniques to achieve the goals requires specification and optimization of both the endpoints and treatment options to be most effective for a given patient situation. In addition to understanding the cellular and subcellular consequences of hypovolemia and the fluid composition and timing elements, it is helpful to consider the more global concepts of oxygen delivery because restoration and maintenance of that system are critical to effecting quality resuscitation. In the overall decision and analysis process, it is also important to appreciate that underlying acute or chronic disease, natural senescence, and pharmacological agents singly or in combination alter normal physiological responses. This is especially true for the cardiopulmonary homeostatic mechanisms (2), the real drivers of oxygen delivery.

CONSEQUENCES OF HEMORRHAGE

Acute hypovolemia from blood loss results in a low flow state, resulting in poor tissue perfusion. Left untreated, inadequate tissue oxygenation and an inability of cells to create energy sources to provide for their basic metabolic and synthetic needs and demands ensue. If uncorrected, this energy deficit eventually results in cell death, the precursor to tissue, organ, and whole body demise. One major consequence of hypovolemia is an alteration in global and organ-specific oxygen delivery; the effects of low flow are manifest clinically and with various degrees of subtlety, biochemically. Covered extensively elsewhere in this book (see Chapter 3), understanding the basic elements of global oxygen delivery is essential to appreciating the consequences of hypovolemia, with implications for treatment.

GLOBAL OXYGEN DELIVERY

Defined as the product of flow and arterial oxygen content, global oxygen delivery is a measure of the overall oxygen delivery to tissues. Flow may be either cardiac output or the normalized cardiac index; arterial oxygen content may be measured or calculated as the product of hemoglobin concentration, arterial oxygen saturation, and a constant, 1.34, plus the amount of oxygen physically dissolved in tissue related to the partial pressure of oxygen:

$$\mathrm{DO_2} = [(1.34 \times \mathrm{Sao_2} \times [\mathrm{Hb}]) + (\mathrm{Pao_2} \times 0.003)] \times \mathrm{CO} = \mathrm{Cao_2} \times \mathrm{CO}$$

GLOBAL OXYGEN CONSUMPTION

Defined as the product of flow and the A–$\mathrm{Vo_2}$ content difference, arterial-mixed venous content, global oxygen consumption represents peripheral tissue oxygen utilization:

$$\mathrm{Vo_2} = (\mathrm{Cao_2} - \mathrm{CMVo_2}) \times \mathrm{Co}$$

OXYGEN EXTRACTION RATIO

This is the ratio of oxygen consumed to oxygen delivered and represents, globally, the functioning aerobic and anaerobic metabolism at the cellular level. It is a reflection of adequate flow to tissues and is maintained between 0.25 and 0.30 under normal conditions:

$$\mathrm{OER} = \frac{\mathrm{Vo_2}}{\mathrm{Do_2}}$$

NORMAL PHYSIOLOGICAL RANGES

Attainment of these levels is a reasonable resuscitative goal:

- Hb Saturation: $\mathrm{Sao_2}$, 95–99%;
- A-MV $\mathrm{Vo_2}$: $\mathrm{C(a\text{-}v)O_2}$, 4–5.5 mL $\mathrm{O_2}$/dL;
- $\mathrm{O_2}$ Del: $\mathrm{Do_2}$, 570–720 mL $\mathrm{O_2}$/min/$\mathrm{M^2}$;
- $\mathrm{O_2}$ Consumption: $\mathrm{Vo_2}$, 100–180 mL $\mathrm{O_2}$/min/$\mathrm{M^2}$;
- OER: OER, 0.22–0.30.

CONCEPT OF OXYGEN DEBT

Deprived of oxygen, most cells switch to anaerobic metabolism, thereby creating an energy deficit directly attributed to a lack of oxygen. If the cells survive the low flow/poor perfusion state, before they can be considered "normal," the energy state must be restored to at least baseline levels. The amount of oxygen needed to restore the cell's metabolic function to normal represents cellular oxygen debt. Failure to repay this debt promptly and efficiently may be related to poor patient outcome. Some argue that it is essential to restore this deficit rapidly and effectively as a goal of hemorrhagic hypovolemia resuscitation, and there is some clinical evidence to support this concept (6, 7). It is not clear that measures of global oxygen delivery and consumption or even serum lactate levels reflect this concept with sufficient sensitivity for widespread clinical use. However, the concept is logically sound and the argument physiologically based with supporting experimental and clinical data. Support for use of a rapid intravascular volume resuscitation is available (1, 4, 5). Counterarguments for minimal volume resuscitation and avoidance of hemodilution with increased bleeding potential have been made; this approach, counter to the accepted paradigm, should be carefully considered and further explored before being universally applied (8).

CLINICAL MANIFESTATIONS OF HYPOVOLEMIA ASSOCIATED WITH HEMORRHAGE

The anesthetized patient may not be able to respond to acute changes in intravascular volume nor manifest some of the important compensatory signs in an expected or predictable fashion; the anesthetic and associated pharmacological treatment, by inhibiting normal homeostatic mechanisms, may simply mask the usual clinical signs of acute hypovolemia. Then again, in the operating room, significant bleeding is rarely subtle; the objective of resuscitation remains provision of adequate tissue perfusion, independent of location. Recognition of modulation of the expected response is a key element in designing the resuscitation effort and evaluating its efficacy.

Associated with decreased tissue perfusion is increased sympathetic and adrenal activity. In combination with poor tissue perfusion, these factors explain many clinical manifestations of hemorrhagic hypovolemia. Table 14.1 shows some physiological and clinical manifestations of various gradations of hemorrhagic hypotension. These manifestations would clearly be tempered by age, intercurrent disease, drug therapy, and rate of blood loss; however, the general patterns would be expected after a given insult. The patient's failure to demonstrate a compensatory response could reflect a more serious insult, greater blood loss, or a longer period of hypovolemia than initially. All factors are to be considered in assessing patient status and response to initial therapy.

Some responses and clinical signs are, as noted, dependent on the rate of loss and other factors, especially in the unanesthetized patient. Orthostatic hypotension tested by sitting the patient up is present with a circulating blood volume loss of ap-

TABLE 14.1. MANIFESTATIONS OF HEMORRHAGIC HYPOVOLEMIA

	Class 1	Class 2	Class 3	Class 4
Blood loss, mL[a]	≤750	750–1250	1250–1800	1800–3000
Blood loss/circulatory volume change, %	up to 15	15–25	25–40	>40
Respiratory rate	14–20 N	20–30	30–35	>35
Pulse rate	70–90 N	>100 N	>120 Inc	>140 Inc
Blood pressure	165/88 N	110/80 N	70–90/50–60 Low	<50/60 sq Low
Urine output; mL/hr	30–35	25–30	5–15	Negative
Gastrointestinal		Anorexia	Anorexia, vomiting	Ileus
Central nervous system: mental status	Anxious	Mildly anxious	Lethargic, confusion	Confusion, lethargy with coma, stupor
Serum	N	N, ↑	↑↑	↑↑↑

All groups have low Co, ↓CVR, ↓PCWP, and ↑PVR.
[a]Based on 70-kg individual, 6.5–7% body weight as blood volume estimate.

proximately 20%. However, because of increased sympathetic and adrenal activity secondary to trauma and stress, it is not uncommon to see a young individual with a relatively normal blood pressure and slight tachycardia who has suffered significant blood loss. Frequently, in the operating room, these individuals drop their systemic blood pressure upon induction of anesthesia with its associated vasodilatation. This most likely results from an assumption of normal volume status related to the vital signs measurement that may, in fact, not reflect true intravascular volume status. Routine use of beta-blockers predisposes older patients to not respond to hypovolemia with tachycardia.

COMPENSATORY MECHANISMS AND THEIR RESPONSE TO HYPOVOLEMIA

Loss of intravascular volume leads to an initial increase in vascular tone reflected in an increased peripheral resistance. This vasoconstriction produces a redistribution of blood flow to those organs with high oxygen consumption, little reserve capacity, and a high-level autoregulatory system (e.g., heart and brain); of necessity, the flow redistribution deprives other organs and tissues, less oxygen sensitive, of adequate and sufficient blood flow. Acute hypovolemia is a general vasoconstricting event affecting arterial and venous circulation alike; venous constriction is really a functional loss of venous capacitance, the objective end result being an increase in cardiac preload to obtain or maintain sufficient cardiac output.

The increased sympathetic tone response to acute hypovolemia produces a tachycardia and increased myocardial contractility; both serve to increase cardiac output, which is one means of increasing global oxygen delivery. Increases in myocardial effort or work to improve cardiac output are not without cost, however. To increase cardiac output, greater cardiac work is required; the production of increased cardiac work requires increased myocardial oxygen consumption. It is likely that a significant portion of any increased "global oxygen delivery" is actually consumed by the myocardium in creating this increased cardiac output (9). Thus, an increased peripheral delivery of oxygen may not be effected. This concept may be important when planning resuscitation; optimization of cardiac output and hemodynamics seem a reasonable first approach to increasing global oxygen delivery and should be considered before adding oxygen-carrying capacity in the form of red cells. It must be recognized that at some point, a portion of the additional global oxygen delivery is consumed by the heart without a concomitant increase in oxygen delivery to the periphery.

Hydrostatic pressures too change with hypovolemia. A hallmark of hypovolemia is the reequilibration, over time, of total body water into the defined fluid compartments. With hemorrhagic hypovolemia, interstitial fluid appears to be the most mobile, rapidly entering the intravascular space and providing first volume and then perhaps an element of dilution for the concentrated cellular blood components. A reasonable body of evidence supports viscosity changes as being detrimental. This is especially true of red blood cells sludging in capillaries and white blood cell occlusion along with platelet aggregation as culprits in tissue ischemic injury and direct endothelial damage (1, 4, 10).

The early acidosis of hypovolemia effects a functional increase in oxygen off-loading capacity by shifting the P_{50} (partial pressure of oxygen at which 50% of the oxygen will off-load) to the right. The clinical implications of this shift fit with the goal of improving oxygen delivery to tissue; acidotic red cells containing hemoglobin with a lower affinity for oxygen allow an increased oxygen off-load (2, 11).

The hypoxia associated with hypovolemia induces a compensatory increase in respiratory rate; this is an additional initial means of increasing oxygen delivery and a mechanism for dealing with the volume-induced metabolic acidosis by creating compensatory respiratory alkalosis. There are two additional consequences: 2,3-DPG increases to elevate the P_{50} and an erythropoietic stimulus begins the production of new red blood cells. Both consequences and compensations take effect in a delayed manner, usually hours and days. The renal hypoxia inducing the erythropoietin response is associated with blood flow redistribution. Renal blood flow redistribution has the purpose of preserving and conserving both salt and water losses, but if renal perfusion is restricted for a prolonged period of time or the perfusion pressure is minimal, renal damage ensues.

The overall physiological response to hypovolemia is the compensation for a decreased oxygen-carrying capacity at the expense of flow to some tissues. In addition, glucose metabolism is altered and the need for new efficient fuel substrates results in mobilization of glycogen and fat.

A host of endocrine and humoral mediators are released in association with acute hemorrhagic hypovolemia (1, 4, 5). It is important to appreciate that these mediators are interrelated, having different effects singly or in combination on hemodynamics and secondary effects on baseline metabolism. Catecholamines inhibit insulin secretion while enhancing glucagon release. Thus, the primary effect appears to be the provision of glucose to those cells that can use it independent of insulin (e.g., heart and brain) while depriving other cells of the necessary glucose fuel (1, 4, 5, 12–14).

Other hormones and mediators are released in response to hypovolemia and decreased tissue oxygen delivery. Corticotropin (ACTH), growth hormone, and arginine vasopressin, also known as antidiuretic hormone, are secreted in direct response to the hypovolemia or the secondary effects mediated via osmolality changes. The renin-angiotensin system is also activated in response to sympathetic stimulation and a decreased renal perfusion and changes in tubular renal urine composition (14).

Once angiotensin renin is released in the lungs, prostaglandin production is stimulated; there is also release of ACTH and aldosterone. Aldosterone secretion is an additional means of sodium conservation allowing loss of excess hydrogen and potassium through a renal mechanism, obviously a means of off-loading unwanted byproducts of anaerobic metabolism and cell damage.

Thus, the metabolic regulatory hormones are linked to the compensatory responses initiated by hypovolemia and tissue hypoxia. Governed in some way by catecholamines, these regulatory agents act and counteract to preserve the organismic integrity. It must be recognized that these systems are all highly related, yet an intercurrent illness or the presence of pharmacological agents could block or augment any of the interacting physiology with a blunting or exaggeration of the clinical events. Recognizing this as a possibility is, in some way, the integration of science and the art of medicine applied at the clinical level.

Other mediators, usually operating at the micro level, are also released in response to hypovolemia and hypoxia. Some of these are generally considered beneficial and homeostatic when seen alone; they can potentiate ill effects when taken in combination, and the net result may be greater insult to tissue. The whole story of the prostaglandin-thromboxane interaction, eicosanoids, endorphins, leukotrienes, and other cytokines and their various roles in response to hypovolemia continues to be a mystery, although the secrets are slowly being revealed to persistent scientists. For now, it is intriguing physiology with the potential for providing a means of exploring new pharmacological approaches to what appear to be persistent, not easily solved problems.

CELLULAR RESPONSE TO HYPOVOLEMIA

Normally, tissue metabolism is aerobic, and few cells have energy reserves to compensate for a decreased adenosine triphosphate synthesis associated with poor perfusion, the end effect of hemorrhagic hypovolemia. Different tissues have varying oxygen requirements, and some are more sensitive to changes in oxygen delivery than others (15). Local and systemic homeostats and regulators, as a rule, serve as protective mechanisms. It is important to consider these normal processes and the effects of pharmacological agents on altering the responsiveness of the systems, especially in the anesthetized patient or in the intensive care unit context, where polypharmacy is commonplace.

As cellular aerobic glycolysis decreases, the sodium potassium cell membrane pump begins to fail; sodium enters the cell more freely and the cell expands as it osmotically draws water from the extracellular space. This swelling of the cell makes it dysfunctional. More critically, this loss of water from the extracellular space (the interstitial compartment) means that this water is not readily available to move into the intravascular space when a colloid or hypertonic resuscitation fluid is used. This process has a relatively defined time course; and from a clinical vantage, the duration of hypovolemia would reflect this equilibration time, and the loss of this water must be taken into consideration in designing resuscitation plans. When a prolonged period of underperfusion and hypovolemia is present, some resuscitation fluids may be less effective because the fluid required for them to be effective is not readily available.

Associated with the onset of anaerobic metabolism and the oxygen debt is an accumulation of pyruvate that is readily converted to lactate. This results in intracellular acidosis, which interferes with normal cellular metabolic activity. Moreover, with breakdown of the cellular membrane, an influx of calcium occurs, resulting in activation of intracellular proteases. These activated enzymes further limit the restorative cellular processes.

The microcirculation and cell metabolism are controlled by many independent and dependent factors normally working in a regulatory "check and balance" manner. Although many are clearly protective mechanisms when stimulated and not adequately shut down or downregulated beyond the immediate need, an excess of any one or combination of many can produce additional systemic problems that can hamper the resuscitation effort and potentially alter the identification of endpoints.

WHAT HAPPENS TO THE BODY FLUID DISTRIBUTION WITH HYPOVOLEMIA?

The response to hypovolemia is well characterized in the classic work by Shires et al. (16) and must be recognized. At different grades of hypovolemic hemorrhage, they determined the distribution of total body red cell mass, plasma volume, and interstitial fluid volume using an elegant triple-isotope method. Once the blood volume loss exceeded 25%, evidence of poor tissue perfusion was present and there was an extra loss of extracellular fluid "beyond the withdrawn blood volume that could be accounted for assuming an internal redistribution of extracellular fluid. . . ." Furthermore, when the shed blood was reinfused, the extracellular volume deficit persisted *unless* additional balanced salt solution was infused (17). Survival was significantly enhanced when balanced salt solutions (e.g., Ringer's lactate, mimics of interstitial fluid) were infused with the shed blood volume. Shires and colleagues later go on to argue (18) that the only feasible and logical explanation is the movement of interstitial fluid into the cellular mass to account for the "additional reduction of extracellular fluid volume. . . ."

If one assumes that maintenance of normal tissue perfusion and fluid compartments are required for function, then restoration of these elements to their preinsult state is the essential therapeutic objective. These two aspects of hemorrhagic hypovolemia are clearly bound; it is at times difficult to tease out the components of each that contribute to the deviations observed for specific directed therapeutic intervention to be possible. Hypovolemia induces fluid shifts between compartments, which make the underlying cell mass more vulnerable to injury. Hypoxia induces changes in cellular metabolism that, if left uncorrected, result in cell death. As a result of the hypovolemia, compensatory mechanisms at both the systemic and cellular levels are evoked. These compensatory mechanisms may not always be in harmony or appropriately coordinated to achieve the best patient outcome. Our current knowledge base, as broad as it appears, would seem to indicate a lack of appreciation of the critical details. However, as our understanding of the pathophysiology of hemorrhagic hypovolemia, hemorrhagic shock, grows increasingly more sophisticated, the likelihood of newer and better therapeutic interventions approaches reality.

RESUSCITATION OPTIONS

If the primary goal of resuscitation in hemorrhagic hypovolemia is the prompt and effective restoration of tissue perfusion and adjustments in vascular volume and hemodynamics, a host of therapeutic options, predicated on understanding the pathophysiology, are available. Indeed, over the years, many approaches have been tried; a few have proven to be conceptually and clinically sound and are now represented as routine standards of patient care.

Therapeutic options to restore vascular volume and tissue perfusion in hemorrhagic hypovolemia include pharmacological manipulation of hemodynamic parameters and replacement of intravascular volume using solutions with or without increased oxygen-carrying capacity. Each unique approach has obvious limitations tempered by patient and situational factors. It would be ideal to match a resuscitation plan for each individual situation. Unfortunately, that approach is neither feasible nor practical because of time constraints associated with the acuity of the resuscitation decisions.

The idealized model/paradigm is difficult to implement because the patient particulars are not always known. An "optimized decision" implemented on best probability of success, with assumptions about missing data, is the next best approach. This form of decision-making applies a general therapeutic principle to the generic state, hypovolemic hemorrhage. For the most part, given the basic pathophysiology, this empiric approach has been safe and effective across the population of similar patients.

If the goals of the resuscitation can be stated and are reasonable, defined endpoints that reflect achievement of these objectives can be established. In the acute hemorrhage situation, there is usually not enough time to establish invasive monitoring techniques so that physiologically defined endpoints can be reached. There must then be reliance on clinical parameters that, as previously noted, are subject to compromise from a number of associated cofactors. Few trauma patients are really candidates for placement of major invasive monitoring lines to obtain measurements of oxygen delivery/utilization parameters, the physiologically useful endpoints (Table 14.2). Although desirable, it may be impractical to resuscitate patients to defined physiological endpoints in the absence of readily available, reliable, potentially noninvasive measurement technologies. On the other hand, patients in the operating room and intensive care unit are frequently subjected to full invasive monitoring; if they experience significant hypovolemic hemorrhage, resuscitations could and should be directed to specific physiological endpoints. Of course, in these situations, the full range of pharmacological and volume resuscitation options can obviously be exercised because there is less reliance on empiric information.

PHARMACOLOGICAL APPROACH TO HYPOVOLEMIC HEMORRHAGE

It must be recognized immediately that this insult is not a primary blood pressure problem. The underlying insult is a defect in tissue oxygenation independent of the etiology. Treatment is therefore directed at optimizing systemic and regional oxygen delivery. Pharmacological modulation of the cellular response may be neither reasonable nor effective depending on the insult, extent of oxygen debt, and other factors. There is great interest in developing pharmacological agents to block or inhibit the production, distribution, or action of cytokines, cell-cell messengers, or various regulatory or controlling proteins and peptides believed involved in the response. If one assumes these mediators to be part of a general homeostatic regulatory mechanism, with significant redundancy and multiple sites of interaction, the logic behind blocking or inhibiting a single one seems flawed. If "the system" is already out of balance because of the hypoxic insult

TABLE 14.2. IDEAL PHYSIOLOGICALLY BASED ENDPOINTS OF RESUSCITATION

Systolic blood pressure	≥90 mm Hg
Diastolic blood pressure	≥50 mm Hg
Global oxygen delivery[a]	1.2–1.5 times normal values Normal values: 120–160mL O_2/min/m^2BSA >10–12 mL O_2/min/kg body weight
Oxygen extraction ratio	≤0.30
Arterial O_2 saturation	≥90%
Urine output	>0.5 mL/kg/hr
Improved mental status	Compared with initial observations
Heart rate decrease	Compared with initial observations
Respiratory rate decrease	Compared with initial observations

[a]Achievable by a combination of cardiac output manipulations and the addition of oxygen-carrying capacity.

and initiation of a cytokine cascade—inflammatory or otherwise—it is possible that a specific interdiction would further unbalance the system, allowing the protective homeostatic mechanisms to become detrimental, destructive, uncountered, and perhaps generally out of control.

Despite the many efforts aimed at developing pharmacological agents to block specific identified effects of the hypoxic injury, there appears to be a lack of both efficacy and specificity. This form of pharmacological intervention, inhibition of mediators and regulatory proteins, is perhaps for the future and is not generally applicable today.

Pharmacological manipulation of various oxygen delivery parameters (cardiac output, preload, contractility, afterload), on the other hand, is both realistic and achievable. Various inotropic agents and vasodilators can be used to increase cardiac output in selected patients to achieve increases in global oxygen delivery and tissue perfusion. However, restoration of vascular volume is essential for this approach to be functional. Tissue perfusion and oxygen delivery are functions of both cardiac output and oxygen content (2, 4, 19); restoration of vascular volume increasing effective cardiac filling pressure (preload) is the reasonable first step in resuscitation before inotropic support or other pharmacological manipulation of central or peripheral hemodynamics is attempted.

VOLUME CONSIDERATION

The mainstay of the treatment of acute hemorrhagic hypovolemia is rapid restoration of vascular volume. Recent developments have challenged this notion; it has been proposed that minimal volume resuscitation or no volume resuscitation could be used with good results. These concepts cannot be readily dismissed because the preliminary results tend to support at least a wider exploration and validation/verification of the concept (8, 20). The idea of "scoop and run" with prompt control of the bleeding site followed by effective volume restitution and tissue resuscitation has some appeal. Models of resuscitation with uncontrolled hemorrhage show a variety of detrimental effects in response to aggressive intravascular volume expansion (21, 22). The idea behind low volume or no volume resuscitation in hemorrhagic hypovolemia is based on studies that show increased blood loss from uncontrolled sites with full volume resuscitation. Thus, it is logical to assume that low volume solutions of many compositional possibilities may have a positive effect, minimizing blood loss.

Two essential attributes of resuscitation fluids to consider when planning vascular space replacement are volume and composition. The actual volume and composition (electrolytes, colloids, osmolality, osmolarity, pH) of resuscitation fluids determine the effective intravascular volume expansion possible and to a lesser degree the duration of the effect. Rapid intravascular volume expansion depends on the volume of distribution of the solution used. The three primary spaces are total body water, the extracellular space, and the intravascular space. The goal is expansion of the extracellular space, especially the extracellular fluid compartment. The extracellular fluid space, variously between 2.5 and 3.5 times greater than the intravascular space, is the primary area of fluid equilibration. It follows that complete restoration of this space requires more fluid than would be lost from the intravascular volume (23). Thus, whole blood could expand the intravascular volume, assuming no ongoing hemorrhage, on a 1:1 basis, but crystalloids require a 3:1 infusion to attain the same effect. Various other solutions, colloids, crystalloids, hypertonic, and/or hyperoncotic formulations, will expand the intravascular volume at a ratio somewhere between these two extremes.

Resuscitation fluids that rely on movement of interstitial fluid into the vascular space (hypertonic, hyperoncotic, and many colloid-based solutions) depend on the availability of interstitial fluid to be effective. Thus, in a patient who has been volume-depleted and dehydrated for a while—long enough for fluid reequilibration to occur—these resuscitation fluids may be less effective.

In a recent study of resuscitation using a hypertonic/hyperoncotic solution in hemorrhaged euhydrated and dehydrated sheep, the "test solution" was effective in restoring hemodynamic parameters to baseline in both groups. However, the dehydrated animals had a lower stroke volume and greater heart rate—primary determinants of cardiac output—indicating increased cardiac work with the potential for increased cardiac stress. These observations imply caution is indicated when considering this technique in older patients with coronary vascular or cardiac compromise (24).

Tradition dictates a discussion of resuscitation fluids in terms of their crystalloid and colloid composition. Crystalloids are osmotically active agents, whereas colloids tend to be oncotically active. Crystalloids are hypo-, iso-, or hypertonic and thus draw water from tissue or provide excess free water; colloids are iso- or hyperoncotic, draw fluid from tissue, but do not supply free water. In addition, colloids can be natural (e.g., albumin, proteins) or synthetically derived compounds. Crystalloids and colloids do not transport oxygen except for a minor physically dissolved amount.

Oxygen-carrying resuscitation fluids fall into two classes: blood and blood products and red cell substitutes. Blood, or more properly packed red blood cells, is available in a variety of forms and storage modalities. The decision to use red cells in the active acute phase of resuscitation determines the form administered, usually dictated by the urgency of the situation. Clearly, fully cross-matched allogeneic units are considered preferable if available; the temporal demands of a specific clinical situation could allow use of type-specific red cells. There are inherent risks in these approaches relating to delays, risks, and tradeoffs to be considered in the decision process. These issues are covered in detail in other chapters in this volume (see Chapters 2–4).

Deciding between uncross-matched type-specific red cells, fully cross-matched units, or type O blood illustrates the role of risk assessment in the resuscitation-transfusion decision. Whenever the decision not to transfuse is made, there is an implied risk assessment; the patient is assumed to have the physiological cardiac reserve to withstand an acute decrease in oxygen delivery without detrimental effects. The risk of transfusion (see Chapter 3, 7) must be weighed against the risk of not transfusing on a patient specific basis.

The importance of an adequate intravascular volume in maintaining homeostasis and affording a rapid and effective restoration of oxygen delivery cannot be overemphasized. The basic characteristics of the various resuscitation solutions with respect to real and effective plasma volume expansion are shown in Table 14.3. The hyperoncotic and/or hypertonic solutions expand the vascular volume by "a hydrated volume" with fluid mobilized from the interstitium. If that body compartment is depleted or dehydrated because of prior compensatory mobilization of fluid, an effective predictable response to hypertonic and/or hyperoncotic fluids may be preempted. The dehydrated patient needs restoration of both vascular volume and total body water to achieve the clinical and physiological endpoints of resuscitation. In fact, one critical element missing in the resuscitation process and

TABLE 14.3. COMPOSITION OF COMMONLY USED RESUSCITATION FLUIDS

Solution	pH	Osmolality (mOsm/L)	Colloid osmotic pressure	Approximate ratio infusion to volume expansion	Na	Cl	K	Ca	Mg
D5%/W	5	253	0	8:1	0	0	0	0	0
D10%/W	4	560	0	3:1	0	0	0	0	0
D5%/W	4.2	2526	0	2:1	0	0	0	0	0
Ringer's lactate	6.7	270	0	3:1	130	109	7	3	0
0.9%NaCl	5.7	308	0	3:1	154	154	0	0	0
Normosol-R[a]	7.4	295	0	3:1	140	98	5	0	3
7.5% NaCl	4.0	2400	0	1:3	1280	1280	0	0	0
Plasma	7.0	290	24	1:1					
5% Albumin	6.6	290	20	1:1	130–160	130–160			
25% Albumin	6.9	310	100	1:3	130–160	130–160			
10% Dextran-40/Dextran	6.7	320	68	1:1	0	0			
10% Dextran-40/saline	6.7	320	68	1:1	154	154			
Hetastarch	5.5	310	70	1:1	154	154			

[a]Is representative of "balanced electrolyte."

endpoint assessment is an inability to determine, on clinical or even subtle biochemical or physiological grounds, changes indicative of significant dehydration. Measurements of hemoglobin and hematocrit and plasma oncotic pressure aid in the assessment but are imprecise (25). Detection of an increased colloid osmotic pressure should reflect dehydration, potentially allowing a more precise decision about the specific composition of the resuscitation fluid.

The history of hypertonic and hyperoncotic resuscitation is rather short; there are some data to support the concept. Using small volumes of resuscitation fluids allow some vital organ perfusion that, in theory, could decrease or even obviate the "reperfusion injury" associated with reoxygenation of anoxic tissue. By providing a low-level tissue perfusion, hypoxia and not anoxia is induced. The tissue response to reoxygenation may therefore be modulated and the various cytokine/mediator cascades with their associated clinical manifestations minimized.

CONTROVERSIES IN RESUSCITATION FLUID COMPOSITION

Since the 1960s, rapid large-volume intravascular resuscitation has been the de facto standard of treatment for acute hemorrhagic hypovolemia. The arguments made previously challenging this concept not withstanding—minimal or no resuscitation until definitive control of the hemorrhagic site is effected—the type and composition of fluid used for resuscitation has been widely debated. Two major controversies continue to be discussed. The first is the "crystalloid-colloid" argument and the second is the "hypertonic-hypertonic/hyperoncotic" discussion.

When assessing the literature dealing with these controversies, both experimental and clinical studies, the heterogenicity of situations and the model variations must be appreciated. Critical factors to consider in evaluating animal models include presence or absence of anesthesia, the type and form of anesthesia, extent of hypovolemia, duration of hypovolemia, controlled or uncontrolled hemorrhage, how cell injury is documented, definition of control groups, comparative solutions, and physiological and survival endpoints. Extrapolation from animal models to use in the clinical situation does not necessarily follow. These criteria could be generally used when reviewing the data that support all proposed resuscitation fluid compositions.

The clinical literature has an even more pronounced heterogenicity. Because all forms of shock share an element of altered tissue perfusion, there is a tendency to group all patients when evaluating specific resuscitation fluids. Comparison of fluids used in elective volume replacement during surgery may have little relevance to resuscitation from hemorrhagic hypovolemia, especially if the study is performed in an operating room where the likelihood of a tissue ischemic event is minimized even in high-risk surgical patients. Endpoints must also be clearly defined for both the solution and clinical outcome; simple survival statistics may be too crude a measure of efficacy to be useful.

These controversies are clearly not resolved and data continue to accumulate. When there is a sufficient body of knowledge to support routine use of any of these solutions as evidenced in appropriately done randomized control trials, the medical community should embrace the concepts and begin using them.

COLLOID VERSUS CRYSTALLOID

It is generally agreed that resuscitation of acute hypovolemic hemorrhage, especially associated with trauma, should be instituted with crystalloid solutions. This approach takes into account the systemic nature of the response to trauma, shifts in body fluid compartments, release of mediators, and initiation of homeostatic mechanisms. It then follows that colloids can be added to obtain a longer duration of expanded intravascular volume and prevent dilutional hypoproteinemia, with potential effects on coagulation and tissue edema. Crystalloids are safe and inexpensive when compared with colloids.

Because crystalloids equilibrate into the extracellular space, larger volumes are required to effect the desirable hemodynamic and intravascular volume effects. The decrease in the intravascular oncotic pressure, presumably resulting from dilution, could induce a net flow of fluid to the interstitial space, resulting in tissue edema. This excess tissue water could ultimately manifest itself as organ dysfunction. The lungs are most sensitive to fluid accumulation, and pulmonary edema with respiratory failure is a possible adverse outcome. However, the active pulmonary lymphatic system usually handles the excess fluid, and few problems are encountered (26). In trauma patients, no difference in outcome or, specifically, the incidence of pulmonary failure could be detected when crystalloid was compared with colloid (27, 28). In other groups of patients, failure to restore the interstitial fluid defect and a variety of other hemodynamic, organ dysfunction, and metabolic defects was associated with colloid resuscitation (29–31). Albumin was the colloid of choice in these studies, and questions have been raised about the volume and sodium load of this particular resuscitation effort.

The cost of crystalloid is far more reasonable than colloid when used for resuscitation. Studies have shown a cost between $8.00 and $45.13 per life saved for crystalloid compared with $1040 and $1493.60 for colloid (28, 32).

The arguments for and against colloid and crystalloids have been summarized and reviewed by others (1, 3, 4, 19, 23, 32–34). More importantly, a meta-analysis of appropriate studies demonstrated a 12% margin of superiority for crystalloid resuscitation compared with colloid efforts (35).

There is no evidence in clinical studies that appropriate volume restitution with crystalloids—balanced salt solutions—is associated with harmful effects. The qualifying caveat, however, is that resuscitation must be directed at achieving appropriate hemodynamic endpoints and viewed to be surrogate clinical measures.

HYPERTONIC RESUSCITATION—ASSETS AND LIABILITIES

Hypertonic saline, with or without colloid solutions, has been proposed as an initial resuscitation fluid for acute hemorrhagic hypovolemia. Because it can be administered in small volumes to achieve an expanded intravascular volume, provided there is sufficient interstitial fluid for mobilization and associated increases in blood pressure and cardiac output, the concept has some appeal.

A growing body of evidence, both experimental and clinical, has shown the small-volume resuscitation to be initially effective, in terms of hemodynamic response (36–40). In some animal studies of uncontrolled hemorrhage and resuscitation, the adverse effects of aggressive crystalloid resuscitation have been demonstrated, showing both increased bleeding and decreased survival, but this is not uniformly nor consistently demonstrated (41, 42).

An additional benefit attributed to hypertonic solution resuscitation is a decrease in intracranial pressure (43). If this laboratory observation can be demonstrated clinically, it may be an indication for the use of hypertonic solutions in the combined hypovolemic head-injured patient (44).

Hypertonic saline solution resuscitation has a short duration of action and response, typically 1–2 hours. The addition of colloids prolongs the beneficial hemodynamic response by a factor of 2 or so. Thus, it is possible to effect a reasonable hemodynamic resuscitation with small volumes and then rapidly transport the patient to a site for definitive care.

At this time, the efficacy of hypertonic saline, with or without colloid, has not been demonstrated in clinical trials. There are suggestions of effectiveness when considered part of an overall resuscitation scheme (8, 40). Additional clinical trials are needed to identify the patient populations most likely to benefit from this potentially useful and applicable technique (45).

A PRACTICAL APPROACH TO RESUSCITATION IN THE HEMORRHAGING PATIENT

The resuscitative effort must be goal-directed with specific objectives (Table 14.2). The goal is restoration of effective oxygen delivery to tissues. The secondary objectives include restoration of adequate circulation and correction of the pathophysiological responses initiated by the acute hemorrhagic hypovolemia. With restoration, cellular aerobic metabolic homeostasis is reestablished. Resuscitation is temporizing therapy, a necessary process before initiation of definitive therapy to control bleeding. In the hemorrhaging surgical patient, resuscitation by and of itself is not the end, rather it is part of a continuous process leading to definitive therapy.

If a patient has sustained significant intravascular blood loss, venous access must be secured. Standard techniques invoke two large-bore upper extremity intravenous access sites as essential. The questions about venous access are many: peripheral versus central, which central site is better (i.e., subclavian versus internal jugular), catheter or needle size, and material; these issues aside, intravenous access is required. Each access site has benefits and potential liabilities and risks of complications immediate or delayed that could potentially compromise the patient. These factors must be considered in the selection of access site.

Using the clinical guidelines of the American College of Surgeons Committee on Trauma (46), the initial resuscitation and restoration of vascular volume should be effected with crystalloid. One liter of lactated Ringer's solution is infused rapidly and vital signs monitored to look for specific responses toward the normal range. Because the clinical presentation of hemorrhagic hypovolemia roughly correlates to the extent of intravascular volume depletion, it is possible to estimate early in the resuscitation based on clinical information alone whether the patient is likely to require red cells as part of the initial resuscitation effort (Table 14.1).

Exactly how the clinical endpoints in Table 14.1 were derived appears lost in the abyss of clinical practice, the art of medicine, and in the depths of standards of care definitions. It is unlikely that there was a scientific basis to explain the observations; rather, the observations were likely to be based on experience that correlated to a beneficial outcome. Analytically, it is clear that these observations can possibly be supported by explanations derived from oxygen delivery physiology data. Assumptions of clinical observations related to decreases in oxygen delivery are quite realistic; a causal relationship remains, however, to be established.

It is important to emphasize that an individual patient's response to hemorrhagic hypovolemia will be modified/altered by preexisting disease, acute pathology, pharmacological agents (legal and illegal), extent of blood loss and intercurrent injury (number of organs), rate of blood loss, duration of hypovolemia, and ambient temperature conditions, to note a few. Interestingly, many of these factors are also general correlates of outcome, making it somewhat problematic to compare and evaluate different resuscitation fluids for efficacy. Part of the problem in establishing the efficacy of resuscitation fluids relates to the general overall improvement in trauma systems, anesthesia generally, surgical techniques, the modern intensive care unit, and overall patient care. If these significant improvements have resulted in improved outcome, is it possible to determine the exact role of the resuscitation fluid in the process? This rhetorical question is posed because of the unlikely prospect of repeating previous studies; data in support of new resuscitation concepts addressing these issues would be useful in placing the problems in an appropriate context.

The classification of resuscitation fluids and their composition have been broadly stated previously (Table 14.3). Tonicity and electrolyte composition are critical components. Isotonic solutions, which are those without electrolytes (e.g., D5/W), are not useful in replacing lost intravascular fluids; they distribute to the total body water space. Balanced salt solutions are considered the first-line treatment for hemorrhagic hypovolemia. Lactated Ringer's has the widest applicability, most reasonable cost, and an excellent safety profile. Other balanced salt solutions may be as effective but have failed to achieve widespread use and are very expensive.

Colloids (low- and high-molecular-weight dextran, hydroxyethyl starch, pentastarch, albumin) are used in the United States; all have been studied and generally show some efficacy. Each also has some apparent limitations related to toxicity or maximal volumes and none are universally applicable to all patients. Specific contraindications have been identified for each. It should also be noted that some colloid solutions used throughout the world are not available for use in the United States.

CRYSTALLOIDS

In mixtures of physiologically active solutes, the sodium concentration is the most important factor in defining the distribution of the infused solutions. The extracellular distribution of sodium determines the distribution of water in these solutions. Sodium-containing solutions are expected to distribute in the extravascular space primarily outside of the intravascular compartment, where it is needed acutely.

ISOTONIC SALINE

A 0.9% solution of sodium chloride will expand the extracellular fluid compartment. If given in large quantities, a hyperchloremic metabolic acidosis is possible.

RINGER'S LACTATE

This is a balanced electrolyte solution that mimics in some ways the interstitial fluid. The lactate is metabolized to carbon dioxide and water and may not be an effective buffer. The small amounts of potassium and calcium cause some concern; however, there is no evidence for adverse consequences attributable to these anions. Balanced salt solutions with increased buffing capacity are also available. Normosol-R has acetate and gluconate to buffer its pH at 7.4; it also has some magnesium, presumed to counter the vasoconstriction associated with hypovolemia. It and similar solutions are more expensive than the usual crystalloids and have not been shown to be any more effective. Normosol-R represents the class that includes Isolyte and Plasmolyte in various compositions (47).

Dextrose may be added to various isotonic or balanced salt solutions. Its distribution is the entire body water space and thus does not have much effect on volume resuscitation. In concentrations greater than 5%, it serves as an osmotic diuretic and can actually inhibit fluid translocation by limiting the amount of fluid available. Glucose enhances the lactic acid production of ischemic brain, and thus its routine use in patients with cerebral ischemia is not recommended (48). If this observation is validated for other tissues, dextrose should not be added to routine resuscitation fluids.

COLLOIDS

Colloids are large-molecular-weight molecules that are generally retained in the vascular space where they "hydrate," expand their size, and thus keep fluid within the intravascular compartment. Each liter of colloid has an effective increase in vascular volume.

ALBUMIN

Albumin is available in 5 and 25% solutions in saline. The therapeutic effectiveness is between 18 and 30 hours after infusion. Endogenous albumin has a serum half-life of close to 21 days. The difference may be due to the processing of the albumin to make it available for infusion.

DEXTRANS

Two commonly available dextrans, made from glucose polymers, can be used as volume expanders. Basically 10% solutions, they can effectively increase the intravascular volume for a short period of time, usually up to 6 hours. The difference between Dextran 40 and Dextran 70 solutions lies not only in their molecular size distribution but also in their rheological properties and effects on the clotting system. Problems have been encountered with clotting and anaphylaxis as well as renal failure. They are generally not used for acute volume resuscitation.

HETASTARCH

Derived from amylopectin, hetastarch is a highly branched glucose polymer; structurally it is similar to glucagon. Because it is an amyl sugar, it is subject to degeneration by amylase and thus is not indicated in the treatment of acute pancreatitis. A 6% solution in saline is similar in effect to 5% albumin. It has been shown to be effective in resuscitation (49). As with other colloids, there have been some adverse unexplained effects (33).

PENTASTARCH

This is a newer formulation of hetastarch with a more restricted molecular size distribution, giving it distinct properties. Its average molecular weight is about 120,000 Da, less than half the size of hetastarch. It has a half-life of about 10 hours and is slightly hyperoncotic. It is slightly more effective in increasing plasma volume than albumin, the dextrans, or hydroxyethyl starch (50). These studies were done in normal volunteers and thus may not be directly applicable to the resuscitation situation.

The hypotensive patient with obvious blood loss usually receives a 1-L bolus volume of lactated Ringer's and the hemodynamic response (e.g., blood pressure and heart rate) is evaluated; this affords a "clinical assessment" of volume status. If vital signs improve, urinary output increases, and the patient appears to stabilize, 1 L may be a sufficient volume for resuscitation. If vital signs and clinical status do not improve or improve transiently, additional infusions of balanced salt solutions are required. If there is no further improvement in vital signs or other clinical parameters or only a transient response, additional crystalloid is infused while red blood cells are obtained. Although covered elsewhere in detail in this book (see Chapter 4) O negative, O positive, and type-specific red blood cells can be used until typed and cross-matched red blood cells (allogenic blood) have been obtained. It is necessary to obtain a blood specimen before initiation of blood-oriented resuscitation for a reference initial blood type if type-specific red cells are required. Once the patient is in the operating room, options for cell salvage to obtain and use autologous red cells can be exercised if the situation is appropriate. Transfusion avoidance techniques such as autologous predeposit or acute normovolemic hemodilution for the acutely bleeding patient are unlikely scenarios; they are noted only for completeness. Obviously, the use of intraoperative red cell salvage relates to the type and site of injury (see Chapter 22).

CONSEQUENCES OF RESUSCITATION

Are there problems associated with resuscitation generally and specifically attributable to each type and class of solution? The lack of pure homogeneous patient population studies makes this question moot. Outcome is clearly influenced by the combination of initial insult and patient risk factors. Minimizing end-organ damage without initiating the sepsis inflammatory response syndrome mediator cycle results in less overhydration, tissue edema, and cellular damage (51). Resuscitation is clearly an empirically driven process. Without easily measured clinical endpoints or surrogates, it is difficult to know when to stop the resuscitation; overshoot of endpoints is likely and possible because their measurement is not precise. In the interest of maintaining perfusion, an overexpansion of the vascular bed may occur. If the inflammatory mediator cycle is not initiated and the patient initiates appropriate homeostatic responses, the excess fluid is excreted with minimal consequences. Once the patient is stabilized and the hemorrhaging site controlled, effective offloading of any excess fluid is possible. There is general agreement that more problems are associated with underresuscitation than with overresuscitation.

Because the endpoints of empiric volume resuscitation are not clear and the presence of an overshoot cannot be defined, it is possible that underresuscitation will occur. This is the crux of the issue: the definition of resuscitation. From it flows the debate regarding techniques. Because the initial resuscitation is directed at restoring tissue oxygenation and there are few clinical correlates of this state, how do we know the end is achieved? Indeed, if one accepts the proposal that an oxygen debt is both real and an important concept, some readily accessible clinical endpoint, to know the debt is eliminated would be helpful. There is scant evidence to support any clinical or chemical parameters to indicate this situation; further study is required to address the issue (6). Thus, underresuscitation, if it fails to repay the O_2 debt, must be viewed as potentially more compromising than overresuscitation; underresuscitated tissues are not fully functional and therefore are not able to withstand additional insults. This concept certainly underlies the proposed use of red blood cells and oxygen-carrying red cell substitutes now under evaluation for acute resuscitation (11, 19).

REFERENCES

1. Jones WG, Faney TJ III, Shires GT. Surgical intensive care. Boston: Little, Brown, 1993.
2. Renzi RM, Kaye W, Greenburg AG. Surgical intensive care. Boston: Little, Brown, 1993.
3. Greenburg AG. Pathophysiology of shock. In: Miller TA, Rowlands BJ, eds. Physiologic basis of modern surgical care. St. Louis: C.V. Mosby, 1988:154–172.
4. Demling RH. Shock in current practice of surgery. New York: Churchill Livingstone, 1993.
5. Astiz ME, Rackow EC, Weil MH. Pathophysiology and treatment of circulatory shock. Crit Care Clin 1993;9:183–203.
6. Shoemaker WC, Paul PL, Kram HB. Tissue oxygen debt as a determinant of lethal and nonlethal postoperative organ failure. Crit Care Med 1986;16:1117–1120.
7. Shoemaker WC, Paul PL, Kram HB. Hemodynamic and oxygen transport responses in survivors and nonsurvivors of high risk surgery. Crit Care Med 1993;21:977–990.
8. Bickell WH, Wall MJ, Pepe PE, et al. Immediate versus delayed fluid resuscitation for hypotensive patient with penetrating torso injuries. N Engl J Med 1994;331:1105–1109.
9. Thakore GN, Rudowski R, Kaye W, Greenburg AG. Use of cardiac efficiency as an indicator for blood transfusion. Chest 1994;56s. [Abstract]
10. Voermann JH, Groeneveld J. Blood viscosity & circulatory shock. Crit Care Med 1989;15:72–78.
11. Woodson RD. Hemoglobin structure and oxygen transport in principles of transfusion medicine. Baltimore: Williams & Wilkins, 1991.
12. Kaneto A, Kajinuma H, Kosaka K. Effect of splanchnic nerve stimulation on glucagon and insulin output in the dog. Endocrinology 1975;96:143–150.
13. Sherwin RS, Sacca L. Effect of epinephrine on glucose metabolism in humans: contribution of the liver. Am J Physiol 1984;246:E157–165.
14. Woolf PD. Endocrinology of shock. Ann Emerg Med 1986;15: 1401–1405.
15. Greenburg AG. Indications for transfusion in care of the surgical patient. New York: Scientific American Medicine, 1988–1994.
16. Shires GT, Williams J, Brown FJ. A method for simultaneous measurement of plasma volume, red cell mean and extracellular fluid space in man using radioactive $^{35}SO_4$ and ^{51}Cv. J Clin Lab Med 1960;55:776.
17. Shires GT, Coln D, Carrico CJ, Lightfoot S. Fluid therapy in hemorrhagic shock Arch Surg 1964;88:688–693.
18. Illner H, Shires GT. The effect of hemorrhagic shock on potassium transport in skeletal muscle. Surg Gynecol Obstet 1980;150:17–25.
19. Greenburg AG. Alternatives to conventional use of blood products critical care: state of the art. Soc Crit Care Med 1992;14:325–351.
20. Lewis FL. Prehospital intravenous fluid therapy; physiologic computer modeling. J Trauma 1986;26:804–811.
21. Krausz MM, Bar Ziv M, Rabinovici R, Gross D. "Scoop and run" or stabilize hemorrhagic shock by normal saline or small volume hypertonic saline. J Trauma 1992;33:6–10.
22. Gross D, Landau EH, Assalia A, Krausz MM. Is hypertonic saline resuscitation safe in uncontrollable hemorrhagic shock? J Trauma 1988; 28:751–756.
23. Lamke LO, Liljedahl SO. Plasma volume changes after infusion of various plasma expanders. Resuscitation 1976;5:93–102.
24. Sondeen JL, Gunther RA, Dubick MA. Comparison of 7.5%NaCl/6% Dextran-70 resuscitation of hemorrhage between euhydrated and dehydrated sheep. Shock 1995;3:63–68.
25. Cordts PR, Lamorte WW, Fisher JB. Poor predictive valve of hematocrit and hemodynamic parameters for erythrocyte deficits after extensive elective vascular operations. Surg Gynecol Obstet 1992;175: 243–248.
26. Zarins CK, Rice CL, Peters RM, et al. Lymphatic and pulmonary response to isotonic reduction in plasma oncotic pressure in baboons. Circ Res 1978;43:925–930.
27. Lowe RJ, Moss GS, Jilek J, Levine MD. Crystalloid vs colloid in the etiology of pulmonary failure after trauma: a randomized trial in man. Surgery 1977;81:676–683.
28. Moss GS, Lowe RJ, Jilek J, Levine MD. Colloid or crystalloid in the resuscitation of hemorrhagic shock: controlled clinical trial. Surgery 1981;89:434–438.
29. Lucas CE, Weaver D, Higgins RF, et al. Effects of albumin versus nonalbumin resuscitation on plasma volume and renal excretory function. J Trauma 1978;18:564–570.
30. Ledgerwood AM, Lucas CE. Post-Resuscitation hypertension: etiology, morbidity and treatment. Arch Surg 1974;108:531–538.
31. Weaver DW, Ledgerwood AM, Lucas CE, et al. Pulmonary effects of albumin resuscitation for severe hypovolemic shock. Arch Surg 1978; 113:387–392.
32. Bisonni RS, Holtgrav DR, Lawler R et al. Colloids versus crystalloids in fluid resuscitation: an analysis of randomized controlled trials. J. Fam Pract 1991;32:387–390.
33. Imm A, Carlson RW. Fluid resuscitation in circulatory shock. Crit Care Clin 1993;9:313–333.
34. Shires GT, Barber AE, Illner HD. Current status of resuscitation: solutions including hypertonic saline. Adv Surg 1995;28:1133–1170.
35. Velanovich V. Crystalloid versus colloid fluid resuscitation a meta-analysis of mortality. Surgery 1989;105:65–71.
36. Baue AE, Tragus ET, Parkins WM. A comparison of isotonic and hypertonic solutions and blood on blood flow and oxygen consumption in the initial treatment of hemorrhagic shock. J Trauma 1967;7:743–756.
37. Nerlick M, Gunther R, Demling R. Resuscitation from hemorrhagic shock with hypertonic saline or lactated Ringer's. Circ Shock 1983;10: 179–188.
38. Vassar MJ, Perry CA, Holcroft JW. Analysis of potential risks associated with 7.5% sodium chloride resuscitation of traumatic shock. Arch Surg 1990;125:1309–1315.
39. Vassar MJ, Perry CA, Holcroff JW. Hypertonic/hyperoncotic resuscitation and improvement in predicted outcome for trauma patients. Circ Shock 1992;37:1309–1315.
40. Mattox KM, Maningas PA, Moore EE. Prehospital hypertonic saline/ dextran infusion for post-traumatic hypotension.The USA Multicenter Study. Ann Surg 1991;213:482–491.
41. Bickwell WH. Use of hypertonic saline/dextran versus lactated Ringer's solution as a resuscitation fluid after uncontrolled aortic hemorrhage in anesthetized swine. Ann Emerg Med 1992;21:1077–1085.
42. Stern SA. Effect of blood pressure on hemorrhage volume and survival in a near-fatal hemorrhage model incorporating a vascular injury. Ann Emerg Med 1993;22:155–163.
43. Prough DS, Johnson JC, Poole GV Jr, et al. Effects on intracranial pressure of resuscitation from hemorrhagic shock with hypertonic saline versus lactated Ringer's solution. Crit Care Med 1985;13: 407–411.

44. Zhavng J, Shackford SR, Schmoreu JD, Pietropaoli JA. Colloid infusion after brain injury: effect on intracranial pressure, cerebral blood flow and oxygen delivery. Crit Care Med 1995;23: 140–148.
45. Krausz MM. Controversies in shock research: hypertonic resuscitation—pros and cons. Shock 1995;3:69–72.
46. Advanced Trauma Life Support Course, Shock 179–191. American College of Surgeons, 1984.
47. AAHFS Drug Information. American Society of Health Systems Pharmacists Bethesda, Maryland. American Society of Hospital Pharmacists, Inc., 1994.
48. Voll CL, Auer RN. The effect of postischemic blood glucose levels on ischemic brain damage in the rat. Ann Neurol 1988;24:638–646.
49. Shatney CH, Deepika K, Militello PR, et al. Efficacy of hetastarch in the resuscitation of patients with multisystem trauma and shock. Arch Surg 1983;118:804–809.
50. Kohler H, Zschiedrich H, Clasen R, et al. The effects of 500 ml 10% hydroxyethyl starch 200/0.5 and 10% Dextran-40 on blood volume, colloid osmotic pressure and level of function in human volunteers. Anesthesia 1982;31:61–67.
51. Cerra FB. Metabolic response to injury. In: Cerra FB, ed. Manual of critical care. St. Louis: C.V. Mosby, 1987:117–145.

Chapter 15

Approach to Patients with Special Red Cell Disorders: Sickle Hemoglobinopathies, Polycythemia, and Autoimmune Hemolytic Anemia

OSWALDO CASTRO
SOHAIL RANA

INTRODUCTION

The preoperative management of patients with sickle hemoglobinopathies or with polycythemia presents unique problems relating to transfusion medicine. Patients with sickle cell disease are at risk for severe sickling (vaso-occlusive) complications in the postoperative period. The frequency of these complications can be reduced by preoperative transfusions because transfusions reduce the percent of circulating red cells capable of sickling. In the polycythemias, especially polycythemia vera, surgery is often complicated by episodes of thrombosis and/or hemorrhage probably due to increased blood viscosity and abnormal platelet function. For this reason, patients with uncontrolled polycythemia require preoperative phlebotomies to reduce blood viscosity by lowering the hematocrit. Anemias of most etiologies are corrected preoperatively with specific measures, such as iron for iron deficiency. Transfusions are used in anemic patients when specific treatment for their anemia is unavailable or when it is not likely to raise the hemoglobin level in time for surgery. Autoimmune hemolytic anemia is discussed as a special red cell disorder because it can present the difficult problem of identifying compatible units when transfusions are required. Preoperative management of the three red cell conditions discussed in this chapter requires close and continued collaboration between the surgeon and the hematologist, the anesthesiologist, and the transfusion medicine specialist.

SICKLE HEMOGLOBINOPATHIES

SICKLE CELL DISEASE

Sickle cell disease consists of a group of genetic disorders characterized by the presence of sickle hemoglobin (Hb S) in the red blood cells (RBCs). Sickle hemoglobin is a structural hemoglobin variant that aggregates or polymerizes when deoxygenated. The most common and also the most severe form of sickle cell disease is sickle cell anemia (homozygous sickle cell disease, Hb SS) in which almost all intracellular hemoglobin is Hb S. Other forms of sickle cell disease are sickle cell-Hb C disease (Hb SC disease), in which Hb S and Hb C are present in equal amounts (each 50%), and the various types of sickle cell-β-thalassemias, which have 70–95% intracellular Hb S (1, 2). The main hematological (3) and clinical characteristics of the various sickle cell genotypes are summarized in Table 15.1.

When Hb S is present in large enough amounts, it forms intracellular polymers at low but still physiological oxygen

TABLE 15.1. CHARACTERISTICS OF THE SICKLING DISORDERS

Genotype	Hb S (%)	Hb C (%)	Hb F (%)	Hb A (%)	Usual Hematocrit (%)	Clinical Severity
Sickle cell anemia (homozygous sickle cell disease, Hb SS)	80–95	0	1–15	0	20–30	++++
Sickle cell-hemoglobin C disease (Hb SC)	~50	~50	1–7	0	26–42	+to+++
Sickle cell-β^+-thalassemia (Hb Sβ^+ thal.)	70–90	0	2–10	10–30	30–42	+to++
Sickle cell-β^0-thalassemia (Hb Sβ^0 thal.)	70–95	0	2–20	0	20–35	++to++++
Sickle cell-$\delta\beta$-thalassemia (Hb S$\delta\beta$ thal.)	75–85	0	15–20	0	26–39	+to+++

tensions (4). These polymers are rigid, liquid, crystal-like structures that markedly decrease red cell deformity and ultimately result in membrane damage and erythrocyte sickling. The pathophysiological consequences of erythrocyte rigidity and sickling are twofold: a chronic hemolytic anemia due to premature destruction of the abnormal red cells and episodes of tissue injury, called vaso-occlusive, or painful, crises. The vaso-occlusive crises are thought to result from ischemia or necrosis due to impaired microvascular flow of the rheologically abnormal cells. The red cells of people with the sickle cell trait, the carrier state for the Hb S gene (Hb AS), have only 30–45% Hb S. This concentration is too low for Hb S polymerization to occur under physiological conditions. For this reason, people with sickle cell trait have no hemolytic anemia or vaso-occlusive crises. They are considered healthy and have no problems from their hemoglobin type except under very special conditions (5).

Sickle cell patients frequently develop complications requiring surgical intervention. Surgery and anesthesia are themselves risk factors for postoperative vaso-occlusive events and for significant morbidity and mortality. As discussed below, the most common complications are postoperative sickle cell chest syndrome and postoperative vaso-occlusive crisis. The Cooperative Study of Sickle Cell Disease (CSSCD) followed prospectively 3765 patients during the period from 1979 to 1988 (6). Koshy et al. (7) reported the surgery and anesthesia experience in 717 CSSCD patients (77% with Hb SS, 14% with Hb SC) who underwent 1079 operative procedures. There were 12 deaths (1.1%) within 30 days after surgery, 3 (0.3%) of which were attributed directly to the surgery and/or anesthesia. No deaths occurred in patients younger than 14 years of age. Mortality rates of up to 3% were reported in earlier retrospective studies (8, 9), whereas more recent series encountered little morbidity and no mortality (10–13). In all but one (13) recent series, preoperative transfusions were used routinely. Factors that could be responsible for the perioperative vaso-occlusive complications in sickle cell patients are hypoxia, hypoperfusion, stasis, acidosis, dehydration, and hypothermia (14, 15).

Preoperative Transfusions

Experience from the above series suggests, but does not prove, that preoperative transfusions decrease the frequency of postoperative sickling complications. Other experimental and clinical observations also support the concept that in general blood transfusions improve tissue perfusion and tend to prevent sickle cell vaso-occlusion:

1. Adding even small quantities of Hb A red cells to Hb SS red cells in vitro improves the rheological characteristics of the mixture (16).
2. The hyposthenuria and functional asplenia characteristic of children with sickle cell anemia can be reversed temporarily by transfusions (17, 18).
3. Exchange transfusions improve exercise capacity in sickle cell patients without substantially raising their hematocrit (19), suggesting that addition of Hb A red cells improves blood rheology and tissue perfusion also in vivo. This interpretation, however, has been challenged (20).
4. Vaso-occlusive complications such as pain crises, chest syndrome, and priapism are rare in children with sickle cell anemia who are on long-term transfusion programs.
5. A prospective randomized trial showed that prophylactic transfusions reduced the incidence of vaso-occlusive crises in pregnant patients with sickle cell anemia (21).

For these reasons, most hematologists recommend preoperative transfusions at least for patients with the more severe forms of sickle cell disease: sickle cell anemia and sickle cell β^0-thalassemia. The transfusion objective is not necessarily to raise the blood oxygen-carrying capacity. Most patients with sickle cell anemia in the steady state have adapted to their low hemoglobin level and ordinarily do not need "correction" of their anemia. Preoperative transfusions are recommended mainly to improve tissue perfusion during surgery and anesthesia by lowering the proportion of red cells capable of sickling.

Simple Versus Exchange Transfusions. Simple transfusions are easy to perform and they lower the proportion of sickling cells in the recipient. This effect is more pronounced over time because the transfused red cells have a longer intravascular survival than the patient's own red cells and because simple transfusions raise the hematocrit, thus inhibiting endogenous erythropoiesis (22). Simple transfusions are the most practical option when the patient's anemia is severe, as is the case with Hb SS disease. On the other hand, because simple transfusions raise the hemoglobin level by approximately 1 g/dL per red cell unit (in adults), they are not appropriate for sickle cell patients with higher hematocrits, such as those with Hb SC disease or Hb S β^+-thalassemia (Table 15.1). In these patients, simple transfusions will raise the hematocrit to levels that could increase blood viscosity. Exchange transfusions are preferable because they rapidly lower the proportion of sickling cells without substantially raising the hematocrit. Other advantages of exchange transfusions for all sickle cell patients are

1. A more physiological (lower) posttransfusion hematocrit;
2. A faster and more efficient reduction in the percent of sickling cells;
3. A much lower amount of iron loading per unit than with simple transfusions.

Disadvantages of exchange transfusions are a higher cost, exposure to more blood donors, and their need for adequate vascular access, which is a problem for many patients.

Exchange transfusions can be accomplished by various manual methods (23) or with the use of automated equipment (erythrocytapheresis) (24). A simple method for manual exchange transfusion in sickle cell patients with an Hb level of at least 7 g/dL or a hematocrit of at least 20% is described below. For lower Hb or hematocrit values, 1 unit of RBCs (adults) or 5 mL/kg RBCs (children) can be administered before the exchange transfusion. Alternatively, if 1 unit (or 5 mL/kg) of RBCs is not expected to raise the Hb level to at least 7 g/dL, one can prepare the patient for surgery using simple transfusions instead of exchange transfusions.

The method for manual exchange transfusion is as follows:

1. Withdraw 1 unit of blood (450 mL) for adults or 7.5 mL/kg of blood for children from an arm vein.
2. Replace blood volume by rapidly infusing normal saline: 500 mL for adults or 8 mL/kg for children.
3. Repeat step 1.
4. Transfuse 2 units of packed RBCs for adults or 10 mL/kg packed RBCs for children.
5. Repeat steps 1–4 once more for patients with sickle cell anemia. Repeat steps 1–4 twice for patients with higher hematocrits (e.g., Hb SC disease).

With this method, 4 units of blood (adults) are removed and replaced with 4 units of packed RBCs plus 1000 mL of normal saline. In adults with higher hematocrits, such as those with Hb SC disease, 6 units of blood are removed and replaced with 6 units of packed RBCs plus 1500 mL of normal saline. After this manual exchange, the proportion of Hb A should exceed 50% and the proportion of Hb S (for sickle cell anemia) or of Hb S plus Hb C (for Hb SC disease) should be lower than 50%.

If automated equipment (blood cell processor, cell separator) is available, a red cell exchange, or erythrocytapheresis (25), can be performed. As with manual exchanges, 4 RBC units should be exchanged in adult patients with sickle cell anemia and 6 units in those with Hb SC disease. Automated red cell exchanges accomplish this objective while keeping the extracorporeal blood volume at about 250 mL (in adults). In contrast, the extracorporeal volume in manual exchanges can be up to 500 mL.

Aggressive Versus Conservative Transfusion Regimen. Vichinsky et al. (26) recently reported the results of a prospective, multicenter, randomized clinical trial comparing two approaches to preoperative transfusions in sickle cell anemia. Over 600 surgical procedures in 551 Hb SS patients were randomized preoperatively to an "aggressive" or "conservative" transfusion regimen. The aim of the aggressive regimen was to achieve a preoperative Hb level of at least 10 g/dL and an Hb S fraction of 30% or less. This regimen usually required exchange transfusions. The objective of the conservative regimen was to maintain an Hb level of 10 g/dL (range 10–11) regardless of the percent Hb S. Most patients in this regimen received simple transfusions. A "no-transfusion" randomization arm was not included because most investigators agreed that some form of preoperative transfusions were necessary in patients with sickle cell anemia undergoing surgery. Both children and adults participated in the trial, and elective and emergency surgical interventions were performed. The anesthesia risk score was 3 in 51% of the patients and 2 in 47% of the patients.

The most common operations were cholecystectomy, ENT (ear, nose, and throat), and orthopedic procedures. Over 80% of the procedures were carried out using a combination of inhalation and intravenous anesthesia, and the average duration of the anesthesia was 2.5 hours. Table 15.2 shows that the aggressive regimen was no better than the conservative regimen in preventing postoperative sickling complications, the most common of which was sickle cell chest syndrome (10% of the cases in both treatment arms). The frequencies of postoperative fever or infection and pain crises ranged from 4 to 7% and were not affected by the preoperative transfusion regimen. In contrast, the frequency of transfusion complications was much higher in the aggressive transfusion arm, presumably because of exposure to a larger number of RBC units. The appearance of new RBC alloantibodies was twice as likely in the aggressive transfusion arm (10% versus 5% in the conservative regimen; $P = .01$). Hemolytic transfusion reactions occurred in 6% of cases managed with aggressive transfusions. Only 1% of patients in the conservative transfusion arm developed this problem.

TABLE 15.2. CLINICAL TRIAL OF CONSERVATIVE VERSUS AGGRESSIVE PREOPERATIVE TRANSFUSION REGIMENS IN SICKLE CELL ANEMIA

	Conservative (77% with simple transfusions)	Aggressive (57% with exchange transfusions)
Patients/operations	273/301	278/303
Mean pretransfusion Hb (g/dL)	7.9	8.0
Mean number RBC units transfused		
Children (birth to 9 yr)	1.5	3.8
Adults	3.3	6.1
Mean posttransfusion Hb (g/dL)	10.6	11
Mean posttransfusion Hb S (%)	59	31
Postoperative complications		
Chest syndrome (%)	10	10
Fever or infection (%)	5	7
Pain crisis (%)	7	4
Transfusion complications		
Hemolytic transfer reaction (%)	1	6
New RBC alloantibody (%)	5	10

Adapted from Vichinsky EP, Halurkern CM, Neumayr L, et al. A comparison of conservative and aggressive transfusion regimens in the perioperative management of sickle cell disease. N Engl J Med 1995;333:206–213.

Multivariate analysis showed that a higher surgical risk category and a history of pulmonary disease were independent risk factors for the most severe postoperative complication, the sickle cell chest syndrome. Age greater than 10 years and over five previous hospitalizations were associated with the development of postoperative pain crisis.

This controlled study (26) indicates that, contrary to expectation, exchange transfusions, or other intensive transfusion regimens that lower the Hb S fraction to less than 50%, are no better than simple transfusions in preventing postoperative vaso-occlusive events. Therefore, simple transfusions are at present preferable in the preoperative preparation of sickle cell anemia patients. Limited exchange transfusions might still be required preoperatively for those few SS patients with higher hematocrits. Furthermore, once a perioperative vaso-occlusive complication has developed, therapeutic exchange transfusions are indicated.

The above clinical trial also raises the question of whether SS patients could undergo surgery and anesthesia without any preoperative transfusions and still have no more complications than in transfused patients. A new prospective randomized study with a no-transfusion arm will be required to answer this question definitively. Based on the rationale for preoperative transfusions discussed above, our prediction is that significantly greater postoperative morbidity and mortality would be found in nontransfused SS patients.

Preoperative Transfusions in Hb SC Disease and Other Less Severe Genotypes. The clinical course of Hb SC disease is variable (27, 28). In general, however, patients with this or with other genotypes that have less hemolysis and less anemia also tend to have a lower vaso-occlusive severity. In the report from the CSSCD (7), 102 Hb SC patients had surgical procedures, and preoperative transfusions were associated with lower rates of postoperative crises and chest syndrome. At our center, we recommend preoperative exchange transfusions in Hb SC disease and sickle cell β^{+}-thalassemia when at least one of the following conditions is present:

1. Ophthalmological procedures, usually vitrectomy, with risk of anterior segment ischemia and/or secondary glaucoma (29);
2. High-risk procedures such as cardiopulmonary bypass (30);
3. Surgery in which substantial blood loss is expected, such as total hip arthroplasty (31); in these cases, perioperative transfusions are likely to occur anyway;
4. Patients with particularly severe clinical course, such as those with three or more hospitalizations for vaso-occlusive crises and/or chest syndrome per year;
5. Presence of risk factors that have been shown to predict postoperative chest syndrome in Hb SS disease in the controlled study discussed above (26).

Recommendations. Because sickle cell disease has a wide spectrum of severity, preoperative transfusion management has to be individualized. Hemoglobin electrophoresis should always be obtained preoperatively because some sickle cell patients may not have been previously diagnosed. If the patient has sickle cell disease (Table 15.1), hematological consultation should be sought for joint perioperative management (32), particularly for decisions involving transfusion. Transfusions are indicated for all surgical interventions requiring general anesthesia, even those that are not particularly invasive such as laparoscopic surgery and débridement or skin grafting of leg ulcers. The same probably applies for procedures requiring regional anesthesia. In fact, the CSSCD series reported more complications in patients operated under regional anesthesia. The estimated odds ratio was 2.32 when compared with general anesthesia (7). On the other hand, this study was not randomized, and patients could have been selected for regional anesthesia because they were believed to have a higher anesthesia risk. Table 15.3 summarizes the preoperative transfusion recommendations for the various forms of sickle cell disease. These recommendations are based on the best currently available information but are not meant to substitute for informed clinical judgment in the individual patient.

Avoidance of Transfusion Reactions. The prevalence of RBC alloimmunization in sickle cell disease is about 20% (33), and these patients have a high risk for delayed transfusion reactions (34). Obtaining an alloimmunization history before any transfusions are given is essential to avoid these reactions. The patient should be asked about transfusion history, transfusion reactions, and known alloantibodies. The patient's primary physician and hospitals where transfusion records might be available also should be contacted to obtain or verify an alloimmunization history. If the patient has a history of having formed a red cell alloantibody, RBC units that are negative for the corresponding antigen should be requested even if the current antibody screen no longer shows that antibody. This is because as many as one-half of the RBC alloantibodies formed by sickle cell patients (33) and by other patients (35) become serologically undetectable within a year. When such a patient is then transfused with RBCs bearing the antigen(s) responsible for the primary immunization, a strong anamnestic antibody response occurs and a life-threatening delayed hemolytic transfusion reaction can develop. In preoperatively transfused patients, these reactions typically take place during the postoperative period.

TABLE 15.3. RECOMMENDATIONS FOR PREOPERATIVE TRANSFUSIONS IN THE SICKLING DISORDERS

Sickle cell anemia, sickle cell-β^0-thalassemia, or sickle cell-$\delta\beta$-thalassemia (Hb SS, Hb S-β^0 thal., or Hb S-$\delta\beta$ thal.)
Hematocrit 20–30%[a]
Simple transfusion 3 units RBCs (adults)
Simple transfusion 15 mL/kg RBCs (children)
Hematocrit >30%
Exchange transfusion 4–6 units RBCs (adults)
Exchange transfusion 15 mL/kg RBCs (children)
Sickle cell-hemoglobin C disease or sickle cell-β^+-thalassemia (Hb SC or Hb Sβ^+ thal.)
Hematocrit <25%
Simple transfusion 3 units RBCs (adults)
Simple transfusion 15 mL/kg RBCs (children)
Hematocrit >25%
Individual consideration (see text)
If transfusions needed use
Exchange transfusion 4–6 units RBCs (adults)
Exchange transfusion 15 mL/kg RBCs (children)

[a]For lower pretransfusion hematocrits, additional units should be used.

Types of RBCs Units to be Used. Sickle-negative RBC units should be used because interpretation of posttransfusion Hb S levels can be problematic in patients transfused with RBCs from sickle cell trait donors. Patients should be given leukodepleted RBC units to avoid febrile transfusion reactions or to avoid primary immunization to leukocyte antigens.

Because of the high risk of alloimmunization (see above), the use of extended RBC antigen matching for all sickle cell patients, regardless of transfusion history, has been recommended (26, 36, 37). The arguments in favor of this recommendation are that transfusion history may be unreliable or unavailable and that screening donors for most antigens against which sickle cell patients form antibodies is relatively simple. Prospective randomized studies to assess the risk-to-benefit ratio of this approach to solve the alloimmunization problem have not been conducted (38). One can predict that matching for the common RBC antigens will still fail to prevent alloimmunization in as many as 25% of sickle cell patients (39). Furthermore, requesting antigen-matched RBCs for preoperative transfusions in nonalloimmunized sickle cell patients could lead to unnecessary delays in the surgical procedure. For these reasons, we believe that requesting antigen-matched RBCs for preoperative transfusion of nonalloimmunized patients is justified only if such a request does not delay transfusion and/or surgery.

SICKLE CELL TRAIT

People with the sickle cell trait (Hb AS) do not have sickle cell disease. They have no hemolysis or anemia because the fraction of Hb S in their red cells is too low for polymerization to occur in vivo. An excellent review of the few medical risks thought to be associated with sickle cell trait was published recently (40). Increased surgical risk has not been demonstrated (41, 42), and preoperative transfusions in sickle cell trait are not needed unless the patient is anemic from an unrelated illness. Based on rare adverse events (43–45), some recommend exchange transfusions for procedures where hypoxia or hypoperfusion may occur, including open heart and intrathoracic surgery (14, 32). Reports from other investigators, however, do not support the need for this recommendation (46). At our institution, we do not use preoperative transfusions in sickle cell trait even in open heart procedures.

AUTOLOGOUS TRANSFUSIONS

An increasing number of preoperatively deposited autologous units are being transfused to surgical patients without sickle cell disease (566,000 units in the United States in 1992 [47]). As stated earlier, however, the objective of transfusions in sickle cell patients is to lower the proportion of red cells capable of sickling to prevent postoperative complications. Replacement of intraoperative blood losses by previously collected autologous RBCs would increase the percent circulating SS RBCs and work against the protective effect of the preoperatively transfused isologous (Hb AA) RBCs. Therefore, autologous units should not be used. There is a report of a fatality, presumably from widespread sickle cell sequestration and disseminated intravascular coagulation, after intraoperative transfusion of autologous Hb SC RBCs (48).

Transfusion of intraoperatively salvaged RBCs is possible but is likely to be safe only in sickle cell patients who have undergone preoperative isologous exchange transfusions. Under these circumstances, the salvaged RBCs are mostly isologous (Hb AA type) and only a small proportion of them (less than 50%) are really autologous (Hb SS). The safety of transfusing autologous RBCs salvaged during surgery in patients who have not received preoperative isologous RBCs has not been shown. The salvage procedure also could pose technical difficulties. Sickle RBCs that are not "diluted" by isologous (Hb AA) RBCs have a tendency to clump in centrifugation bowls (49) and may do the same in the cell saver. At our center we recommend "autotransfusion" of RBCs salvaged during surgery only if the proportion of SS cells has been lowered to less than 50% via preoperative isologous (Hb AA) transfusions. A published case report suggests that this is probably a safe strategy (50).

The situation is quite different in sickle cell trait. Surgical patients with Hb AS should take advantage of alternatives to isologous transfusions (51) just like patients without sickle hemoglobin. There are no studies of autologous transfusions in people with sickle cell trait. However, some of the half million autologous units transfused yearly in the United States (45) must have been given to subjects with sickle trait, and we are unaware of any reports of untoward effects. Liquid storage of Hb AS red cells does not appear to affect their intravascular survival in autologous (52) or homologous (53, 54) recipients. Frozen storage of Hb AS red cells, however, requires special procedures during the deglycerolization process to avoid hemolysis (55, 56). Also, there may be problems when using filters for leukodepletion of sickle trait units after their liquid storage (57). It should be possible to use the cell saver for intraoperative autotransfusion in sickle cell trait. However, there is a report of sickling of Hb AS RBCs after their collection in the cell saver so that autotransfusion was not carried out and its safety was questioned (58).

THE FUTURE: HYDROXYUREA AND OTHER NEW THERAPIES

Fetal hemoglobin (Hb F) inhibits Hb S polymerization and sickling of Hb SS erythrocytes (59). The antineoplastic agent hydroxyurea increases Hb F and thus improves the anemia in homozygous sickle cell disease (60). In a recently published clinical trial, Charache et al. (61) showed that this drug also reduced the frequency of painful crises, chest syndrome, and transfusions in sickle cell anemia all by about 50%. Participants in this trial were adult SS patients who had at least three crises per year so that they had moderate to severe sickle cell disease (56% of them had over six crises in the year preceding the study). The beneficial effect of hydroxyurea in these severely ill patients is encouraging even though the drug has potentially serious side effects and is not expected to help all patients. In many patients on hydroxyurea, the clinical course improves substantially so that it resembles that of the milder genotypes such as Hb SC disease. Whether SS patients treated successfully with hydroxyurea will benefit from transfusions before surgery and anesthesia is a matter of speculation.

Other drugs that can increase fetal hemoglobin in sickle cell anemia are under investigation (62). If proven clinically effective, their use could dramatically reduce the need for all transfusions, including preoperative transfusions. Finally, it should be mentioned that allogeneic bone marrow transplantation may one day be shown to be safe and curative in sickle cell disease (63) as is the case in many patients with thalassemia major (64). The treatment of sickle cell disease is changing, and the outlook for the future in these patients is now brighter.

POLYCYTHEMIA

Polycythemia or erythrocytosis denotes an elevated hemoglobin concentration and packed red cell volume (hematocrit). The increased hemoglobin concentration can be due to absolute erythrocytosis, in which there is an elevated red cell mass, or to relative erythrocytosis (spurious erythrocytosis, spurious polycythemia), in which there is reduced plasma volume. Only absolute erythrocytoses are discussed in this chapter.

CLASSIFICATION

The polycythemias can be classified pathophysiologically into two categories.

Polycythemias Caused by Increased Erythropoietin (Secondary Polycythemias)

A variety of clinical conditions leading to blood or tissue hypoxia (e.g., residence at high altitude, pulmonary diseases, cyanotic congenital heart diseases, high oxygen affinity hemoglobins, and carbon monoxide intoxication) are associated with erythrocytosis (65). Neonates have high red cell volume in response to intrauterine hypoxia and the high oxygen affinity of fetal hemoglobin. The increased erythropoietin secretion responsible for these polycythemias is appropriate because it represents a physiological response to hypoxia. Other secondary polycythemias are due to inappropriate release of erythropoietin or erythropoietin-like substances from abnormal, predominantly neoplastic tissues. Examples include polycythemias due to renal cysts and tumors, hepatomas, and cerebellar hemangiomas.

Polycythemias Without Increased Erythropoietin (Primary Polycythemias)

Polycythemia vera (P. vera) is by far the most common and important type of primary polycythemia. This condition and its preoperative management are discussed below. Other forms of primary polycythemia are rare. Familial forms could be due to increased sensitivity of erythroid progenitor cells to erythropoietin.

Definition and Incidence. P. vera is a neoplastic clonal stem cell disorder characterized by excessive marrow hemopoiesis in the presence of low erythropoietin levels (66). The annual incidence of P. vera in the United States is approximately 5–17 cases per million (67, 68). The average age at diagnosis is 60 years, and the disease is extremely rare before 30 years of age.

Clinical Feature, and Course of the Disease. Most patients with P. vera have a prolonged survival (69). Patients may present without any symptoms, and on routine examination they may have erythrocytosis, thrombocytosis, or splenomegaly. However, the clinical picture in untreated patients then evolves into a long symptomatic phase due to excessive production of blood cells of various lineages. Symptoms are frequently nonspecific and may be related to impaired cerebral blood flow from increased blood viscosity. Headache, weakness, weight loss, pruritus, visual disturbances, paresthesias, excessive sweating, and joint pain are frequent complaints. Venous and arterial thromboses are the most common serious complications. The physical findings in P. vera include ruddy cyanosis, conjunctival plethora, hepatomegaly, splenomegaly, and hypertension (66, 70). The "proliferative" phase of P. vera is frequently followed by a stage, postpolycythemic myeloid metaplasia (71), in which the patient no longer suffers from the consequences of erythrocytosis but is now anemic or pancytopenic, has gross splenomegaly, and is cachectic. This phase (spent polycythemia) resembles the terminal stage of a malignant tumor (72). In fact, a number of P. vera patients will ultimately go on to develop acute myeloid leukemia (73).

Diagnosis. The criteria for diagnosis of P. vera have been defined by the Polycythemia Vera Study Group (74). The diagnostic criteria have been classified into two categories based on their relative significance:

1. Category A
    - A1. Increased red cell volume (measured with ^{51}Cr-labeled red cells): men at least 36 mL/kg and women at least 32 mL/kg;
    - A2. Normal arterial oxygen saturation (at least 92%);
    - A3. Splenomegaly.
2. Category B
    - B1. Thrombocytosis: platelets at least 400×10^9/L;
    - B2. Leukocytosis: white cells at least 12×10^9/L;
    - B3. Elevated leukocyte alkaline phosphatase score (greater than 100) in absence of fever or infection;
    - B4. Elevated serum vitamin B_{12} level or B_{12} binding capacity: B_{12} more than 900 pg/ml; $UB_{12}BC$ (binding capacity) more than 2200 pg/mL.

The diagnosis of P. vera can be made if all three criteria in category A are present or the combination of an elevated red cell volume and a normal oxygen saturation is present with any two parameters from category B.

Thrombotic and Hemorrhagic Complications. Untreated patients with polycythemia are at a high risk of both thrombosis and hemorrhage. Thrombosis was listed as a cause of death in as many as 37% of fatalities in P. vera (69, 75). Patients may develop deep venous thrombosis of the lower extremities and cerebral, coronary, or peripheral artery occlusion (76). Erythromelalgia with burning pain in the digits is a common symptom. Painful ulcerating lesions of the toes and fingers may develop. Other vascular events include Budd-Chiari syndrome; pulmonary embolism; and thrombosis of mesenteric, hepatic, or splenic arteries (77). Transient ischemic episodes, cerebral infarction or hemorrhage, dementia, choreic syndromes, and paresthesias occur in a large percentage of untreated patients with P. vera (78). Bleeding complications are a cause of death in 5–10% of P. vera patients and as many as 30–40% of patients may experience serious hemorrhagic events (79). Epistaxis, gingival hemorrhages, gastrointestinal bleeding, or hematomas involving vital organs may develop. Patients with uncontrolled P. vera have a very high risk (79%) of complications during and after surgery (80–82). Thrombosis, hemorrhage, or both may develop.

Treatment of P. Vera and Secondary Polycythemias. Phlebotomy is the initial treatment recommended for P. vera. Patients who are less than 40 years of age should be managed with phlebotomies alone (83). If phlebotomies cannot control the increased hematocrit or if thrombocytosis with its associated thrombosis risk is present, myelosuppression with hydroxyurea is indicated. Radioactive phosphorus is used to achieve myelosuppression in patients over 70 years of age. It is not used in younger subjects because of its leukemogenesis risk. The immunomodulatory agent interferon α-2b, anagrelide (a selective inhibitor of platelet production), and antiplatelet medications have all been used to treat P. vera. The choice of therapy remains a subject of active debate. Therapy should be individualized, and a combination of different approaches is often necessary (84, 85). The goal of therapy is to maintain the hematocrit at 42–45% and to prevent thrombotic complications.

The main therapeutic goal in secondary polycythemia is to correct, if possible, the condition responsible for the increased erythropoietin production. Phlebotomies are used to lower the hematocrit and prevent hyperviscosity while the primary condition is being corrected or when it is untreatable. Some have reported successful management of the polycythemia of cyanotic congenital heart disease using hydroxyurea instead of phlebotomies (86). Neonates who are small for gestational age and those born to diabetic mothers can have hyperviscosity due to an excessively high hematocrit (more than 65%) and may require treatment with exchange transfusion.

RECOMMENDATIONS FOR PREOPERATIVE MANAGEMENT

In patients with uncontrolled P. vera, surgical procedures are associated with development of serious complications due to hemorrhage, thrombosis, or both. As many as 75% of patients may develop these complications and approximately one-third could die as a result (80–82). The frequency of these complications can be reduced to 28% by preoperative measures that normalize the hematological parameters. Treatment should be individualized. The following recommendations are offered as a general guideline for preoperative management of patients with P. vera:

1. Elective surgery and dental procedures should be postponed until the red cell mass and the platelet count have been normalized for at least 2 months. The longer the hematological control has been in effect, the lower the frequency of complications in the postoperative period.
2. In case the patient requires an emergency procedure, intensive phlebotomy treatment accompanied by replacement with plasma should be carried out. The rate of blood removal will depend on the patient's hemodynamic status. The goal is to reduce the hematocrit to around 42–45%. The platelet count may be reduced using plateletpheresis. The value of antiplatelet agents such as aspirin in preventing thrombosis is questionable.

Therapeutic venesection to improve cerebral blood flow and increase exercise tolerance may also be indicated in patients with secondary polycythemias such as those due to pulmonary disease and cyanotic congenital heart disease (87, 88). In these secondary polycythemias, the hematocrit should be maintained at about 50% and 55–60%, respectively. In neonates, partial exchange transfusion may be needed to decrease the hematocrit to acceptable levels (55–60%).

AUTOIMMUNE HEMOLYTIC ANEMIA

Autoimmune hemolytic anemias (AIHA) (89) are characterized by the presence of an autoantibody directed against antigens on the red cell membrane and by shortened red cell life span occurring as a result of this antibody. The autoantibodies are of three general types: cold agglutinins, virtually always IgM, which cause clumping of red cells at cold temperatures; warm antibodies of IgG type, which bind to red cells at 37°C but do not agglutinate them; and Donath-Landsteiner antibodies, rare antibodies of IgG isotype, which fix to the red cell membrane at cold temperatures and activate the hemolytic complement pathway when the cells are warmed to 37°C. AIHA can be due to an underlying disease (secondary AIHA) or can develop without such diseases (idiopathic AIHA).

AIHA has an annual incidence of approximately 1 in 80,000. It affects all age and ethnic groups but is more common in midlife and in women. Most cases of AIHA are due to warm antibodies (70–80%). Cold agglutinin disease (CAD) is less common (10–20%) and paroxysmal cold hemoglobinuria (PCH) due to a Donath-Landsteiner antibody accounts for a small percentage of all patients with AIHA (2–5%). Approximately half the cases are secondary to an underlying disease, most commonly a lymphoproliferative disorder. Other cases are induced by drugs, and in some patients, AIHA is a component of an autoimmune disease such as systemic lupus erythematosus.

CLINICAL FINDINGS

The disease can present acutely or may be discovered incidentally by a positive antiglobulin (Coombs') test when a patient is referred for transfusion therapy. Clinical features include jaundice, symptoms and signs of anemia, and splenomegaly. Jaundice is usually mild, and splenomegaly is present in approximately one-third of the patients. The presence of lymphadenopathy, petechiae, fever, hypertension, or renal failure should point to the possibility of an underlying disease in a patient with AIHA. Intravascular hemolysis with accompanying hemoglobinuria and hemosiderinuria occurs in both CAD and PCH.

DIAGNOSIS

A positive direct Coombs' test (antiglobulin test) in the presence of hemolysis is the hallmark of AIHA. The direct Coombs' test detects autoantibodies on the red cells. These antibodies destroy red cells either by intravascular complement-mediated hemolysis or, more frequently, by opsonization and reticuloendothelial system phagocytosis. A positive indirect Coombs' test is due to the presence of antibodies in the serum. In 80% of patients with the warm antibody type of AIHA, both direct and indirect Coombs' tests are positive. A positive indirect Coombs' with a negative direct Coombs' test usually indicates the presence of alloantibodies induced by prior transfusions or pregnancies. Alloantibodies bind only to red cell antigens not present on the patient's red cells.

A Coombs' test is frequently positive during the acute attacks of PCH, and a Coombs' test done with anti-C3 or anti-C3dg is often positive in CAD (90). Cold antibodies are generally present in very high titers but are not detected by the antiglobulin test because the IgM antibodies easily dissociate from the erythrocytes during the washing procedures and at warmer temperatures. The Coombs' test can be falsely positive in 8% of patients and may be falsely negative in 2–4% of all cases of AIHA. More sensitive tests such as the antiglobulin consumption test or tests with ^{125}I-staphylococcal protein A may be needed (91, 92). Patients with AIHA can have both autoantibodies and alloantibodies (from recent or remote transfusions), causing difficulties in identifying the antibody responsible for hemolysis. Specialized reference laboratories may be required for accurate diagnosis in such cases.

TREATMENT OF AIHA

When an underlying disease is responsible for the production of the autoantibody, treatment is directed to the management of the primary problem. The prognosis is dependent on the primary disease and its response to therapy. In patients with postinfectious PCH and CAD, hemolysis is generally self-limited. In those with idiopathic forms of CAD, the disease is generally mild, and avoidance of cold is often sufficient to prevent severe anemia. Plasmapheresis, cytotoxic chemotherapy, or interferon may be used in patients with CAD who have severe anemia. In idiopathic PCH, red cell destruction can be marked and transfusions may be required (see below).

Steroids are the preferred initial treatment for AIHA of the warm antibody type. Patients with severe disease may require transfusions. Most children with AIHA will achieve a complete remission with steroids. However, permanent remissions are unusual in adults. Splenectomy is indicated in patients who do not respond to steroids or who relapse during or after decreases in the dosage of prednisone (93). If possible, patients should be immunized with pneumococcal vaccine several weeks before splenectomy. Patients who do not respond to splenectomy may benefit from immunosuppressive therapy, danazol, or high-dose intravenous immune globulin. Occasional dramatic responses have been reported with plasma exchange in patients who were being prepared for surgery (94).

TRANSFUSIONS IN PATIENTS WITH AIHA

In AIHA, transfusions are reserved for those patients with severe symptomatic anemia. Severe anemia may cause high-output cardiac failure, pulmonary edema, tachycardia, lightheadedness, chest pain, and restlessness or somnolence. Patients with these problems need to be transfused, but transfusions pose special problems in AIHA (95–99). The patients may have to be transfused with in vitro "incompatible" or "least incompatible" red cell units. Also, as mentioned above, alloantibodies may be present because of previous transfusions or maternal-fetal incompatibility (100, 101). These alloantibodies can be difficult to identify in the presence of AIHA so that an alloimmunization history is crucial (see *Avoidance of Transfusion Reactions,* Sickle Cell Disease, above). Oxygen (100%) may be beneficial because the plasma

TABLE 15.4. GENERAL GUIDELINES FOR TRANSFUSING PATIENTS WITH AUTOIMMUNE HEMOLYTIC ANEMIA

1. If cardiac or cerebral function is threatened, transfuse without delay even before all the serological testing is complete.
2. In patients without a history of previous transfusions or pregnancy, ABO and Rh-compatible red cells are generally safe to administer.[a]
3. In patients who have been pregnant or transfused previously, testing for alloantibodies is essential. Give red cells as described in item 2 above. These units should be negative for the antigen(s) against which the alloantibody(ies) is directed.
4. Transfuse relatively small amounts of red cells (0.5–1 unit of packed RBCs in adults and 2–5 mL/kg in children). These quantities are often sufficient to alleviate signs and symptoms of anemia. Overtransfusion can precipitate or worsen cardiac failure.
5. Patients with CAD and PCH should receive prewarmed and preferably washed red cells.
6. Blood should be administered slowly and leukocyte filters should be used to prevent reactions, which may be confused with hemolytic reactions.
7. Administer furosemide after transfusion and observe the patient closely for 6–12 hours for signs and symptoms of fluid overload.
8. Monitor patients for hemolytic transfusion reactions. Acute intravascular hemolysis can occur in the absence of any serological incompatibility.
9. In preparation for surgery, transfuse to increase the hemoglobin concentration to approximately 8 g/dL.

Jefferies LC. Transfusion therapy in autoimmune hemolytic anemia. Hematol Oncol Clin North Am 1994;8:1087–1104.

[a]Sometimes autoantibodies react less strongly in vitro with cells lacking specific antigens (e.g., Rh antigens in warm type AIHA and I or M antigens in CAD). In such cases, RBC units that are negative for these antigens may be selected, if available.

is capable of carrying a small amount (0.3 mL/dL) of oxygen, but it is no substitute for red cells. The clinician must work closely with the blood bank in making the decision to transfuse these patients. Table 15.4 lists general guidelines for transfusing patients with AIHA.

REFERENCES

1. Yang YM, Brigham S, Liu PI. Diagnosis of sickle cell disease and related hemoglobin disorders. In: Mankad VN, Moore RB, eds. Sickle cell disease. Pathophysiology, diagnosis and management. Westport, CT: Praeger, 1992:201–220.
2. Adams JG III. Clinical laboratory diagnosis. In: Embury SH, Hebbel RP, Mohandas N, Steinberg MH, eds. Sickle cell disease. Basic principles and clinical practice. New York: Raven Press, 1994:457–468.
3. West MS, Wethers D, Smith J, Steinberg MH, Cooperative Study of Sickle Cell Disease. Laboratory profile of sickle cell disease: a cross-sectional analysis. J Clin Epidemiol 1992;45:893–909.
4. Noguchi CT, Schechter AN. The intracellular polymerization of sickle hemoglobin and its relevance to sickle cell disease. Blood 1981;58:1057–1068.
5. Kark JA, Ward FT. Exercise and hemoglobin S. Semin Hematol 1994;31:181–225.
6. Gaston M, Rosse WF: The Cooperative Study of Sickle Cell Disease: review of study design and objectives. Am J Pediatr Hematol 1982;4:197.
7. Koshy M, Weiner SJ, Miller ST, et al. Surgery and anesthesia in sickle cell disease. Blood 1995;86:3676–3684.
8. Homi J, Reynolds J, Skinner A, Hanna W, Serjeant GR. General anaesthesia in sickle-cell disease. Br Med J 1979;1:1599–1601.
9. Oduro KA, Searle JF. Anaesthesia in sickle cell states: a plea for simplicity. Br Med J 1972;4:596–598.
10. Janik J, Seeler RA. Perioperative management of children with sickle hemoglobinopathies. 1980;15:117–120.
11. Morrison JC, Whybrew WD, Bocovaz ET. Use of partial exchange transfusion preoperatively in patients with sickle cell hemoglobinopathies. Am J Obstet Gynecol 1978;132:59–63.
12. Fullerton MW, Philippart AI, Sarnaik S, Lusher JM. Preoperative exchange transfusion in sickle cell anemia. 1981;16:297–300.
13. Griffin TC, Buchanan GR. Elective surgery in children with sickle cell disease without preoperative blood transfusion. J Pediatr Surg 1993;28:681–685.
14. Scott-Conner CEH, Brunson CD. Surgery and anesthesia. In: Embury SH, Hebbel RP, Mohandas N, Steinberg MH, eds. Sickle cell disease. Basic principles and clinical practice. New York: Raven Press, 1994:809–827.
15. Sharon BI. Transfusion therapy in congenital hemolytic anemias. Hematol Oncol Clin North Am 1994;8:1053–1086.
16. Lessin LS, Kurantsin-Mills J, Klug PP, Weems HB. Determination of rheologically optimal mixtures of AA and SS erythrocytes for transfusion. Prog Clin Biol Res 1978;20:124–134.
17. Statius van Eps LW, Schouten H, Ter Haar Romeny-Wachter CH, La Porte-Wysman LW. The relation between age and urine concentrating capacity in sickle cell disease and hemoglobin C disease. Clin Chim Acta 1970;27:501–511.
18. Pearson HA, Cornelius EA, Schwartz AD, Zelson JH, Wolfson SL, Spencer RP. Transfusion reversible asplenia in young children with sickle-cell anemia. N Engl J Med 1970;283:334–337.
19. Miller DM, Winslow RM, Klein HG, et al. Improved exercise performance after exchange transfusion in subjects with sickle cell anemia. Blood 1980;56:1127–1131.
20. Charache S, Bleecker ER, Bross DS. Effects of blood transfusion on exercise capacity in patients with sickle-cell anemia. Am J Med 1983;74:757–764.
21. Koshy M, Burd L, Wallace D, Moawad A, Baron J. Prophylactic red-cell transfusions in pregnant patients with sickle cell disease: a randomized cooperative study. N Engl J Med 1988;319:1447–1452.
22. Zinkham WH, Seidler AJ, Kickler TS. Variable degrees of suppression of hemoglobin S synthesis in subjects with hemoglobin SS disease on a long-term transfusion regimen. J Pediatr 1994;124:215.
23. Wayne AD, Kevy SV, Nathan DG. Transfusion management of sickle cell anemia. Blood 1993;81:1109–1123.
24. Castro O, Finke-Castro H, Coats D. Improved method for automated red cell exchange in sickle cell disease. J Clin Apheresis 1986;3:93–99.
25. Kim HC, Dugan NP, Silber JH, et al. Erythrocytapheresis therapy to reduce iron overload in chronically transfused patients with sickle cell disease. Blood 1994;83:1136–1142.

26. Vichinsky EP, Haberkern CM, Neumayr L, et al. A comparison of conservative and aggressive transfusion regimens in the perioperative management of sickle cell disease. N Engl J Med 1995;333:206–213 .
27. Ballas SK, Lewis CN, Noone AM, Kransnow SH, Kamurulzaman E, Burka ER. Clinical, hematological and biochemical features of Hb SC disease. Am J Hematol 1982;13:37–51.
28. Serjeant GR. Sickle cell disease. Oxford: Oxford University Press, 1985:296–304.
29. Jampol LM, Green JL, Goldberg MF, et al. An update on vitrectomy surgery and retinal detachment repair in sickle cell disease. Arch Ophthalmol 1982;100:591–593.
30. Balasudaram S, Duran CG, al-Halees Z, Kassay M. Cardiopulmonary bypass in sickle cell anaemia. J Cardiovasc Surg 1991;32:271–274.
31. Clarke HJ, Jinnah RH, Brooker AF, Michaelson JD. Total replacement of the hip for avascular necrosis in sickle cell disease. J Bone Joint Surg [B]1989;71:465–470.
32. Mankad AV. Anesthetic management of patients with sickle cell disease. In: Mankad VN, Moore RB, eds. Sickle cell disease. Pathophysiology, diagnosis and management. Westport, CT: Praeger, 1992:351–363.
33. Rosse WF, Gallagher D, Kinney TR, et al. Transfusion and alloimmunization in sickle cell disease. Blood 1990;76:1431–1437.
34. Vichinsky EP, Earles A, Johnson RA, Hoag MS, Williams A, Lubin B. Alloimmunization in sickle cell anemia and transfusion of racially unmatched blood. N Engl J Med 1990;322:1617–1621.
35. Ramsey G, Smietana SJ. Long-term follow-up testing of red cell alloantibodies. Transfusion 1994;34:122–124.
36. Tahhan HR, Holbrook CT, Braddy LR, Brewer LD, Christie JD. Antigen-matched donor blood in the transfusion management of patients with sickle cell disease. Transfusion 1994;34:562–569 .
37. Ambruso DR, Githens JH, Alcorn R, et al. Experience with donors matched for minor blood group antigens in patients with sickle cell anemia who are receiving chronic transfusion therapy. Transfusion 1987; 27:94–98.
38. Ness PM. To match or not to match: the question for chronically transfused patients with sickle cell anemia. Transfusion 1994;34:558–560.
39. Castro O, Sandier SO. Estimating the effect of donor-recipient phenotype matching for transfusions in sickle cell patients [abstract]. Blood 1995;86(Suppl 1):644a.
40. Sears DA. Sickle cell trait. In: Embury SH, Hebbel RP, Mohandas N, Steinberg MH, eds. Sickle cell disease. Basic principles and clinical practice. New York: Raven Press, 1994:381–394.
41. Atlas SA. The sickle cell trait and surgical complications. A matched pair patient analysis. JAMA 1974;229:1078–1080.
42. Searle JF. Anesthesia in sickle cell states. Anesthesia 1973;28:48–58.
43. Leachman RD, Miller WT, Atlas IM. Sickle cell trait complicated by sickle cell thrombi after open heart surgery. Am Heart J 1967;74: 268–270.
44. Dunn A, Davies A, Eckert G, et al. Intraoperative death during caesarean section in a patient with sickle cell trait. Can J Anaesth 1987;34: 67–70.
45. Heiner M, Teasdale SJ, Dvid T, Scott AA, Glynn MFX. Aorto-coronary bypass in a patient with sickle cell trait. Can Anaesth Soc J 1979;26: 428–434.
46. Metras D, Ouezzin Colibaly A, Ouattara K, Longechaud A, Millet P, Chauvet J. Open-heart surgery in sickle-cell haemoglobinopathies: report of 15 cases. Thorax 1982;37:486–491.
47. Wallace EL, Churchill WH, Surgenor DM, et al. Collection and transfusion of blood and blood components in the United States, 1992. Transfusion 1995;35:802–812.
48. DeChristopher PJ, Orlina AR. Sudden death associated with autologous transfusion in a surgical patient with hemoglobin SC disease [abstract]. Abstract book, Meeting of the American Association of Blood Banks, 1990:119.
49. Klein HG, Garner RJ, Miller DM, et al. Automated partial exchange transfusion in sickle cell anemia. Transfusion 1980;20:578–584.
50. Cook A, Hanowell LH. Intraoperative autotransfusion for a patient with homozygous sickle cell disease. Anesthesiology 1990;75:177–179.
51. Romanoff ME, Woodward DG, Bullard WG. Autologous blood transfusion in patients with sickle cell trait. Anesthesiology 1988;68: 820–821.
52. Ray RN, Cassell BS, Chaplin H Jr. In vitro and in vivo observations on stored sickle cell trait red blood cells. Am J Clin Pathol 1959;32: 430–435.
53. Kaufman M, Stier W, Applewhaite F, Ruggiero S, Ginsberg V. Sickle-cell trait in blood donors. Am J Med Sci 1965;249:56–61.
54. Ahmed MAM, Al-Ali AK, Al-Idrissi HY, Al-Sibai MH, Al-Mutairy AR, Knox-Macaulay H. Sickle cell trait and G6PD deficiency in blood donors in Eastern Saudi Arabia. Vox Sang 1991;61:69–70.
55. Meryman HT, Hornblower M. Freezing and deglycerolizing sickle-trait red blood cells. Transfusion 1976;16:627–632.
56. Kelleher JF Jr, Luban NLC. Transfusion of frozen erythrocytes from a donor with sickle trait. Transfusion 1984;24:167–168.
57. Bodensteiner D. White cell reduction in blood from donors with sickle cell trait. Transfusion 1994;34:84.
58. Brajtbord D, Johnson D, Ramsay M, et al. Use of the cell saver in patients with sickle cell trait. Anesthesiology 1989;70:878–879.
59. Nagel RL, Bookchin RM, Johnson J, et al. Structural bases of the inhibitory effects of hemoglobin F and hemoglobin A2 on the polymerization of hemoglobin S. Proc Natl Acad Sci USA 1979;76:670–672.
60. Charache S, Dover GJ, Moore RD, et al. Hydroxyurea: effects on Hb F production in patients with sickle cell anemia. Blood 1992;79: 2555–2565.
61. Charache S, Terrin ML, Moore R, et al. Effect of hydroxyurea on the frequency of painful crises in sickle cell anemia. N Engl J Med 1995;332:1317–1322.
62. Liakopoulou E, Blau CA, Li Q, et al. Stimulation of fetal hemoglobin production by short chain fatty acids. Blood 1995;86:3227–3235.
63. Walters MC, Sullivan KM, Bernaudin F, et al. Neurologic complications after allogeneic marrow transplantation for sickle cell anemia. Blood 1995;85:879–884 .
64. Lucarelli G, Giaradini C, Baronciani D. Bone marrow transplantation in thalassemia. Semin Hematol 1995;32:297–230.
65. Erslev AJ. Secondary polycythemia (erythrocytosis). In: Williams WJ, Beutler E, Erslev AJ, Lichtman MA, eds. Hematology. 4th ed. New York: McGraw-Hill, 1990:705–715.
66. Berlin NI. Diagnosis and classification of the polycythemias. Semin Hematol 1975;12:339–351.
67. Modan B. An epidemiologic study of polycythemia vera. Blood 1965; 26:657–667.
68. Silverstein MN, Lanier AP. Polycythemia vera, 1935–1969: an epidemiologic survey in Rochester, Minnesota. Mayo Clin Proc 1971;4b:751–753.
69. Gruppo Italiano Studio Policitemia. Polycythemia vera: the natural history of 1213 patients followed for 20 years. Ann Intern Med 1995;123: 656–664.
70. Chievitz E, Thiede T. Complications and causes of death in patients with polycythemia vera. Acta Med Scand 1962;172:513–523.
71. Silverstein MH. Postpolycythemia myeloid metaplasia. Arch Intern Med 1974;134:113–115.

72. Najean Y, Arrago JP, Rain JD, et al. The "spent" phase of polycythemia vera: hypersplenism in the absence of myelofibrosis. Br J Haematol 1984;56:163–170.
73. Landaw SA. Acute leukemia in polycythemia vera. Semin Hematol 1986;23:156–165.
74. Spivak JL. Erythrocytosis. In: Hoffman R, Benz EJ, Shattil SJ, Furie B, Cohen HJ, Silberstein LE, eds. Hematology: basic principles and practice. New York: Churchill Livingstone, 1995:84–91.
75. Pearson TC, Wetherley-Mein G. Vascular occlusive episodes and venous haematocrit in primary proliferative polycythemia. Lancet 1978;2: 1219–1222.
76. Edwards EA, Cooley MH. Peripheral vascular symptoms as the initial manifestation of polycythemia vera. JAMA 1970;215:1463–1467.
77. Mitchell MC, Boitnott JK, Kaufman S, et al. Budd-Chiari syndrome: etiology, diagnosis, and management. Medicine 1982;61:199–218.
78. Silverstein A, Gilbert H, Wasserman LR. Neurologic complications of polycythemia. Ann Intern Med 1962;57:909–916.
79. Schafer AI. Bleeding and thrombosis in myeloproliferative disorders. Blood 1984;64:1–12.
80. Wasserman LR, Gilbert HS. Surgical bleeding in polycythemia vera. Ann NY Acad Sci 1964;115:122–138.
81. Rigby PG, Leavell BS. Polycythemia vera: a review of fifty cases with emphasis on risk of surgery. Arch Intern Med 1960;106:622–627.
82. Fitts WT, Erde A, Peskin GW, et al. Surgical implications of polycythemia vera. Ann Surg 1960;152:548–558.
83. Wasserman LR. Polycythemia Vera Study Group. A historical perspective. Semin Hematol 1986;23:183–187.
84. Berk PD, Goldberg JD, Donovan PB, Fruchtman SM, Berlin NI, Wasserman LR. Therapeutic recommendations in polycythemia vera based on Polycythemia Vera Study Group protocols. Semin Hematol 1986;23:132–143.
85. Bilgrami S, Greenberg BR. Polycythemia rubra vera. Semin Oncol 1995;22:307–326.
86. Triadu P, Maier-Redelsperger M, Krishnamoorty R, et al. Fetal hemoglobin variations following hydroxyurea treatment in patients with cyanotic congenital heart disease. Nouv Rev Fr Hematol 1994;36: 367–372.
87. Chetty KG, Brown SE, Light RW. Improved exercise tolerance of the polycythemic lung patient following phlebotomy. Am J Med 1983;74: 415–420.
88. Wallis PJW, Skehan JD, Newland AC, et al. Effects of erythropheresis on pulmonary haemodynamics and oxygen transport in patients with secondary polycythemia and cor pulmonale. Clin Sci 1986;70:91–98.
89. Engelfriet CP, Overbeeke MAM, von dem Borne AKGK. Autoimmune hemolytic anemia. Semin Hematol 1992;29:3–12.
90. Djulbegovic B, ed. Reasoning and decision making in hematology. New York: Churchill Livingstone, 1992:51–56.
91. Gilliland BC, Baxter E, Evans RS. Red-cell antibodies in acquired hemolytic anemia with negative serum antiglobulin tests. N Engl J Med 1971;285:252–254.
92. Salama A, Mueller-Eckhardt C, Bhakdi D. A two stage immunoradiometric assay with ^{125}I-staphylococcal protein A for the detection of antibodies and complement on human blood cells. Vox Sang 1985;48: 239–245.
93. Coon WW. Splenectomy in the treatment of hemolytic anemia. Arch Surg 1985;120:625–628.
94. Kutti J, Wadenvik H, Safai-Kutti S, et al. Successful treatment of refractory autoimmune hemolytic anemia by plasmapheresis. Scand J Haematol 1984;32:149–152.
95. Rosenfield RE, Jagathambal K. Transfusion therapy for autoimmune hemolytic anemia. Semin Hematol 1976;13:311–321.
96. Jefferies LC. Transfusion therapy in autoimmune hemolytic anemia. Hematol Oncol Clin North Am 1994;8:1087–1104.
97. Petz LD. Red cell transfusion problems in immunohematologic disease. Annu Rev Med 1982;33:355–361.
98. Plapp FV, Beck ML. Transfusion support in the management of immune haemolytic disorders. Clin Haematol 1984;13:167–183.
99. Sokol RJ, Hewitt S, Booker DJ, Morris BM. Patients with red cell autoantibodies: selection of blood for transfusion. Clin Lab Haematol 1988;10:257–264.
100. Wallhermfechtel MA, Polhl BA, Chaplin H. Alloimmunization in patients with warm autoantibodies. Transfusion 1984;24:482–485.
101. Laine ML, Beattie KM. Frequency of alloantibodies accompanying autoantibodies. Transfusion 1985;25:545–546.

Chapter 16

Perioperative Coagulation Monitoring

BRUCE D. SPIESS

INTRODUCTION

Coagulation function is reviewed in Chapter 6. Some concepts from that chapter are repeated and interpreted here in the context of rational monitoring both preoperatively and in the perioperative period. The data and concepts of coagulation function have changed radically over the last 10 years. Unfortunately, the available clinical coagulation monitoring devices have not changed as radically, although there are now some schemes and algorithms that may be incorporating some of these changes (1, 2). This chapter discusses coagulation as an event occurring at the site of endothelial injury or dysfunction. It examines the limitations placed on our monitoring and the individual tests available. Finally, it looks at combining those tests in the most appropriate way to guide therapy. One thing is clear: there is no perfect coagulation monitor that can detect all coagulopathies or guide all therapies.

REVIEW OF THE CONCEPT OF COAGULATION

As was just stated, coagulation occurs at a site of endothelial injury (3–6). Blood is maintained in a liquid form by a very active process involving plasma proteins (alpha-2-antitrypsin, antithrombin III, other antithrombins), prostaglandins (E_1), heparan, protein C and S with thrombomodulin, tissue plasminogen activator, nitric oxide, and proteoglycan (7–12). There may well be a number of other inducible compounds that are antithrombotic as well. Many of these are produced by endothelial cells to maintain blood in its liquid form. Damage to the endothelial cell leads to a loss of inhibition to coagulation. Unfortunately, we have no method of assessing local endothelial cell function. There may be a way in the future to examine "whole body" endothelial health. But, if one views coagulation as an event that occurs at a site of endothelial injury, then one of the first limitations of coagulation monitoring becomes obvious. The changes that occur at the site of injury are diluted in the circulating blood volume. The concentration of proteins and cell lines as they change undergoes a number of dynamic controls that may not become visible to monitoring technology for a considerable length of time. If a thrombus is forming in an organ or an extremity, at the site of endothelial injury, rather profound changes must take place before a blood sample drawn from an artery or vein quite remote from the site of injury can reflect a coagulopathy. Such is the limitation of coagulation monitoring, because for most problems we have no ability to sample blood or fluid draining directly from the site of injury. Another limitation of our coagulation monitoring is that it is at best a snapshot in time. A blood sample is obtained at a specific time, and to date we do not have continuous monitoring devices such as we have for hemodynamics. Also, the coagulation data require some time to acquire. For many of the coagulation tests, that amount of time required for data acquisition has become a limiting factor in their utility. If, for example, a critical coagulation test is very accurate and is also quite predictive of hemorrhage but it takes 60 or 90 minutes to run in the laboratory when a patient is hemorrhaging in surgery and changing blood volume every 30 minutes, by the time the result is acquired, it has become obsolete. Timely, as close to real time, data acquisition is a key limitation. Attempts have been made to increase the speed of data acquisition, and "on-site" coagulation analyzers now exist that allow "bedside" testing or operating room testing (1, 13, 14). Other "systems" improvements allow routine laboratories to control the testing and provide timely data (15).

The present day limitations to testing speed should therefore rarely provide such an impediment that "clinical judgment" is necessary to treat a coagulopathy.

Even though coagulation has been well described, there are some concepts that should be reviewed and expanded for the reader so that they are fresh in mind before discussing the individual tests used. The reader could visualize coagulation as a wave of activity occurring at the site of blood and endothelial interface (Fig. 16.1). Coagulation is triggered by the endothelium becoming dysfunctional or destroyed, thereby decreasing the local anticoagulant potential and potentially exposing collagen or basement membrane. Extravascular tissue destruction will lead to tissue thromboplastin (tissue factor) release, and new data are arising that show endothelial cells can be triggered to increase RNA encoding and production of their own tissue factor (3). The early stimulus for coagulation might be appropriately called the initiation phase (16).

Once the initiation phase has occurred, there is a rapid movement to the acceleration phase. This is the point at which platelets become of key importance. Platelets are activated by exposure to collagen, tissue factor, and a wide range of other agents potentially released either from damaged tissue or from dysfunctional or damaged endothelium. Once activated, these cells are attached to abnormal surfaces (basement membrane, other tissues, dead endothelial cells, cardiopulmonary bypass circuit, etc.) with a protein glue-like substance—von Willebrand factor (vWF). The glycoprotein 1B (GPIB) binding site is where vWF attaches to the surface of platelets. Once activated, the platelets undergo a phase change that allows them to spread over the surface of injury, become more spiculated, less spherical, and release granules. This is an ATP-dependent process that requires the internal release of calcium and actin and myocin contraction. As granule contents are released, other platelets are attracted, and the formation of a platelet plug occurs. The platelet plug is of critical importance to stopping the "oozing" of surgical wound edges. Platelet plug formation is the body's initial step toward controlling microvascular (less than 50 μm vessel diameter) hemorrhage. However, the platelet-to-platelet interaction does not form a stable shear-resistant clot. It will hold together for only about 10 minutes and will certainly break down quicker if there are flow patterns or blood pressure to push it off its site of adherence.

Platelets are of key importance to the normal functioning of coagulation. Again, one is referred to Chapter 6 for extensive discussions of platelet morphology and biochemistry.

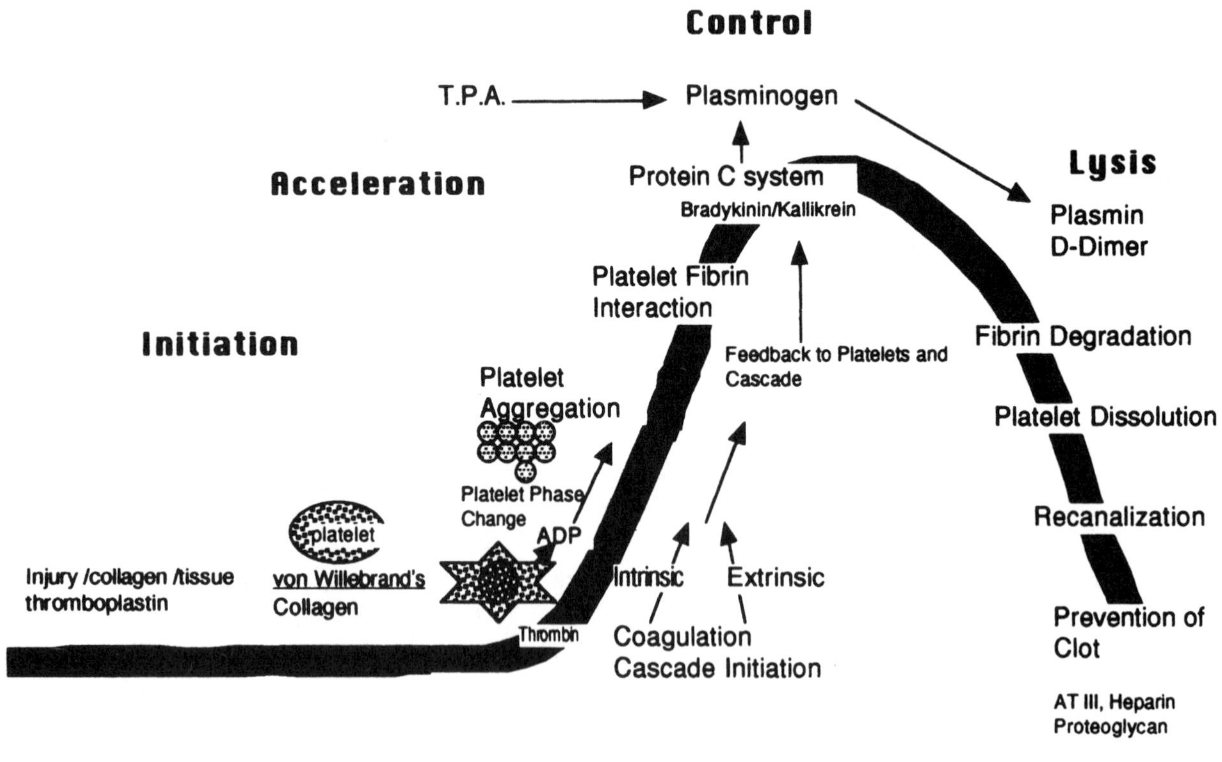

Figure 16.1. The coagulation events are limited to a localized area of dysfunctional endothelium. The events occur as a wave of activity brought on by activation, furthered by acceleration, limited by control, and eventually leading to lysis. (Reprinted by permission from Spiess BD. Perioperative coagulation concerns: function, monitoring and therapy. Clin Anesth Updates 1993;4:1–6.)

Throughout this chapter, stress is placed on the interaction of platelets with the rest of the coagulation proteins and cofactors. It is after the initiation phase or simultaneous to platelet initiation that protein coagulation begins. Indeed, platelet and protein coagulation may begin in parallel, but they become interdependent very quickly. The platelet surface with its glycoprotein binding sites is the place where the coagulation cascade moves from one reaction to another (17–21). GPIB is the site for vWF (later incorporated into factor VIII). It is also the site for factor XIa to bind and then trigger factor IX, leading to the macromolecular complex of factors X and VIII calcium and platelet factor 3. Immediately adjacent to the GPIB binding site is the glycoprotein IIB/IIIA (GPIIB/IIIA) binding site. GPIIB/IIIA is the binding site for fibrinogen/fibrin (17–21). There may be 50,000 or greater GPIIB/IIIA binding sites per platelet membrane when they are fully expressed (20). Each fibrinogen molecule can bind up to six GPIIB/IIIA binding sites. Therefore, the possibilities for molecular interaction and cross-linking seem nearly infinite when one realizes that fibrin-to-fibrin interactions are possible between multiple molecules.

The monitoring of coagulation should take into account all of the above concepts of coagulation. Unfortunately, the tests most often performed are not designed to make the assessments of platelet-to-fibrin interactions. The prothrombin time (PT), activated partial thromboplastin time (aPTT), and thrombin time (TT) all examine the proteins as they are artificially stimulated in plasma. Therefore, these tests, although very useful, provide little or no information regarding the way in which in vivo human coagulation proceeds.

Once the protein cascade has been activated, the platelet plug may become stabilized with fibrin deposition and attachment of fibrin to platelets, thereby creating a more resilient and maturing clot. However, the clot still has considerable processes to go through. Fibrin is cross-linked and further stabilized by factor XIII (21). Factor XIII also incorporates alpha-2 antiplasmin, thereby building into the matrix a protection from fibrinolysis (22, 23). The platelets continue to undergo cytoskeletal contraction, and this in conjunction with the covalent cross-linking creates clot retraction. The acceleration phase of coagulation would continue unimpeded if it was not for the control phase of the wave of coagulation (16). Indeed, in some disease states such as vasculitis, sepsis, and endothelial intoxication from drug overdose, there is no ability to control coagulation and diffuse intravascular coagulation does occur.

The control phase of coagulation is begun once again as soon as initiation and acceleration are well underway. As platelets are stimulated and they interact with the protein cascade, certain controlling proteins are released that downregulate the coagulation reactions. As thrombin is formed and as platelets are activated, thrombomodulin is released. This in turn activates the protein C and S axis that leads to decreased production of thrombin (24). Endothelial cells respond to thrombin by releasing tissue plasminogen activator, which in turn catalyzes the production of plasmin from its inactive zymogen plasminogen. Plasmin not only causes the breakdown of fibrinogen and fibrin but also has profound effects on the glycoprotein binding sites of platelets. As mentioned earlier, it is the GPIB and GPIIB/IIIA binding sites on platelets that control adherence to basement membrane, protein cascade function, and fibrin platelet adhesion. Plasmin, at normothermia, destroys or renders nonfunctional GPIIB/IIIA binding sites (25–27). It also appears to both cleave vWF and attack the GPIB binding site (28). The end product is hypocoagulability and platelet inability to adhere. It may also be responsible for making the platelet plug more friable if the number of glycoprotein binding sites or their affinity for their protein cofactors is reduced.

Nearby normal functioning endothelial cells not involved in the site of tissue injury will also act to limit the spread of coagulation by continuing to manufacture and export their normal surface anticoagulants.

After the predominance of activity within the developing clot has shifted from acceleration to control, eventually a much longer and slower lysis phase will prevail. This is the lysis phase, and plasminogen slowly breaks the bonds of fibrin. Plasmin's initial effects are to cleave fibrinogen, releasing fibrinopeptide A and B. Both of these are prothrombotic and create feedbacks to activation of thrombin. The fibrin molecule will break down eventually to D-dimer, which itself is an anticoagulant, inhibiting some of the serine proteases of the intrinsic cascade. Depending on the blood flow, level of cross-linking by factor XIII, and the amount of alpha-1 antitrypsin incorporated, the amount of time for clot lysis may be hours to several days in normal healthy organisms.

THE COAGULATION PROFILE

No amount of coagulation monitoring will replace a good history and physical; however, history is by far the more important. A few moments asking probing questions couched from the point of an informed examiner will be so much more cost-effective than widely applied screening tests. Patients with a rare congenital coagulopathy most often will not be discovered at the time of surgery but will be known from prior experiences. Hemophilia, vonWillebrand's disease, and Christmas disease patients generally have had a long family history and an adequate workup by a hematologist. However, if one asks about bleeding with dental hygiene, abnormal menses, and bleeding with otherwise minor or incidental trauma, you may uncover a patient who has not had a workup. For infants and small children, it is worthwhile to ask the parents about family history; however, remember that many of these are recessive and therefore it is entirely possible that both parents have not had a bleeding history or are from point mutations in one chromosome and have a recessive characteristic from the other parent. The reader is referred to Chapter 6 regarding the congenital coagulopathies. Many of these patients may have recent administrations of factor replacement (factors VIII and IX) or D-8-amino arginine vasopressin (DDAVP) therapy. Repeat factor levels should be assessed in advance of a major surgery to ensure that appropriate levels are still circulating.

Platelet function or early platelet lysis abnormalities can occur because of idiopathic thrombocytopenia and drug-induced or associated poorly understood viral syndromes. Very often these will present with spontaneous subcutaneous petechiae. Rarely do such abnormalities create as their first manifestation a bleeding into a hollow viscus, brain, or joint. However, if a patient does complain of one or more of these undiagnosed problems, it is certainly worth delaying elective surgery and asking for the hematologist to assist in the diagnosis.

The coagulation profile is sometimes referred to as "routine coagulation testing." However, it should be realized that not all tests considered in the coagulation profile are always performed, and by calling them routine it may infer that some tests not included are not routine. Those tests may be routine at another institution, so one should avoid this terminology and simply stick to designating this group of tests as a coagulation profile. Most often the coagulation profile consists of a platelet count, fibrinogen concentration, PT, aPTT, and TT. Sometimes a fibrin degradation products level and a euglobulin lysis time may be included. Of note, there is no platelet function test. Each test is reviewed here regarding how it is performed and what that means in terms of the risk of perioperative bleeding. Using a coagulation profile for patients to screen for abnormal bleeding is simply not cost-effective. Each test costs somewhere between $5 and $20 individually. The entire coagulation profile may be $25–75 depending on the institution and the exact tests included. There are no data to say that any given level of these tests connotes an inordinate risk of bleeding, and there are certainly no data in the face of a negative history to suggest that it is cost-effective to screen the large population (more than 20 million operations per year).

Platelet count can be very reliably obtained today using automated cell counters. This test had previously been performed manually by a technician by counting platelets in a special slide well that had a defined volume and a grid pattern to allow identification of known size areas. The manual technique, as one might expect, has a considerable amount of intratechnician variability and is therefore simply not very reliable. The present-day automated counters use laser technology to size the various cells or particles, and some have the ability to classify intracellular organelles such that they define a cell type not only by size but also by morphology. Automated flow also is used in the newest models to identify cell lines by the type of cell adhesion molecules.

Platelet counts are normally between 150,000 and 250,000/mL. However, thrombocythemia is not defined until the levels of platelet concentration exceed 400,000/mL. It is unclear at what level there is an increased risk of thrombosis or embolic phenomenon. Perhaps the interaction of the platelets with endothelial cells and fibrinogen is more important than simply the number expressed per milliliter. Hypercoagulability has been shown recently with certain genetic alleles of platelet surface GPIIB/IIIA ligands (29). This may result in an increased risk of early myocardial infarction, but such discoveries are so new that we do not know the implications for this group of patients and surgery.

Thrombocytopenia exists, by definition, if the platelet count drops below 150,000/mL. However, in the cancer chemotherapy patient, leukemics, and so on, spontaneous bleeding is not seen until the platelet count is well below 5000/mL. Therefore, it is possible that bleeding may not be an issue until such low levels are reached if all other factors are normal. Most anesthesiologists and surgeons would prefer not to be at the absolute limit of normal coagulation, and the standard recommendations in texts are a minimum of 20,000–50,000/mL for elective surgery. For cardiopulmonary bypass, the number quoted is more often approximately 100,000/mL (30). However, as this chapter is being written, there are no studies to quote to give the reader an increased risk index for each incremental fall in platelet count. Of course, if the platelet function is abnormal, a platelet count of 150,000 or greater may be insufficient to ensure normal coagulation.

There is no level of blood loss or euvolemic hemodilution at which a prophylactic platelet transfusion should be given (31, 32). Indeed, the platelet count is incredibly well preserved. Every surgery has some element of euvolemic hemodilution that does occur. As blood is lost and intravenous crystalloid or colloid is administered, there is a slow and often predictable level of hemodilution that does occur. Several studies have examined the predicted level of platelet count (32, 33). There have been computed slopes for platelet count reduction as hemodilution occurs. However, the actual measured platelet count never fits that expected by hemodilution alone. Rather, the actual count always exceeds that level as platelets are released from marrow, splenic, and hepatic stores in response to stress. Therefore, there is no reason to transfuse platelets for any given amount of blood lost. If the platelet count has been normal or is assumed to be before surgery or before a traumatic event, then one can expect at least one blood volume to be lost before the platelet count reaches levels that may be critical. In studies of patients suffering massive trauma, most patients who had undergone a blood volume blood loss still had a platelet count in excess of 100,000/mL (32, 33). Platelet counts can now be performed so rapidly that there is very little if ever a reason to transfuse patients on "clinical" indications for suspected low platelet counts. Platelet function abnormalities may be a different problem and are dealt with later in this chapter.

The measures of protein cascade function are generally broken down into three major tests: aPTT, PT, and TT. These three tests classically examine the intrinsic and extrinsic cascades and the final common pathway (i.e., fibrinogen to fibrin). These tests should be considered as screening tests for overall protein function, and one must realize that they are highly contrived to serve a certain purpose. When these tests were invented, the motivation for their creation was to find ways to ferret out congenital coagulation defects or to follow problems of hepatic failure. They were created at the time when the coagulation cascades were being described and characterized. They were not initially intended to find any particular risk for coagulopathic bleeding after surgery.

The classic teaching of the coagulation mechanism has focused on the trisection of the protein cascades. Perhaps it is easier to learn if one has a schematic that nicely compartmentalizes certain protein reactions. Unfortunately, this teaching is so ingrained into the medical school curriculum that it has led generations of surgeons and anesthesiologists to practice that if these three tests are normal, then the patient will not bleed; if they are abnormal, they should be treated before surgery, and other tests are not necessary or are less meaningful. Nothing could be further from the truth.

These three screening tests of protein coagulation function do not mimic in vivo coagulation; however, they will do what they were designed to do. That is, they will pick up congenital abnormalities and the effects of hepatic failure. Furthermore, the aPTT is useful for following the dosing of low- or moderate-dose heparin therapy and the PT is useful for following Coumadin or warfarin therapy. One should understand how each test is performed to get an appreciation for their limitations and clinical worth.

The aPTT is performed in an automated system that stimulates plasma with a contact activator. Most often this is either Kaolin (aluminum silicate) or cellite-diatomaceous earth (sodium silicate). Other contact activators can be used as well. Aluminum silicate is an artificial product that has the potential for being standardized more readily than diatomaceous earth. Cellite is isolated from clay deposits that are heavily laden with the microskeletons of diatoms (prehistoric protozoan-like creatures). Either one of these stimulating agents causes the initial activation of Hageman factor and leads to factor IX and then factor Xa production. The assay does require the competency of the final common pathway as an automated fibrometer detects the earliest formation of fibrin strands. Therefore, the entire test looks only at the time to initial fibrin strand formation when isolated plasma is artificially stimulated for contact activation. Hypofibrinogenemia (no more than 50–75 mg/dL), dysfibrinogenemia, or excesses of fibrin degradation products may prolong this test (predominately D-dimer); D-dimer will inhibit the function of factor IX. The test is sensitive to heparin activity in low to moderate dosages because heparin is an antithrombin that blocks thrombin's action on fibrin and also has weak effects on certain serine proteases (most notably factor IXa) (34). The aPTT has a reproducible sensitivity range up to about 100–129 seconds. Beyond that level, the data become much less reproducible, and if heparin has been administered such that the aPTT is prolonged beyond that range, then some other test must be used to follow it (perhaps the activated clotting time [ACT], a titrated heparin level [Hepcon, Medtronic Inc.], or a heparin assay) (34).

What is a safe aPTT for patients to undergo surgery? Unfortunately, there is no easy answer to that question, because the circumstances are always different. Perhaps a level of 1.5–1.8 times normal should be considered an appropriate level above which the risk of bleeding may increase. However, a linear relationship has not been shown between the relative abnormality of the test (aPTT) and the amount of post- or intraoperative bleeding. Remember, heparin can be relatively easily reversed with protamine administration, and if rapid restoration of the aPTT to baseline is necessary, that is the way to proceed. There are also no data to suggest that placement of either a spinal or epidural block is safe or unsafe with any given level of increased aPTT. Clearly, we will never know because clinicians are not willing to take the risk of a neurological injury of potentially catastrophic proportion in the face of abnormal coagulation testing. But just because it is not done does not connote any particular risk.

The PT like the aPTT is performed by automated equipment using isolated plasma. It is interesting that this test examines the extrinsic coagulation cascade as bovine thromboplastin or tissue factor is used as an activator for the factor VII activation. This test, like the aPTT, proceeds from the time of active stimulation until the first strands of fibrin are formed. It is also a timed test. The PT is a screening test for the relative activity of the vitamin K-dependent hepatically produced coagulation proteins (factors II, V, VII, and X). Therefore, it is useful in following drugs that directly influence these factor's production and the synthetic capabilities of the liver. Indeed, in end-stage liver failure and in hepatic transplantation, it can be used to follow organ function. The PT is an interesting example of how these tests, although useful, do not mimic normal human coagulation. A significant number of crossovers in activation occur in vivo between the intrinsic and extrinsic cascade. For example, factor VII can activate factor IX and in turn lead to activation of factor XIa. However, this activation must occur on the surface of activated platelets at the GPIB binding site. The PT test has no platelets and hence no glycoprotein binding sites allow this cross-activation. What does the PT mean then in the context of the intact human that has functional platelet surfaces? That question is hard to answer because, like the aPTT, there are no data to correlate any given PT with a certain risk of hemorrhage. But once again, if the PT is 1.5–2 times normal, then the risk of hemorrhage may indeed be elevated (33).

This is the time to discuss the concept of the International Normalized Ratio (INR) (35, 36). Because the activator for the PT is derived from a biological source and therefore each batch may have a different activity profile, it is necessary to run a standard for comparison. The INR is a method of comparing the patient's activity with a known standard run each day with the batch of activator to be used for that run of samples. This may also limit the variability from laboratory to laboratory, and if one speaks of INR, then it is easier to compare. An INR of 1.5 at one institution should be the same as an INR of 1.5 at another, although the actual PT numbers may differ considerably. Therefore, when we consider the risk of hemorrhage, an INR of 1.5–2 could represent an increased risk for hemorrhage.

The aPTT is used to follow low- to moderate-dose heparin, usually given in the intensive care unit and routine nursing floors either for deep vein thrombosis (DVT), myocardial ischemia, or other embolic prophylaxis or treatment. Therapeutic ranges for the aPTT and heparin dosing differ again from center to center, but usually raising it to 1.5–2 times normal seems appropriate. One can argue about how much of a risk for bleeding during surgery such therapy causes, but if the heparin is turned off 2–4 hours before surgery, usually the aPTT will return to normal. The heparin is cleared by combined hepatic and renal clearance and should have a $t_{1/2}$ of 90 minutes to 4 hours. One can always reverse residual heparin with protamine, but simply performing an ACT alone and finding it normal will not mean that all amounts of trace heparin are reversed. Either a repeat aPTT or a TT can be used to prove that trace heparin has been neutralized. A test of whole blood clot strength, the thromboelastograph (TEG), may be the most sensitive to trace heparin, but this is not available at many centers.

Another potential prolongation of the aPTT exists with lupus anticoagulant (37). This is really a misnomer, because there is not truly any effect on coagulation function. Rather, an immunoglobulin is present in the serum that binds to the activator in the aPTT and therefore, depending on the affinity of the particular immunoglobulin and its concentration, the aPTT will be elevated and unreliable as an indicator of abnormal intrinsic cascade function. Lupus anticoagulant will also affect the ACT and make it unreliable for monitoring heparinization during cardiopulmonary bypass. Lupus anticoagulant can be found as an isolated finding but most often is associated with some malignancy that has the body producing immunoglobulins as a reaction.

Congenital coagulopathies of the intrinsic cascade may be discovered and followed with the aPTT (38–40). Most important might be factor XI deficiency seen in some Eastern European Jewish populations. In one study among this population, 10 cases were found in 1148 patients screened and coming to surgery. It is possible for bleeding to result after surgery when this is undiagnosed. However, in other populations, the disease is so rare that it may not be cost-effective to screen for it blindly with the aPTT. Others that the aPTT can find are von Willebrand's disease, classic hemophilia or hemophilia A (decreases amount of factor VIII), and Christmas disease (factor IX deficiency). If the aPTT is normal, this is an effective screen for these congenital deficiencies, because only 20–30% of normal circulating levels of these proteins are needed, if every other protein is normal, for there to be a normal aPTT. Restoration of the aPTT to normal before major surgery in the face of these congenital abnormalities makes sense, but more often, once the abnormality is identified, assays for the levels of the particular protein will be followed.

The TT tests the final common pathway and is performed in some ways similarly to the aPTT. That is, the plasma is separated from the red cells, platelets, and white cells using centrifugation and then the plasma is artificially stimulated. Once activated, the time until initial fibrin formation is timed using a fibrometer (now completely automated). The activator is usually bovine thrombin, and this directly activates fibrinogen to polymerize into fibrin. Clearly, if heparin and antithrombin III complexes are present, then the TT will be prolonged because the thrombin is bound to these complexes. Also, if dysfibrinogenemia exists such that the fibrinogen is congenitally dysfunctional, a prolongation will exist also. If the fibrinogen concentration is extremely low, the TT will also be prolonged (probably less than 25–30 mg/dL). At this low range of fibrinogen, diffuse and potentially severe bleeding during surgery is possible as well. If heparin is present and the amount of final common pathway function needs to be assessed, then a reptilase time can be performed. This test uses a viper serum to activate the fibrinogen to fibrin reaction, and unlike thrombin, that serum protein is not able to attach to heparin-ATIII complexes.

The fibrinogen concentration can be assayed by either a dilutional technique, again using thrombin as an activator to different dilutions of plasma or by immunoassay. Fibrinogen concentrations greater than 100 mg/dL are sufficient to have normal clot function, if every other function of the clotting system is normal. Usually, if there has been enough dilution to decrease fibrinogen to this concentration, then diffuse abnormalities exist such as factor V and VIII depression and thrombocytopenia. If hypofibrinogenemia exists from hepatic failure or from drug effects, then again multiple other problems probably exist and the fibrinogen level will not be the only risk for bleeding. Following fibrinogen as an indicator of the amount of hemodilution is not necessarily accurate, because fibrinogen is released from hepatic stores in response to stress. This release is nowhere near the same potential effect as seen with platelet release. If one is transfusing packed red cells, one should remember that these carry very small amounts of plasma and therefore fibrinogen will decrease. Cell salvaged blood (from washed processing systems) carries no plasma at all and that from nonwashed systems may have variable amounts of fibrinogen and fibrin degradation products present, because this blood usually has undergone some element of coagulation and fibrinolysis before collection. Modified whole blood has had cryoprecipitate removed and therefore its fibrinogen concentration is about one-half normal.

Many other tests of individual procoagulant protein precursors can be assayed for particular concentrations. Some are performed using dilutions of plasma with the activators used in the PT and aPTT and yet others require chromogenic, ELISA, and radioimmunoassay tests. It is beyond the scope of this chapter and not necessary for the surgical/anesthesia practitioner to know how each of these assays is performed. Usually, if a particular factor level is low, a hematology consultation should be involved to follow the patient. There is no need to assay the levels of the protein's intrinsic or extrinsic cascade if the aPTT or PT is prolonged, provided a reasonable explanation exists. These tests are often very expensive and cannot be run quickly and routinely. Therefore, they are not of great use during the dynamic events of surgery but may be useful after some of the congenital or iatrogenically caused isolated abnormalities before surgery. As well as levels of coagulation, procoagulants rare immunological effects can happen wherein an immunoglobulin cross-reacts with a protein and causes an isolated coagulopathy (i.e., IgG to factor V or VII). Again, an expert hematologist will be required to guide diagnosis and therapy for such patients before and during surgery, but the suspicion of such a diagnosis may begin with a history of bleeding or an abnormal aPTT or PT. In yet another study examining 2000 patients screened preoperatively with the aPTT and PT, only 0.5% of tests had an abnormality not expected by clinical history (39). Other studies have shown that the most common cause of abnormal studies when the history is negative is laboratory error (41).

All of the above-mentioned tests of coagulation have focused on the protein cascade in isolation from other elements of the blood. As stated, a great deal of useful information can be gleaned from these tests, but they also have considerable limitations. Whole "blood point of care" testing has now become available for the aPTT and PT (1). Using a capillary tube system that draws blood forward through a convoluted tubing system by capillary action, these systems measure the speed of advancement of a small drop of blood through the capillary tube system. When a drop of whole blood is placed on the disposable cartridge for one of these tests, the blood first mixes with a reagent before moving forward into the capillary tubes. The time until the leading edge of the advancing blood column stops is noted and using an algorithm to correct that time for a known compared standard, the aPTT or PT is reported. In other words, the whole blood aPTT or PT in time until the advancing column stops is not exactly the same amount of time as that for a laboratory plasma aPTT or PT. That is probably due to the fact that when whole blood is present and activated, the platelets become activated and release a number of compounds that amplify the coagulation reactions. The accuracy of these "point of care" systems has been compared with laboratory "gold standards" and the PT has very good correlation coefficients, whereas the aPTT seems to have more variability (42). They are, however, useful even with these variations, and one cannot know which should be considered the most appropriate because blood coagulation in vivo occurs with all the elements interacting.

As noted previously in this chapter, the individual protein coagulation tests in isolation are not very predictive of abnormal bleeding at surgery; certainly not until they reach levels of 1.5–2 times normal. This makes sense, as the human body has a wide range of redundancies, and although there may be an isolated abnormality in one test, the ways in which coagulation can be activated go beyond one pathway. However, an approach looking at prediction of bleeding using an algorithm for these tests has been proposed and tested in relation to postcardiopulmonary bypass bleeding (Fig. 16.2) (1). By using aPTT, PT, and fibrinogen concentration, a

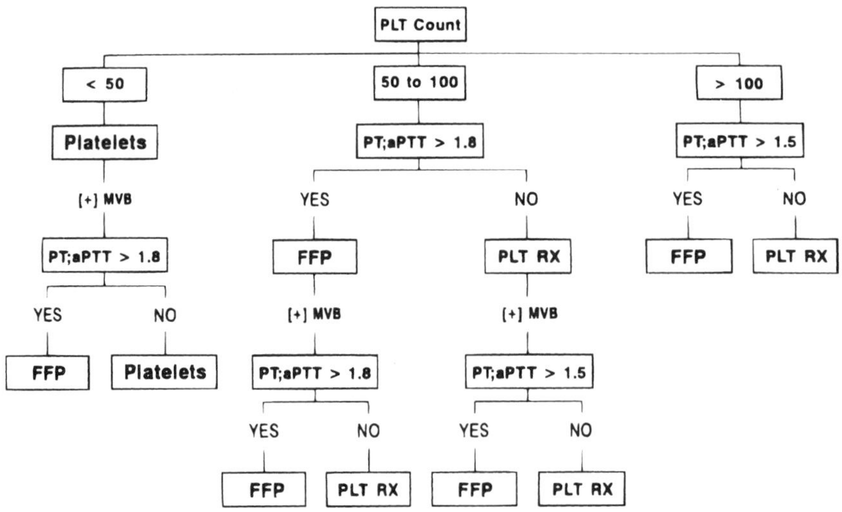

Figure 16.2. An algorithm for treating coagulopathies based on PT, aPTT, and platelet count. Note that this system attempts to discern platelet dysfunction by a process of elimination. (Reprinted by permission from Despotis GJ, Santoro SA, Spitznagel E, et al. Prospective evaluation and clinical utility of on-site monitoring of coagulation in patients undergoing cardiac operations. J Thorac Cardiovasc Surg 1994;107:271.)

branching algorithm for treatment of abnormalities has been tested. Using this algorithm, the use of blood products was decreased in one trial. However, because the utilization of any rational approach to transfusion in cardiopulmonary bypass patients would be better than "clinical judgment," it is hard to say at this time if this algorithm is "the best" way to approach all patients. Essentially, the algorithm uses the protein coagulation tests, along with platelet number, to isolate platelet function abnormalities by process of elimination.

Another test of whole blood clot function looking at protein function is the ACT (43). This test uses either cellite or kaolin to activate the intrinsic cascade. The concentration of activator is so high that it overcomes low- and moderate-dose heparin and gives a dose-dependent relationship to higher dose heparin. For cardiopulmonary bypass at the dosages of heparin used, the aPTT is prolonged beyond the range of its usable readings; therefore, the ACT is used for gauging heparin administration and dosing during cardiopulmonary bypass. The ACT was originally devised by Bull et al. (44) as a modification of a LEE-White whole blood clotting time. Essentially, whole blood is placed either in a glass test tube (either kaolin or cellite) with premeasured activator or into a plastic well also containing activator (kaolin). If the test tube system is used, the tube rotates with a magnetic indicator-stirrer in the whole blood until the first gel formation occurs and the magnet is caught in the gel, triggering a detector that the clot has formed. If the well system is used, a plunger is lifted once every second and allowed to drop by gravity back through the whole blood. When the speed of descent of the plunger is slowed, again due to initial gel formation, then the system is triggered and the time in seconds reported. The ACT produces a straight-line relationship between heparin administered and prolongation of the ACT, in seconds as long as certain criteria are met. These include normal AT-III concentrations, normal factor XII activity, normothermia, platelet number greater than 50,000/mL, reasonable platelet function, and fibrinogen concentration greater than 100 mg/dL (45). These qualifiers do not always exist in the postbypass situation, particularly the presence of reasonable platelet function, platelet number, and fibrinogen concentration. The ACT warms the cuvettes to 37°C, but with very cold blood from deep hypothermic patients or if the warming system is not allowed to warm the test tube or wells before introduction of the blood sample, temperature can introduce a significant prolongation. Therefore, not every prolonged ACT represents heparin presence or incomplete reversal of heparin with protamine. At our institution, a dose-response curve is hand-drawn for each patient before cardiopulmonary bypass (Fig. 16.3). A sample of blood is taken as a baseline before heparin and an ACT are conducted; after heparin administration, another sample is run. A straight-line (two-point) dose-response curve is drawn. If the ACT does not reach the institutional acceptable level for bypass (ACT of 450 seconds), then the dose-response curve may be useful in judging how much additional heparin to administer. Also, the dose-response curve can be used during cardiopulmonary bypass to judge how much extra heparin is needed to maintain the ACT greater than 450 seconds.

There is nothing magical about 450 seconds because some institutions use levels below and others use levels above. The ACT during and after cardiopulmonary bypass may well have a different slope of dose-response because hemodilution and the other factor just mentioned may play roles in changing that slope. However, it is impossible to continuously create new individual dose-response curves. The ACT after cardiopulmonary bypass should return to normal or actually below the number obtained for baseline if protamine is administered. If the ACT is still prolonged above baseline, then one of the six reasons mentioned above has occurred or an excess of protamine has been administered. Again, at our institution, the ACT dose-response curve drawn before cardiopulmonary bypass is used to calculate a protamine dosage (Fig. 16.3). The last ACT before separation from cardiopulmonary bypass is translated into a protamine dose based on an arbitrary titration of 1:1 heparin activity to protamine administration. The in vitro work with protamine has showed that it is capable of reversing in ratios as little as 0.33 protamine for heparin dosage (46). If the ACT is mildly prolonged and extra protamine is given in an attempt to neutralize any remaining heparin, the ACT should get shorter. If it stays the same or gets mildly longer, then a protamine interaction with thrombin is probably present and further administration of protamine will only cause more anticoagulation. Once again, all prolongations of the ACT are not from heparin, and worshiping some specific number of the ACT is not born out by research as a measure of safety.

The ACT is not a predictor of abnormal bleeding. Clearly, moderate prolongations of the ACT after cardiopulmonary bypass might suggest an increased risk of bleeding, but a normal ACT is meaningless in terms of the risk. The ACT is an insensitive test for trace amounts of heparin, and some argument can be made that trace or reheparinization can occur even with normal ACT levels (47). How much these events contribute to chest tube bleeding is unclear. Unfortunately, the aPTT is mildly prolonged by cardiopulmonary bypass alone, and it may well be that the heparin-protamine complex partially inhibits the activators or that the platelet inhibition found in cardiopulmonary bypass decreases the amplification capability of the platelets to the intrinsic cascade stimulation. ACT levels of 1.5–1.8 times normal may well be the mean level after cardiopulmonary bypass and do not connote any increased risk of hemorrhage. The TT and TEG may be followed for trace heparin levels.

The ACT gives a bioassay of heparin activity in whole blood. However, one can get chromogenic heparin levels (the gold standard) if circulating heparin concentration is needed. These are expensive, not done at every institution, time-consuming, and are therefore not of practical value for routine surgery (cardiopulmonary bypass). They should be reserved for research. However, a heparin assay is available (Hepcon, Medtronic Inc.). This automated system uses a lot of the ACT technology previously discussed. Wells with premeasured activator (kaolin) are placed into the machine and heated to 37°C. One group of cartridges has none, heparin, and then small measured amounts of heparin. With the differences in time to clot formation between these wells, the machine can construct a heparin dose-response curve and will tell the practitioner how much heparin to administer to achieve a given ACT. Other cartridges have different aliquots of protamine in them, and when blood from the patient is put into these, the differences in time to formation of clot will allow the machine to detect a close estimate of circulating heparin concentration. Several different cartridges are available with ranges of possible circulating heparin concentration. If one targets the patient to have a stable heparin level of 3.4 mg/mL of circulating blood and considerably more or less is present, then a second cartridge will have to be run. There is some debate as to whether it is more favorable to have patients managed for cardiopulmonary bypass using a target heparin level in the blood or whether it is better to use the ACT. Because the target heparin level looks at the relative time for coagulation from one well to another, it does not strictly examine the functionality of heparin and AT-III complexes.

As we have already discussed, there are considerable variables that can affect the ACT. Comparisons of Hepcon-managed versus routine-managed coagulation during cardiopulmonary bypass have shown some improvement with the Hepcon system for perioperative bleeding (48–51). However, these studies compared the Hepcon system to heparin management that used ACT but did not do so with dose-response curves but rather gave protamine based on a recipe of 1.3 times the total heparin dose. That may well reflect a relative overdose of protamine compared with dose-response curve managed therapy. In one study at our institution where the Hepcon system was used for research and therapy was based on the maintenance of a constant level of heparin circulating at 3.4 mg/mL, we gave more heparin and therefore more protamine than we would have given otherwise. Notably, the placebo (this was an aprotinin study) patients in this group bled more than our routine patients from our database using our hand-drawn dose-response curve. The Hepcon automated dosing system is effective if persons are not willing to spend the time doing the hand-drawn dosing or if stable circulating levels of heparin are important to the team managing the patients. However, this system is considerably more costly than the routine ACT management. The inserts for testing heparin levels are more than $10.00, and the cost for an entire case to manage therapy may be in excess of $100.00.

Platelet counts are readily available using automated devices with laser technology. These "Coulter counters" size particles in the blood and separate out the populations based on size. Computer programming of the systems means that

PRE-BYPASS DATA						
PT	PTT	TT	Fib	Plat	Hgb/Hct	OTHER

TEG				
R	K	α	MA	A_{60}

MEDICATIONS

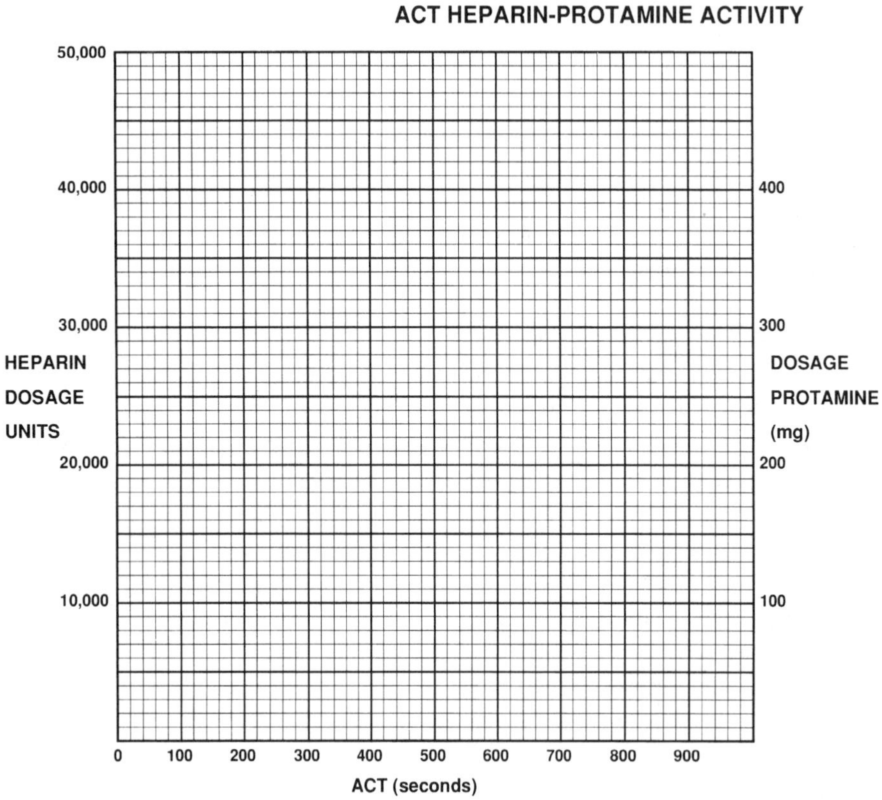

TIME:

$ACT_{baseline}$ ______ ______

$ACT_{postheparin}$ ______ ______

ACT CPB_1 ______ ______

ACT CPB_2 ______ ______

ACT CPB_3 ______ ______

ACT CPB_4 ______ ______

ACT CPB_5 ______ ______

HEPARIN INITIAL ____________

TOTAL HEPARIN ____________

PROTAMINE ____________

POST CPB					
ACT	TEG				
	R	K	α	MA	A_{60}

POST OPERATIVE												
ACT	TEG											
	R	K	α	MA	A_{60}	PT	PTT	Fib	FSP	TT	Plat	Hgb

PT.NO.

NAME

D.O.B.

UNIVERSITY OF WASHINGTON MEDICAL CENTERS
HARBORVIEW MEDICAL CENTER - UW MEDICAL CENTER
SEATTLE, WASHINGTON

CARDIOPULMONARY BYPASS
COAGULATION REPORT

* U 0 9 3 6 *

UH N 0936 REV JUN 94

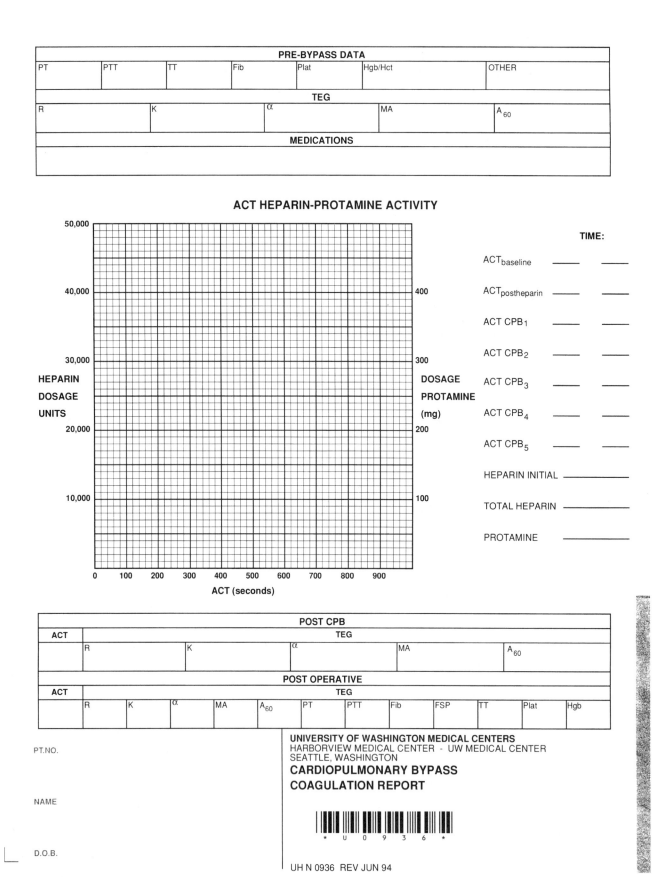

Figure 16.3. The heparin dose-response curve used as a modification of a standard "Bull" wave. Of note is that the protamine dose can be calculated in a 1:1 dosing schema from the last activated clotting time before weaning from cardiopulmonary bypass.

certain sized particles will be deemed platelets, others white cells, and still others erythrocytes. The newest technology not only sorts the cell types by size but also uses methods to detect intracellular organelles and in some flow-cytometry to differentiate cell membrane ligands. As we move into the future and some type of artificial oxygen-carrying media becomes available (either hemoglobin based or perfluorocarbon), a challenge may be presented to separate these iatrogenically administered solutions from normal human cell lines. It appears that the newest cell counters can distinguish between perfluorocarbon emulsions (no intracellular inclusions) and platelets.

We can count platelets, and a good clinical laboratory should be able to give rapid turnaround from sample collection to data, reporting such that the dynamic situation in the operating room can use these data. However, the real-time ability to follow platelet function has always been more of a challenge. Platelet aggregometry can be performed to work up certain platelet function abnormalities. These tests use the patient's plasma to which a certain known and closely controlled concentration of the patient's own platelets has been added back. An aggregometer is a warmed chamber through which a light is shined, thereby measuring the turbidity of the system. When a stimulating chemical is added to the system, the platelets will begin to clump and precipitate, leaving a change in turbidity as a curve. One can perform a spontaneous platelet aggregometry without any in vitro stimulus. Recently, it has been shown that if patients have an abnormally fast spontaneous platelet aggregometry, then their risk for myocardial infarction and unstable angina may be increased (52). That means that spontaneous platelet aggregometry may be a test for increased platelet activity or "stickiness." Many other compounds can be added as stimuli for platelet aggregometry, including ADP, collagen, epinephrine, serotonin, ristocetin, platelet activating factor, fibrinogen, and thromboxane. Although abnormalities may be demonstrated in one or more of these artificially stimulated platelet aggregation tests, it is very difficult to infer from any one test a certain increased risk of bleeding. Because these require precise measurement of platelet concentration and resuspension of platelets in plasma, the amount of technician time required to perform these tests prohibits them from being of utility during surgery.

The bleeding time is a very crude test of platelet plug formation that has been of historical interest mostly. A small controlled cut is made by a spring-loaded template either on the inner surface of the forearm (Ivy) or on the pinna of the ear (Duke). If the arm is used, a tourniquet is inflated to 40 mm Hg above the site of the template scratch and maintained that way until the test is completed. Filter paper is used to blot (not wipe) the wound every 30 seconds until the bleeding stops. It is considered stopped when the filter paper no longer absorbs blood. As such, the test would appear to examine the speed of formation of the initial platelet plug, but a wide range of problems exist with this test. In healthy young volunteers, a number of studies demonstrate that if the bleeding time was normal before the administration of a particular medication known to influence platelets (nonsteroidal anti-inflammatory drugs) and another bleeding time is then performed, the second one will be prolonged. From these data, practitioners have assumed that they will then be able to detect platelet dysfunction in other groups of patients. The fallacy behind that argument is that if one tries to apply the bleeding time to patient populations that might be at risk for bleeding from platelet dysfunction, other problems inherent in those patient populations lead to prolongation of the bleeding time.

Temperature of the skin, volume status or presence of extra cellular fluid (edema), skin blood flow, the use of catecholamine or vasodilator drips, and muscle tone may all affect the bleeding time. In patients during surgery, the skin temperature has wide fluctuations as does skin blood flow. One can see that these other variables may be present to create either spuriously prolonged or shortened bleeding times. Several recent reviews of the literature on the bleeding time have been written, and they have concluded that the bleeding time has no use in predicting a risk for abnormal hemorrhage during or after surgery (53). Furthermore, some institutions will perform a bleeding time before the placement of certain regional blocks in the face of preeclampsia or eclampsia. It seems unreasonable to expect that a small lance cut on the forearm would have anything to do with the risk of a bleed from a 17- or 18-gauge needle inside a body cavity with a closed space that is warmed to core temperature. There are no data at all in the literature supporting the use of a bleeding time in deciding whether a patient can or cannot receive an epidural. The bleeding time in cardiopulmonary bypass patients, a group with universal platelet dysfunction, has had no predictive value in most studies. Only if the bleeding time is massively prolonged does the specificity of the test become reasonable. The logistical problems alone make performing the bleeding time prohibitive for most surgeries. It can also leave a small telltale scar on the forearm, and if one is performing several of these, in each case one may find patients quite unhappy to have a series of little scars.

The Hepcon system has just released a new test (Hemostat, Medtronic Inc., Minneapolis, MN) for platelet function using similar wells filled with differing concentrations of activator (in this case, platelet activating factor). When whole blood is placed in this well and the platelets are stimulated to aggregate, the relative amount of time to initial clot formation between the different wells is noted. The results are reported out in percentage of normal platelet function. It is possible to have normal platelet function and thrombocytopenia or severe hypofibrinogenemia and have the machine report out depressed platelet function. Third-party validation of this technology is just now beginning. Much work is yet to be done with this system before we can say how useful it is in part of the coagulation management schema. It does look appealing simply because it is easy to use, requires little maintenance, and provides data quickly at the "point of care" in the operating rooms. However, for it to be useful, the numbers must mean something in terms of bleeding and guiding transfusion.

Whole blood clot testing for viscoelastic properties has gained popularity in the perioperative period (54). Two tests presently exist to test such properties, but others are in the design phase. The properties of clot strength change over time, and viscosity changes may well be quite important in predicting hemorrhage. In the end analysis, clot is merely the interaction of platelet surfaces with fibrin. Of course, fibrin cross-linking the presence of other cell types such as white cells and erythrocytes enmeshed within the clot may have importance. The screening tests of protein clot function are all quite contrived in vitro tests that examine only one small part of the coagulation process. As stated earlier, the protein cascades do not exist separated from the platelet surfaces in vivo. Therefore, although we may be able to demonstrate abnormalities in the aPTT or PT, when these prolongations are mild to moderate, it is hard to find any increased risk of bleeding. Fibrinogen has six binding sites for GPIIB/IIIA. The interaction of fibrin with these surface receptors is key to the strength of a clot. The interactions of platelet to platelet stimulation (formation of the platelet plug) in an acceleration phase of coagulation and with the protein cascades are very important. These events lead to the rapidity with which clot strength grows.

The TEG is a test of whole blood clot strength and was first invented in 1947 by a German hematologist (55). Its mechanism uses a warmed cup or crucible previously made of stainless steel but now made of disposable plastic. Suspended inside the cup is a piston that does not touch the walls of the cup. The cup moves through an arc of 4.5 degrees once every second, pauses for 1 second, and then moves back through the arc in the opposite direction. There is no connection between the cup and the piston until whole blood is placed in the cup and coagulation begins. A very small amount of blood is needed to perform this test (0.35 mL). In routine TEG, coagulation begins with spontaneous stimulation of the intrinsic cascade (59). This is used only with the old stainless steel cups and pistons. With the new plastic systems, some type of stimulus is needed because the onset to coagulation is quite variable, probably due to imperfections in the plastic. With the new system, either cellite or, potentially in the future, tissue factor may be used.

The TEG measures clot strength over time by maintaining the piston stable in an electromagnetic field. A paper tracing relates the amount of power necessary to maintain that as the rotational motion of the cup is transferred to the piston. This paper tracing has an amplitude at any given time and is displayed in Figure 16.4. Standard parameters can be measured from the TEG tracing (Fig. 16.5). Probably, most important is the maximum amplitude (MA) and that measurement is the paper representation of the maximum clot strength. Clot strength is related to amplitude by the equation $G = 5000\,(A)/\,100 - A$, where G is measured in dynes/cm^2 and A is the amplitude at any given time. The relationship of G to MA is curvilinear and logarithmic because the MA is measured on a scale of 0–100 mm, whereas G goes from 0 to in-

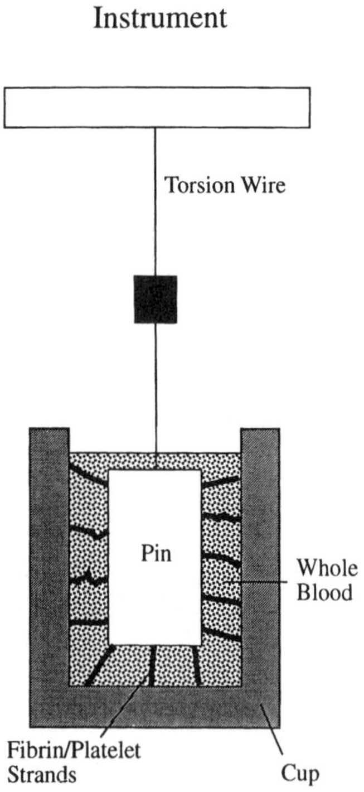

Figure 16.4. The TEG mechanism uses a cuvette warmed to 37°C that rotates through a 4.5° arc. Suspended inside that cuvette is a piston. Whole blood (0.35 mL) is placed into the cuvette and as coagulation progresses, platelet/fibrin strands form between the cuvette and the piston. An electromagnetic field holds the piston steady and the paper trace then reflects the energy necessary to hold the piston stable. The TEG simply tests clot strength over time. (Reprinted by permission from Chandler W. The thromboelastograph and the thromboelastograph technique. Semin Thromb Hemost 1995;21(Suppl 4):1–6.)

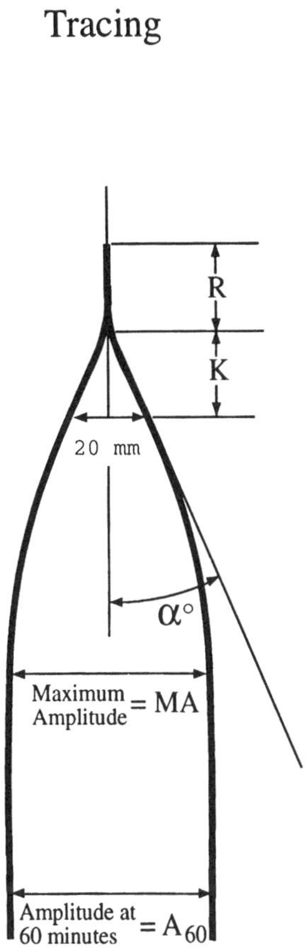

Figure 16.5. The TEG tracing has standard parameters that can be measured, including R value (onset of test until amplitude is 2 mm); K value, from the end of R until amplitude = 20 mm; α angle, a measure of the angle to the upslope of the TEG trace; A_{60}, the amplitude 60 minutes after the MA. (Reprinted by permission from Chandler WL. The thromboelastograph and the thromboelastograph technique. Semin Thromb Hemost 1995;21(Suppl 4):1–6.)

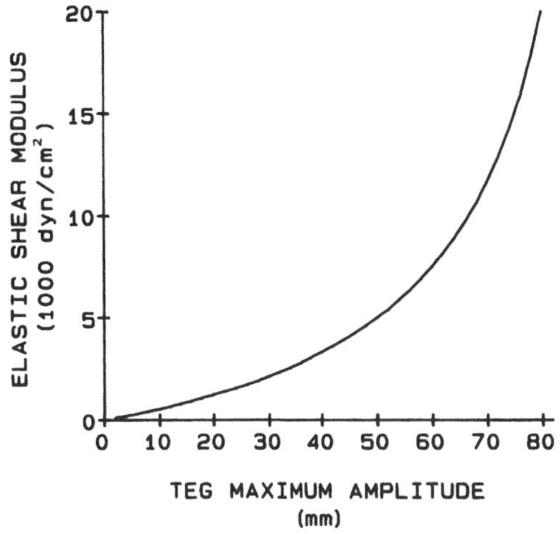

Figure 16.6. The maximum amplitude is related to clot strength (G) as a logarithmic function. The mean for the population is approximately 5000 dynes/cm² or 50-mm amplitude. Notice that if the amplitude decreases from 50 to 35 mm, a 30% reduction in MA, the force is decreased by 50% or more. (Reprinted by permission from Chandler WL. The thromboelastograph and the thromboelastograph technique. Semin Thromb Hemost 1995;21:1–6.)

finity (Fig. 16.6). Therefore, small or moderate changes in MA may translate into considerably larger changes in actual clot strength (G force). Most papers report the MA, but one wonders if it is not more appropriate to speak in terms of physical force.

The TEG examines whole blood coagulation from the time of initiation through acceleration, control, and eventual lysis. It can tell us essentially only four major things about coagulation: how fast the clot forms, the speed of clot growth, clot strength, and whether clot strength is maintained or breaks down early. These four facts about clot function are the key elements in whether a patient bleeds or not. If they are all normal, a significant coagulopathy cannot exist.

The physical strength of clot is dependent on the interaction of platelets and fibrin. Work has shown that platelets have about twice as much effect on the MA as does the fibrinogen concentration alone (56). Recent work with glycoprotein-blocking agents have shown that the TEG MA relates very closely to the dosage of blocking agent administered, whereas the TEG MA has little or no relationship to changes in ADP platelet aggregation (57, 58). There have never been any data showing that a given change in ADP platelet aggregation has any relationship to the risk of bleeding. The TEG is relatively insensitive to the changes found with aspirin therapy (59). Aspirin blocks thromboxane production in platelets as they are generated. However, there are multiple pathways by which platelets are activated, and if one supposes that the blood sample in the TEG is activated by the intrinsic pathway, then thrombin will be the chief mechanism for platelet activation, not thromboxane.

The TEG was first used in surgery for the monitoring of coagulation in hepatic transplantation (60). On-site rapid coagulation assessment was necessary because the changes of coagulation during these long and complex cases were profound. TEG technology has also been applied to cardiopulmonary bypass patients, with at least seven studies showing it to be the single best predictor of abnormal postoperative hemorrhage (61–67). One particular study examined the sensitivity and specificity of the TEG test as compared with other protein coagulation tests, platelet counts, and the bleeding time (67). The TEG had the best sensitivity and specificity of any coagulation test examined. Only one study has disagreed with these other seven studies, and if one examines that study very closely, it actually does show that the TEG MA has a highly significant predictability for excess coagulation (68). This study tried to correlate chest tube output to TEG MA and showed a rather poor correlation coefficient. The TEG MA is a linear representation of the G force, and as previously noted, the relationship is logarithmic. Chest tube bleeding is not a straight-line relationship but is a non-Gaussian data form with population clusters of routine bleeding and a small population of very severe bleeding. A simple Pearson R correlation coefficient should not be expected to show a relationship. However, in this study, the TEG MA was almost as predictive as platelet count, and the authors noted that if the TEG was normal and the patient was bleeding, a surgical bleeder was always found. The efficacy of the TEG for predicting surgical bleeding (a normal TEG) is greater than 90%.

The TEG is the best predictor for hemorrhage with percutaneous renal biopsy as well in patients with end-stage renal failure (69). Its use in guiding coagulation therapy has been demonstrated with the use of DDAVP (61). This compound increases the release of vWF in patients with end-stage renal failure or those with hemophilia. It has been used in trials in cardiopulmonary bypass patients with mixed success. However, in one study wherein the TEG was used as a method to sort out populations with normal platelet function (MA greater than 50 mm) and those with depressed platelet function (MA less than 50 mm), the patients who had depressed platelet function and received DDAVP had the same chest tube output after surgery as those who had normal platelet function. Those patients with depressed platelet function who did not receive DDAVP had considerably greater chest tube drainage and those patients who had normal platelet function, whether they received DDAVP or not, had reasonable amounts of chest tube output (Fig. 16.7). This is one of the strongest studies in support of the fact that TEG can be used effectively to not only guide therapy but also access platelet function (at least the overall function important to the risk of bleeding). The routine application of TEG coagulation assessment in cardiac surgery has reduced blood utilization by approximately 33% in one study (62). Subsequent to that study, an algorithm for blood replacement has been created based on the TEG and the platelet count and the fibrinogen concentration (Fig. 16.8). That algorithm is yet to be tested against the one previously outlined in this chapter, but the TEG algorithm does directly identify platelet function abnormalities rather than find them by process of elimination. By using the TEG, not only can blood product administrations be cut down, but the reexploration rate, a major cause of morbidity, some mortality, and certainly cost, has been considerably decreased (Table 16.1).

Most anesthesia departments run the TEG systems themselves, and this has been a source of some considerable dis-

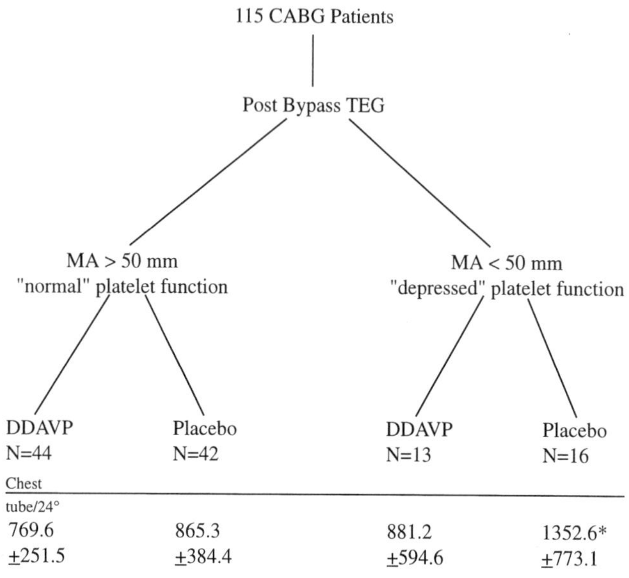

Figure 16.7. The TEG was used to segregate groups of patients with normal or depressed platelet function. Note that patients in the abnormal platelet function group who then received DDAVP had the same (normalized) chest tube output as those in the normal platelet function group. *Significantly different, $P \leq .05$. (Adapted from Mongan PD, Hosking MP. The role of desmopressin acetate in patients undergoing coronary artery bypass surgery. Anesthesiology 1992;77:38–46.)

satisfaction and criticism of the technology. The TEG must be critically quality-controlled, and new government regulations state that it must be done every 8–24 hours. A bioassay system using plasma with a known concentration of fibrinogen has been published (56). Maintenance of the technology is critical for reliable data acquisition. A cooperative effort with the laboratory medicine department has been published that allows quick data return and all the proper maintenance and quality control of the machines. TEG has been criticized for being slow in giving data; however, if the MA is the most important piece of information, then it can be obtained usually within 15–20 minutes. With new technology just being written about today, it seems that the TEG MA may be obtained in under 5 minutes (the speed of an ACT). Another approach to obtaining timely and predictive data has been to reverse heparin with either heparinase or protamine while patients are still on cardiopulmonary bypass and therefore predict bleeding and guide therapy before separating from cardiopulmonary bypass and administering protamine systemically.

The TEG is the best predictor of trace amounts of heparin. It also is the best test for overall hypercoagulability. Several articles show that it follows hypercoagulability after surgery very well (70–72). Large studies are necessary to demonstrate whether it can predict patients at risk for pulmonary

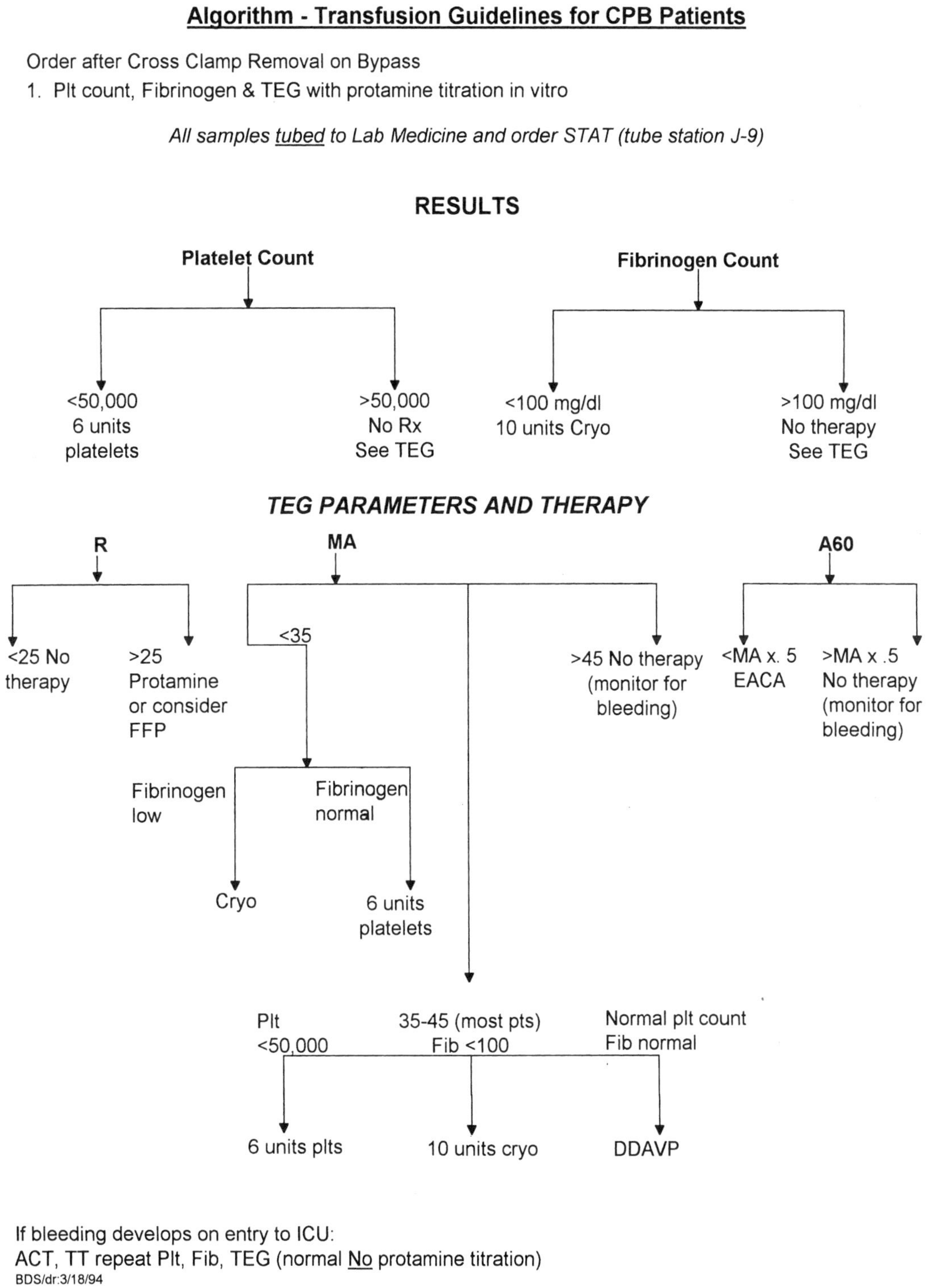

Figure 16.8. The algorithm based on TEG, platelet count, and fibrinogen concentration. This algorithm, although used largely for cardiac surgery, should be universally applicable to other surgeries. (Reprinted by permission from Spiess BD. Coagulation dysfunction after cardiopulmonary bypass. In: Williams JP, ed. Postoperative management of the cardiac surgical patient. New York: Churchill Livingstone, 1996;175–197.)

TABLE 16.1. CHANGES IN BLOOD UTILIZATION AND TRANSFUSION BEFORE AND AFTER TEG-GUIDED THERAPY

Transfusion practice per surgical case type[a]	Group 1 (N = 488)	Group 2 (N = 591)	p
CABG (%)			
Total	87.6	77.7	.001
RBC	84.5	73.1	.001
Plt	57.2	42.7	.001
FFP	31.6	19.6	.001
Cryo	4.5	3.3	.392
Open ventricle or complex (%)			
Total	82.7	81.1	NS
RBC	79.7	76.4	NS
Plt	64.7	64.9	NS
FFP	48.1	46.6	NS
Cryo	11.28	18.9	NS

Mediastinal reexploration rates[b]	Group 1 (N = 488)	Group 2 (N = 591)	p
Mediastinal reexploration (n)	28	9	0.0001
Total %	5.7	1.5	
CABG			
Number	16/355	6/443	0.007
Percent	4.5	1.4	
Complex			
Number	12/133	3/148	0.009
Percent	9.0	2.0	

[a]Overall decreases in blood utilization were made because of changes in the needs for transfusion in CABG patients. Open ventricle procedures did not change during this time.

[b]The use of TEG-guided therapy and decision making (reexploration of the mediastinum) has influenced both blood utilization and reoperation rates.

CABG, coronary artery bypass graft; RBC, red blood cell count; Plt, platelet; FFP, fresh frozen plasma; cryo, cryoprecipitate; NS, not significant.

Adapted from Spiess BD, Gillies BSA, Chandler W, Verrier E. Changes in transfusion therapy and reexploration rate after institution of a blood

emboli, graft thrombosis, and other hypercoagulable catastrophes (myocardial infarction and stroke).

The Sonoclot (Sienco, Denver, CO) is a similar device to the TEG in that it assesses whole blood coagulation function as it goes from a liquid to a gel (73, 74). It uses a cup with a suspended piston warmed to 37°C; however, the piston in this system vibrates up and down very rapidly and the impedance to vibration is measured. As clot forms from the wall of the cup to the piston, the impedance to vibration increases. Essentially, this system provides a continuous assessment of viscosity. Viscosity and clot strength are related, but one might be more easily convinced that clot strength is the physical force that is necessary to stop capillary bleeding. A Sonoclot signature has been described (Fig. 16.9), and some variations with expected coagulopathies have also been described. The Sonoclot signature has several inflection points, and the time to these inflection points and the height of the tracing at these inflections can be measured. What those inflection points mean in terms of actual biological clot function is not known. Some authors have ascribed certain platelet-mediated events to these inflection points, but scientific corroboration has not been forthcoming. There are also no widely published normals for when and at what height these inflection points should occur.

The Sonoclot does appear to follow changes in coagulation with cardiopulmonary bypass, and at least in one comparative study with TEG and other coagulation tests, it was almost equally predictive of bleeding with TEG (73). However, much less research has been conducted with Sonoclot than with TEG, and therefore we simply know less about what factors affect the changes in clot viscosity compared with TEG.

Presently, we are learning more about the basic science of what factors contribute to the whole blood clot strength. Development is underway to produce other whole blood viscoelastic clot-monitoring technologies. We have certainly learned from the TEG that clot strength is a valuable parameter. The use of these data along with other coagulation data (fibrinogen and platelet number) seems to be very useful. The coagulation profile is sometimes referred to as routine coagulation monitoring as opposed to viscoelastic monitoring. This misnomer should no longer be used because the TEG and Sonoclot have become routine in some institutions.

SUMMARY

Coagulation function is dependent on the action of the protein cascades and the surface ligands of platelets, leading to the eventual formation of a gel that is in the final analysis an interaction of platelets and fibrin. Coagulation monitoring is complex, with a large number of potential in vitro studies that can be performed on any given blood sample. With a rational approach focused on the key interaction of platelets and fibrin, it is now possible to perform timely coagulation monitoring that has predictive value toward patient hemor-

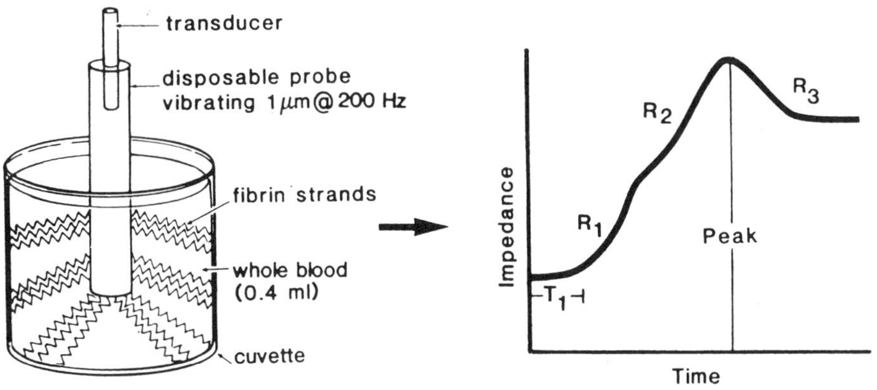

Figure 16.9. The Sonoclot analyzer uses a vertically vibrating probe lowered into a stable cuvette. It tests viscosity over time, and the typical signature is shown with multiple inflection points as viscosity increases. (Reprinted by permission from Tuman KJ, Spiess BD, McCarthy RJ, Ivankovich AD. Comparison of viscoelastic measures of coagulation after cardiopulmonary bypass. Anesth Analg 1989;69:69–75.

rhage. In the future, creative solutions, creation of algorithms, and possibly new technologies should be helpful in following coagulation changes in the perioperative period.

REFERENCES

1. Despotis GJ, Santoro SA, Spitznagel E, et al. Prospective evaluation and clinical utility of on-site monitoring of coagulation in patients undergoing cardiac operation. J Thorac Cardiovasc Surg 1994;107: 271–279.
2. Spiess BD. Coagulation dysfunction after cardiopulmonary bypass. In: Williams JP, ed. Postoperative management of the cardiac surgical patient. New York: Churchill Livingstone, 1996:175–197.
3. Boyle E, Verrier ED, Spiess, BD. Endothelial cell injury in cardiovascular surgery: the procoagulant response. Ann Thorac Surg 1996;62: 1–9.
4. Bevilacqua MP, Schleef RR, Grimbrone MA, Loskutoff DJ. Regulation of the fibrinolytic system of cultured human vascular endothelium by interleukin 1. J Clin Invest 1986;78:587–591.
5. McEver RP, Beckstead JH, Moore KL, et al. GMP-140, a platelet alpha-granule membrane protein, is also synthesized by vascular endothelial cells and is localized in Weibel-Palade bodies. J Clin Invest 1989;84: 92–99.
6. Boldt J, Schindler E, Knothe C, et al. Does aprotinin influence endothelial-associated coagulation in cardiac surgery? J Cardiothorac Vasc Anesth 1994;8:527–531.
7. Nachman RL, Hajjar KA, Silverstein RL, Dinarello CA. Interleukin 1 induces endothelial cell synthesis of plasminogen activator inhibitor. J Exp Med 1986;163:1595–1600.
8. Johnson M, Haddix T, Pohlman T, Verrier ED. Hypothermia reversibly inhibits endothelial cell expression of E-selectin and tissue factor. J Cardiol Surg 1995;10:428–435.
9. Foreman KE, Vaporciyan AA, Bonish BK, et al. C5a-induced expression of P-selectin in endothelial cells. J Clin Invest 1994;94:1147–1155.
10. Lucore C. Regulation of fibrinolysis by vascular endothelium. Coron Artery Dis 1991;2:157–166.
11. Luchtman-Jones L, Broze GJ. The current status of coagulation. Ann Med 1995;27:47–52.
12. Parry GC, Mackman N. Transcriptional regulation of tissue factor expression in human endothelial cells. Arterioscler Thromb Vasc Biol 1995;15:612–621.
13. Ammar T, Reich DL. Bedside coagulation monitoring [editorial]. J Cardiothorac Vasc Anesth 1995;9:353–361.
14. Reich DL, Yanakakis MJ, Vela-Cantos FP, DePerio M, Jacobs E. Comparison of bedside coagulation monitoring tests with standard laboratory tests in patients after cardiac surgery. Anesth Analg 1993;77: 673–679.
15. Sane DC, Gresalfi NJ, Enney-O'Mara LA, et al. Exploration of rapid bedside monitoring of coagulation and fibrinolysis parameters during thrombolytic therapy. Blood Coagul Fibrinol 1992;3:47–54.
16. Spiess BD. Perioperative coagulation concerns: function, monitoring and therapy. Clin Anesth Updates 1993;4:1–16.
17. Plow E, Ginsberg MH. Cellular adhesion: GPIIB-IIIA as a prototypic adhesion receptor. Prog Hemost Thromb 1989:9:117–156.
18. Coller BS. Blockade of platelet GPIIB/IIIA receptors as an antithrombotic strategy. Circulation 1995;92:2373–2380.
19. Nachman RL, Leung LL. Complex formation of platelet membrane glycoproteins IIB and IIIA with fibrinogen. J Clin Invest 1982;69: 263–269.
20. Lefkovits J, Plow EF, Topol EJ. Platelet glycoprotein IIB/IIIA receptors in cardiovascular medicine. N Engl J Med 1995;332:1553–1559.
21. Nurden AT, Caen JP. An abnormal platelet glycoprotein pattern in three cases of Glanzmann's thrombasthenia. Br J Haematol 1974;28: 253–260.
22. Karges HE, Clemens R. Factor XIII: enzymatic and clinical aspects. Behring Ins Mitt 1988;82:43–58.
23. Shainoff JR, Estafanous FG, Yared JP, et al. Low factor XIIIA levels are associated with increased blood loss after coronary artery bypass grafting. J Thorac Cardiovasc Surg 1994;108:437–445.
24. Koster T, Rosendaal FR, Briet E, et al. Protein C deficiency in a controlled series of unselected outpatients: an infrequent but clear risk factor for venous thrombosis (Leiden Thrombophilia Study). Blood 1995; 85:2756–2761.
25. Gouin I, Lecompte T, Morel MC. In vitro effect of plasmin on human platelet function in plasma. Inhibition of aggregation caused by fibrinogenolysis. Circulation 1992;85:935–941.
26. Rinder CS, Bohnert J, Rinder HM, et al. Platelet activation and aggregation during cardiopulmonary bypass. Anesthesiology 1991;75: 388–393.

27. Kestin AS, Valeri CR, Khuri SF, et al. The platelet function defect of cardiopulmonary bypass. Blood 1993;82:107–117.
28. Rinder CS, Mathew JP, Rinder HM, Bonan J, Ault KA, Smith BR. Modulation of platelet surface adhesion receptors during cardiopulmonary bypass. Anesthesiology 1991;75:563–570.
29. Weiss EJ, Bray PF, Tayback M, et al. A polymorphism of a platelet glycoprotein receptor as an inherited risk factor for coronary thrombosis. N Engl J Med 1996;334:1090–1094.
30. Goodnough LT, Johnston MF, Ramsey G, et al. Guidelines for transfusion support in patients undergoing coronary artery bypass grafting. Ann Thorac Surg 1990;50:675–683.
31. Simon TL, Akl BF, Murphy W. Controlled trial of routine administration of platelet concentrates in cardiopulmonary bypass surgery. Ann Thorac Surg 1984;37:359–364.
32. Counts RB, Haisch C, Simon TL, Maxwell NG, Heimbach DM, Carrico CJ. Hemostasis in massively transfused trauma patients. Ann Surg 1979;190:91–99.
33. Ciavarella D, Reed RL, Counts RB, et al. Clotting factor levels and the risk of diffuse microvascular bleeding in the massively transfused patient. Br J Haematol 1987;67:365–368.
34. Gravlee G, Goldsmith J, Low J, Harrison G, Barch J. Heparin sensitivity comparison of the ACT, SCT, and APTT. Anesthesiology 1989;71: A4.
35. Loeliger EA. ICSH/ISTH recommendations for reporting prothrombin time in oral anticoagulant control. Thromb Haemost 1985;53:155–160.
36. WHO Expert Committee on Biological Standardization 28th Report. WHO Technical Report Series 610. Geneva: World Health Organization, 1977:14:45.
37. Clagett GP. Preoperative assessment of hemostasis. In: Rossi EC, Simon TL, Moss GS, eds. Principles of transfusion medicine. Baltimore: Williams & Wilkins, 1991:453–460.
38. Sidi A, Seligsohn U, Jonas P, Many M. Factor XI deficiency: detection and management during urological surgery. J Urol 1978;119:528–530.
39. Kaplan EB, Sheiner LB, Boeckmann AJ. The usefulness of preoperative laboratory screening. JAMA 1985;253:3576–3581.
40. Eika C, Havig O, Godal HC. The value of preoperative haemostatic screening. Scand J Haematol 1978;21:349–354.
41. Eisenberg JM, Clarke JR, Sussman SA. Prothrombin and partial thromboplastin times as preoperative screening tests. Arch Surg 1982;117: 48–51.
42. Despotis GJ, Santoro SA, Spitznagel E, et al. On-site prothrombin time, activated partial thromboplastin time, and platelet count. A comparison between whole blood and laboratory assays with coagulation factor analysis in patients presenting for cardiac surgery. Anesthesiology 1994;80:338–351.
43. Jobes DR, Schwartz AJ, Ellison N, et al. Monitoring heparin anticoagulation and its neutralization. Ann Thorac Surg 1981;31:161–166.
44. Bull BS, Korpman RA, Huse WM, et al. Heparin therapy during extracorporeal circulation. I. Problems inherent in existing heparin protocols. J Thorac Cardiovasc Surg 1975;69:674–684.
45. Gravlee GP, Whitaker CL, Mark LJ, et al. Baseline activated coagulation time should be measured after surgical incision. Anesth Analg 1990;71:549–553.
46. Ellison N, Ominsky AJ, Wollman H. Is protamine a clinically important anticoagulant? Anesthesiology 1971;35:621–629.
47. Gravlee GP, Rogers AT, Dudas LM, et al. Heparin management protocol for cardiopulmonary bypass influences postoperative heparin rebound but not bleeding. Anesthesiology 1992;76:393–401.
48. Gravlee GP, Haddon WS, Rothberger HK, et al. Heparin dosing and monitoring for cardiopulmonary bypass: a comparison of techniques with measurement of subclinical plasma coagulation. J Thorac Cardiovasc Surg 1990;99:518–527.
49. Despotis GJ, Joist JH, Joiner-Maier D. Effect of aprotinin on activated clotting time, whole blood and plasma heparin measurements. Ann Thorac Surg 1995;59:106–111.
50. Groce JB, Gal B, Douglas JB, Steuterman MC. Heparin dosage adjustment in patients with deep-vein thrombosis using heparin concentrations rather than activated thromboplastin time. Clin Pharmacol 1987;6: 216–222.
51. van den Besselaar AM, Meeuwisse-Braun J, Bertina RM. Monitoring heparin therapy: relationships between the activated partial thromboplastin time and heparin assays based on ex-vivo heparin samples. Thromb Haemost 1990;63:16–23.
52. Elwood PC, Beswick AD, Sharp DS, et al. Whole blood impedance platelet aggregometry and ischemic heart disease. The Caerphilly Collaborative Heart Disease Study. Arteriosclerosis 1990;10:1032–1036.
53. Rodgers RP, Levin J. A critical reappraisal of the bleeding time. Semin Thromb Hemost 1990;16:1–20.
54. Caprini JA, Traverso CI, Walenga JM, Arcelus JI, Fareed J, Spiess BD. Thromboelastography. Semin Thromb Hemost 1995;21(Suppl 4):21–26.
55. Hartert H. Blutgerinnungsstudien unit der thromboelastographie, einen neven untersuchungsverfahren. Klin Wochenschr 1948;26:577–583.
56. Chandler W. The thromboelastograph and the thromboelastograph technique. Semin Thromb Hemost 1995;21(suppl 4):1–6.
57. Khurana S. Thromboelastography can rapidly bioassay fibrinogen. Anesthesiology 1996;85:A457.
58. Sharma S, Philip J, Perez B, Wiley J. Thromboelastography using tissue factor and cellulite: normal measurements in pregnant and postpartum women. Anesthesiology 1996;85:A905.
59. Trentalange MJ, Walts LF. A comparison of thromboelastogram and template bleeding time in the evaluation of platelet function after aspirin ingestion. J Clin Anesth 1991;3:377–381.
60. Kang YG, Martin DJ, Marquez J, et al. Intraoperative changes in blood coagulation and thromboelastographic monitoring in liver transplantation. Anesth Analg 1985;64:888–896.
61. Mongan PD, Hosking MP. The role of desmopressin acetate in patients undergoing coronary artery bypass surgery. Anesthesiology 1992;77:38–46.
62. Spiess BD, Gillies BSA, Chandler W, Verrier E. Changes in transfusion therapy and reexploration rate after institution of a blood management program in cardiac surgical patients. J Cardiothorac Vasc Anesth 1995; 9:168–173.
63. Spiess BD, Tuman K, McCarthy R, et al. Thromboelastography as an indicator of post-cardiopulmonary bypass coagulopathies. J Clin Monit 1987;3:25–30.
64. Spiess BD, Logas W, Tuman K, et al. Thromboelastography (TEG) used for the detection of perioperative fibrinolysis. A report of four cases. J Cardiothorac Anesth 1988;2:666–672.
65. Whitten CW, Allison PM, Latson TW, et al. Evaluation of laboratory coagulation and lytic parameters resulting from autologous whole blood transfusion during primary aortocoronary artery bypass grafting. J Clin Anesth 1996;8:229–235.
66. Tuman KJ, McCarthy RJ, Djuric M, Rizzo V, Ivankovich AD. Evaluation of coagulation during cardiopulmonary bypass with a heparinase-modified thromboelastographic assay. J Cardiothorac Vasc Anesth 1994;8:144–149.
67. Essell JH, Martin TJ, Salinas J, et al. Comparison of thromboelastography to bleeding time and standard coagulation tests in patients after

cardiopulmonary bypass. J Cardiothorac Vasc Anesth 1993;7:410–415.

68. Wang JS, Lin CY, Hung WT, et al. Thromboelastogram fails to predict postoperative hemorrhage in cardiac patients. Ann Thorac Surg 1992; 53:435–439.
69. Davis CL, Chandler WL. Thromboelastography for the prediction of bleeding after transplant renal biopsy. J Am Soc Nephrol 1995;6:1250–1255.
70. Gibbs NM, Crawford GP, Michalopoulos N. Thromboelastographic patterns following abdominal aortic surgery. Anaesth Intensive Care 1994;22:534–538.
71. Francis JL, Francis DA, Gunathilagan GJ. Assessment of hypercoagulability in patients with cancer using the Sonoclot Analyzer and thromboelastography. Thromb Res 1994;74:335–346.
72. Tuman KJ, McCarthy RJ, March RJ, et al. Effects of epidural anesthesia and analgesia on coagulation and outcome after major vascular surgery. Anesth Analg 1991;73:696–704.
73. LaForce WR, Brudno DS, Kanto WP, et al. Evaluation of the SonoClot Analyzer for the measurement of platelet function in whole blood. Ann Clin Lab Sci 1992;22:30–33.
74. Tuman KJ, Spiess BD, McCarthy RJ, Ivankovich AD. Comparison of viscoelastic measures of coagulation after cardiopulmonary bypass. Anesth Analg 1989;69:69–75.

Chapter 17

Implications of Anticoagulant Therapy in Anesthesia and Surgery

PHILIP COMP

INTRODUCTION

The use of both acute and chronic anticoagulation is changing rapidly in clinical practice. Ever increasing numbers of patients are receiving chronic oral anticoagulation or chronic antiplatelet therapy. The development of new low-molecular-weight heparin compounds has improved the prevention of thrombophlebitis and pulmonary embolism in the postoperative period. The treatment of deep vein thrombosis and pulmonary embolism is also undergoing significant changes that are aimed at safely establishing an effective level of anticoagulation as rapidly as possible. These areas are discussed in this chapter.

INCREASED USE OF CHRONIC ANTICOAGULATION AND ANTIPLATELET THERAPY

The use of long-term oral anticoagulation with warfarin is increasing rapidly. This is particularly evident in the prevention of stroke in older patients with chronic atrial fibrillation. An impressive body of data supporting the use of oral anticoagulation to prevent stroke in patients with atrial fibrillation has led to the prescription of warfarin to many older patients who previously would not have been considered for such long-term therapy. Between 5% and 6% of people in their 70s have atrial fibrillation; this can occur in the absence of underlying mitral valve disease or congestive heart failure (1). The risk of stroke in patients with atrial fibrillation is approximately six times higher than in patients without atrial fibrillation (2). Warfarin has been shown in six large collaborative trials to reduce the incidence of stroke by approximately 60% (3). This has prompted the recommendation that all patients over age 65 years who have atrial fibrillation and an associated risk factor, such as prior transient ischemic attack or stroke, hypertension, heart failure, diabetes, clinically evident coronary artery disease, mitral stenosis, prosthetic heart valves, or thyrotoxicosis, should receive long-term oral anticoagulation with warfarin (4). This means that potentially 5% of patients in their 70s will be receiving oral anticoagulation, which will need to be safely discontinued before elective surgery and restarted after surgery.

IMPROVED MONITORING IN ORAL ANTICOAGULATION

The development of a new system of monitoring oral anticoagulation has helped to ensure the safety and convenience of using warfarin therapy. This involves the use of the International Normalized Ratio (INR) to monitor oral anticoagulation (5). The INR is essentially a normalized measure of the intensity of oral anticoagulation. The prothrombin time (PT) is dependent on the type of coagulation reagent and the type of blood clotting instrument used in the hospital laboratory. If the same sample of plasma from an anticoagulated patient is measured in different laboratories, different PTs may be obtained. This makes maintenance of a given intensity of oral anticoagulation difficult. For example, a patient may have a PT of 18 seconds just before discharge from the hospital and a PT of 14 seconds 1 day later as an outpatient. Although the significant shortening of the PT may reflect a decrease in the intensity of anticoagulation, it may just as easily reflect a difference in the sensitivity of the instrument and reagents used to do the test.

The INR is a mathematical normalization of the PT that corrects for the various machines and reagents used (Fig. 17.1). For a given patient sample, similar INR results are obtained between laboratories. This has significantly improved monitoring of oral anticoagulation. The adoption of the INR has also allowed improved comparison of the results of various clinical trials because all results of these studies can be expressed in a comparable manner, regardless of the types of laboratory reagents used.

The development of the INR system has permitted the development of very specific recommendations, based on solid clinical evidence, for the intensity of treatment of both venous and arterial thrombotic conditions (5). These recommendations vary from relatively low INR levels of 2–3 for the treatment of deep vein thrombosis and prevention of stroke in atrial fibrillation to higher levels in prevention of thrombotic stroke in mechanical heart valve patients (4, 6). Physicians no longer need to make approximate calculations of the level of anticoagulation based on the simple ratio of the patient's PT to a laboratory control time.

INHERITED CONDITIONS PREDISPOSING TO VENOUS THROMBOSIS

Recognition of inherited conditions that predispose to risk of developing deep vein thrombosis has increased the number of patients who receive long-term oral anticoagulation (7, 8). Antithrombin III deficiency has been recognized for a number of years as an inherited cause of recurrent venous thrombosis and pulmonary embolism. A family of anticoagulant plasma proteins that comprise the protein C pathway has now been recognized as the major protein system in the plasma that prevents the formation of intravenous thrombi (9), and abnormalities of this system have been found to predispose to venous thrombosis. During the normal operation of this anticoagulant system, protein C is converted to activated protein C. With the help of protein S, activated protein C destroys the activity of clotting factor V, thus preventing the formation of intravascular thrombi. More recently, a new inherited abnormality, activated protein C resistance, which also predisposes to venous thrombosis, has been described (10). With this condition, a specific amino acid in the factor V molecule has mutated, rendering the factor V resistant to the anticoagulant effect of activated protein C. The abnormal factor V molecule is able to perpetuate intravenous clotting despite what is a normally functioning protein C system. As tests for conditions such as activated protein C resistance become increasingly available, more patients with venous thrombosis will be tested, and it is inevitable that many with positive tests will receive indefinite oral anticoagulation.

EMERGING AREAS OF CHRONIC ORAL ANTICOAGULATION

The use of chronic anticoagulants is expected to rise even further in the next decade. Two major trials are now underway in North America to test the efficacy of combined aspirin and warfarin in preventing reinfarction after an initial cardiac ischemic event. One trial, the Coumadin Aspirin Reinfarction Study, being conducted in the United States and Canada, ex-

The International Normalized Ratio (INR) corrects the prothrombin time for differences between laboratories

INR = (Patient's PT/ Mean Normal PT)^{ISI}

In this example, a split sample of patient plasma may have very different prothrombin times in two different laboratories, but will have the same INR. The patient has a prothrombin time at laboratory 1 of 16 seconds and a prothrombin time of 24 seconds at laboratory 2, but the INR is the same (2.6) at both laboratories, e.g.,

$$INR_{Lab\ 1} = (16\ sec/\ 12\ sec)^{3.2} = 2.6$$

$$INR_{Lab\ 2} = (24\ sec/\ 11\ sec)^{1.2} = 2.6$$

(Mean Normal PT = average prothrombin time for 20 normal volunteers determined using the laboratory's reagents and clotting instrument. ISI = International Sensitivity Index, which is known for a given coagulation reagent and clotting instrument combination being used and corrects the determination for relative sensitivity.)

Figure 17.1.

amines a fixed dose of warfarin (3 mg) in conjunction with 80 mg aspirin versus 160 mg aspirin alone (11, 12). The other study, the Combination Hemotherapy and Monitoring Prevention Study, being conducted in the Veterans Administration medical centers, will determine if an adjusted dose of warfarin combined with aspirin is superior to aspirin alone to prevent reinfarction (3, 13). If either or both of these studies demonstrate the efficacy of such therapy, many or perhaps most patients who have suffered a myocardial infarction will receive combined aspirin/warfarin anticoagulation.

LOW-MOLECULAR-WEIGHT HEPARINS

The development of various low-molecular-weight heparin compounds is having an increasing impact on postoperative surgical care. At present, two low-molecular-weight heparin compounds are approved in the United States, Lovenox and Fragmin (Table 17.1). Lovenox is currently approved for prevention of thrombophlebitis after elective hip or knee replacement surgery, and Fragmin is approved for prophylaxis after abdominal surgery. Low-molecular-weight heparins have advantages over other methods of preventing postoperative thrombophlebitis (14–17). Unlike warfarin, these low-molecular-weight heparins do not require adjustment based on laboratory monitoring. This eliminates the need for daily PTs or partial thromboplastin times (PTTs) in the postoperative period. The route of administration with low-molecular-weight heparin is subcutaneous. The compounds have a sustained release for the subcutaneous injections site and thus permits twice daily, or as is the case for Fragmin, once daily subcutaneous dosing. Additionally, the low-molecular-weight heparins may not carry the hemorrhagic risk or risk of heparin-induced thrombocytopenia that has been associated with unfractionated heparin. Unfortunately, the optimal duration of use of the low-molecular-weight heparins after surgery is not known. Two clinical trials are presently underway that will determine if home administration of once daily low-molecular-weight heparin will significantly reduce the incidence of thrombophlebitis after hip and knee replacement. This information is critical because the typical 4-day postoperative hospital stay does not allow adequate time for sufficient prophylaxis in these high-risk surgical patients. Home administration of low-molecular-weight heparin involves teaching the patient to self-administer the low-molecular-weight heparin or arranging for home health agencies to perform this task.

TABLE 17.1. LOW-MOLECULAR-WEIGHT HEPARINS

Generic Names	U.S. Trade Name	Manufacturer
Licensed in the United States[a]		
Enoxaparin	Lovenox	Rhone Poulenc Rorer
Dalteparin	Fragmin	Pharmacia-Upjohn
Pending licensing in the United States		
Ardeparin	Normiflo	Wyeth Ayerst
Tinzaparin	Logiparin	Novo-Nordisk, Leo
Nadroparin	Fraxiparine	Sanofi Winthrop
Certiparin	Sandoparin	Sandoz
Reviparin	Clivarin	Knoll AG
Parnaparin	Fluxum	Opocrin
Heparanoids		
Danaparoid[b]		Organon

[a]Enoxaparin is currently approved for elective hip and knee replacement surgery, and dalteparin is approved for general surgery.
[b]Danaparoid is not a low-molecular-weight heparin; it is a mixture of heparin sulfate, dermatan sulfate, and chondroitin sulfate.
Adapted from Raskob GE. Low molecular weight heparin, heparin and warfarin. Curr Opin Cardiol 1995;2:372–379.

Within the next 5 years, as many as six low-molecular-weight heparins and heparanoid compounds will be available for a variety of indications, ranging from treatment of acute thrombosis to prevention of myocardial infarction (14). The use of these agents virtually eliminates the need for laboratory testing because the low-molecular-weight heparins have little or no effect on the PT or PTT. In clinical trials, single daily administration of low-molecular-weight heparin has proven effective in the treatment of established deep vein thrombosis (18). This advance will eventually make treatment of uncomplicated deep vein thrombosis in an outpatient setting a reality.

PATIENTS WITH PRIOR POSTOPERATIVE DEEP VEIN THROMBOSIS

Many clinical trials using low-molecular-weight heparins to prevent postoperative thrombophlebitis have specifically excluded patients with a previous history of thrombophlebitis or pulmonary embolism. Until good evidence is presented to demonstrate that the low-molecular-weight heparins alone are effective in these very high risk patients, it is prudent to use at least two methods of prophylaxis. This could involve a low-molecular-weight heparin postoperatively with simultaneous introduction of warfarin therapy. After the INR reaches 2.0–3.0, the low-molecular-weight heparin can be stopped and the warfarin continued for a minimum of 6 weeks. This combined use of prophylactic methods may significantly reduce the risk that high-risk patients will develop thrombophlebitis.

TREATMENT OF THROMBOPHLEBITIS

Advances have been made in the use of anticoagulation to treat postoperative thrombophlebitis, as well as thrombophlebitis occurring in the nonoperative setting (19). The current emphasis is on establishing a therapeutic level of intravenous heparin in a safe and expeditious manner. A 5000-unit bolus of heparin is recommended, with institution of a continuous infusion of heparin (Table 17.2). The initial dose of the continuous heparin infusion of approximately 1300 unit/hr is suggested. This is significantly higher than the traditional 1000-unit/hr dose. The level of anticoagulation is checked in 4–6 hours using the activated partial thromboplastin time (aPTT); adjustments in the infusion rate are made at that time. The desired therapeutic range is approximately 55–80 seconds. The use of the 1300-unit/hr infusion rate helps to ensure that a therapeutic level of anticoagulation will be obtained. This can be further ensured by frequent monitoring using the aPTT. Institution of warfarin is now recommended at the initiation of heparin therapy; an initial dose of 5–10 mg is used. Although the length of overlap of warfarin and heparin is debated, heparin is generally discontinued after the INR reaches 2–3.

CURRENT INDICATIONS FOR ANTICOAGULANTS AND ANTITHROMBOTIC AGENTS

ASPIRIN

Aspirin is widely used as an antithrombotic agent to prevent arterial thrombotic events other than stroke in atrial fibrillation patients. Aspirin is indicated in patients with stable angina, unstable angina, acute myocardial infarction, transient ischemic attacks, thrombotic stroke, and peripheral vascular disease (20). Aspirin will reduce the incidence of stroke in patients with chronic atrial fibrillation by approximately one-third and is recommended for those patients with atrial fibrillation who cannot take warfarin therapy (21).

TABLE 17.2. TREATMENT OF POSTOPERATIVE DEEP VEIN THROMBOSIS

1. Objective diagnosis of deep vein thrombosis or pulmonary embolism (venogram, lung scan, etc.)
2. Start warfarin therapy
3. 5000-unit heparin bolus IV
4. 1300-unit/hr continuous heparin infusion
5. Check aPTT in 4–6 hr and adjust infusion rate to keep aPTT in 55- to 80-sec range. Repeat aPTT every 4–6 hr as needed to reach therapeutic range and then daily
6. When INR = 2–3, stop heparin.
7. Continue warfarin at least 6 weeks with INR 2–3.

Compelling data indicate that aspirin is effective in prevention of stroke in patients with transient ischemic attacks (22–24), prevention of stroke in patients with nonvalvular atrial fibrillation (25, 26), and in the prevention of myocardial infarction (27–29). The relatively low cost and lack of need for therapeutic monitoring have been significant factors leading to the use of aspirin.

WARFARIN

Warfarin has enjoyed long use in the prevention and treatment of venous thrombosis and pulmonary emboli, as well as the prevention of stroke in patients with rheumatic valve disease and thrombogenic prosthetic heart valves (30–33). The recognition that lower intensity oral anticoagulation is effective in preventing a number of thrombotic events while not causing an intolerable increase in bleeding risk has enhanced the use of long-term oral anticoagulation. The potential value of warfarin in preventing myocardial infarction is receiving increased recognition by the medical community.

DIPYRIDAMOLE

Dipyridamole is approved for use in conjunction with warfarin to prevent thromboembolism in patients with prosthetic heart valves. Persantine is also used in patients who are particularly sensitive to the gastrointestinal or hemorrhagic side effects of aspirin (34, 35). The relatively high cost and the lack of data on clinical indications have limited the use of this drug.

ANTICOAGULANTS AND SURGICAL BLEEDING

Surgical procedures are discussed in terms of the hemorrhagic complications of concomitant use of aspirin, warfarin, and dipyridamole. Much of the available data is derived from retrospective case reviews. Few prospective clinical trials have been conducted in which patients are randomly allocated to receive the anticoagulant drug or placebo before surgery. The quantitation of surgical blood loss remains a difficult problem. Very little information, even anecdotal in nature, is available on the hemorrhagic surgical complications of the newer antithrombotic agents such as ticlopidine.

CORONARY ARTERY BYPASS SURGERY

In a prospective study, patients receiving 325 mg aspirin 12 hours before bypass surgery have increased operative blood loss and receive more packed blood cells and more blood products than do patients who are not treated with aspirin (36). Additional prospective studies have found similar results (37). The dosing and timing of aspirin before surgery appears to be critical because a retrospective examination of a cohort of patients who received aspirin within 1 week of admission for bypass surgery did not find significantly increased homologous blood requirements (38). A case-control study examining 90 patients who underwent reoperation for bleeding after coronary artery concluded that aspirin exposure within 7 days before bypass surgery is associated with an increased rate of reoperation for bleeding and increased use of blood products (39). The increased blood loss that is seen with perioperative aspirin use must be weighed against improved early graft patency rates (40) and patency rates at 1 year (41, 42).

It would appear rather clearcut that aspirin use before cardiopulmonary bypass increases chest tube bleeding. However, two studies underway are demonstrating some controversy. In one study of patients undergoing repeat coronary revascularization, in a group at high risk for bleeding, chest tube output was no different if patients had aspirin up until surgery, aspirin and heparin, or no anticoagulation at all. A total of 241 patients were involved (43). In an unpublished series of over 2400 patients, the use of aspirin within 3–7 days of surgery had no effect on bleeding, transfusion, or reoperation (Multicentered Study of Perioperative Ischemia Hematology Subgroup, unpublished data).

ORTHOPEDIC SURGERY

Recognition of the risks of thrombophlebitis and pulmonary embolism after both knee and hip arthroplasty has significantly increased the use of heparin and warfarin in the perioperative period (44–46). A number of low-molecular-weight heparin compounds and heparin-like compounds are being tested for the prevention of venous thrombosis after orthopedic surgery (47) (Table 17.1).

Generally, low-molecular-weight heparin has proven more effective than intermittent pneumatic compression stockings after hip replacement surgery (78% versus 57% reduction in risk of thrombophlebitis) and less effective than intermittent pneumatic compression stockings after knee replacement (44% versus 82% reduction in risk) (48). These results contrast to general surgery where pooled data suggest that low-molecular-weight heparins are more effective (80% risk reduction) than intermittent pneumatic compression stockings (60% risk reduction) (48). What remains to be determined is the relative effectiveness of combined methods to prevent deep vein thrombosis. These could include the combination of low-molecular-weight heparin, intermittent pneumatic compression stockings, and elastic hose or low-molecular-weight heparin and warfarin.

The initiation of anticoagulation before surgery to prevent thrombophlebitis and pulmonary embolism has been of interest for at least the last decade. Two-step warfarin therapy has been used in knee and hip replacement to prevent venous thrombosis (49). Very-low-dose warfarin therapy is initiated 10 days to 2 weeks before surgery and the PT is regulated to 1.5–3 seconds longer than control. In contemporary laboratory parlance, these values could reflect INRs of 1.1–1.6. After surgery, warfarin dosage was increased to bring the PTs to 1.5 times control. The overall incidence of venous thrombosis was 21% in the treated group and 51% in the dextran treatment control subjects; femoral or popliteal clots were 2% versus 16%, respectively. There was no significance in blood loss in the perioperative period. This small ($n = 50 + 50$) prospective study demonstrated the safety of performing orthopedic surgery in patients with a measurable level of oral anticoagulation. Unfortunately, large secondary studies of this form of therapy are not available to help determine if the results are generally applicable, nor is information available on how many centers are successfully using this form of clot prevention (49, 50).

Low-dose heparin, administered before or after surgery, has been used extensively in knee and hip surgery. Although meta-analyses show an increase in the incidence of wound hematoma, there is not a significant increase in blood loss or an increased need to reoperate in patients receiving such treatment (51). This relative lack of bleeding may reflect the mechanism of action of the low-molecular-weight heparins. These compounds inhibit the clotting cascade at the level of factor X, whereas unfractionated heparin inhibits clotting at the level of factor X and the level of thrombin, the last step in the clotting cascade.

Low-molecular-weight heparin compounds are being used extensively in Europe and increasingly so in North America to prevent thrombophlebitis after hip and knee surgery. Even when administered preoperatively, these heparins do not significantly increase operative blood loss (47, 52). The low-molecular-weight heparins have several advantages over unfractionated heparin. They are given once (Fragmin) or twice (Lovenox) daily subcutaneously. The bioavailability of these compounds allows a gradual release from the subcutaneous tissue into the bloodstream. Heparin-induced thrombocytopenia is a recognized complication of unfractionated heparin (53–55); the low-molecular-weight heparins appear to carry a much lower risk of this serious complication. The heparinoid danaparoid may be particularly useful in this regard (56).

Although not anticoagulants, nonsteroidal anti-inflammatory drugs may increase operative blood loss in orthopedic surgery (57–59). Unfortunately, the bulk of evidence is based on retrospective case reviews and may favor the identification of cases in which significant hemorrhage occurred. Well-controlled prospective studies are needed because of the frequent use of these drugs in patients with rheumatoid arthritis and the orthopedic surgery patient population in general.

OTHER TYPES OF SURGERY

In general surgery, low-molecular-weight heparin does not significantly increase surgical blood loss (60). Newer surgical techniques may decrease blood loss in the presence of low-dose heparin even further. Relatively little information is available on the effects of aspirin or warfarin on ophthalmologic surgery. As an increasing number of patients are on chronic warfarin for conditions such as atrial fibrillation, the need for controlled studies in this area will become increasingly apparent.

Surgery in Patients on Chronic Oral Anticoagulation

Patients, such as those with thrombogenic heart valves, need relatively high-intensity oral anticoagulation and are at significant risk of stroke when that therapy is interrupted. When elective surgery is a necessity, oral anticoagulation is stopped for the shortest possible period of time. On the third day before surgery, the patient is instructed to stop taking the oral anticoagulant. On the second day before surgery, the patient enters the hospital and is placed on full-dose intravenous heparin. This is continued until the morning of surgery when the heparin is stopped 3 hours before the procedure. After surgery, full-dose heparin therapy is reinstituted as soon as possible with concomitant reinstitution of oral anticoagulation. The administration of vitamin K is avoided because its use can make the subsequent use of oral anticoagulation difficult and can prolong the time required to reattain a therapeutic level of oral anticoagulation. If emergency surgery is necessary, the use of large doses of vitamin K should be avoided. A dose of 3–5 mg given subcutaneously should have a maximal effect in correcting PT. The use of fresh-frozen plasma immediately before surgery may be necessary. However, because the effects of fresh-frozen plasma are dependent on the short half-life of factor VII, the plasma must be given as shortly before surgery as cardiovascular status permits. An adequate dose of fresh-frozen plasma is often about one-third of the plasma volume or typically 800–1000 mL (3–5 units).

Unfortunately, there are no controlled studies examining the risks of bleeding in patients receiving differing intensities of oral anticoagulation. The amount of blood loss cannot be predicted exactly based on the PT or INR. Physicians can only assume that the more closely the PT or INR is to normal, the less operative blood loss there will be.

LOW-MOLECULAR-WEIGHT HEPARINS AND SPINAL AND EPIDURAL ANESTHESIA

There is considerable concern about the risk of epidural or spinal anesthesia in patients receiving low-molecular-weight heparin. As more low-molecular-weight heparins become available and the indications for their use broaden, this will be an issue of major interest.

Using an extensive European database, Wolf (61) reviewed 9006 patients who received epidural or spinal anesthesia while receiving low-molecular-weight heparin. None of these patients experienced any neurological complications due to hemorrhage at the puncture site. Bergqvist (52) performed an extensive review of the literature in this area and concluded that neurological complications after epidural or spinal anesthesia in patients receiving postoperative thromboprophylaxis with low-molecular-weight heparin in low doses and low-dose unfractionated heparin are extremely rare. It was concluded that the use of these prophylactic measures is safe in this setting. After their extensive review of the literature, Vandermuelan et al. (62) concluded that the benefits of low-molecular-weight heparin use outweigh the risk of local hemorrhage after spinal and epidural anesthesia. They suggested that subcutaneous low-molecular-weight heparin should be started 10–12 hours before the anesthesia, or at least 1 hour after the spinal or epidural anesthesia is initiated. They further suggested that epidural or spinal catheters should be removed at least 10–12 hours after the last dose of low-molecular-weight heparin. Unfortunately, given the infrequency of hemorrhage complications after this type of anesthesia, controlled studies to resolve the correct timing of the anesthesia and low-molecular-weight heparin administration are not possible due to the number of patients required.

SUMMARY

The use of chronic anticoagulation is becoming more common in general medical practice. More and more patients will be receiving long-term anticoagulation. Surgeons need to become increasingly familiar with the monitoring of oral anticoagulation and must be familiar with the discontinuation of anticoagulation before and reinstitution after surgery. The appearance of low-molecular-weight heparin compounds is simplifying the prevention of postoperative deep vein thrombosis. Improved methods of anticoagulating patients who develop postoperative deep vein thrombosis and pulmonary embolism are now in practice. All these recent changes in the use of anticoagulants will have a direct effect on future surgical practice.

REFERENCES

1. Nattel S. Newer developments in the management of atrial fibrillation. Am Heart J 1995;130:1094–1106.
2. Wheeldon NM. Atrial fibrillation and anticoagulant therapy. Eur Heart J 1995; 16:302–312.
3. Ukani ZA, Ezekowitz MD. Contemporary management of atrial fibrillation. Med Clin North Am 1995;79:1135–1152.
4. Laupacis A, Albers G, Dalen J, Dunn M, Feinberg W, Jacobson A. Antithrombotic therapy in atrial fibrillation. Chest 1995;108:352S–359S.
5. Hirsh J, Dalen JE, Deykin D, Poller L, Bussey H. Oral anticoagulants. Mechanism of action, clinical effectiveness, and optimal therapeutic range. Chest 1995;108:231S–246S.
6. Stein PD, Alpert JS, Copeland J, Dalen JE, Goldman S, Turpie AG. Antithrombotic therapy in patients with mechanical and biological prosthetic heart valves. Chest 1995;108:371S–379S.
7. Alving BM, Comp PC. Recent advances in understanding clotting and evaluating patients with recurrent thrombosis. Am J Obstet Gynecol 1992;167:1184–1191.
8. Comp PC. Congenital and acquired hypercoagulable states. In: Hull R, Pineo GF, eds. Disorders of thrombosis. Philadelphia: WB Saunders, 1996:339–347.
9. Dahlback B. The protein C anticoagulant system: inherited defects as basis for venous thrombosis. Thromb Res 1995;77:1–43.
10. Dahlback B. Molecular genetics of thrombophilia: factor V gene mutation causing resistance to activated protein C as a basis of the hypercoagulable state. J Lab Clin Med 1995;125:566–571.
11. Raskob GE, Durica SS, Morrissey JH, Owen WL, Comp PC. Effect of treatment with low-dose warfarin-aspirin on activated factor VII. Blood 1995;85:3034–3039.
12. Goodman SG, Langer A, Durica SS, et al. Safety and anticoagulation effect of a low-dose combination of warfarin and aspirin in clinically stable coronary artery disease. Coumadin Aspirin Reinfarction (CARS) Pilot Study Group. Am J Cardiol 1994;74:657–661.
13. Ezekowitz MD, James KE, Nazarian SM, et al. Silent cerebral infarction in patients with nonrheumatic atrial fibrillation. The Veterans Affairs Stroke Prevention in Nonrheumatic Atrial Fibrillation Investigators. Circulation 1995;92:2178–2182.
14. Weitz J. New anticoagulant strategies. Current status and future potential. Drugs 1994;48:485–497.
15. Hirsh J, Levine MN. Low molecular weight heparin: laboratory properties and clinical evaluation. A review. Eur J Surg 1994;571(Suppl): 9–22.
16. Jorgensen LN, Wille-Jorgensen P, Hauch O. Prophylaxis of postoperative thromboembolism with low molecular weight heparins. Br J Surg 1993;80:689–704.
17. Barrowcliffe TW. Low molecular weight heparin(s). Br J Haematol 1995;90:1–7.
18. Tapson VF, Hull RD. Management of venous thromboembolic disease. The impact of low-molecular-weight heparin. Clin Chest Med 1995;16: 281–294.
19. Hyers TM, Hull RD, Weg JG. Antithrombotic therapy for venous thromboembolic disease. Chest 1995;108:335S–351S.
20. Hirsh J, Dalen JE, Fuster V, Harker LB, Patrono C, Roth G. Aspirin and other platelet-active drugs. The relationship among dose, effectiveness, and side effects. Chest 1995;108:247S–257S.
21. Anonymous. Collaborative overview of randomised trials of antiplatelet therapy. III. Reduction in venous thrombosis and pulmonary embolism by antiplatelet prophylaxis among surgical and medical patients. Antiplatelet Trialists' Collaboration. BMJ 1994;308:235–246.
22. Barnett HJ, Eliasziw M, Meldrum HE. Drugs and surgery in the prevention of ischemic stroke. N Engl J Med 1995;332:238–248.
23. Deantonio HJ, Movahed A. Atrial fibrillation: current therapeutic approaches. Am Fam Physician 1992;45:2576–2584.
24. Nelson KM, Talbert RL. Preventing stroke in patients with nonrheumatic atrial fibrillation. Am J Hosp Pharm 1994;51:1175–1183.
25. Hart RG. Prevention of stroke in atrial fibrillation: an update. Health Rep 1994;6:126–131.
26. Falk RH. Current management of atrial fibrillation. Curr Opin Cardiol 1994;9:30–39.
27. Flapan AD. Management of patients after their first myocardial infarction. BMJ 1994;309:1129–1134.
28. Flaker GC, Singh VN. Prevention of myocardial reinfarction. Recommendations based on results of drug trials. Postgrad Med 1993;94: 94–98, 102–104.
29. Yusuf S, Lessem J, Jha P, Lonn E. Primary and secondary prevention of myocardial infarction and strokes: an update of randomly allocated, controlled trials. J Hypertens 1993;11(Suppl):S61–S73.
30. Goldhaber SZ. Venous thrombosis: prevention, treatment, and relationship to paradoxical embolization. Cardiol Clin 1994;12:505–516.
31. de Bono D. Management of thrombosis in coronary heart disease. Br Med Bull 1994;50:904–910.
32. Stein PD, Grandison D, Hua TA, et al. Therapeutic level of oral anticoagulation with warfarin in patients with mechanical prosthetic heart valves: review of literature and recommendations based on international normalized ratio. Postgrad Med J 1994;70(Suppl 1):S72–S83.
33. Kondo NI, Maddi R, Ewenstein BM, Goldhaber SZ. Anticoagulation and hemostasis in cardiac surgical patients. J Cardiol Surg 1994;9: 443–461.
34. Green D, Miller V. The role of dipyridamole in the therapy of vascular disease. Geriatrics 1993;48:46, 51–53, 57–58.
35. Hirsh J, Dalen JE, Fuster V, Harker LB, Salzman EW. Aspirin and other platelet-active drugs. The relationship between dose, effectiveness, and side effects. Chest 1992;102:327S–336S.
36. Sethi GK, Copeland JG, Goldman S, Moritz T, Zadina K, Henderson WG. Implications of preoperative administration of aspirin in patients undergoing coronary artery bypass grafting. Department of Veterans Affairs Cooperative Study on Antiplatelet Therapy. J Am Coll Cardiol 1990;15:15–20.
37. Kallis P, Tooze JA, Talbot S, Cowans D, Bevan DH, Treasure T. Preoperative aspirin decreases platelet aggregation and increases postoperative blood loss—a prospective, randomised, placebo controlled, double-blind clinical trial in 100 patients with chronic stable angina. Eur J Cardiothorac Surg 1994;8:404–409.
38. Reich DL, Patel GC, Vela-Cantos F, Bodian C, Lansman S. Aspirin does not increase homologous blood requirements in elective coronary bypass surgery. Anesth Analg 1994;79:4–8.
39. Puga FJ. Risk of preoperative aspirin in patients undergoing coronary artery bypass surgery. J Am Coll Cardiol 1990;15:21–22.
40. Goldman S, Copeland J, Moritz T, et al. Improvement in early saphenous vein graft patency after coronary artery bypass surgery with antiplatelet therapy: results of a Veterans Administration Cooperative Study. Circulation 1988;77:1324–1332.

41. Goldman S, Copeland J, Moritz T, et al. Saphenous vein graft patency 1 year after coronary artery bypass surgery and effects of antiplatelet therapy. Results of a Veterans Administration Cooperative Study. Circulation 1989;80:1190–1197.
42. Anonymous. Collaborative overview of randomised trials of antiplatelet therapy. I. Prevention of death, myocardial infarction, and stroke by prolonged antiplatelet therapy in various categories of patients. Antiplatelet Trialists' Collaboration. BMJ 1994;308:81–106.
43. McCarthy RJ, O'Conner CJ, McCarthy WE, Tuman KJ, Ivankovich AD. Interaction of preoperative aspirin and heparin therapy on allogenic blood requirements after repeat CABG. Anesthesiology 1995; 83:A100.
44. Merli GJ. Update. Deep vein thrombosis and pulmonary embolism prophylaxis in orthopedic surgery. Med Clin North Am 1993;77:397–411.
45. Yen D. Current concepts in the prevention, detection, and treatment of deep vein thrombosis in total hip and knee replacement. Curr Opin Rheumatol 1992;4:210–215.
46. Swayze OS, Nasser S, Roberson JR. Deep venous thrombosis in total hip arthroplasty. Orthop Clin North Am 1992;23:359–364.
47. Leizorovicz A, Haugh MC, Chapuis FR, Samama MM, Boissel JP. Low molecular weight heparin in prevention of perioperative thrombosis. BMJ 1992;305:913–920.
48. Clagett GP, Anderson FA Jr, Heit J, Levine MN, Wheeler HB. Prevention of venous thromboembolism. Chest 1995;108:312S–334S.
49. Francis CW, Marder VJ, Evarts CM, Yaukoolbodi S. Two-step warfarin therapy. Prevention of postoperative venous thrombosis without excessive bleeding. JAMA 1983;249:374–378.
50. Mader VJ, Francis CW. Two-step warfarin therapy for the prophylaxis of venous thrombosis after elective surgery. Adv Exp Med Biol 1987; 214:159–163.
51. Collins R, Scrimgeour A, Yusuf S, Peto R. Reduction in fatal pulmonary embolism and venous thrombosis by perioperative administration of subcutaneous heparin. Overview of results of randomized trials in general, orthopedic, and urologic surgery. N Engl J Med 1988;318: 1162–1173.
52. Bergqvist D. Perioperative hemorrhagic complications in patients on low molecular weight heparins. Semin Thromb Hemost 1993;19(Suppl 1):128–130.
53. Hirsh J, Raschke R, Warkentin TE, Dalen JE, Deykin D, Poller L. Heparin: mechanism of action, pharmacokinetics, dosing considerations, monitoring, efficacy, and safety. Chest 1995;108:258S–275S.
54. Borris LC, Lassen MR. A comparative review of the adverse effect profiles of heparins and heparinoids. Drug Saf 1995;12:26–31.
55. Chong BH. Heparin-induced thrombocytopenia. Br J Haematol 1995; 89:431–439.
56. Magnani HN. Heparin-induced thrombocytopenia (HIT): an overview of 230 patients treated with orgaran (Org 10172). Thromb Haemost 1993;70:554–561.
57. Fauno P, Petersen KD, Husted SE. Increased blood loss after preoperative NSAID. Retrospective study of 186 hip arthroplasties. Acta Orthop Scand 1993;64:522–524.
58. Robinson CM, Christie J, Malcolm-Smith N. Nonsteroidal antiinflammatory drugs, perioperative blood loss, and transfusion requirements in elective hip arthroplasty. J Arthroplasty 1993;8:607–610.
59. An HS, Mikhail WE, Jackson WT, Tolin B, Dodd GA. Effects of hypotensive anesthesia, nonsteroidal antiinflammatory drugs, and polymethylmethacrylate on bleeding in total hip arthroplasty patients. J Arthroplasty 1991;6:245–250.
60. Clagett GP, Reisch JS. Prevention of venous thromboembolism in general surgical patients. Results of meta-analysis. Ann Surg 1988;208:227–240.
61. Wolf H. Experience with regional anesthesia in pateints receiving low molecular weight heparins. Semin Thromb Hemost 1993;19:152–154.
62. Vandermuelen EP, Van Aken H, Vermylen J. Anticoagulants and spinal-epidural anesthesia. Anesth Analg 1994;79:1165–1177.

Chapter 18

Surgical Management of Congenital Clotting Factor Deficiencies

ARTHUR R. THOMPSON

INTRODUCTION

Congenital bleeding disorders are sometimes readily apparent with a history of spontaneous bleeding episodes or of major bleeding evoked by minimal trauma. More often, however, they are sufficiently mild that their presence is difficult to recognize. Mild disorders in particular require a high level of suspicion and careful historical and laboratory screening strategies to recognize their presence and diagnose the specific defect. Regardless of their severity, however, a hallmark of congenital bleeding disorders is excessive intraoperative and especially postoperative bleeding in the absence of specific treatment.

Effective therapy requires correction of the defect, usually with a concentrated form of the deficient clotting factor. A variety of plasma-derived or recombinant factor concentrates are now available, and the optimal treatment is dictated by the risk of complications in addition to efficacy and cost. For surgical patients, a deficient factor level is best raised to the midnormal range with an infusion just before the procedure. Additional infusions are required to prevent rebleeding for 10–14 days. Prolonged therapy is necessary to prevent oozing until there is sufficient wound healing and collagen formation to prevent dehiscence. Understanding the kinetics of the various factors in vivo is necessary to predict both the dosage and frequency of infusions. It is essential to monitor the clinical response to verify that hemostatically effective levels have been achieved and maintained.

Several salient features of the surgical management of patients with congenital clotting factor deficiencies are outlined in Table 18.1. As mentioned above, most congenital bleeding tendencies are mild and may not be easily recognized. Personal and family histories should consider how various challenges to the patient's hemostatic mechanism have been met, including the extent to which it has been challenged. In general, a careful history is the most sensitive way to screen for mild disorders, but a negative history will be encountered in some patients, especially if they have only been exposed to limited trauma. The bleeding pattern is often that of prolonged oozing for several days or partial healing with rebleeding up to 2 weeks later. Tooth extractions are more likely to produce abnormal bleeding than are superficial cuts and injuries. Frequent epistaxis or prolonged menstrual bleeding may be useful, but these are less specific because abnormal bleeding is more frequently related to local or hormonal changes than to an underlying bleeding tendency. For any suspicious history, laboratory screening is necessary to identify the type of hemostatic defect present, and a diagnosis is made with specific factor assays.

In patients with hemophilia, spontaneous bleeding episodes usually indicate a severe bleeding tendency and are associated with a factor VIII or IX level of less than 1%. Those with a moderately severe or mild tendency will have prolonged bleeding after varying degrees of trauma and usually have levels of 1–5% and from greater than 5–30%, respectively; together these nonsevere types represent over half of the patients with hemophilia. The absence of a family history cannot exclude hemophilia, because it is isolated in about half of the families. Occasionally, women who are carriers will have such sufficiently low levels themselves (e.g., less than 30%) that they will have a mild bleeding tendency.

TABLE 18.1. MANAGING CONGENITAL CLOTTING FACTOR DISORDERS

Principle	Considerations, Rationale, or Comment
Consider mild defects	
Preoperative	History of response to prior trauma or surgery
Intraoperative	Amount of bleeding from "typical" lesions or surgical wounds
Establish correct diagnosis	Treatment differs in type, amount, and frequency
Exclude inhibitors (e.g., alloantibodies)	For hemophilia A, 2-hr incubated inhibitor screen necessary
Administer preoperative "loading" dose	Maximal level achieved immediately postadministration; half-lives vary
Maintain factor levels >30%, with repeat doses	Obtain post-op, then periodic "trough" levels (i.e., before A.M. dose)
Continue therapy until wound is collagen stabilized (~10 days)	Rebleeding as likely to occur 3–7 days post-op as immediately
Monitor clinical response to therapy	Oozing may be early sign of ↓ recovery and/or survival; noninhibiting alloantibodies occur

Alloantibodies occur in 10–30% of patients with severe hemophilia A and are found less frequently in patients with other factor deficiencies. Before elective surgery, it is prudent to screen known hemophilic patients to exclude inhibitors. Factor VIII inhibitors may not be present with the typical features of other inhibitors in that the partial thromboplastin time (PTT) may correct significantly after mixing equal volumes of patient and normal plasmas; to demonstrate the inhibition of the factor VIII in normal plasma, a 2-hour preincubation of the mixture (at 37°C) before the assay is often required. Some alloantibodies predominantly affect recovery and survival of infused factor and are not detected in inhibitor assays. Although this type is usually not high titer or boost responding, its presence will require larger and often more frequent doses to maintain surgical hemostasis.

In preparing a patient for surgery, the typical recoveries and half-lives of infused factors (Table 18.2) and the availability of concentrates need to be considered. When a concentrate is selected, a *loading dose* is administered immediately preoperatively. When available, and particularly after surgeries with significant blood loss and transfusions, a postoperative factor activity assay will both verify the predicted response and screen for excessive factor loss due to surgical bleeding. Follow-up doses are required to maintain *minimum* levels above those required for normal hemostasis, as shown in Figure 18.1. For most factors, this means a level that is greater than 30–40% of normal just before the next interval dose. The duration of *maintenance therapy* depends on the extent of surgical trauma. For a simple incision through muscle layers, there is a significant risk of wound hematomas for about 10 days; thus, 10 days of treatment is recommended for an uncomplicated cholecystectomy or hernia repair. Two weeks of replacement therapy are recommended for most major and orthopedic surgeries; additional infusions may be necessary for rehabilitation. At any time in the operative period or up to 2 weeks postoperatively, increased oozing can occur and usually indicates that the factor level is below the minimum necessary for hemostasis. An additional dose should be administered after a sample is drawn to confirm a suboptimal response.

COMPONENTS AND CLOTTING FACTOR CONCENTRATES

For nearly half a century, blood centers have had plasma available. Type-specific, fresh-frozen plasma can provide clotting factors to congenitally deficient patients. A major difficulty with plasma transfusion, however, is the volume required. To even transiently reach a hemostatic level of factor VIII, for example, a minimum of 4–6 units or bags (1–1.5 L) of plasma would need to be infused. For a prolonged infusion, the 10-hour half-life of factor VIII would require frequent additional units, along with diuresis or partial plasma exchange to achieve and maintain hemostatic levels.

Clinical concentrates of the clotting factors were prepared on a small-scale in Europe some 30–35 years ago, but large-scale preparations were not available until the advent of the cryoprecipitation technique developed by Pool and Shannon (1). By 1970, commercial manufacturers of factor VIII and factor IX produced a variety of lyophilized products that were derived from large pools of paid donors. Thus, in the United States, factor VIII and IX concentrates have been widely available to hemophilic patients for about 25 years.

The types of concentrate preparations have undergone several changes in the past three decades (2). Initially, simple precipitation and large-scale fractionation techniques for

TABLE 18.2. PROPERTIES OF CLOTTING FACTORS

Factor	Size (mol wt)	Plasma Level µg/mL	Plasma Level Molality	Plasma Level Minimum[a] (%)	Intravascular Recovery (%)	Posttransfusion Half-life (hr)
Cofactors; stabilizer						
Factor VIII	300,000	0.1	0.3 nM	30	80–100	10
Factor V	350,000	0.2	0.5 nM	15–20	80–100	12
vWF monomer[b]	240,000	10	35 nM	40	80–100	~72
Vitamin K-dependent zymogens						
Factor IX	55,000	5	90 nM	25–30	30–50	20
Factor VII	50,000	0.5	10 nM	10	30–50	6
Factor X	55,000	10	180 nM	15–20	30–50	50
Prothrombin	70,000	100	1.5 µM	~40	50–60	60
Other, multimeric factors						
Factor XI (dimer)	160,000	6	40 nM	~30	80–100	50–60
Fibrinogen $(A\alpha,B\beta,\delta)_2$	340,000	3000	9 µM	25–30	80–100	75
Factor XIII (A_2B_2)	320,000	20	60 nM	5	80–100	250

Values are approximate.

[a]Minimum levels for hemostasis reflect lowest or "trough" levels at or below which abnormal surgical bleeding is likely to occur.

[b]vWF circulates as 800,000 to 12×10^6 mol wt multimers; only the highest mol wt multimers function in platelet adhesion.

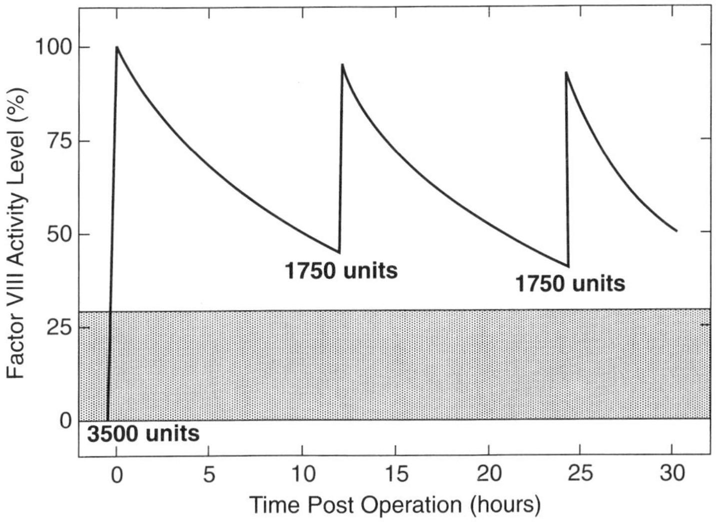

Figure 18.1. Response to intermittent bolus factor VIII infusions in severe hemophilia A. Theoretically, a 70-kg severe hemophilia A patient has a plasma volume of 2800 mL (40 mL/kg × 70 kg). A preoperative dose of 3500 factor VIII units (50 units/kg) should raise the level acutely to 100%, assuming an 80% recovery (0.8 × 3500 units = 2800 units in 2800 mL plasma or 1 unit/mL; 100%). Survival is calculated for a 10-hour half-life, and the level should be 45% at 12 hours just before the first postoperative dose and 42% before the next dose. Infusions of half the initial dose (1750 units in this example) every 12 hours will ensure that the minimum level remains above the minimum for normal hemostasis (above the shaded area, greater than 30%). Thus, the risk of bleeding should be no greater than that of a non-hemophilic patient. In practice, it is advisable to first examine the patient's plasma before surgery to exclude detectable inhibitors. Second, a factor activity level drawn postoperatively allows one to verify the expected response, excluding either a low initial recovery of the factor or significant dilution from intraoperative blood loss and fluid replacement. Subsequent factor assays are most informative if drawn just before a dose; one drawn the morning of the first postoperative day will exclude shortened survival. Doses are adjusted accordingly. As an alternative to intermittent bolus infusions, continuous infusion can be begun after the initial bolus (10). Overall, continuous infusions result in less total factor infused but require an accurate delivery system and more frequent monitoring.

factor VIII or factor IX were used. More sophisticated chromatographic purifications were introduced providing concentrates of greater purity; in particular, immunoaffinity chromatography has been used to prepare some of the highest purity concentrates available. In the last few years, recombinant technology has begun to provide materials that are not plasma-derived and as such should be free of human viral contamination.

Since the introduction of component therapy and concentrate use, it has been appreciated that plasma-derived products, even from small pools of volunteer donors, carried a high risk of transfusion-transmitted hepatitis, namely hepatitis B and C virus infections. From 1979 until 1985, there was also a major risk of contamination with human immunodeficiency virus (HIV), especially in concentrates made from large numbers of donors. During 1984, it was appreciated that heating the lyophilized concentrates to 68°C for 72 hours (but not 60°C) was an effective means of inactivating HIV. This, along with donor screening for HIV antibodies introduced in the early part of 1985, has virtually eliminated the risk of HIV viral transmission and (more recently) hepatitis B and C infections from concentrates given to hemophilic patients. Products and their viral inactivation methods are summarized in Table 18.3.

In a technique developed at the New York Blood Center, it was found that treatment of plasma before its fractionation with a solvent and detergent inactivated HIV and also hepatitis B and C viruses (3). Several manufacturers have incorporated this process into their purification or plasma fractionation schemes. For lyophilized concentrates, 68°C heating for 72 hours kills HIV but not hepatitis viruses. Dry heating to 80°C for 72 hours is necessary to inactivate hepatitis B and C viruses. Factor VIII is largely inactivated at the higher temperature. Therefore, this procedure is only useful in concentrates of vitamin K-dependent or other more stable factors. To kill HIV and hepatitis B and C viruses with wet heat treatment, the only effective procedures are pasteurization or a two-stage vapor heat treatment, the latter developed by Immuno in Austria. Because the solvent-detergent method and dry or wet heating treatments are most effective against lipid-envelope viruses, it is known that they do not inactivate hepatitis A or parvovirus B19 (4). Hepatitis A has been found in a limited number of lots of factor VIII manufactured in Europe. It should be assumed that parvovirus is present in virtually all plasma-derived concentrates; fortunately, it is rarely pathogenic. Overall, the viral safety of concentrates has improved tremendously in the past decade (5).

Isohemagglutinins are present in cryoprecipitate and intermediate purity concentrates, but amounts infused are low unless the cryoprecipitate is dissolved in donor plasma instead of saline or a donor has an inordinately high titer of anti-A, for example. Clinically significant hemolysis is quite uncommon and is usually seen when large doses are given, as with attempts to overwhelm a low level inhibitor. The various factor concentrates in clinical use as discussed are presented in Table 18.3.

FACTOR VIII CONCENTRATES

Cryoprecipitate

A relatively simple closed-bag system is used by local blood centers to prepare cryoprecipitate. The plasma is rapidly frozen and then thawed at 4°C. Under optimal conditions, about two-thirds of the factor VIII and von Willebrand factor (vWF) and one-third of the fibrinogen remain insoluble at 2–4°C, whereas most other plasma proteins are dissolved. The precipitate is then centrifuged and the cryo-poor plasma removed. Cryoprecipitate can be frozen at −20°C for at least 1 year. Before use, it is thawed in a small volume of normal saline (or plasma) providing six- to eightfold concentrations of factor VIII over those in plasma. To reduce donor exposure, some centers have also prepared single-donor cryoprecipitate. For example, a relative of a young hemophilia A patient (who has a normal factor VIII level) can receive desmopressin (DDAVP) to raise the circulating level of factor VIII and be plasmapheresed, removing 2–3 L of plasma (receiving his or her own cryo-poor plasma from a previous donation). The equivalent of 20–30 bags of cryoprecipitate can be made from a single individual, thus limiting the donor exposure of a young hemophilic patient.

Intermediate Purity Factor VIII Concentrates

Factor VIII prepared by precipitation methods has specific activities from 2 to 5 units/mg protein; at least one preparation contains a significant amount of functional vWF (active high-molecular-weight multimers) (6). Chromatographically purified factor VIII concentrates are of variably greater purity (15–150 units/mg) and do not contain functional vWF.

High Purity Concentrates

The highest level of purity of factor VIII is from immunoaffinity chromatography. This procedure uses adsorption to and elution from insolubilized, monoclonal antibodies with epitopes for either vWF or factor VIII. The eluted factor VIII is highly purified (2000–3000 units/mg) but is quite unstable in solution unless a high concentration of pasteurized human albumin is added (final "specific activity" is approximately 10 units/mg protein). Upon infusion, factor VIII is stabilized by binding to the recipient's vWF. Immunoaffinity purified concentrates contain trace amounts of murine monoclonal antibody, but this contaminant has not been associated with adverse reactions.

TABLE 18.3. CURRENTLY AVAILABLE COMPONENTS AND FACTOR CONCENTRATES

Concentrate (Manufacturer)	Virucidal Treatment	Purification or Comment
Factor VIII		
Low purity		
Cryoprecipitate	None	Random or single, volunteer donor; also contains vWF and fibrinogen
Intermediate purity		
Koate-HP (Bayer/Miles)	Solvent-detergent[a]	Chromatographic purification
Alphanate (Alpha)	Solvent-detergent[a]	
Humate-P (Behring/Armour)	Pasteurized	Glycine/salt precipitation; contains functional vWF
High purity		
Monoclate-P (Armour/Rhone)	Pasteurized	Immunoaffinity purification; >98% albumin (pasteurized) added to stabilize
Hemophil-M (Baxter/Hyland)	Solvent-detergent[a]	
Method M (ARC/Baxter)	Solvent-detergent[b]	
Recombinant		
Kogenate (Bayer/Miles)	None	Free of known pathogenic human viruses; immunoaffinity purification; >98% albumin (pasteurized) added to stabilize
Helixate (Armour by Bayer)	None	
Recombinate (Baxter/Hyland)	None	
Bioclate (Armour, by Baxter)	None	
Porcine		
Hyate-C (Speywood/Porton)	None	For hemophilia A inhibitor patients; polyelectrolyte fractionation
Factor IX		
Low purity		DEAE fractionation; risk of thrombosis present; contain factors IX, X, and prothrombin
Konyne-80 (Bayer/Miles)	80°C, 72hr (dry)	
Bebulin (Immuno, Vienna)	Vapor heat	
High purity		Low risk of thrombosis;
Alphanine-SD (Alpha)	Solvent-detergent[a]	Chromatographic purification
Mononine (Armour/Rhone)	Thiocyanate and ultrafiltration	Immunoaffinity purification
Activated		"Controlled" activation, no thrombin;
Autoplex (Baxter/Hyland)	60°C, 6d[b] (dry)	Calcium phosphate fractionation
FEIBA-VH (Immuno AG)	Vapor heat	DEAE fractionation
Other and experimental preparations		
Fresh-frozen plasma (New York Blood Center)	Solvent-detergent[a]	Volunteer donor pool; type-specific
Recombinant factor IX (Genetics Institute, Boston)	None	Affinity purification (no albumin); clinical trials begun, 1995
Factor XI (Bioproducts, UK)	80°C, 72hr (dry)	Chromatography; ? thrombogenic (UK contains antithrombin III)
(Biotransfusion, Lille, FR)	Solvent-detergent[a]	
Factor XIII (Behring AG)	Pasteurized	Salt extraction
(Bioproducts, Elstree, UK)	Pasteurized	EtOH & citrate extractions; + albumin
vWF (Biotransfusion/ARC)	Solvent-detergent[a]	Low factor VIII
Factor VII (Immuno AG; Bioproducts; Biotransfusion)	Vapor heat; 80°C, 72hr; solvent detergent	DEAE-Sephadex fractionation; relatively short half-life
Recombinant Factor VIIa (Novo Nordisk, Copenhagen)	None	Immunoaffinity purification; used in hemophilic inhibitor patients

ARC, American Red Cross; aa, amino acid.

[a]Solvent (*t*-*N*-butyl phosphate) and Detergent (Tween-80, polysorbate, or Triton X-100, octoxynol) treatment of pooled plasma before purification.

[b]Does not necessarily inactivate hepatitis B or C viruses.

Recombinant Factor VIII

Two concentrates were licensed by the U.S. Food and Drug Administration (FDA) by early 1993. A major advantage is their low risk of viral contamination. After immunoaffinity purification, they require albumin for stabilization. The albumin is plasma-derived and pasteurized. As the recombinant factor VIII is made in nonhuman, mammalian cells that have been transfected with the cDNA for factor VIII, the synthesized protein has minor differences (e.g., in carbohydrate sequences) compared with plasma-derived factor VIII (i.e., that synthesized by a human liver). Although a rather high incidence of inhibitor formation in previously untransfused patients has been observed (up to about 30%), it is not yet clear whether this is due to any conformational differences within the recombinant factor VIII protein or to more thorough screening for inhibitor development. Most inhibitors observed are low titer and are often transient.

Porcine Factor VIII

Crude preparations of porcine or bovine factor VIII were studied in the United Kingdom over 30 years ago but were found to induce profound thrombocytopenia. By introducing polyelectrolyte fractionation to the porcine preparation, an intermediate purity concentrate results that minimizes this side effect; mild thrombocytopenia is still occasionally observed. The major indication for porcine factor VIII is in hemophilic patients that develop high-titer inhibitors (alloantibodies) to factor VIII or, as more frequently effective, in acquired hemophilia (autoantibodies). The inhibitor's titer against the porcine protein is often much lower than it is to human factor VIII such that hemostasis can be achieved, at least transiently, with the porcine preparation. Experimentally, recombinant hybrid factor VIII proteins are being prepared because one may need to have only two of factor VIII's six domains with the porcine sequence to avoid inactivation by most human allo- or auto-anti-factor VIII inhibitors.

FACTOR IX CONCENTRATES

Low Purity Factor IX Concentrates

When plasma is adsorbed by positively charged insoluble salts or resins, the vitamin K-dependent proteins in particular require high salt concentrations for elution. This interaction is largely dependent on intact gamma-carboxyglutamyl (Gla) domains that are strongly negatively charged. Early concentrates were often referred to as "prothrombin complex concentrates" because they contained factor IX, prothrombin, factor X, and varying degrees of factor VII. When tricalcium phosphate was used, for example, the yield of factor VII was reasonable; use of DEAE-Sephadex or Sepharose beads, however, resulted in low factor VII recovery. There is no evidence that these different factors associate with one another or form a "complex," however.

Between 1979 and 1985, the risks of HIV transmission from products derived from large pools of paid donor plasma were high, but it was somewhat less (i.e., 40–50%) in hemophilia B patients than in hemophilia A patients receiving commercial factor VIII concentrates (80–90%). The risk of transmitting hepatitis B and C viruses has been high since the concentrates were first released. Within the last few years, known pathogenic viruses have been eliminated from factor IX concentrates. This has been accomplished by more careful donor selection and screening and treatment with higher temperatures (either dry or vapor heated) or with solvent-detergent treatment. However, as with factor VIII, factor IX concentrates may not be totally free of plasma-derived viruses.

Soon after the factor IX concentrates were introduced, it was noted that the low purity concentrates had a definite risk of venous or arterial thrombosis and, occasionally, disseminated intravascular coagulation. Since improvements in the manufacturing procedures by the late 1970s, the thrombotic risk has largely been confined to patients with liver disease or those receiving large (e.g., 75 factor IX units/kg) or repetitive doses, the latter as required for surgical patients.

Purified Factor IX Concentrates

Factor IX can be more highly purified by large-scale chromatographic or immunoaffinity procedures. Purification reduces the thrombotic risk considerably. Infusion of very large doses (up to 200 units/kg) into animal models or of therapeutic doses (e.g., 50 units/kg) into hemophilia B patients results in a marked reduction of biochemical markers of thrombosis such as the prothrombin fragment 1.2 (2, 7).

Recombinant Factor IX

A "synthetic" factor IX began clinical trials in 1995 (8). It is chromatographically purified from conditioned media. Compared with factor VIII, factor IX is quite stable after isolation so there is no requirement for addition of albumin to high purity preparations.

Activated Factor IX Concentrates

Two preparations are available, but only the vapor-heated process is sufficient to inactivate hepatitis viruses. Partial activation of clotting proteases (without thrombin generation) renders the low purity concentrates more thrombogenic, and they have been used in attempts to "bypass" inhibitors. High doses (50–75 units/kg) of the routine low purity factor IX products are also used in attempts to promote hemostasis during bleeding episodes in patients with inhibitors.

OTHER FACTOR PREPARATIONS

Fresh-Frozen Plasma

Plasma is routinely prepared by blood centers as single units (about 250 ml per bag) from volunteer donors and the average content is 1 unit/ml of each clotting factor. Type-specific single donor pheresed plasma can be used for some patients to limit donor exposure; this is most useful for factors with high intravascular recoveries and long half-lives such as factor XI or XIII. A preparation from a limited pool of volunteer donor plasma that has been solvent-detergent treated (3) is in clinical trials in congenitally deficient patients and may have a broader role in acquired deficiency states.

von Willebrand Factor Concentrates

For functional vWF, cryoprecipitate has been the primary concentrate available for many years. Salt-fractionated, low purity factor VIII concentrates retain variable quantities of functional vWF (high-molecular-weight multimers) and are treated to inactivate viruses. Of the products available, the largest experience has been with a pasteurized product, Humate-P, which is effective (6). In addition, a concentrate has been developed in France by a process that optimizes recovery of functional vWF; it is currently in clinical trials in the United States, sponsored by the American Red Cross. The French product may be more uniform in supporting platelet adhesion, although it has little factor VIII. Thus, in a severely affected von Willebrand disease patient, a "priming" dose is given several hours before surgery to achieve normal factor VIII levels; alternatively, a factor VIII concentrate can be administered acutely with the initial vWF dose.

Factor VII Concentrates

Preparations of factor VII are made from DEAE-adsorbed plasma proteins because this factor elutes more readily (at lower salt concentrations) than factors IX and X and prothrombin. Three products have been used in Europe for patients with congenital deficiencies and, on a compassionate use basis, in the United States. Each manufacturer uses a different viral-inactivation step. Half-lives after infusion have, in general, been short (3–4 hours). This could be explained if partial activation had occurred, giving an apparent clotting activity level that is higher than the amount of factor VII protein present.

Recombinant Factor VIIa

When recombinant factor VII is purified from conditioned media, near quantitative activation occurs during immunoaffinity chromatography. This is presumably due to cleavage by low levels of contaminant proteases in the insolubilized murine antibody preparation. In high doses and at frequent intervals, factor VIIa has achieved hemostasis in most patients with high-titer factor VIII or IX inhibitors, even during and after major surgery. The half-life is at least several minutes, and patient prothrombin times are fast, being shortened below the normal range.

Factor XI Concentrates

Two preparations are manufactured in Europe and each is partially purified by adsorption of cryoprecipitate and chromatography. When heparin-sepharose is used for the chromatography, significant amounts of antithrombin III are copurified. Viral inactivation varies with the preferred method of the manufacturer. Factor XI concentrates have been widely used in Europe, but there are occasional reports of thrombotic episodes in susceptible patients that are temporally associated with the infusion. The degree of thrombogenicity and its clinical significance, however, remain to be established.

Factor XIII Concentrates

There are two pasteurized concentrates available in Europe. Both are prepared from normal plasma. After ethanol precipitation, factor XIII is sodium citrate-extracted, heated, concentrated, and lyophilized.

CONGENITAL CLOTTING FACTOR DISORDERS

The different types of clotting factor deficiencies were distinguished from each other as the ability of the plasma from one patient to correct the prolonged clotting time of another. Inasmuch as the physical and chemical properties of these factors differ, different concentrates are required as indicated in Table 18.4. It also follows from the differences in the minimum levels necessary for hemostasis and infusion kinetics of the clotting factors (Table 18.2) that the frequency and size of doses necessary to maintain levels above the minimum level for hemostasis will vary. Hemophilias A and B are relatively frequent and in the more severe forms more likely to require surgical intervention for chronic complications such as hemophilic arthropathy. Milder disorders, including the common type of von Willebrand disease, are important to recognize because, untreated, they will lead to excessive surgical and postoperative morbidity from bleeding.

HEMOPHILIA A

Classical hemophilia A accounts for 75–80% of hemophilic patients and is due to an X-linked deficient factor VIII clotting activity. About 1 in every 10,000 males is affected. One-third of the patients have a severe bleeding dis-

TABLE 18.4. CONGENITAL CLOTTING FACTOR DISORDERS

Disorder	Therapy for Surgical Procedures
Hemophilia A	Factor VIII concentrate (plasma derived or recombinant)
Mild (>10–20%)	Factor VIII concentrate (+/− DDAVP[a] supplemented)
Inhibitor	Porcine factor VIII; recombinant factor VIIa+
Hemophilia B	High purity factor IX concentrate
von Willebrand Disease	Some factor VIII concentrates (e.g., Humate-P), cryoprecipitate, or vWF concentrate[b]
Mild, type 1	DDAVP
Other disorders	
Factor V deficiency	Plasma[c] (platelets)
Factor X deficiency	Low purity factor IX concentrate
Factors VII, XI, or XIII deficiencies	Plasma[c]; concentrate[b]
Afibrinogenemia	Cryoprecipitate (volunteer or single donor)

[a]DDAVP can be substituted for some postoperative doses in mild hemophilia A patients or used exclusively before dental extraction (with a postextraction course of an oral fibrinolytic inhibitor in the latter), or used in mild responsive von Willebrand disease patients.

[b]Investigational preparations with limited availability in United States.

[c]ABO type-specific plasma from either volunteer or "single" donors or a solvent-detergent treated pool.

order. This is recognized by frequent spontaneous bleeding episodes and a clotting activity that is less than 1% of that in a plasma pool from normal donors. Moderately severe and mild bleeding tendencies require increasing amounts of trauma to be manifest as prolonged bleeding episodes or poor wound healing; these types are somewhat arbitrarily divided into patients with factor VIII clotting activity levels from 1–5% and greater than 5–30%, respectively. The clinical phenotype is generally the same among different patients within a family. However, hemophilia is "sporadic" in up to half of the families such that there is often no family history. Some women who are carriers will have sufficiently low levels to be symptomatic. Individuals with baseline levels above 30% usually have normal hemostatic responses to trauma or surgery. Levels can be elevated with strenuous exercise, acute stress, chronic inflammation, or estrogen effects.

Infusion Kinetics

Because of its high molecular weight, infused factor VIII is essentially all recovered in the intravascular or plasma compartment. Half-lives average about 10 hours and are essentially the same for all factor VIII products. Once infused, the hemophilic patient's own circulating vWF binds factor VIII to provide the same degree of stability as seen in normal persons. If recovery and survival are diminished, alloantibodies should be suspected.

Replacement Therapy for Surgery

Factor VIII concentrates are indicated to control or prevent abnormal bleeding in hemophilia A patients (9). For surgery, a dose is administered just before the operation to raise the patient's level to 80–100%. This requires around 50 factor VIII units/kg or about 3500 units for a 70-kg patient. Alternatively, one can calculate the dose required recognizing that 1 unit of factor VIII per kg will increase the plasma level about 2%. For procedures with large amounts of surgical blood loss, it may be necessary to add a supplementary dose. After major surgical procedures, a recovery room sample for factor VIII activity will determine whether or not the expected recovery and initial survival are as predicted. Otherwise, about half of the original dose (e.g., 25 units/kg) is infused every 12 hours to maintain a level that before the next dose will sustain normal hemostasis (i.e., above 40%) (Fig. 18.1). Some centers switch to continuous infusion postoperatively, monitoring factor VIII activity levels daily (10); continuous infusions can minimize the total postoperative dose. Although most concentrates do not have FDA approval for prolonged storage at room temperature after reconstitution, it appears that several factor VIII preparations are sufficiently stable in solution to allow an 8- to 12-hour dose for infusion. For bolus infusions every 12 hours, monitoring assays on samples drawn just before a morning dose are usually performed less frequently, with doses adjusted accordingly.

The *duration* of treatment is dependent on the extent of surgical trauma. Minor procedures such as percutaneous biopsies have been successfully managed with 3–5 days of therapy. For most "routine" surgeries, however, wound hematomas and poor healing can occur up to 10 days postoperatively, and major operations will require 14 days of full replacement therapy. For physical therapy after orthopedic procedures, additional doses are often necessary to prevent bleeding, and a single daily dose (just before the most vigorous therapy session) will usually be sufficient.

Mild Hemophilia A

Patients with mild hemophilia may be unaware of their bleeding tendency until they have been challenged by major trauma or surgery. Nevertheless, their requirement for postoperative replacement therapy is nearly the same as with more severe forms, especially for the duration of factor VIII coverage. Delayed bleeding or wound hematomas are likely to occur if therapy is stopped early (e.g., before about 10 days for a laparotomy).

When a patient's baseline factor VIII level is above 10%, and especially when it is 20–30%, DDAVP (11) will often raise the level sufficiently to achieve hemostasis. DDAVP appears to act by releasing endogenous "stores," doubling or tripling the baseline circulating factor VIII level. The best explanation of this effect is that endothelial-bound vWF-factor VIII complexes are released; a similar change is observed with epinephrine. The half-life of released factor VIII is the same as that of infused factor VIII, about 10 hours. Patients are refractory to additional doses for 24–48 hours; tachyphylaxis is sometimes observed. Because most surgical procedures require prolonged elevation of factor VIII above the minimum level for hemostasis, concentrate infusions are needed; for mild hemophilia, some postoperative doses can be supplemented with DDAVP. An exception to concentrate use in DDAVP-responsive patients is oral surgery. Before tooth extractions, a single dose of DDAVP is usually sufficient, provided a fibrinolytic inhibitor is given orally for 7–10 days. Doses of DDAVP are 0.3 μg/kg as a 15- to 20-min infusion in saline. Alternatively, a nasal formulation may be substituted, but only if the patient has previously been shown to have an excellent response to this form. Although more convenient for home therapy, the nasal spray often gives lower responses than intravenous administration and is more expensive unless frequent use is anticipated. Should rebleeding from the socket occur, it is usually 3–5 days later such that a repeat dose of DDAVP will usually suffice. Two fibrinolytic inhibitors are available and begun orally postextraction. Epsilon-aminocaproic acid (Amicar) is given every 6 hours as 40–50 mg/kg (3 g per dose in a 70-kg person); tranexamic acid (Cyklokapron) is given every 8 hours in a 25-mg/kg dose.

Hemophilic Patients with Inhibitors

Alloantibodies to factor VIII occur in up to 30% of severe hemophilia A patients. They may be low level and even noninhibitory; in these patients, larger more frequent doses of factor VIII concentrate provide normal hemostasis. Low-titer alloantibodies are occasionally seen in patients with moderately severe hemophilia.

Some 5–10% of patients with severe hemophilia A develop high-titer, boost responding inhibitors that preclude effective therapy with infusions of human factor VIII concentrates. For these patients, a simple bleeding episode may extend into a potential surgical emergency. For example, a deep muscle hematoma may continue to ooze and present with symptoms of an impending compartment syndrome. Unless hemostasis can be achieved, however, surgical intervention will only lead to major external bleeding. If hemostasis can be achieved, then surgery may not be necessary. Thus, it is important to evaluate the remaining therapeutic options, namely to attempt to lower the titer, to acutely "overwhelm" the inhibitor, or to "bypass" it with activated factors (12).

Hemophilic alloantibodies are usually resistant to common immunosuppressive agents such as prednisone or cyclophosphamide. Adjunctive use of intravenous immunoglobulin or plasmapheresis in an acute setting has only occasionally been helpful. About 75% of high titer inhibitors (especially in children) will respond to daily factor VIII infusions, and in 3–6 months the inhibitor is either undetectable or the titer is sufficiently low (e.g., less than 5 Bethesda units/mL) that patients respond to large doses of factor VIII concentrates. Alternatively, porcine factor VIII can be considered (13). The cross-reactivity of most alloantibodies with factor VIII from other species is often only about one-tenth the titer, allowing hemostasis to be achieved with lower doses of factor VIII. Some patients with inhibitors tolerate repeated doses of porcine factor VIII and even use it for home therapy. For really high titer inhibitors, however, a boost response usually occurs within a few days. The titer against porcine and human factor VIII soars, precluding effective therapy. In some patients, the subsequent alloantibodies shift in their epitope specificity, indicating a direct response to porcine factor VIII epitopes. Surgical hemostasis in this setting can only be achieved for a few days and the initial bleeding is then complicated by bleeding into the site of the surgical wound.

The third option is to promote hemostasis by infusing activated factors. Low purity factor IX concentrates contain variable amounts of procoagulants and high doses (e.g., about 75 units/kg) stop or slow bleeding about half the time. Similar results are seen with activated factor IX concentrates and doses have been repeated up to every 6–8 hours. There is a risk of thrombosis at other sites, however, as seen with repeated doses of low purity factor IX concentrates in hemophilia B patients without inhibitors. In the last few years, a recombinant factor VIIa preparation has been available on a compassionate use basis, and FDA licensure is pending. When high doses are administered frequently (every 2–4 hours), hemostasis is usually achieved in these patients (14); therapy has usually been maintained for at least 3 weeks. Even several elective surgeries have been supported with recombinant factor VIIa. Fortunately, although experience has been limited, major thrombotic complications have not been encountered. This is presumably because factor VIIa requires tissue factor for extrinsic clotting activation and tissue factor is found predominantly at sites of tissue injury or wounds.

Surgery in HIV-Positive Hemophilic Patients

Immunosuppression is usually considered a risk factor for postoperative infections. In a retrospective study of 83 hemophilic patients undergoing 169 procedures, however, Buehrer et al. (15) found no differences in infection rates in those that were HIV positive from those known to be HIV negative subsequent to the surgery. The lack of difference held for operations on contaminated as well as "clean" sites; the only wound infections occurred in one HIV-positive patient and a second who tested positively on subsequent screening. Most patients were asymptomatic, although 24 procedures were performed on HIV-positive patients when their CD4 lymphocyte counts were below 200. There does not appear to be any undue risk of postoperative infectious complications. The potential benefits of elective surgeries, including joint replacement, should take into account both the patient's history of infectious acquired immunodeficiency syndrome (AIDS) complications and the fact that several infected hemophilic patients are long-term survivors. In HIV-positive patients, platelet counts should be obtained because thrombocytopenia is a frequent complication of the infection or therapy; management is as discussed in Chapter 5.

A second issue among HIV-positive hemophilia A patients is the choice of concentrates. During clinical trials, there was suggestive evidence that highly purified factor VIII concentrates were associated with a slower rate of progression of CD4 lymphocyte decline than that seen in patients treated with intermediate purity concentrates. In a small randomized trial of heavily transfused patients, Seremetis et al. (16) found essentially no decline among 20 patients (of 30 entered) treated with a monoclonal-purified product compared with 15 (of 30 entered) treated with various intermediate purity concentrates with a 3-year follow-up. An intermediate rate of decline was found in a similar number of patients receiving recombinant factor VIII (17). In contrast, prospectively collected data from the Transfusion Safety Study showed no difference in progression of falling CD4 counts in hemophilic patients given intermediate purity concentrates when the amount of treatment (varying from none to heavy) per time interval was considered (18). Furthermore, Goedert et al. (19) found no significant correlation between the CD4 count and progression to clinically significant AIDS or death among hemophilic patients. The issue of a potential benefit of high purity concentrates in asymptomatic HIV-infected hemophilia A patients remains unresolved at this point.

HEMOPHILIA B

Factor IX deficiency is X-linked and clinically indistinguishable from hemophilia A, although hemophilia B is about one-fifth as prevalent. Both types have a similar range of severities and are due to a variety of mutations. Alloantibody inhibitors occur less frequently in severely affected hemophilia B patients than in those with hemophilia A. When they occur, their management is similar to that of factor VIII inhibitors discussed above. For most hemophilia B patients, factor IX concentrates are needed for hemostasis (7).

Infusion Kinetics

Factor IX is somewhat smaller than albumin; thus, it is distributed in the intra- and extravascular spaces. The intravascular recovery is 30–50% after infusion, and disappearance rates fit a two-compartment open model. The average second or beta-phase of disappearance is 20–24 hours. There is no evidence that different types of concentrates have any differences in infusion kinetics.

Concentrate Purity Versus Thrombogenicity

When low purity factor IX concentrates are given in large or frequent (including daily) doses, there is a high risk of a thrombotic complication. Until purified concentrates were released in 1990, the only alternative was to supplement with plasma. Particularly in very mild hemophilia B, one could achieve surgical hemostasis. However, diuretics and occasional partial plasma exchange were usually needed. Animal studies and surgical experience to date strongly argue that this complication is considerably reduced if not eliminated by further purification of factor IX using either chromatographic or immunoaffinity procedures. Clinical trials of a high-purity recombinant factor IX preparation are underway and the preparation appears safe and effective (8).

Replacement Therapy for Surgery

With low purity concentrates, it is essential to use only the minimal amount of factor IX concentrates needed to achieve hemostasis. Even then, there is a significant issue of safety. Now that high purity concentrates are available, it appears safe to raise the immediate preoperative level to 80–100 instead of 50%. This is accomplished by infusing about 70–80 units/kg, or about 5000 factor IX units into a 70-kg patient. An alternative calculation assumes a 50% recovery and is that 1 unit factor IX/kg will raise the plasma factor IX level about 1%. As with hemophilia A, a recovery room sample for factor IX clotting activity will allow adjustments for unanticipated shortened survival or excessive intraoperative loss. Subsequent doses are usually about half of the initial dose and given every 12 hours. After a few days, therapeutic levels can usually be maintained with somewhat higher daily doses. Continuous infusion might be an alternative providing there is no significant activation occurring during prolonged storage at room temperature; stability of factor IX under these conditions should be less of a concern than with factor VIII.

VON WILLEBRAND DISEASE

von Willebrand disease is the most common inherited bleeding disorder. It is usually associated with a clinically mild bleeding tendency (20). Typically, there is autosomal dominant inheritance, and the two major functions of vWF, namely to support adhesion of platelet glycoprotein Ib to the subendothelium and to stabilize factor VIII, are both mildly reduced. The platelet dysfunction is manifest as a prolonged template bleeding time and, in vitro, by an abnormal ristocetin cofactor assay. The concentration of vWF antigen present is assessed by immunoassays. In the common type, type 1, both antigen and functional assays are comparably reduced. The circulating factor VIII is likewise mildly below normal such that the PTT is mildly prolonged. The diagnosis may be confounded, however, by acquired effects that can stimulate vWF and factor VIII levels masking the deficiency. Moreover, many individuals with low in vitro levels actually have asymptomatic variants, and their bleeding tendencies are only manifest when they are homozygous, compound heterozygous, or inherit or acquire a second hemostatic defect. Parents that are carriers of severe, recessive type 3 von Willebrand disease are often asymptomatic. Type 3 patients are rarely encountered and have very low to undetectable levels of vWF, markedly prolonged bleeding times, and factor VIII clotting activities that are less than 5%.

Several variants of von Willebrand disease have been identified and most of them have dysfunctional vWF present. In such type 2 patients, the circulating level of vWF antigen is normal or near normal, whereas the ristocetin cofactor activity is reduced and the bleeding time is prolonged. In most of these type 2 patients, there is alteration of the multimeric pattern of vWF (as observed on large-pore gel electrophoresis) with reduction of the high-molecular-weight forms that are most active in supporting platelet adhesion. Factor VIII binding and activity may be relatively spared. However, in another variant type, the mutation selectively interferes with factor VIII binding. In patients with this "Normandy" variant, platelet function is normal but the factor VIII activity is low, creating an autosomally inherited hemophilic disorder. The variability and complexity of inheritance of clinical phenotypes are important to recognize as they influence therapeutic options.

Infusion Kinetics

vWF circulates as a large series of multimers with molecular weights from the 440,000 dimer to 20 million. Recovery approaches 100%, although proteolysis of the largest multimers can occur, decreasing the specific activity in terms of platelet adhesion. The half-life is variably reported depending on which assay is followed. After infusion of vWF into patients with severe type 3 disorders, the platelet function abnormality is only transiently corrected over the first 4–6 hours. This suggests that survival of the largest multimers is transient. Factor VIII, however, remains elevated for up to 48 hours, indicating sufficient residual vWF protein for stabilization of the patient's endogenous protein.

Therapy for Surgery

For patients with mild (type 1) deficiencies, it is useful to have demonstrated before surgery the degree to which they respond to DDAVP. For major surgical procedures, the drug (0.3 μg/kg in saline) is administered intravenously within 1 hour of the operation. Some centers recommend follow-up doses at 12 and 24 hours postoperatively daily through the third to fifth postoperative day and then every 48 hours or at any sign of increasing pain or bleeding. Tachyphylaxis is less common than with mild hemophilia A but can occur; less frequent postoperative dosing may also be effective (6, 20). DDAVP is contraindicated in children under 2 years old because hyponatremia occurs, especially after repeated dosing. Mild, transient flushing or hypertension is a common side effect. A few patients have experienced acute myocardial infarctions during or shortly after the infusion (11) such that arteriosclerotic coronary disease should be considered a relative contraindication. Replacement therapy with concentrated vWF should be considered for any operative or postoperative bleeding that does not respond to DDAVP.

Cryoprecipitate contains functional large vWF multimers that are six- to eightfold concentrated over plasma. Until recently, volunteer or single donor products have been the mainstay of therapy for DDAVP-unresponsive patients, including those that are moderately or severely affected and some with type 2 variants. Selected donors given DDAVP and then plasmapheresed can provide sufficient cryoprecipitated vWF for several treatment doses and limit donor exposure. Intermediate purity factor VIII preparations have variable amounts of high-molecular-weight multimers, and one product, Humate-P (Table 18.3), has been effective in treating bleeding episodes and providing surgical hemostasis. The recommended dose just before major surgeries is 30–40 equivalent factor VIII units/kg of Humate-P or cryoprecipitate. Half of the initial dose is administered in 12 and 24 hours to provide platelet function activity, and it is recommended to maintain every 12-hour dosing for 3 days and daily for an additional 3–5 days (6). Over 20 years of experience with highly functional cryoprecipitate preparations suggests that after the first postoperative day, less frequent therapy is required (Counts, Clements-Johnson, and Thompson, unpublished observations). Although the bleeding time correction may not be complete and lasts only 4–6 hours in type 3 patients, surgical wound healing correlates with maintaining the factor VIII level above 50%.

OTHER CONGENITAL PLATELET FUNCTION DISORDERS

Platelet membrane defects can lead to other types of platelet dysfunction (21). *Bernard-Soulier syndrome* is a rare recessive defect of the glycoprotein Ib/IX/V receptor of vWF. It mimics von Willebrand disease but is unresponsive to transfused vWF. *Glanzmann's thrombasthenia* is due to mutations in glycoprotein IIb/IIIa that impair platelet aggregation. For membrane defects, platelet transfusions are necessary to achieve hemostasis. Apheresis platelets are preferred because they will limit exposure to different donors and reduce the risk of alloimmunization.

Defects of *storage pools* in dense or alpha granules within platelets or of the release of granule contents (e.g., of ADP that recruits other platelets in aggregation) can lead to a mild bleeding tendency. The bleeding time is usually mildly prolonged (e.g., 10–15 min) but, in the clinical laboratory, the diagnosis is usually based on excluding acquired platelet dysfunction, a technical problem in performing the bleeding time test, or von Willebrand disease. Several of these patients have been shown to respond (nonspecifically) to intravenous DDAVP.

OTHER CONGENITAL CLOTTING FACTOR DISORDERS

Factor V Deficiency

Because of its role in prothrombin activation in the "common path" of clotting, low levels of factor V prolong both the prothrombin time and PTT. Congenital factor V deficiency is a rare autosomal recessive disorder that can be quite severe. Although factor V's infusion kinetics are similar to its homologous cofactor, factor VIII, the minimum level required for hemostasis is only about half that of factor VIII (Table 18.2). Thus, most bleeding episodes and even surgery can be managed with plasma replacement therapy, providing the patients have not developed alloantibody inhibitors. Solvent-detergent treated plasma is being studied as a means to protect against exposure to lipid enveloped viruses, but allergic reactions might be more frequent to patients receiving plasma repeatedly from donor pools compared with single donors. There is no factor V concentrate available, although platelets are enriched with bound factor V and the latter is sometimes more effective than plasma in patients with inhibitors.

Factor X Deficiency

Factor X is another common path factor, but some patients have their prothrombin or PTTs disproportionately prolonged, depending on the type of mutation involved. Deficiency is a rare autosomal recessive disorder that presents with variable severity comparable with that in hemophilia B. Factor X has a longer half-life than its vitamin K-dependent homologue, factor IX, and somewhat lower levels are required for hemostasis (Table 18.2). A low purity factor IX concentrate (Konyne-80) has been treated to inactivate HIV and hepatitis B and C viruses and contains comparable levels of factors IX and X. With lower and less frequent doses required for factor X than IX deficiency, the risk of thrombosis is decreased; it is also possible on alternate postoperative days to use fresh-frozen plasma instead of concentrate to further reduce the thrombotic risk.

Factor VII Deficiency

This rare autosomal recessive disorder of another vitamin K-dependent zymogen likewise results from a variety of mutations. In nonconsanguineous occurrences, it is usually due to compound heterozygosity. Although the minimum level for normal hemostasis is low, the low recovery and short half-life of factor VII complicate effective therapy by plasma, especially in patients with severe defects. Factor VII concentrates are available in Europe (22) (Table 18.3), and have been approved for compassionate clinical trials in the United States.

Factor XI Deficiency

There is a high frequency of this autosomal recessive disorder in persons of Ashkenazi Jewish descent, but it is rare in most other populations. Bleeding with surgical procedures is unpredictable, even in some patients homozygous for a premature stop codon (and thus with undetectable factor XI). Excessive blood loss is most likely to occur in operations associated with mucosal injury such as with prostatic surgeries in men or uterine operations in women. Once postoperative bleeding occurs, however, it is more difficult to achieve hemostasis than to have prevented it. The latter is relatively simple for factor XI-deficient patients because of the large size of this protein and long half-life after infusion (Table 18.2). Plasma or concentrates prepared in Europe (22) (Table 18.3) and under study in some centers in the United States are options for replacement therapy. Until more experience with the concentrates has accrued to address a question of possible thrombogenicity, patients with known arteriosclerotic coronary artery disease should receive plasma.

Afibrinogenemia

Because fibrinogen plays a dual role as the structural component of a clot and the bridge between platelet glycoprotein IIb/IIIa molecules in platelet aggregation, the bleeding pattern in patients with this rare autosomal recessive disorder is distinct from that in the hemophilias. Spontaneous intracerebral hemorrhages and prolonged oozing from minor cuts in the skin are common without prophylactic replacement therapy. Cryoprecipitate is the only available source of concentrated fibrinogen, and because of its large size and half-life of 3–4 days, a single dose (e.g., 15 bags) can provide protection for up to 2–3 weeks and doses every 3–4 days can maintain levels above 80 mg/dL postoperatively. A plasmapheresed single donor is preferred to multiple random donors to limit potential viral exposure.

Factor XIII Deficiency

Fibrin stabilization by cross-linking occurs after fibrin polymers are formed, and thus all kinetic clinical clotting tests are normal even in severe deficiencies. For normal clotting in vivo, only about 5% of the average normal level is required; the half-life of factor XIII is on the order of 11 days (Table 18.2). In addition to acute bleeding, severely affected patients frequently have a history of prolonged oozing from the umbilical stump. Keloids often form after skin lacerations or incisions and are due to recurrent dehiscence and poor wound healing. Relatively little treatment is required, and single preoperative doses of plasma or concentrate (as prepared in Europe) (22) (Table 18.3) can be sufficient for normal hemostasis and wound healing.

FUTURE APPROACHES AND PROSPECTS FOR GENE THERAPY

Greater understanding of the hemostatic mechanisms in vivo is leading to development of reagents that can selectively promote hemostasis in a variety of acquired and congenital deficiencies. Fibrin glue is a topical preparation that facilitates clot formation and wound healing (see Chapter 32). Preliminary reports of fibrin glue packing of the sockets of hemophilic patients after tooth extraction suggest that bleeding is controlled in most patients without factor concentrate coverage. Some patients did require postextraction clotting factor replacement, however. Some experience with topical use of recombinant factor VIIa to control surgical bleeding or systemic use in hemophilic patients without inhibitors is accruing; although effective in anecdotal cases, it is unclear if the clot formed and wound healing in hemophilic wounds is comparable with that when their hemostatic system is normalized by infusion therapy. Recombinant tissue factor is another procoagulant considered, but experiments in animals have suggested that the thrombotic risk is too high. Currently, it appears that a generalized procoagulant approach may be developed that would, at least in part, contribute to hemostasis and wound healing in patients with congenital clotting factor disorders. Different reagents may have different indications and topical adjunctive hemostatic agents are promising. Recombinant factors and nonplasma-derived stabilizing reagents are most desirable to avoid the risk of viral transmission.

Gene therapy has been proposed as a means to cure the hemophilias and some success has been reported in animal models (23). Once a safe effective procedure is established, it would seem most prudent to reserve it for the most severely affected hemophilic patients. By synthesizing their own factor, the therapeutic effect would be comparable with continuous prophylactic infusions; even partial success would alleviate spontaneous bleeding episodes. Transfer of DNA into host cells is accomplished by a vector, and both in vitro (cultured cells) and in vivo (infused) transduction of somatic cells has been tried. A variety of vectors and host cell types are being tried, and each has its advantages and disadvantages. Hepatocytes, for example, are best transduced in vivo because it is difficult to culture the human cells. Retroviral vectors require dividing cells for transduction. Thus, for hemophilia B dogs, long-term expression (over 5 months) of canine factor IX required a partial hepatectomy to induce hepatocyte cell division (24). The number of transduced cells was limited, and the levels achieved were detectable but too low to be clinically significant. On the other hand, adenoviral vectors insert multiple copies in nondividing cells and portal infusion resulted in normal factor IX levels (25). Because the adenoviral vectors do not integrate into the host cell's genome, the effect only lasted several days and the animals developed immune-mediated resistance to subsequent vector challenges. There is considerable research interest in improving vectors and cellular expression, and it is likely that a clinically useful combination of vector and host cells will be developed in the near future. A related approach that may be effective is using implanted immune-isolation chambers in which implanted transduced allogeneic cells can grow. Because factor IX is a smaller gene and a more stable protein is expressed, patients with hemophilia B will likely be the first to undergo studies of gene transfer.

REFERENCES

1. Pool JG, Shannon AE. Production of high-potency concentrates of antihemophilic globulin in closed-bag system. N Engl J Med 1965;273: 1443–1447.

2. Kasper CK, Lusher JM. Recent evolution of clotting factor concentrates for hemophilia A and B. Transfusion 1993;33:422–434.
3. Horowitz B, Bonomo R, Prince AM, et al. Solvent/detergent-treated plasma: a virus-inactivated substitute for fresh frozen plasma. Blood 1992;79:826–831.
4. Zakrzewska K, Azzi A, Patou G, Morfini M, Rafanelli D, Pattison JR. Human parvovirus B19 in clotting factor concentrates: B19 DNA detection by the nested polymerase chain reaction. Br J Haematol 1992;81: 407–412.
5. Fricke WA, Lamb MA. Viral safety of clotting factor concentrates. Semin Thromb Hemostas 1993;19:54–61.
6. Scott JP, Montgomery RR. Therapy of von Willebrand disease. Semin Thromb Hemostas 1993;19:37–47.
7. Thompson AR. Factor IX concentrates for clinical use. Semin Thromb Hemostas 1993;19:25–36.
8. White GC, Shapiro AD, Ragni MV, et al. A pharmacokinetic evaluation of recombinant human factor IX in patients with severe hemophilia B. Thrombos Hemostas 1995;73:1015.
9. Gill JC. Therapy of factor VIII deficiency. Semin Thromb Hemostas 1993;19:1–12.
10. Martinowitz U, Shulman S, Gitel S, et al. Adjusted dose continuous infusion of factor VIII in patients with haemophilia A. Br J Haematol 1992;82:729–734.
11. Shulman S. DDAVP—the multipotent drug in patients with coagulopathies. Trans Med Rev 1991;5:132–144.
12. Macik BG. Treatment of factor VIII inhibitors: products and strategies. Semin Thromb Hemostas 1993;19:13–24.
13. Brettler DB, Forsberg AD, Levine PH, et al. The use of porcine factor VIII concentrate (Hyate:C) in the treatment of patients with inhibitor antibodies to factor VIII. Arch Intern Med 1989;149:1381–1385.
14. Hedner U, Glazer S, Falch J. Recombinant activated factor VII in the treatment of bleeding episodes in patients with inherited and acquired bleeding disorders. Transfusion Med Rev 1993;7:78–83.
15. Buehrer JL, Weber DJ, Meyer AA, et al. Wound infection rates after invasive procedures in HIV-1 seropositive versus HIV-1 seronegative hemophiliacs. Ann Surg 1990;11:492–498.
16. Seremetis SV, Aledort LM, Bergman GE, et al. Three year randomised study of high-purity or intermediate-purity factor VIII concentrates in symptom-free HIV-positive haemophiliacs: effects on immune status. Lancet 1993;342:700–703.
17. Mannucci PM, Brettler DB, Aledort LM, et al. Immune status of human immunodeficiency virus seropositive and seronegative hemophiliacs infused for 3.5 years with recombinant factor VIII. Blood 1994;83: 1958–1962.
18. Gjerset GF, Pike MC, Mosley JW, et al. Effect of low- and intermediate purity clotting factor therapy on progression of human immunodeficiency virus infection in congenital clotting disorders. Blood 1994;84: 1666–1671.
19. Goedert JJ, Cohen AR, Kessler CM, et al. Risks of immune deficiency, AIDS, and death by purity of factor VIII concentrates. Lancet 1994;344: 791–792.
20. Rick ME. Diagnosis and management of von Willebrand's syndrome. Med Clin North Am 1994;78:609–623.
21. Bray PF. Inherited diseases of platelet glycoproteins: considerations for rapid molecular characterization. Thrombos Hemostas 1994;72:492–502.
22. Stirling D, Ludlam CA. Therapeutic concentrates for the treatment of congenital deficiencies of factors VII, XI, and XIII. Semin Thromb Hemostas 1993;19:48–53.
23. Thompson AR. Progress towards gene therapy for the hemophilias. Thrombos Hemostas 1995;74:45–51.
24. Kay MA, Rothenberg S, Landen CN, et al. In vivo gene therapy for hemophilia B: sustained partial correction in factor IX deficient dogs. Science 1993;262:117–119.
25. Kay MA, Landen CN, Rothenberg SR, et al. In vivo hepatic gene therapy: complete albeit transient correction of factor IX deficiency in hemophilia B dogs. Proc Natl Acad Sci USA 1994;91:2353–2357.

Chapter 19

Perioperative Assessment and Management of the Hypercoagulable Patient

MICHAEL M. MILLENSON
KENNETH A. BAUER

INTRODUCTION

The perioperative period has long been recognized as a time when patients are particularly prone to complications such as deep venous thrombosis (DVT) and pulmonary embolism. The perioperative period is often characterized by major alterations in vascular homeostasis that may culminate in the formation of endovascular clot at an inappropriate time and place in the vascular tree (thrombosis). In recent decades, a great deal has been learned about the pathogenesis of thrombosis in the perioperative period, and effective strategies for preventing thrombotic complications related to surgery have been devised and incorporated into clinical practice. These include the use of graduated compression stockings; intermittent pneumatic calf compression devices; and anticoagulants such as warfarin, minidose unfractionated heparin, adjusted-dose unfractionated heparin, and, more recently, the low-molecular-weight heparins.

Ideally, the choice among preventive strategies should be made based on a preoperative assessment of the risk of thrombosis in the individual patient. Unfortunately, such risk assessment is difficult to quantify and has proved only partially successful when applied to individual patients (1). The likelihood that an individual patient will develop perioperative thrombotic complications depends not only on the type of surgery and the duration of the postoperative convalescence, but is also determined by features unique to the patient. Certain individuals appear to be unusually predisposed to thrombosis (i.e., are "prethrombotic" or "hypercoagulable"), and for these patients, surgical procedures may represent a more serious thrombotic risk. This chapter provides an overview of the hypercoagulable states and discusses in detail the perioperative evaluation and management of such patients with preexisting problems of hypercoagulability.

PATHOGENESIS OF THROMBOSIS IN THE PERIOPERATIVE PERIOD

Thrombosis in the perioperative period results from a disturbance in the equilibrium that normally exists between prothrombotic and antithrombotic forces within the bloodstream (2). The nature of this disturbance was originally conceptualized by Virchow (3), who in 1856 described three common alterations in vascular homeostasis that may result in thrombus formation. These three features, referred to as *Virchow's Triad,* consist of alterations in blood flow (stasis or turbulence), alterations in the vessel wall, and alterations in the coagulability of blood (hypercoagulability). Abnormalities of all three components of Virchow's triad appear to play a role during the perioperative period.

ALTERATIONS IN BLOOD FLOW

Altered venous blood flow (stasis) may result from immobilization associated with the induction of anesthesia, the operative procedure itself, positioning, and the postoperative convalescence. There is substantial evidence to suggest that induction of general anesthesia itself directly causes venodilation in the deep veins of the lower extremities, with subsequent stasis of venous blood flow (4, 5). Venous stasis may also result from physical obstruction to venous outflow, as in the case of a pelvic tumor or a gravid uterus causing compression of the iliac veins or residual luminal obstruction related to a prior thrombus. Alternatively, venous stasis may result from elevation of venous pressures related to severe congestive heart failure or to incompetent venous valves related to prior thrombotic injury and the postphlebitic syndrome. Each condition is a well-known risk factor for venous thrombosis.

The importance of venous stasis in the pathogenesis of perioperative venous thromboembolism cannot be overstated, although the precise underlying pathophysiological mechanisms remain to be fully elucidated. Under normal circumstances, the luminal flow of blood helps to dilute and clear the local accumulation of activated clotting factors at the endothelial surface. As a consequence of the normal luminal flow of blood, the interactions of activated clotting factors and platelets with the vessel wall are minimized, and the activated clotting factors are mixed with the various physiological anticoagulants, resulting in neutralization of local procoagulant activity. The loss of these features in the setting of slow or absent flow (venous stasis) creates a permissive environment for local thrombus formation (6). Experimental models of venous thrombosis using venous ligation suggest that stasis alone does not generally result in thrombus formation but that an additional prothrombotic stimulus is necessary for thrombosis to occur (7, 8).

There is also some evidence to suggest that venous flow is an important determinant of fibrinolytic activity, because luminal blood flow appears to stimulate release of tissue plasminogen activator from endothelial cells. Loss of flow (stasis) may therefore result in diminished fibrinolytic activity at the endothelial surface (9, 10). Flow may also promote release of an endogenous nitrovasodilator, such that loss of flow (stasis) may result in vasoconstriction and loss of antiaggregatory effect on platelets (11).

Although the precise biochemical mechanisms by which venous stasis promotes thrombogenesis remain poorly defined, the epidemiological evidence supporting a causal association is overwhelming. Perioperative immobilization results in the absence of normal muscular contraction in the lower extremities, with resultant loss of the normal pumping action that promotes blood flow centrally out of the venous sinuses of the calf and thigh. As a consequence, blood may pool in the soleal venous plexi, where local activation of blood coagulation by a variety of thrombogenic stimuli may result in the formation of small deposits of fibrin. This process is readily demonstrated in the deep veins of the calf using radiolabeled fibrinogen scanning (12). These small deposits of fibrin may serve as a nidus for thrombus growth, and if the thrombus extends proximally and grows to sufficient size, the patient may experience pain and swelling in the affected limb as a result of venous engorgement and inflammation due to obstruction to venous outflow.

Other epidemiological studies confirm the association between venous stasis and thromboembolism. There appears to be a direct correlation between the prevalence of venous thrombosis found at autopsy and the duration of immobilization antemortem (13). Perhaps the most compelling evidence comes from studies comparing the frequencies of venous thrombosis in patients with immobilized limbs secondary to hemiplegia and paraplegia. Venous thrombosis occurs with equal frequency in the paralyzed limbs of paraplegic patients, but the frequency is up to 10-fold greater in the paralyzed compared with the unaffected limb in stroke patients with hemiplegia (14, 15). Finally, the preponderance of evidence from interventional studies in humans supports an important role of stasis in the pathogenesis of venous thrombosis. As discussed in detail below, interventions designed to combat venous stasis, such as early patient mobilization, with use of intermittent pneumatic calf compression devices and/or graduated compression stockings, have been shown to effectively reduce the frequency of venous thromboembolism (16–18).

On the arterial side of the circulation, altered blood flow (turbulence) may promote thrombus formation by virtue of local endothelial injury and platelet activation associated with high shear stress forces. Arterial grafts are at particular risk because of the high degree of associated turbulence at sites of anastomosis. Most arterial thrombi are found to occur within abnormal vessels, typically in areas where atherosclerotic plaque or stenosis results in a significant hemodynamic disturbance with interruption of the normal laminar flow of blood. As a consequence of high shear stress, the endothelial layer may be denuded, and platelets may become activated and subsequently adhere to the exposed subendothelial matrix, resulting in formation of a platelet-rich thrombus. The common observation that arterial thrombi are platelet-rich and venous thrombi are platelet-poor reinforces the notion that platelet-vessel wall interactions resulting from turbulent flow are of preeminent importance in causing arterial thrombosis and are probably of lesser significance in the pathogenesis of venous thrombosis (6, 19).

ALTERATIONS IN THE VESSEL WALL

Under normal circumstances, the intact endothelial surface is nonthrombogenic by virtue of the fact that it does not activate platelets or coagulation proteins to a sufficient degree to cause thrombus formation in the absence of prothrombotic stimuli. The intact endothelium prevents platelets and clotting proteins from interacting with components of the subendothelial matrix, and the vessel wall elaborates both prostacyclin and endothelial-derived nitric oxide, which act as potent vasodilators and inhibitors of platelet aggregation (20, 21). The normal vessel wall is also endowed with a number of anticoagulant and fibrinolytic mechanisms that prevent the deposition of fibrin on the endothelial surface. The endothelium may be converted from a nonthrombogenic to a prothrombogenic surface by a variety of factors, including direct injury from trauma and by exposure to various cytokines such as tumor necrosis factor and interleukin-1, which may be elaborated in the setting of perioperative tissue injury or sepsis (22).

Abnormalities in the vessel wall undoubtedly play an important role in the pathogenesis of thrombosis for certain patients in the perioperative period. Direct injury to the iliofemoral veins may occur with a variety of surgical procedures known to have a high risk of DVT of the lower extremities, such as pelvic surgery or orthopedic surgery. Twisting of the iliofemoral veins during total hip arthroplasty may account in part for the very high rate of venous thrombosis encountered in patients undergoing this procedure (23). In most patients who develop venous thromboembolism, however, detailed pathological studies have failed to reveal consistent evidence of abnormalities within the vessel wall. This suggests that on the venous side of the circulation, the other two components of Virchow's triad contribute more significantly to the pathogenesis of thrombosis.

In contrast, thrombosis on the arterial side of the circulation usually occurs within diseased blood vessels where alterations in the vessel wall appear to play a prominent role pathophysiologically. The association between acute arterial thrombosis and atherosclerotic vascular disease is particularly compelling because of the finding that a stenotic atheromatous lesion is almost always present when a native artery becomes occluded with thrombus (24). The relative contributions of alterations in blood flow (turbulence) versus alterations in the vessel wall to the development of thrombosis at sites of stenotic lesions remains undefined, because the two processes usually coexist. This association is most clearly manifest in the setting of vascular bypass surgery, where thromboses of autogenous venous bypass grafts almost always occur at sites of critical stenosis either in the body of the graft or at one of the anastomoses (25). Nonetheless, there appear to be instances where acute arterial thrombosis develops in the setting of an otherwise trivial arterial defect, suggesting that other factors, such as the coagulability of blood, may be of overriding importance in determining graft patency in certain patients undergoing bypass surgery.

ALTERATIONS IN THE COAGULABILITY OF BLOOD (HYPERCOAGULABILITY)

The term "hypercoagulability" refers to an alteration in the normal biochemical balance between prothrombotic and antithrombotic forces within the bloodstream, resulting in a heightened tendency for activation of the coagulation system (2). This is manifest clinically by the observation that certain patients appear to develop thrombotic events in response to fairly trivial thrombogenic stimuli or even in the absence of recognizable stimuli (i.e., "spontaneously").

A number of pathophysiological changes occur in the perioperative period that may result in hypercoagulability and may account in part for the strong epidemiological association between surgery and thrombosis. Various procoagulant cytokines such as tumor necrosis factor (26) and interleukin-1 (27) may be released as a result of perioperative tissue injury or sepsis. The activity of the fibrinolytic system may be dampened because of the release of a major inhibitor of fibrinolysis (plasminogen activator inhibitor-1) (28) occurring as part of the perioperative acute-phase response. Finally, the natural anticoagulant mechanisms that normally resist thrombin generation and fibrin clot formation may become disrupted in the postoperative setting. There is some evidence that the plasma levels of certain natural anticoagulant proteins, particularly protein C (29) and free protein S (30), may fall during the postoperative period, resulting in an acquired hypercoagulable state. The fact that thrombosis often occurs in patients lacking evidence of vessel wall injury or altered blood flow suggests that hypercoagulability of blood may be a critical factor in the pathogenesis of thrombosis as originally conceptualized by Virchow.

OVERVIEW OF THE HYPERCOAGULABLE STATES

In clinical practice, patients who are suspected of having a thrombotic tendency are grouped into two general pathophysiologic categories—the primary and the secondary hypercoagulable states (31–33). These are listed in Tables 19.1 and 19.2. The primary hypercoagulable states consist of those disorders in which a specific inherited defect in one of the natural anticoagulant mechanisms is identified. These are usually inherited in an autosomal dominant fashion, and a careful history may lead to identification of other affected family members. In general, affected individuals begin to develop symptomatic (usually venous) thromboses sometime

TABLE 19.1. THE PRIMARY (INHERITED) HYPERCOAGULABLE STATES

Activated protein C (APC) resistance
Protein C deficiency
Protein S deficiency
Antithrombin III deficiency
Dysfibrinogenemias

TABLE 19.2. THE ACQUIRED (SECONDARY) HYPERCOAGULABLE STATES

Lupus anticoagulant and the antiphospholipid antibody syndrome
The postoperative state
Chronic venous stasis (venous varicosities, prior deep venous thrombosis)
Prolonged immobilization, trauma
Pregnancy and the postpartum state
Exogenous estrogens and oral contraceptive agents
Malignancy (occult or overt)
Advanced age
Advanced congestive heart failure
Morbid obesity
The nephrotic syndrome
Hyperviscosity syndromes
Polycythemia vera
Dysproteinemias (multiple myeloma, Waldenström's macroglobulinemia)
Elevated fibrinogen in chronic inflammatory states
Various hematological disorders
Myeloproliferative disorders (P. vera, essential thrombocytosis)
Thrombotic thrombocytopenic purpura
Paroxysmal nocturnal hemoglobinuria
Heparin-induced thrombocytopenia with thrombosis

beyond the age of puberty, often in the context of superimposed risk factors such as surgery or pregnancy. For many of the primary hypercoagulable states, the cumulative lifetime risk of symptomatic venous thromboembolism approaches 50% or higher, and recurrence of thrombotic events is common.

The secondary hypercoagulable states consist of a heterogeneous array of clinical conditions that are widely recognized on epidemiological grounds as being associated with an increased risk of thrombosis (Table 19.2). In fact, these conditions account for most patients with thrombotic disease encountered in clinical practice. In contrast to the primary hypercoagulable states, however, the pathophysiological basis of thrombogenesis in these disorders is poorly understood for the most part. It is important to emphasize that the primary and secondary hypercoagulable states are not mutually exclusive categories. In fact, patients with any of the primary hypercoagulable states may be particularly prone to developing thrombosis when exposed to the high-risk conditions comprising the secondary hypercoagulable states, especially major surgery and the postoperative state. Similarly, many disorders regarded as secondary hypercoagulable states may coexist in the same patient, making the cumulative risk of perioperative thrombosis that much greater. Although most of the discussion to follow focuses on the perioperative evaluation and management of the primary hypercoagulable states, specific interventions aimed at correcting selected abnormalities among the secondary hypercoagulable states are also discussed.

PRIMARY HYPERCOAGULABLE STATES

The pathophysiological mechanisms underlying the thrombotic tendency in the primary hypercoagulable states are fairly well understood and are reviewed briefly. A thrombotic tendency resulting from inherited abnormalities of the natural anticoagulant pathways is predictable based on an understanding of the biochemical functions of the involved proteins. These are depicted schematically in Figures 19.1 and 19.2. A fibrin clot is formed when the coagulation mechanism becomes activated in conjunction with the activation of platelets. This results in the formation of fibrin strands with entrapment of platelet aggregates and red blood cells, together constituting the evolving thrombus. The generation of thrombin appears to be a critical step in this process, because thrombin enzymatically converts fibrinogen to fibrin and is itself a potent platelet agonist. Thrombin is the principal end product of the blood coagulation cascade, a series of linked proteolytic reactions in which inactive zymogens are serially converted to their active serine proteases (Fig. 19.1). Most of these reactions take place on or near phospholipid surfaces on platelets, endothelial cells, and white blood cells.

Under normal circumstances, several natural anticoagulant mechanisms exist which ensure the maintenance of blood fluidity or, in the event of vascular injury, serve to limit and localize thrombus formation to the site of such injury. The most important natural anticoagulant pathways in vivo are the heparin-antithrombin III pathway and the protein C-thrombomodulin-protein S pathway. The biochemical interactions of these natural anticoagulants with their target substrates within the coagulation cascade are illustrated in Figure 19.2.

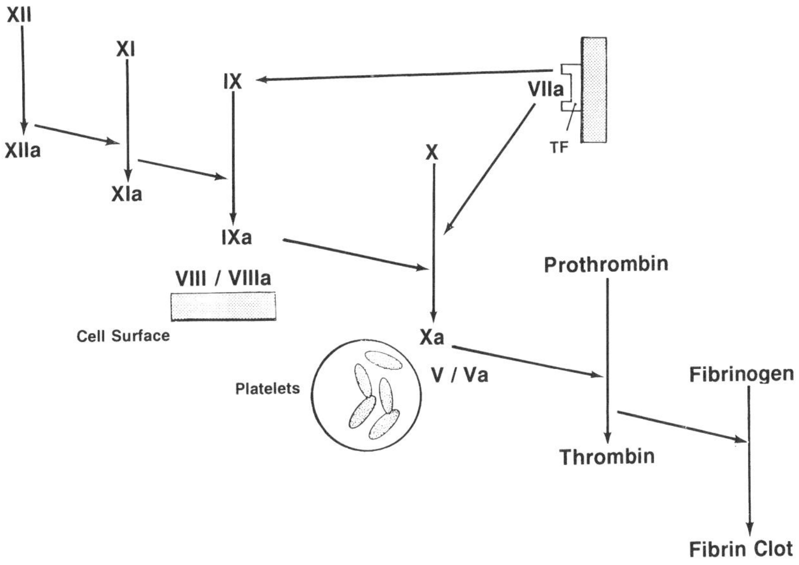

Figure 19.1. The coagulation cascade is a series of linked proteolytic reactions in which inactive zymogens are serially converted to their active serine proteases. The phospholipid-bound tissue factor-factor VIIa complex (TF-VIIa) is the major initiator of the coagulation mechanism in vivo. TF-VIIa exhibits substrate specificity for both factor IX (FIX) and factor X (FX). TF-VIIa may generate FXa via the *extrinsic pathway* by directly converting FX to FXa or may do so via the *intrinsic pathway* by first converting FIX to FIXa that, in association with its cofactor (FVIIIa), may then convert FX to FXa. FXa then combines with its cofactor (FVa) on activated platelets to form the "prothrombinase complex," itself a serine protease that mediates the conversion of prothrombin to thrombin. Thrombin then plays a critical role in generating fibrin clot by further activating platelets and by enzymatically converting fibrinogen to fibrin.

ANTITHROMBIN III DEFICIENCY

Antithrombin III (ATIII) is an important member of the general class of plasma proteins known as serine protease inhibitors (serpins) and functions as the predominant physiological inhibitor of thrombin in vivo (34). ATIII also inhibits the other serine proteases of the coagulation cascade (factors XIIa, XIa, IXa, and Xa). The interaction between ATIII and thrombin is accelerated up to 1000–10,000-fold in the presence of heparin (thus accounting for the known antithrombotic properties of heparin). Recent studies suggest that heparin sulfate molecules associated with the vascular endothelium may serve to enhance the local anticoagulant activity of ATIII at the endothelial surface (35).

Based on an understanding of the function of ATIII, one would predict that an inherited defect in ATIII would allow for the unopposed action of thrombin in vivo. This would result in increased fibrin formation along with platelet activation, ultimately translating into a clinical thrombotic tendency. This prediction is born out by the well-known association between congenital deficiencies of ATIII and the occurrence of venous thrombosis (36). The most common sites of involvement are the deep veins of the legs (with or without pulmonary emboli) and the mesenteric veins. ATIII deficiency is inherited in an autosomal dominant fashion, with affected heterozygotes having functional ATIII levels in plasma of 30–60% of normal. Biochemically affected individuals generally have a lifetime risk of thrombosis of over 50%, with thrombotic events usually beginning to occur sometime after puberty and increasing in frequency with advancing age. The initial thrombotic events occur spontaneously in about 40% of affected individuals, with the remaining 60% experiencing episodes in the context of an inciting event such as surgery, trauma, or pregnancy (37). Approximately 2–3% of carefully studied patients with recurrent idiopathic thromboses will be found to be ATIII deficient (38, 39).

PROTEIN C DEFICIENCY

The protein C pathway functions in parallel with the other natural anticoagulant pathways to regulate the thrombotic process in vivo, as shown in Figure 19.2. Protein C is a vitamin K-dependent zymogen that requires conversion to its serine protease, activated protein C (APC), to function as an anticoagulant. APC serves as an anticoagulant by enzymatically cleaving and thereby inactivating the activated cofactors factor Va and factor VIIIa, thus inhibiting the activation of factor X and prothrombin, respectively (40, 41). In light of this biochemical function of APC, one would anticipate that a defect in the protein C pathway would result in excessive activation of factor X and prothrombin, with a heightened potential for clinical thrombosis.

In fact, there is an association between inherited deficiencies of protein C and the occurrence of venous thrombosis (42–44). Many large kindreds have been identified in which

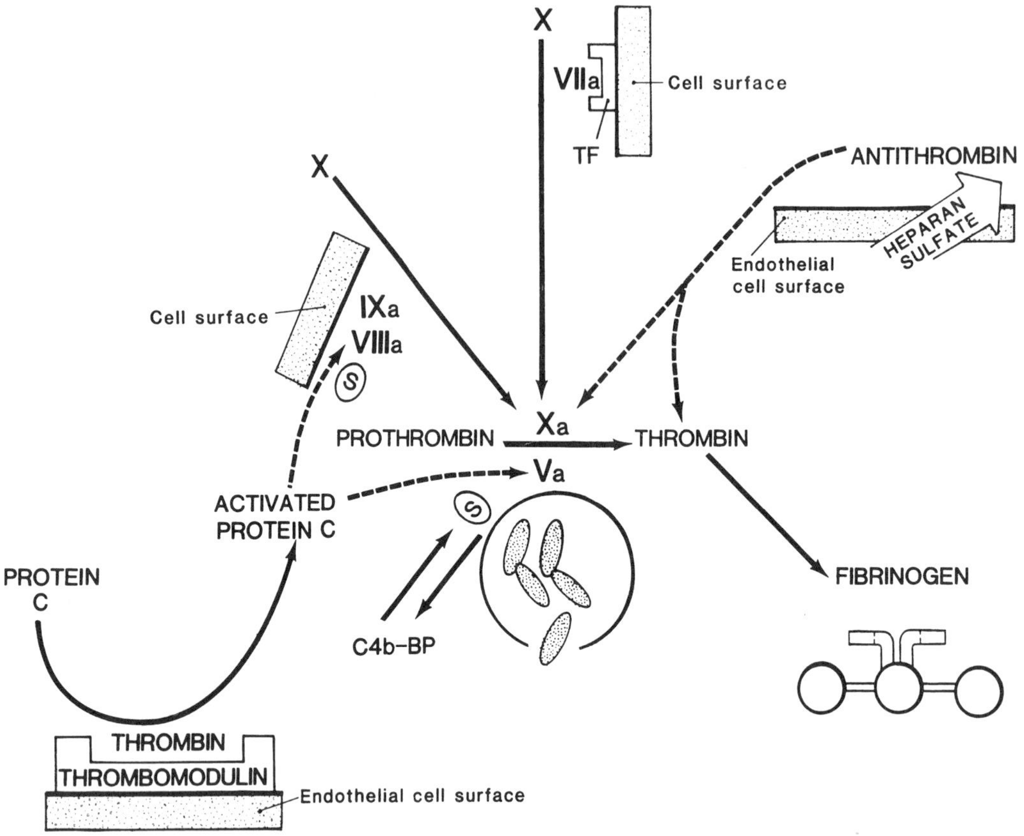

Figure 19.2. Antithrombin III (ATIII) functions as an anticoagulant by complexing with and inactivating thrombin and several other serine proteases in the coagulation cascade (including factor Xa). The inactivation of thrombin by ATIII is greatly accelerated in the presence of heparan sulfate molecules associated with the endothelial surface. Protein C functions as an anticoagulant by first undergoing conversion to activated protein C (APC) by thrombin bound to the endothelial receptor thrombomodulin. APC serves as an anticoagulant by inactivating factors VIIIa and Va. Protein S functions as a cofactor for APC by enhancing its binding to phospholipid surfaces, thereby accelerating APC-mediated inactivation of surface-bound factors VIIIa and Va. Protein S functional activity may be modulated by binding to C4b-binding protein (C4b-BP), a component of the complement system, because only the free (unbound) form of protein S is active as a cofactor for APC.

several individuals having protein C levels of approximately 50% of normal have experienced thromboembolic events. Protein C deficiency follows an autosomal dominant mode of inheritance and has clinical features that are quite similar to those of hereditary ATIII deficiency. The most common sites for thrombosis are the deep veins of the legs and the mesenteric veins, although other manifestations have been reported, including superficial thrombophlebitis, cerebral vein thrombosis, and the phenomenon of warfarin-induced skin necrosis. Skin necrosis appears to be from thrombosis of dermal blood vessels resulting from the transient suppressive effect of warfarin on protein C anticoagulant activity relative to the other vitamin K-dependent procoagulant clotting factors (45–47). Individuals with severe protein C deficiency (either homozygotes or double heterozygotes) may present during the neonatal period with a syndrome of purpura fulminans, with skin findings that are clinically and pathologically similar to those seen with warfarin-induced skin necrosis (48, 49).

Biochemically affected individuals from thrombosis-prone families with heterozygous protein C deficiency appear to have a lifetime risk of thrombosis approaching 75%. As is the case for ATIII deficiency, patients who are heterozygous for protein C deficiency are usually asymptomatic until the third decade of life, after which time the cumulative risk of thrombosis increases substantially with advancing age. Many of these initial thrombotic events occur at the time of the patient's first major surgical or obstetrical challenge. Careful laboratory evaluation of patients with recurrent, idiopathic venous thrombosis will reveal a diagnosis of protein C deficiency about 3–5% of the time (38, 39).

PROTEIN S DEFICIENCY

Protein S contributes to the normal functioning of the protein C anticoagulant pathway by serving as a cofactor for the APC-dependent inactivation of factors Va and VIIIa (50), as illustrated schematically in Figure 19.2. Protein S is a vitamin K-dependent protein that forms a stoichiometric complex with APC in the presence of calcium ions on a phospholipid surface. It accelerates APC-mediated cleavage of factors Va and VIIIa by enhancing the binding of APC to cell membranes where these reactions take place (51, 52). Given this mechanism of action, one would anticipate that a deficiency of protein S would result in excessive factors Va and VIIIa cofactor activity, culminating in a clinical thrombotic tendency.

The association between inherited protein S deficiency and venous thrombotic disease is also well established. Several kindreds have been described in which individuals with reduced plasma levels of protein S have exhibited a marked tendency to develop recurrent venous thrombosis (53–55). The clinical features of patients with heterozygous protein S deficiency are quite similar to those of ATIII or protein C deficiency. The usual sites of involvement are the deep veins of the legs (with or without pulmonary emboli), although axillary, mesenteric, and cerebral vein thrombosis have all been described. Superficial thrombophlebitis also appears to be common. A case report has described purpura fulminans in a neonate with homozygous protein S deficiency (56).

Individuals with heterozygous protein S deficiency from thrombosis-prone kindreds appear to have a cumulative lifetime risk of thrombosis of approximately 75% (57). As with the other inherited hypercoagulable states, biochemically affected individuals begin to develop thrombotic episodes sometime beyond puberty, with the incidence rising thereafter. About 50% of these episodes occur spontaneously, with the remainder occurring in association with a recognizable precipitating event such as surgery or trauma. Approximately 3–5% of carefully studied patients with recurrent, idiopathic thromboses will be found to be protein S deficient (38, 39).

INHERITED RESISTANCE TO APC

In the past few years, investigators have identified another inherited disorder within the protein C anticoagulant pathway that is associated with venous thromboembolism. The existence of this hereditary defect was initially predicted based on the finding of a poor anticoagulant response to the addition of purified APC to plasmas from unrelated thrombophilic patients (58). Subsequent studies have identified this defect in 20–60% of thrombophilic patients with no other identifiable laboratory abnormality, making it 5–10 times more prevalent than any of the other inherited hypercoagulable states (59–61).

APC resistance has been shown to be due to the presence of an abnormal factor V molecule (62–64). The overwhelming majority of patients with hereditary resistance to APC have inherited a mutant factor V resulting from substitution of an arginine by a glutamine at position 506 (referred to as factor V Leiden). This site is the initial APC cleavage site of factor Va, and the Arg506Gln substitution makes the mutant factor Va molecule relatively resistant to inactivation by APC. Approximately 5% of the general population in the United States are heterozygotes for the factor V Leiden mutation, which suggests that other factors, as yet unidentified, likely play a role in causing the phenotypic expression of thrombosis in these individuals. Patients who are homozygous for the factor V Leiden mutation have been described, and their relative risk of developing clinical thrombosis is higher than that for heterozygotes (approximately 80 times that of the general population as compared with 7 times, respectively) (64). The clinical presentation of biochemically affected individuals is quite similar to that seen with the other inherited hypercoagulable states, with thrombosis of the deep veins of the legs and pulmonary embolism being the most common sites of involvement.

ABNORMALITIES OF FIBRINOGEN AND FIBRINOLYSIS

Several patients and their families have been described in which inheritance of an abnormal fibrinogen molecule has been associated with a clinical thrombotic diathesis. These qualitatively abnormal fibrinogens have usually manifested an autosomal dominant pattern of inheritance. Many of these inherited dysfibrinogenemias result in formation of fibrin that is relatively resistant to normal endogenous fibrinolytic mechanisms (65, 66). Fewer than 20 cases of variant fibrinogens have been reported in association with thrombotic complications, and a dysfibrinogenemia will be found in well less than 1% of patients with familial idiopathic venous thrombosis (38, 39).

The extent to which inherited abnormalities of fibrinolysis contribute to a thrombotic tendency remains uncertain. Several individuals have been identified with recurrent venous thrombosis and inherited abnormalities of plasminogen (67, 68), the plasma protein whose activated counterpart, plasmin, is the major plasma enzyme responsible for lysis of cross-linked fibrin in vivo. However, family members found to have the same biochemical abnormality have not demonstrated a thrombophilic tendency, raising serious doubt as to the causal association between thrombosis and abnormalities of plasminogen (69). Several other families with recurrent thromboses have been characterized in which abnormalities of other components of the fibrinolytic system have been identified (70). However, given the weak causal association between these laboratory tests and thrombosis, routine testing of fibrinolytic function is generally not warranted.

SECONDARY HYPERCOAGULABLE STATES

The clinical conditions comprising the acquired hypercoagulable states (Table 19.2) are very common in clinical practice and are often readily apparent to the treating physician. As discussed earlier, the precise pathophysiological mechanisms by which these conditions contribute to a thrombotic tendency are not fully known and have proved difficult to substantiate scientifically. Many disorders listed in Table 19.2 have in common the tendency to cause impairment of venous blood flow in the lower extremities. For instance, elderly patients or those who are morbidly obese may have poor overall mobility, with loss of muscular contraction in the lower extremities resulting in venous stasis. These patients may be especially prone to immobility during the period of postoperative convalescence. Severe congestive heart failure may likewise result in loss of mobility and, together with elevated venous pressures, may result in stagnant venous outflow from the lower extremities. Blood flow through the iliofemoral veins may be impeded as a result of venous compression by a gravid uterus or by an abdominal or pelvic tumor. Prolonged limb immobilization resulting from a prior cerebrovascular accident or from recent trauma or surgery may also result in venous pooling in the affected limb due to loss of the pumping action associated with muscle contraction.

Many acquired hypercoagulable states have also been associated with biochemical alterations in the normal balance between procoagulant and anticoagulant forces within the bloodstream (6). The extent to which these biochemical changes contribute to the thrombotic tendency in these conditions remains uncertain. For example, ingestion of exogenous estrogens and oral contraceptive agents may result in a significant decline in levels of protein S and ATIII (71–73), and pregnancy has been associated with a substantial drop in both free and total levels of protein S (73, 74). Patients with the nephrotic syndrome, who are known to be at increased risk of renal vein thrombosis, have been found to have reduced levels of ATIII, presumably as a consequence of urinary protein loss (75). Multiple biochemical changes have also been identified during the postoperative state itself, including a reduction in protein C levels (29) and a significant decline in overall fibrinolytic activity (76–78). The postoperative decline in fibrinolytic activity may be due to increased synthesis or release of plasminogen activator inhibitor from endothelial cells during the early postoperative period.

Patients with underlying malignancies have been found to have biochemical evidence of activation of the hemostatic system (79, 80), and these patients must be regarded as having a particularly high risk for perioperative thrombosis. Similar changes in biochemical markers of coagulation activation have also been seen in patients with anticardiolipin antibodies (81) and in patients who are very elderly (82).

LUPUS ANTICOAGULANTS AND THE ANTIPHOSPHOLIPID ANTIBODY SYNDROME

Antibodies directed against phospholipids have been identified in the plasmas of certain patients with a history of thrombosis, and this unique clinical syndrome warrants special discussion. Two specific types of antibodies against phospholipids have been identified, defined by the laboratory methods by which they are detected—the lupus anticoagulant and antiphospholipid antibodies. Lupus anticoagulants are immunoglobulins that bind to a variety of phospholipids and are often, although not exclusively, found in patients with systemic lupus erythematosus (SLE). They are usually detected because of interference with phospholipid-dependent clotting assays in vitro, resulting in prolongation of the clotting time (most commonly the activated partial thromboplastin time [APPT]). For this reason, they are often referred to as lupus *inhibitors*. In contrast, antiphospholipid antibodies are immunoglobulins that bind to negatively charged phospholipids such as cardiolipin and that are usually defined by their ability to bind to immobilized cardiolipin in an enzyme-linked immunoassay (83).

Although these two types of antibodies share many characteristics, they do not necessarily coexist in individual patients with this syndrome. About one-third of thrombosis-prone individuals with antibodies directed against phospholipids will have the lupus anticoagulant alone, one-third will have antiphospholipid antibody only, and one-third will have both (84, 85). These antibodies have been detected in a variety of patients, including those with a history of SLE, malignancy, infection, recurrent fetal loss, exposure to certain medications, and recurrent arterial and venous thrombosis (86). They are also seen in a small percentage of otherwise normal individuals.

The risk of thrombosis in individuals with either of these antibodies is difficult to quantify, because many initial reports were retrospective and subject to overreporting and selection bias. More recent studies suggest that the association of antiphospholipid antibodies with thrombosis is strongest in patients with SLE and that the risk of thrombosis may correlate better with a high-titer antiphospholipid antibody than with a positive lupus anticoagulant alone (87–89). Patients with persistent antiphospholipid antibodies and a known thrombotic history appear to be at increased risk for recurrent thrombosis, with a recurrence rate approaching 50% over a 5-

year period (90, 91). Aggressive perioperative thromboembolic prophylaxis should therefore be considered mandatory in such patients.

HEPARIN-INDUCED THROMBOCYTOPENIA WITH THROMBOSIS

The development of a thrombotic diathesis occurring in the context of heparin-induced thrombocytopenia represents a well-recognized type of acquired hypercoagulable state that is commonly encountered in surgical patients. Heparin administration is associated with mild thrombocytopenia in approximately 5% of treated patients, typically developing after 5–7 days of treatment (92). Most patients have a benign clinical course, and the mild thrombocytopenia that accompanies heparin administration in these patients may be the result of nonimmune platelet aggregation by heparin. In fact, many patients with the benign variant of heparin-induced thrombocytopenia will experience resolution of the thrombocytopenia despite continued administration of the drug.

A small subset of patients, however, will develop more severe thrombocytopenia, presumably due to heparin-dependent IgG antibody-mediated activation of platelets in vivo (93). This subset of patients appears to be at substantial risk of developing arterial and venous thrombosis, often with devastating clinical consequences. The clinical manifestations of thrombosis in these patients includes lower limb ischemia, digital necrosis, myocardial infarction, cardiac arrest, ischemic neurological events, and skin or bowel necrosis. Although the diagnosis of heparin-induced thrombocytopenia with thrombosis can often be made based on clinical grounds, laboratory confirmation is often helpful (94). The laboratory tests having the best sensitivity and specificity measure ^{14}C-serotonin release in mixtures of the patient's serum with normal platelet-rich plasma in the presence and absence of heparin (95, 96).

Because of the potentially devastating nature of this syndrome, it is imperative that platelet counts are carefully monitored in all patients receiving heparin therapy and that heparin is promptly discontinued in any patient suspected of having heparin-induced thrombocytopenia. Platelet transfusions should be avoided if possible because they may theoretically worsen the thrombotic diathesis. In patients with demonstrable heparin-dependent platelet aggregation who require ongoing acute anticoagulant therapy, there are several newer agents that may be considered. These include ancrod, a rapidly acting defibrinogenating agent (97), and heparinoid Org 10172, a commercial mixture of heparin-like compounds (98). Unfortunately, both the heparinoids and the newly available low-molecular-weight heparins, although less reactive than unfractionated heparins, are still sufficiently cross-reactive with heparin-dependent antiplatelet antibodies that they may not be safe alternatives in patients with thrombosis caused by unfractionated heparins. The newer specific thrombin inhibitors, such as hirudin and hirulog, may yet prove to be useful in maintaining anticoagulation in patients with this syndrome. Other specific treatment measures, such as use of streptokinase (99) and platelet-inhibiting drugs (100), have met with anecdotal success in reversing or preventing the thrombotic diathesis. Future use of heparin should be considered contraindicated in patients with a prior history of heparin-induced thrombocytopenia with thrombosis.

DIAGNOSTIC APPROACH TO THE HYPERCOAGULABLE PATIENT

It is important during the preoperative evaluation of patients with a positive thrombotic history to maintain a high index of suspicion for one of the recognizable hypercoagulable states discussed above. It is helpful to take a thorough family history, because the primary hypercoagulable states generally conform to an autosomal dominant pattern of inheritance within affected kindreds. Affected patients may be diagnosed either because of prior development of symptomatic thromboembolism or because of identification through family studies undertaken as part of the evaluation of a blood relative with a history of symptomatic thromboembolism. Because of the low frequency of most of these disorders in the general population, along with the poor predictive value of a positive screening test for the subsequent development of symptomatic thrombosis, it is not recommended that testing for the primary hypercoagulable states be performed as a routine preoperative screen in all patients. However, the potential benefits of correctly diagnosing patients with one of the inherited thrombotic disorders may be substantial, because appropriate perioperative prophylaxis may prevent considerable morbidity and mortality. This is likely to be increasingly important in the future as specific replacement therapies such as protein concentrates become more widely available.

It is not currently practical to attempt to identify most patients with one of the primary hypercoagulable states before the development of their first thrombotic event. The challenge to physicians involved in the perioperative care of such patients is to establish a specific diagnosis and initiate appropriate management to prevent additional symptomatic thromboses after the initial thrombotic event. Achievement of this goal requires careful history taking during the preoperative assessment of the patient, with particular attention to the circumstances surrounding the initial thrombotic event.

It is important to establish the age of the patient at the time of prior thrombotic events, along with the presence or absence of any identifiable risk factors for thrombosis that fall within the category of the acquired hypercoagulable states. The number and severity of prior thrombotic events should be ascertained, along with the response to prior anticoagulant therapy. In the course of evaluating a thrombosis-prone individual, it is often difficult to determine whether recurrent symptoms in an extremity that previously sustained a venous thrombosis are truly indicative of a recurrent clot. For instance, patients with iliofemoral DVT may develop a postphlebitic syndrome characterized by episodic pain and swelling in the affected limb as a result of previous damage to the vein. It is mandatory that recurrent episodes be thoroughly evaluated with the appropriate objective diagnostic tests before being labeled as a recurrent thrombosis.

Patients should be questioned in detail about possible adverse outcomes occurring in association with prior surgery or trauma, including limb fractures with cast immobilization. Women should specifically be questioned about adverse obstetrical outcomes and history of oral contraceptive or exogenous estrogen use. A detailed family history that focuses on outcomes after significant surgical and obstetrical challenges in blood relatives is mandatory.

If the history reveals that a patient has experienced severe, recurrent, "idiopathic" (i.e., spontaneous or unprovoked) venous thromboembolism beginning early in life, the clinician should have a high index of suspicion for one of the primary hypercoagulable states. In the absence of a recognizable secondary hypercoagulable state upon presentation with a first thrombotic episode, the clinician must decide whether to evaluate a given thrombosis-prone patient for the presence of a primary hypercoagulable state. At present, there are no firmly established guidelines for screening for the inherited hypercoagulable states, although the British Society for Haematology has put forth a series of recommendations. These are summarized in Table 19.3 (70).

TABLE 19.3. GUIDELINES ON THE INVESTIGATION OF THROMBOPHILA: CLINICAL FEATURES THAT SHOULD PROMPT A LABORATORY EVALUATION

1. Venous thrombosis at an early age (generally <45 years).
2. Recurrent thrombosis, especially without apparent precipitating factors.
3. Thrombosis occurring at unusual sites (mesenteric veins, cerebral veins).
4. Unexplained neonatal thrombosis.
5. Warfarin-induced skin necrosis.
6. Arterial thrombosis < age 30.
7. Relatives of patients with thrombophilic abnormality.
8. Family history of thromboembolic disease.
9. Unexplained prolonged APTT.
10. History of recurrent fetal loss, idiopathic thrombocytopenia, or SLE.

Reprinted with permission from The British Committee for Standards in Haematology. Guidelines on the investigation and management of thrombophilia. J Clin Pathol 1990;43:703–709.

LABORATORY EVALUATION

If a detailed preoperative history suggests that the patient may have a thrombotic tendency, then further evaluation, including laboratory testing, is warranted. This is often undertaken with input from hematologists having a particular interest and expertise in thrombosis. Until recently, the yield of such a laboratory evaluation was quite low, with only 5–15% of unselected thrombosis-prone patients having an identifiable laboratory abnormality. This yield increases to as high as 30% if one selects young patients with recurrent thromboembolic events and a strongly positive family history (39). However, with the recent identification of APC resistance as the major identifiable cause of inherited thrombophilia, the yield is now much higher, accounting for up to 60% of patients with recurrent unexplained venous thrombosis (59–61).

Several routine laboratory studies are usually undertaken as part of the initial evaluation of patients suspected of having an underlying hypercoagulable state. An APTT should be done in all patients as a screen for a lupus anticoagulant and the antiphospholipid antibody syndrome. Serum for anticardiolipin antibody titers should also be drawn, because some patients with the antiphospholipid antibody syndrome will have a normal APTT. The identification of a lupus anticoagulant or positive anticardiolipin antibody titer should always be confirmed by repeat testing 2–3 months later to verify the diagnosis (88). Additional routine laboratory studies may be pursued as guided by clues obtained in the history or on physical examination. For instance, patients with splenomegaly or a history of portal or hepatic vein thrombosis should have a complete blood count with examination of the peripheral smear, as this may provide evidence for an underlying myeloproliferative disorder.

The recommended screening laboratory studies for evaluation of patients suspected of having a primary (inherited) hypercoagulable state are listed in Table 19.4. No formal guidelines have been established for prioritizing the laboratory evaluation for the thrombosis-prone individual. Because the prevalence of APC resistance is 5–10 times greater than that for the other inherited thrombophilic states, we believe that testing

TABLE 19.4. SCREENING LABORATORY EVALUATION AND EXPECTED YIELD[a] FOR THE INHERITED PROTEIN ABNORMALITIES RESULTING IN THE PRIMARY (INHERITED) HYPERCOAGULABLE STATES

Studies	Percent
Poor anticoagulant response to exogenous APC in an APTT assay OR PCR-based assay for the factor V Leiden mutation	30–50
Functional and immunological assays of protein C	4–5
Functional and immunological assays of free and total protein S	4–5
Functional assay of ATIII (heparin-cofactor assay)	2–3
Screen for dysfibrinogenemia (functional and immunological assays of fibrinogen, thrombin time, reptilase time)	<1

[a]Reported as the percentage of patients with recurrent, unexplained, or idiopathic venous thromboembolism who will have the identified laboratory abnormality.

for APC resistance should be undertaken in all cases. The diagnosis is suggested by the demonstration of a poor anticoagulant response in the APTT when exogenous APC is added to the patient's plasma. The diagnosis may be confirmed by genotypic analysis using a polymerase chain reaction- (PCR) based assay for the factor V Leiden mutation. The APTT-based assay used for detecting APC resistance requires careful standardization because it may be affected by the characteristics of the specific PTT reagent used and the amount of APC added to the test plasma (101, 102). Furthermore, this assay may only be used in patients who are not receiving anticoagulants because these drugs will result in marked prolongation of the clotting times in the presence of APC. The PCR-based assay for detection of factor V Leiden may be used to establish the diagnosis of APC resistance in patients who are receiving anticoagulants but will miss up to 10% of APC-resistant patients who have other factor V mutations (103).

In practice, plasma samples are usually drawn and sent for all studies listed in Table 19.4, with many specialized coagulation laboratories having their own algorithms for the sequence in which these studies are performed. In general, functional assays are preferred over immunological assays as screening tools, because many individuals with these disorders have been described in which normal amounts of a dysfunctional protein are found. The clinician must understand and anticipate certain diagnostic pitfalls that may arise when interpreting the results of the various assays listed in Table 19.4. For instance, a variety of pathophysiological conditions may result in reduced plasma levels of ATIII, each of which could potentially lead to an erroneous diagnosis of hereditary deficiency (104). These include acute thrombosis, concurrent heparin therapy, disseminated intravascular coagulation, severe liver disease, and estrogen or oral contraceptive use. Similar caution must be used when interpreting the laboratory investigation in patients receiving oral anticoagulants, because both protein C and protein S are vitamin K-dependent proteins whose functional levels may drop substantially in response to anticoagulation with warfarin.

Because of these confounding variables, the laboratory evaluation for the primary hypercoagulable states is best undertaken when the acute thrombotic event has completely resolved and the patient has ceased taking anticoagulants for at least 1 week. Patients whose laboratory results are compatible with a deficiency state should undergo repeat testing to confirm the diagnosis, and family members of such patients should also be studied.

PERIOPERATIVE MANAGEMENT OF THE THROMBOPHILIC PATIENT

The management of the thrombosis-prone patient during the perioperative period should be individualized. The treating physician must take into account both the inherent risk of the proposed surgical operation and the specific clinical risk factors unique to the individual patient. The overall risk of DVT in untreated control patients undergoing general surgery is approximately 20–25%, with a 1–2% incidence of clinically recognized pulmonary embolism (105). The incidence of fatal pulmonary embolism in this group of patients is approximately 0.5–1.0%. These risks are substantially higher in patients undergoing orthopedic or trauma surgery, where the risk of DVT in patients not receiving thromboprophylaxis is in the range of 40–60%, with fatal pulmonary embolism occurring in up to 6% of patients (106). These risk estimates are likely to be much higher in patients with one of the known hypercoagulable states discussed in the sections above.

The prophylactic strategies that are commonly used for routine prevention of perioperative thromboembolism include both mechanical and pharmacological methods. The mechanical interventions include use of graduated compression stockings and/or intermittent pneumatic compression devices. Both interventions appear to prevent venous stasis by increasing the velocity of venous blood flow in the lower extremities (107, 108), and pneumatic compression may also augment local fibrinolytic activity (109). These mechanical methods are moderately effective at preventing postoperative thromboembolism, with a risk reduction of approximately 60% in patients at intermediate risk (110). These methods are recommended in low-risk patients or as an adjunct to pharmacological methods in higher risk patients, but they are not of sufficient efficacy to be used alone in high-risk patients with known thrombophilia.

The pharmacological strategies for preventing perioperative thromboembolism include use of warfarin, unfractionated heparin (either fixed or adjusted dose), or the low-molecular-weight heparins. In general, each is effective in reducing the risk of postoperative DVT and pulmonary embolism, although this benefit is partially offset by a small but significant increase in bleeding complications, especially wound hematomas (111). Use of these agents may be contraindicated in patients with active bleeding or in those at high risk of complications secondary to bleeding.

Dextran is a high-molecular-weight glucose polymer that exerts its antithrombotic effect by reducing platelet adhesiveness and aggregation and by reducing red cell aggregation. Its use is relatively limited because of side effects such as volume overload and allergic reactions, including anaphylaxis. Fixed low-dose unfractionated heparin is moderately effective in patients at intermediate risk of thromboembolism, with reduction in the relative risk by approximately 60% (105, 112). For patients at high risk, however, more aggressive pharmacological alternatives such as warfarin, adjusted-dose unfractionated heparin, or low-molecular-weight heparin are warranted. Studies involving direct comparisons of these alternatives have generally been performed in patients undergoing orthopedic procedures such as total hip or total knee replacement surgery. These studies suggest that low-molecular-weight heparins are at least as effective as either warfarin (113) or unfractionated heparin (114, 115) in preventing perioperative thromboembolism and may be associated with a lower risk of bleeding. To date, there have been no studies specifically comparing these various pharmacological approaches in patients with known thrombophilic states such as inherited deficiencies of ATIII, protein C, or protein S who are undergoing surgery.

RECOMMENDATIONS FOR PATIENTS WITH THE INHERITED THROMBOPHILIC STATES

Given these general management strategies, several specific perioperative measures are recommended for patients with thrombophilia resulting from the inherited disorders discussed earlier in this chapter. Most patients who are known to have one of the primary hypercoagulable states and who have had two or more thrombotic events are advised to undertake lifelong anticoagulation with warfarin. These patients must be considered to be at very high risk for perioperative venous thromboembolism and should be managed accordingly. When such patients are planning elective surgery, we usually recommend that warfarin be discontinued 1 week before the scheduled surgery, allowing the prothrombin time to subsequently drift toward the normal range to achieve acceptable perioperative hemostasis. In patients with a severe thrombotic tendency, in whom the clinician is concerned about withholding anticoagulation even briefly, the patient may be given adjusted-dose heparin subcutaneously as an outpatient during this preoperative period, and the heparin dose may be held on the morning of surgery in preparation for the procedure. Low-molecular-weight heparin could also be used for this purpose, although its safety and efficacy in this setting have not been adequately studied.

These patients should generally be mobilized as soon as possible after surgery, and mechanical thromboprophylactic measures such as use of graduated compression stockings and intermittent pneumatic compression devices should be routinely used. We usually recommend that patients with a severe thrombotic tendency be fully anticoagulated with continuous intravenous heparin beginning as soon as is safely possible after surgery, aiming to achieve a partial thromboplastin time of 2.0–2.5 times the control value. Oral warfarin should be resumed once the patient is able to tolerate medications by mouth, and the daily dose should be titrated to achieve an International Normalized Ratio (INR) of 2–3 (116). Warfarin requirements during the immediate postoperative period may be significantly less than the patient's preoperative requirements, due to perioperative alterations in the bioavailability of vitamin K and due to suppression of hepatic synthesis of the coagulation proteins. We generally recommend that heparin and warfarin therapy be overlapped in these high-risk patients and that the heparin not be discontinued until the INR is stably maintained within the desired therapeutic range. Certain high-risk patients, such as those with lupus anticoagulants and a history of recurrent thromboembolism, may require a greater intensity of anticoagulation, and many of these patients will be maintained chronically at INRs above 2–3 (91, 117).

Beyond the general prophylactic measures mentioned above, several newer strategies aimed at correcting the underlying deficiencies in patients with inherited thrombophilia are emerging. Specific replacement therapy using ATIII concentrate is currently licensed for use in North America as adjunctive therapy for patients with hereditary ATIII deficiency (118). Although no controlled clinical trials have been performed, several studies suggest that administration of ATIII concentrate to congenitally deficient patients, with or without heparin, is effective in preventing thrombosis after surgery (118–121). The infusion of 50 units/kg body weight of ATIII concentrate (with 1 unit defined as the amount of ATIII present in 1 mL of normal human plasma) raises the plasma level of ATIII to approximately 120% in a congenitally deficient patient with a baseline level of 50% (32, 121). Because the biological half-life of ATIII is approximately 48 hours, the plasma levels of ATIII must be monitored serially in patients receiving replacement therapy. Most investigators recommend maintaining ATIII levels between 80 and 120%, which usually requires administration of 60% of the initial loading dose of ATIII concentrate at 24-hour intervals. Most studies that have demonstrated the efficacy of this approach have maintained ATIII levels between 80 and 120% for a period of at least 1 week postoperatively (118), but the optimum duration of replacement therapy remains undefined.

Highly purified concentrates of protein C are also now available, although their use remains investigational in North America. Protein C concentrates have been used to successfully treat patients with warfarin-induced skin necrosis (122) and neonatal purpura fulminans due to severe (homozygous) protein C deficiency (123). Recent studies have also shown that the elevated level of activity of the hemostatic mechanism in patients with severe protein C deficiency is lowered into the normal range by administration of purified protein C concentrate (124). Whether prophylactic replacement of protein C will be useful in the perioperative management of patients with inherited abnormalities in the protein C pathway remains to be established by future investigations.

REFERENCES

1. Carter CJ. Epidemiology of venous thromboembolism. In: Hull R, Pineo GF, eds. Disorders of thrombosis. Philadelphia: WB Saunders, 1996: 159–174.
2. Bauer KA, Rosenberg RD. The pathophysiology of the prethrombotic state in humans: insights gained from studies using markers of hemostatic system activation. Blood 1987;70:343–350.
3. Virchow R. Phlogese und thrombose in GefaBsystem. In: Virchow R, ed. Gesammelte Abhandluger zur Wissenschaftlichen Medicin. Frankfurt: von Meidinger Sohn, 1856:458–636.
4. Comerota AJ, Stewart GJ, Alburger PD, Smalley K, White JV. Operative venodilation: a previously unsuspected factor in the cause of postoperative deep venous thrombosis. Surgery 1989;106:301–309.
5. Poikolainen E, Hendolin H. Effects of lumbar epidural analgesia and general anesthesia on flow velocity in the femoral vein and postoperative deep vein thrombosis. Acta Chir Scand 1983;149:361–364.
6. Millenson MM, Bauer KA. Pathogenesis of venous thromboembolism. In: Hull R, Pineo GF, eds. Disorders of thrombosis. Philadelphia: WB Saunders, 1996:175–190.
7. Schaub RG, Simmons CA, Koetz MH, Romano PJ II, Stewart GJ. Early events in the formation of venous thrombus following local trauma and stasis. Lab Invest 1984;51:218–224.
8. Pescador R, Porta R, Conz A, Mantovani M. A quantitative venous thrombosis model with stasis based on vascular lesion. Thromb Res 1989;53:197–201.
9. Slack SM, Cui Y, Turitto VT. The effect of flow on blood coagulation and thrombosis. Thromb Haemost 1993;70:129–134.
10. Diamond SL, Eskin SG, McIntire LV. Fluid flow stimulates tissue plasminogen activator secretion by cultured human endothelial cells. Science 1989;243:1483–1485.
11. Cooke JP, Rossitch E Jr, Andon NA, Loscalzo J, Dzau VJ. Flow activates an endothelial potassium channel to release an endogenous nitrovasodilator. J Clin Invest 1991;88:1663–1671.
12. Kakkar VV. The diagnosis of DVT using the ^{125}I-fibrinogen test. Arch Surg 1972;104:152–159.
13. Gibbs NM. Venous thrombosis of the lower limb with particular reference to bedrest. Br J Surg 1957;45:209.
14. Warlow C, Ogston D, Douglas AS. Deep venous thrombosis of the legs after stroke. Br Med J 1976;1:1178–1183.
15. Bors E, Conrad CA, Massell TB. Venous occlusion of the lower extremities in paraplegic patients. Surg Gynecol Obstet 1954;99:451.
16. National Institutes of Health Consensus Development Conference. Prevention of venous thrombosis and pulmonary embolism. JAMA 1986; 256:744–749.
17. Scurr JH, Coleridge-Smith PD, Hasty JH. Regimen for improved effectiveness of intermittent pneumatic compression in deep venous thrombosis prophylaxis. Surgery 1987;102:816–820.
18. Colditz GA, Tuden RL, Oster G. Rates of venous thrombosis after general surgery: combined results of randomized clinical trials. Lancet 1986;2:143–146.
19. Carter CJ. Pathogenesis of arterial thrombosis. In: Hull R, Pineo GR, eds. Disorders of thrombosis. Philadelphia: WB Saunders, 1996:18–30.
20. Palmer RM, Ferrige AG, Moncada S. Nitric oxide release accounts for the biological activity of endothelium-derived relaxing factor. Nature 1987;327:524–526.
21. Vane JR, Anggard EE, Botting RM. Regulatory functions of the vascular endothelium. N Engl J Med 1990;323:27–36.
22. Salzman EW, Hirsh J. The epidemiology, pathogenesis, and natural history of venous thrombosis. In: Colman RW, Hirsh J, Marder VJ, Salzman EW, eds. Hemostasis and thrombosis: basic principles and clinical practice, 3rd ed. Philadelphia: J.B. Lippincott, 1994:1275–1296.
23. Stamatakis JD, Kakkar VV, Sagar S, Lawrence D, Nairn D, Bentley PG. Femoral vein thrombosis and total hip replacement. Br Med J 1977;2:223–225.
24. Ouriel K, Marder VJ. Acute arterial obstruction. In: Hull R, Pineo GF, eds. Disorders of thrombosis. Philadelphia: WB Saunders, 1996:135–142.
25. Donaldson MC, Mannick JA, Whittemore AD. Causes of primary graft failure after in situ saphenous vein bypass grafting. J Vasc Surg 1992; 15:113–120.
26. Bevilacqua MP, Pober JS, Majean GR, Fiers W, Cotran RS, Gimbrone MA Jr. Recombinant tumor necrosis factor induces procoagulant activity in cultured human vascular endothelium: characterization and comparison with action of interleukin 1. Proc Natl Acad Sci USA 1986;83: 4533–4537.
27. Bevilacqua MP, Pober JS, Majean GR, Cotran RS, Gimbrone MA Jr. Interleukin 1 (IL-1) induces biosynthesis and cell surface expression of procoagulant activity in human vascular cells. J Exp Med 1984;160: 618–623.
28. Sorensen JV, Lassen MR, Borris LC, et al. Postoperative deep vein thrombosis and plasma levels of tissue plasminogen activator inhibitor. Thromb Res 1990;60:247–251.

29. Mannucci PM, Vigano S. Deficiencies of protein C, an inhibitor of blood coagulation. Lancet 1982;2:463–467.
30. D'Angelo A, Vigano-D'Angelo S, Esmon CT, Comp PC. Acquired deficiencies of protein S: protein S activity during oral anticoagulation, in liver disease, and in disseminated intravascular coagulation. J Clin Invest 1988;81:1445–1454.
31. Schafer AI. The hypercoagulable states. Ann Intern Med 1985;102: 814–828.
32. Bauer KA. Pathobiology of the hypercoagulable states: clinical features, laboratory evaluation, and management. In: Hoffman J, Benz EJ, Shattil SJ, Furie B, Cohen HJ, eds. Hematology: basic principles and practice, 2nd ed. New York: Churchill Livingstone, 1994:1781–1795.
33. Nachman RL, Silverstein RL. Hypercoagulable states. Ann Intern Med 1993;119:819–827.
34. Rosenberg RD. Actions and interactions of antithrombin and heparin. N Engl J Med 1975;292:146–151.
35. Marcum JA, McKenney JB, Rosenberg RD. The acceleration of thrombin-antithrombin complex formation in rat hindquarters via heparin-like molecules bound to the endothelium. J Clin Invest 1984;74:341–350.
36. Demers C, Ginsberg JS, Hirsh J, Henderson P, Blajchman MA. Thrombosis in antithrombin III-deficient persons: report of a large kindred and literature review. Ann Intern Med 1992;116:754–761.
37. Thaler E, Lechner K. Anithrombin III deficiency and thromboembolism. Clin Haematol 1981;10:369–390.
38. Malm J, Laurell M, Nilsson IM, Dahlback B. Thromboembolic disease—critical evaluation of laboratory investigation. Thromb Haemost 1992;68:7–13.
39. Heijboer H, Brandjes DPM, Buller HR, Sturk A, ten Cate JW. Deficiencies of coagulation-inhibiting and fibrinolytic proteins in outpatients with deep venous thrombosis. N Engl J Med 1990;323:1512–1516.
40. Fulcher CA, Gardiner JE, Griffin JH, Zimmerman TS. Proteolytic inactivation of human factor VIII procoagulant protein by activated human protein C and its analogy with factor V. Blood 1984;63:486–489.
41. Marlar RA, Kleiss AJ, Griffin JH. Mechanism of action of human activated protein C, a thrombin-dependent anticoagulant enzyme. Blood 1982;59:1067–1072.
42. Griffin JH, Evatt B, Zimmerman TS, Kleiss AJ. Deficiency of protein C in congenital thrombotic disease. J Clin Invest 1981;68:1370–1373.
43. Broekmans AW, Veltkamp JJ, Bertina RM. Congenital protein C deficiency and venous thromboembolism: a study of three Dutch families. N Engl J Med 1983;309:340–344.
44. Bovill EG, Bauer KA, Dickerman JD, Callas P, West B. The clinical spectrum of heterozygous protein C deficiency in a large New England kindred. Blood 1989;73:712–717.
45. McGehee WG, Klotz TA, Epstein DJ, Rapaport SI. Coumarin necrosis associated with hereditary protein C deficiency. Ann Intern Med 1984; 100:59–60.
46. D'Angelo SV, Comp PC, Esmon CT, D'Angelo A. Relationship between protein C antigen and anticoagulant activity during oral anticoagulation and in selected disease states. J Clin Invest 1986;77:416–425.
47. Conway EM, Bauer KA, Barzegar S, Rosenberg RD. Suppression of hemostatic system activation by oral anticoagulants in the blood of patients with thrombotic diatheses. J Clin Invest 1987;80:1535–1544.
48. Branson HE, Katz J, Marble R, Griffin JH. Inherited protein C deficiency and coumarin-responsive chronic relapsing purpura fulminans in a newborn infant. Lancet 1983;2:1165–1168.
49. Seligsohn U, Berger A, Abend M, et al. Homozygous protein C deficiency manifested by massive venous thrombosis in the newborn. N Engl J Med 1984;310:559–562.
50. Walker FJ. The regulation of activated protein C by a new protein: a possible function for bovine protein S. J Biol Chem 1980;255:5521–5524.
51. Walker FJ. Regulation of protein C by protein S: the role of phospholipid in factor Va inactivation. J Biol Chem 1981;256:11128–11131.
52. Walker FJ, Chavin SI, Fay PJ. Inactivation of factor VIII by activated protein C and protein S. Arch Biochem Biophys 1987;252:322–328.
53. Comp PC, Esmon CT. Recurrent venous thromboembolism in patients with partial deficiency of protein S. N Engl J Med 1984;311:1525–1528.
54. Schwarz HP, Fischer M, Hopmeier P, Batard MA, Griffin JH. Plasma protein S deficiency in familial thrombotic disease. Blood 1984;64: 1297–1300.
55. Comp PC, Nixon RR, Cooper MR, Esmon CT. Familial protein S deficiency in association with recurrent thrombosis. J Clin Invest 1984;74: 2082–2088.
56. Mahasandana C, Suvatte V, Chuansumrit A, et al. Homozygous protein S deficiency in an infant with purpura fulminans. J Pediatr 1990;117: 750–753.
57. Engesser L, Broekmans AW, Briet E, Brommer EJP, Bertina RM. Hereditary protein S deficiency: clinical manifestations. Ann Intern Med 1987;106:677–682.
58. Dahlback B, Carlsson M, Svensson PJ. Familial thrombophilia due to a previously unrecognized mechanism characterized by poor anticoagulant response to activated protein C: prediction of a cofactor to activated protein C. Proc Natl Acad Sci USA 1993;90:1004–1008.
59. Koster T, Rosendaal FR, de Ronde H, Briet E, Vandenbroucke JP, Bertina RM. Venous thrombosis due to poor anticoagulant response to activated protein C: Leiden thrombophilia study. Lancet 1993;342: 1503–1506.
60. Griffin JH, Evatt B, Wideman C, Fernandez JA. Anticoagulant protein C pathway defective in majority of thrombophilic patients. Blood 1993;82:1989–1993.
61. Svensson PJ, Dahlback B. Resistance to activated protein C as a basis for venous thrombosis. N Engl J Med 1994;330:517–522.
62. Dahlback B, Hildebrand B. Inherited resistance to activated protein C is corrected by anticoagulant cofactor activity found to be a property of factor V. Proc Natl Acad Sci USA 1994;91:1396–1400.
63. Bertina RM, Koeleman BPC, Koster T, et al. Mutation in factor V associated with resistance to activated protein C. Nature 1994;369:64–67.
64. Rosendaal FR, Koster T, Vandenbroucke JP, Reitsma PH. High risk of thrombosis in patients homozygous for factor V Leiden (activated protein C resistance). Blood 1995;85:1504–1508.
65. Carrell N, Gabriel DA, Blatt PM, Carr ME, McDonagh J. Hereditary dysfibrinogenemia in a patient with thrombotic disease. Blood 1983;63: 439–447.
66. Soria J, Soria C, Caen JP. A new type of congenital dysfibrinogenemia with defective fibrin lysis—Dusart syndrome: possible relation to thrombosis. Br J Haematol 1983;53:575–586.
67. Aoki N, Moroi M, Sakata Y, Yoshida N, Matsuda M. Abnormal plasminogen: a hereditary molecular abnormality found in a patient with recurrent thrombosis. J Clin Invest 1978;61:1186–1195.
68. Miyata T, Iwanaga S, Sakata Y, Aoki N. Plasminogen Tochigi:Inactive plasmin resulting from replacement of alanine-600 by threonine in the active site. Proc Natl Acad Sci USA 1982;79:6132–6136.
69. Prins MH, Hirsh J. A critical review of the evidence supporting a relationship between impaired fibrinolytic activity and venous thromboembolism. Arch Intern Med 1991;151:1721–1731.
70. The British Committee for Standards in Haematology. Guidelines on the investigation and management of thrombophilia. J Clin Pathol 1990;43:703–709.

71. Caine YG, Bauer KA, Barzegar S, et al. Coagulation activation following estrogen administration to postmenopausal women. Thromb Haemost 1992;68:392–395.
72. Boerger LM, Morris PC, Thurnau GR, Esmon CT, Comp PC. Oral contraceptives and gender affect protein S status. Blood 1987;69:692–694.
73. Malm J, Laurell M, Dahlback B. Changes in the plasma levels of the vitamin K-dependent proteins C and S and of C4b-binding protein during pregnancy and oral contraception. Br J Haematol 1988;68:437–443.
74. Comp PC, Thurnau GR, Welsh J, Esmon CT. Functional and immunologic protein S levels are decreased during pregnancy. Blood 1986;68: 881–885.
75. Kauffman RH, Veltkamp JJ, Van Tilburg NH, Van Es LA. Acquired antithrombin III deficiency and thrombosis in the nephrotic syndrome. Am J Med 1978;65:607–613.
76. Comp PC, Jacocks RM, Taylor FB Jr. The dilute whole blood clot lysis assay:A screening method for identifying post-operative patients with a high incidence of deep venous thrombosis. J Lab Clin Med 1979;93:120–127.
77. Crandon AJ, Peel KR, Anderson JA, Thompson V, McNicol GP. Postoperative deep vein thrombosis: identifying high risk patients. Br Med J 1980;281:343–344.
78. Kluft C, Jie AFH, Lowe GDO, Blamey SL, Forbes CD. Association between post-operative hyperresponse to tPA-inhibition and deep vein thrombosis. Thromb Haemost 1986;56:107.
79. Bick RL. Coagulation abnormalities in malignancy: a review. Semin Thromb Haemost 1992;18:353–372.
80. Luzzato G, Schafer AI. The prethrombotic state in cancer. Semin Oncol 1990;17:147–159.
81. Ginsberg JS, Demers C, Brill-Edwards P, et al. Increased thrombin generation and activity in patients with systemic lupus erythematosus and anticardiolipin antibodies: evidence for a prethrombotic state. Blood 1993;81:2958–2963.
82. Mari D, Mannucci PM, Coppola R, Bottasso B, Bauer KA, Rosenberg RD. Hypercoagulability in centenarians: the paradox of successful aging. Blood 1995;85:3144–3149.
83. Comp PC. Congenital and acquired hypercoagulable states. In: Hull R, Pineo GF, eds. Disorders of thrombosis. Philadelphia: WB Saunders, 1996:339–347.
84. Triplett DA, Brandt JT, Musgrave KA, Orr CA. The relationship between lupus anticoagulants and antibodies to phospholipid. JAMA 1988;259:550–554.
85. Triplett DA, Brandt J. Laboratory identification of the lupus anticoagulant. Br J Haematol 1989;73:139–142.
86. Kunkel LA. Acquired circulating anticoagulants. Hematol Oncol Clin North Am 1992;6:1341–1357.
87. Long AA, Ginsberg JS, Brill-Edwards P, et al. The relationship of antiphospholipid antibodies to thromboembolic disease in systemic lupus erythematosus: a cross-sectional study. Thromb Haemost 1991;66: 520–524.
88. Ginsberg JS, Brill-Edwards P, Johnston M, et al. Relationship of antiphospholipid antibodies to pregnancy loss in patients with systemic lupus erythematosus:A cross sectional study. Blood 1992;80:975–980.
89. Love PE, Santoro SA. Antiphospholipid antibodies:Anticardiolipin and the lupus anticoagulant in systemic lupus erythematosus (SLE) and in non-SLE disorders. Ann Intern Med 1990;112:682–698.
90. Triplett DA. Protean clinical presentation of antiphospholipid-protein antibodies (APA). Thromb Haemost 1995;74:329–337.
91. Rosove MH, Brewer PMC. Antiphospholipid thrombosis: clinical course after the first thrombotic episode in 70 patients. Ann Intern Med 1992; 117:303–308.
92. Wartenkin TE, Kelton JG. Heparin-induced thrombocytopenia. Prog Hemost Thromb 1991;10:1–34.
93. George JN. Heparin-associated thrombocytopenia. In: Hull R, Pineo GF, eds. Disorders of thrombosis. Philadelphia: WB Saunders, 1996: 359–373.
94. Chong BH, Burgess J, Ismail F. The clinical usefulness of the platelet aggregation test for the diagnosis of heparin-induced thrombocytopenia. Thromb Haemost 1993;69:344–350.
95. Sheridan D, Carter C, Kelton JG. A diagnostic test for heparin-induced thrombocytopenia. Blood 1986;67:27–30.
96. Greinacher A, Michels I, Kiefel V, Mueller-Eckhardt C. A rapid and sensitive test for diagnosing heparin-associated thrombocytopenia. Thromb Haemost 1991;66:734–736.
97. Demers C, Ginsberg JS, Brill-Edwards P, et al. Rapid anticoagulation using ancrod for heparin-induced thrombocytopenia. Blood 1991;78: 2194–2197.
98. Chong BH, Ismail F, Cade J, Gallus AS, Gordon S, Chesterman CN. Heparin-induced thrombocytopenia: studies with a new low molecular weight heparinoid, Org 10172. Blood 1989;73:1592–1596.
99. Mehta DP, Yoder EL, Appel J, Bergsman KL. Heparin-induced thrombocytopenia and thrombosis: reversal with streptokinase A case report and review of literature. Am J Hematol 1991;36:275–279.
100. Walls JT, Curtis JJ, Silver D, Boley TM. Heparin-induced thrombocytopenia in patients who undergo open heart surgery. Surgery 1990;108: 686–693.
101. de Ronde H, Bertina RM. Laboratory diagnosis of APC-resistance. A critical evaluation of the test and the development of diagnostic criteria. Thromb Haemost 1994;72:880–886.
102. Rosen S, Johansson K, Lindberg K, Dahlback B (for the APC Resistance Study Group). Multicenter evaluation of a kit for activated protein C resistance on various coagulation instruments using plasmas from healthy individuals. Thromb Haemost 1994;72:255–260.
103. Dahlback B. New molecular insights into the genetics of thrombophilia: resistance to activated protein C caused by Arg^{506} to Gln mutation in factor V as a pathogenic risk factor for venous thrombosis. Thromb Haemost 1995;74:139–148.
104. Millenson MM, Bauer KA. Hypercoagulable states and thrombotic disease. In: Bone R, ed. Current practice of medicine. Vol. 3. Philadelphia: Current Medicine, 1996:25.1–25.8.
105. Clagett GP, Reisch JS. Prevention of venous thromboembolism in general surgical patients: results of meta-analysis. Ann Surg 1988;208: 227–240.
106. Haake DA, Berkman SA. Venous thromboembolic disease after hip surgery. Clin Orthop 1989;242:212–231.
107. Lawrence D, Kakkar VV. Graduated, static, external compression of the lower limb: a physiological assessment. Br J Surg 1980;67:119–121.
108. Blackshear WM, Prescott C, LePain F, Benoit S, Dickstein R, Seifert KB. Influence of sequential pneumatic compression on postoperative venous function. J Vasc Surg 1987;5:432–436.
109. Summaria L, Caprini J, McMillan R, et al. Relationship between postsurgical fibrinolytic parameters and deep vein thrombosis in surgical patients treated with compression devices. Am Surg 1988;54:156–160.
110. Well PS, Lensing AWA, Hirsh J. Graduated compression stockings in the prevention of postoperative venous thromboembolism: a metaanalysis. Arch Intern Med 1994;154:67–72.
111. Clagett GP, Anderson FA, Levine MN, Salzman EW, Wheeler HB. Prevention of venous thromboembolism. Chest 1992;102:391S–407S.
112. Collins R, Scrimgeour A, Yusuf S, Peto R. Reduction in fatal pulmonary and venous thrombosis by perioperative administration of

subcutaneous heparin: overview of randomized trials of general and ortheopaedic and urological surgery. N Engl J Med 1988;318: 1162–1173.
113. Hull R, Raskob G, Pineo G, et al. A comparison of subcutaneous low-molecular-weight heparin with warfarin sodium for prophylaxis against deep-vein thrombosis after hip or knee implantation. N Engl J Med 1993;329:1370–1376.
114. Nurmohamed MT, Rosendaal FR, Buller HR, et al. Low molecular weight heparin versus standard heparin in general and orthopaedic surgery: a meta-analysis. Lancet 1992;340:152–156.
115. Leyvraz PF, Bachmann F, Hoek J, et al. Prevention of deep vein thrombosis after hip replacement: randomized comparison between unfractionated heparin and low molecular weight heparin. Br Med J 1991;303:543–548.
116. Hirsh J. Oral anticoagulant drugs. N Engl J Med 1991;324:1865–1875.
117. Derksen RHWM, DeGroot PG, Kater L, Niewenhuis HK. Patients with antiphospholipid antibodies and venous thrombosis should receive long term anticoagulant treatment. Ann Rheum Dis 1993;52:689–692.
118. Menache D. Antithrombin III concentrates. Hematol Oncol Clin North Am 1992;6:1115–1119.
119. Menache D, O'Malley JP, Schorr JB, Wagner B, Williams C, the Co-operative Study Group. Evaluation of the safety, recovery, half-life, and clinical efficacy of antithrombin III (human) in patients with hereditary antithrombin III deficiency. Blood 1990;75:33–39.
120. Mannucci PM, Boyer C, Wolf M, Triposi A, Larrieu MJ. Treatment of congenital antithrombin III deficiency with concentrates. Br J Haematol 1982;50:531–535.
121. Schwartz RS, Bauer KA, Rosenberg RD, Kavanaugh EJ, Davies DC, Bogdanoff DA. Clinical experience with anithrombin III concentrate in treatment of congenital and acquired deficiency of antithrombin. Am J Med 1989;87:53S-60S.
122. Schramm W, Spannagl M, Bauer KA, et al. Treatment of coumarin-induced skin necrosis with a monoclonal antibody purified protein C concentrate. Arch Dermatol 1993;129:753–756.
123. Dreyfus M, Magny JF, Bridey F, et al. Treatment of homozygous protein C deficiency and neonatal purpura fulminans with a purified protein C concentrate. N Engl J Med 1991;325:1565–1568.
124. Conard J, Bauer KA, Gruber A, et al. Normalization of markers of coagulation activation with a purified protein C concentrate in adults with homozygous protein C deficiency. Blood 1993;82:1159–1164.

Section IV
Operative Transfusion Management

Chapter 20

Intraoperative Monitoring of Oxygen Supply and Consumption

IAN H. WRIGHT

Tissue oxygenation depends on a sequence of processes: oxygen uptake in the lungs, transport in blood (bound to hemoglobin [Hgb] and dissolved in the blood), delivery of oxygenated blood to the tissues (involving global and regional distribution of blood flow), diffusion from capillaries into the cells, and intracellular utilization of delivered oxygen. Monitoring the first two of these processes is straightforward and outside the scope of this chapter. The relationship between oxygen delivery ($\dot{D}O_2$) and consumption ($\dot{V}O_2$) and how best to monitor that relationship is controversial. This chapter is therefore limited to this aspect of the oxygen cascade. To rationally discuss monitoring, it is necessary to understand how $\dot{D}O_2$ and $\dot{V}O_2$ are related in health and disease. Only then can the indications for, and limitations of, current monitoring modalities be recognized.

PHYSIOLOGICAL OXYGEN SUPPLY DEPENDENCY

Global $\dot{D}O_2$ is equal to the volume of oxygen delivered from the heart each minute and is calculated as the product of cardiac output (CO) and arterial oxygen content (CaO_2). Oxygen consumption is the amount of oxygen consumed by the tissues. It too may be calculated by the inverse Fick method and is equal to the product of the CO and the difference between CaO_2 and the mixed venous oxygen content ($C\bar{v}O_2$). Alternatively, $\dot{V}O_2$ may be measured directly by measuring minute volume ($\dot{V}$, the volume of gas inhaled and exhaled per minute) and inspired and expired gas concentrations (see below). The fraction of delivered oxygen that is consumed is termed the extraction ratio (ERO_2). Table 20.1 gives the standard formulae and normal ranges for these calculated values.

Under normal circumstances, $\dot{D}O_2$ exceeds tissue oxygen demands. $\dot{V}O_2$ depends on the metabolic requirements of the cells and is independent of $\dot{D}O_2$. The relationship between the two variables is a "demand-led" system, so that if oxygen demand increases (e.g., during exercise), $\dot{D}O_2$ will increase as necessary. If $\dot{D}O_2$ falls, ERO_2 increases, maintaining $\dot{V}O_2$ (1). As $\dot{D}O_2$ falls further, however, ERO_2 reaches a maximum and a so-called critical point is reached. If $\dot{D}O_2$ is reduced further, $\dot{V}O_2$ also falls (Fig. 20.1). Below the critical point, $\dot{V}O_2$ becomes supply-dependent. This was first demonstrated experimentally in dogs (2). Samsel and Schumacker (3) reviewed animal studies and noted that supply dependency occurs at an ERO_2 of 60–75% and that this figure is constant between species, even though the critical point may vary considerably when measured by oxygen delivery. For example, rats have a metabolic rate approximately three times higher than dogs (15 versus 5 mL/kg/min), and their critical oxygen delivery is approximately three times higher (23 versus 8 mL/kg/min). Both species have a critical ERO_2 of 68–74%.

When $\dot{D}O_2$ falls below the critical point, cellular oxygen supply becomes insufficient to sustain aerobic metabolism. Anaerobic metabolism occurs, resulting in lactate and hydrogen ion production (4).

It is currently unclear whether oxygen uptake by the cells is limited by defects in convective or diffusive oxygen transport (5). Convective transport refers to the bulk transport of oxygen by the circulation and microcirculation, whereas diffusive transport refers to the transport of oxygen from the capillaries to the cells. Some studies have suggested that $\dot{V}O_2$ is diffusion limited when $\dot{D}O_2$ falls due to hypoxemia (6),

TABLE 20.1. STANDARD FORMULAE AND NORMAL RANGES

Variable	Formula	Normal value
Oxygen delivery, $\dot{D}O_2$	$CO \times CaO_2 \times 10$	500–750 mL/min/m^2
Oxygen consumption, $\dot{V}O_2$	$CO \times C(a\text{-}v)O_2 \times 10$	100–180 mL/min/m^2
Arterial oxygen content, CaO_2	$1.34 \times Hgb \times SaO_2 + (0.003 \times PaO_2)$	16–22mL/dL
Mixed venous oxygen content, $C\bar{v}O_2$	$1.34 \times Hgb \times S\bar{v}O_2 + (0.003 \times P\bar{v}O_2)$	12–17mL/dL
Oxygen extraction ratio, ERO_2	$(CaO_2 - C\bar{v}O_2)/CaO_2$	0.23–0.30

whereas others have suggested that the mechanism of reduction of $\dot{D}O_2$ (anemia, hypoxemia, or low flow) was irrelevant (2, 7). Schumacker and Samsel (8) used the Krogh tissue cylinder model to examine this question. If the intercapillary distances were less than 80 μm, the critical point was the same irrespective of the mechanism of reduced $\dot{D}O_2$. When intercapillary distances exceeded 80 μm, the critical point was reached at a higher $\dot{D}O_2$ during hypoxemia. It follows that in organs with decreased capillary density, during tissue edema, or in diseases where patchy defects in microcirculation occur (such as sepsis), diffusion defects are more important. This distinction may have therapeutic implications that may underlie some of the inconsistencies in experimental data in critically ill patients. Clearly, if convective transport is impaired, measures designed to improve global $\dot{D}O_2$ are appropriate, and a relationship will be seen between increasing $\dot{D}O_2$ and increasing $\dot{V}O_2$. Conversely, if diffusive oxygen transport is impaired, increasing $\dot{D}O_2$ would not be expected to affect $\dot{V}O_2$; treatment aimed at the underlying pathological process would be warranted (9).

Reviewing the available theoretical and animal evidence,

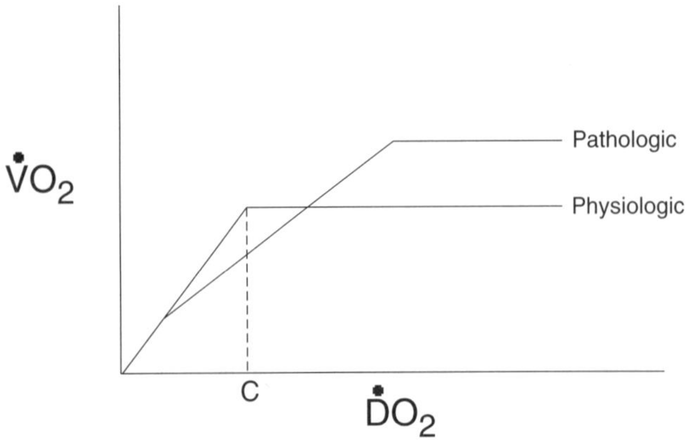

Figure 20.1. The biphasic relationship between oxygen delivery ($\dot{D}O_2$) and oxygen consumption ($\dot{V}O_2$) is similar in physiological and pathological situations. C, critical oxygen delivery.

the relationship between $\dot{D}O_2$ and $\dot{V}O_2$ seems to be clearcut. However, human experience in health and disease is more heterogeneous, and conclusions are difficult to draw for a number of reasons. First, the relationship between the two variables is demand-led, and $\dot{D}O_2$ will increase if possible to match increases in $\dot{V}O_2$. Pooling data from numerous patients with differing levels of sedation/anesthesia, differing diseases, differing temperatures, differing nutritional states, and differing respiratory work (in other words, grossly different metabolic requirements) is fraught with hazard. Furthermore, monitoring global indices of $\dot{D}O_2$ and $\dot{V}O_2$ may be inaccurate, whatever method is chosen (see below). Finally, global measures may not reflect what is happening at the microcirculatory or cellular level.

Shibutani et al. (10) studied anesthetized patients before cardiopulmonary bypass (CPB). A biphasic relationship (Fig. 20.1) was noted between $\dot{D}O_2$ and $\dot{V}O_2$ with a critical point at 330 mL/min/m^2 and with an ERO_2 of 0.33, and the same group showed similar results post-CPB (11). However, there were very few data points per patient, the ERO_2 was much lower than that seen in animals, and there was no attempt to account for differences between patients. A critical point has been identified in other patients. Ronco et al. (12) studied critically ill patients during withdrawal of life support and found a critical point of 150–170 mL/min/m^2, with an ERO_2 of 0.75–0.80. Van Woerkens et al. (13) studied a Jehovah's Witness during extreme hemodilution and found a critical point of 184 mL/min/m^2 at an ERO_2 of 0.44. Although the figures vary, presumably because of different metabolic and pathological states, the basic concept of a biphasic response with a critical point below which supply-dependent $\dot{V}O_2$ is seen was confirmed.

PATHOLOGICAL OXYGEN SUPPLY DEPENDENCY

By contrast, studies in critically ill patients have shown a different relationship between $\dot{D}O_2$ and $\dot{V}O_2$ in which no critical point and no plateau of $\dot{V}O_2$ with increasing $\dot{D}O_2$ could be demonstrated. This is termed pathological supply dependency and has been demonstrated in a wide range of disease processes including sepsis, adult respiratory distress syndrome, heart failure, and chronic obstructive pulmonary disease (14–17). Other investigators have suggested that pathological supply dependency is associated with increased lactate levels (18–21). This body of experimental evidence implies that in patients with a range of different pathologies, $\dot{D}O_2$ is less than that needed to supply the metabolic needs of the body, even though absolute levels may be normal or supranormal. It also implies that increasing $\dot{D}O_2$ further would allow $\dot{V}O_2$ to increase, potentially leading to decreased mortality by improving cellular oxygenation. Bihari et al. (22) studied critically ill patients, comparing them with normal volunteers, and measured $\dot{D}O_2$ and $\dot{V}O_2$. Having maximized $\dot{D}O_2$ and $\dot{V}O_2$ by conventional treatment in the critically ill patients, they then gave prostacyclin, an arterial vasodilator. Control subjects and survivors increased their $\dot{V}O_2$ by about 5%, whereas nonsurvivors increased their $\dot{V}O_2$ by about 19%. This was interpreted as showing that control subjects and survivors were on the plateau portion of a biphasic $\dot{D}O_2$–$\dot{V}O_2$ relationship, whereas nonsurvivors exhibited pathological supply dependency. The question remained, however, as to whether manipulating oxygen flux variables would lead to a survival benefit or whether pathological supply dependency was a marker for advanced disease processes with a high mortality.

Vincent and De Backer (23) reviewed the arguments against the concept of pathological supply dependency. First, the observed covariance between $\dot{D}O_2$ and $\dot{V}O_2$ is expected physiologically. As noted above, $\dot{D}O_2$ increases as oxygen demand increases physiologically in response to stress, exercise, infection, and so on. It is therefore important to ensure in studies that patients are strictly comparable (with respect to degree of sedation and paralysis, whether ventilated or not, etc.). Studies using pooled data from many patients should be interpreted with caution. Second, inotropic agents may alter cellular metabolism directly (24, 25). However, dobutamine does not cause significant increases in $\dot{V}O_2$ when given to critically ill patients who are hemodynamically stable (26–28). Finally, it has been said that measurement errors may cause false correlation between $\dot{D}O_2$ and $\dot{V}O_2$, and the whole concept of pathological supply dependency is a chimera. Specifically, doubt has been cast on the validity of the reverse Fick method of calculating $\dot{V}O_2$, because the use of CO as a common variable in the calculation of $\dot{D}O_2$ and $\dot{V}O_2$ may cause mathematical "coupling" (i.e., a spurious association between the variables). These issues are considered below. Vincent and De Backer (23) concluded that pathological supply dependency did exist, but caution in applying the concept to patient treatment was warranted.

Pinsky (29) took the opposite view. He noted three principles that should be adhered to in any research on this topic. The issue of mathematical coupling and demand-led changes in oxygen supply can be resolved by minimizing muscular and sympathetic activity and measuring $\dot{D}O_2$ and $\dot{V}O_2$ by independent means. Finally, to ascertain true covariance, multiple data pairs should be collected for each subject over a wide range of $\dot{D}O_2$ values. Few studies adhere to the above principles (30–32), and none demonstrates pathological supply dependency.

How to resolve these conflicting positions? It is apparent that when tissue hypoperfusion occurs, anaerobic metabolism supervenes and lactate is produced. A degree of "oxygen debt" occurs, which can be reversed if resuscitation occurs before cell death. $\dot{V}O_2$ will rise to supranormal levels, as will $\dot{D}O_2$, if possible, according to the normal physiological linkage noted above. This physiological relationship may be interpreted as "pathological supply dependency" until $\dot{V}O_2$ returns to normal levels (33). These changes in global indices of oxygen flux obscure the fact that the critical $\dot{D}O_2$ varies depending on which organ is studied, the disease state, and extent of treatment (34–38). In other words, some areas of the body, notably the gut, may exhibit supply dependency even though global indices are normal (37) or supranormal.

THERAPEUTIC IMPLICATIONS OF OXYGEN SUPPLY DEPENDENCY

GLOBAL OXYGEN FLUX

Many studies have addressed the therapeutic implications of the above experimental data. The underlying theory is that by raising $\dot{D}O_2$ to "supranormal" levels, not only will global oxygen demand be satisfied, but regional hypoperfusion will be mitigated. Shoemaker et al. (39) first noted physiological variables, including oxygen flux variables, that correlated with outcome. Subsequently, the same group prospectively tested a treatment algorithm in postoperative patients designed to achieve supranormal oxygen flux variables (40). They showed a marked reduction in mortality. A later study from the same group (41) randomized surgical patients into three groups: one group received postoperative therapy based on hemodynamic data derived from a central venous pressure (CVP) catheter, one group had a pulmonary artery catheter (PAC) placed and therapy was titrated to achieve normal values, and the third group had a PAC placed and therapy titrated to supranormal values. The third group had lower mortality, fewer complications, less duration of ventilation, and a shorter intensive care unit stay. No difference was seen between the first two groups. This study was criticized because no severity of illness score was used, making it difficult to compare groups. Some control patients achieved supranormal values anyway, and even in the protocol group, supranormal oxygen flux variables were achieved for only short time periods. This may suggest that rather than demonstrating pathological supply dependency, survivors merely repaid the oxygen debt accumulated during the initial insult and the increased $\dot{V}O_2$ and $\dot{D}O_2$ were physiological, not pathological.

In any case, a number of studies in surgical, medical, and critically ill patients were performed over the next 4 years. They were reviewed comprehensively by Erstad (42), who noted a survival advantage in only two studies (41, 43). Both studies involved high-risk surgical patients, and therapy was often instituted preoperatively. The other studies showed no survival advantage when supranormal therapy was used. Typical was Yu et al.'s study (44) that showed no difference between groups on an intention to treat basis. However, subset analysis showed significantly reduced mortality in those patients who achieved supranormal goals, irrespective of treatment. In other words, the ability to increase $\dot{D}O_2$ and $\dot{V}O_2$ was a marker for survival rather than the cause. More recently, a large trial in 56 intensive care units in Italy (45) demonstrated no mortality difference between groups when standard hemodynamic therapy, therapy designed to achieve supranormal goals, and therapy designed to achieve normal mixed venous oxygen saturation ($S\bar{v}O_2$) were compared.

The relationship between $\dot{D}O_2$ and $\dot{V}O_2$ is complex. It is apparent from animal and human experiments that a biphasic relationship exists, with a critical $\dot{D}O_2$ below which $\dot{V}O_2$ is supply-dependent. In some patients, this supply dependency occurs at much higher values of $\dot{D}O_2$. Whether this is a physiological response to increased oxygen demand (either because of a "hypermetabolic" state or to repay an oxygen debt) or is truly a "pathological" supply dependency caused by disrupted conductive or diffusive oxygen transport systems is a moot point. If $\dot{D}O_2$ does not increase to meet demand, anaerobiosis occurs, and mortality is increased.

REGIONAL OXYGEN FLUX

Although $\dot{D}O_2$ must be increased to match demand, no consistent therapeutic benefit has been shown in clinical trials when supranormal oxygen flux variables have been achieved. This may be a reflection that regional hypoperfusion can be present when global indices are normal. Monitoring regional perfusion by measuring gut intramucosal pH (pHi) has been suggested to be a more accurate endpoint to allow therapy to be titrated. Multiple studies (46–51) have demonstrated that gastric pHi predicts outcome after cardiac surgery, trauma, acute circulatory failure, orthotopic liver transplantation, and in critically ill patients. Ivatury et al. (52) compared pHi with global indicators of oxygen flux as outcome predictors in patients undergoing major trauma surgery. Although there was no difference in mortality between the groups (the study being too small to show such a difference), it was noteworthy that 44 of 57 patients had pHi optimized within 24 hours. Of these, 3 died of multiple organ failure compared with 7 of 13 whose pHi remained persistently low. Again, the restoration of pHi served as a marker of, and not an explanation for, survival. The study was started after entry to the intensive care unit, which was 10.5–11.5 hours after admission, and after (prolonged) surgery. Perhaps earlier monitoring to allow more aggressive treatment would be beneficial.

From the above discussions, the importance of global and regional indices of oxygen flux is obvious in a broad range of operative and postoperative patients. Multiple studies have failed to show prognostic benefit from monitoring common hemodynamic variables, such as CO, heart rate, and blood pressure (39, 53–55). By contrast, it has been suggested that measurement of oxygen flux variables and evidence of global hypoperfusion (such as lactic acidosis) or regional hypoperfusion (gastric intramucosal pH) are more accurate prognostic indicators. The advantage of monitoring these variables is that if they truly reflect survival, it may be possible to intervene early during resuscitation, perioperatively or postoperatively, to titrate therapy that would minimize hypoperfusion, causing irreversible cellular damage. The evidence for and against this concept was reviewed earlier. The remainder of this chapter deals with a critical evaluation of monitors of global and regional hypoperfusion.

MONITORING OF OXYGEN FLUX VARIABLES

GLOBAL INDICES BY CALCULATION

The Fick principle states that the uptake or release of a substance by an organ is the product of the blood flow to the organ and the arterial-venous concentration difference of the substance. This principle is used to calculate CO when $\dot{V}O_2$ and the arterial-venous oxygen content differences are measured. Alternatively, the formula may be rearranged in the so-called "reverse Fick" manner (Table 20.1) to give $\dot{V}O_2$ if the other variables are measured. The various techniques of CO measurement have been well described (56) and are outside the scope of this chapter.

The most common intraoperative method to measure CO is by thermodilution after insertion of a PAC, first described in

Ganz et al. (57). Its accuracy is affected by arrhythmias, low CO states, intracardiac shunts, tricuspid regurgitation, and the phase of positive pressure ventilation and at best is ±10% (58, 59).

The most common method of measuring arterial and venous oxygen saturation (SaO_2, $S\bar{v}O_2$) is by measuring arterial or mixed venous partial pressure of oxygen (PaO_2, $P\bar{v}O_2$) in a blood gas analyzer and using standard nomograms to convert these values to SaO_2 or $S\bar{v}O_2$. This method is inaccurate because it assumes a normal position of the oxygen dissociation curve that may be shifted to the right or left by changes in temperature, acid-base balance, and 2,3-diphosphoglycerate levels (60). More accurate $SaO_2/S\bar{v}O_2$ estimations may be obtained by direct measurement using a co-oximeter, accurate to ±2%. Hgb values are measured to an accuracy of ±5%. It can be seen that the combined inaccuracy of calculated $\dot{V}O_2$ using the reverse Fick method may be about ±15%, and it has therefore been estimated that changes in $\dot{V}O_2$ of less than 20% cannot be reliably detected (61). It should also be noted that pulmonary oxygen consumption is not measured by this method. In health, pulmonary $\dot{V}O_2$ accounts for less than 5% of total $\dot{V}O_2$, but inflammatory conditions such as adult respiratory distress syndrome or pneumonia may increase that figure to 20% (62, 63).

Obviously, because the same variables are used to derive $\dot{D}O_2$ (Table 20.1), similar inaccuracies will arise. In addition to the obvious, however, mathematical coupling will occur if the same variable (in this case CO) is used when two values are compared (64). This may give spurious correlations between the two values and may explain some of the discrepancies between studies (12, 31, 65–67). Coupling as an explanation has been analyzed by Stratton et al. (68), who noted that if the change in the measured variables exceeds the error in their measurement, then it is possible to conclude that a real change has occurred. They reanalyzed the data of Powers et al. (69) and Danek et al. (15) using a correcting coefficient and found that the relationship between $\dot{D}O_2$ and $\dot{V}O_2$ held true even if the measurement errors were doubled. It is reasonable to conclude that studies in which $\dot{D}O_2$ is increased by greater than 15% are probably accurate. In addition, Vincent and De Backer (23) pointed out that a number of studies have recorded oxygen supply dependency in some patients but not others, despite similar methodologies of measurement. They noted that some studies show good agreement between direct and indirect measurements of $\dot{V}O_2$, even in critically ill patients (70–72) and concluded that coupling is a theoretical explanation for the correlation of $\dot{D}O_2$ versus $\dot{V}O_2$ but is less important than first thought.

GLOBAL INDICES BY MEASUREMENT

To avoid this controversy, it is useful to look at studies where $\dot{D}O_2$ has been calculated and $\dot{V}O_2$ has been measured directly. A number of commercially available systems use similar methodology to measure inspired and expired oxygen concentrations, carbon dioxide concentrations, and expired gas volumes, thus allowing derivation of $\dot{V}O_2$. Devices such as the Deltatrac monitor (Deltatrac, Datex, Helsinki, Finland) use paramagnetic oxygen sensors, infrared CO sensors, and volume measurements. They are accurate at high inspired oxygen fractions, high inflation pressures, and high humidity. There are multiple potential sources of error (measurements of gas concentrations, volumes, and in the complex calculations to give $\dot{V}O_2$ from the measured variables), and patients should also be "metabolically" stable for 15–20 minutes, making it less useful in rapidly changing environments. The system has been shown to be useful and accurate, with $\dot{V}O_2$ measured to an accuracy of −7–3% (mean −2.1%) (12, 63, 73). Some groups (71) found good agreement between measured and calculated oxygen flux variables. By contrast, Cohen et al. (74), using similar methodology, noted good agreement between calculated and measured $\dot{V}O_2$ during a steady state. However, when patients immediately after release of aortic cross-clamping were studied, significant disagreement was seen because of rapidly changing respiratory quotient. Hanique and colleagues (75) studied measured versus calculated oxygen flux variables in a well-designed study in the intensive care unit. The patients were metabolically and cardiovascularly stable and had $\dot{D}O_2$ increased by at least 45 mL/min/m^2 by volume loading. There was poor correlation between measured and calculated variables. Indeed, measured $\dot{V}O_2$ remained constant, whereas calculated $\dot{V}O_2$ increased (artifactually, the authors concluded). The same group (76) studied a different group of patients and concluded that although measured and calculated values for $\dot{V}O_2$ agreed well in aggregate, individual values could vary by as much as 45%. Usually, the calculated values underestimated the measured values; although pulmonary oxygen consumption has been said to explain these differences, the magnitude of the differences makes this unlikely. Also, $\dot{V}O_2$ measurements were shown to be 1.74 times more reproducible when measured rather than calculated. Although indirect calorimetry may be more accurate, its applicability to rapidly changing circumstances may be limited (74). Feustel et al. (77) attempted to evaluate continuous $\dot{D}O_2$ and CO measurements by application of the Fick principle. $S\bar{v}O_2$ was measured continuously by fiber optic PACs, SaO_2 from pulse oximetry, and $\dot{V}O_2$ by indirect calorimetry. From these measurements, CO and $\dot{D}O_2$ may be calculated using standard formulae (Table 20.1). The authors assumed that PaO_2, $P\bar{v}O_2$, and Hgb were constant. They showed (theoretically) that changes in Hgb produced little effect on $\dot{D}O_2$ values (a 10% change in Hgb produced a 0.2% change in $\dot{D}O_2$). Measurement errors are more important; errors in $\dot{V}O_2$ measurement are directly reflected in $\dot{D}O_2$ calculation, whereas a 10% error in $S\bar{v}O_2$ measurement results in a 33% error in $\dot{D}O_2$. These errors are magnified if the arteriovenous difference in oxygen content is small. The advantage of using this technique is that within-patient correlation between $\dot{D}O_2$ and $\dot{V}O_2$ may be demonstrated. This study shows that a sufficiently large reliability coefficient can be achieved only with a large range of deliveries, a high arteriovenous oxygen content difference (i.e., a low $S\bar{v}O_2$) and low error in $\dot{V}O_2$ and $S\bar{v}O_2$ measurement. Such conditions are hard to achieve clinically, and the authors recommend independent measurement of $\dot{D}O_2$.

The above methods (reverse Fick or indirect calorimetry) are both complex and invasive. Noninvasive monitoring is most commonly used intraoperatively to assess routine hemodynamic and respiratory variables. Pulse oximetry is now a standard intraoperative monitor. It has been shown to reliably indicate hypoxemia (78), although limitations due to loss of signal, abnormal Hgbs, or other factors are well known (79–81). Shoemaker et al. (82) assessed more comprehensive noninvasive monitoring of oxygen flux variables. They studied 71 high-risk surgical patients undergoing major surgery and compared bioimpedance CO, transcutaneous oxygen tension, and saturation from pulse oximetry with invasive monitoring using a PAC. They demonstrated good agreement between invasive and noninvasive CO measurements and showed temporal patterns of noninvasive measurements that differed between survivors and nonsurvivors. They suggested that there are clear distinctions appearing early in the natural history of these patients that may identify those patients in whom aggressive and invasive monitoring may be warranted.

REGIONAL INDICES

As shock progresses, autoregulation maintains blood flow to the vital organs, at the expense of less "important" tissues such as the skin and splanchnic organs, particularly the gut. Astiz and Rackow (83) reviewed many of the lesser known (and less significant) techniques. Subcutaneous, transcutaneous, and conjunctival oxygen tension are readily measured. Values fall with either hypoxemia or tissue hypoperfusion, and trends may be used to assess adequacy of resuscitation. Quantitation is difficult, however, especially in hyperdynamic states such as sepsis. More promising is the role of gastric pHi.

The importance and scope of pHi monitoring have been covered previously. The technique involves passage of a nasogastric tube with a silicone, gas-permeable balloon attached into the stomach. The balloon is filled with saline, and after 30–60 minutes to allow equilibration, the saline is aspirated and the partial pressure of CO_2 that has diffused into the saline is measured. A conversion factor accounts for incomplete equilibration, and the corrected PCO_2 value is substituted into the Henderson-Hasselbalch equation to give a value for pHi. There are significant problems with this method, including the long time period necessary for equilibration, the requisite medical and nursing effort involved, errors in measuring PCO_2 in saline, errors introduced by systemic bicarbonate administration, and the presence of acid, bacteria, and stool in the stomach (84). Knichwitz et al. (85) attempted to address many of these problems using a new device to measure pHi by incorporating a fiber optic PCO_2 sensor into a nasogastric tube to measure intraluminal PCO_2 directly and continuously. They found that measured values reached actual values very rapidly. Interestingly, the difference between directly measured PCO_2 and that measured simultaneously with tonometry was almost exactly equivalent to the correction factor alluded to above. Further studies are necessary to define its utility in the critically ill patient with mesenteric hypoperfusion, but the concept of low cost, reusable, minimally invasive measurement of the adequacy of gut perfusion remains intriguing.

BALANCE BETWEEN $\dot{D}O_2$ AND $\dot{V}O_2$

The above techniques measure $\dot{D}O_2$ and $\dot{V}O_2$ with varying degrees of accuracy, but as is clear from the earlier discussion, it is not absolute levels of oxygen flux variables that matter but rather their temporal course and whether $\dot{D}O_2$ is able to satisfy oxygen demand.

One way is to measure oxygen flux variables as above and then perform an "oxygen flux" challenge, in which the response of $\dot{V}O_2$ to an increase in $\dot{D}O_2$ is seen. $\dot{D}O_2$ may be increased by fluid loading, alterations in positive end expiratory pressure, or using vasoactive or inotropic drugs (86). Obviously, factors affecting oxygen demand such as temperature, sedation, paralysis, and so on must be kept constant; if $\dot{V}O_2$ increases in response to an increase in $\dot{D}O_2$, particularly if there is lactic acidosis, further increases in $\dot{D}O_2$ may be warranted.

Measurement of $S\bar{v}O_2$ levels may also be helpful. Theoretically, if oxygen demand is held constant, then $S\bar{v}O_2$ is inversely related to $\dot{D}O_2$, and levels above 60% are indicative of adequate tissue perfusion. Critical levels of $S\bar{v}O_2$ are higher with severe anemia than with hypoxemia (presumably because of viscosity-related improvements in microvascular flow) (2, 7). However, inaccuracies may arise in sepsis, arterial-venous fistulae, cirrhosis, left-to-right cardiac shunts, peripheral shunts, cyanide poisoning, hypothermia, unintentional wedging of the PAC, and rapid withdrawal of arterialized blood from the PAC (87), causing high $S\bar{v}O_2$ despite hemodynamic compromise. In the sick patient, too many variables are involved to allow precise diagnosis with a low $S\bar{v}O_2$, and it may be best regarded as an early warning of an imbalance between $\dot{D}O_2$ and $\dot{V}O_2$ (88–91). This is particularly so where defects in peripheral oxygen extraction occur such as septic shock and liver failure, where evidence of lactic acidosis may be seen with high $S\bar{v}O_2$ levels (92, 93).

When $\dot{D}O_2$ is insufficient to meet oxygen needs, anaerobic metabolism supervenes. Mizock and Falk (4) reviewed the current body of knowledge concerning lactic acidosis in critical illness. They noted that either global or regional hypoperfusion may cause lactic acidosis. Numerous studies have documented increased mortality with increased lactate levels; for example, Weil and Afifi (94) noted mortality increased from 10% to 90% as lactate levels at presentation increased from 2.0 to 8.0 μmol/L. Falling lactate levels also correlate with effective treatment. Vincent et al. (95) showed that those patients whose lactate fell by more than 5% in the first hour of treatment had a better prognosis than did those patients whose lactate did not fall. However, for lactic acidosis to occur, the production of lactic acid must exceed the metabolic capacity of the liver, kidneys, and skeletal muscle. If this does not occur, significant regional hypoperfusion may be present with normal lactate levels.

SUMMARY

In summary, the relationship between $\dot{D}O_2$ and $\dot{V}O_2$ is complex. In health, the homeostatic system is "demand-led." If oxygen demand increases, either $\dot{D}O_2$, oxygen extraction, or both increase to supply oxygen needs. Much controversy has been engendered over the years by the concept of pathological supply dependency. Studies that used independent measures of $\dot{D}O_2$ and $\dot{V}O_2$ have mostly failed to show such a relationship, and therapeutic trials using supranormal goals have given equivocal results. However, it is clear that in many surgical and critically ill patients, $\dot{V}O_2$ is raised above normal, presumably reflecting either hypermetabolism or repayment of an "oxygen debt" from a period of hypoperfusion. It is key in managing patients to intervene early and effectively to match $\dot{D}O_2$ with oxygen demand.

Oxygen flux variables may be measured noninvasively, as a trend, or invasively with varying degrees of accuracy. It is important to understand the limitations of the monitoring devices and use them appropriately. Global monitoring is useful, but newer devices are being developed that will allow measurement of regional tissue perfusion (e.g., pHi) in selected patients.

REFERENCES

1. Vincent JL. The relationship between oxygen demand, oxygen uptake, and oxygen supply. Intensive Care Med 1990;16(Suppl. 2):S145-S148.
2. Cain SM. Oxygen delivery and uptake in dogs during anemic and hypoxic hypoxia. J Appl Physiol 1977;42:228–234.
3. Samsel RW, Schumacker PT. Oxygen delivery to tissues. Eur Respir J 1991;4:1258–1267.
4. Mizock BA, Falk JL. Lactic acidosis in critical illness. Crit Care Med 1992;20:80–93.
5. Leach RM, Treacher DF. The relationship between oxygen delivery and consumption. Dis Mon 1994;40:301–368.
6. Gutierrez G, Pohil RJ, Strong R. Effect of flow on oxygen consumption during progressive hypoxemia. J Appl Physiol 1988;65:601–607.
7. Cain SM. Appearance of excess lactate in anesthetized dogs during anemic and hypoxic hypoxia. J Appl Physiol 1965;209:604–610.
8. Schumacker PT, Samsel RW. Analysis of oxygen delivery and uptake relationships in the Krogh tissue model. J Appl Physiol 1989;67: 1234–1244.
9. Knox JB. Oxygen consumption-oxygen delivery dependence on adult respiratory distress syndrome. New Horiz 1993;1:381–387.
10. Shibutani K, Komatsu T, Kubal K, Sanchala V, Kumar V, Bizzarri DV. Critical level of oxygen delivery in anesthetized man. Crit Care Med 1983;11:640–643.
11. Komatsu K, Shibutani K, Okamoto K, et al. Critical level of oxygen delivery after cardiopulmonary bypass. Crit Care Med 1987;15:194–197.
12. Ronco JJ, Fenwick JC, Tweeddale MG, et al. Identification of the critical oxygen delivery for anaerobic metabolism in critically ill septic and non-septic humans. JAMA 1993;270:1724–1730.
13. Van Woerkens EC, Trouwborst A, van Lanschot JJ. Profound hemodilution: what is the critical level of hemodilution at which oxygen delivery-dependent oxygen consumption starts in an anesthetized human? Anesth Analg 1992;75:818–821.
14. Haupt MT, Gilbert EM, Carlson RW. Fluid loading increases oxygen consumption in septic patients with lactic acidosis. Am Rev Respir Dis 1985;131:912–916.
15. Danek SJ, Lynch JP, Weg JG, Dantzker DR. The dependence of oxygen uptake on oxygen delivery in the adult respiratory distress syndrome. Am Rev Respir Dis 1980;122:387–395.
16. Mohsenifar Z, Amin D, Jasper AC, Shah PK, Koerner SK. Dependence of oxygen consumption on oxygen delivery in patients with chronic congestive cardiac failure. Chest 1987;92:447–450.
17. Brent BN, Matthay RA, Mahler DA, Berger HJ, Zaret BL, Lister G. Relationship between oxygen uptake and oxygen transport in stable patients with chronic obstructive pulmonary disease. Am Rev Respir Dis 1984;129:682–686.
18. Gilbert EM, Haupt MT, Mandanas RY, Huaringa AJ, Carlson RW. The effect of fluid loading, blood transfusion and catecholamine infusion on oxygen delivery and consumption in patients with sepsis. Am Rev Respir Dis 1986;134:873–878.
19. Vincent JL, Roman A, De Backer D, Kahn RJ. Oxygen uptake/supply dependency: effects of short term dobutamine infusion. Am Rev Respir Dis 1990;142:2–7.
20. Fenwick JC, Dodek PM, Ronco JJ, Phang PT, Wiggs B, Russell JA. Increased concentrations of lactate predict pathological dependence of oxygen consumption on oxygen delivery in patients with adult respiratory distress syndrome. J Crit Care 1990;5:81–87.

21. Kruse JA, Haupt MT, Puri VK, Carlson RW. Lactate levels as predictors of the relationship between oxygen delivery and oxygen consumption in ARDS. Chest 1990;98:959–962.
22. Bihari D, Smithies M, Gimson A, Tinker J. The effects of vasodilation with prostacyclin on oxygen delivery and uptake in critically ill patients. N Engl J Med 1987;317:397–403.
23. Vincent JL, De Backer D. Oxygen uptake/oxygen supply dependency: fact or fiction? Acta Anaesthesiol Scand 1995;39(Suppl. 107):229–237.
24. Bhatt SB, Hutchinson RC, Tomlinson B, Oh TE, Mak M. Effect of dobutamine on oxygen supply and uptake in healthy volunteers. Br J Anaesth 1992;69:298–303.
25. Green CJ, Frazer RS, Underhill S, Maycock P, Fairhurst JA, Campbell IT. Metabolic effects of dobutamine in normal man. Clin Sci 1992;82:77–83.
26. Silverman HJ, Tuma P. Gastric tonometry in patients with sepsis. Effects of dobutamine infusions and packed red blood cell transfusions. Chest 1992;102:184–188.
27. De Backer D, Berre J, Zhang H, Vincent JL. Relationship between oxygen uptake and oxygen delivery in septic patients: effects of prostacyclin vs dobutamine. Crit Care Med 1993;21:1658–1664.
28. Ronco JJ, Fenwick JC, Wiggs BR, Phang PT, Russell JA, Tweeddale MG. Oxygen consumption is independent of increases in oxygen delivery by dobutamine in septic patients who have normal or increased concentration of plasma lactate. Am Rev Respir Dis 1993;147:25–31.
29. Pinsky MR. Beyond global oxygen supply-demand relations: in search of measures of dysoxia. Intensive Care Med 1994;20:1–3.
30. Annat G, Viale J-P, Percival C, Froment M, Motin J. Oxygen delivery and uptake in the adult respiratory distress syndrome. Am Rev Respir Dis 1986;133:999–1001.
31. Ronco JJ, Phang PT, Walley KR, Wiggs B, Fenwick JC, Russell JA. Oxygen consumption is independent of changes in oxygen delivery in severe adult respiratory distress syndrome. Am Rev Respir Dis 1991;143: 1267–1273.
32. Vermeij CG, Feenstra BW, Adrichem WJ, Bruining HA. Independent oxygen uptake and oxygen delivery in septic and post-operative patients. Chest 1991;99:1438–1443.
33. Fahey JT, Lister G. Oxygen transport in low cardiac output states. J Crit Care 1987;2:288–305.
34. Pinsky MR, Matuschak GM. Cardiovascular determinants of the hemodynamic response to acute endotoxemia in the dog. J Crit Care 1986;1: 18–31.
35. Rasmussen I, Arvidsson D, Zak A, Haglund U. Splanchnic and total body oxygen consumption in experimental fecal peritonitis in pigs: effects of dextran and Iloprost. Circ Shock 1992;36:299–306.
36. Schlichtig R, Klions HA, Kramer DJ, Nemoto EM. Hepatic dysoxia commences during oxygen supply dependence. J Appl Physiol 1992;72: 1499–1505.
37. Fink MP, Kaups KL, Wang H, Rothschild HR. Maintenance of superior mesenteric arterial perfusion prevents increased intestinal permeability in endotoxic pigs. Surgery 1991;110:154–161.
38. Kobayashi S, Clemens MG. Kupffer cell exacerbation of hepatocyte hypoxia/reoxygenation injury. Circ Shock 1992;37:245–252.
39. Shoemaker WC, Montgomery ES, Kaplan E, Elwyn DH. Physiologic patterns in surviving and non-surviving shock patients. Arch Surg 1973;106:630–636.
40. Shoemaker WC, Appel PL, Waxman K, Schwartz S, Chang P. Clinical trial of survivors' cardiorespiratory patterns as therapeutic goals in critically ill postoperative patients. Crit Care Med 1982;10:398–403.
41. Shoemaker WC, Appel PL, Kram HB, Waxman K, Lee TS. Prospective trial of supranormal values of survivors as therapeutic goals in high risk surgical patients. Chest 1988;94:1176–1186.
42. Erstad BL. Oxygen transport goals in the resuscitation of critically ill patients. Ann Pharmacother 1994;28:1273–1284.
43. Boyd O, Grounds RM, Bennet ED. A randomized clinical trial of the effect of deliberate perioperative increase of oxygen delivery on mortality in high-risk surgical patients. JAMA 1993;270:2699–2707.
44. Yu M, Levy MM, Smith P, Takiguchi SA, Miyasaki A, Myers SA. Effect of maximizing oxygen delivery on morbidity and mortality rates in critically ill patients: a prospective, randomized, controlled study. Crit Care Med 1993;21:830–838.
45. Gattinoni L, Brazzi D, Pelosi P, et al. A trial of goal-oriented hemodynamic therapy in critically ill patients. N Engl J Med 1995;333: 1025–1032.
46. Marik PE. Gastric intramucosal pH. A better predictor of multiorgan dysfunction syndrome and death then oxygen derived variables in patients with sepsis. Chest 1993;104:225–229.
47. Fiddian-Green RG, Baker S. Predictive value of the stomach wall pH for complications after cardiac operations. Comparison with other monitoring. Crit Care Med 1987;15:153–156.
48. Chang MC, Cheatham ML, Nelson LD, Rutherford EJ, Morris JA. Gastric tonometry supplements information provided by systemic indicators of oxygen transport. J Trauma 1994;37:488–494.
49. Maynard N, Bihari D, Beale R, et al. Assessment of splanchnic oxygenation by gastric tonometry in patients with acute circulatory failure. JAMA 1993;270:1203–1210.
50. Downing A, Cottam S, Beard C, Potter D. Gastric intramucosal pH predicts major morbidity following orthotopic liver transplantation. Transplant Proc 1993;25:1804.
51. Gutierrez G, Palizas F, Doglio G, et al. Gastric intramucosal pH as a therapeutic index of tissue oxygenation in the critically ill. Lancet 1992;339:195–199.
52. Ivatury RR, Simon RJ, Islam S, Fueg A, Rohman M, Stahl WM. A prospective randomized study of the end points of resuscitation after major trauma: global oxygen transport indices versus organ-specific gastric mucosal pH. J Am Coll Surg 1996;183:145–154.
53. Shoemaker WC, Czer LS. Evaluation of the biological importance of various hemodynamic and oxygen transport variables. Which variables should be measured in postoperative shock? Crit Care Med 1979;7: 424–431.
54. Bland R, Shoemaker WC, Shabot M. Physiologic monitoring goals for the critically ill patient. Surg Gynecol Obstet 1987;147:833–841.
55. Gutierrez G, Bismar H, Dantzker D, Silva N. Comparison of gastric intramucosal pH with measures of oxygen transport and consumption in critically ill patients. Crit Care Med 1992;20:451–457.
56. Stanley TE III, Reves JG. Cardiovascular monitoring. In: Miller RD, ed. Anesthesia, 4th ed. New York: Churchill Livingstone, 1994:1161–1228.
57. Ganz W, Donoso R, Marcus HS, Forrester JS, Swan HJ. A new technique for measurement of cardiac output by thermodilution in man. Am J Cardiol 1971;27:392–396.
58. Levitt JM, Repolge RI. Thermodilution cardiac output: a critical analysis and review of the literature. J Surg Res 1979;27:392–404.
59. Runciman WB, Ilsely AH, Roberts JG. Thermodilution cardiac output: systematic error. Anaesth Intensive Care 1981;9:135–139.
60. Myburgh JA. Derived oxygen saturations are not clinically useful for the calculation of oxygen consumption. Anaesth Intensive Care 1992;20: 460–463.

61. Takala J, Ruokonen E. Assessment of systemic and regional oxygen delivery and consumption. In: Vincent J-L, ed. 1993 yearbook of intensive care and emergency medicine. Berlin: Springer-Verlag, 1993:413–421.
62. Light RB. Intrapulmonary oxygen consumption in experimental pneumococcal pneumonia. J Appl Physiol 1988;64:2490–2495.
63. Smithies MN, Royston B, Makita K, Konieczko K, Nunn JF. Comparison of oxygen consumption measurements: indirect calorimetry versus reversed Fick method. Crit Care Med 1991;19:1401–1406.
64. Archie JP Jr. Mathematical coupling of data: a common source of error. Ann Surg 1981;193:296–303.
65. Vermeij CG, Feenstra BW, Bruining HA. Oxygen delivery and oxygen uptake in postoperative and septic patients. Chest 1990;98:415–420.
66. Carlile PV, Gray BA. Effect of opposite changes in cardiac output and arterial PO_2 on the relationship between mixed venous PO_2 and oxygen transport. Am Rev Respir Dis 1989;140:891–898.
67. Wysocki M, Besbes M, Roupie E, Brun-Buisson C. Modification of oxygen extraction ratio by change in oxygen transport in septic shock. Chest 1992;102:221–226.
68. Stratton HH, Feustel PJ, Newell JC. Regression of calculated variables in the presence of shared measurement error. J Appl Physiol 1987;62: 2083–2093.
69. Powers SR Jr, Mannal R, Neclerio M, et al. Physiologic consequences of positive end expiratory pressure. Ann Surg 1973;178:265–272.
70. Chappell TR, Rubin LJ, Markham RV, Firth BG. Independence of oxygen consumption and systemic oxygen transport in patients with either stable pulmonary hypertension or refractory left ventricular failure. Am Rev Respir Dis 1983;128:30–33.
71. Hankeln KB, Gronemeyer R, Held A, Bohmert F. Use of continuous noninvasive measurement of oxygen consumption in patients with adult respiratory distress syndrome following shock of various etiologies. Crit Care Med 1991;19:642–649.
72. De Backer D, Moraine JJ, Berre J, Kahn RJ, Vincent JL. Effects of dobutamine on oxygen consumption in septic patients: direct vs indirect determinations. Am J Respir Crit Care Med 1994;150:95–100.
73. Ronco JJ, Phang PT.Validation of an indirect calorimeter to measure oxygen consumption in critically ill patients. J Crit Care 1991;6:36–41.
74. Cohen IL, Roberts KW, Perkins RJ, Feustel PJ, Shah DM. Fick-derived hemodynamics. Oxygen consumption measured directly vs oxygen consumption calculated from CO_2 production under steady state and dynamic conditions. Chest 1992;102:1124–1127.
75. Hanique G, Dugernier T, Laterre PF, Dougnac A, Roeseler J, Reynaert MS. Significance of pathologic oxygen supply dependency in critically ill patients: comparison between measured and calculated methods. Intensive Care Med 1994;20:12–18.
76. Hanique G, Dugernier T, Laterre PF, Roeseler J, Dougnac A, Reynaert MS. Evaluation of oxygen uptake and delivery in critically ill patients: a statistical reappraisal. Intensive Care Med 1994;20:19–26.
77. Feustel PJ, Perkins RJ, Oppenlander JE, Stratton HH, Cohen IL. Feasibility of continuous oxygen delivery and cardiac output measurement by application of the Fick principle. Am J Respir Crit Care Med 1994;149:751–758.
78. Zaune U, Knarr C, Kruselmann M, Pauli MH, Boeden G, Martin E. Value and accuracy of dual oximetry during pulmonary resections. J Cardiothorac Anesth 1990;4:441–452.
79. Severinghaus JW, Naifeh KH. Accuracy of response of six pulse oximeters to profound hypoxia. Anesthesiology 1987;67:551–558.
80. Tremper KK, Barker SJ. Pulse oximetry. Anesthesiology 1989;70: 98–108.
81. Moon RE, Camporesi EM. Respiratory monitoring. In: Miller RD, ed. Anesthesia, 4th ed. New York: Churchill Livingstone, 1994:1253–1292.
82. Shoemaker WC, Wo CC, Bishop MH, et al. Noninvasive physiologic monitoring of high risk surgical patients. Arch Surg 1996;131:732–737.
83. Astiz ME, Rackow EC. Assessing perfusion failure during circulatory shock. Crit Care Clin 1993;9:299–312.
84. Garrett SA, Pearl RG. Improved gastric tonometry for monitoring tissue perfusion: the canary sings louder. Anesth Analg 1996;83:1–3.
85. Knichwitz G, Rotker J, Brussel T, Kuhmann M, Mertes N, Mollhof T. A new method for continuous intramucosal PCO_2 measurement in the gastrointestinal tract. Anesth Analg 1996;83:6–11.
86. Soni N, Fawcett WJ, Halliday FC. Beyond the lung: oxygen delivery and tissue oxygenation. Anaesthesia 1993;48:704–711.
87. Birman H, Haq A, Hew E, Aberman A. Continuous monitoring of mixed venous oxygen saturation in hemodynamically unstable patients. Chest 1984;86:753–756.
88. Schmidt C, Frank L, Forsythe S, et al. Continuous $S\bar{v}O_2$ measurement and oxygen transport patterns in cardiac surgery patients. Crit Care Med 1984;12:523–527.
89. Norfleet EA, Watson CB. Continuous mixed venous oxygen saturation measurement: a significant advance in hemodynamic monitoring? J Clin Monit 1985;1:245–258.
90. Schweiss JF. Mixed venous hemoglobin saturation: theory and application. Int Anesthesiol Clin 1987;25:113–136.
91. Vaughn S, Puri VK. Cardiac output changes and continuous mixed venous oxygen saturation measurement in the critically ill. Crit Care Med 1988;16:495–498.
92. Astiz ME, Rackow EC, Kaufman B, Falk JL, Weil M. Relationship of oxygen delivery and mixed venous oxygenation to lactic acidosis in patients with sepsis and acute myocardial infarction. Crit Care Med 1988; 16:655–658.
93. Bakker J, Coffernils M, Leon M, Gris P, Vincent JL. Blood lactates are superior to oxygen derived variables in predicting outcome in human septic shock. Chest 1991;99:956–962.
94. Weil MH, Afifi AA. Experimental and clinical studies on lactate and pyruvate as indicators of the severity of acute circulatory failure (shock). Circulation 1970;41:989–1001.
95. Vincent JL, Dufaye B, Berre J, et al.. Serial lactate determinations during circulatory shock. Crit Care Med 1983;11:449–451.

Chapter 21

Blood Conservation Techniques in Anesthesia

JAN HEMSTAD

INTRODUCTION

There is a growing body of knowledge suggesting that the choice of anesthetic technique has an influence on surgical mortality and morbidity. One such area of concern is the influence of anesthetic choice on perioperative blood loss. The focus on blood loss has been heightened during the past decade because of a greater awareness of the risk of transferring infectious agents during homologous blood transfusion. Out of this heightened awareness has developed an attempt to evaluate the benefit of techniques, or combination of techniques, to reduce blood loss and the need for transfusion of blood products. Historically, anesthetic interventions to decrease blood loss were undertaken to improve operating conditions for the surgeon. What originated as an effort to improve the operative field has, consequently, developed into an area of clinical knowledge aimed at improving surgical outcome.

This chapter focuses on the influence of physiological techniques, such as patient positioning and ventilation mode, controlled hypotension, and the role of regional anesthesia in blood conservation.

PHYSIOLOGICAL TECHNIQUES

POSITIONING

Proper positioning of a patient for surgery may play an important role in blood conservation. The role of patient position and blood loss is best seen in spinal surgery. Because spinal surgery is most often performed in the prone position, placing the patient with support below the pelvis and shoulders leaves the abdomen free. It has been shown that by preventing pressure on the abdominal wall, the pressure on the vena cava is minimized, thus reducing blood flow through collateral vertebral venous plexuses, known as Batson's plexus (1). The result is a reduction in blood loss. To assist in minimizing abdominal pressure, it has also been suggested that complete paralysis be maintained (2). An additional technique pertinent to spinal surgery, as well as other surgical procedures, especially those involving the head and neck (3), is raising the operative site above the level of the heart. Venous return is thereby promoted, reducing blood pooling at the surgical site. The risk of venous air embolism, however, must be considered with the latter technique.

VENTILATION

During mechanical ventilation, airway pressure increases, resulting in an increase in mean intrathoracic pressure. Because venous return to the thorax is dependent on the difference between peripheral venous pressure and intrathoracic pressure, venous return is, consequently, impeded during inspiratory cycle of mechanical ventilation (4). There is evidence that elevation in intrathoracic pressures during mechanical ventilation raises the peripheral vascular pressure enough to affect blood loss (5–7). Spontaneous ventilation, on the other hand, assists venous return because of reduced mean intrathoracic pressure with inspiration. The hemodynamic differences, therefore, between spontaneous and mechanical ventilation can reduce intraoperative blood loss (5, 6).

Another aspect of ventilation affecting venous return is expiratory and inspiratory resistance. Maintaining expiratory resistance as low as possible assists venous return by reducing intrathoracic pressure (8). Appropriate management of reactive airway disease, appropriate setting of the inspiratory-to-expiratory ratio, allowing adequate expiration time, and maintaining unobstructed expiratory flows (e.g., avoiding kinks or buildup of secretions in the endotracheal tube) may be beneficial in reducing blood loss. Interestingly, an inspiratory-resistive load that is adapted to an individual patient produces an increase in stroke volume by enhancing venous return and also may be beneficial in blood conservation (8).

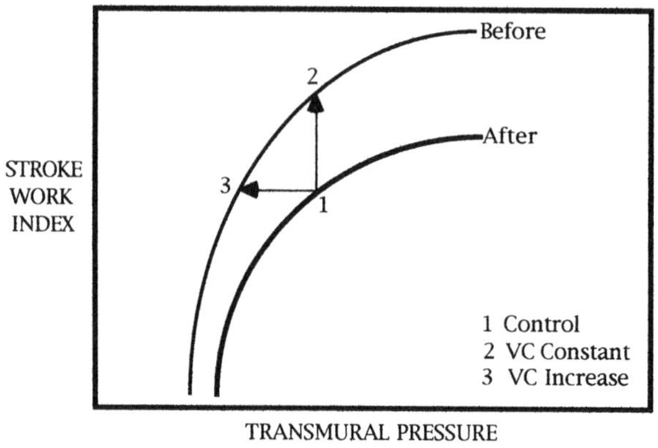

Figure 21.1. Effect of a vasodilator on the Frank-Starling relationship. A decrease in afterload shifts the curve (heavy line) to the left (light line). If transmural pressure (preload) remains constant, the cardiac output will increase; if the decrease in afterload is also associated with a decrease in preload (transmural pressure), then cardiac output will remain constant. VC, venous compliance. (Reprinted by permission from Fahmy NM. Indications and contraindications for deliberate hypotension with a review of its cardiovascular effects. Int Anesth Clin 1979;17:175–187.)

PHARMACOLOGICAL TECHNIQUES

PHYSIOLOGY OF BLOOD LOSS REDUCTION DURING CONTROLLED HYPOTENSION AND REGIONAL ANESTHESIA

In exploring the physiology of controlled hypotension, it is important to determine what aspect of the affected cardiovascular system is responsible for reducing blood loss. Are the beneficial effects of hypotension correlated best with the cardiac output of the heart or the pressure/flow characteristics of the arterial tree and/or venous capacitance system? The question regarding cardiac output was demonstrated by Sivarajan et al. (9). It had previously been suggested that cardiac output correlated with dryness of the surgical field (10). Sivarajan et al. studied 20 subjects undergoing bilateral mandibular osteotomies, randomly assigned to receive trimethaphan or sodium nitroprusside. With no statistical difference in the duration and the extent of mean arterial blood pressure reduction or the total administered intravenous fluids during controlled hypotension (mean arterial pressures of approximately 50–60 mm Hg), blood loss between the two groups was the same. When compared with control values for the same group, however, trimethaphan produced a 37% decrease in cardiac output, whereas sodium nitroprusside produced a 27% increase. Associated with these changes in cardiac output and mean arterial pressure, trimethaphan decreased heart rate and left total peripheral vascular resistance unchanged, whereas sodium nitroprusside caused a significant rise in heart rate and reduced total peripheral vascular resistance. It is apparent, therefore, that mean arterial pressure correlates with reduced blood loss during controlled hypotension and not cardiac output.

As pointed out by Fahmy (11), however, the hemodynamic responses to vasodilators such as sodium nitroprusside or trimethaphan depend on ventricular function as defined by the Frank-Starling relationship (Fig. 21.1) and on the effects of the anesthetic agents used. Controlled hypotension with sodium nitroprusside, for example, has been associated with either no

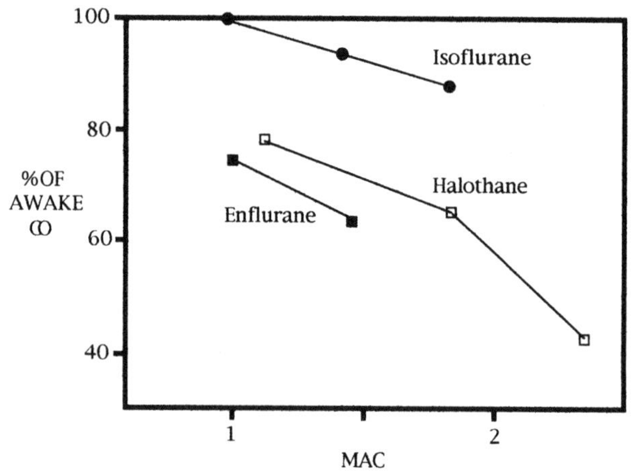

Figure 21.2. Percent change from awake values of cardiac output in anesthetized normocapnic volunteers. CO, cardiac output; MAC, minimum alveolar concentration. (Reprinted by permission from Eger EI. Isoflurane: review. Anesthesiology 1981;55:559.)

change (12, 13) or an increase in cardiac output (9). The discrepancies can be explained by the dose response of halothane on cardiac output and baroreceptor reflexes. Halothane not only decreases cardiac output in a dose-dependent fashion (Fig. 21.2) but also attenuates baroreceptor reflexes. Depending on the dosing, therefore, halothane may affect the reflex increase in heart rate produced by sodium nitroprusside (11). Further insight can be gained by looking at the cardiovascular effects of sodium nitroprusside in the awake and halothane-anesthetized states as shown in Fig. 21.3.

In a similar fashion, μ-receptor opiods, such as fentanyl, which have central vagal effects (14), may also offset the re-

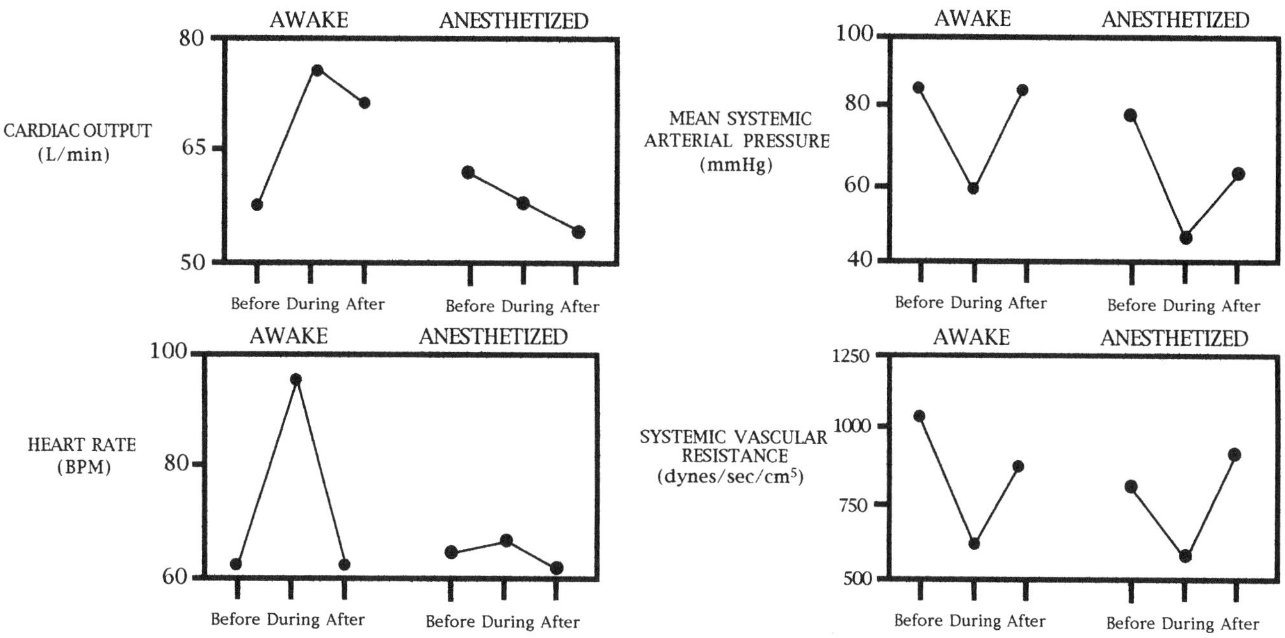

Figure 21.3. Systemic hemodynamic effects of sodium nitroprusside in the awake state and during anesthesia (halothane-oxygen). (Reprinted by permission from Fahmy NM. Indications and contraindications for deliberate hypotension with a review of its cardiovascular effects. Int Anesth Clin 1979;17:175–187.)

flex increase heart rate of sodium nitroprusside. The resultant cardiac outputs, therefore, will depend not only on the lowered afterload and/or preload caused by the hypotensive agent but also on the changes in heart rate, peripheral vascular hemodynamics, and myocardial effects caused by the dosage and selection of anesthetic agents.

The effect of cardiac output on blood loss has also been evaluated by Sharrock et al. (15) under epidural hypotensive anesthesia. Under equally hypotensive epidural anesthesia with mean arterial pressures of 50–60 mm Hg, Sharrock et al. (15) found in 30 patients undergoing total hip arthroplasty and randomly assigned to low-dose epinephrine infusions significantly higher cardiac outputs than those assigned to phenylephrine infusions. Blood loss, however, was not significantly different between groups.

The literature seems to have established that cardiac output is not associated with reduction in intraoperative blood loss. The other proposed explanations are reductions in arterial and/or venous pressure. Mean arterial pressure, however, is most likely the main hemodynamic change influencing blood loss during surgery (6, 15–17). The importance of arterial pressure is demonstrated by Sharrock et al. (16) where intraoperative blood loss was found to be significantly related to average systolic pressure. In this study, 40 patients undergoing total hip arthroplasty during epidural anesthesia were randomly assigned to two pressure categories: 50 ± 5 or 60 ± 5 mm Hg. Both by quantitative and qualitative measurement, blood loss was significantly greater in the 60-mm Hg group. Blood loss, however, was not significantly related to average intraoperative central venous pressure in the two groups. As pointed out by Sharrock et al. (16), although they demonstrated a difference in blood loss with the two degrees of hypotension, the relationship of mean arterial pressure to blood loss is still not entirely clear. Whether the relationship is linear or curvilinear needs yet to be demonstrated.

The relationship, however, between mean arterial pressure reduction and blood loss is not always consistent. The studies mentioned above involve orthopedic surgery where the best documentation of blood conservation with controlled hypotension has been made due to the extent of blood loss associated with these procedures. Fromme et al. (18) evaluated two levels of hypotension (75–85 and 55–60 mm Hg) compared with a control group with a mean arterial blood pressure of 90–100 mm Hg in orthognathic surgery. No reduction in blood loss at the two levels of hypotension compared with the control group was demonstrated. It is likely, therefore, that other factors, such as type of surgery and positioning, may be more important in determining blood loss in certain types of surgery.

Blood loss during controlled hypotension is at least in part dependent on venous pressure (5, 19). Fahmy (19) studied 91 patients undergoing total hip replacement under general anesthesia who received either nitroglycerine or sodium nitroprusside to induce hypotension. In his study, systolic blood pressures were decreased to comparable levels with the two drugs (73–76 mm Hg); mean and diastolic pressures, however, were significantly higher with nitroglycerine (60–63 and 52–55 mm Hg, respectively) than with sodium nitroprusside (52–54 and 42–44 mm Hg, respectively). On the other hand, right atrial pressure was significantly lower with nitroglycerin than with sodium nitroprusside, the difference most likely due to the greater dilatation of venous capacitance induced by nitroglycerine. Despite the slightly higher mean arterial pressure in the nitroglycerine group, the mean intraoperative blood loss was 578 ± 82 mL in the nitroglycerine group compared with 762 ± 93 mL in the sodium nitroprusside group. This difference was statistically significant. In a similar study comparing isoflurane and sodium nitroprusside as hypotensive agents (17) where mean hypotensive arterial pressures and right atrial pressures were comparable, blood loss was the same.

The potential contribution of venous pressure to blood loss can be further understood from studies using epidural anesthesia. Modig et al. (5, 6) demonstrated that both intraoperative and postoperative blood loss is significantly lower during epidural anesthesia compared with general anesthesia in patients undergoing total hip replacement. Within their study, two general anesthesia subgroups were also compared: an inhalation (spontaneous ventilation) anesthesia group and an intermittent positive pressure ventilation (IPPV) group. The inhalation anesthesia group had a significantly lower blood loss than the IPPV group. The differences in blood loss are attributed to the greater drop in mean arterial pressure associated with epidural anesthesia and a significant reduction in right atrial and peripheral venous pressures—the epidural group having the largest reductions and the inhalation anesthesia group having a greater reduction than the IPPV group. The reduction in arterial pressure is thought to result in reduced arterial bleeding. Likewise, the reduction in central venous and peripheral venous pressure lessens venous oozing at the surgical site. The differences in spontaneous and controlled ventilation are considered the result of elevated intrathoracic pressures with IPPV. In conjunction with reduced central and peripheral venous pressures during epidural anesthesia, it has also been shown that arterial and venous flow and venous capacitance are increased (20–23). It is likely, therefore, that pressure and not flow is the major determinant of blood loss.

The venous pressure, however, will be influenced by other factors besides the vasodilator effects of anesthetics and hypotensive agents. In total hip arthroplasty, for example, the lateral decubitus position places the surgical site above the level of the right atrium. The actual peripheral venous pressure at the surgical site will consequently be less than central venous pressure. This may account for the lack of correlation between central venous pressure and blood loss observed in some studies (16). It has also been suggested that regional anesthesia reduces blood loss more than general anesthesia despite similar reductions in blood pressure (24, 25). This observation, however, is not a consistent finding (26).

CONTROLLED HYPOTENSION

History

The clinical practice of controlled hypotension in surgery was first introduced in the 1940s by Gardner (27) in which he used the technique of hemorrhagic hypotension. Hypotension with the use of high subarachnoid block was also proposed (28). Attempts to achieve a practical approach to controlling blood loss were actively sought at this time in anesthetic and surgical history to improve operative conditions. Anesthesia at the time was maintained with agents such as chloroform, ether, cyclopropane, or trichloroethylene. Hypertension with systolic blood pressures above 200 mm Hg was not uncommon (29). It was not until the 1950s, however, with the introduction of ganglionic blockers and the 1960s with direct acting vasodilators that controlled hypotension became a practical and accepted approach to reducing intraoperative blood loss (30). In current anesthesia practice, many pharmacological techniques are used to induce controlled hypotension (Table 21.1).

Blood Conservation in Surgical Subspecialties

The best documentation that the technique of controlled hypotension reduces blood loss has come from studies in orthopedic surgery, particularly total hip replacement. Sollevi (31) in 1988 reviewed the literature for controlled prospective studies back to 1974. Thirteen studies were cited in his review. The collective findings were that patients undergoing total hip replacement, irrespective of the anesthetic technique, had a reduction in blood loss of approximately 50%. He also noted that there were no major differences in blood loss despite the variability in hypotensive levels used in the various studies. In his review, Sollevi also looked at studies involving scoliosis, orthognathic, and cancer (cystectomy) surgeries. All demonstrated significant blood loss reductions except one evaluating orthognathic procedures.

The result of hypotensive techniques to control blood loss in spinal surgery is similar to that found in total hip arthroplasty. In both prospective (32, 33) and retrospective (34–36) studies between 1982 and 1992, reduction in blood loss using controlled hypotension has been demonstrated between 27% and 42%.

In pelvic surgery, the benefits of controlled hypotension in blood conservation are also apparent. In a retrospective study of patients undergoing radical cystectomy, Ahlering et al. (37)

TABLE 21.1. PHARMACOLOGICAL TECHNIQUES IN CONTROLLED HYPOTENSION

- Neuraxial blockade
  - Subarachnoid block
  - Epidural block
- Inhalation anesthetics
  - Isoflurane
  - Halothane
  - Enflurane
- Intravenous medications
  - Beta-adrenergic blockers
    - Esmolol
    - Propranolol
    - Labetalol
  - Alpha-adrenergic blocking agents
    - Phentolamine
  - Calcium channel blockers
    - Nicardipine
    - Diltiazem
  - Direct vasodilators
    - Arterial and venous vasodilators
      - Nitroglycerine
      - Sodium nitroprusside
    - Arterial vasodilators
      - Hydralazine
  - Ganglionic blocking agents
    - Trimethaphan
  - Purine derivatives
    - Adenosine
  - Prostaglandins
    - PGE_1

demonstrated a 53% reduction in intraoperative blood loss in patients receiving trimethaphan for controlled hypotension. In another retrospective study of patients undergoing radical hysterectomy and pelvic lymphadenectomy, the use of nitroglycerine to reduce mean arterial blood pressure to approximately 60 mm Hg resulted in a 70% reduction in blood loss compared with the control group (38). Pelvic floor repair under controlled hypotensive anesthesia with trimethaphan was shown by Donald (39) to reduce blood loss by 50%.

Clinical Considerations

Indications and Contraindications

The use of controlled hypotension during anesthesia must be based on clinical judgment. Knowledge of the extent of the potential benefits based on the surgical procedure must be measured in relationship to the pharmacology of the hypotensive medication used and to the patient's pathophysiology. Those procedures thought to benefit most with regard to blood conservation are listed in the Table 21.2. The contraindications or relative contraindications to the use of controlled hypotension focus on the concern for inadequate perfusion of vital organs. Table 21.3 lists those commonly accepted contraindications to controlled hypotension.

The major clinical intention of deliberate hypotension is to control intraoperative blood loss for the purpose of both improving the surgeon's operative field and reducing the need for homologous blood transfusions with its associated risks. Other benefits of the technique have also been proposed such as decreased incidence of infection due to reduced cauterized and ligated tissue, improved skin flap viability secondary to reduced oozing, reduced anesthetic needs, and modified systemic effects of acrylic bone cement in hip arthroplasty (11).

Controlled hypotension is usually defined as reducing mean arterial pressure to 50–75 mm Hg. Reduced systolic blood pressure in the range of 80–90 mm Hg is also used (31).

Complications

Mortality. Evaluation of mortality related to controlled hypotension has been a concern since the inception of the ef-

TABLE 21.2. INDICATIONS FOR CONTROLLED HYPOTENSION

- Head and neck surgery
  - Middle ear surgery
  - Orthognathic procedures
  - Oncological surgery
  - Craniofacial procedures
- Orthopedic surgery
  - Hip arthroplasty
  - Spinal fusion
- Neurosurgery
  - Aneurysm
  - Arteriovenous malformation
  - Vascular tumors
- Pelvic surgery
  - Radical prostatectomy
  - Cystectomy
  - AP resection
  - Radical hysterectomy
- Chest wall surgery
  - Radical mastectomy
- Transfusion restrictions
  - Patient refusal

TABLE 21.3. CONTRAINDICATIONS TO CONTROLLED HYPOTENSION

Cardiovascular disease
- Uncontrolled hypertension
- Coronary artery disease

Cerebral vascular disease
Severe pulmonary disease
Renal disease
Hepatic disease
Pregnancy
Anemia
Hypovolemia

TABLE 21.4. MORTALITY IN CONTROLLED HYPERTENSION

Investigators	Years	Patients	Deaths (%)
Hampton and Little(40)	1950–1953	27,930	96(0.34)
Enderby(41)	1950–1960	9107	9(0.10)
Larson(42)	1958–1964	13,264	113(0.10)
Enderby(43)	1960–1976	9256	2(0.02)
Pasch and Huk(44)	1977–1984	1802	1(0.06)
Enderby(45)	1950–1979	20,558	10(0.04)

Reprinted with permission from Van Aken H, Miller ED. Deliberate hypotension. In: Miller RD, ed. Anesthesia. New York: Churchill Livingstone, 1994:1481–1503.

fective clinical use of the technique. Most studies looking at mortality indicate that the mortality associated with controlled hypotension is infrequent (Table 21.4). With advancing anesthetic technique and monitoring plus better knowledge of the physiology and pharmacology of controlled hypotensive techniques, the incidence of complications has decreased. Sollevi (31) in his review of the subject found no mortality in 13 prospective randomized studies of 764 total hip arthroplasties from 1974 to 1986. Of these studies, only one noted a single complication of reduced Pa_{O_2}.

Morbidity. *Central Nervous System.* Morbidity associated with controlled hypotension usually focuses on the potential threat of reduced perfusion to vital organs. Of utmost concern is cerebral perfusion. Theoretically, if mean arterial pressure is maintained above central venous pressure plus oncotic pressure (calculated at approximately 30–40 mm Hg), then cerebral perfusion should be adequate (11) in a healthy individual. As a margin of safety, most define the lower limits of pressure in a healthy individual as 50 mm Hg. The rationale for using a mean arterial pressure of 50 mm Hg is that this value represents the lowest pressure at which autoregulation of cerebral blood flow occurs. Below this level, cerebral blood flow becomes pressure-dependent. The margin of safety may be greater in healthy individuals where normal cerebral oxygen metabolism has been shown to persist with cerebral blood flow as low as 18 mL/100 g/min; this corresponds to a mean arterial perfusion pressure of 30–40 mm Hg (46). Other determinants of cerebral blood flow, specifically, carbon dioxide and oxygen tensions, must also be taken into account (Fig. 21.4). In normal brain at normotension, cerebral blood flow changes approximately 2 mL/100 g/mm Hg in Pa_{CO_2} (47). This relationship, however, is modified by controlled hypotension. The slope of this relationship between Pa_{CO_2} and cerebral blood flow is progressively reduced as blood pressure drops such that when mean arterial pressure falls below 50 mm Hg, cerebral blood flow does not

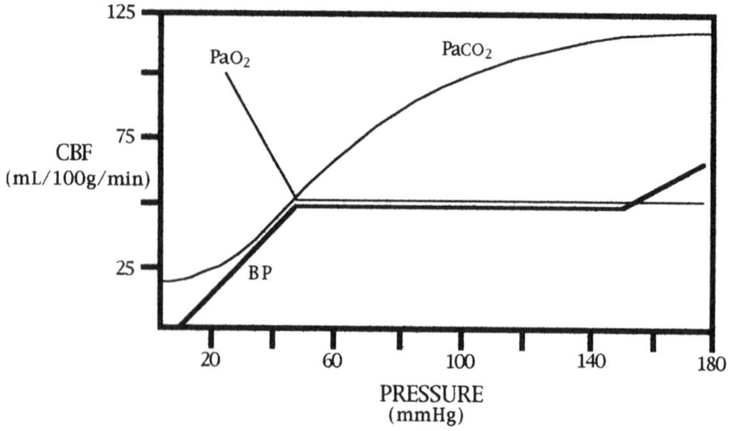

Figure 21.4. Cerebral blood flow changes due to alterations in Pa_{CO_2} and blood pressure. The other two variables remain stable at normal values when the remaining value is altered. (Reprinted by permission from Shapiro HM. Physiology and pharmacologic regulation of cerebral blood flow. In: ASA Refresher Courses in Anesthesiology. J.B. Lippincott, 1977:161–178.)

change in response to changes in Pa_{CO_2} (48). Additionally, the influence of the hypotensive agent chosen to induce controlled hypotension will further modify the response of the cerebral vasculature.

In patients with cerebrovascular disease or chronic hypertension, the margin of safety may require a higher lower limit of blood pressure. Pasch and Huk (44) reviewed 1802 patients undergoing otorhinolaryngological procedures under controlled hypotension from 1977 to 1984. Four patients suffered postoperative cerebral events, with one death. Two patients had preoperatively unrecognized cerebrovascular disease: one had a stenotic internal carotid artery and sustained an intraoperative stroke and one had a hypoplastic vertebral artery and died on the seventh postoperative day of generalized ischemic brain injury. The latter injury was thought to be related to positioning, although controlled hypotension may have had a contributing effect. The other cerebral injuries occurred late in the postoperative period. The morbidity related to controlled hypotension in this study was 2 of 1802 (0.11%) and the mortality, 1 of 1802 (0.06%).

Cerebral blood flow is also a concern in patients with hypertension. Hypertension resets the lower limits of cerebral blood flow autoregulation. Strandgaard (49) evaluated cerebral blood flow autoregulation in awake patients with untreated or ineffectively treated hypertension during controlled hypotension using trimethaphan and reverse Trendelenburg. He compared this patient population with a previously hypertensive group with well-controlled hypertension on medical therapy and a normotensive group. The resting mean arterial blood pressures, the lower limit of cerebral blood flow, and the lowest tolerated blood pressures are listed for the three groups in Table 21.5. The data demonstrate that a reduction in mean arterial pressure of approximately 25% was required to reach the lower limit of cerebral blood flow autoregulation. Additionally, a reduction of approximately 55% was required to reach the mean arterial pressure at which symptoms of brain hypoperfusion occurred. The associated cerebral blood flow studies demonstrate that the autoregulation curve in the uncontrolled hypertensive patients is shifted to the right (Fig. 21.5). The autoregulation curves in the well-controlled hypertensive patients, however, were highly variable. The variability ranged from normal curves to curves shifted to the right as much as untreated hypertensive patients. It is also important to point out that in the uncontrolled hypertensive group given long-term antihypertensive therapy (8–12 months follow-up), cerebral blood flow autoregulation varied from normal to no evidence of change. The application of controlled hypotension, therefore, in the patient with well-treated hypertension as well as the poorly controlled hypertensive must be used with caution because the cerebral autoregulatory mechanism may or may not be normal.

In another study concerning patients with hypertension, Sharrock et al. (50) evaluated the safety of controlled hypoten-

TABLE 21.5. AUTOREGULATION AND CEREBRAL BLOOD FLOW

	Mean Arterial Blood Pressure (mm Hg)		
Group	Rest	Limit of Autoregulation	Lowest BP Tolerated
Group 1	145 ± 17	113 ± 13	65 ± 10
Group 2	116 ± 18	96 ± 17	53 ± 18
Group 3	98 ± 10	73 ± 9	43 ± 8

Group 1, uncontrolled hypertensives; group 2, well-controlled hypertensives; group 3, normotensives. Values are given as mean ± SD. Reprinted with permission from Strandgaard S. Autoregulation of cerebral blood flow in hypertensive patients. Circulation 1976;53:723–724.

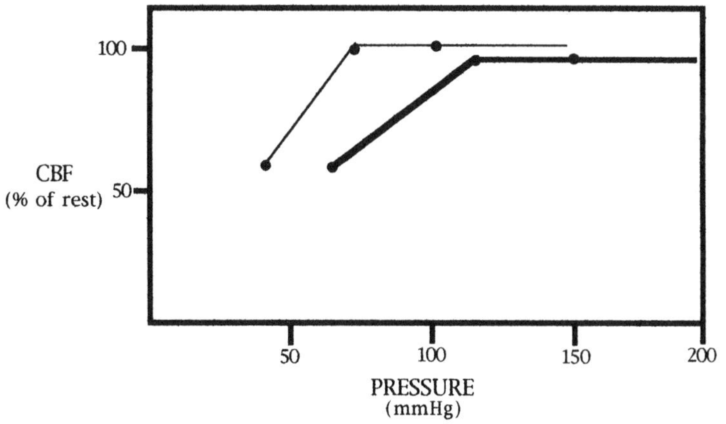

Figure 21.5. Mean curves of autoregulation of cerebral blood flow (CBF) in normotensive (light line) and severely hypertensive (heavy line) human subjects. Each curve is defined by the mean values of resting blood pressure, the lower limit of CBF autoregulation, and the lowest tolerated blood pressure. The curve from the hypertensive patients is shifted to the right on the blood pressure axis. (Reprinted by permission from Strandgaard S. Autoregulation of cerebral blood flow in hypertensive patients. Circulation 1976;53:723–724).

sion using epidural anesthesia in controlled hypertensive patients undergoing total hip replacement. He found no increased incidence of cerebral hypoperfusion, myocardial infarct, or renal failure in comparing the response of induced hypotension to 52–55 mm Hg in nonhypertensive or controlled hypertensive groups. He also noted that no observed signs or symptoms of cerebral hypoperfusion as seen by Strandgaard (49) occurred at mean arterial pressures of 50 mm Hg as long as cardiac output was maintained (cardiac index greater than 2.0 L/min/m). The symptoms noted by Strandgaard (49) may in part be due to reduced cardiac output because the technique of reverse Trendelenburg preload reduction plus trimethaphan afterload reduction is known to reduce cardiac output (50). In the Sharrock et al. (50) study of extradural induced hypotension to 50 mm Hg, cardiac output and stroke volume remained unchanged in both the nonhypertensive and the controlled hypertensive group. Maintenance of cardiac output is, therefore, probably of great importance for the safety of controlled hypotension in patients with a history of hypertension.

Another area of concern with regard to the central nervous system occurs during instrumentation of the spinal column. Spinal cord injury may occur during distraction of the vertebral column for fracture stabilization or spinal deformity correction, a technique frequently performed with controlled hypotensive anesthesia to reduce blood loss. It has been shown that the spinal cord is more sensitive to distraction and/or compression during controlled hypotension than at normotension as measured by reduction in somatosensory evoked potentials (33, 51, 52). The effect of controlled hypotension on somatosensory evoked potentials may also depend on the agent used for inducing hypotension. In the canine model, different agents have variable effects on spinal cord blood flow. For instance, sodium nitroprusside reduces spinal cord blood flow initially with associated hypotension and then blood flow returns to normal as autoregulatory mechanisms come into play. With trimethaphan-induced hypotension, no autoregulatory compensation is seen until it is discontinued. Nitroglycerine, on the other hand, has been shown to maintain control levels of blood flow throughout the hypotensive period (53). The potential for an additive effect of spinal cord distraction and controlled hypotension emphasizes the importance of intraoperative evoked potential monitoring when using controlled hypotension during these surgical procedures.

The effect of controlled hypotension on brain function as measured by neuropsychological tests has also been evaluated. In healthy individuals undergoing controlled hypotensive anesthesia, there has been no demonstration of impairment of memory or mental functions compared with patients undergoing normotensive anesthesia (54, 55).

Cardiac. The primary concern with the use of controlled hypotension in relation to the heart is the supply of adequate oxygen to meet myocardial oxygen demand. Like the cerebral arterial system, progressive hypotension elicits a local autoregulatory response in the coronary arteries, resulting in vasodilatation and increased blood flow. Because the myocardium maximally extracts oxygen, an increase in myocardial oxygen requirements necessitates an increase in coronary blood flow by means of a vasodilatory response. Hypotension, therefore, reduces the coronary vasodilatory reserve.

Patients with atherosclerotic coronary artery disease have an existing impaired vasodilatory reserve due to compensatory arteriolar vasodilatation, resulting from epicardial flow impairment (56). Systemic hypotension in the presence of coronary artery stenosis will directly reduce myocardial perfusion and, depending on the extent, may result in ischemia (57). The pharmacological techniques for inducing controlled hypotension reduce ventricular work by cardiac unloading, resulting in a reduction in myocardial oxygen uptake (58). This may increase the therapeutic index of controlled hypotension in patients with coronary artery disease. However, when the pharmacological techniques used involve coronary arteriolar vasodilators such as sodium nitroprusside, adenosine, and possibly isoflurane, the potential for coronary steal exists (56, 59). In contrast, medications such as nitroglycerine, which primarily cause epicardial vasodilatation as well as unloading the heart, will reduce the potential for myocardial ischemia (56). Additionally, the use of beta-1 antagonists in controlled hypotension to reduce myocardial metabolic requirements may also be beneficial in reducing the potential for ischemia (60).

Pulmonary. The effects of controlled hypotension on pulmonary function and oxygenation involve two main areas of concern: the effect on dead space and on the inhibition of hypoxic pulmonary vasoconstriction. Initial studies suggested that controlled hypotension may contribute to an increase in dead space (61). Later studies, however, found that if cardiac output is maintained, then dead space is not affected by controlled hypotension (62–64).

Vasodilators used to induce hypotension may affect oxygenation by inhibiting hypoxic pulmonary vasoconstriction. Significant reductions in PaO_2 have been observed with nitroglycerine, sodium nitroprusside, trimethaphan, and prostaglandin E_1 (65–67). A significant deterioration in gas exchange with increased intrapulmonary shunting, however, has not been observed with isoflurane-induced hypotension (64). Sparing of significant pulmonary shunting is also observed in patients with chronic obstructive pulmonary disease (67). It is proposed that patients with chronic obstructive pulmonary disease have destructive vascular changes that increase pulmonary arterial pressures, preventing significant decreases in pulmonary vascular resistance by vasodilators. Other vasodilators also result in increased pulmonary shunting such as calcium channel blockers. Nicardipine (68) and nifedipine (69) have both been shown to increase intrapulmonary shunt. Little or no change has been observed with diltiazem (69). Similarly, little or no change has been observed with labetolol (69, 70). Because of the potential reductions in arterial oxygenation resulting from the use of vasodilators for inducing controlled hypotension, arterial blood gas monitoring is a prerequisite for using this technique in blood conservation.

Renal. The rate of blood flow through the kidney is maintained relatively constant with arterial pressures between 80 and 180 mm Hg; a similar autoregulatory pattern holds for glomerular filtration rate (71). Below 80 mm Hg, effective renal blood flow and glomerular filtration rate fall. During controlled hypotension with mean arterial pressures reduced to 50–60 mm Hg urine flow rate, endogenous creatinine clearance and osmolar clearance fall; these values return to normal with discontinuation of hypotension (72–76). Because of the return of normal renal parameters after discontinuation of hypotension, the use of controlled hypotension is not considered to be detrimental to renal function if normovolemia is maintained.

Controlled hypotension leads to the stimulation of the renin-angiotensin system in response to decreased renal perfusion. It also results in a reflex activation of the autonomic nervous system. These responses are in addition to the stress response induced by surgery itself and are variable depending on the agents used to produce hypotension. Sodium nitroprusside-induced hypotension results in the release of catecholamines and activation of the renin-angiotensin system compared with trimethaphan, which inhibits the renin-angiotensin response and release of catecholamines by ganglionic blockade (77). Isoflurane, or isoflurane with labetalol, induced hypotension attenuates the stress response, reducing catecholamine release and minimizing renin activity (78, 79). Adenosine triphosphate, nitroglycerine, and prostaglandin E_1 all increase plasma renin activity during hypotensive anesthesia. Norepinephrine is also significantly elevated by adenosine triphosphate, nitroglycerine, and prostaglandin E_1; however, epinephrine is elevated by nitroglycerine and prostaglandin E_1 but not adenosine triphosphate (80).

Discontinuation of hypotensive anesthesia may result in a transient period of rebound hypertension due to persistence of the effects of the activated renin-angiotensin system. Sodium nitroprusside is the only drug with which this is a significant problem. The use of beta-blockade in conjunction with sodium nitroprusside, however, can attenuate this response and reduce the required dosage and reflex tachycardia associated with sodium nitroprusside (81, 82). Captopril, which prevents the conversion of angiotensin I to angiotensin II, may also be beneficial in preventing rebound (83).

Hepatic. Total liver blood flow is the sum of portal venous and hepatic arterial blood flows. Total liver blood flow is held fairly constant by fluctuations in hepatic arterial flow to compensate for variations in portal vein blood flow from the splanchnic bed (84). Controlled hypotension (mean arterial pressures of 35–60 mm Hg) with sodium nitroprusside and trimethaphan has been shown not to change total liver blood flow (85, 86). The hepatic oxygen supply, however, is largely determined by the arterial fraction from the hepatic artery (87). Concern has been raised regarding the ratio of hepatic arterial to portal venous blood flow during controlled hypotension because of the greater contribution of oxygen supplied by the hepatic arterial circulation (88). In a study by Sivarajan et al. (86), evaluation of controlled hypotension with sodium nitroprusside and trimethaphan showed no significant differences in total liver blood flow or the ratio of hepatic artery blood flow to total blood flow. In patients with normal hepatic function, therefore, controlled hypotension maintained within normal autoregulatory limits is probably not detrimental to the liver.

MONITORING

Arterial catheter monitoring is standard care for controlled hypotension. It not only allows for beat-to-beat measurement of the patient's blood pressure, but also allows for efficient access to obtain laboratory data (especially arterial blood gases and hematocrits) helpful in managing controlled hypotensive anesthesia. Radial artery catheters are preferred because mean arterial pressures during controlled hypotension obtained from the dorsal pedal artery are variable. With the use of sodium nitroprusside, mean arterial pressure is higher at the dorsal pedal artery than at the radial artery; with isoflurane the opposite is true (89). Direct blood pressure measurement is also preferred over oscillometry because of a tendency in the latter to overestimate blood pressure below a mean arterial pressure of 80 mm Hg (90).

Central venous pressure monitoring may also be helpful to guide fluid replacement in procedures where significant blood loss can be anticipated. Maintenance of normovolemia during controlled hypotension allows cardiac output to remain at baseline values despite a reduction in arterial pressures. The use of a urometer to track urine output is beneficial during controlled hypotension where reduced renal perfusion can be anticipated. Temperature monitoring is especially important where the vasodilator effects of hypotensive agents and epidural anesthesia contribute to reductions in body temperature. Electrocardiography and pulse oximetry should be routine. Capnography will be helpful as a trend monitor, but it must be remembered that the end tidal and arterial CO_2 difference may be affected by controlled hypotension with its potential effect on physiological dead space and cardiac output.

REGIONAL ANESTHESIA

Meta-Analysis of Blood Loss Reduction

It is a generally held observation that regional anesthetic techniques, specifically neuraxial blockade, are associated with a reduction in blood loss during surgery. This benefit has also been shown to extend to the postoperative period (91). Epidural anesthesia has been associated with lower mean arterial pressures, right atrial pressures, mean pulmonary artery pressures, and peripheral venous pressures compared with patients undergoing general anesthesia (91). Recently, several meta-analyses of the literature evaluating regional versus general anesthesia have been performed. Pitner et al. (92) evaluated 11 studies meeting the criteria of randomized controlled trials comparing regional versus general anesthesia where intraoperative blood loss was recorded. The selection of studies was compiled from review of the literature from 1966 to 1993. The pooled studies included total hip replacement ($n = 6$), hip fracture ($n = 4$), and open prostatectomy ($n = 1$). The meta-analysis revealed a significant benefit of regional anesthesia in only the total hip replacement group with a mean overall difference of 414 mL of reduced blood loss over general anesthesia (Table 21.6). Similar results were obtained in a second independent meta-analysis (93). In this analysis, the mean greater blood loss was 384 mL. Also, there was a 20% greater incidence of deep venous thrombosis and a 14% greater incidence of pulmonary embolism in the general anesthesia group compared with the regional group (both epidural and subarachnoid anesthesia). In contrast to the two meta-analyses discussed above, another meta-analysis by Sorenson et al. (94), looking at regional (epidural and subarachnoid blocks) and general anesthesia during the surgical repair of femoral neck fractures, found no difference in estimated operative blood loss. Of the 13 randomized control trials evaluated, however, only 9 reported the estimated blood loss and only 4 gave quantitative values.

Epidural Anesthesia

The benefit of spinal or epidural anesthesia in reducing intraoperative blood loss was demonstrated as early as 1967. Madsen and Madsen (95) found a reduction in blood loss in patients undergoing prostatectomies with neuraxial block compared with general anesthesia. With abdominal prostatectomies, the literature indicated a reduction in blood loss in patients receiving regional as opposed to general anesthesia (96, 97). In these studies, the reduction in blood loss averaged 30–40%. The reduction in blood loss was observed with the use of epidural anesthesia even in the presence of equivalent mean arterial blood pressures to those found in the general anesthesia group (97). More profound blood conservation has been observed when the epidural anesthesia is associated with reduced blood pressure compared with general anesthesia. In a study by Thorud et al. (96), they noted a 69% reduction in blood loss in comparing neuroleptic with epidural anesthesia where epidural anesthesia averaged lower systolic and diastolic blood pressures during the operation, although their statistical analysis failed to show a significant correlation between blood pressure and blood loss. In transurethral prostatectomy (TUR-P), however, there is disagreement. Significant reductions in operative blood loss with spinal and epidural anesthesia were reported by Abrams et al. (98) in patients undergoing TUR-P. They observed a 43% reduction in blood loss in the regional group with no significant relationship between blood pressure and blood loss. Others have found no significant benefit to regional anesthetic techniques (99). Other major pelvic surgical pro-

TABLE 21.6. META-ANALYSIS OF REGIONAL VERSUS GENERAL ANESTHESIA: MEASURE OF BLOOD LOSS CHANGE

Surgery	No. Studies Positive/ Negative	Summary Effect Size	Mean Overall Difference (mL)	95% Confidence Limits (mL)	Power of Negative Studies (%)
Total hip replacement	4/2	−0.89	−414	−533 to −330	24 40 6
Hip fracture	1/3	−0.08	−20	−81 to 41	5
Open prostatectomy	1/0	−1.44	N/A	N/A	N/A

Reprinted with permission from Pitner R, Crews J, Mathieu A. Is regional anesthesia more effective than general anesthesia in reducing intraoperative blood loss [abstract]. Anesthesiology 1993;79(Suppl. 3A):A1070.

cedures have also demonstrated the blood-conserving effects of epidural anesthesia, including pelvic floor operations (100, 101), cystectomy (102), hypospadias repair (103), and cesarean section (104, 105).

The benefit in blood conservation with the use of epidural anesthesia, however, has not been a significant observation in major vascular procedures. In three large prospective randomized studies of general versus epidural anesthesia in patients undergoing major revascularization of the abdominal aorta and lower extremities, no significant differences were noted regarding blood loss (26, 106, 107). Similar observations have been described in other vascular procedures. Muskett et al. (108) studied 75 consecutive patients undergoing either deep cervical plexus blocks or general anesthesia for carotid endarterectomy. Blood loss between the two groups was similar, and there was no significant difference in blood pressures between the two groups. The absence of benefit to blood conservation in vascular surgery may relate to the surgical technique where most blood loss is related to arteriotomy and flushing of grafts.

The benefits of blood conservation in total hip replacement observed with controlled hypotension are also quite apparent with the use of epidural anesthesia (5, 6, 16, 24, 25, 109). The question may then arise as to which is the better technique for blood conservation: epidural anesthesia or general anesthesia with controlled hypotension? Rosberg et al. (25) prospectively studied 157 consecutive patients for total hip replacement. Their study evaluated four groups of anesthesia: halothane/N_2O with sodium nitroprusside controlled hypotension, halothane/N_2O without hypotension, neuroleptic anesthesia, and epidural anesthesia. The greatest reduction in blood loss occurred in the controlled hypotensive group, followed by epidural anesthesia, halothane/N_2O anesthesia, and neuroleptic anesthesia (Table 21.7). Mean intraoperative blood loss for the controlled hypotension group was 660 mL, epidural blood loss was 35% greater, halothane/N_2O blood loss was 46% greater, and neuroleptic anesthesia resulted in a 63% greater blood loss. The study sheds some insight into the importance of different anesthetic techniques with regard to surgical blood loss. In a similar study by Keith (109) without a controlled hypotensive group, a 47% increase in blood loss was seen in the halothane/N_2O group and a 54% increase in the neuroleptic group over the epidural anesthesia group.

Postoperative blood loss has also been evaluated, although the results are less consistent. There is evidence to suggest, however, that if epidural analgesia is maintained postoperatively, blood loss can be reduced further (110).

In spinal surgery where controlled hypotension has proven to be an effective measure to reduce blood loss, epidural anesthesia may also play a role. In a retrospective review of 80 patients undergoing lumbar spine surgery, Greenbarg et al. (111) found a reduction in operative blood loss of 35% in patients receiving lumbar epidural anesthesia compared with general anesthesia.

Subarachnoid Anesthesia

The relationship of subarachnoid anesthesia to intraoperative blood loss is similar to that of epidural anesthesia. In a review of general versus subarachnoid anesthesia by Covino (112), 11 studies were analyzed. Of the 11 there were 4 studies of total hip arthroplasty performed with subarachnoid or general anesthesia. The average blood loss for the general anesthesia group was 1167 mL compared with 765 mL in the subarachnoid group. The findings in hip fracture surgery,

TABLE 21.7. ANESTHETIC TECHNIQUE AND SURGICAL BLOOD LOSS

Group	Intraoperative Blood Loss	Postoperative Blood Loss	Total Blood Loss	Perioperative Blood Loss	Mean Arterial Pressure (mm Hg)	Operative Time (min)
Hypotensive anesthesia(I)	0.66 ± 0.07	0.60 ± 0.11	1.27 ± 0.11	1.12 ± 0.15	61 ± 1.2	105 ± 4.8
Halothane anesthesia(II)	1.22 ± 0.13	0.74 ± 0.13	1.96 ± 0.11	1.66 ± 0.23	85 ± 2.1	108 ± 5.6
Epidural anesthesia(III)	1.02 ± 0.10	0.58 ± 0.04	1.59 ± 0.10	1.62 ± 0.10	92 ± 4.5	103 ± 3.0
NLA(IV)	1.78 ± 0.35	0.84 ± 0.20	2.62 ± 0.49	2.22 ± 0.46	101 ± 3.6	109 ± 8.0

Values are mean ± SD.

Reprinted with permission from Rosberg B, Fredin H, Gustafson C. Anesthetic techniques and surgical blood loss in total hip arthroplasty. Acta Anaesth Scand 1982;26:189–193.

however, are variable. In a meta-analysis by Sorenson and Pace (94) of anesthetic techniques during the surgical repair of femoral neck fractures, there were 11 of 13 randomized controlled trials performed under subarachnoid anesthesia. The other two used epidural anesthesia. The study found no difference in the estimated operative blood loss. However, as Covert and Fox (113) pointed out in their review of anaesthesia for hip surgery in the elderly, the variability may be due to the operative approach and type of hip fracture. They noted that the intraoperative blood loss for internal fixation of femoral neck fractures is less than that for intertrochanteric fractures and hemiarthroplasty procedures. Further insight into this question is obtained by looking again at Sorenson and Pace's meta-analysis (94). Although the exact numbers are not discussed, they state that the vast majority of the patients had surgical repair by open reduction with internal fixation of femoral neck fractures. In two of those studies, however, where most patients had intertrochanteric fractures, intraoperative blood loss was significantly less in the subarachnoid anesthesia group (114, 115).

The benefits of regional anesthesia, specifically subarachnoid block, regarding intraoperative blood conservation have also been demonstrated in transurethral prostatectomy (95, 116), lower extremity vascular surgery (117), and colectomy (118).

Effect of Regional Anesthesia on Coagulation

Epidural anesthesia and analgesia have been associated with both direct and indirect effects on hemostasis (107, 110, 119, 120). Surgery performed with general anesthesia results in hypercoagulability manifested by an increase in fibrinogen and platelet activation; the opposite is true for epidural anesthesia alone or combined with general anesthesia (107, 119, 120). Epidural anesthesia is associated with an increase in the level of plasminogen activators and an increase in the capacity of the venous endothelium to release these activators. This effect extends to the third postoperative day (119). The benefit of such an effect is the reduction in thrombotic events in peripheral arterial grafts and the coronary arteries and the reduction in deep venous thrombosis and pulmonary embolism (26, 107, 121). The potential for increased blood loss might be considered given the effects of epidural anesthesia on coagulation. In actuality, there is no difference in blood loss (26, 107), or possibly there may even be a reduction in blood loss (91).

Additionally, local anesthetics have been shown to exert an effect on hemostasis by inhibiting platelet aggregation (119). This effect occurs at clinically relevant concentrations and in a dose-dependent fashion. As pointed out by Borg and Modig (120), local anesthetics are thought to have a stabilizing effect on all blood cells, including inhibition of leukocyte locomotion and response to endothelial injury. The effects in relation to surgical blood loss, however, are not clinically relevant.

SUMMARY

Much of the blood loss that occurs during surgery is largely dependent on the type and extent of the operative procedure. The anesthesiologist's intervention, however, can modify the degree of blood loss in many circumstances. The benefit to the surgeon is an improved surgical field, allowing greater efficiency and consequently the potential for further reduction in blood loss. The benefit to the patient resides in the reduced exposure to the need for blood transfusion with its inherent risks.

REFERENCES

1. Relton J, Hall J. Reduction of haemorrhage during spinal fusion combined with internal metallic fixation using a new scoliosis operating frame. Br J Bone Joint Surg 1967;49B:327–332.
2. Tate DE, Friedman RJ. Blood conservation in spinal surgery. Review of current techniques. Spine 1992;17:1450–1456.
3. Washburn MC, Hyer RL. Deliberate hypotension for elective major maxillofacial surgery: a balanced halothane and morphine technique. J Maxillofac Surg 1982;10:50–55.
4. West JB. Pulmonary pathophysiology—the essentials. 2nd ed. Baltimore: Williams & Wilkins, 1982:187–201.
5. Modig J. Beneficial effects on intraoperative and postoperative blood loss in total hip replacement when performed under lumbar epidural anesthesia. Acta Chir Scand 1988;550(Suppl.):95–103.
6. Modig J, Karlstrom G. Intra- and post-operative blood loss and haemodynamics in total hip replacement when performed under lumbar epidural versus general anaesthesia. Eur J Anaesth 1987;4:345–355.
7. Wildsmith JA, Sinclair CJ, Thorn J, MacRae WR, Fagan D, Scott DB. Haemodynamic effects of induced hypotension with a nitroprusside-trimethaphan mixture. Br J Anaesth 1983;55:381–389.
8. Bertrand D, Hannhart B, Laxenaire MC. Haemodynamic effects of inspiratory and expiratory resistances in anaesthetic breathing systems during induced hypotension. Eur J Anaesth 1985;2:353–359.
9. Sivarajan M, Amory DW, Everett GB, Buffington C. Blood pressure, not cardiac output, determines blood loss during induced hypotension. Anesth Analg 1980;59:203–206.
10. Didier EP, Clagett OT, Theye RA. Cardiac performance during controlled hypotension. Anesth Analg 1965;44:379–386.
11. Fahmy NM. Indications and contraindications for deliberate hypotension with a review of its cardiovascular effects. Int Anesthesiol Clin 1979;17:175–187.
12. Porter SS, Asher M, Fox DK. Comparison of intravenous nitroprusside-captopril, and nitroglycerine for deliberate hypotension during posterior spine fusion in adults. J Clin Anesth 1988;1:87–95.
13. Styles M, Coleman AJ, Leary WP. Some hemodynamic effects of sodium nitroprusside. Anesthesiology 1973;38:173–176.
14. Bailey PL, Stanely TH. Narcotic intravenous anesthetics. In: Miller RD, ed. Anesthesia. 3rd ed. New York: Churchill Livingston, 1990:281–366.

15. Sharrock NE, Mineo R, Go G. The effect of cardiac output on intraoperative blood loss during total hip arthroplasty. Reg Anesth 1993;18: 24–29.
16. Sharrock NE, Mineo R, Urquhart B, Salvati EA. The effect of two levels of hypotension on intraoperative blood loss during total hip arthroplasty performed under lumbar epidural anesthesia. Anesth Analg 1993;76:580–584.
17. Bernard JM, Pinaud M, Ganansia MF, Chatelier H, Souron R. Letenneur J. Systemic haemodynamic and metabolic effects of deliberate hypotension with isoflurane anaesthesia or sodium nitroprusside during total hip arthroplasty. Can J Anaesth 1987;34:135–140.
18. Fromme GA, MacKenzie RA, Gould AB Jr, Lund BA, Offord KP. Controlled hypotension for orthognathic surgery. Anesth Analg 1986;65: 683–686.
19. Fahmy NR. Nitroglycerin as a hypotensive drug during general anesthesia. Anesthesiology 1978;49:17–20.
20. Modig J, Malmberg P, Karlstrom G. Effect of epidural versus general anaesthesia on calf blood flow. Acta Anaesth Scand 1980;24:305–309.
21. Haljamae H. Effects of anesthesia on leg blood flow in vascular surgical patients. Acta Chir Scand 1989;550(Suppl.):81–87.
22. Holm J, Frid I, Akerstrom G, Haljamae H. Ankle-brachial index (ABI) and leg blood flow following epidural anaesthesia. Int Angiol 1988:7: 26–31.
23. Haljamae H, Frid I, Holm J, Akerstrom G. Epidural vs general anaesthesia and leg blood flow in patients with occlusive atherosclerotic disease. Eur J Vasc Surg 1988;2:395–400.
24. Chin SP, Abou-Madi MN, Eurin B, Witvoet J, Montagne J. Blood loss in total hip replacement: extradural v. phenoperidine analgesia. Br J Anaesth 1982;54:491–495.
25. Rosberg B, Fredin H. Gustafson C. Anesthetic techniques and surgical blood loss in total hip arthroplasty. Acta Anaesth Scand 1982;26: 189–193.
26. Chrisopherson R, Beattie C, Frank SM, et al. Perioperative morbidity in patients randomized to epidural or general anesthesia for lower extremity vascular surgery. Anesthesiology 1993;79:422–434.
27. Gardner WJ. The control of bleeding during operation by induced hyptension. JAMA 1946;132:572–574.
28. Griffiths HWC, Gillies J. Thoraco-lumbar splanchnicectomy and sympathectomy: anaesthetic procedure. Anaesthesia 1948;3:134–136.
29. Leigh JM. The history of controlled hypotension. Br J Anaesth 1975; 47:745–749.
30. Petrozza PH. Induced hypotension. Int Anaesth Clin 1990;28:223–229.
31. Sollevi A. Hypotensive anesthesia and blood loss. Acta Anaesth Scand 1988;32(Suppl. 89):39–43.
32. Brodsky JW, Dickson JH, Erwin WD, Rossi CD. Hypotensive anesthesia for scoliosis surgery in Jehovah's Witnesses. Spine 1991;16: 304–306.
33. Grundy BL, Nash CL, Brown RH. Deliberate hypotension for spinal fusion: prospective randomized study with evoked potential monitoring. Can Anaesthetists Soc J 1982;29:452–462.
34. Lawhon SM, Kahn A, Crawford AH, Brinker MS. Controlled hypotensive anesthesia during spinal surgery: a retrospective study. Spine 1984;9:450–453.
35. Patel NJ, Patel BS, Paskin S, Laufer S. Induced moderate hypotensive anesthesia for spinal fusion and Harrington-rod instrumentation. J Bone Joint Surg 1985;67A:1384–1387.
36. Ullrich PF, Keene JS, Hogan KJ, Roecker EB. Results of hypotensive anesthesia in operative treatment of thoracolumbar fractures. J Spinal Dis 1990;3:329–333.
37. Ahlering TE, Henderson JB, Skinner DG. Controlled hypotensive anesthesia to reduce blood loss in radical cystectomy for bladder cancer. J Urol 1983;129:953–954.
38. Powell JL, Mogelnicki SR, Franklin EW, Chambers DA, Burrell MO. A deliberate hypotensive technique for decreasing blood loss during radical hysterectomy and pelvic lymphadenectomy. Am J Obstet Gynecol 1983;147:196–202.
39. Donald JR. The effect of anaesthesia, hypotension, and epidural analgesia on blood loss in surgery for pelvic floor repair. Br J Anaesth 1969;41:155–165.
40. Hampton LJ, Little DM Jr. Complications associated with the use of "controlled hypotension" in anesthesia. Arch Surg 1953;67:549.
41. Enderby GEH. A report on mortality and morbidity following 9,106 hypotensive anaesthetics. Br J Anaesth 1961;33:109.
42. Larson AG. Deliberate hypotension. Anesthesiology 1964;25:682.
43. Enderby G. Hypotensive anesthesia. In: Gray TC, Nunn JF, Utting JE, eds. General anesthesia. 4th ed. London: Butterworths, 1980:1140.
44. Pasch T, Huk W. Cerebral complications following induced hypotension. Eur J Anaesth 1986;3:299–312.
45. Enderby G. Safe hypotensive anaesthesia. In: Enderby G, eds. Hypotensive anesthesia. New York: Churchill Livingstone, 1985:262.
46. Van Aken H, Miller ED Jr. Deliberate hypotension. In: Miller RD, ed. Anesthesia. 4th ed. New York: Churchill Livingstone, 1994:1481–1503.
47. Shapiro HM. Physiology and pharmacologic regulation of cerebral blood flow. In: ASA Refresher Coures in Anesthesiology. Philadelphia: J.B. Lippincott, 1977:161–178.
48. Harper AM, Glass HI. Effects of alterations in the arterial carbon dioxide tension on the blood flow through the cerebral cortex at normal and low arterial blood pressures. J Neurol Neurosurg Psychiatry 1965;28: 449.
49. Strandgaard S. Autoregulation of cerebral blood flow in hypertensive patients. The modifying influence of prolonged antihypertensive treatment on the tolerance to acute, drug-induced hypotension. Circulation 1976;53:720–727.
50. Sharrock NE, Mineo R, Urquhart B. Haemodynamic effects and outcome analysis of hypotensive extradural anaesthesia in controlled hypertensive patients undergoing total hip arthroplasty. Br J Anaesth 1991;67:17–25.
51. Yeoman PM, Gibson MJ, Hutchinson A, Crawshaw C, Bradshaw K, Beattie A. Influence of induced hypotension and spinal distraction on feline spinal somatosensory evoked potentials. Br J Anaesth 1989;63: 315–320.
52. Krengel WF III, Robinson LR, Schneider VA. Combined effects of compression and hypotension on nerve root function: a clinical case. Spine 1993;18:306–309.
53. Phillips WA, Hensinger RN. Control of blood loss during scoliosis surgery. Clin Ortho Related Res 1988;229:88–93.
54. Townes BD, Dikmen SS, Bledsoe SW, Hornbein TF, Martin DC, Janesheski JA. Neuropsychological changes in a young, healthy population after controlled hypotensive anesthesia. Anesth Analg 1986;65: 955–959.
55. Toivonen J, Kuikka P, Kaukinen S. Effects of deliberate hypotension induced by labetalol with isoflurane on neuropsychological function. Acta Anaesth Scand 1993;37:7–11.
56. Sill JC. Pharmacology of the coronary circulation. Can J Anaesth 1987;34:S2-S11.
57. Hickey RF, Verreir ED, Baer RW, Vlahakes GJ, Fein G, Hoffman JI. A canine model of acute coronary artery stenosis: effects of deliberate hypotension. Anesthesiology 1983;59:226–236.

58. Bloor BC, Fukunaga AF, Ma C, et al. Myocardial hemodynamics during induced hypotension: a comparison between sodium nitroprusside and adenosine triphosphate. Anesthesiology 1985;63:517–525.
59. Hartman JC, Kampine JP, Schmeling WT, Warltier DC. Steal-prone coronary circulation in chronically instrumented dogs: isoflurane versus adenosine. Anesthesiology 1991;74:744–756.
60. Braunwald E, Muller JE, Kloner RA, Maroko PR. Role of beta-adrenergic blockade in the therapy of patients with myocardial infarction. Am J Med 1983;74:113–123.
61. Echenhoff JE, Enderby GEH, Larson A, et al. Pulmonary gas exchange during deliberate hypotension. Br J Anaesth 1963;35:750.
62. Khambatta HJ, Stone JG, Matteo RS. Effect of sodium nitroprusside-induced hypotension on pulmonary deadspace. Br J Anaesth 1982;54: 1197–1200.
63. Suwa K, Hedley-Whyte J, Bendixen HH. Circulation and physiologic dead space changes on controlling the ventilation of dogs. J Appl Physiol 1966;21:1855–1859.
64. Nicholas JF, Lam AM. Isoflurane-induced hypotension does not cause impairment in pulmonary gas exchange. Can Anaesthetists Soc J 1984; 31:352–358.
65. Yamakage M, Iwasaki H, Satoh K, Namiki A. Effects of induced hypotension on arterial blood-gases under spontaneous breathing. Acta Anaesth Scand 1994;38:368–371.
66. Wildsmith JA, Drummond GB, MacRae WR. Blood-gas changes during induced hypotension with sodium nitroprusside. Br J Anaesth 1975;47:1205–1211.
67. Casthely PA, Lear S, Cottrell JE, Lear E. Intrapulmonary shunting during induced hypotension. Anesth Analg 1982;61:231–235.
68. Bernard JM, Passuti N, Pinaud M. Long-term hypotensive technique with nicardipine and nitroprusside during isoflurane anesthesia for spinal surgery. Anesth Analg 1992;75:175–185.
69. Casthely PA, Villanueva R, Rabinowitz L, Gandhi P, Litwak B, Fyman PN. Intrapulmonary shunting during deliberate hypotension with nifedipine, diltiazem and labetalol in dogs. Can Anaesth Soc J 1985;32:119–123.
70. Saarnivaara L, Klemola UM, Lindgren L. Labetalol as a hypotensive agent for middle ear surgery. Acta Anaesth Scand 1987;31:196–201.
71. Vander AJ. Renal physiology. 3rd ed. New York: McGraw-Hill, 1985: 70–85.
72. Toivonen J, Kaukinen S, Oikkonen M, Hannelin M. Effects of deliberate hypotension induced by labetalol on renal function. Eur J Anaesth 1991;8:13–20.
73. Lessard MR, Trepanier CA. Renal function and hemodynamics during prolonged isoflurane-induced hypotension in humans. Anesthesiology 1991;74:860–865.
74. Behnia R, Martin A, Koushanpour E, Brunner EA. Trimethaphan-induced hypotension: effect on renal function. Can Anaesth Soc J 1982; 29:581–586.
75. Behnia R, Siqueira EB, Brunner EA. Sodium nitroprusside-induced hypotension: effect on renal function. Anesth Anesth 1978;57:521–526.
76. Thompson GE, Miller RD, Stevens WC, Murray WR. Hypotensive anesthesia for total hip arthroplasty: a study of blood loss and organ function (brain, heart, liver, kidney). Anesthesiology 1978;48:91–96.
77. Knight PR, Lane GA, Hensinger RN, Bolles RS, Bjoraker DJ. Catecholamine and renin-angiotension response during hypotensive anesthesia induced by sodium nitroprusside or trimethaphan camsylate. Anesthesiology 1983;59:248–253.
78. Macnab MS, Manninen PH, Lam AM, Gleb AW. The stress response to induced hypotension for cerebral aneurysm surgery: a comparison of two hypotensive techniques. Can J Anaesth 1988;35:111–115.
79. Toivonen J. Plasma renin, catecholamines, vasopressin and aldosterone during hypotension induced by labetalol with isoflurane. Acta Anaesth Scand 1991;35:496–501.
80. Fukayama H, Ito H, Shimada M, Kubota Y, Fukunaga AF. Effects of hypotensive anesthesia on endocrine systems in oral surgery. Anesth Prog 1989;36:169–177.
81. Khambatta HJ, Stone JG, Khan E. Propranolol alters renin release during nitroprusside-induced hypotension and prevents hypertension on discontinuation of nitroprusside. Anesth Analg 1981;60:569–573.
82. Fahmy NR, Milelakos PT, Battit GE, Lappas DG. Propranolol prevents hemodynamic and humeral events after abrupt withdrawal of nitroprusside. Clin Pharmacol Ther 1984;36:470–477.
83. Woodside J Jr, Garner L, Bedford RF, et al. Captopril reduces the dose requirement for sodium nitroprusside induced hypotension. Anesthesiology 1984;60:413–417.
84. Maze M. Hepatic physiology. In: Miller RD, ed. Anesthesia. New York: Churchill Livingstone, 1990:585–600.
85. Chauvin M, Bonner B, Montembault C, Lafay M, Curet P, Viars P. Hepatic plasma flow during sodium nitroprusside-induced hypotension in humans. Anesthesiology 1985;63:287–293.
86. Sivarajan M, Amory DW, McKenzie SM. Regional blood flows during induced hypotension produced by nitroprusside or trimethaphan in the rhesus monkey. Anesth Analg 1985;64:759–766.
87. Greenway CV, Stark RD. Hepatic vascular bed. Physiol Rev 1971;51: 23–65.
88. Gelman S. Hepatic blood flow during controlled hypotension [letter]. Anesth Analg 1986;65:423–424.
89. Abou-Madi M, Lensi S, Archer D, Ravussin P, Trop D. Comparison of direct blood pressure measurements at the radial and dorsalis pedis arteries during sodium nitroprusside- and isoflurane-induced hypotension. Anesthesiology 1986;65:692–695.
90. Gourdeau M, Martin R. Lamarche Y. Tetreault L. Oscillometry and direct blood pressure: a comparative study during deliberate hypotension. Can Anaesthetists Soc J 1986;33:300–307.
91. Modig, J. Regional anesthesia and blood loss. Acta Anaesth Scand 1988;32(Suppl. 89):44–48.
92. Pitner R, Crews J, Mathieu A. Is regional anesthesia (RA) more effective than general anesthesia (GA) in reducing intraoperative blood loss? A meta-analysis. Anesthesiology 1993;79(Suppl. 3A):A1070.
93. Bradway JA, Pace NL. A meta-analysis of regional vs. general anesthesia in total hip arthroplasty. Anesthesiology 1993;79(Suppl. 3A): A1064.
94. Sorenson RM, Pace NL. Anesthetic techniques during surgical repair of femoral neck fractures: a meta-analysis. Anesthesiology 1992;77: 1095–1104.
95. Madsen RE, Madsen PO. Influence of anesthesia form on blood loss in transurethral prostatectomy. Anesth Analg 1967;46:330–332.
96. Thorud T, Lund I, Holm I. The effect of anesthesia on intraoperative and postoperative bleeding during abdominal prostatectomies: a comparison of neurolept anesthesia, halothane anesthesia and epidural anesthesia. Acta Anaesth Scand 1975;57(Suppl.):83–88.
97. Malhorta V, Stout R, Girardi SC. Comparison of epidural anesthesia, general anesthesia, and combined epidural general anesthesia for radical prostatectomy. Anesthesiology 1994;81(Suppl. 3A): A973.
98. Abrams PH, Shah PJR, Bryning K, Gaches CGC, Green NA. Blood loss during transurethral resection of the prostate. Anaesthesia 1982;37: 71–73.
99. Nielsen KK, Andersen K, Asbjorn J, Vork F, Ohrt-Nissen A. Blood loss in transuretheral prostatectomy: epidural versus general anaesthesia. Internat Urol Neph 1987;19:287–292.

100. Donald JR. The effect of anaesthesia, hypotension, and epidural analgesia on blood loss in surgery for pelvic floor repair. Br J Anaesth 1969;41:155–165.
101. Donald DM. Blood loss during major vaginal surgery. Br J Anaesth 1968;40:233–239.
102. Ryan DW. Anaesthesia for cystectomy. Anaesthesia 1982;37:554–560.
103. Gunter JB, Forestner JE, Manley CB. Caudal epidural anesthesia reduces blood loss during hypospadias repair. J Urol 1990;144: 517–519.
104. Andrews WW, Ramin SM, Maberry MC, Shearer V, Black S, Wallace DH. Effect of type of anesthesia on blood loss at elective repeat cesarean section. Am J Perinatol 1992;9:197–200.
105. Gilstrap LC III, Hauth JC, Hankins DV, Patterson AR. Effect of type of anesthesia on blood loss at cesarean section. Obstet Gynecol 1987;69:328–813.
106. Davies MJ, Silbert BS, Mooney PJ, Dysart RH, Meads AC. Combined epidural and general anaesthesia versus general anaesthesia for abdominal aortic surgery: a prospective randomized study. Anaesth Intersive Care 1993;21:790–794.
107. Tuman KJ, McCarthy RJ, March RJ, DeLaria GA, Patel RV, Ivankovich AD. Effects of epidural anesthesia and analgesia on coagulation and outcome after major vascular surgery. Anesth Analg 1991;73:696–704.
108. Muskett A, McGreevy J, Miller M. Detailed comparison of regional and general anesthesia for carotid endarterectomy. Am J Surg 1986;152: 691–694.
109. Keith I. Anaesthesia and blood loss in total hip replacement. Anaesthesia 1977;32:444–450.
110. Modig J, Borg T, Karlstrom G, Maripuu E, Sahlstedt B. Thromboembolism after total hip replacement: role of epidural and general anesthesia. Anesth Analg 1983;62:174–180.
111. Greenbarg PE, Brown MD, Pallares VS, Tompkins JS, Mann NH. Epidural anesthesia for lumbar spine surgery. J Spinal Disord 1988;1: 139–143.
112. Covino BG. Rationale for spinal anesthesia. Int Anesth Clin 1989; 27:8–12.
113. Covert CR, Fox GS. Anaesthesia for hip surgery in the elderly. Can J Anesth 1989;36:311–319.
114. Davis FM, Laurenson VG. Spinal anaesthesia or general anaesthesia for emergency hip surgery in elderly patients. Anaesth Intens Care 1981;9:352–358.
115. Valentin N, Lomholt B, Jensen JS, Hejgaard N, Kreiner S. Spinal or general anaesthesia for surgery of fractured hip? A prospective study of mortality in 578 patients. Br J Anaesth 1986;58:284–291.
116. Mackenzie AR. Influence of anaesthesia on blood loss in transurethral prostatectomy. Scot Med J 1990;35:14–16.
117. Cook PT, Davies MJ, Cronin KD, Moran P. A prospective randomised trial comparing spinal anaesthesia using hyperbaric cinchocaine with general anaesthesia for lower limb surgery. Anaesth Intens Care 1986; 14:373–380.
118. Worsley MH, Wishart HY, Peebles Brown DA, Aitkenhead AR. High spinal nerve block for large bowel anastomosis. Br J Anaesth 1988; 60:836–840.
119. Modig J, Borg T, Baage L, Saldeen T. Role of extradural and of general anaesthesia in fibrinolysis and coagulation after total hip replacement. Br J Anaesth 1983;55:625–629.
120. Borg T, Modig J. Potential anti-thrombotic effects of local anaesthetics due to their inhibition of platelet aggregation. Acta Anaesthesiol Scand 1985;29:739–742.
121. Modig J, Hjelmstedt A, Sahlstedt B, Maripuu E. Comparative influences of epidural and general anaesthesia on deep venous thrombosis and pulmonary embolism after total hip replacement. Acta Chir Scand 1981;147:125–130.

Chapter 22

Intraoperative Techniques to Conserve Autologous Blood: Red-Cell Salvage, Platelet-Rich Plasma, and Acute Normovolemic Hemodilution

MARK H. ERETH
WILLIAM C. OLIVER, JR.
PAULA J. SANTRACH

INTRODUCTION

Heightened awareness in the medical community and among the public over the risks associated with the transfusion of allogeneic blood products has generated renewed interest in strategies to reduce allogeneic blood product transfusion. The risks of transfusion of blood products have been recognized for many years; recently, however, increased concerns about the transmission of viral pathogens in banked blood have motivated many physicians to reevaluate their transfusion practices and to search for alternatives to transfusion. In a recent editorial, Dodd (1) estimated the current risk of serious or fatal transfusion-transmitted disease to be about 3 in 10,000 blood recipients. Transfusion-associated morbidity includes hemolysis, posttransfusion hepatitis, transfusion-related acute lung injury, anaphylaxis, and acquired immunodeficiency syndrome (Table 22.1). A detailed discussion of infectious risks and transfusion safety can be found in Chapter 7. Although banked blood is relatively safe, we must continue to develop strategies and techniques to further reduce the exposure and complications associated with allogeneic blood transfusion.

The second reason to reduce transfusion requirements is that a greater number of hospitals are transfusing more blood, thereby rapidly increasing the demand for blood products. This factor necessitates judicious use of the banked blood supply. From 1979 to 1984 alone, the transfusion of red blood cells (RBCs) and blood components to patients at Mayo Clinic increased 27% and 77%, respectively (2). Furthermore, over two-thirds of all RBC transfusions in the United States are given in the perioperative period, emphasizing the sizable impact that perioperative transfusion practices (primarily guided by anesthesiologists and surgeons) can have on the demand for banked blood (3).

Perioperative allogeneic blood transfusion can be decreased by the use of autologous blood procedures. Transfusion of autologous blood eliminates the risk of transfusion-transmitted viral disease and isoimmunization directed at foreign RBC, platelet, and leukocyte antigens (4). The use of autologous blood is also desirable for patients with multiple RBC antibodies or a rare blood phenotype. Autologous blood can be collected preoperatively as whole blood or blood components; intraoperatively as fresh whole blood, acute normovolemic hemodilution (ANH), salvaged RBCs, or platelet-rich plasma (PRP); and postoperatively from chest-tube or joint drains. Advances in the development of autotransfusion equipment have greatly contributed to the expanded clinical application of blood salvage procedures.

Physicians must use multidisciplinary resources to evalu-

TABLE 22.1. ADVERSE EFFECTS ASSOCIATED WITH TRANSFUSION OF BLOOD AND BLOOD COMPONENTS

	Approximate Frequency[a]	
Effect	**Ratio**	**%**
Immediate		
Acute hemolytic transfusion reaction	1/25,000	0.004
Febrile, nonhemolytic transfusion reaction	1/200	0.500
Allergic reactions	1/100 to 300	0.200
Hypervolemia	Variable	
Noncardiogenic pulmonary edema	1/5,000	0.020
Bacterial sepsis	Rare	
Anaphylactic hypotensive reactions	1/150,000	0.0007
Complications of massive transfusions (hemostatic defect, hypothermia and metabolic abnormalities	Unknown	
Delayed		
Delayed hemolytic transfusion reaction	1/1500 to 9000	0.020
Red blood cell alloimmunization	1/100	1.000
Leukocyte/platelet alloimmunization	1/10	10.000
Hemosiderosis	Unknown	
Graft-versus-host disease	Rare	
Posttransfusion purpura	Rare	
Viral hepatitis	1/1500	0.006
Transfusion-associated AIDS	1/36,000 to 300,000	0.0007
Transfusion-associated malaria	Rare	

Reprinted with permission from Menitove JE. How safe is blood transfusion? In: Smith DM Jr, Dodd RY, eds. Transfusion-transmitted infections. Chicago: ASCP Press, 1991:10. By permission of the American Society of Clinical Pathologists.

[a]Frequency, risk per unit transfused.

AIDS, acquired immunodeficiency syndrome.

ate the exposure risks, benefits, and expenses of autologous and allogeneic transfusion for the best patient outcomes. This chapter focuses on the options available to physicians to reduce the amount of transfused allogeneic blood products. We focus on techniques such as preoperative, intraoperative, and postoperative cell salvage, PRP, and ANH that conserve autologous blood or blood components. Other techniques, including hemofiltration devices and heparin-coated cardiopulmonary bypass (CPB) circuits and oxygenators, that facilitate red-cell mass conservation are also briefly reviewed. Much of the chapter will be directed toward the cardiac-surgery setting, but most of these techniques can be applied to a wide variety of surgical procedures.

AUTOLOGOUS BLOOD SALVAGE

Autologous blood transfusion involves the harvesting of blood or blood products for subsequent administration to the same patient. Autologous transfusion was originally used to secure blood replacement when circumstances made conventional transfusion of banked blood impossible. However, safety has become the driving force behind further development and implementation of autologous transfusion procedures.

The concept of autologous blood transfusion was introduced into medical practice in 1818. Blundell (5) has been credited with performing the first such autotransfusion of blood recovered during postpartum hemorrhage. He also published a series of experiments in which he demonstrated that autologous blood transfusion in animals with a syringe-infusion technique was safe, minimized air embolism, and was preferable to allogeneic blood transfusion (6). The apparent first instance of transfusion of blood collected intraoperatively was carried out by Duncan in 1885 (7). In that case, a small amount of blood collected from an amputated limb was anticoagulated with sodium phosphate and injected into the patient intravenously. Published in the 1920s and 1930s, a series of small case reports described blood that was collected from various abdominal cavities, strained through sterile gauze, citrated, and then reinfused to the patient. At this time, adverse reactions, including hemoglobinuria, were recognized and documented. Suction apparatuses were eventually used to facilitate the collection of salvaged blood for reinfusion (8). Even in the 1940s, when transfusion-transmitted disease was not an issue, the cost-effectiveness and benefits of autotransfusion were recognized. In 1968, Wilson and Taswell (9) introduced a new apparatus that permitted blood collection, processing, washing, and reinfusion in a continuous process. This development rapidly transformed intraoperative salvage techniques. With the apparatus, blood was collected from the surgical field via a suction aspirator; the blood was then fed into a continuous-flow centrifugation bowl in which the erythrocytes were selectively separated and extracted from the waste supernatant. These washed RBCs were then resuspended for infusion back to the patient. In 1970, Klebanoff (10) introduced a modified disposable autotransfusion apparatus that was considered to be safe, simple, and efficient. Further refinements in the development of washing with intermittent-flow centrifugation devices resulted in a decrease in the coagulopathy associated with intraoperative blood salvage. The removal of thromboplastic material by washing decreased the hemorrhagic complications but also resulted in removing all plasma proteins, including procoagulants (11, 12). For safety, contemporary autotransfusion practices rely on a combination of reservoirs for collection and washing procedures. The typical components of a modern autotransfusion device are depicted in Figure 22.1.

INTRAOPERATIVE RED-CELL SALVAGE

Intraoperative blood salvage can be accomplished through a variety of configurations. In cases where a large volume of blood loss is anticipated, shed blood, along with an added anticoagulant solution, is aspirated into a reservoir that contains a filter to remove blood clots and tissue debris. The collected blood is pumped into a centrifuge-based cell-salvage instrument that then concentrates the erythrocytes and washes them with 1–2 L of saline. After such processing, the red-cell concentrate is available for reinfusion to the patient. In situations of rapid hemorrhage, high-speed cell-salvage instruments can process a unit of RBCs in less than 5 minutes. When bleeding is slow, the blood can be held in the reservoir and then processed by a portable, table-top instrument or sent to a central processing area when sufficient quantities have been collected. Alternatively, shed blood can be collected, filtered, and reinfused without any concentration or washing. This method is typically used during surgical procedures

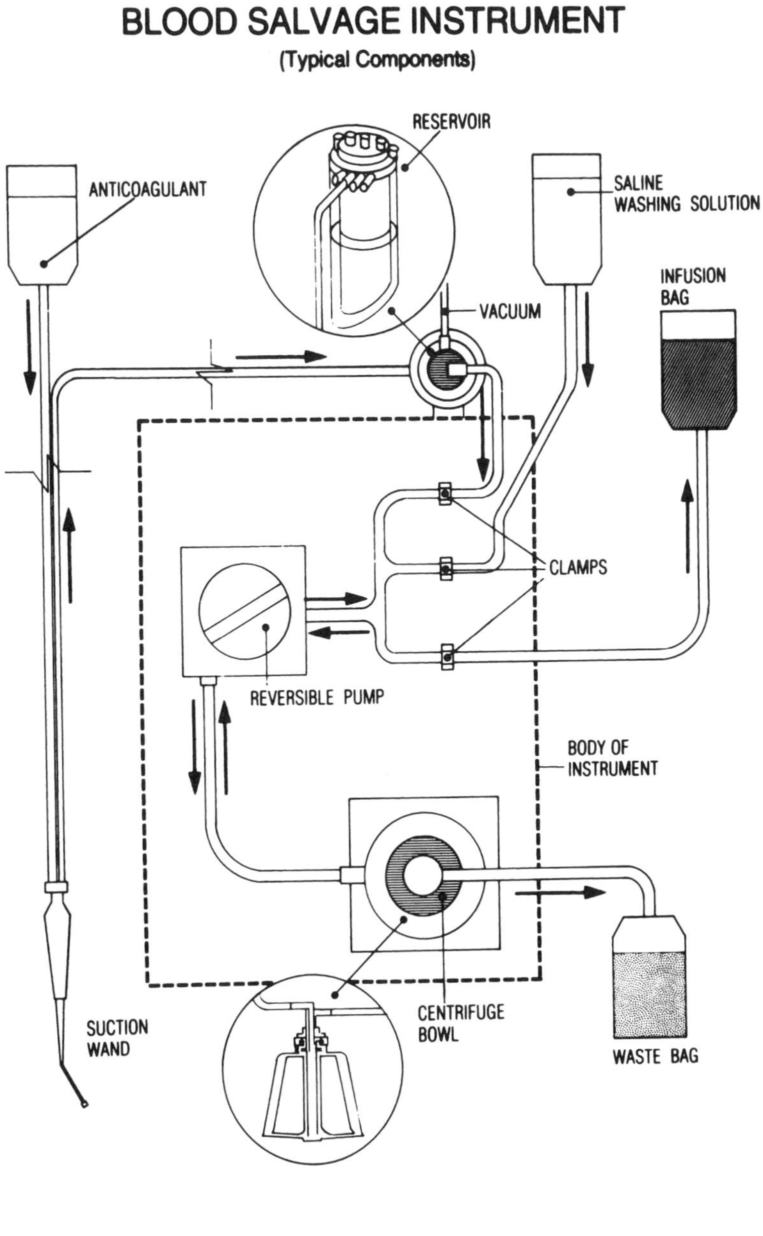

Figure 22.1. Diagram of components of a typical centrifuge-based blood salvage instrument. (Reprinted with permission from Williamson KR, Taswell HF, Rettke SR, Krom RAF. Intraoperative autologous transfusion: its role in orthotopic liver transplantation. Mayo Clin Proc 1989;64:340–345.)

with low volumes of blood loss, and a number of commercially available devices use this approach. Blood salvage can be extended for a limited time into the postoperative period in situations where continued bleeding occurs through a drain or chest tube. Postoperative systems can provide a washed or unwashed product for direct reinfusion.

The controversial decision to wash or not wash salvaged blood is often made at the institution level or even by the anesthesiologist, surgeon, or both physicians together. Issues to be considered include the type of surgical procedure, the estimated blood loss and salvaged-blood volume, the composition of the shed blood, and the rapidity of bleeding. Proponents of washing believe that it removes potentially harmful substances and that the simultaneous concentration of salvaged red cells is advantageous. Others claim that such processing is unnecessary, adding only time and expense to the procedure.

Salvaged blood is known to have low initial hematocrits (Hct), elevated free hemoglobin (Hgb), decreased coagulation factors, increased fibrin-degradation products (FDPs), and significant amounts of anticoagulant (13). Before processing, the Hct of shed blood is typically 20–30%, with lower levels seen in orthopedic cases (13) and in the later stages of postoperative drainage (14). Cell-salvage instruments can increase the Hct to 45–65%. Some hemolysis of RBCs occurs secondary to surgical trauma and aspiration from the wound. Resultant free Hgb levels are commonly less than 300 mg/dL but may be as high as 2000 mg/dL (15). Despite these high levels of free Hgb, erythrocyte indices and morphology are normal. Washing can remove most free Hgb while producing only mild morphological changes in erythrocytes. Both processed and unprocessed salvaged RBCs have been shown to have acceptable survival in vivo (16–18). Variable numbers of platelets and leukocytes are present in salvaged blood. With processing, platelet counts decrease and platelet and white-cell function are impaired.

Because thrombosis and fibrinolysis are activated during and after operations, shed blood contains decreased amounts of coagulation factors and increased levels of FDPs (19). Fibrinogen levels are typically very low in mediastinal and joint drainage; such blood does not usually clot and anticoagulation may not be needed during collection. Concern about the reinfusion of unwashed salvaged blood has focused on FDP potential to initiate coagulopathy. de Haan and colleagues (20) have also suggested that fibrin monomers and tissue-type plasminogen activator-stimulating activity in shed mediastinal blood potentiate the platelet dysfunction seen after CPB and lead to increased postoperative bleeding. Processing salvaged chest-tube blood will further decrease coagulation factors but also effectively remove FDPs and fibrin.

Schaff et al. (21) studied patients receiving shed mediastinal blood and control subjects and found no difference between the groups in the prothrombin time, activated partial thromboplastin time, fibrinogen, and FDPs. Others have found increases in fibrinolytic products in the reinfused blood, but the effect on patients was transient (19). Griffith et al. (22) found extremely high titers of FDPs in mediastinal blood. They compared the level of FDP in mediastinal blood that was both washed and unwashed. FDP titers were significantly elevated in the unwashed mediastinal blood, but no differences were found in the bleeding or coagulation parameters of the patients. Characteristics of shed mediastinal and pleural blood are summarized in Table 22.2 (23–26).

Unprocessed blood has also been shown to contain elevated levels of C3a, C5a, and terminal complement complexes (27); an altered lipid profile (28, 29); measurable

TABLE 22.2. CHARACTERISTICS OF SHED MEDIASTINAL AND PLEURAL BLOOD

	Pleural Blood	Mediastinal Blood			
Variable	Stored Whole Blood	Symbas (23)	Thurer et al. (24)	Hauer et al. (25)	Adan et al. (26)
Hematocrit value, %	38	17.5	19.9	25.1	21
Platelets, no. × $10^3/\mu L$	0	0	67.8	63.3	132
Plasma-free Hemoglobin, mg/dL	14	13	315	77.4	224
Fibrinogen, mg/dL	155	23	—	10	<100

Reprinted with permission from Chavez AM, Tarazi RY, Cosgrove DM III. Postoperative blood salvage. In: Taswell HF, Pineda AA, eds. Autologous transfusion and hemotherapy. Boston: Blackwell Scientific Publications, 1991:155–163.

amounts of methylmethacrylate (orthopedic bone cement); and fat particles (30). The presence of these materials raises concern regarding the safety of infusing unwashed salvaged blood. Faris et al. (31) reported a 22% incidence of febrile reactions accompanying the transfusion of unwashed autologous blood that was collected from joint drainage 6–12 hours after operations. However, unprocessed shed blood has been administered to many groups of patients in numerous studies with minimal ill effects. Much of this success may be related to the limited amount of unprocessed blood that is infused (usually less than 1 L) and to the limited collection periods (usually less than 6 hours). This risk of complications must be addressed in the context of the amount of mediastinal or drained blood that is directly transfused. Caution should be exerted if over 1 L of blood is being retransfused or if the patient appears to be bleeding more; with less than 1 L, reinfusion of unwashed blood is likely safe.

CLINICAL APPLICATIONS

Blood salvage has been applied most extensively in cardiac operations, such as coronary artery bypass grafting (CABG), valve replacement, repair of congenital heart disease, and other complex cardiac surgical procedures. Blood is typically collected intraoperatively and washed before reinfusion; blood from the CPB circuit may be added to the salvaged blood. As documented by Giordano and colleagues (32), significant amounts of autologous blood can be harvested in this manner. In their review of 6 years of experience with 9918 patients, the median amount of blood salvaged was equivalent to over 3 units of RBCs, with 59% coming from the operative field, 34% from the CPB circuit, and less than 10% from postoperative drainage. Larger amounts of blood are collected in reoperations and in combined CABG and valve-replacement operations. Multiple studies have suggested that the use of intraoperative (33–36) and postoperative (37, 38) blood salvage significantly decreases allogeneic transfusion requirements.

The use of intraoperative salvage in cardiac operations is well accepted. Postoperative salvage is more controversial; however, because the blood is usually unwashed and according to some recent studies, postoperative salvage may not reduce the need for allogeneic transfusions (39–42). The assessment of such efficacy has been problematic because of numerous other changes in transfusion practices over the last decade. These changes include improved surgical technique, the use of pharmacological agents to decrease blood loss, increased availability of preoperatively donated autologous blood, altered criteria for allogeneic transfusion, and the use of ANH. Controlled, randomized, and blinded trials are also difficult to perform. Thus, conclusions regarding effectiveness in today's clinical setting may be different from those found in earlier investigations. Determinations of efficacy may also need to be done, at least to some degree, at the local level.

Orthopedic surgeons have also been using perioperative blood salvage for spinal operations and hip and knee arthroplasties. In orthopedic procedures, smaller amounts of blood are lost over a longer period of time, and the collected blood contains tissue and bone debris, fat, and methylmethacrylate. The use of a tourniquet in total knee arthroscopy shifts blood loss into the postoperative period. Because of these characteristics, only 50–70% of the shed blood is salvaged (16), and the yield is often equivalent to less than 1 unit of RBCs (32), particularly in the postoperative drainage of replaced joints (43). Because most bleeding in joint arthroplasty occurs postoperatively, intense interest has arisen in the use of simple salvage devices to collect and reinfuse this drainage without further processing. Recent prospective randomized trials of this technique have had mixed results (44–49). One of the confounding factors in such studies is the availability of preoperatively donated autologous blood, a practice that is common in today's orthopedic surgery practices. The concurrent use of these predonated units tends to minimize or negate the effectiveness of blood salvage in reducing allogeneic transfusions (43–45).

Significant amounts of autologous blood have also been salvaged in vascular, liver transplant, neurosurgical, and trauma operations. Although aortic aneurysm repair commonly uses cell-salvage instruments to provide for greater than 50% of the transfusion needs of these patients (50–52), reinfusion of unprocessed shed blood has also been reported to be effective (53). Surgeons performing aorta bifemoral bypass grafting procedures frequently use intraoperative blood salvage, but its efficacy in this setting has recently been questioned (54). During liver transplantation procedures, blood loss can be both rapid and massive. High-speed cell-salvage instruments have been used to provide an average of 4–9 units of RBCs per case and 29–45% of the intraoperative transfusion needs (55–57). In these instances, blood salvage plays an important role in conserving the allogeneic blood supply. In neurosurgery, shed blood can be salvaged during the resection of intracranial arteriovenous malformations. An average of 3.1 units and as many as 16 units have been washed, concentrated, and reinfused in these cases (58).

The use of blood salvage techniques in patients with traumatic injuries has been accomplished but is somewhat challenging. Systems using washed or unwashed blood have been used in cases of hemothorax and hemoperitoneum where large amounts (1–4 L) of blood have been reinfused, but these amounts account for less than half of the total transfusion needs (59–62). Difficulties arise in trying to predict which patients will need the procedure and which patients will have bacterial contamination from intestinal injuries. Such bacterial contamination is generally a contraindication to blood salvage because of concerns of producing sepsis. However, salvaged blood that is known to be culture-positive has been infused into trauma patients with concurrent antibiotic administration and has not resulted in an increased risk of infectious complications (61, 63).

Intraoperative blood salvage has also been used in cases of ruptured ectopic pregnancy (15). It has not been routinely applied to other obstetrical patients because of concerns about the potential for amniotic fluid embolism. Recent in vitro work by Rutherford et al. (64) suggested that amniotic fluid is effectively removed from salvaged blood by washing with saline. This finding is supported, however, by limited clinical experience. A brief report describes a lack of amniotic fluid embolism or any other adverse reactions in 64 patients who received 136 units of salvaged and washed blood after cesarean section (65).

Many Jehovah's Witnesses, who refuse allogeneic blood on religious grounds, will accept intraoperative blood salvage using a high-speed cell-salvage instrument in either a modified (continuous circuit) or conventional configuration (66). Patients with multiple or high-frequency RBC alloantibodies may also benefit from blood salvage because it provides a source of compatible blood for transfusion.

CONTRAINDICATIONS AND COMPLICATIONS

Conditions thought to be contraindications to blood salvage include the use of microfibrillar collagen materials and infection or malignancy at the operative site. Microfibrillar collagen is not removed from the salvaged blood during the washing procedure, and infusion of units containing this material has caused significant morbidity and mortality in animals (67). Microfibrillar collagen is also not completely removed by passage through the typical 20-μm filter (68, 69), but recent evidence suggests that leukocyte-depletion filters do eliminate this compound (69).

Washing of salvaged blood does not reliably remove contaminating microorganisms. Therefore, aspiration of blood from an infected wound or one contaminated by bowel contents has been considered a risk for subsequent sepsis. However, as previously described, blood salvage, usually with the concurrent administration of broad-spectrum antibiotics, has been used successfully with penetrating abdominal injuries. Even when obtaining cultures from obviously noninfected operative sites, a significant number of routine surveillance cultures of salvaged blood from a wide variety of surgical procedures will be positive. The vast majority of these cases involve very low numbers of organisms (less than 1–2 colony-forming units/mL), which are recognized as skin and environmental contaminants (coagulase-negative staphylococci, diphtheroids, and other nonpathogens) (70–73). Clinical infections resulting from the infusion of culture-positive salvaged blood have not been seen.

Malignant cells are also known to survive processing and routine filtering of salvaged blood (74–77). No consistent correlation exists between the presence of circulating tumor cells and subsequent metastatic disease (78); furthermore, there have been no reports of cancer dissemination secondary to hematogenous spread by intraoperatively salvaged blood. Studies of the application of blood salvage procedures in urological cancer operations are ongoing and, thus far, have shown no evidence of increased malignancy recurrence or dissemination (79–80). Similar favorable results have been seen in cases of hepatic malignancies (81) and in renal carcinomas with intravascular extension (82).

The process of blood salvage is associated with few complications. Air embolism is a concern if the reinfusion bag of the cell-salvage circuit is directly connected to the patient's vascular access (15). However, this complication can be prevented by simply transferring the RBCs into a separate blood bag before administration. Antibiotics not intended for intravenous use may also end up in salvaged blood if irrigating solutions are aspirated into the collection reservoirs. Topical antibiotics placed in orthopedic wounds can also reach significant levels in postoperative drainage intended for direct reinfusion (83). Blood salvaged during removal of pheochromocytomas has been shown to cause hypertension in patients after reinfusion (84), because extensive washing does not eliminate epinephrine and norepinephrine. The direct reinfusion of shed mediastinal blood has been associated with increased serum enzymes (creatine kinase, lactate dehydrogenase, aspartate aminotransferase), and myoglobin and troponin levels in patients undergoing cardiac operations (85, 86). These elevated laboratory parameters may obscure the diagnosis of postoperative myocardial ischemia. The myocardial band (MB) fraction of creatine kinase is not elevated, however.

The development of a clinically significant coagulopathy after the infusion of salvaged blood has been a persistent concern. Although it occurred frequently in the past with the administration of large volumes of unwashed blood, coagulopathy is much less common now that modern cell-salvage instruments are in use. However, dilutional coagulopathy may still be seen in patients receiving large amounts of washed RBCs. Yawn (87) reported consistent decreases in platelet counts and coagulation-factor levels when more than 6 units of washed RBCs were given to patients undergoing complex aortic-aneurysm repairs. Moderate to severe abnormalities in the prothrombin time and the partial thromboplastin time were seen in 31% of trauma patients in one large series (88). In these patients, the coagulopathies developed in patients undergoing massive transfusion (greater than 15 units of salvaged and washed blood, greater than 10 units of salvaged and washed blood in patients with bowel injuries, or greater than 50 units of salvaged and allogeneic blood). Frank disseminated intravascular coagulation has also been noted, even in patients receiving only 1–2 units of salvaged and washed RBCs (89).

Bull and Bull (90) described the salvaged-blood syndrome in which patients develop manifestations of increased capillary permeability (such as adult respiratory distress syndrome or anasarca), intravascular coagulation, or a combination of these complications. Their investigations found deposits of platelets and leukocytes in the centrifuge bowls and reinfusion bags of such patients. They postulated that platelets are activated during blood salvage, particularly if the blood has been diluted with significant amounts of saline before aspiration. During the concentration phase of processing, these platelets deposit on the walls of the centrifuge bowl, degranulate, and release procoagulant and leukoattractant substances. The activated leukocytes also adhere to the platelet deposits. With reinfusion, the procoagulant platelet phospholipid and activated phagocytes may initiate disseminated intravascular coagulation, adult respiratory distress syndrome, and anasarca. Fortunately, salvaged blood syndrome is rare. In some cases of coagulopathy, additional factors such as acidosis, hypotension, hypothermia, and tissue trauma may contribute to the hemostatic abnormalities. Many of these patients will require supplemental transfusions of platelets and fresh-frozen plasma.

In summary, the ultimate goal of perioperative blood salvage is to minimize the use of allogeneic blood products by providing autologous blood for transfusion. The ability of salvage procedures to achieve this goal was discussed earlier in this chapter. Recent debate has now shifted to the cost-effectiveness of the procedure. At which point do the benefits of decreased risk and expense of allogeneic transfusion outweigh the risks and costs of blood salvage? This question has been approached from the view of the transfusion costs of allogeneic blood versus salvaged blood and the determination of a break-even point. For procedures using dedicated cell-salvage instruments, that point is 2–4 units of salvaged blood (52, 91). For canister- or reservoir-based systems with subsequent processing, it is around 2 units (2, 91), and for direct reinfusion devices, it may be as low as 1 unit (45). However, the concurrent availability of preoperatively donated autologous blood, its increased costs compared with allogeneic blood, and the risks of allogeneic transfusion have not been factored into previous analyses. One recent retrospective study of patients with spinal operations (49) suggests no benefit to the use of blood salvage when preoperatively donated autologous blood is available in sufficient quantities. Further work needs to be done to better define the most appropriate and cost-effective combinations of autologous blood sources for a variety of surgical procedures. Each institution will also have to perform its own cost-benefit analyses when examining the effectiveness of specific autologous programs.

AUTOLOGOUS PRP

Therapeutic plasmapheresis was first used in the early 1900s to treat uremia and to procure antibodies from animals (92, 93). Not until the 1950s, however, was plasmapheresis used on a larger scale to collect plasma for fractionation (94). Separation of various blood constituents is accomplished largely by the sedimenting characteristics of the constituents under the influence of centrifugal force. Centrifugation is the preferred means of blood cell and plasma separation. The development of two centrifugation systems, the intermittent-flow system and the continuous-flow system, interestingly originated from the first open continuous flow centrifuge for separating cream from milk, which revolutionized the dairy industry after it was introduced in 1878 (95). Intermittent-flow autotransfusion bowls were further developed for platelet washing and glycerolizing and deglycerolizing erythrocytes for plasma removal (96). Additional refinements have resulted in the production of a variety of blood cell separators that are in use today.

Developed in 1968, the plateletpheresis technique allows selective collection of large quantities of platelets from a single donor (97). Used in cardiac operations over the past decade, this procedure may have applications outside cardiac surgery in cases such as major aortic reconstruction and instrumented spine procedures.

After anesthetic induction (before CPB), the patient's blood is diverted (usually through a dedicated 8-Fr internal jugular catheter) into a centrifuge-based instrument that separates the RBCs from the platelets and plasma, including the buffy coat. The RBCs are immediately returned to the patient; the PRP product is stored at room temperature in a transfer pack containing anticoagulant citrate phosphate dextrose-A (ACD-A) and then administered at the completion of bypass. Through a series of draw-process-return cycles, the appropriate quantity of PRP, usually 10–30% of the patient's estimated plasma volume, is collected. The collection process, which may require 30–45 minutes to complete, is carried out after anesthetic induction during the initial opening steps of the surgical procedure and is usually completed shortly after sternotomy. During the PRP draw, an intravenous infusion of colloid (5% albumin or hetastarch) or crystalloid is used to minimize any untoward hemodynamic responses. The goal of the PRP procedure is to minimize postbypass bleeding by providing the patient with autologous functional platelets and coagulation factors that have not been exposed to the CPB circuit.

The deleterious effects of CPB on coagulation are well appreciated. In the first 5 minutes of CPB, a protein monolayer is laid down on the nonbiological surfaces of the circuit and oxygenator. It is the nature and interaction of this protein layer that will result in untoward effects on thrombosis and fibrinolysis. Even in the presence of adequate anticoagulation with heparin, thrombosis and fibrinolysis are activated. Platelet activation, sequestration, and dysfunction; dilution and consumption of coagulation factors; and fibrinolysis all occur when blood is exposed to the nonbiological extracorporeal circuit during CPB (98–101). These hemostatic defects can contribute to excessive post-CPB bleeding, and there is a theoretical advantage in limiting the exposure of platelets and plasma to the bypass circuit.

This exposure accelerates contact activation and activates high-molecular-weight kininogen, complement, and prekallikrein, which also contribute to the total body inflammatory response (99). Coagulation factors are diluted by the CPB prime, and their enzymatic reaction rates are reduced by hypothermia. After CPB, the prothrombin time, activated partial thromboplastin time, and bleeding time are prolonged. The primary clinically significant coagulation defect after CPB is likely a thrombocytopathy and relative thrombocytopenia (98). CPB also depletes various platelet glycoprotein receptors. The receptor for the von Willebrand factor, glycoprotein Ib (GpIb), is inactivated, and the platelet cross-linking fibrinogen receptors GpIIb/IIIa are depleted (100). The net result is a functional platelet defect that may significantly contribute to post-CPB bleeding and coagulopathy. Limiting the activation of thrombosis, fibrinolysis, and the inflammatory response to CPB with a procedure like PRP may help prevent post-CPB coagulopathy and reduce allogeneic transfusion requirements.

EARLY CLINICAL TRIALS

The success of this procedure in limiting allogeneic blood transfusion has been mixed (102–114). Some of the variability in results may be related to the dose of platelets collected and to differences in study designs (115). Table 22.3 summarizes the pertinent and clinically significant PRP studies, which vary greatly in their methodological approaches. The studies are arranged temporally.

Giordano and colleagues (105, 106) published the first two clinically important trials of PRP. The first study was prospective and demonstrated impressive reductions in transfusion requirements. However, they compared patients receiving PRP with historic control subjects and also reported transfusion data in mean values. Transfusion requirements among any group of patients undergoing cardiac operations can be quite skewed, and unevenly distributed data may best be reported as median values with ranges of distribution. In the second study, which included some data from the first study and again reported impressive reductions in transfusion requirements, the authors compared 373 consecutive PRP patients enrolled in 1987–1988 with 147 historical control patients from 1985 to 1986. The PRP treatment was not assigned in a random fashion, and a variety of surgical procedures were included. In the mid 1980s, transfusion practices were beginning to be scrutinized. Important changes in clinical transfusion criteria over these 4 years easily could have adversely affected the results of this study.

Shortly thereafter, Boldt et al. (109) published a small, prospective, and randomized trial of 45 patients undergoing cardiac operations who were assigned to one of three groups: control, platelet-poor plasma, or PRP. The authors did not show a reduction in transfusion requirements but did demonstrate that PRP was associated with reduced polymorphonuclear elastase, a proteolytic enzyme released by polymorphonuclear neutrophils and assumed to be an important mediator in the development of postperfusion lung syndrome. Another trial by Del Rossi et al. (102) demonstrated reduced transfusion requirements and higher platelet counts post-CPB with the use of PRP. However, only nine patients were in each of the PRP and control groups, and transfusion requirements were pooled for each group.

Perhaps the best early trial of PRP was published by Jones et al. in 1990 (110). They enrolled 100 patients scheduled for elective cardiac operations and prospectively and randomly assigned them to PRP or control groups. They standardized transfusion criteria and reported a significant reduction in red cell mass loss and allogeneic transfusion. Although otherwise an excellent study, they did not remove the bias in transfusion decisions by blinding the participating clinicians.

Davies and colleagues (111) believed that additional benefits of using PRP include improvement in postoperative pulmonary function and reduced time to extubation. They published a small unblinded series that also reported reductions in blood loss and transfusion requirements with PRP.

All of these earlier trials demonstrated moderate to impressive results with PRP, but they also had some important methodological limitations. More recent trials with improved methods demonstrate less impressive results.

TABLE 22.3. AUTOLOGOUS PLATELET-RICH PLASMA

Year	Reference	Patient Population	Sample Size	Study Characteristics	Transfusion Requirements	Coagulation Studies	Blood Loss	Median Platelet Yield	Comments
1988	Giordano et al. (102)	CABG/valve/ congenital/mixed surgery/redo surgery	57-Control 65-PRP	Prospective	Reduced 54%[a]	Not reported	NS	1.0–2.0 × 10^{11} platelets	
1989	Giordano et al. (103)	CABG/valve/ congenital/redo surgery	147-Control 373-PRP	Historical control group (1985–1986) PRP study group (1987–1988)	Reduced 59%[a]	Not reported	Reduced 10%[a]	18% of estimated plasma volume	Transfusion practice may have changed significantly between 1985 and 1988
1990	Boldt et al. (106)	CABG	15-Control 15-PPP 15-PRP	Prospective Randomized	NS	Increased platelet count, fibrinogen, and antithrombin-III, postop[a]	Reduced 25%[a]	2.4 × 10^{8} platelets-PRP 2.3 × 10^{7} platelets-PPP	Reduced polymorphonuclear elastase[a]
1990	De Rossi et al. (99)	CABG/valve/mixed surgery	9-Control 9-PRP	Prospective Randomized	Summated group data reduced 51%[a] Per patient-NS	Improved platelet count postbypass[a] Postop-NS	Reduced 25%	Estimated 5.5–7.7 × 10^{11} platelets (220 mL)	Reported group data, not median patient requirements
1990	Jones et al. (107)	CABG	50-Control 50-PRP	Prospective Randomized	Reduced 63%[a]	Not reported	Intraop-reduced 15%[a] Postop-NS Reduced chest tube hematocrit[a]	2.5 × 10^{11} platelets	RBC mass measured by radioiodinated albumin and radiochromium (^{51}Cr) methods
1992	Davies et al. (108)	CABG/redo/CABG	32-Control 32-PRP	Historical control group	Reduced 59%	Not reported	Reduced 46%	3.5 × 10^{11} platelets	Possible improvement in postoperative pulmonary function Some emergency surgery

TABLE 22.3. AUTOLOGOUS PLATELET-RICH PLASMA (*continued*)

Year	Reference	Patient Population	Sample Size	Study Characteristics	Transfusion Requirements	Coagulation Studies	Blood Loss	Median Platelet Yield	Comments
1993	Boey et al. (109)	CABG	20-Control 19-PRP	Prospective Randomized	Reduced 37%[a] (RBCs) Platelets-NS FFP-NS	Reduced fibrinogen[a] Reduced haptoglobin[a]	NS	2.0×10^{11} platelets	Increased fibrinogen consumption and hemolysis in PRP group Cell salvage not used
1993	Boldt et al. (104)	CABG	12-Control 12-PPP 12-PRP	Prospective Randomized	Summated group data reduced[a] Per patient-NS	Higher platelet count postop[a] Increased maximum aggregation and gradient of aggregation of platelets postbypass[a]	NS	1.9×10^{11} platelets-PRP 1.9×10^{10} platelets-PPP	All male patients Platelet aggregation normalized after 24 hrs
1993	Ereth et al. (100)	Redo valve surgery	28-Sham control 28-PRP	Prospective Randomized Blinded	NS	Minor changes intraop Postop-NS	NS	1.5×10^{11} platelets	Sham procedure
1993	Tobe et al. (101)	CABG	27-Sham control 24-PRP	Prospective Randomized Blinded	NS	Reduced prothrombin time Post PRP infusion[a] Postop-NS	NS	Unable to calculate yield 8–10 mL/kg-up to 1 L	Sham procedure Surgeons subjective assessment of coagulation-NS
1994	Wong et al. (110)	CABG/valve/mixed surgery	19-Control 19-PRP	Prospective Randomized	NS	NS	NS (4, 12, and 20 hr postop)	1.25×10^{11} platelets	Strict transfusion criteria likely reduced variability

[a]Statistical difference.

NS, no significance; PPP, platelet-poor plasma.

RECENT CLINICAL TRIALS

Four recently published trials were all prospective, randomized, and well controlled (103, 104, 112, 113). The studies by Boey et al. (112) and Tobe et al. (104) each used a blinding technique that entailed collecting PRP in all patients, immediately returning it in the control group, and returning it to the PRP group after CPB. The study by Ereth et al. (103) used a sham procedure, whereby the collection tubing and equipment were all placed behind blinding curtains. The last of the four studies, by Wong et al. (113), was not blinded but did examine coagulation function more closely than did the others.

Three of these trials were conducted using patients undergoing primary cardiac operations (104, 112, 113). The fourth trial assessed a group of patients undergoing repeat valvular operations (103), a population that has a much greater degree of blood loss and transfusion requirements than does the primary cardiac operation population.

None of these trials demonstrated any reduction in bleeding or transfusion requirements. Only minor changes in coagulation function were noted between groups. In Ereth's series (103), transfusion-related expenses, including the PRP procedure, were actually greater for patients in the treatment group than in the control group, and no improvement in outcome was shown.

Another recent investigation demonstrated that PRP resulted in improvement in platelet function and number immediately post-CPB (107). However, some of the largest and most active platelets are not collected during the PRP procedure because they remain admixed with the RBCs. This finding is consistent with the observation that administration of autologous *fresh* whole blood similarly improves platelet count and function (116). Perhaps collecting and readministering fresh autologous whole blood, thus preserving the largest and presumably most active platelets, would be equal or superior to PRP (117, 118).

A number of reasons account for the discrepancies between the earlier and more recent clinical trials of PRP. Important changes have taken place in the transfusion practices of most clinicians over the past decade. Early trials were not prospective, randomized, or blinded—characteristics all necessary for scientifically sound clinical trials. Transfusion practice is variable and is often influenced by a subjective component; thus, nonblinded studies introduce potentially important bias.

PRP may be ineffective for other reasons. The use of ACD-A as an anticoagulant for PRP storage may be a factor because citrate may damage PRP platelet membranes (119). Centrifugation from the PRP procedure itself may result in the release of platelet-granule contents, with possible impaired hemostatic function (120), and may partially inactivate and thereby decrease the clinical effectiveness of larger platelets in the RBC layer. The initial plateletpheresis may traumatize the blood components, perhaps as CPB does itself, or it may potentiate the platelet functional defects of preoperative aspirin ingestion (121). The RBCs returned to the patient after PRP separation may be fragile, and greater hemolysis may occur during CPB, which has been demonstrated by higher serum haptoglobin concentrations during CPB in PRP groups.

The importance of platelet yield must be considered as well. A standard allogeneic apheresis unit contains 3.0×10^{11} platelets. Only 2 of 11 trials presented in Table 22.3 reached that degree of yield. Yet autologous PRP should contain platelets that are more active than the banked allogeneic unit. In addition, platelet preparation and storage lesions cannot be overlooked. However, Boldt et al. (107) found no adverse effects of PRP on platelet function when using platelet aggregation as a measure of platelet function. Storage lesions are also unlikely with PRP because the product is stored for only a few hours.

In summary, platelet dysfunction is the most predictable defect resulting from cardiac operations and extracorporeal circulation. It seems intuitive that by removing the patient's own platelets from exposure to the CPB circuit and returning them later, platelet function might be preserved. Unfortunately, this may not be the case; recent well-controlled trials of PRP in both primary and repeat cardiac operations do not demonstrate clinical effectiveness in decreasing blood loss or transfusion requirements.

We believe that PRP should not be considered for routine use but rather on an individual basis, and its routine use in low-risk patients having primary CABG procedures is not warranted. The limited likelihood of coagulopathy and the availability of other blood-conservation methods alone or in combination should be considered first. Recent and well-controlled studies have not confirmed the optimistic results of earlier trials. At best, it appears that PRP (in standard form) does little to improve post-CPB coagulation function, exposes the patient to unnecessary hemodynamic risks, and does not reduce transfusion needs. Unless this procedure can be modified to increase true and clinically effective platelet yield, confirmed by well-controlled prospective trials that may include platelet-receptor studies, and is shown to reduce allogeneic transfusion requirements, it should not be in clinical use.

PRP is not an innocuous procedure. Its use requires a second large-bore intravascular catheter and may induce significant volume shifts during the draw and return cycles. Wickey et al. (122) demonstrated heparin resistance in patients who had PRP withdrawn pre-CPB. Significantly more heparin was required to initiate and to maintain anticoagulation for CPB in the PRP group than in the control group. Anticoagulation during CPB can be affected by many parameters and clinicians must be vigilant when using autologous blood procedures that may alter coagulation function.

In the evaluation of this and other blood conservation methods, specific outcome indicators (i.e., postoperative bleeding and blood component use), blinding methods, and specific criteria for transfusion should be used to determine the risks, benefits, and expense of such techniques. We must not be swayed by science based on a subjective assessment of blood banking procedures. Transfusion decisions are inherently subjective and are rarely objective in nature. If autologous PRP offers a benefit in cardiac operations, it is unclear when or in whom. This conclusion is echoed in a recently published review article (123).

ACUTE NORMOVOLEMIC HEMODILUTION

ANH is one of the many options clinicians may use to minimize perioperative exposure to allogeneic blood products. ANH is a single term for a broad therapeutic initiative that involves simultaneously removing the patient's blood and replacing it with a nonblood product. By producing a considerable decrease in the erythrocyte mass and, thus, a decrease in the net erythrocyte loss, ANH often decreases subsequent need for blood products. The volume of blood conserved is directly proportional to the differences between the original and postdilution Hct values. These autologous units have a full complement of coagulation factors and platelets, which may limit but not eliminate the development of coagulopathy in those patients in which it is used. The only blood conservation technique that results in fresh whole autologous blood, ANH is endorsed by the National Institutes of Health Consensus Conference on Perioperative Red Blood Cell Transfusion (3) and the American Society of Anesthesiologists. This accessible and easily institutable technique should be considered for some surgical patients, although its suitability and efficacy will depend on the clinical situation (124, 125).

ANH is based on studies conducted in the 1950s that demonstrated well-maintained compensatory responses to acute anemia when up to 50% of the patient's total circulating Hgb mass was removed (126). Further studies on the rheological, hemodynamic, metabolic, and cardiovascular consequences of hemorrhagic shock provided additional support for the concept of hemodilution (127). A 1972 study found that until an Hct value of 30% was reached, decreased viscosity and increased cardiac output (CO) provided maintenance of a maximal oxygen delivery to the tissues during hemodilution (128). In many situations, ANH is considered to be a viable alternative to transfusion with allogeneic blood products (129) and since the early 1970s has been used for surgical patients.

PROCEDURE DESCRIPTION

ANH is characterized as either moderate or severe hemodilution, depending on whether the Hct is 25–30% (moderate or limited) or 15–20% (severe or extreme). ANH is not simply the administration of nonblood fluid to reduce the Hgb but involves the active withdrawal of the patient's blood and the temporary acceptance of a lower Hgb. The collected blood is temporarily stored and subsequently transfused to the patient as indicated. Severe hemodilution, which may result in significant hemodynamic and physiological compromise that necessitates careful patient monitoring, may be most suitable for patients undergoing the protective effects of hypothermia and extracorporeal circulation.

Before the withdrawal of blood, adequate intravenous access is necessary. A urinary catheter, pulse oximeter for continuous monitoring of Hgb saturation, and an intraarterial catheter should be in place. Some authors have advocated the use of a central venous catheter (130) or pulmonary artery catheter for assessing ventricular filling (131) or approximating the adequacy of tissue oxygenation (132).

The hemodynamic response to phlebotomy of 500–700 mL is often minimal, and larger volumes of 1000–2000 mL have been removed without difficulty (133) but are more likely to elicit a stress response (134). Blood, which is usually withdrawn from a central venous or arterial catheter, drains by gravity into standard blood collection bags containing an anticoagulant such as ACD-A or citrate-phosphate-dextrose. If the blood is drawn from a peripheral vein, an automated blood pressure cuff may facilitate collection. If the patient requires CPB, the blood may be collected before or after heparin exposure (135, 136). Blood that is exposed to heparin may have a weaker hemostatic effect due to the effect of heparin on platelet function (137).

The collection of fresh whole blood should require about 10 minutes per unit. Strict adherence to sterile technique should be maintained. The blood should not leave the operating room so that there is little chance of administering it to the wrong patient. The blood should remain at room temperature in the operating room; if removed from the operating room, it must be appropriately labeled and stored at 4–6°C (124). The blood should be readministered in reverse order of collection, a method that ensures that the most hemodiluted unit is given first and the one with the most clotting factors and RBCs will be given last (138).

The amount of blood withdrawn for ANH, usually between 400 and 2000 mL, depends on the anticipated surgical blood loss and the patient's initial Hgb (136, 139, 140) and may be determined as a percentage of estimated blood volume or body weight. ANH has usually been limited to 20 mL/kg in children (141). In adults, the Hgb will decrease approximately 1 g/dL for each unit of blood removed.

There are several formulas to guide the process of withdrawing the predetermined amount of blood: $V = EBV \times Hct_i - Hct_f$/average Hct, where the average Hct $= (Hct_i - Hct_f)/2 + Hct_f$, where EBV is the estimated blood volume, V is the volume to be collected, Hct_i is the initial Hct, and Hct_f is the final desired Hct. An alternate formula that is an accurate guide to determine the volume of blood to withdraw for ANH is $V = EBV (Hct_i - Hct_f) (3 - \text{avg Hct})$.

During ANH, large amounts of fluid are frequently necessary to maintain normovolemia, although the net fluid increase may be insignificant compared with the usual transfusion requirements (136). Complications associated with the increased fluid include peripheral edema, pulmonary edema, abnormal wound healing, and worsened postoperative pulmonary function (142). Peripheral edema is relatively common with ANH, but pulmonary edema is fortunately not common (131). In most patients with good ventricular function, the increased fluid is well tolerated and usually resolves in 72 hours. Left ventricular hypertrophy or dysfunction reduces the tolerance to the increased fluid volumes. Overall, the benefit of ANH appears to outweigh the problems of the increased intravascular fluid (143).

Because the withdrawn blood must be adequately replaced with crystalloid or colloid fluid (136), comparisons have been performed to determine the optimal type of fluid replacement for ANH. Although crystalloid alone is acceptable, either colloid alone or a combination of crystalloid and colloid is favored (144). Albumin (144), hydroxyethyl starch, and dextran are all colloids that have been successfully used for ANH (145). Dextran provides excellent volume replacement but may cause greater blood loss in certain situations because of alterations in coagulation function (146). As such, dextran should be avoided in cardiac operations (147). Abnormal clotting studies may be seen with hydroxyethyl starch usage, but clinical bleeding has not yet been proven to be associated with this colloid.

Crystalloid is usually given as a 3- to 4-mL replacement per mL of withdrawn blood; colloid is usually given at 1–2 mL per mL of blood withdrawn. Generalized edema is more common with crystalloid than colloid replacement. Colloids have better intravascular retention and are more effective in restoring normovolemia than are crystalloids at four times the volume (148). Colloids are also associated with greater hemodynamic stability. Intravascular crystalloid equilibrates very quickly with the interstitial spaces. Only a small volume of crystalloid remains in the intravascular space with the heart and gastrointestinal tract developing the most edema (149).

The primary indication for ANH in surgical patients is the reduction of allogeneic blood transfusion. Perioperative transfusion of RBC (139, 150–153) and other blood products (154, 155) have been decreased with ANH. As important, the percentage of patients who do not receive any blood products is increased from 13% to 42% if ANH is combined with other blood salvage procedures during cardiac (156) and noncardiac operations (139).

ANH may be used in any type of operative procedure, including emergency procedures, if the patient is hemodynamically stable. In contrast to preoperative donation, infection does not preclude the use of ANH. The stress response is different during blood withdrawal in the awake patient for preoperative donation than it is during ANH in the anesthetized patient (134). Intraoperative ANH is not stress inducing; hormonal markers for stress are not elevated (134). However, preoperative blood donation has resulted in significant hemodynamic fluctuations in elderly patients, leading to more urgent cardiac operations and, perhaps, contributing to perioperative morbidity (157). With intraoperative ANH, invasive and noninvasive hemodynamic monitoring is available. These factors may increase the safety of intraoperative ANH and permit the participation of higher risk patients who would be otherwise rejected for preoperative donation (134). Because intraoperative ANH may be as effective as preoperative donation in reducing blood transfusions (158), ANH may be considered when preoperative blood donation is questionable, unsuitable, unavailable, or urgent.

SAFETY AND PHYSIOLOGICAL IMPLICATIONS OF ANH

Since ANH was introduced, studies have been performed to determine its benefits and risks (131). Unfortunately, no consensus has been established about the safety of ANH. Many physicians support the use of moderate hemodilution (131) yet consider the risks associated with an Hct less than 28% too great. The safety of ANH appears to be a function of various factors that are unique for each patient.

The safety of ANH has been demonstrated in cardiac (147, 153), vascular (139), orthopedic (155, 159), urological (158), and general operations (160). In a well-controlled prospective study involving patients undergoing radical retropubic prostatectomy, ANH was recently determined to be safe and beneficial. An expected blood loss of 1000 mL in this study was associated with the greatest benefit in reducing allogeneic blood transfusion (131). This degree of blood loss may be a good indication for ANH but has not been validated.

Certain factors increase the risk of hemodilution, and ANH may not be suitable for some patients. Contraindications include anemia (preoperative Hgb should at least be 11.1–12.0 g/dL) (145, 156); severe chronic obstructive pulmonary disease (if the baseline oxygenation is significantly impaired) (138); hemoglobinopathy, coagulation abnormalities, hepatic dysfunction, or low plasma-coagulation proteins (138); poor renal function; and severe aortic stenosis, unstable angina, or both.

The indications and consequences of ANH in the patient with coronary artery disease (CAD) for cardiac or noncardiac operations are not clear. The safety of ANH in patients with ischemic heart disease has been questioned recently in light of its potential benefit (161). Numerous animal and human studies concerning CAD and ANH have produced conflicting data. CAD and myocardial dysfunction are probably the two most important factors concerning the safety of ANH.

Johnson et al. (153) studied patients undergoing CABG and ANH and targeted an Hct of 32% or 25% for transfusion. They found no differences between these groups in fluid requirements, hemodynamic profile, or perioperative complications. They were also unable to identify an increased risk associated with a lower Hct in patients with good ventricular function who underwent elective CABG. However, the patient population was not large, and the study will need to be confirmed. In another series of patients undergoing CABG and hemodilution to an Hct of 15%, there was no evidence of myocardial ischemia or inadequate tissue oxygenation (162). Moreover, compared with patients who did not undergo ANH, those who had hemodilution had improved tissue oxygenation before CPB. Recently, patients hemodiluted to 15% before CABG by withdrawal of 1500 mL of blood subsequently had their Hct raised to 20% and then 25% (163). Electrocardiographic or metabolic data at any of the Hct levels did not show evidence of ischemia. In contrast, Weisel et al. (150) looked at myocardial metabolic indices in patients for CABG operations who were hemodiluted to an Hct of 21–24%. They reported delayed myocardial metabolic recovery, yet no mortality, myocardial ischemia or difference in creatinine kinase MB isoenzymes between hemodiluted and control patients. In this study, it is important to note that this delayed metabolic recovery was present long after the metabolic-reducing effects of general anesthesia. The assessment of these patients focused primarily on postoperative risk and hemodilution. Kim et al. (164) did not find postoperative evidence of insufficient myocardial or systemic oxygen supply in patients hemodiluted to an Hct of 23%. These patients had good myocardial baseline function and increased their CO without difficulty.

The use of moderate ANH is safe in noncardiac operations such as aortic-aneurysmal repair (139, 165). Kramer et al. (139) saw no evidence of tissue hypoxia based on the mixed venous oxygen saturation in patients undergoing abdominal aortic operations. Recently, a study using transesophageal echocardiography, a more sensitive indicator of myocardial ischemia, in patients undergoing abdominal-aortic-aneurysm repair with ANH to an Hct of 30% (166) showed no evidence of segmental regional wall motion abnormalities during aortic cross-clamping. These patients with CAD not only tolerated ANH but also had a decreased incidence of myocardial ischemia. Patients undergoing general operations appear to tolerate an Hct of 25% if the left ventricular function is adequate and CAD is not too severe. In contrast, others have found evidence of myocardial ischemia in patients undergoing vascular operations who had a postoperative Hct less than 30% after ANH (167, 168). Some people believe that patients with vascular operations should not undergo ANH because of their high incidence of CAD (142). Concern regarding myocardial injury is valid because anemia may predispose a patient to ischemic injury (150). The mechanism of myocardial ischemia may be a result of the reduced oxygen-carrying capacity (anemia) and the compensatory mechanisms (i.e., tachycardia) that increase myocardial oxygen consumption (169).

Studies in animal models of CAD and ANH have also yielded conflicting results. As Hct is reduced from 43% to 20%, myocardial oxygen demand is greatly increased (169). Below an Hct of 15%, the myocardium is unable to extract further oxygen (170) or increase coronary blood flow enough to satisfy additional oxygen demands. If the heart is unable to increase or maintain CO, and thus coronary perfusion, myocardial ischemia will result.

The consequences of hemodilution in animals or humans with compromised coronary blood flow are not fully appreciated. The pressure gradient across a stenotic artery is a critical determinant of myocardial ischemia. Increased coronary blood flow secondary to hemodilution may increase turbulence that results in a pressure decrease proximal to the coronary stenosis. Because these coronary vessels may be maximally dilated, they are unable to further compensate, which results in a reduced gradient and reduced coronary blood flow distal to the stenosis (171). Therefore, the expected increase in coronary blood flow associated with hemodilution may not occur in stenosed coronary arteries (168, 171). Hemodilution that would normally have increased coronary blood flow by 200% may increase coronary blood flow by only 47% in stenotic arteries (172).

Another potential cause for myocardial ischemia in the patient with ANH and CAD is the distribution of coronary blood flow. Under normal circumstances, endocardial coronary blood flow is slightly greater than epicardial coronary blood flow. With mild hemodilution, the ratio of endocardial to epicardial flow is maintained (169). In two studies (173, 174), electrocardiographic changes and myocardial failure resulted when dogs were hemodiluted. The maintenance of myocardial oxygenation is dependent on adequate perfusion pressure, particularly when the Hct is low (175). Data by Crystal and Salem (175) suggest that myocardial dysfunction occurs with a higher perfusion pressure in the presence of CAD and even moderate hemodilution. Heart failure occurred at a higher Hct in dogs with stenosed coronaries, a factor suggesting that patients with CAD have less reserve and may require a higher Hct.

Spahn et al. (176) found the lowest Hgb without myocardial dysfunction was 7.5 g/dL in dogs with artificially created left anterior descending coronary artery stenosis. The coronary stenosis limited the increase in coronary blood flow that usually follows hemodilution. Perhaps more important is that regional myocardial dysfunction was reversed with blood transfusion or removal of coronary constrictions.

Some animal studies have refuted previous investigations of ANH in CAD models. When Yoshikawa et al. (177) occluded the coronary arteries of dogs during ANH, hemodilution did not worsen ischemia. More recently, dogs hemodiluted to 15% significantly increased coronary blood flow across a stenotic portion of left anterior descending artery (LAD) (171). A large increase in coronary blood flow despite coronary stenosis may explain a lack of morbidity and mortality in many patients who undergo ANH and have CAD. Coronary blood flow in humans has been measured through cannulation of the coronary sinus after hemodilution from an Hct of 37% to 28%. The coronary blood flow increased 59%, and there was no evidence of increased oxygen extraction by the myocardium (178).

The degree of anemia that a patient with CAD can accept is not clear, but the minimal Hgb for sufficient myocardial oxygen supply in a patient with CAD will depend on myocardial oxygen demand. If the coronary blood flow is unable to increase in response to myocardial oxygen demands as the Hct decreases, this is the minimal safe Hct for hemodilution. Some studies suggest that a specific Hct is intolerable; however, tachycardia and decreased coronary driving pressure are important factors and may account for an insufficient balance of myocardial oxygen supply and demand. Patients are frequently hemodiluted to an Hct of 20% at the onset of CPB without widespread morbidity and mortality. Tolerance of a low Hct is quite different during CPB than it is in patients undergoing noncardiac operations.

Because many studies have been unable to reach a conclusion concerning CAD and ANH, some researchers maintain that coronary disease is a relative contraindication to ANH and suggest maintaining an Hct of 30% to achieve optimal myocardial recovery (179). Others will exclude the patient with CAD from ANH if the patient has depressed left ventricular function because that patient may require a higher Hct to avoid ischemia (180). Patients with cardiovascular disease are known to have episodes of silent ischemia. More important is that a certain percentage of patients not considered at risk for CAD have evidence of silent myocardial ischemia that places them at risk. Some people consider this sufficient evidence to argue against the routine use of ANH. As yet, no successful method identifies patients who will be at increased risk for myocardial ischemia with ANH. A patient should be assessed carefully and a determination made as to the benefit and potential risk of ANH based on the degree of hemodilution, ventricular function, and possibility or severity of CAD.

The age of a patient may also limit the degree of hemodilution. Severe hemodilution is usually reserved for younger patients. An Hct of 15–20% is well tolerated in a young healthy patient during cardiac or noncardiac operations (155, 159, 160). ANH has been used in children for major cancer operations, liver resections, and cardiac operations (141, 181). Hemodilution to an Hct of 20% is safe in humans (155).

Many elderly patients tolerate ANH quite well (145). When patients with a mean age of 69 years undergoing major operations with ANH were compared with a group of patients with a mean age of 46 years undergoing major operations, the perioperative outcomes were similar (138). With ANH, the hemodynamic compensatory actions of patients above 60 years of age were similar to those of patients less than 60 years of age (182). Although a patient's age may partially limit the response of compensatory mechanisms to hemodilution, many elderly patients respond effectively to the volume shifts of phlebotomy (183). Unless the patient has CAD, ANH is considered as safe in patients greater than 60 years of age as in those less than 60 years of age. Although the inability of some geriatric patients to increase myocardial blood flow with extreme hemodilution is well documented (155, 157), extremes of age are not contraindications to ANH (145). Older patients may require an Hct greater than 30%, particularly in the postoperative period when anesthesia no longer reduces metabolic oxygen requirements (132).

Animal studies support the finding that the limit of hemodilution for physiological integrity appears to be an Hct of 10% (172, 184). Hcts of 10% have been documented during cardiac operations in children with congenital heart disease who were Jehovah's Witnesses. These children displayed no evidence of neurological sequelae or other complications attributable to hemodilution (141, 181).

The major limiting factor in the tolerance of a low Hct is oxygen demand. The removal of blood causes a reduction in arterial oxygen content (CaO_2). Despite the reduction in oxygen content with a low Hgb, oxygen consumption in humans is such that there is a large margin of safety (169). When oxygen delivery remains sufficient, compensatory mechanisms for anemia are not invoked. Cerebral and myocardial tissues are more vulnerable to reduced oxygen-carrying capacity because they have high oxygen utilization. If oxygen supply is inadequate, compensatory mechanisms will attempt to increase oxygen delivery by increasing perfusion (132).

The major acute compensatory mechanism for maintenance of oxygen delivery during ANH is an increase in CO (138), which increases in direct proportion to a decrease in Hct (132) (Fig. 22.2). The increase in CO is primarily due to increased stroke volume (130, 160, 169) and increased venous return (138). The hemodiluted blood is less viscous; therefore, afterload is reduced and venous return increased (145).

For these compensatory mechanisms to maintain systemic oxygen transport, normovolemia and adequate cardiovascular function are necessary. Compounding intraoperative factors such as hypovolemia, general anesthesia, or hypothermia may limit compensatory increases in CO (155). If the CO is unable to increase in response to hemodilution and decreased arterial oxygen content, increased oxygen extraction is another compensatory mechanism (185).

During ANH, a widening arteriovenous oxygen saturation difference (155) or increased heart rate (138) may indicate that oxygen delivery is marginal or inadequate. An increased heart rate during anesthesia may be a sign of hypovolemia, although tachycardia is not a completely reliable indicator (171). In a patient's awake state, heart rate will increase with blood withdrawal to augment CO; conversely, in the anesthetized state, the stroke volume will increase (186).

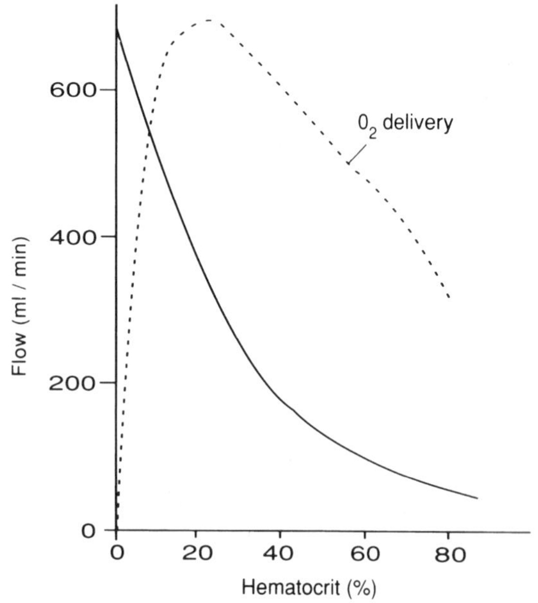

Figure 22.2. Blood flow and O_2 delivery through a glass tube at constant pressure as the hematocrit is varied. (Modified with permission from Crowell JW, Smith EE. Determination of the optimal hematocrit. J Appl Physiol 1967;22:501–504.)

Hemodilution also changes the distribution of blood flow between and within organs. Within a certain range of Hct levels, a constant rate of oxygen delivery will be maintained to vascular beds by vasodilation and vasoconstriction depending on the blood viscosity and oxygen consumption (170). Blood flow to tissues and organs that are supply-dependent, such as the heart and brain, increases significantly with hemodilution to an Hct of 15% (169, 171). These tissues use the greatest amounts of oxygen and have a high near-maximal oxygen-extraction ratio. They are unable to compensate for hemodilution-induced, reduced oxygen delivery by increasing oxygen extraction. Cerebral blood flow increases 500–600% in both animals and humans with hemodilution to an Hct of 10% (169). This increase in cerebral and myocardial blood flow is primarily related to the change in viscosity but is not in the same proportion as the increase in CO. During hypothermia, patients may have higher cerebral oxygen delivery with a 23% Hct than a 28% Hct (187). In fact, Lilleaasen (188) has shown that during CPB, cerebral circulation is maintained as well at an Hct of 18% as at 27%.

Blood flow to the rest of the body is more reflective of the change in CO associated with hemodilution. Blood flow in the vertebral artery, mesenteric artery, and lower aorta matches the change in CO. Direct measurements of oxygen tension in these tissues have shown adequate oxygenation with an Hct of 20%. Blood flow in the hepatic and carotid arteries increased proportionately less (132). In dogs undergoing ANH, renal blood flow remains stable (189), and in patients undergoing aortic vascular reconstruction, renal function may even be preserved (152).

ANH not only results in alteration in oxygen-carrying capacity but may also challenge osmotic and intravascular-interstitial fluid balance. The lungs are at risk for interstitial or frank pulmonary edema with ANH because these patients receive significant fluid challenges. Most patients will exhibit some increase in lung water after CPB, but hemodiluted patients have even more of an increase. Diuretics, fluid restriction, or both can serve to remove this fluid more rapidly, although it may resolve within the first 4 days (143). If the patient receiving crystalloid is supplemented with some colloid to increase intravascular oncotic pressure, renal blood flow is augmented and contributes to more rapid diuresis (152).

Maintaining colloid osmotic pressure during CPB is an important factor in reducing postoperative pulmonary dysfunction (190). Several studies have attempted to determine if the choice of colloid or crystalloid influenced pulmonary dysfunction after CPB with ANH. Compared with patients given crystalloid, patients given colloid tended to have reduced pulmonary complications (190). The use of crystalloid solutions to prime the extracorporeal circuit or replace blood during ANH increases the alveolar-arterial oxygen gradient after CPB (190). If a colloid is used for ANH in patients undergoing CABG, lung water and the pulmonary gas exchange are no different than those in patients who did not undergo ANH (190). With crystalloid compared with colloid use in CABG patients, there is also a greater alveolar-arterial gradient upon extubation (150). Yet others have found no adverse effects after infusing 10 L of crystalloid (186), and some patients undergoing extreme hemodilution tolerate the fluid challenges without developing pulmonary edema (190).

Hypertonic solutions have been used for ANH. Boldt et al. (147) found that a hypertonic hydroxyethyl starch solution was more effective in preserving pulmonary gas exchange, maintaining adequate circulatory volume, and preserving hemodynamics in CABG patients undergoing ANH. The effects of hypertonic solutions on hemodynamic parameters during ANH are not transitory (147), and renal blood flow is well maintained. However, it is important to be aware of the potential complications of hypertonic solutions such as hypernatremia and central pontine myelinolysis.

The physiological implications of ANH are different for each patient. The clinician must be aware of the potential for physiological insult with moderate or severe hemodilution and apply that knowledge to the care and monitoring of each specific patient. In contrast to preoperative blood donation, the procedure of ANH is begun after the induction of anesthesia; therefore, the patient is continuously monitored.

EFFICACY IN REDUCING TRANSFUSION REQUIREMENTS

The blood-saving effect of ANH is attributed to several factors. A major reason is the conservation of RBC mass by decreasing the Hct of shed blood. In a patient with an Hct of 40% and an estimated surgical blood loss of 1000 mL, the RBC loss is 400 mL. If the Hct is only 25%, the RBC loss is reduced to 250 mL. The net RBC mass conservation in this example is 150 mL, which could be even more because a patient's Hct constantly changes during hemodilution (161).

Another explanation for reduced blood product transfusions in cardiac operations with ANH has been credited to a lack of exposure of the withdrawn blood (platelets and coagulation factors) to the deleterious effects of CPB (191). Fresh whole blood collected before CPB improves hemostasis after CPB better than platelet concentrates (192). The hemostatic benefit of a single unit of fresh whole blood has been compared with an allogeneic transfusion of 10 units of platelet concentrates (193). Platelets in fresh whole blood are larger and more hemostatically active (194). Fresh whole blood also contains some clotting factors that may contribute to hemostasis. Autologous fresh whole blood does not undergo certain biochemical processes to the same extent that stored blood does. In contrast to preoperatively donated blood, the fresh whole blood of ANH is stored only briefly at room temperature, a factor that preserves platelet function better than hypothermic storage does.

ANH was used early in the development of cardiac operations because transfusion and excessive blood loss were frequent (195). More recently, ANH is commonly used in many different surgical settings (145). In 1957, Dodrill et al. (135) were one of the first groups to collect heparinized blood intraoperatively and reinfuse it after CPB. ANH has subsequently been shown to reduce allogeneic blood requirements by 25–58% (136, 143, 153). Recently, Ikeda et al. (196), using multiple blood conservation techniques but not pharmacological hemostatic agents or preoperative donation, found a clear difference in the quantity of intraoperative and postoperative blood products transfused in patients who underwent ANH before CPB. ANH is also popular in spinal operations and joint arthroplasty where it reduces allogeneic blood use (131). In a wide range of surgical procedures, ANH has decreased allogeneic transfusion by 18–90% (131). Comparisons of blood use between ANH and historical control subjects reveal a 75% reduction in allogeneic blood use in pediatric spinal fusion (197), hepatic resection (198), major colon operations, and radical cystectomy (186). However, as we point out in our discussion, studies in which a therapeutic intervention is compared with historic control subjects are flawed and must be interpreted with great caution.

In 1977, Lilleaasen (188) found that compared with moderate hemodilution, extreme hemodilution further reduced blood loss and transfusion requirements. A recent report from Dale et al. (199) confirms these findings. Dramatic reductions in blood transfusion are also reported with severe hemodilution in settings apart from cardiac operations. Martin and Ott (155) prospectively studied 26 teenagers undergoing Harrington-rod instrumentation for scoliosis who were hemodiluted to an Hct of 15%. Mean allogeneic transfusion requirements were reduced from 4370 to 750 mL, and, at discharge, total allogeneic blood transfusion in control patients was six times higher than in ANH patients.

Other studies have not found a difference in transfusion requirements with ANH (125, 140). Recently, Vedrinne et al. (140) compared the hemostatic effects of ANH with aprotinin, which significantly reduces transfusion requirements and blood loss in cardiac operations (200). Compared with aprotinin, ANH did not reduce transfusion requirements or mediastinal blood loss. The lack of efficacy was postulated as inadequate storage of the fresh whole blood or insufficient volume of blood withdrawn. Vedrinne et al. (140) collected only 400 mL of blood; other ANH studies collected 700–1500 mL of blood and reported a benefit (136, 201). However, Scott et al. (156) withdrew only 575 mL of blood and reported a reduction in blood transfusion in primary cardiac operations. In a noncardiac surgery setting, a case study analysis of patients undergoing radical prostatectomy demonstrated that the blood conservation benefit of ANH was minimal (125). However, the degree of hemodilution in this study (125) was much less than in other successful trials of ANH. In this trial, dextran, which may adversely affect thrombosis and surgical blood loss, was used as the volume replacement after the blood was withdrawn.

ADDITIONAL BENEFITS AND CONCERNS

Other additional benefits of ANH include a reduced incidence of wound infection (202), an improvement in oxygen delivery to peripheral tissues, and an increase in 2,3-diphosphoglycerate (DPG) (203). Another advantage of ANH over preoperatively donated blood is the fact that ATP and 2,3-DPG are decreased in preoperatively donated blood during hypothermic storage. Once transfused, this preoperatively stored blood does not immediately have the same oxygen delivery capabilities as fresh whole blood collected for ANH.

ANH also improves perfusion and oxygen delivery to the tissues by decreasing blood viscosity. With hemodilution to an Hct of 15%, blood acts like a Newtonian fluid (169). The effect of Hct is greatest at a lower flow rate. At a high flow rate, only an Hct of 40–45% provides optimal oxygenation (145). At a lower flow rate, an Hct of 45% will reduce oxygen transport as a result of the increased viscosity (145). This, then, is the reason that a lower Hct with lower flow rates can still provide adequate oxygenation.

Hemodilution also affects the shear rate (velocity gradient) of the fluid in the microcirculation. Shear rate varies directly with vessel size; the microcirculation has a low shear rate. At a low shear rate, one sees the maximal effect of lowered viscosity and hemodilution in the capillaries and the postcapillary venules. This low rate results in more homogenous flow that provides better perfusion and reduces the chance of anaerobic metabolism (130, 162). In some models, oxygen delivery increases as the Hct decreases to 25% (169) (Fig. 22.3). Even with an Hct of 20% during ANH, oxygen transport is reduced only 10% from its maximal value, yet the mean tissue Po_2 actually increases slightly. These studies illustrate how ANH increases oxygen supply to the tissues

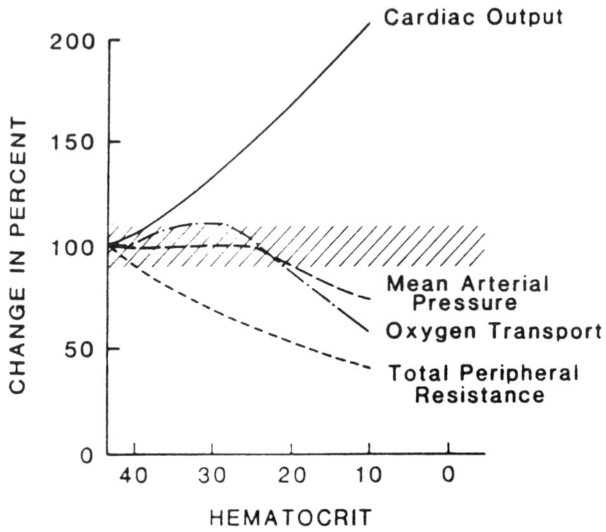

Figure 22.3. Physiological response to isovolumic hemodilution. Increased cardiac output maintains mean arterial pressure and oxygen delivery despite a decreased total peripheral resistance caused by anemia. (Reprinted with permission from Klimberg IW. Autotransfusion and blood conservation in urologic oncology. Semin Surg Oncol 1989;5:286–292.) Reprinted by permission of Wiley-Liss, Inc., a subsidiary of John Wiley & Sons, Inc.

(138). Initiation of hemodilution in tissues that are ischemic results in an increase in oxygen tension (169). Thus, there are numerous theoretical benefits to ANH.

Some clinicians and scientists express concern regarding increased bleeding as a result of hemodilution. However, compared with control subjects, ANH patients undergoing total hip arthroplasty had no increase in surgical bleeding (204). Another concern involves further hemodilution of coagulation factors and thrombocytopenia, but an association of increased bleeding with ANH has yet to be documented. Clotting factors remain within physiological ranges (205).

ANH may be combined with other techniques to reduce blood loss. Induced hypotension has been combined with ANH to safely reduce bleeding and transfusion requirements (204). Recently, 119 patients undergoing spinal fusion were hemodiluted to an Hct of 20%, hypotension was induced with nitroglycerin, and tissue perfusion remained adequate (159). The drug of choice for induced hypotension with ANH is unclear. Adenosine may provide safe and effective induced hypotension (206). Nitroprusside can also be used but is not universally recommended (189). A detailed discussion of induced hypotension is presented in Chapter 21.

In summary, a conclusive statement regarding transfusion requirements and blood loss with ANH is difficult. Because multiple conservation techniques are frequently used, the impact of an individual technique is difficult to ascertain. The effect of ANH on transfusion requirements varies greatly depending on the surgical procedure and study design. Many factors contribute to perioperative transfusion and blood loss (124). The number of blood products transfused is strongly related to the transfusion trigger (151, 207). In the past, patients were generally transfused if the Hgb was below 10.0 g/dL, particularly during anesthesia (208). It is now generally recognized that most patients under general anesthesia tolerate an Hgb of 8.0 g/dL (209). Transfusion of RBC is now being delayed without difficulty in some cases until the Hct is 15% (151, 155, 207). This factor alone will influence transfusion requirements to an extent irrespective of any hemostatic effect of ANH.

There are many practical benefits to using ANH. The intraoperative collection of blood for ANH is simpler than is preoperative autologous donation and does not require any additional equipment or typing and crossmatching. ANH is easy to coordinate and requires minimal preoperative planning. Because the patient is in the operating room, the blood is readily available for immediate transfusion without delay. ANH is free of the risks of transfusion reactions and infection. ANH may slightly increase anesthesia and operative time (165); however, obtaining the same amount of preoperatively donated blood is much more expensive and labor intensive (131, 158).

In conclusion, ANH is a technique that can be used to reduce transfusion requirements associated with operations. Carefully controlled, prospective, randomized clinical trials are needed to further define the risks and benefits. Patient selection and optimal management, particularly in the patient with CAD, will need to be studied further. Hemodynamics must be appropriately managed to reduce the incidence of myocardial ischemia in patients during ANH. The practice of ANH is variable, reflecting the many concerns and issues that still surround its use (131). The risk, benefit, and cost-effectiveness profile of ANH has yet to be determined. Future developments such as artificial oxygen carriers may reduce some negative effects of hemodilution and resulting reduced oxygen-carrying capacity. ANH is a safe therapeutic option to reduce the occurrence of blood transfusion associated with operations.

CPB TECHNIQUES

In the setting of CPB, many other interventions may be helpful in conserving red-cell mass during cardiac operations. The use of a nonblood prime for CPB, heparin-coated CPB oxygenators and circuits, and hemofiltration during CPB may effectively conserve red-cell mass and also reduce transfusion requirements.

NONBLOOD PRIME FOR CPB

Nonblood prime for the CPB circuit has been used for many years with success. With nonblood prime, the Hgb will tend to decrease to 7.0–8.0 g/dL. This range appears to provide the optimal viscosity for maximal perfusion yet ensures acceptable oxygen-carrying capacity. Nonblood prime results in significant reductions in blood requirements in cardiac operations (210) and improves perfusion to end organs. Hemostasis is not adversely affected by the hemodilution despite the fall in fibrinogen level and platelet counts. In one study, platelet adhesiveness was better and patients bled less with the more extreme hemodilution (199).

HEMOFILTRATION

Techniques using cell-salvage instruments may decrease transfusion requirements, but they also result in discarding the plasma fraction of the processed blood. Preserving the plasma fraction of blood can be accomplished with hemofiltration. Hemofiltration (also known as ultrafiltration) is an extracorporeal technique that uses convection transport across a semipermeable membrane under a hydrostatic gradient to remove water and low molecular solutes from blood. Early uses included treating fluid overload due to renal or cardiac failure and when preparing patients for specific surgical procedures. It also enables patients with renal failure to successfully undergo cardiac operations with CPB. Approximately a decade ago, hemofiltration began to be used during and after CPB to remove excess fluid and to concentrate the blood remaining in the CPB circuit at the end of bypass. Hemofiltration removes a renal ultrafiltrate while conserving platelets, plasma, fibrinogen, and other coagulation factors (211). Derangements in colloid osmotic pressure are also reduced with hemofiltration. Cell-salvage and hemofiltration techniques often function comparably with respect to hemoconcentration. Hemofiltration may be indicated during cardiac operations for patients with renal failure and when high volumes of crystalloid cardioplegia are used.

Boldt et al. (212) demonstrated lower fluid balance with hemofiltration techniques in cardiac patients. They also reported that antithrombin III, fibrinogen, platelet number, albumin, total protein, and colloid osmotic pressure were less compromised when hemofiltration was used.

More recently, Journois et al. (213) carefully examined hemostasis, cytokines, and components of complement in patients hemofiltrated during repair of congenital heart disease. They concluded that hemofiltration improved hemodynamics and early postoperative oxygenation and reduced postoperative blood loss and the duration of mechanical ventilation.

The systemic inflammatory response that occurs during CPB may result in a capillary leak syndrome that contributes to morbidity and mortality (214). This process can lead to fluid overload, impede pulmonary gas exchange, and delay separation from mechanical ventilation. In addition, the CPB-associated hemodilution of platelets and coagulation factors promotes the hemostatic impairment that is generally observed in children undergoing cardiac operations (215). Hemofiltration also removes some major mediators of the inflammatory response such as C3a, C5a, interleukin-6, and tumor necrosis factor-α.

The improvement in several biochemical and clinical markers of patient well-being in the early postoperative period when hemofiltration is used is impressive. It is likely that hemofiltration will gain greater scientific and clinical acceptance as an important adjunct in the perioperative care of patients undergoing CPB.

HEPARIN-COATED CPB OXYGENATORS AND TUBING

Reduction or elimination of systemic heparinization during CPB with the use of heparin-coated oxygenators and CPB circuits may decrease the incidence and severity of coagulopathy associated with CPB (216). This area holds great promise; however, definitive outcome studies have not been published.

SUMMARY AND CONCLUSION

In the last two decades, intraoperative blood salvage has advanced into an important tool of proven benefit to the patient, the surgeon, the anesthesiologist, and the transfusion medicine specialist. A high degree of safety now exists in these therapeutic interventions, which can be carried out at increasing speeds and with a decreasing number of personnel and amount of equipment. The heightened awareness of the threat of fatal disease transmission by blood transfusions has served as a catalytic force to accelerate the use and public acceptance of intraoperative blood salvage and all forms of autologous blood transfusion. The increased understanding of the clinical efficacy of intraoperative blood salvage procedures, along with excellent risk:benefit ratios, has established these interventions as important medical therapeutic options.

Unfortunately, underuse of autologous procedures may occur. Transfusion practices vary significantly and are quite subjective at times. Removing transfusion bias in clinical trials is necessary to achieve appropriate conclusions that have direct application to patient care. Studies should be interpreted with caution. Those procedures that have a reliably defined effect or change in outcome, such as reduced bleeding or need for transfusion, cost-effectiveness, and balanced risk:benefit ratio, should continue to be applied to clinical care. Those interventions that do not should be abandoned. In the new era of cost-effective health care, resources must be directed to those activities that truly benefit patients.

When applied appropriately, the use of intraoperative salvage techniques can be very beneficial to patients. Intraoperative or postoperative cell salvage can significantly reduce transfusion requirements. The use of PRP is less likely to provide a benefit to the patient than are the other salvage techniques and, in standard configuration, may only increase transfusion-related expenses. ANH is efficacious in certain clinical situations but is certainly not applicable to all patients and all surgical procedures. Astute clinicians must evaluate published trials, such as those reviewed in this chapter, and apply them to their own practice settings. Appropriate application of these and other perioperative interventions can benefit patients greatly by reducing blood loss, allogeneic transfusion requirements, transfusion-related expenses, and allogeneic transfusion-associated morbidity and mortality.

REFERENCES

1. Dodd RY. The risk of transfusion-transmitted infection [editorial]. N Engl J Med 1992;327:419–421.
2. Popovsky MA, Devine PA, Taswell HF. Intraoperative autologous transfusion. Mayo Clin Proc 1985;60:125–134.
3. Anonymous. Consensus Conference. Perioperative red blood transfusion [review]. JAMA 1988;260:2700–2703.
4. Saarela E. Autotransfusion: a review. Ann Clin Res 1981;13(Suppl. 33):48–56.
5. Allen JG. Discussion. Ann Surg 1963;158:337.
6. Blundell J. Experiments on the transfusion of blood by the syringe. Med Chirg Trans 1818;9:57–92.
7. Duncan J. On re-infusion of blood in primary and other amputations. Br Med J 1886;30:192–193.
8. Davis LE, Cushing H. Experiences with blood replacement during or after major intracranial operations. Surg Gynecol Obstet 1925;40: 310–322.
9. Wilson JD, Taswell HF. Autotransfusion: historical review and preliminary report on a new method. Mayo Clin Proc 1968;43:26–35.
10. Klebanoff G. Early clinical experience with a disposable unit for the intraoperative salvage and reinfusion of blood loss (intraoperative autotransfusion). Am J Surg 1970;120:718–722.
11. Wilson JD, Utz DC, Taswell HF. Autotransfusion during transurethral resection of the prostate: technique and preliminary clinical evaluation. Mayo Clin Proc 1969;44:374–386.
12. Kingsley JR, Valeri CR, Peters H, Cole BC, Fouty WJ, Herman CM. Citrate anticoagulation and on-line cell washing in intraoperative autotransfusion in the baboon. Surg Forum 1973;24:258–260.
13. Yawn DH. Properties of salvaged blood. In: Taswell HF, Pineda AA, eds. Autologous transfusion and hemotherapy. Boston: Blackwell Scientific Publications, 1991:194–206.

14. Eng J, Kay PH, Murday AJ, et al. Postoperative autologous transfusion in cardiac surgery. A prospective, randomised study. Eur J Cardiothorac Surg 1990;4:595–600.
15. Williamson KR, Taswell HF. Intraoperative blood salvage: a review. Transfusion 1991;31:662–675.
16. Ray JM, Flynn JC, Bierman AH. Erythrocyte survival following intraoperative autotransfusion in spinal surgery: an in vivo comparative study and 5-year update. Spine 1986;11:879–882.
17. Kent P, Ashley S, Thorley PJ, Shaw A, Parkin A, Kester RC. 24-hour survival of autotransfused red cells in elective aortic surgery: a comparison of two intraoperative autotransfusion systems. Br J Surg 1991; 78:1473–1475.
18. Davis RJ, Agnew DK, Shealy CR, Friedman SE. Erythrocyte viability in postoperative autotransfusion. J Pediatr Orthop 1993;13:781–783.
19. Fuller JA, Buxton BF, Picken J, Harris RA, Davies MJ. Haematological effects of reinfused mediastinal blood after cardiac surgery. Med J Aust 1991;154:737–740.
20. de Haan J, Schonberger J, Haan J, van Oeveren W, Eijgelaar A. Tissue-type plasminogen activator and fibrin monomers synergistically cause platelet dysfunction during retransfusion of shed blood after cardiopulmonary bypass. J Thorac Cardiovasc Surg 1993;106:1017–1023.
21. Schaff HV, Hauer J, Gardner TJ, et al. Routine use of autotransfusion following cardiac surgery: experience in 700 patients. Ann Thorac Surg 1979;27:493–499.
22. Griffith LD, Billman GF, Daily PO, Lane TA. Apparent coagulopathy caused by infusion of shed mediastinal blood and its prevention by washing of the infusate. Ann Thorac Surg 1989;47:400–406.
23. Symbas PN. Extraoperative autotransfusion from hemothorax. Surgery 1978;84:722–727.
24. Thurer RL, Lytle BW, Cosgrove DM, Loop FD. Autotransfusion following cardiac operations: a randomized, prospective study. Ann Thorac Surg 1979;27:500–507.
25. Hauer JM, Schaff HV, Bell WR, et al. Reinfusion of shed mediastinal tube blood following open heart surgery: a prospective study [abstract]. Circulation 1977:56(Suppl.):III–250.
26. Adan A, Brutel de la Riviere A, Haas F, van Zalk A, de Nooij E. Autotransfusion of drained mediastinal blood after cardiac surgery: a reappraisal. Thorac Cardiovasc Surg 1988;36:10–14.
27. Bengtson JP, Backman L, Stenqvist O, Heideman M, Bengtsson A. Complement activation and reinfusion of wound drainage blood. Anesthesiology 1990;73:376–380.
28. Langton SR, Sieunarine K, Lawrence-Brown MMD, Goodman MA, Prendergast FJ, Hellings M. Lipolytic enzyme and phospholipid level changes in intraoperative salvaged blood. Transfusion Med 1991;1: 263–267.
29. Sieunarine K, Lawrence-Brown MM, Goodman MA, Prendergast FJ, Rocchetta S. Plasma levels of the lipid mediators, leukotriene B_4 and lyso platelet-activating factor, in intraoperative salvaged blood. Vox Sang 1992;63:168–171.
30. Healy WL, Wasilewski SA, Pfeifer BA, et al. Methylmethacrylate monomer and fat content in shed blood after total joint arthroplasty. Clin Orthop Res 1993;286:15–17.
31. Faris PM, Ritter MA, Keating EM, Valeri CR. Unwashed filtered shed blood collected after knee and hip arthroplasties: a source of autologous red blood cells. J Bone Joint Surg [Am] 1991;73:1169–1178.
32. Giordano GF, Giordano DM, Wallace BA, Giordano KM, Prust RS, Sandler SG. An analysis of 9,918 consecutive perioperative autotransfusions. Surg Gynecol Obstet 1993;176:103–110.
33. Keeling MM, Gray LA Jr, Brink MA, Hillerich VK, Bland KI. Intraoperative autotransfusion. Experience in 725 consecutive cases. Ann Surg 1983;197:536–541.
34. Breyer RH, Engelman RM, Rousou JA, Lemeshow S. Blood conservation for myocardial revascularization. Is it cost effective? J Thorac Cardiovasc Surg 1987;93:512–522.
35. McCarthy PM, Popovsky MA, Schaff HV, et al. Effect of blood conservation efforts in cardiac operations at the Mayo Clinic. Mayo Clin Proc 1988;63:225–229.
36. Hall RI, Schweiger IM, Finlayson DC. The benefit of the Haemonetics cell saver apparatus during cardiac surgery. Can J Anaesth 1990;37: 618–623.
37. Schaff HV, Hauer JM, Bell WR, et al. Autotransfusion of shed mediastinal blood after cardiac surgery: a prospective study. J Thorac Cardiovasc Surg 1978;75:632–641.
38. Morris JJ, Tan YS. Autotransfusion: is there a benefit in a current practice of aggressive blood conservation? Ann Thorac Surg 1994;58: 502–507.
39. Roberts SR, Early GL, Brown B, Hannah H III, McDonald HL. Autotransfusion of unwashed mediastinal shed blood fails to decrease banked blood requirements in patients undergoing aortocoronary bypass surgery. Am J Surg 1991;162:477–480.
40. Ward HB, Smith RRA, Landis KP, Nemzek, TG, Dalmasso AP, Swaim WR. Prospective, randomized trial of autotransfusion after routine cardiac operations. Ann Thorac Surg 1993;56:137–141.
41. Axford TC, Dearani JA, Ragno G, et al. Safety and therapeutic effectiveness of reinfused shed blood after open heart surgery. Ann Thorac Surg 1994;57:615–622.
42. Bouboulis N, Kardara M, Kesteven PJ, Jayakrishnan AG. Autotransfusion after coronary artery bypass surgery: is there any benefit? J Card Surg 1994;9:314–321.
43. Umlas J, Foster RR, Dalal SA, O'Leary SM, Garcia L, Kruskall MS. Red cell loss following orthopedic surgery: the case against postoperative blood salvage. Transfusion 1994;34:402–406.
44. Majkowski RS, Currie IC, Newman JH. Postoperative collection and reinfusion of autologous blood in total knee arthroplasty. Ann R Coll Surg Engl 1991;73:381–384.
45. Kristensen PW, Sorensen LS, Thyregod HC. Autotransfusion of drainage blood in arthroplasty: a prospective, controlled study of 31 operations. Acta Orthop Scand 1992;63:377–380.
46. Heddle NM, Brox WT, Klama LN, Dickson LL, Levine MN. A randomized trial on the efficacy of an autologous blood drainage and transfusion device in patients undergoing elective knee arthroplasty. Transfusion 1992;32:742–746.
47. Gannon DM, Lombardi AV Jr, Mallory TH, Vaughn BK, Finney CR, Niemcryk S. An evaluation of the efficacy of postoperative blood salvage after total joint arthroplasty: a prospective randomized trial. J Arthroplasty 1991;6:109–114.
48. Mauerhan DR, Nussman D, Mokris JG, Beaver WB. Effect of postoperative reinfusion systems on hemoglobin levels in primary total hip and total knee arthroplasties. J Arthroplasty 1993;8:523–527.
49. Simpson MB, Georgopoulos G, Eilert RE. Intraoperative blood salvage in children and young adults undergoing spinal surgery with predeposited autologous blood: efficacy and cost effectiveness. J Pediatr Orthop 1993;13:777–780.
50. Yawn DH. Autologous transfusion in the context of aneurysm surgery. Presented at a Symposium on Intraoperative Blood Recovery and Autologous Transfusion (Thur Cardiovascular Systems), Houston, Texas, November 23, 1985.
51. Hallett JW Jr, Popovsky M, Ilstrup D. Minimizing blood transfusions

during abdominal aortic surgery: recent advances in rapid autotransfusion. J Vasc Surg 1987;5:601–606.
52. Reddy DJ, Ryan CJ, Shepard AD, et al. Intraoperative autotransfusion in vascular surgery. Arch Surg 1990;125:1012–1016.
53. Ouriel K, Shortell CK, Green RM, DeWeese JA. Intraoperative autotransfusion in aortic surgery. J Vasc Surg 1993;18:16–22.
54. Kelley-Patteson C, Ammar AD, Kelley H. Should the Cell Saver Autotransfusion Device be used routinely in all infrarenal abdominal aortic bypass operations? J Vasc Surg 1993;18:261–265.
55. Dzik WH, Jenkins R. Use of intraoperative blood salvage during orthotopic liver transplantation. Arch Surg 1985;120:946–948.
56. Dale RF, Lindop MJ, Farman JV, Smith MF. Autotransfusion, an experience of seventy six cases. Ann R Coll Surg Engl 1986;68:295–297.
57. Williamson KR, Taswell HF, Rettke SR, Krom RAF. Intraoperative autologous transfusion: its role in orthotopic liver transplantation. Mayo Clin Proc 1989;64:340–345.
58. Santrach PJ, Williamson KR, Taswell HF, Cucchiara RF, Piepgras DG. Intraoperative blood salvage in neurosurgery [abstract]. Transfusion 1989;29(Suppl.):23s.
59. Jacobs LM, Hsieh JW. A clinical review of autotransfusion and its role in trauma. JAMA 1984;251:3283–3287.
60. Jurkovich GJ, Moore EE, Medina G. Autotransfusion in trauma. A pragmatic analysis. Am J Surg 1984;148:782–785.
61. Timberlake GA, McSwain NE Jr. Autotransfusion of blood contaminated by enteric contents: a potentially life-saving measure in the massively hemorrhaging trauma patient? J Trauma 1988;28:855–857.
62. Plaisier BR, McCarthy MC, Canal DF, Solotkin K, Broadie TA. Autotransfusion in trauma: a comparison of two systems. Am Surg 1992;58: 562–566.
63. Ozmen V, McSwain NE Jr, Nichols RL, Smith J, Flint LM. Autotransfusion of potentially culture-positive blood (CPB) in abdominal trauma: preliminary data from a prospective study. J Trauma 1992;32:36–39.
64. Rutherford CJ, Thornhill ML, O'Leary AJ, Lussos SA, Johnson MD. Assessment of amniotic fluid removal from human blood by cell saver processing [abstract]. Transfusion 1991;31:22s.
65. Jackson SH, Lonser RE. Safety and effectiveness of intracesarean blood salvage. Transfusion 1993;33:181.
66. Spence RK, Alexander JB, DelRossi AJ, et al. Transfusion guidelines for cardiovascular surgery: lessons learned from operations in Jehovah's Witnesses. J Vasc Surg 1992;16:825–831.
67. Robicsek F, Duncan GD, Born GVR, Wilkinson HA, Masters TN, McClure M. Inherent dangers of simultaneous application of microfibrillar collagen hemostat and blood-saving devices. J Thorac Cardiovasc Surg 1986;92:766–770.
68. Niebauer GW, Oz MC, Goldschmidt M, Lemole G. Simultaneous use of microfibrillar collagen hemostat and blood saving devices in a canine kidney perfusion model. Ann Thorac Surg 1989;48:523–527.
69. Orr MD, Ferdman AG, Maresh JG. Removal of avitene microfibrillar collagen hemostat by use of suitable transfusion filters. Ann Thorac Surg 1994;57:1007–1011.
70. Williamson KR, Anhalt JP, Koehler LC, Willis EA, Taswell HF. Cultures of intraoperatively salvaged blood in light of FDA guidelines [abstract]. Transfusion 1989;29(Suppl.):23s.
71. Kang Y, Aggarwal S, Virji M, et al. Clinical evaluation of autotransfusion during liver transplantation. Anesth Analg 1991;72:94–100.
72. Ezzedine H, Baele P, Robert A. Bacteriologic quality of intraoperative autotransfusion. Surgery 1991;109:259–264.
73. Bland LA, Villarino ME, Arduino MJ, et al. Bacteriologic and endotoxin analysis of salvaged blood used in autologous transfusions during cardiac operations. J Thorac Cardiovasc Surg 1992;103: 582–588.
74. Yaw PB, Sentany M, Link WJ, Wahle WM, Glover JL. Tumor cells carried through autotransfusion. Contraindication to intraoperative blood recovery? JAMA 1975;231:490–491.
75. Homann B, Zenner HP, Schauber J, Ackermann R. Tumor cells carried through autotransfusion. Are these cells still malignant? Acta Anaesthesiol Belg 1984;35:51–59.
76. Miller GV, Ramsden CW, Primrose JN. Autologous transfusion: an alternative to transfusion with banked blood during surgery for cancer. Br J Surg 1991;78:713–715.
77. Karczewski DM, Lema MJ, Glaves D. The efficiency of an autotransfusion system for tumor cell removal from blood salvaged during cancer surgery. Anesth Analg 1994;78:1131–1135.
78. Salsbury AJ. The significance of the circulating cancer cell. Cancer Treat Rev 1975;2:55–72.
79. Klimberg I, Sirois R, Wajsman Z, Baker J. Intraoperative autotransfusion in urologic oncology. Arch Surg 1986;121:1326–1329.
80. Hart OJ III, Klimberg IW, Wajsman Z, Baker J. Intraoperative autotransfusion in radical cystectomy for carcinoma of the bladder. Surg Gynecol Obstet 1989;168:302–306.
81. Zulim RA, Rocco M, Goodnight JE Jr, Smith GJ, Krag DN, Schneider PD. Intraoperative autotransfusion in hepatic resection for malignancy. Is it safe? Arch Surg 1993;128:206–211.
82. Dzik WH, Sherburne B. Intraoperative blood salvage: medical controversies. Tranfusion Med Rev 1990;4:208–235.
83. Lux PS, Martin JW, Whiteside LA. Reinfusion of whole blood following addition of tobramycin powder to the wound during total knee arthroplasty. J Arthroplasty 1993;8:269–271.
84. Smith DF, Mihm FG, Mefford I. Hypertension after intraoperative autotransfusion in bilateral adrenalectomy for pheochromocytoma. Anesthesiology 1983;58:182–184.
85. Wahl GW, Feins RH, Alfieres G, Bixby K. Reinfusion of shed blood after coronary operation causes elevation of cardiac enzyme levels. Ann Thorac Surg 1992;53:625–627.
86. Hannes W, Keilich M, Koster W, Seitelberger R, Fasol R. Shed blood autotransfusion influences ischemia-sensitive laboratory parameters after coronary operations. Ann Thorac Surg 1994;57:1289–1294.
87. Yawn DH. Autologous blood salvage during elective surgery. Transfusion Sci 1989;10:107–116.
88. Horst HM, Dlugos S, Fath JJ, Sorensen VJ, Obeid FN, Bivins BA. Coagulopathy and intraoperative blood salvage (IBS). J Trauma 1992;32: 646–653.
89. Murray DJ, Gress K, Weinstein SL. Coagulopathy after reinfusion of autologous scavenged red blood cells. Anesth Analg 1992;75: 125–129.
90. Bull BS, Bull MH. The salvaged blood syndrome: a sequel to mechanochemical activation of platelets and leukocytes? Blood Cells 1990;16:5–23.
91. Solomon MD, Rutledge ML, Kane LE, Yawn DH. Cost comparison of intraoperative autologous versus homologous transfusion. Transfusion 1988;28:379–382.
92. Fleig C. L'auto-transfusion de globules lavés comme procédé de lavage aus ang dans les toxhémies: L'hétéro-transfusion de globules lavés dans les anémies. Bull Mens Acad Sci Montp 1909;1:4–6.
93. Abel JJ, Rowntree LG, Turner BB. Plasma removal with return of corpuscles (plasmapheresis). J Pharmacol Exp Ther 1914:5:625–641.
94. Grifols-Lucas JA. Use of plasmapheresis in blood donors. Br Med J 1952;1:854.

95. Judson G, Jones A, Kellogg R, et al. Closed continuous-flow centrifuge. Nature 1968;217:816–818.
96. Tullis JL, Tinch RJ, Gibson JB II, Baudanza P. A simplified centrifuge for the separation and processing of blood cells. Transfusion 1967;7: 232–242.
97. Tullis JL, Eberle WG II, Baudenza P, Tinch R. Platelet-pheresis: description of a new technic. Transfusion 1968;8:154–164.
98. Holloway DS, Summaria L, Sandesara J, Vagher JP, Alexander JC, Caprini JA. Decreased platelet number and function and increased fibrinolysis contribute to postoperative bleeding in cardiopulmonary bypass patients. Thromb Haemost 1988;59:62–67.
99. Kirklin JK, Westaby S, Blackstone EH, Kirklin JW, Chenoweth DE, Pacifico AD. Complement and the damaging effects of cardiopulmonary bypass. J Thorac Cardiovasc Surg 1983;86:845–857.
100. Wenger RK, Lukasiewicz H, Mikuta BS, Niewiarowski S, Edmunds LH Jr. Loss of platelet fibrinogen receptors during clinical cardiopulmonary bypass. J Thorac Cardiovasc Surg 1989;97:235–239.
101. Zilla P, Fasol R, Groscurth P, Klepetko W, Reichenspurner H, Wolner E. Blood platelets in cardiopulmonary bypass operations. Recovery occurs after initial stimulation, rather than continual activation. J Thorac Cardiovasc Surg 1989;97:379–388.
102. DelRossi AJ, Cernaianu AC, Vertrees RA, et al. Platelet-rich plasma reduces postoperative blood loss after cardiopulmonary bypass. J Thorac Cardiovasc Surg 1990;100:281–286.
103. Ereth MH, Oliver WC Jr, Beynen FMK, et al. Autologous platelet-rich plasma does not reduce transfusion of homologous blood products in patients undergoing repeat valvular surgery. Anesthesiology 1993;79: 540–547.
104. Tobe CE, Vocelka C, Sepulvada R, et al. Infusion of autologous platelet rich plasma does not reduce blood loss and product use after coronary artery bypass. A prospective, randomized, blinded study. J Thorac Cardiovasc Surg 1993;105:1007–1014.
105. Giordano GF, Rivers SL, Chung GKT, et al. Autologous platelet-rich plasma in cardiac surgery: effect on intraoperative and postoperative transfusion requirements. Ann Thorac Surg 1988;46:416–419.
106. Giordano GF Sr, Giordano GF Jr, Rivers SL, et al. Determinants of homologous blood usage utilizing autologous platelet-rich plasma in cardiac operations. Ann Thorac Surg 1989;47:897–902.
107. Boldt J, Zickmann B, Ballesteros M, Oehmke S, Stertmann F, Hempelmann G. Influence of acute preoperative plasmapheresis on platelet function in cardiac surgery. J Cardiothorac Vasc Anesth 1993;7:4–9.
108. Noon GP, Jones J, Fehir K, Yawn DH. Use of pre-operatively obtained platelets and plasma in patients undergoing cardiopulmonary bypass. J Clin Apheresis 1990;5:91–96.
109. Boldt J, von Bormann B, Kling D, Jacobi M, Moosdorf R, Hempelmann G. Preoperative plasmapheresis in patients undergoing cardiac surgery procedures. Anesthesiology 1990;72:282–288.
110. Jones JW, McCoy TA, Rawitscher RE, Lindsley DA. Effects of intraoperative plasmapheresis on blood loss in cardiac surgery. Ann Thorac Surg 1990;49:585–590.
111. Davies GG, Wells DG, Mabee TM, Sadler R, Melling NJ. Platelet-leukocyte plasmapheresis attenuates the deleterious effects of cardiopulmonary bypass. Ann Thorac Surg 1992;53:274–277.
112. Boey SK, Ong BC, Dhara SS. Preoperative plateletpheresis does not reduce blood loss during cardiac surgery. Can J Anaesth 1993;40:844–850.
113. Wong CA, Franklin ML, Wade LD. Coagulation tests, blood loss, and transfusion requirements in platelet-rich plasmapheresed versus nonpheresed cardiac surgery patients. Anesth Analg 1994;78:29–36.
114. Wells DG, Davies GG. Platelet salvage in cardiac surgery. J Cardiothorac Vasc Anesth 1993;7:448–451.
115. Gravlee GP. Autologous platelet-rich plasma in cardiac surgery: aesthetics versus virtue [editorial]. J Cardiothorac Vasc Anesth 1993;7:1–3.
116. Mohr R, Goor DA, Yellin A, Moshkovitz Y, Shinfeld A, Martinowitz U. Fresh blood units contain large potent platelets that improve hemostasis after open heart operations. Ann Thorac Surg 1992;53:650–654.
117. Mohr R, Sagi B, Lavee J, Goor DA. The hemostatic effect of autologous platelet-rich plasma versus autologous whole blood after cardiac operations: is platelet separation really necessary [letter]? J Thorac Cardiovasc Surg 1993;105:371–373.
118. Mohr R, Martinowitz U, Lavee J, Amroch D, Ramot B, Goor DA. The hemostatic effect of transfusing fresh whole blood versus platelet concentrates after cardiac operations. J Thorac Cardiovasc Surg 1988;96: 530–534.
119. Wallace HW, Brooks H, Stein TP, Zimmerman NJ. The contribution of anticoagulants to platelet dysfunction with extracorporeal circulation. J Thorac Cardiovasc Surg 1976;32:735–741.
120. Anderson NAB, Pamphilon DH, Tandy NJ, Saunders J, Fraser ID. Comparison of platelet-rich plasma collection using the Haemonetics PCS and Baxter Autopheresis C. Vox Sang 1991;60:155–158.
121. Ferraris VA, Ferraris SP, Lough FC, Berry WR. Preoperative aspirin ingestion increases operative blood loss after coronary artery bypass grafting. Ann Thorac Surg 1988;45:71–74.
122. Wickey GS, Keifer JC, Larach DR, Diaz MR, Williams DR. Heparin resistance after intraoperative platelet-rich plasma harvesting. J Thorac Cardiovasc Surg 1992;103:1172–1176.
123. Boldt J. Acute platelet-rich plasmapheresis for cardiac surgery. J Cardiothorac Vasc Anesth 1995;9:79–88.
124. Anonymous. The use of autologous blood. The National Blood Resource Education Program Expert Panel. JAMA 1990;263:414–417.
125. Goodnough LT, Grishaber JE, Monk TG, Catalona WJ. Acute preoperative hemodilution in patients undergoing radical prostatectomy: a case study analysis of efficacy. Anesth Analg 1994;78:932–937.
126. Wise W, Head LR, Morse M, Allen JG. The physiological effects of acute anemia produced by the replacement of serial hemorrhages with dextran, plasma, and whole blood. Surg Forum 1957;8:18–22.
127. Replogle RL, Merrill EW. Hemodilution: rheologic, hemodynamic, and metabolic consequences in shock. Surg Forum 1967;18:157–159.
128. Messmer K, Lewis DH, Sunder-Plasmann L, Klövekorn WP, Mendler N, Holper K. Acute normovolemic hemodilution. Changes of central hemodynamics and microcirculatory flow in a skeletal muscle. Eur Surg Res 1972;4:55–70.
129. Hardesty RL, Bayer WL, Bahnson HT. A technique for the use of autologous fresh blood during open-heart surgery. J Thorac Cardiovasc Surg 1968;56:683–688.
130. Landow L. Perioperative hemodilution. Can J Surg 1987;30:321–325.
131. Stehling L, Zauder HL. Controversies in transfusion medicine. Perioperative hemodilution: pro [review]. Transfusion 1994;34:265–268.
132. Robertie PG, Gravlee GP. Safe limits of isovolemic hemodilution and recommendations for erythrocyte transfusion [review]. Int Anesthesiol Clin 1990;28:197–204.
133. Hughes GS Jr, DeSmith VL, Locker PK, Francom SF. Phlebotomy of 500 or 750 milliliters of whole blood followed by isovolemic hemodilution or autologous transfusion yields similar hemodynamic, hematologic, and biochemical effects. J Lab Clin Med 1994;123:290–298.
134. Atallah MM, Abdelbaky SM, Saied MM. Does timing of hemodilution influence the stress response and overall outcome? Anesth Analg 1993;76:113–117.

135. Dodrill FD, Marshall N, Nyboer J, Hughes CH, Derbyshire AJ, Stearns AB. The use of the heart-lung apparatus in human cardiac surgery. J Thorac Cardiovasc Surg 1957;33:60–73.
136. Hallowell P, Bland JH, Buckley MJ, Lowenstein E. Transfusion of fresh autologous blood in open-heart surgery. A method for reducing blood bank blood requirements. J Thorac Cardiovasc Surg 1972;64: 941–948.
137. Kestin AS, Valeri CR, Khuri SF, et al. The platelet function defect of cardiopulmonary bypass. Blood 1993;82:107–117.
138. Messmer K. Hemodilution-possibilities and safety aspects [review]. Acta Anaesthesiol Scand 1988;89(Suppl.):49–53.
139. Kramer AH, Hertzer NR, Beven EG. Intraoperative hemodilution during elective vascular reconstruction. Surg Gynecol Obstet 1979;149: 831–836.
140. Vedrinne C, Girard C, Jegaden O, et al. Reduction in blood loss and blood use after cardiopulmonary bypass with high-dose aprotinin versus autologous fresh whole blood transfusion. J Cardiothorac Vasc Anesth 1992;6:319–323.
141. Stein JI, Gombotz H, Rigler B, Metzler H, Suppan C, Beitzke A. Open heart surgery in children of Jehovah's Witnesses: extreme hemodilution on cardiopulmonary bypass. Pediatr Cardiol 1991;12:170–174.
142. Gillon J. Controversies in transfusion medicine. Acute normovolemic hemodilution in elective major surgery: con [review]. Transfusion 1994;34:269–271.
143. Scott WJ, Kessler R, Wernly JA. Blood conservation in cardiac surgery [review]. Ann Thorac Surg 1990;50:843–851.
144. Brinkmeyer S, Safar P, Motoyama E, Stezoski W. Superiority of colloid over electrolyte solution for fluid resuscitation (severe normovolemic hemodilution). Crit Care Med 1981;9:369–370.
145. Stehling L, Zauder HL. Acute normovolemic hemodilution. Transfusion 1991;31:857–868.
146. Kallos T, Smith TC. Replacement for intraoperative blood loss. Anesthesiology 1974;41:293–295.
147. Boldt J, Kling D, Weidler B, et al. Acute preoperative hemodilution in cardiac surgery: volume replacement with a hypertonic saline-hydroxyethyl starch solution. J Cardiothorac Vasc Anesth 1991;5: 23–28.
148. Shoemaker WC. Comparison of the relative effectiveness of whole blood transfusions and various types of fluid therapy in resuscitation. Crit Care Med 1976;4:71–78.
149. Utley JR, Wachtel C, Cain RB, Spaw EA, Collins JC, Stephens DB. Effects of hypothermia, hemodilution, and pump oxygenation on organ water content, blood flow and oxygen delivery, and renal function. Ann Thorac Surg 1981;31:121–133.
150. Weisel RD, Charlesworth DC, Mickleborough LL, et al. Limitations of blood conservation. J Thorac Cardiovasc Surg 1984;88:26–38.
151. Jones JW, Rawitscher RE, McLean TR, Beall AC Jr, Thornby JI. Benefit from combining blood conservation measures in cardiac operations. Ann Thorac Surg 1991;51:541–546.
152. Welch M, Knight DG, Carr HM, Smyth JV, Walker MG. The preservation of renal function by isovolemic hemodilution during aortic operations. J Vasc Surg 1993;18:858–866.
153. Johnson RG, Thurer RL, Kruskall MS, et al. Comparison of two transfusion strategies after elective operations for myocardial revascularization. J Thorac Cardiovasc Surg 1992;104:307–314.
154. Milam JD, Austin SF, Nihill MR, Keats AS, Cooley DA. Use of sufficient hemodilution to prevent coagulopathies following surgical correction of cyanotic heart disease. J Thorac Cardiovasc Surg 1985;89: 623–629.
155. Martin E, Ott E. Extreme hemodilution in the Harrington procedure. Bibl Haematol 1981;47:322–337.
156. Scott WJ, Rode R, Castlemain B, et al. Efficacy, complications, and cost of a comprehensive blood conservation program for cardiac operations. J Thorac Cardiovasc Surg 1992;103:1001–1007.
157. Spiess BD, Sassetti R, McCarthy RJ, Narbone RF, Tuman KJ, Ivankovich AD. Autologous blood donation: hemodynamics in a high-risk patient population. Transfusion 1992;32:17–22.
158. Ness PM, Bourke DL, Walsh PC. A randomized trial of perioperative hemodilution versus transfusion of preoperatively deposited autologous blood in elective surgery. Transfusion 1992;32:226–230.
159. Hur SR, Huizenga BA, Major M. Acute normovolemic hemodilution combined with hypotensive anesthesia and other techniques to avoid homologous transfusion in spinal fusion surgery. Spine 1992;17: 867–873.
160. Laks J, Pilon RN, Klovekorn WP, Anderson W, MacCallum JR, O'Connor NE. Acute hemodilution: its effect of hemodynamics and oxygen transport in anesthetized man. Ann Surg 1974;180:103–109.
161. Brecher ME, Rosenfeld M. Mathematical and computer modeling of acute normovolemic hemodilution. Transfusion 1994;34:176–179.
162. Niinikoski J, Laaksonen V, Meretoja O, Jalonen J, Arstila M, Inberg MV. Oxygen transport and tissue oxygenation under moderate and extreme hemodilution during coronary bypass surgery. Ann Clin Res 1981;33(Suppl. 13):59–64.
163. Mathru M, Kleinman B, Blakeman B, Sullivan H, Kumar P, Dries DJ. Myocardial metabolism and adaptation during extreme hemodilution in humans after coronary revascularization. Crit Care Med 1992;20: 1420–1425.
164. Kim YD, Katz NM, Ng L, Nancherla A, Ahmed SW, Wallace RB. Effects of hypothermia and hemodilution on oxygen metabolism and hemodynamics in patients recovering from coronary artery bypass operations. J Thorac Cardiovasc Surg 1989;97:36–42.
165. Paty PS, Shah DM, Chang BB, Kaufman JL, Feustel PJ, Leather RP. Immediate preoperative phlebotomy with autologous blood donation for aortic replacement. Surg Gynecol Obstet 1990;171:326–330.
166. Catoire P, Saada M, Liu N, Delaunay L, Rauss A, Bonnet F. Effect of preoperative normovolemic hemodilution on left ventricular segmental wall motion during abdominal aortic surgery. Anesth Analg 1992; 75:654–659.
167. Rao TLK, Montoya A. Cardiovascular, electrocardiographic and respiratory changes following acute anemia with volume replacement in patients with coronary artery disease. Anesthesiol Rev 1985;12:49–54.
168. Christopherson R, Frank S, Norris E, Rock P, Gottlieb S, Beattie C. Low postoperative hematocrit is associated with cardiac ischemia in high-risk patients. Anesthesiology 1991;75:A99.
169. Tuman KJ. Tissue oxygen delivery: the physiology of anemia. Anesthesiol Clin North Am 1990;8:451–469.
170. Fan F, Chen RY, Schuessler GB, Chien S. Effects of hematocrit variations on regional hemodynamics and oxygen transport in the dog. Am J Physiol 1980;238:H545–H522.
171. Spahn DR, Smith LR, Veronee CD, et al. Acute isovolemic hemodilution and blood transfusion. Effects on regional function and metabolism in myocardium with compromised coronary blood flow. J Thorac Cardiovasc Surg 1993;105:694–704.
172. Hagl S, Heimisch W, Meisner H, Erben R, Baum M, Mendler N. The effect of hemodilution on regional myocardial function in the presence of coronary stenosis. Basic Res Cardiol 1977;72:344–364.
173. Brazier J, Cooper N, Buckberg G. The adequacy of subendocardial oxygen delivery: the interaction of determinants of flow, arterial oxy-

gen content and myocardial oxygen need. Circulation 1974;49: 968–977.
174. Crystal GJ, Levy PS, Eckel PK, Kim S-J, Chavez R. Effect of coronary stenosis on cardiac compensation during hemodilution. Anesthesiology 1991;75:A516.
175. Crystal GJ, Salem MR. Myocardial oxygen consumption and segmental shortening during selective coronary hemodilution in dogs. Anesth Analg 1988;67:500–508.
176. Spahn DR, Smith LR, McRae RL, Leone BJ. Effects of acute isovolemic hemodilution and anesthesia on regional function in left ventricular myocardium with compromised coronary blood flow. Acta Anaesthesiol Scand 1992;36:628–636.
177. Yoshikawa H, Powell WJ Jr, Bland JH, Lowenstein E. Effect of acute anemia on experimental myocardial ischemia. Am J Cardiol 1973;32: 670–678.
178. Gisselsson L, Rosberg B, Ericsson M. Myocardial blood flow, oxygen uptake and carbon dioxide release of the human heart during hemodilution. Acta Anaesthesiol Scand 1982;26:589–591.
179. Messmer KF. Acceptable hematocrit levels in surgical patients [review]. World J Surg 1987;11:41–46.
180. Estafanous FG, Smith CE, Selim WM, Tarazi RC. Cardiovascular effects of acute normovolemic hemodilution in rats with disopyramide-induced myocardial depression. Basic Res Cardiol 1990;85:227–236.
181. Henling CE, Carmichael MJ, Keats AS, Cooley DA. Cardiac operation for congenital heart disease in children of Jehovah's Witnesses. J Thorac Cardiovasc Surg 1985;89:914–920.
182. Vara-Thorbeck R, Guerrero-Fernandez Marcote JA. Hemodynamic response of elderly patients undergoing major surgery under moderate normovolemic hemodilution. Eur Surg Res 1985;17:372–376.
183. Kuchel GA, Avorn J, Reed MJ, Fields D. Cardiovascular responses to phlebotomy and sitting in middle-aged and elderly subjects. Arch Intern Med 1992;152:366–370.
184. Wilkerson DK, Rosen AL, Sehgal LR, Gould SA, Sehgal HL, Moss GS. Limits of cardiac compensation in anemic baboons. Surgery 1988;103:665–670.
185. Roseberg B, Wulff K. Hemodynamics following normovolemic hemodilution in elderly patients. Acta Anaesth Scand 1981;25:402–406.
186. Rose D, Coutsoftides T. Intraoperative normovolemic hemodilution. J Surg Res 1981;31:375–381.
187. Roy RC, Prough DS, Rogers AT, Stump DA, Cordell AR. Higher hematocrit limits cerebral oxygenation during hypothermic, nonpulsatile cardiopulmonary bypass [abstract]. Anesthesiology 1989;71:A75.
188. Lilleaasen P. Moderate and extreme haemodilution in open-heart surgery: blood requirements, bleeding and platelet counts. Scand J Thorac Cardiovasc Surg 1977;11:97–103.
189. Crystal GJ, Salem MR. Myocardial and systemic hemodynamics during isovolemic hemodilution alone and combined with nitroprusside-induced controlled hypotension. Anesth Analg 1991;72:227–237.
190. Boldt J, Bormann BV, Kling D, Scheld H, Hempelmann G. Influence of acute normovolemic hemodilution on extravascular lung water in cardiac surgery. Crit Care Med 1988;16:336–339.
191. Harker LA, Malpass TW, Branson HE, Hessel EA II, Slichter SJ. Mechanism of abnormal bleeding in patients undergoing cardiopulmonary bypass: acquired transient platelet dysfunction associated with selective alpha-granule release. Blood 1980;56:824–834.
192. Mohr R, Martinowitz U, Lavee J, Amroch D, Ramot B, Goor DA. The hemostatic effect of transfusing fresh whole blood versus platelet concentrates after cardiac operations. J Thorac Cardiovasc Surg 1988;96: 530–534.
193. Lavee J, Martinowitz U, Mohr R, et al. The effect of transfusion of fresh whole blood versus platelet concentrates after cardiac operations. A scanning electron microscope study of platelet aggregation on extracellular matrix. J Thorac Cardiovasc Surg 1989;97:204–212.
194. Mohr R, Goor DA, Yellin A, Moshkovitz Y, Shinfeld A, Martinowitz U. Fresh blood units contain large potent platelets that improve hemostasis after open heart operations. Ann Thorac Surg 1992;53:650–654.
195. Bick RL. Hemostasis defects associated with cardiac surgery, prosthetic devices, and other extracorporeal circuits. Semin Thromb Hemost 1985;11:249–280.
196. Ikeda S, Johnston MF, Yagi K, Gillespie KN, Schweiss JF, Homan SM. Intraoperative autologous blood salvage with cardiac surgery: an analysis of five years' experience in more than 3,000 patients. J Clin Anesth 1992;4:359–366.
197. Haberkern M, Dangel P. Normovolemic haemodilution and intraoperative auto-transfusion in children: experience with 30 cases of spinal fusion. Eur J Pediatr Surg 1991;1:30–35.
198. Sejourne P, Poirier A, Meakins JL, et al. Effect of haemodilution on transfusion requirements in liver resection. Lancet 1989;2:1380–1382.
199. Dale J, Lilleaasen P, Erikssen J. Hemostasis after open-heart surgery with extreme or moderate hemodilution. Eur Surg Res 1987;19: 339–347.
200. Royston D. High-dose aprotinin therapy: a review of the first five years' experience. J Cardiothorac Vasc Anesth 1992;6:76–100.
201. Kaplan JA, Cannarella C, Jones EL, Kutner MH, Hatcher CR Jr, Dunbar RW. Autologous blood transfusion during cardiac surgery. A reevaluation of three methods. J Thorac Cardiovasc Surg 1977;74:4–10.
202. Murphy P, Heal JM, Blumberg N. Infection or suspected infection after hip replacement surgery with autologous or homologous blood transfusions. Transfusion 1991;31:212–217.
203. Sunder-Plassmann L, Kessler M, Jesch F, Dieterle R, Messmer K. Acute normovolemic hemodilution. Changes in tissue oxygen supply and hemoglobin-oxygen affinity. Bibl Haematol 1975;41:44–53.
204. Barbier-Bohm G, Desmonts JM, Couderc E, Moulin D, Prokocimer P, Oliver H. Comparative effects of induced hypotension and normovolaemic haemodilution on blood loss in total hip arthroplasty. Br J Anaesth 1980;52:1039–1043.
205. Rosberg B. Blood coagulation during and after normovolemic hemodilution in elective surgery. Ann Clin Res 1981;33(Suppl. 13):84–88.
206. Crystal GJ, Rooney MW, Salem MR. Myocardial blood flow and oxygen consumption during isovolemic hemodilution alone and in combination with adenosine-induced controlled hypotension. Anesth Analg 1988;67:539–547.
207. Cosgrove DM, Loop FD, Lytle BW, et al. Determinants of blood utilization during myocardial revascularization. Ann Thorac Surg 1985; 40:380–384.
208. Czer LS, Shoemaker WC. Optimal hematocrit value in critically ill postoperative patients. Surg Gynecol Obstet 1978;147:363–368.
209. Rose D, Forest R, Coutsoftides T. Acute normovolemic hemodilution. Anesthesiology 1979;51:S91.
210. Greer AE, Carey JM, Zuhdi N. Hemodilution principle of hypothermic perfusion: a concept obviating blood priming. J Thorac Cardiovasc Surg 1962;43:640–648.
211. Boldt J, Kling D, von Bormann B, Züge M, Scheld H, Hempelmann G. Blood conservation in cardiac operations. Cell separation versus hemofiltration. J Thorac Cardiovasc Surg 1989;97:832–840.
212. Boldt J, Kling D, Zickmann B, Jacobi M, Dapper F, Hempelmann G. Acute preoperative plasmapheresis and established blood conservation techniques. Ann Thorac Surg 1990;50:62–68.

213. Journois D, Pouard P, Greeley WJ, Mauriat P, Vouhé P, Safran D. Hemofiltration during cardiopulmonary bypass in pediatric cardiac surgery. Anesthesiology 1994;81:1181–1189.
214. Kirklin JK, Blackstone EH, Kirklin JW. Cardiopulmonary bypass: studies on its damaging effects. Blood Purif 1987;5:168–178.
215. Kern FH, Morana NJ, Sears JJ, Hickey PR. Coagulation defects in neonates during cardiopulmonary bypass. Ann Thorac Surg 1992;54: 541–546.
216. von Segesser LK, Weiss BM, Garcia E, von Felten A, Turina MI. Reduction and elimination of systemic heparinization during cardiopulmonary bypass. J Thorac Cardiovasc Surg 1992;103: 790–799.

Chapter 23

Massive Transfusion

ALEXANDER P. REINER

INTRODUCTION

Massive blood transfusion, generally defined as transfusion of at least one blood volume (10 or more units of blood) within 24 hours, can occur in a number of surgical and critical care settings. In a tertiary care hospital containing a level I trauma center, the frequency of massive transfusion was reported as 125 of 20,000 or approximately 0.6% of all surgical procedures (1). Trauma accounted for 29% of these cases, whereas gastrointestinal hemorrhage accounted for 31%, cardiovascular surgery 12%, neoplastic disease 9%, and obstetrical emergencies 4%. In this center, 0.6% of patients accounted for approximately 15% of the total blood component use (1). Another common setting of massive transfusion is liver transplantation. At the University of Pittsburgh between 1981 and 1985, liver transplantation surgery was performed in only 0.01% of all hospital admissions but accounted for 20% of all red cell transfusions (2).

The physiological effects of massive hemorrhage can be severe and far-reaching. Improvements in resuscitative, critical care, anesthetic, and surgical techniques have significantly reduced the overall morbidity and mortality associated with massive blood loss. Overall survival is currently in the range of 50% (1, 3–5), and survival has been reported in patients receiving 100 or more units of blood (6, 7). Adverse prognostic factors include cirrhosis, prolonged hypotension, severe brain trauma, and advanced patient age (1, 3–5). Although the hospital recovery course can be prolonged and costly, most massively transfused patients who survive have an excellent long-term outcome and are able to return to work.

The pathophysiology underlying the morbidity and mortality associated with massive transfusion is complex. Acutely, patients can develop severe physiological and metabolic abnormalities, which can be related to the patient's underlying condition or injury, the consequences of hemorrhagic shock (i.e., tissue hypoperfusion, acidosis, and hypoxia), and the transfused blood components. Thus, prompt institution of appropriate resuscitative measures such as intravenous fluids and blood component therapy is imperative. Furthermore, the recognition of potential adverse consequences of the transfusion of massive amounts of blood and fluids is important to minimize morbidity. This chapter reviews the composition of fluids and blood components used during massive transfusion, the appropriate use of these components, several unique complications of massive transfusion, and some possible alternative therapies that decrease the risks of massive transfusion therapy. It is important to keep in mind that in most massive transfusion situations, the cause of bleeding is a wound so extensive that it requires primary surgical treatment to achieve hemostasis. Blood component therapy is usually supportive rather than primarily therapeutic, even with regard to securing hemostasis. Thus, the goals of transfusion therapy are to maintain physiological support of the circulation and oxygen transport while avoiding deficiencies of hemostatic factors or other physiological deficits.

FLUIDS AND BLOOD COMPONENTS USED IN THE MANAGEMENT OF THE MASSIVELY BLEEDING PATIENT

FLUIDS USED FOR VOLUME REPLACEMENT

Initial replacement therapy in the massively bleeding patient involves the infusion of asanguinous fluids to restore intravascular volume. Two types of solutions are available: salt (i.e., "crystalloid") solutions and colloid (protein- or starch-containing) solutions.

Salt Solutions

Isotonic salt solutions are the most common fluids used during early resuscitation of massively bleeding patients. The most widely used solutions are normal saline (0.9% NaCl) or lactated Ringer's solution. Lactated Ringer's contains physiological concentrations of sodium, potassium, and calcium, as well as lactate as a buffer. Normal saline is the only salt solution that may be mixed directly with blood components, because lactated Ringer's contains calcium, which may induce blood coagulation. Because isotonic salt solutions have a relatively low colloid oncotic pressure, approximately 80% of the infused volume rapidly equilibrates into the extravascular space and only 20% remains within the intravascular space. Thus, a volume of normal saline or lactated Ringer's approximately three to four times that of the patient's blood loss must be infused to maintain intravascular volume.

Hypertonic salt solutions such as 7.5% saline transiently result in greater expansion of intravascular volume compared with isotonic solutions. Infusion of 250 mL of 7.5% saline, for example, can increase intravascular volume up to 1 L. In a recent prospective randomized study of prehospital resuscitation of trauma patients, hypertonic saline compared favorably with lactated Ringer's with respect to survival rates in patients with relatively low Glasgow scale scores (8). Thus, because of the smaller volume required, hypertonic saline is potentially useful in the prehospital phase of fluid resuscitation. Hypertonic saline should be avoided in the later stages of resuscitation, however, because of potential adverse effects on hemostasis (9). Hypotonic glucose solutions such as 5% dextrose should not be infused in large quantities during massive blood transfusion because of inadequate intravascular volume expansion and the potential for hemolysis of simultaneously infused red blood cells.

Colloid Solutions

Colloid solutions have a greater oncotic pressure than isotonic salt solutions and thus result in greater volume expansion with less volume infused. The major disadvantages of colloid compared with salt solutions are cost and availability. The most commonly used colloid is a 5% solution of human albumin. A hyperoncotic 25% albumin preparation is also available. These albumin solutions are produced from pooled human plasma and are pasteurized to inactivate viruses. The intravascular half-life of infused albumin is approximately 24 hours. Because of increased vascular permeability in patients with shock, chest trauma, and adult respiratory distress syndrome (ARDS), the differential expansion of intravascular volume with albumin or plasma may often be less than one would theoretically estimate from the protein concentration, because equilibration of the infused protein with the extracellular space may occur much more rapidly than in normal subjects.

Other colloid solutions are also available for volume expansion. Plasma protein fraction contains 83% albumin and 17% globulins. Rapid administration of plasma protein fraction was initially associated with transient hypotension (10), but current preparations appear to be safe. Other available colloid solutions include hydroxyethyl starch (hetastarch), a synthetic starch-like polymer available as a 6% solution in saline, and dextran, a glucose polymer of varying molecular weight. Both hetastarch and dextran can maintain intravascular volume expansion for up to 24 hours. Large doses of either product, however, can impair hemostasis. In addition, dextran can interfere with red blood cell compatibility testing and has occasionally been associated with anaphylactic reactions (11).

RED BLOOD CELL COMPONENTS

Restoration of oxygen-carrying capacity is accomplished by the transfusion of red cell-containing blood components. Two types of red cell-containing blood products are generally available: whole blood and red blood cells.

Whole Blood

Whole blood contains both the red blood cells and plasma derived from a single blood donor. One unit of whole blood contains approximately 200 mL of red cells and 250 mL of plasma in about 60 mL of an anticoagulant-preservative solution called CPDA-1 (citrate, phosphate, dextrose, and adenine). The hematocrit of a unit of whole blood is therefore in the range of 35–45%. CPDA-1 allows storage of whole blood up to 35 days under refrigeration (1–6°C).

Whole blood stored for more than approximately 24 hours does not contain functional platelets or leukocytes. Whole blood from which platelets have been removed as a platelet concentrate must be labeled "modified whole blood." However, the number of functional platelets in modified whole blood is the same as in unmodified whole blood that has been stored in the refrigerator, namely, nil. Levels of most coagulation factors, on the other hand, are relatively well maintained during storage of whole blood (12) (Table 23.1). Although there is a progressive decline of factor V and VIII levels during storage, the practical significance of these is limited for several reasons. The decline in factor V level to approximately 35% by 21 days of storage is still adequate for surgical hemostasis. Although factor VIII levels decline more precipitously (reaching approximately 5% by 21 days of storage), factor VIII is an acute-phase protein that is rapidly released in response to stress or injury. Thus, endogenous factor VIII levels are generally *elevated* in trauma and surgical patients.

Because whole blood contains adequate amounts of plasma coagulation factors to prevent dilution, it is the preferred

TABLE 23.1. HEMOSTASIS COMPONENTS PROVIDED IN WHOLE BLOOD

Clotting Factor	Probable Minimum Level for Surgical Hemostasis (% of normal)	Activity in Blood Stored 21 Days at 4°C (% of normal)
Prothrombin	15–25	70
V	15–20	35
VII	10	66
VIIII	30	5
IX	25–30	97
X	15–20	85
XI	5–20	107
Fibrinogen, mg/dL	80–100	150–300
Platelets /μL	50,000–80,000	No functional platelets

Reprinted with permission from Counts RB, Haisch C, Simon TL, Maxwell NG, Heimbach DM, Carrico CJ. Hemostasis in massively transfused trauma patients. Ann Surg 1979;190:91–99.

blood component during massive transfusion. Replacement of red cells, plasma volume, and coagulation factors occurs simultaneously. Furthermore, because the red cells and plasma are derived from the same blood donor, patient exposure to potential transmissible agents is minimized.

Whole blood must be ABO identical with the transfusion recipient. Emergency uncrossmatched group O whole blood should *not* be transfused to patients of unknown blood type; because units of group O whole blood contain significant amounts of plasma, the potential exists for transfusion of a high-titered anti-A or -B isohemagglutin that may cause intravascular hemolysis of patient red cells in a patient subsequently identified as group A, B, or AB.

Red Blood Cells

Red blood cells, or packed red blood cells, are prepared by centrifugation of a unit of donated whole blood followed by removal of most of the plasma. A unit of red blood cells in CPDA-1 contains approximately 200 mL of red cells and 50 mL of residual plasma and can be stored for up to 35 days at 1–6°C; the hematocrit value thus ranges from 70 to 80%. Newer red cell storage solutions (e.g., adenine saline-1 (AS-1)) contain higher concentrations of adenine and saline and allow extended storage up to 42 days. The removal of all plasma and the addition of saline reduce the hematocrit of AS-1 red cell units to 50–60% and somewhat decrease the viscosity, which allows more rapid infusion.

TABLE 23.2. ACCEPTABLE BLOOD GROUP SUBSTITUTIONS FOR RED BLOOD CELLS AND PLASMA

	Donor Type	
Patient Type	Red Blood Cell Transfusion	FFP Transfusion
O	O only	O, A, B, AB
A	A, O	A, AB
B	B, O	B, AB
AB	AB, A, B, O	AB only

Red blood cells are the component of choice when replacing oxygen-carrying capacity in patients with a stable blood volume (or expected blood loss and replacement of less than one blood volume) and normal coagulation status. One unit of red blood cells (or whole blood) should raise the hematocrit by 2–3%. Because units of red blood cells are relatively plasma poor, adequate amounts of coagulation factors are absent. As with stored whole blood, red blood cells do not contain functional platelets or leukocytes.

Because red blood cells, unlike whole blood, contain minimal amounts of plasma, transfusion of significant amounts of ABO isoantibodies is much less of a concern. Thus, red blood cells can be either ABO identical or ABO compatible with the recipient (Table 23.2). For emergency transfusion, type O red blood cells should be used if the patient's blood type is not known with certainty.

HEMOSTATIC BLOOD COMPONENTS

Massively transfused patients may require the replacement of specific hemostatic components, including platelets, plasma coagulation factors, and/or fibrinogen.

Platelet Concentrates

Platelets may be prepared either from units of whole blood or by apheresis from a single platelet donor. One unit of whole blood platelets contains at least 5.5×10^{10} platelets along with variable numbers of red cells and leukocytes suspended in approximately 50 mL of plasma. The usual adult dose of whole blood platelets is 6 units (or approximately 1 unit/10 kg body weight) that are pooled into one bag before transfusion. Apheresis platelets contain at least 30×10^{10} platelets suspended in 200–400 mL of plasma. Thus, 6 units of pooled whole blood platelets are approximately equivalent to a single donor apheresis platelet transfusion. Apheresis platelets contain markedly fewer leukocytes than whole blood platelets. The potential benefits of apheresis platelets thus include reduced donor exposure and reduced leukocyte content. Both whole blood and apheresis platelet components are stored at room temperature under continuous gentle agitation for up to 5 days.

Platelets transfusions are indicated in the massively bleeding patient with significant thrombocytopenia (platelet count less than 50,000–70,000/μL) or platelet dysfunction (as indicated by a significantly prolonged bleeding time of more than10–15 minutes). In patients undergoing liver transplantation monitored by thromboelastography (TEG), platelet transfusions are often guided by the maximum amplitude (13). Recent data indicate that the maximum amplitude of the TEG is a function of both platelet count and fibrinogen level (14). In the absence of significant platelet consumption or immune destruction, 1 unit of whole blood platelets should raise the platelet count by 5000–10,000/μL. It should be noted that 6 units of pooled whole blood platelets or a single apheresis platelet transfusion each contains approximately 200–400 mL of plasma, which includes the equivalent amount of coagulation factors as 1–2 units of fresh-frozen plasma (FFP) (15).

In the setting of massive transfusion, ABO compatibility is preferred but not required for platelet transfusions. Because platelet concentrates can contain enough red cells for Rh sensitization, Rh-negative recipients should receive platelets from Rh-negative donors.

Fresh-Frozen Plasma

FFP is the plasma derived from a unit of whole blood by centrifugation; the plasma is frozen within 6 hours of collection. Each unit contains approximately 250 mL of plasma containing normal amounts of all coagulation factors including the labile coagulation factors V and VIII. FFP can be stored at −20°C for up to 1 year. Plasma transfusion is indicated for replacement of coagulation factor deficits in patients with specific underlying coagulation abnormalities such as liver disease, disseminated intravascular coagulation (DIC), emergency reversal of warfarin therapy, or congenital coagulation factor deficiencies (16). In the setting of massive transfusion, plasma transfusion is indicated in actively bleeding patients with laboratory evidence of significant coagulation factor deficiency as determined by a prothrombin time (PT) or partial thromboplastin time (PTT) greater than 1.5 times the control value. The usual dose is 2–6 units of plasma depending on the severity of the coagulation abnormality. One unit of plasma should raise coagulation factor levels by approximately 2–3%.

Before transfusion, frozen plasma must be thawed at 37°C, which can take up to 30–45 minutes. FFP must be ABO compatible with the recipient's red cells (Table 23.2). If the patient's ABO type is unknown, type AB plasma may be administered. If used to provide labile clotting factors (e.g., factor V), plasma should be transfused within 12 hours of thawing. Fibrinogen and factors VII, IX, and X and prothrombin are stable for several days when plasma is kept at 4°C after thawing.

Cryoprecipitate

Cryoprecipitate is prepared by thawing frozen plasma at 4°C and recovering the precipitated material. On average, each bag of cryoprecipitate derived from a unit of whole blood contains 80–100 units of factor VIII and von Willebrand factor (vWF) and at least 150 mg of fibrinogen in less than 15 mL of plasma. Thus, cryoprecipitate contains factor VIII, vWF, and fibrinogen concentrated approximately 10-fold over plasma. Cryoprecipitate is stored at −20°C for up to 1 year. Cryoprecipitate is used for factor VIII or vWF replacement in patients with hemophilia type A or von Willebrand disease, respectively. In the setting of massive transfusion, cryoprecipitate is indicated in patients with significant hypofibrinogenemia. If the plasma fibrinogen level falls below 100 mg/dL, 10–20 bags of cryoprecipitate are pooled, reconstituted with a small amount of plasma or saline, and transfused into an average-size adult. One unit of cryoprecipitate should raise the plasma fibrinogen level by 5–7 mg/dL. In the United States, cryoprecipitate is also used as a source of fibrinogen for a surgical hemostatic agent known as "fibrin glue." Fibrin glue may be efficacious as a topical hemostatic agent in several massive transfusion settings, such as open heart surgery or abdominal trauma.

Because of the minimal volume of residual plasma, ABO compatibility is generally not required for cryoprecipitate transfusion. Thawing, pooling, and processing of cryoprecipitate for transfusion can take up to 30–45 minutes. Thawed cryoprecipitate should be kept at room temperature and transfused within 6 hours of thawing or 4 hours of pooling.

MANAGEMENT OF THE MASSIVELY BLEEDING PATIENT

The management of a patient with massive hemorrhage can be physiologically and temporally divided into three stages: initial fluid resuscitation, which begins to replete intravascular volume; restoration of tissue oxygenation with red blood cell transfusion; and replacement of hemostatic components. Although all three stages are interrelated and may overlap in time, they are discussed separately.

INITIAL FLUID RESUSCITATION

Initial replacement of intravascular volume with asanguinous solutions is important in patients with acute blood loss to prevent irreversible tissue injury and organ damage.

Initial fluid resuscitation is particularly critical in the prehospital setting, such as trauma. Salt or colloid solutions may be used, but salt solutions are generally preferred as initial therapy because of availability and cost. Traditionally, patients in hemorrhagic shock are given three to four times the volume of isotonic salt solution (i.e., normal saline or lactated Ringer's) than their estimated blood loss.

Recently, the traditional concept of initial management of acute blood loss with crystalloid or colloid solutions has come into question. Although the aim of immediate fluid resuscitation in acutely bleeding patients is to maintain adequate tissue perfusion and organ function, there has been recent concern that immediate fluid administration may actually be detrimental in patients with uncontrolled hemorrhage. Potential deleterious effects include fluid overload that leads to the development of pulmonary edema and accentuation of hemorrhage by disruption of clot formation due to increased intravascular pressure (17). A recent prospective study indicated that hypotensive patients with penetrating torso injuries who were given delayed intravenous fluid therapy had a better survival rate than patients who received traditional immediate fluid resuscitation before surgery (18). Whether this practice is applicable in other clinical situations (i.e., older patients, other types of injuries, longer prehospitalization times) remains to be determined.

Monitoring of the patient's volume and hemodynamic status is essential during the initial stages of management of the massively bleeding patient. In the prehospital setting, the patient's vital signs are the most important indicators of intravascular volume. Tachycardia and hypotension indicate hypovolemia, and normalization of pulse and blood pressure correlates with volume resuscitation. In the emergency room or operating room, more invasive monitoring of central venous pressure, arterial blood pressure, urine output, and pulmonary capillary wedge pressure may be indicated. The extent of blood loss may be more or less apparent depending on the nature of the injury or surgical procedure. Intraabdominal or retroperitoneal bleeding may be much more difficult to monitor than external hemorrhage. The amount of fluid infused also depends on the patient's underlying condition. Patients with congestive heart failure or significant renal disease will poorly tolerate excess fluid administration. Extensive tissue trauma or end-stage liver disease will result in significant "third spacing" of administered fluid.

Replacement fluids should be administered through at least two large-bore (14 gauge or larger) intravenous catheters, preferably in an uninjured part of the body with known intact venous drainage. As volume replacement therapy is initiated, baseline laboratory values for electrolytes, hematocrit, and coagulation screening assays should be obtained. The hematocrit, however, is a less reliable indicator of acute red cell transfusion requirement than hemodynamic measurements. As a rule, patients who respond hemodynamically to 1–2 L of crystalloid solution have not sustained significant blood loss. An absent or transient hemodynamic response, on the other hand, suggests massive or ongoing blood loss and the need for immediate blood transfusion.

RESTORATION OF OXYGEN-CARRYING CAPACITY

Although infusion of asanguinous solutions will begin to restore intravascular volume in patients with massive blood loss, red blood cell volume must also be replenished to maintain adequate tissue oxygenation. The type of red cell component transfused depends on the clinical situation and the local availability of red cell components. If available, whole blood is preferable to packed red blood cells for massive transfusion therapy, because the former contains not only red blood cells but plasma coagulation factors as well. Packed red blood cells should be used as the initial component therapy only if whole blood is unavailable or if type O blood is transfused emergently before the patient's blood type is known (see below).

Before routine (nonemergent) red cell or whole blood transfusion, certain serological tests are performed. These include ABO and Rh typing of the donor and recipient, screening the recipient for unexpected red cell alloantibodies, and performing a cross match between donor red cells and patient serum. In an emergency setting in which the patient is hemodynamically unstable, blood may be transfused before routine pretransfusion testing is completed (Table 23.3). If the patient's blood type is unknown, uncrossmatched type O red blood cells should be transfused (19, 20). In acute severe hemorrhagic shock where the patient's ABO and Rh type are unknown, group O Rh-negative red blood cells are generally transfused to minimize the risk of Rh sensitization in the approximately 15% of patients who are Rh negative. This is of particular concern in women of childbearing age who are at risk of developing hemolytic disease of the newborn. Group O Rh-negative blood is often in short supply, however, because only 6% of blood donors are O Rh negative. For this reason, group O Rh-positive red blood cells can be used for emergency transfusions in patients of unknown blood type, particularly in men and older women in whom the development of Rh antibody is less of a concern (21). This is particularly relevant in the setting of trauma, in which approximately 70–80% of recipients are young males.

If the patient's blood type is known, ABO type-specific blood can be transfused, even before completion of the routine cross-match testing. If a patient initially received uncross-

TABLE 23.3. RED CELL COMPONENTS USED DURING MASSIVE TRANSFUSION

Component	WB/RBC	Availability (min)	Indication	Risks
Emergency group O[a] (uncross matched)	RBC only	0–5	• Emergency transfusion in hemodynamically unstable patient of uncertain blood type	• Hemolytic transfusion reaction (usually extravascular) due to unexpected (e.g., Rh, Kell, Kidd) patient red cell alloantibody
ABO type-specific (uncross matched)	WB or RBC	10–15	• Less emergent transfusion in unstable patient of uncertain blood type, or • Emergency transfusion in unstable patient of known blood type	• Same risk of extravascular hemolytic transfusion reaction due to unexpected red cell alloantibody as above • Small risk of potentially fatal intravascular hemolytic reaction due to ABO incompatibility if transfusion error occurs because of emergency setting (e.g., clerical error, patient or blood component misidentification).
Cross match compatible ABO type-specific	WB or RBC	30–60[b]	• Hemodynamically stable patient • Patient with known red cell alloantibody(ies)	

[a]Group O Rh-negative RBC are generally used, particularly for women of childbearing age. Group O Rh-positive RBC may be used for men and older women, particularly if group O Rh-negative RBC are in short supply.
[b]If an unexpected RBC alloantibody is identified during pretransfusion testing, availability of antigen-compatible units may take up to several hours. If the clinical situation warrants immediate transfusion, the decision to transfuse incompatible or untested units of blood should be made in consultation with the transfusion service director.
WB, whole blood; RBC, red blood cells.

matched group O red blood cells and his or her blood type subsequently is identified as other than group O, the decision to switch the patient to type-specific blood should be based on several factors, including the amount of blood already transfused, the total estimated transfusion requirement, the availability of the particular blood type, and a cross-match sample using a recently drawn patient serum sample. Although some transfusionists advocate using uncrossmatched ABO type-specific blood as soon as it becomes available, the use of type O red cells in emergency situations is advantageous in that the possibility of a patient erroneously receiving ABO-incompatible blood is minimized. Acute intravascular hemolytic reactions due to ABO incompatibility are usually the result of clerical or technical errors that are most likely to occur at times of increased urgency or emotional stress (e.g., multiple trauma). These intravascular hemolytic reactions are the most common cause of acute mortality related to blood transfusion (22) but are usually preventable because they are almost always due to human error.

It should also be noted that recipients of emergency uncrossmatched group O red cells, or even ABO type-specific uncrossmatched blood, may occasionally develop acute hemolytic reactions caused by unexpected non-ABO recipient red cell alloantibodies that were undetected because of the abbreviated compatibility testing. These unexpected (e.g., Rh, Kell, Duffy, Kidd) alloantibodies occur in approximately 1% of transfusion recipients (23). In contrast to intravascular hemolytic reactions caused by ABO incompatibility, however, these unexpected alloantibodies generally result in extravascular hemolysis and thus are not usually life-threatening.

Rapid infusion of relatively large volumes of blood can be accomplished by using large-bore intravenous catheters and tubing, multiple infusion sites, and infusion under pressure (24, 25). The rate of infusion of red blood cells can also be increased by either direct addition of normal saline or mixing of the red cells with normal saline before infusion via a Y transfusion set. Using these techniques, a unit of blood can be infused as rapidly as 20 seconds. The volume of blood transfused should be determined by careful hemodynamic monitoring and frequent determinations of the patient's hematocrit. Otherwise healthy young adults can easily tolerate a hematocrit in the range of 20–25%. The presence of coexisting cardiopulmonary or cerebrovascular disease may dictate a higher target hematocrit value.

PREVENTION AND CORRECTION OF HEMOSTATIC ABNORMALITIES

Abnormalities of platelets and/or coagulation factors can complicate massive transfusion and occasionally contribute to bleeding during or after resuscitation. In theory, these hemostatic abnormalities may occur because of either a dilutional effect of massive transfusion or the patient's underlying condition (e.g., consumption due to DIC).

Pathophysiology of Hemostatic Abnormalities

Because stored whole blood and packed red blood cells are deficient in certain hemostatic elements, some dilutional effect would be expected during massive transfusion. Both whole blood and packed red cells stored for more than 24 hours do not contain viable platelets. Stored whole blood contains relatively normal levels of most plasma coagulation factors, with the exception of the labile coagulation factors V and VIII, which decline during storage (see Table 23.1). Packed red blood cells, on the other hand, contain only a small volume of plasma and thus do not provide plasma coagulation factors. Based on mathematical models of continuous exchange transfusion, however, the variability in platelet counts between massively transfused patients cannot be explained by simple dilution alone (26).

The second, and probably more important, pathophysiological process contributing to the coagulopathy associated with massive transfusion is consumption of coagulation elements due to DIC. If a patient experiences massive tissue injury or if repletion of intravascular volume, tissue perfusion, and oxygen-carrying capacity is inadequate, a cycle of hypotension, tissue injury or ischemia, and acidosis will result in the release of tissue factor into the circulation. This results in systemic activation of the coagulation system. The resulting pathological process of DIC is characterized by coagulation factor and platelet activation and consumption, intravascular thrombi formation, and activation of the fibrinolytic system. This leads to thrombocytopenia, depletion of plasma coagulation factors and fibrinogen, and elevated levels of fibrinogen/fibrin degradation products (FDPs). Circulating FDPs interfere with normal clot formation and thus exacerbate the hemostatic defect. Studies that indicate a correlation between the development of coagulation abnormalities and the duration of hypotension in massively transfused patients indirectly suggest that consumption contributes significantly to the coagulopathy associated with massive transfusion (27, 28).

Other factors may contribute to the development of coagulation abnormalities during massive transfusion. Massive crystalloid or colloid fluid infusion may have a dilutional effect. Recent evidence suggests that hypothermia can adversely affect platelet function (29) and coagulation enzymatic reactions (30, 31). Finally, certain underlying hemostatic abnormalities, such as heparin, liver disease, or uremia, can contribute to bleeding. In patients undergoing liver transplantation, there are multiple possible causes of abnormal hemostasis, including defective synthesis and clearance of coagulation proteins, platelet sequestration, DIC, increased fibrinolysis, and release of heparin-like substances from the donor liver (Chapter 32).

Development of Hemostatic Abnormalities in Massively Transfused Patients

THROMBOCYTOPENIA

When whole blood is used for red cell replacement, thrombocytopenia is the most common hemostatic laboratory abnormality in massively transfused patients (12, 26, 32). Significant thrombocytopenia (platelet count less than 50,000–100,000) frequently develops after transfusion of 15–20 units of whole blood or packed red blood cells (12, 33) (Fig. 23.1). The variability in the correlation between platelet counts and number of units of blood transfused, however, indicates that other factors in addition to dilution (such as DIC or release of platelets into the circulation from the spleen or bone marrow) are also involved. Thus, there is no benefit of prophylactic or formula-based supplemental platelet transfusions in massively transfused patients; most patients with moderate platelet dilution do not develop microvascular bleeding, and unfortunately no reliable method exists to predict which patients will develop this complication (26, 34). Furthermore, many patients who develop thrombocytopenia and microvascular bleeding also have platelet consumption and thus require repeated doses of platelets.

COAGULATION FACTOR DEFICIENCY

The development of laboratory coagulation test abnormalities during massive blood transfusion depends in part on whether whole blood, packed red blood cells, or cell saver washed red blood cells are transfused. In studies using whole blood, significant coagulation screening test abnormalities are uncommon, and there is little relationship between amount of blood transfused and the levels of various coagulation factors (12). Studies involving the use of plasma-poor red blood cells, on the other hand, indicate that significant prolongations of the PT and PTT frequently develop in patients receiving 10–12 or more units of red blood cells (33, 35–37). The risk of microvascular bleeding correlates poorly with coagulation screening test abnormalities, unless the PT and PTT are significantly prolonged (more than1.5 times control) or fibrinogen level is less than 75 mg/dL (37, 38).

Other factors that influence the development of coagulopathy in massively transfused patients are related to the extent of

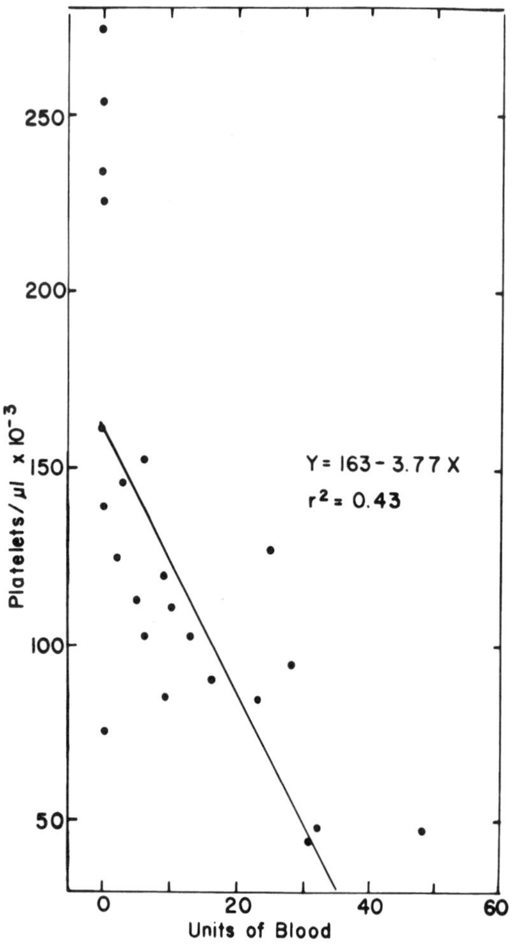

Figure 23.1. Inverse relationship of platelet count to number of units of blood transfused in massively transfused platelets. (Reprinted with permission from Counts RB, Haisch C, Simon TL, Maxwell NG, Heimbach DM, Carrico CJ. Hemostasis in massively transfused trauma patients. Ann Surg 1979;190:91–99.)

the patient's injury or underlying conditions. In patients with severe acute blood loss due to cardiac surgery, ruptured aortic aneurysm, upper gastrointestinal hemorrhage, or trauma, coagulation abnormalities correlate with the duration of hypotension (28). In particular, patients with brain injury are at a much higher risk for development of coagulopathy (particularly hypofibrinogenemia) due to DIC (35, 39).

Hemostatic Component Therapy

Based on the preceding considerations, the following approach to hemostatic component therapy during massive transfusion can be recommended (Fig. 23.2). Appropriate hemostasis screening tests (platelet count, PT, PTT, thrombin time, fibrinogen, and/or whole blood TEG) should be performed at the initiation of therapy, and at frequent intervals until hemorrhage is controlled. *There is no justification for the prophylactic use of platelets or FFP in the massively transfused patient* (26). If generalized microvascular bleeding occurs, initial treatment should consist of platelet transfusion, because a platelet count below the range of 50,000–100,000/μL is the most frequent hemostatic abnormality observed in massively transfused patients. If the platelet count falls below 50,000/μL, platelets should also be considered even in the absence of microvascular bleeding, because this degree of thrombocytopenia has historically been deemed the lower limit for adequate surgical hemostasis. Six units of pooled platelets or one bag of apheresis platelets should raise the platelet count by 30,000–60,000/μL, although in actively bleeding patients or ongoing DIC, the rise may not be sustained for long. In liver transplantation, the presence of splenomegaly may render the administration of platelet concentrates quite ineffective. To determine the effect, a posttransfusion platelet count should be obtained. If microvascular bleeding persists despite a platelet count of at least 90,000–100,000/μL, either platelet dysfunction (e.g., due to hypothermia or FDPs) or coagulation factor abnormalities can be presumed.

Transfusion of coagulation components generally should be guided by frequent monitoring of coagulation laboratory assays (platelet count, PT, PTT, thrombin time, fibrinogen and/or TEG) and/or the response of microvascular bleeding to platelet transfusions. Patients with significant tissue injury (particularly brain injury), significant endothelial disruption (e.g., ruptured aortic aneurysm), or prolonged hypotension and tissue hypoxia are particularly at risk for combined consumption of platelets and fibrinogen due to DIC. Thus, the presence of microvascular bleeding in these patients may warrant, in addition to platelets, the transfusion of cryoprecipitate (10–20 units in an adult) to replete fibrinogen. Supplemental cryoprecipitate transfusion is also advised if the fibrinogen level is less than 80–100 mg/dL.

Before assessing the patient's coagulation status based on the PT and PTT, it is important to know the fibrinogen level and thrombin time. It should be noted that severe hypofibrinogenemia (i.e., less than 50–70 mg/dL) can result in prolongation of the PT and PTT independently of levels of the other coagulation factors. Furthermore, a prolonged thrombin time in the presence of a fibrinogen level greater than 100 mg/dL indicates the presence of a circulating coagulation inhibitor (e.g., FDP or heparin). With heparin, the thrombin time is usually markedly prolonged (more than 50 seconds) and can be corrected by the addition of protamine. If the adequacy of heparin neutralization is in question, a trial dose of 50 mg protamine should be administered and the thrombin time repeated to determine its effect. Recent data suggest that an intensive release of heparin or heparin-like substances may occur during liver transplantation (40). During the donor liver preservation phase, heparin sulfate may be released

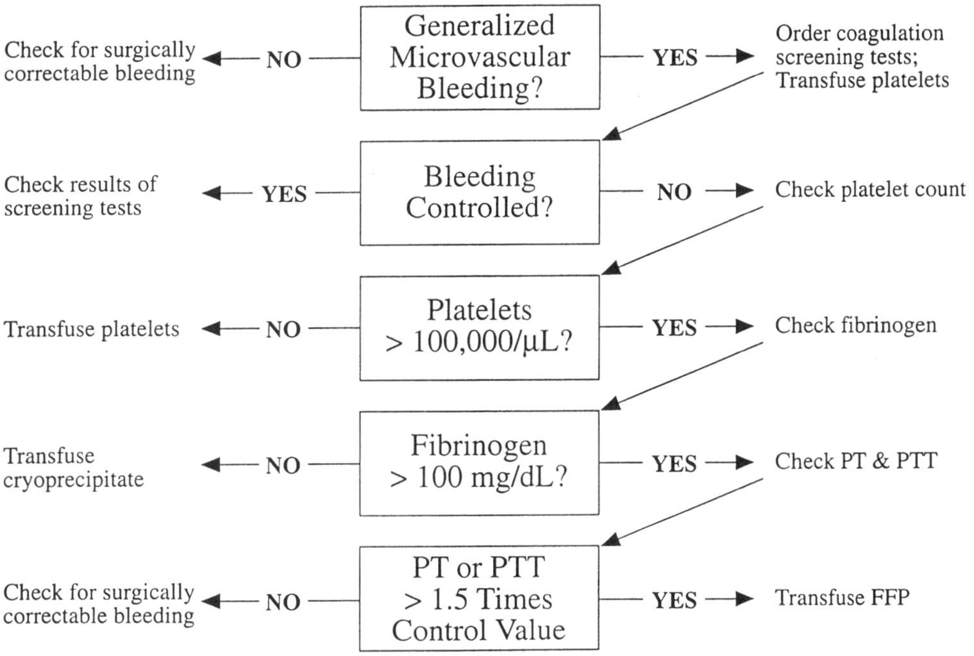

Figure 23.2. Algorithm for management of bleeding during massive transfusion.

from endothelial cell surfaces and, upon reestablishment of hepatic circulation, may be washed into the liver recipient. TEG has shown a straight-line response in such patients and is reversed by heparinase. Treatment of such patients with protamine (20–50 mg) may be useful. The activated clotting time is particularly insensitive to heparin and therefore is of little use in detecting low-level endogenous heparin or intrinsic heparan release. The R-wave of the TEG is much more sensitive to low-dose heparin (Chapter 17).

When the thrombin time is normal and the fibrinogen is greater than 100 mg/dL, a significantly prolonged PT and/or PTT (more than 1.5 times control) is a reliable indicator of significant coagulation factor deficit(s). Transfusion of FFP (2–6 units) should generally be reserved for patients with prolongation of the PT and/or PTT that exceed this level. Plasma transfusion is more likely to be required, however, in patients who receive packed red blood cells rather than whole blood, patients undergoing surgical procedures in which washed salvaged blood is returned to the patient, and patients with an underlying coagulopathy such as liver disease. Replacement of vitamin K-dependent clotting factors with FFP is also indicated for the emergency reversal of warfarin therapy.

METABOLIC COMPLICATIONS OF MASSIVE TRANSFUSION

A number of complications of massive blood transfusion are related to the rapid infusion of constituents of the preservative solutions used for blood storage, the biochemical changes that occur during blood storage, and/or the temperature (4°C) at which blood is stored. Many of these metabolic effects of massive transfusion are interrelated. In addition, the development of any one of these adverse effects is determined by a complex interaction of the rate and amount of blood infused and the underlying condition and acute metabolic status of the patient. Thus, the diagnosis and management of these metabolic abnormalities should be guided by frequent biochemical and hemodynamic monitoring of the massively transfused patient.

POTASSIUM ABNORMALITIES

Because of the extracellular shift of potassium from red blood cells to plasma that occurs during blood storage, whole blood and red blood cells accumulate up to approximately 40 mEq/L and approximately 80 mEq/L of potassium, respectively, after 3–4 weeks of storage. Once red cells are transfused into a more "physiological" environment, the biochemical changes that occur during storage are rapidly reversed. Rapid infusion of large volumes of red blood cells may result in a transient hyperkalemia that is usually clinically insignificant (41–43). Significant hyperkalemia, however, can depress myocardial function and also result in fatal cardiac arrhythmias, particularly when accompanied by hypocalcemia (44, 45). Therefore, in patients with defective potassium excretion (i.e., neonates or adults with significant underlying renal disease), it may be important to minimize the potassium load during massive transfusion by using either relatively fresh blood or washed red blood cells (which are relatively free of plasma potassium).

Hypokalemia actually occurs even more commonly in massively transfused patients than does hyperkalemia and may require potassium supplementation (42, 46). The development of hypokalemia during massive transfusion may be related to other metabolic disturbances such as hypotension, alkalosis, and catecholamine release, causing reentry of potassium into the red blood cells. Because the development of potassium abnormalities is unpredictable and may depend on other coexisting factors, potassium levels should be monitored closely in massively transfused patients.

CITRATE TOXICITY

Citrate is universally used as an anticoagulant for blood storage because it effectively binds ionized calcium that is required for the coagulation cascade. During routine blood transfusion, citrate is rapidly diluted by the recipient's blood volume. During massive transfusion, citrate is rapidly metabolized and excreted primarily by the liver and kidney, respectively. The rate of citrate clearance can be impeded, however, by hypotension, hypothermia, alkalosis, or hepatic or renal ischemia (47). During the anhepatic phase of liver transplantation, for example, there is a marked increase in serum citrate levels associated with a decrease in ionized calcium levels. Transfusion of massive amounts of citrated blood can result in significant hypocalcemia, which can cause hypotension, depressed cardiac function, cardiac arrhythmia, hypocoagulability, and potentially death (47). Calcium levels, although capable of falling precipitously during massive transfusion, never reach such low levels that they cause a coagulopathy. Hypotension due to loss of vascular tone and depression of cardiac output occurs at levels of 0.7–0.8 mg/dL; however, coagulopathy does not occur until 0.1–0.2 mg/dL.

Empiric supplemental calcium administration is generally not required in massively transfused adults with normal liver function and, in fact, can result in lethal hypercalcemia (47). Most normothermic, normovolemic adults with normal liver function can tolerate transfusion of up to 1 unit of blood every 5 minutes without adverse clinical consequence. Furthermore, unnecessary ionized calcium administration may lead to bradycardia, prolongation of atrial ventricular conduction, and hypotension.

Calcium supplementation during massive transfusion is generally required only in neonates or patients with significant liver disease or those undergoing liver transplantation and should be guided by frequent monitoring of serum ionized calcium levels. If serum-ionized calcium levels drop to below 50% of normal, intravenous calcium chloride should be administered (48). Calcium solution should *not,* however, be added to blood components. In liver transplantation during massive transfusion, 5–10 g of ionized calcium may be required over rather short periods of time. Calcium chloride is the preferred solution for severe acute changes in calcium levels because it is immediately biologically available. Calcium gluconate contains almost no ionized calcium and therefore is useful only in situations with normal liver function and relatively slow decreases/losses of ionized calcium.

ACID–BASE ABNORMALITIES

During storage, whole blood or red blood cells accumulate acid that is mostly in the form of lactate and citrate. By the end of 5 weeks of storage, pH ranges from approximately 6.5–6.7. This acid load may contribute to an initial metabolic acidosis during the resuscitation of massively bleeding patients. Significant acidosis, however, is more likely the result of the consequences of uncontrolled hemorrhage, i.e., severe hypovolemia and poor tissue perfusion (49). Thus, prompt restoration of intravascular volume and oxygen-carrying capacity is much more important than supplemental sodium bicarbonate administration in avoiding metabolic acidosis during massive transfusion. In fact, many massively transfused patients develop a slight metabolic alkalosis during the recovery phase after massive transfusion (41, 49, 50), as the citrate is rapidly metabolized to sodium bicarbonate in the liver. Because severe alkalosis can result in reduced myocardial function and respiration and increased hemoglobin oxygen affinity, empiric bicarbonate administration during massive transfusion to prevent acidosis is generally not advised.

In the patient undergoing liver transplantation or in end-stage hepatic failure, metabolic acids may not be metabolized, and acidosis is more prevalent, severe, and prolonged. Acidosis combined with hypocalcemia creates a particularly lethal combination because catecholamine hormones require a very narrow range for normal activity.

Hemoglobin Oxygen Affinity

During blood storage, red blood cell 2,3-diphosphoglycerate (DPG) levels decline significantly, reaching less than 10% of the initial value by 5 weeks of storage. Like alkalosis, reduced levels of 2,3-DPG are associated with increased hemoglobin oxygen affinity and thus may theoretically impair tissue oxygen delivery in massively transfused patients. Once stored blood is transfused, however, 2,3-DPG levels are restored within 24 hours (51). Furthermore, patients with adequate myocardial function can compensate for any transient change in hemoglobin oxygen affinity by increasing cardiac output. Thus, the clinical significance of the increased hemoglobin oxygen affinity of stored blood in massively transfused patients has never been demonstrated. In patients with severe underlying cardiopulmonary disease, it may be desirable to compensate for any theoretical detrimental effect by maintaining a higher hematocrit value (approximately 30%). Exogenous administration of 2,3-DPG has not been of any benefit nor has its addition to red cell products immediately before administration; 2,3-DPG is rapidly degraded in plasma and is only effective if contained in red cells attached to hemoglobin.

HYPOTHERMIA

Rapid infusion of large amounts of blood stored at 4°C can result in hypothermia. Patients particularly at risk are those with severe trauma, advanced age, or prolonged hypotension and those undergoing open thoracic or abdominal surgery who are at additional risk of heat loss. The potential adverse effects of hypothermia include depressed myocardial function, increased hemoglobin oxygen affinity, and decreased hepatic metabolism of citrate (52). Myocardial contractility is severely depressed by 32°C, and ventricular tachycardia/fibrillation occurs between 28 and 30°C. Asystole is commonly seen with myocardial temperatures below 28°C. Rapid infusion of cold blood in a severely hypovolemic heart may cause direct cooling of the conduction system in the right atrium and intraventricular septum. Streaming of blood and incomplete mixing may mean that cold blood actually does find its way to coronary arteries. Direct infusion of 4°C blood into the central circulation is extremely dangerous, especially when one considers that in cardiac surgery, attempts to stop the heart are carried out with 4°C cardioplegia solution.

Hypothermia can also adversely affect platelet function (29) and the coagulation cascade (30, 31) and thus contribute to the bleeding associated with massive transfusion (53). Not only are systemic temperatures important, but the temperature at which the wound is expected to coagulate is critical (54). It is not uncommon during surgery to find a patient's bladder or rectal temperature at 35°C and the wound edge (where coagulation is expected to take place) at 27–28°C. That temperature is a level at which coagulation is quite dysfunctional (see Chapter 26).

Warming of intravenous fluids and blood products to 37°C can ameliorate hypothermia during massive transfusion (55). Several high-flow blood-warming devices are available for warming transfused blood to 37°C, but temperature must be carefully controlled, because hemolysis will occur if the temperature is greater than 42°C. The most effective is the Haemonetics Rapid Infusion System (Haemonetics, Braintree, MA). This roller pump-based system can deliver up to 1500 mL/min warmed from 4 to 37°C. Other systems such as the Level One (Level One Technology, Marshfield, MA) can deliver 500–700 mL/min warmed to 37°C for considerably less cost. Other measures to prevent hypothermia include keeping the resuscitation room or operating room heated to approximately 30°C and insulating the patient's head and extremities. Extracorporeal rewarming using an arteriovenous or venovenous bypass circuit may be required in patients with severe hypothermia (56, 57).

PULMONARY COMPLICATIONS

Pulmonary edema can complicate massive transfusion, particularly in the setting of trauma. The pathophysiology of this complication is unclear and may be related to either the transfused blood or the patient's underlying injury and its associated complications. Studies in severely injured combat victims in Vietnam suggested that this complication is probably related more to the nature and extent of the patient's injury than to the volume of blood transfused (58). Potential factors relating to the patient or the underlying injury include aspiration or bacterial pneumonia, sepsis resulting in ARDS, and renal failure. In many cases, however, volume overload may play a significant role. Therefore, the volume and rate of resuscitative fluids and blood components should be monitored carefully in massively transfused patients, particularly in patients with underlying cardiac, pulmonary, or renal disease or those with underlying infection.

The effects of substances that damage the lungs, such as blood microaggregates, have been studied frequently with conflicting results. Stored blood accumulates microaggregate particles composed of cellular fragments and fibrin that may escape standard 170-μm^3 blood transfusion filters. Evidence of a beneficial effect on pulmonary function by removal of these microaggregates using filters of smaller pore size, however, is equivocal (59). Furthermore, these micropore filters can become easily obstructed during rapid blood infusion and thus may impede resuscitation.

An uncommon but increasingly recognized cause of post-transfusion pulmonary edema is the passive transfer of donor antileukocyte antibodies that react with human leukocyte antigen or neutrophil-specific antigens on recipient leukocytes (60). These leukocyte antigen-antibody complexes activate the complement system and lead to leukocyte accumulation in the pulmonary capillaries. Release of inflammatory mediators is thought to result in pulmonary vascular endothelial injury and thus extravasation of fluid into the alveoli. Clinically, acute respiratory distress and hypoxemia due to noncardiogenic pulmonary edema usually develop within 6 hours of the transfusion and may be accompanied by fever and hypotension (60). Acute respiratory symptoms and hypoxemia generally resolve within 2–3 days but may require aggressive respiratory support. In massively transfused patients, this syndrome may be mistaken for volume overload or cardiogenic pulmonary edema; thus, hemodynamic monitoring (central venous and pulmonary capillary wedge pressures) can be helpful in evaluating pulmonary edema in the massive transfusion setting.

ALTERNATIVE APPROACHES TO MASSIVE TRANSFUSION

In addition to the potential metabolic complications specifically associated with massive transfusion, transfusion of blood components in any setting carries certain risks. As discussed in Chapter 7, the transmission of infectious diseases is a well-recognized complication of homologous blood transfusion. In addition, various immunological complications of blood transfusions exist; these include hemolytic, febrile, and allergic transfusion reactions and a possible immunosuppressive effect of blood transfusion itself. Reducing the number of allogeneic blood components to which a patient is exposed can help to reduce these risks. Several alternative methods of restoring intravascular volume and oxygen-carrying capacity are currently available or under study. Three such approaches are discussed below.

AUTOTRANSFUSION AND CELL SALVAGE DEVICES

Donation of autologous blood in advance of elective surgery has become increasingly popular as a means of reducing homologous blood exposure in patients undergoing surgical procedures. In the setting of massive blood loss, related to either emergency surgery or trauma, such an approach is not feasible. The use of intraoperative cell salvage devices, on the other hand, can be effective in reducing the need for homologous blood transfusion in patients undergoing certain surgical procedures. Using these devices, blood lost from the surgical or traumatic bleeding site can be reinfused into the patient. This technique has been successful in cardiovascular surgery, orthopedic surgery, liver transplantation, and trauma surgery (61). Although generally contraindicated in patients with sepsis or malignancy, autotransfusion of blood from a bacterially contaminated field (e.g., traumatic bowel injury) may be appropriate if the blood is washed before reinfusion (36, 62).

In general, two different types of cell salvage devices are available. The Haemonetics Cell Saver (Haemonetics Corp.) collects shed autologous blood and then washes the red cells to remove patient plasma before reinfusion. In this type of system, there is thus a potential for dilution of coagulation factors that may contribute to development of coagulopathy (36). Other types of devices such as the Autotransfusor (Abbott Laboratories, Chicago, IL) collect shed blood by gravity and return both cells and plasma to the patient.

ACUTE NORMOVOLEMIC HEMODILUTION

Acute normovolemic hemodilution is another technique that has been used to reduce intraoperative blood transfusion (63). In this procedure, several units of autologous blood are removed preoperatively and replaced with crystalloid and/or colloid solutions to restore intravascular volume. The autologous blood is anticoagulated, stored at room temperature, and reinfused into the patient during the operation as needed. This procedure may be useful in operations in which a significant amount of blood loss is anticipated, but the benefit of this technique in reducing the need for homologous blood transfusion is equivocal. In addition, this procedure is obviously not useful in an emergency setting.

RED BLOOD CELL SUBSTITUTES

The availability of a biological or synthetic material capable of acting as a substitute oxygen carrier would presumably eliminate the problems of infectious disease transmission and sensitization to cellular antigens that can complicate standard transfusion therapy. In general, two different types of red cell substitutes have been studied. The first group consists of synthetic substances such as perfluorocarbons. Although efficient oxygen carriers, these substances require an inspired oxygen concentration of 100% for complete saturation to occur. Thus, success in clinical studies has been limited (64). However, second-generation compounds capable of carrying up to four times as much perfluorocarbon may prove useful (see Chapter 10b.) The other class of agents currently under study is hemoglobin or modified hemoglobin solutions. Solutions of nonantigenic stroma-free hemoglobin have been studied but are limited by low oxygen-carrying capacity, a relatively short half-life, and renal toxicity. Chemical modification of hemoglobin has included polymerization, pyridoxylation, or encapsulation of the unmodified hemoglobin tetramer molecule to increase circulating half-life and eliminate toxicity. Clinical studies of some of these stroma-free modified hemoglobin solutions in massively transfused patients are currently under way (see Chapter 10a).

SUMMARY

Massive transfusion most often occurs in patients with trauma or gastrointestinal hemorrhage or in patients undergoing cardiovascular surgery or liver transplantation. The overall survival rate of massively transfused patients is in the range of 50%. Primary replacement therapy involves initial repletion of intravascular volume with salt and/or colloid solutions and restoration of oxygen-carrying capacity with red blood cell-containing components (whole blood and/or packed red blood cells). Whole blood should be used, if available, and has the advantage of simultaneous replacement of both red blood cells and plasma coagulation factors (both derived from the same blood donor). If urgent transfusion is required and the patient's blood type is unknown, uncrossmatched group O packed RBC may be transfused.

Hemostatic abnormalities are common in massively transfused patients and may warrant the transfusion of platelet concentrates, cryoprecipitate, and/or FFP. Thrombocytopenia is the most common hemostatic abnormality in massively transfused patients transfused with whole blood. More recent data suggest that coagulation factor deficits are more likely if relatively plasma-poor red blood cells are used exclusively for red cell replacement. In any event, there is no indication for empiric or formula-based transfusion of hemostatic components in massively transfused patients. Hemostatic component therapy should be guided by frequent monitoring of coagulation screening tests and careful observation for clinical evidence of microvascular bleeding.

Aside from the well-recognized complications of transfusion reactions and infectious disease transmission, massively transfused patients may also develop certain metabolic complications, including potassium and acid–base disturbances, hypocalcemia, hypothermia, and pulmonary edema. The development of these abnormalities often depends on both the transfusion of massive amounts of stored blood and the patient's underlying clinical condition. To minimize the adverse effects of massive transfusion, alternatives to allogeneic transfusion, such as intraoperative autologous transfusion, should be used whenever indicated. Other transfusion alternatives, such as perfluorocarbons and stroma-free hemoglobin solutions, are currently under study.

REFERENCES

1. Sawyer PR, Harrison CR. Massive transfusion in adults: diagnoses, survival and blood bank support. Vox Sang 1990;58:199–203.
2. Nusbacher J. Blood transfusion support in liver transplantation. Transfus Med Rev 1991;5:207–213.
3. Wudel JH, Morris JA, Yates K, Wilson A, Bass SM. Massive transfusion: outcome in blunt trauma patients. J Trauma 1991;31:1–7.
4. Phillips TF, Soulier G, Wilson RF. Outcome of massive transfusion exceeding two blood volumes in trauma and emergency surgery. J Trauma 1987;27:903–910.
5. Wilson RF, Dulchavsky SA, Soullier G, Beckman B. Problems with 20 or more blood transfusions in 24 hours. Am Surg 1987;53:410–417.
6. Brotman S, Lamonica C, Cowley RA. Massive transfusion without major complications after trauma. Am J Emerg Med 1986;4:514–515.
7. Michelsen T, Salmela L, Tigerstedt I, Mäkeläinen, Linko K. Massive blood transfusion: is there a limit? Crit Care Med 1989;17:699–700.
8. Vassar MJ, Fischer RP, O'Brien PE, et al. A multicenter trial for resuscitation of injured patients with 7.5% sodium chloride. Arch Surg 1993;128:1003–1011.
9. Reed RL II, Johnston TD, Chen Y, Fischer RP. Hypertonic saline alters plasma clotting times and platelet aggregation. J Trauma 1991;31:8–14.
10. Alving BM, Hojima Y, Pisano JJ, et al. Hypotension associated with prekallikrein activator (Hageman-factor fragments) in plasma protein fraction. N Engl J Med 1978;299:66–70.
11. Paull J. A Prospective Study of dextran-induced anaphylactoid reactions in 5745 patients. Anaesth Intens Care 1987;15:163–167.
12. Counts RB, Haisch C, Simon TL, Maxwell NG, Heimbach DM, Carrico CJ. Hemostasis in massively transfused trauma patients. Ann Surg 1979;190:91–99.
13. Kang YG, Martin DJ, Maquez J, et al. Intraoperative changes in blood coagulation and thromboelastographic monitoring in liver transplantation. Anesth Analg 1985;64:888–896.
14. Chandler WL. The thromboelastograph and the thromboelastograph technique. Semin Thromb Hemost 1995;21(Suppl. 4):1–6.
15. Simon TL, Henderson R. Coagulation factor activity in platelet concentrates. Transfusion 1979;19:186–189.
16. Tullis JL, Alving B, Bove JR, et al. Fresh-frozen plasma: indications and risks [Consensus Development Conference]. JAMA 1985;253:551–553.
17. Stern SA, Dronen SC, Birrer P, Wang X. Effect of blood pressure on hemorrhage volume and survival in a near-fatal hemorrhage model incorporating a vascular injury. Ann Emerg Med 1993;22:155–163.
18. Bickell WH, Wall MJ Jr., Pepe PE, et al. Immediate versus delayed fluid resuscitation for hypotensive patients with penetrating torso injuries. N Engl J Med 1994;331:1105–1109.
19. Schwab CW, Shayne JP, Turner J. Immediate trauma resuscitation with type O uncrossmatched blood: a two-year prospective experience. J Trauma 1986;26:897–902.
20. Lefebre J, McLellan BA, Coovadia AS. Seven years experience with group O unmatched packed red blood cells in a regional trauma unit. Ann Emerg Med 1987;16:1344–1349.
21. Schmidt PJ, Leparc GF, Samia CT. Use of Rh positive blood in emergency situations. Surg Gynecol Obstet 1988;167:229–233.
22. Sazama K. Reports of 355 transfusion-associated deaths: 1976 through 1985. Transfusion 1990;30:583–590.
23. Giblett ER. Blood group alloantibodies: an assessment of some laboratory practices. Transfusion 1977;17:299–308.
24. Millikan JS, Cain TL, Hansbrough J. Rapid volume replacement for hypovolemic shock: a comparison of techniques and equipment. J Trauma 1984;24:428–431.
25. Floccare DJ, Kelen GD, Altman RS, et al. Rapid infusion of additive red blood cells: alternative techniques for massive hemorrhage. Ann Emerg Med 1990;19:129–133.
26. Reed RL II, Heimbach DM, Counts RB, et al. Prophylactic platelet administration during massive transfusion: a prospective, randomized, double-blind clinical study. Ann Surg 1986;203:40–48.
27. Harke H, Rahman S. Haemostatic disorders in massive transfusion. Bibl Haemat 1980;46:179–188.
28. Hewson JR, Neame PB, Naresh K, et al. Coagulopathy related to dilution and hypotension during massive transfusion. Crit Care Med 1985;13:387–391.

29. Valeri CR, Cassidy G, Khuri S, Feingold H, Ragno G, Altschule MD. Hypothermia-induced reversible platelet dysfunction. Ann Surg 1987; 205:175–181.
30. Rohrer MJ, Natale AM. Effect of hypothermia on the coagulation cascade. Crit Care Med 1992;20:1402–1405.
31. Johnston TD, Chen Y, Reed RL II. Functional equivalence of hypothermia to specific clotting factor deficiencies. J Trauma 1994;37: 413–417.
32. Miller RD, Robbins TO, Tong MJ, Barton SL. Coagulation defects associated with massive blood transfusions. Ann Surg 1971;174: 794–801.
33. Leslie SD, Toy PTCY. Laboratory hemostatic abnormalities in massively transfused patients given red blood cells and crystalloid. Am J Clin Pathol 1991;96:770–773.
34. Harrigan C, Lucas CE, Ledgerwood AM, Walz DA, Mammen EF. Serial changes in primary hemostasis after massive transfusion. Surgery 1985;98:836–843.
35. Faringer PD, Mullins RJ, Johnson RL, Trunkey DD. Blood component supplementation during massive transfusion of AS-1 red cells in trauma patients. J Trauma 1993;34:481–487.
36. Horst HM, Dlugos S, Fath JJ, Sorensen VJ, Obeid FN, Bivins BA. Coagulopathy and intraoperative blood salvage (IBS). J Trauma 1992; 32:646–652.
37. Murray DJ, Olson J, Strauss R, Tinker JH. Coagulation changes during packed red cell replacement of major blood loss. Anesthesiology 1988; 69:839–845.
38. Ciavarella D, Reed RL, Counts RB, et al. Clotting factor levels and the risk of diffuse microvascular bleeding in the massively transfused patient. Br J Haematol 1987;67:365–368.
39. Goodnight SH, Kenoyer G, Rapaport SI, Patch MJ, Lee JA, Kurze T. Defibrination after brain-tissue destruction: a serious complication of head injury. N Engl J Med 1974;290:1043–1047.
40. Bayly PJ, Thick M. Reversal of post-reperfusion coagulopathy by protamine sulphate in orthotopic liver transplantation. Br J Anaesth 1994; 73:840–842.
41. Linko K, Saxelin I. Electrolyte and acid-base disturbances caused by blood transfusions. Acta Anaesth Scand 1986;30:139–144.
42. Reddy SVG, Sein K. Potassium and massive blood transfusion. Singapore Med J 1991;32:29–30.
43. Wilson RF, Binkley LE, Sabo FM, et al. Electrolyte and acid-base changes with massive blood transfusions. Am Surg 1992;58:535–544.
44. Linko K, Tigerstedt I. Hyperpotassemia during massive blood transfusions. Acta Anaesth Scand 1984;28:220–221.
45. Jameson LC, Popic PM, Harms BA. Hyperkalemic death during use of a high-capacity fluid warmer for massive transfusion. Anesthesiology 1990;73:1050–1052.
46. Carmichael D, Hosty T, Kastl D, Beckman D. Hypokalemia and massive transfusion. Southern Med J 1984;77:315–317.
47. Dzik WH, Kirkley SA. Citrate toxicity during massive blood transfusion. Transfus Med Rev 1988;2:76–94.
48. Martin TJ, Kang Y, Robertson KM, et al. Ionization and hemodynamic effects of calcium chloride and calcium gluconate in the absence of hepatic function. Anesthesiology 1990;73:62–65.
49. Collins JA, Simmons RL, James PM, Bredenberg CE, Anderson RW, Heisterkamp CA III. Acid-base status of seriously wounded combat casualties: II. Resuscitation with stored blood. Ann Surg 1971;173:6–18.
50. Driscoll DF, Bistrian BR, Jenkins RL, et al. Development of metabolic alkalosis after massive transfusion during orthotopic liver transplantation. Crit Care Med 1987;15:905–908.
51. Beutler E, Wood L. The in vivo regeneration of red cell 2,3-diphosphoglyceric acid (DPG) after transfusion of stored blood. J Lab Clin Med 1969;74:300–304.
52. Collins JA. Problems associated with the massive transfusion of stored blood. Surgery 1974;75:274–295.
53. Ferrara A, MacArthur JD, Wright HK, Modlin IM, McMillen MA. Hypothermia and acidosis worsen coagulopathy in the patient requiring massive transfusion. Am J Surg 1990;160:515–518.
54. Valeri CR, Khabbaz K, Khuri SF, et al. Effect of skin temperature on platelet function in patients undergoing extracorporeal bypass. J Thorac Cardiovasc Surg 1992;104:108–116.
55. Iserson KV, Huestis DW. Blood warming: Current applications and techniques. Transfusion 1991;31:558–570.
56. Gentilello LM, Cobean RA, Offner PJ, Soderberg RW, Jurkovich GJ. Continuous arteriovenous rewarming: rapid reversal of hypothermia in critically ill patients. J Trauma 1992;32:316–325.
57. Gregory JS, Flancbaum L, Smead WL, Reilley TE, Jonasson O. Extracorporeal venovenous recirculation for the treatment of hypothermia during elective aortic surgery: A phase I study. Surgery 1993;114: 40–45.
58. Collins JA, James PM, Bredenberg CE, Anderson RW, Heisterkamp CA, Simmons RL. The relationship between transfusion and hypoxemia in combat casualties. Ann Surg 1978;188:513–519.
59. Snyder EL, Bookbinder M. Role of microaggregate blood filtration in clinical medicine. Transfusion 1983;23:460–470.
60. Popovsky MA, Chaplin HC, Moore SB. Transfusion-related acute lung injury: a neglected, serious complication of hemotherapy. Transfusion 1992;32:589–592.
61. Williamson KR, Taswell HF. Intraoperative blood salvage: a review. Transfusion 1991;31:662–675.
62. Ozmen V, McSwain NE Jr, Nichols RL, Smith J, Flint LM. Autotransfusion of potentially culture-positive blood (CPB) in abdominal trauma: preliminary data from a prospective study. J Trauma 1992;32:36–39.
63. Stehling L, Zauder HL. Acute normovolemic hemodilution. Transfusion 1991;31:857–868.
64. Gould SA, Rosen AL, Sehgal L, et al. Fluosol-DA as a red-cell substitute in acute anemia. N Engl J Med 1986;314:1653–1656.

Chapter 24

Hypothermia and Hemorrhage

R. LAWRENCE REED II
LARRY M. GENTILELLO

INTRODUCTION

Hypothermia is defined as a core body temperature below normal in a homeothermic organism and is considered present in humans when core temperature drops below 35°C (1). In a study performed at Harborview Medical Center in Seattle, the average initial temperature of intubated trauma victims upon arrival to the emergency department was 35°C, with no seasonal variation, and 23% of patients had an initial core temperature of 34°C or less (2). Even in the temperate climate of San Diego, hypothermia was reported to occur in 21% of seriously injured patients, and as many as 46% of trauma victims that require laparotomy leave the operating room with some degree of hypothermia (3, 4).

A multicenter review of 401 cases of hypothermia due to exposure reported that mortality was only 21% in patients admitted with a core temperature between 28 and 32°C, with virtually all deaths attributable to underlying diseases rather than to the hypothermia (5). In contrast, studies on outcome from hypothermia in injured patients indicate that a core body temperature of 32°C or less carries a very high mortality rate and that any hypothermia is a poor prognostic sign (2, 6, 7).

Uncontrollable hemorrhage, often compounded by coagulopathy, is the most frequent cause of early death in these patients. The primary factors thought to contribute to coagulopathic bleeding are dilution with volume expanders deficient in clotting factors and platelets (8, 9), acidosis (10, 11), hypoperfusion (12, 13), tissue trauma (14–17), and hypothermia (18–20). Hemodilution is usually cited as the primary cause of coagulopathic bleeding when these patients undergo massive transfusion; however, the prophylactic administration of platelets or fresh-frozen plasma has failed to demonstrate any beneficial effects (10–12, 21). Therefore, increasing attention to the potential roles played by some of these other factors is warranted.

The initial surge of interest in the effects of hypothermia on coagulation occurred in the late 1950s as a result of the development of hypothermic cardioplegia for cardiac surgery. Reports of coagulation abnormalities in patients with apparently normal clotting factor levels surfaced shortly after its introduction (22, 23). Renewed interest occurred in the 1980s as a part of efforts to unravel the coagulopathy that often accompanied major injuries.

The extent to which hypothermia causes coagulation problems is often underestimated because of the multiplicity of potential etiologies for coagulation impairment in these patients, which makes it difficult to assess its relative contribution (8, 9). Theoretically, hypothermia could affect each of the three major components of the clotting process: vascular, platelet, and clotting factor function.

VASCULAR EFFECTS

The initial response of vessels to vascular injury is vasoconstriction. Systemic hypothermia has also long been known to provoke cutaneous vasoconstriction. No doubt because of this observation, the topical application of cold has been advocated as a means of controlling bleeding. Hippocrates, for example, listed hemorrhage control as one of the primary uses of cold application (24). It is a common practice to use ice packs to control nosebleeds or to limit hematoma formation, and for over two decades, iced saline lavage was advocated as a technique for controlling upper gastrointestinal hemorrhage (25–27). Unfortunately, many of these practices were used without objective scientific evidence of efficacy.

Although systemic hypothermia causes vasoconstriction, topical exposure to cold appears to have quite different effects.

Local cooling elicits skin and skeletal muscle vasodilation at 33°C in both innervated and denervated forelimbs (28). At more profound levels of hypothermia (28°C), there is only a slight increase in skin and skeletal muscle vascular resistance, perhaps due to a rise in blood viscosity.

This phenomenon makes sense from a physiological standpoint. In homeothermic animals, systemic hypothermia produces serious adverse consequences for the entire organism, and efforts are directed toward conserving body heat by diminishing cutaneous circulation. On the other hand, topical administration of cold produces a regional hypothermia that stimulates local measures designed to improve the flow of warm blood into the affected region through vasodilation. An example of this response is the redness of the ears and cheeks when exposed to cold weather. Interestingly, locally induced vasodilatation appears to override the powerful vasoconstrictor response caused by systemic cooling and appears to be an active rather than passive vasodilatation (28). Hypothermia-induced topical vasoconstriction either does not exist or cannot be relied on to stop bleeding.

PLATELET EFFECTS

Normal coagulation requires adequacy of both platelet count and function. Studies have demonstrated that deep hypothermia is associated with a decrease in platelet count (29). Helmsworth and associates (30, 31) found an 82% reduction in platelets in dogs cooled to 18–26° C, and Couves and colleagues (32) noted platelet counts of 40,000 or less in dogs when core temperature dropped below 20°C. Studies using ^{32}P-labeled platelets demonstrated that the portal circulation was the primary site of platelet sequestration and that 80% of platelets returned to the circulation upon rewarming (29, 33).

Ellis et al. (35) in 1957 and Wensel and Bigalow (34) in 1959 noted that heparin administration (2–3 mg/kg) can reduce the degree of thrombocytopenia seen during hypothermia, which is fortuitous, because patients receiving controlled hypothermia typically receive heparin.

The response of platelets to exposed collagen or basement membrane substances is characterized initially by adhesion and subsequently by aggregation. Human platelets exposed to cold undergo morphological changes that affect adherence, including loss of shape, cytoplasmic swelling, and dissolution of cytoplasmic microtubules necessary for normal motility. These changes also result in spontaneous platelet aggregation, or "clumping" (36).

Although significant effects of hypothermia on platelet count have not been demonstrated during milder degrees of hypothermia, levels of hypothermia commonly encountered in clinical practice do have a significant effect on platelet function. Platelets contain granules with a variety of components necessary for normal aggregation, including adenosine diphosphate (ADP), which is released within seconds of platelet activation. Platelet activation is also associated with activation of cell-membrane phospholipase, which hydrolyzes phospholipids to arachidonic acid. Arachidonic acid is in turn converted to prostaglandin endoperoxides, which are converted by thromboxane synthetase to thromboxane A_2, a potent vasoconstrictor necessary for normal platelet function (37).

At moderate degrees of hypothermia (29.5°C), platelet aggregation is minimally influenced when aggregation is stimulated by ADP, ristocetin, or collagen. However, a roughly 50% impairment of epinephrine-stimulated aggregation has been identified, suggesting a potential alteration in the platelet's alpha-receptor (36). Interestingly, ADP improves aggregation slightly in a hypothermic environment, whereas epinephrine stimulates platelets most effectively in a normothermic environment.

In coagulopathic patients, the amount of nonsurgical blood loss correlates closely with the bleeding time (Duke or Ivy method), which is primarily a measure of platelet function (38). Valeri and associates (39) induced systemic hypothermia to 32°C in baboons but kept one forearm warm using heating lamps and a warming blanket. Simultaneous bleeding time measurements in the warm and cold arm were 2.4 and 5.8 minutes, respectively. This effect, which was reversible with rewarming, appeared to be mediated by cold-induced slowing of the enzymatic reaction rate of thromboxane synthetase, which resulted in decreased production of thromboxane A_2. The authors concluded that warming to restore wound temperature to normal should be tried before resorting to transfusion therapy with platelets and clotting factors when treating hypothermic platelets with nonsurgical bleeding.

CLOTTING FACTORS

In contrast to the effects of hypothermia on platelet count and function, the effect of hypothermia on clotting factors has been harder to specify. Wilson and colleagues (40) studied dogs with rectal temperatures ranging from 21 to 26°C, and there were minimal effects on Lee-White glass tube clotting times, clot retraction times, prothrombin times, and circulating fibrinogen levels. In a similar study, Couves and coworkers (32) studied dogs kept at temperatures from 18 to 25°C for 1–4 hours and found no significant changes in a variety of coagulation assays.

Fisher and colleagues (41) produced a prolonged model of cold exposure in dogs and maintained a body temperature between 22.5 and 24.5°C for up to 26 hours. They found an increase in the Lee-White clotting time in all animals after 4 hours of exposure, whereas an increase in prothrombin time was not seen until 6 hours of exposure had elapsed. These prolongations were minor, however, and severe deteriorations in coagulation were not observed until after 10–15 hours of hypothermia.

Because of the controlled nature of hypothermia during cardiopulmonary bypass, studies of clotting function have also been performed on humans undergoing open-heart surgery. Bunker and Goldstein (42) studied clotting tests during hypothermia (29–31°C) in 10 cardiac patients and failed to find significant alterations in the levels of any clotting factors. In a more extensive analysis, von Kaulla and Swan (42) studied eight patients who underwent hypothermic anesthesia for open-heart surgery and found variable results in the clotting tests performed. The whole blood recalcification time was slightly decreased, and minimal changes were seen in prothrombin consumption, although there was a drop in prothrombin activity. Overall, the findings of these studies were so variable that it was not possible to identify any significant effect of hypothermia on coagulation.

These findings would suggest that hypothermia to the extent usually found in general surgical operating rooms should not adversely affect standard clotting tests, particularly because it is rare for patients to exhibit core temperatures below 32°C (2, 6, 19). However, many patients with mild degrees of hypothermia appear clinically coagulopathic, and core temperature appears inversely related to the severity of the coagulopathy.

This apparent paradox has been investigated in recent studies that demonstrated that coagulation during hypothermia is disturbed more from enzymatic dysfunction than from altered clotting factor levels. Clinical tests of coagulation are temperature standardized to 37°C. As with blood gas machines, fibrometers that measure coagulation contain a thermal block that heats the plasma and reagents to 37°C before initiating the assay. Thus, tests of coagulation provide quantitative information about clotting factor depletion but are corrected for any potential effect of hypothermia on clotting factor function. This is not necessarily improper, because the primary therapeutic approach toward coagulopathy is replacement of components that have become deficient, and temperature standardized clotting tests will reflect clotting factor deficiencies.

However, this explains the lack of correlation between experimental data and clinical experience, because coagulation tests in the abovementioned studies were performed at 37°C instead of at the subject's actual core temperature. Sincar (44) first considered this issue in 1954, when dogs were made hypothermic and coagulation assays were performed at the actual temperature of the animal. Still, only severe hypothermia (23–25°C) was studied, and the only clotting test used was the capillary tube method using the undersurface of the tongue.

Bunker and Goldstein (42), in a study of controlled hypothermia in 10 patients, performed coagulation tests at the actual temperature of the patient and at 37°C. Although they found no significant changes in coagulation times performed at 37°C, they stated that "prolongation of the clotting times for all coagulation tests except whole blood clotting times was consistently observed when performed at the hypothermic temperatures." Unfortunately, they provided no data to describe the degree of the disturbance seen at the hypothermic testing temperatures. They postulated that depression of clotting factor enzymatic activity during hypothermia may be a fortuitous event, preventing intravascular thrombosis during circulatory slowing.

A more detailed study of the kinetic effects of hypothermia on clotting factor function has been undertaken by Reed et al. (45). By connecting a fibrometer to a thermally controlled external power source, clotting tests (prothrombin time, partial thromboplastin time, and thrombin time) were performed on reference human plasma containing normal levels of all clotting factors at temperatures ranging from 25 to 37°C. The results showed a significant slowing of clotting factor function at temperatures of 35°C or less that was proportional to the degree of hypothermia.

The prolongation of clot formation that occurred at clinically relevant levels of hypothermia was equivalent to that seen in normothermic patients with significant clotting factor depletion. For example, assays of plasma with normal clotting factor levels conducted at 35, 33, and 31°C prolonged the partial thromboplastin time to the same extent as would occur with a reduction in factor IX levels to 66%, 32%, and 7% of normal in a euthermic patient (Table 24.1).

Interestingly, slowing of the multienzymatic pathways such as the partial thromboplastin time and the prothrombin time was more pronounced than the slowing of a single enzymatic pathway such as the thrombin time. This probably represents the cumulative effect of enzymatic slowing on the multistage clotting cascade.

In many seriously injured patients, clotting factor depletion exists in conjunction with hypothermia. The additional effect of hypothermic enzymatic inhibition on factor-depleted plasma was recently analyzed by Gubler et al. (46). A modified fibrometer was used to analyze both normal human volunteer plasma and clotting factor-depleted plasma taken from critically ill patients (Fig. 24.1). The study demonstrated a potentiating effect of hypothermia on coagulation dysfunction in plasma with deficient clotting factor levels, although there did not appear to be synergy between the two conditions.

TABLE 24.1. PLASMA WITH NORMAL CLOTTING FACTOR LEVELS

Temperature °C	Percentage of Factor							
	II	V	VII	VIII	IX	X	XI	XII
25°	5	3	5	0	0	4	2	1
27°	7	5	7	0	0	6	2	1
29°	10	8	12	3	3	10	4	1
31°	17	22	34	16	7	20	16	10
33°	24	50	60	59	32	44	60	17
35°	82	75	82	79	66	81	85	65
37°	100	100	100	100	100	100	100	100

Reprinted with permission from Johnston TD, Chen Y, Reed RL II. Functional equivalence of hypothermia to specific clotting factor deficiencies. J Trauma 1994;37:413–417.

When assayed at hypothermic temperatures, plasma behaves as if clotting factor deficient. At temperatures less than 37°C, hypothermia prolongs clotting to the same extent as a reduction in the various clotting factors to the level shown here.

The importance of the effect of temperature on the coagulation cascade was further refined in a follow-up study by Reed et al. (47). Blood coagulation was studied in three groups of rats. In the first group, hypothermia to one of seven different core temperatures (25, 27, 29, 31, 33, 35, and 37°C) was induced for 2 hours, after which blood was withdrawn and clotting tests performed at 37°C, regardless of the animal's core temperature. Any abnormalities in clotting times would represent a hypothermia-induced alteration in clotting factor levels, because coagulation tests were performed at a normothermic temperature. All clotting results were normal in this group, demonstrating the absence of any effect of hypothermia on clotting factor levels or clotting factor viability.

The second group was maintained in a euthermic state at 37°C for the 2-hour study duration, but the clotting tests were performed at each of the seven different study temperatures. This group of rats would represent the effect of hypothermia upon clotting enzyme function and would also control for any effects produced by the cold water immersion. A marked prolongation occurred in all clotting tests performed below 35°C (Fig. 24.2). The degree of abnormality was inversely proportional to the temperature at which the assay was conducted, indicating that the effect of hypothermia on coagulation is not due to a systemic effect of hypothermia but is due to a temperature-related effect on enzymatic reaction rates.

Hypothermia to each of the seven temperatures was induced in the remaining group of animals, and clotting tests were performed at the animals' actual core temperature. This group provided an assessment of any interactive effect between systemic hypothermia and the effect of hypothermia on clotting factor enzyme kinetics. There was no difference in clotting times in plasma taken from the warm animals in group 2 and the cold animals in group 3 for assays conducted at the same temperature. This indicates that hypothermia-induced clotting factor enzymatic dysfunction is simply due to temperature-related effects on enzymatic function and that standard 37°C hospital coagulation tests are insensitive to this effect. Furthermore, because systemic hypothermia did not appear to influence the integrity of clotting factors or their concentration, coagulopathic bleeding in cold patients will respond to warming measures.

DISSEMINATED INTRAVASCULAR COAGULATION

Fibrinolytic activity is markedly higher in dogs subjected to hypothermia, and rewarming may accelerate the activity of enzymes responsible for fibrinolysis and coagulation. One study

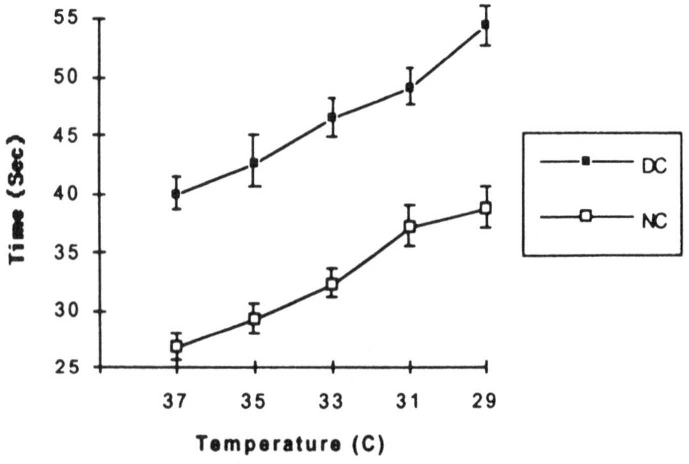

Figure 24.1. The effect of temperature on coagulation assays in human plasma taken from patients with normal clotting factor levels (NC) and with dilutional coagulopathy. (Reprinted with permission from Gubler KD, Gentilello LM, Hassantash SA, et al. The impact of hypothermia on dilutional coagulopathy. J Trauma 1994;36:847–851.)

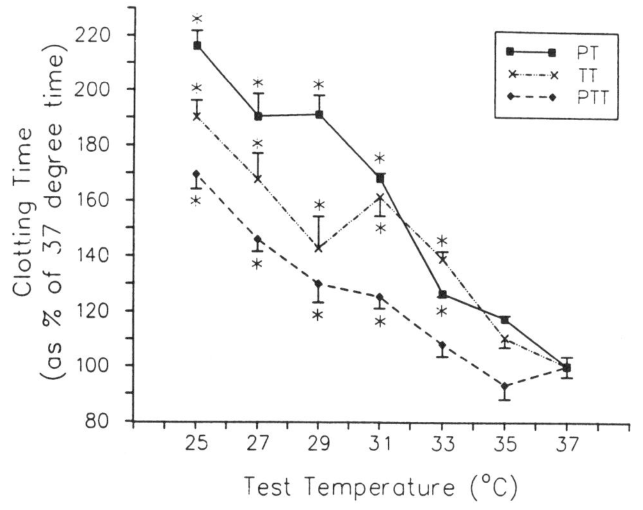

Figure 24.2. Clotting times for normothermic rats when the clotting tests are performed at hypothermic temperatures. Results are expressed as a percentage of the clotting time observed when the test is performed at 37°C. PT, prothrombin time; TT, thrombin time; PTT, partial thromboplastin time. (Reprinted with permission from Reed RL II, Johnston TD, Hudson JD, et al. The disparity between hypothermic coagulopathy and clotting studies. J Trauma 1992;33:465–470.)

indicated that fibrinolytic processes are accelerated during rewarming at a greater rate than procoagulant processes. In experimental studies, several investigators have also detected the presence of a heparin-like factor released from platelets and mast cells during hypothermia (48–50). Originally described in neonates and subsequently reported in adults, the causes of the syndrome of disseminated intravascular coagulation after rewarming are probably multifactorial and probably include tissue damage produced by hypothermia, associated hypoxia and hypotension, and release of tissue thromboplastin that activates coagulation pathways (51–53).

SUMMARY

Hypothermia is a clinical condition that occurs in association with transfusion of cold fluids or blood products, environmental exposure, multiple trauma, and exposed body cavities. In many of these situations, patients will simultaneously have a moderate to severe coagulopathy, and the potential contribution of hypothermia to this process is significant. Much of the clinical experience has been reported in the way of anecdotal observations, whereas the basic science laboratories have made efforts to identify the particular contributions of hypothermia to coagulation by isolating the variables of interest.

However, a major distinction between recently performed studies and those performed during the 1950s and 1960s is that earlier studies on the effect of hypothermia performed the clotting tests under normothermic conditions, resulting in part in an underestimation of the effect of hypothermia on coagulation. Recent studies demonstrate a profound effect of hypothermia on coagulation due to enzymatic inhibition of platelets and clotting factors through temperature-induced alterations in their kinetic activities.

REFERENCES

1. Report of Committee on Accidental Hypothermia. London: Royal College of Physicians, 1966.
2. Luna GK, Maier RV, Pavlin EG, et al. Incidence and effect of hypothermia in seriously injured patients. J Trauma 1987;27:1014–1017.
3. Steinemann S, Shackford SR, Davis JW. Implications of admission hypothermia in trauma patients. J Trauma 1990;30:200–202.
4. Gregory JS, Flancbaum L, Townsend C, et al. Incidence and timing of hypothermia in trauma patients undergoing operations. J Trauma 1991; 31:795–800.
5. Danzl D. Pozos RS, Auerbach PS, et al. Multicenter hypothermia survey. Ann Emerg Med 1987;16:1042–1055.
6. Jurkovich GJ, Greiser WB, Luterman A, et al. Hypothermia in trauma victims: an ominous predictor of survival. J Trauma 1987;27:1019–1024.
7. Psarras P, Ivatury RR, Rohman M, et al. Presented at the Eastern Association for the Surgery of Trauma, Longboat Key, Florida, 1988.
8. Gralnick HR. Massive transfusion. In: Colman RW, Hirsch J, Marder VJ, Salzman EW, eds. Hemostasis and thrombosis: basic principles and clinical practice. Philadelphia: J.B. Lippincott, 1982:612–622.
9. Broema RI, Bullm GD, Mammen EF. Acidosis induced disseminated intravascular microthrombosis and its dissolution by streptokinase. Thromb Diath Haemorrh 1969;36(Suppl.):171–176.
10. Broersma RI, Bullemer GD, Mammen EF. Blood coagulation changes in hemorrhagic shock and acidosis. Thromb Diath Haemorrh 1969;36 (Suppl.):171–176.
11. Nagasue N, Iwaki A, Yukaya H, Koyanagi N, Kobayashi M, Inokuchi K. Disseminated intravascular coagulation and refractory shock induced by splanchnic metabolic acidosis. Surg Gynecol Obstet 1977; 144:519–524.
12. Harke H, Rahman S. Coagulation disorders in massively injured patients. Prog Clin Biol Res 1982:18:213–224.
13. Bergentz SE, Leandoer L. Disseminated intravascular coagulation in shock. Ann Chir Gynaecol 1971;60:175–179.
14. Brinkhous KM, Scarborough DE. Some mechanisms of thrombin formation and hemorrhage following trauma. J Trauma 1969;9:684–691.
15. String T, Robinson AJ, Blaisdell FW. Massive trauma: effect of intravascular coagulation on prognosis. Arch Surg 1971;102:406–410.
16. Hirsch EF, Fletcher JR, Moquin R, Dostalek R, Lucas S. Coagulation changes after combat trauma and sepsis. Surg Gynecol Obstet 1971; 133:393–396.
17. Goodnight SH, Kenoyer G, Rapaport SI. Defibrination after brain tissue destruction: a serious complication of head injury. N Engl J Med 1974;290:1043–1047.
18. Gentilello LM, Cortes V, Moujaes S, et al. Continuous arteriovenous rewarming: experimental results and thermodynamic model simulation of treatment for hyopthermia. J Trauma 1990;30:1436.
19. Gentilello LM, Cobean R, Offner PJ, et al. Continuous arteriovenous rewarming: rapid reversal of hypothermia in critically ill patients. J Trauma 1992;2:316.

20. Gentilello LG, Jurkovich GJ, Moujaes S. Hypothermia and injury: thermodynamic principles of prevention and treatment. In: Levine B, ed. Perspectives in surgery. Vol. 2. St. Louis: Quality Medical Publishers, 1991:25–55.
21. Reed RL, Ciavarella D, Heimbach DM, Baron L, Pavlin E, Counts RB, Carrico CJ. Prophylactic platelet administration during massive transfusion: a prospective, randomized, double-blind clinical study. Ann Surg 1986;203:40–48.
22. Bachmann F, McKenna, Cole ER, Najafi H. The hemostatic mechanism after open heart surgery. I. Studies on plasma coagulation factors and fibrinolysis in 512 patients after extracorporeal circulation. J Thorac Cardiovasc Surg 1975;79:76–85.
23. Harker LA, Malpass TW, Branson HE, Hellel EA, Slichter SJ. Mechanism of abnormal bleeding in patients undergoing cardiopulmonary bypass: acquired transient platelet dysfunction associated with selective-granule release. Blood 1980;56:824–834.
24. Adams F. The genuine works of Hippocrates. New York: William Wood, 1886.
25. Law D, Gregory D. Gastrointestinal bleeding. In: Sleisinger M, Fordtran JS, eds. Gastrointestinal diseases. Philadelphia: WB Saunders, 1973:199.
26. Boboch H. Hematemesis and melena. In: Bockus HL, ed. Gastroenterology. 3rd ed. Philadelphia: WB Saunders, 1974:814.
27. Lekagul S, Smyth NP, Brooks MH, et al. The control of upper gastrointestinal hemorrhage in the dog by peritoneal cooling. J Surg Res 1970;10:421–431.
28. Major TC, Schwinghamer JM, Winston S. Cutaneous and skeletal muscle vascular response to hypothermia. Am J Physiol 1981;240:H868–H873.
29. Villalobos TJ, Adelson E, Riley PA, et al. A cause of the thrombocytopenia and leukopenia that occur in dogs during deep hypothermia. J Clin Invest 1958;37:1–7.
30. Helmsworth JA, Stiles WJ, Elstun W. Leukopenic and thrombocytopenic effect of hypothermia in dogs. Proc Soc Exp Biol Med 1955; 90:474–476.
31. Helmsworth JA, Stiles WJ, Elstun W. Changes in blood cellular elements in dogs during hypothermia. Surgery 1955;38:843–846.
32. Couves CM, Overton RC, Eaton WL. Hematologic changes in hypothermic dogs. Surg Forum 1955;6:102–106.
33. Hessel EA, Schner G, Dillar DH. Platelet kinetics during deep hypothermia. J Surg Res 1980;28:23–34.
34. Wensel RH, Bigelow WG. The use of heparin to minimize thrombocytopenia and bleeding tendency during hypothermia. Surgery 1959;45: 223–228.
35. Ellis PR, Kleinsasser LJ, Speer RI. Changes in coagulation occurring in dogs during hypothermia and cardiac surgery. Surgery 1957;41:198–210.
36. Kattlove HE, Alexander B. The effect of cold on platelets: 1. Cold-induced platelet aggregation. Blood 1971;38:39–47.
37. Patt Anita, McCroskey BL, Moore EE. Hypothermia-induced coagulopathies in trauma. Surg Clin North Am 1988;68:775–789.
38. Czer L, et al. Prospective trial of DDAVP in treatment of severe platelet dysfunction and hemorrhage after cardiopulmonary bypass. Circulation 1985;72:III–130.
39. Valeri CR, Feingold H, Cassidy G, et al. Hypothermia induced reversible platelet dysfunction. Ann Surg 1987;205:175–181.
40. Wilson JT, Miller WR, Eliot TS. Blood studies in the hypothermic dog. Surgery 1958;43:979–989.
41. Fisher B, Russ C, Fedor E, et al. Experimental evaluation of prolonged hypothermia. Arch Surg.
42. Bunker JP, Goldstein R. Coagulation during hypothermia in man. Proc Soc Exp Biol Med 1958;97:199–202.
43. von Kaulla KN, Swan H. Clotting deviations in man associated with open-heart surgery during hypothermia. J Thorac Surg 1958;36: 857–868.
44. Sincar P. Plasma volume, bleeding and clotting times on hypothermic dogs. Proc Soc Exp Biol Med 1954;87:194–195.
45. Reed RL, Bracey AW, Hudson JD, et al. Hypothermia and blood coagulation: dissociation between enzyme activity and clotting factor levels. Circ Shock 1990;32:141–152.
46. Gubler KD, Gentilello LM, Hassantash SA, et al. The impact of hypothermia on dilutional coagulopathy. J Trauma 1994;36:847–851.
47. Reed RL, Johnston TD, Hudson JD, et al. The disparity between hypothermic coagulopathy and clotting studies. J Trauma 1992;33: 465–470.
48. Yoshihara H, Takatoshi Y, Mihara H. Changes in coagulation and fibrinolysis occurring in dogs during hypothermia. Thromb Res 1985;37: 503–512.
49. Beller BK, Archer LT, Kosanke SD, et al. Extracorporeal perfusion without anticoagulation and the response to endotoxin. Surg Gynecol Obstet 1979;148:679–684.
50. Paul J, Cornillon B, Baquet J, et al. In vivo release of a heparin-like factor in dogs during profound hypothermia. J Thorac Cardiovasc Surg 1981;82:45–48.
51. Mahajan SL, Myers TJ, Baldini MG. Disseminated intravascular coagulation during rewarming following hypothermia. JAMA 1981;245: 2517–2518.
52. Chadd MA, Gray OP. Hypothermia and coagulation defects in the newborn. Arch Dis Child 1972;47:819–821.
53. Cohen IJ. Cold injury in early infancy: relationship between mortality and disseminated intravascular coagulation. Isr J Med Sci 1977;13: 405–409.

Chapter 25

Fresh-Frozen Plasma: Indications for Use

LINDA STEHLING
HOWARD L. ZAUDER

INTRODUCTION

A single unit of whole blood served the needs of only one patient before the introduction of plastic blood bags with integral tubing and satellite bags. These bags, together with high-speed refrigerated centrifugation, facilitated component preparation and significantly expanded transfusion therapy options. Separation of whole blood into its components makes it possible for 1 unit to be used for multiple therapeutic applications tailored to each patient's specific needs. One unit of whole blood can yield red blood cells (RBCs), platelets, plasma, and cryoprecipitate.

PLASMA PREPARATIONS

Plasma is derived from anticoagulated whole blood obtained from a single, uninterrupted, nontraumatic venipuncture. Separation is accomplished by centrifugation after which the primary bag is placed in a plasma expressor and 200–250 mL of plasma is transferred into a satellite bag that is then sealed and separated from the primary bag.

FRESH-FROZEN PLASMA

Plasma that is separated from RBCs and placed at −18°C or lower within 8 hours of collection has a 1-year shelf life. A number of factors, including the time from collection to freezing, the rate of freezing, storage temperature, and type of anticoagulant, can affect the level of coagulation factors present after thawing (1). Properly prepared, a single unit of fresh-frozen plasma (FFP) should contain 400 mg of fibrinogen and about 1 unit of activity/mL of each clotting factor. In addition, a typical unit with a pH of 7.2–7.4 contains sodium 170 mmol/L, potassium 4 mmol/L, glucose 22 mmol/L, citrate 20 mmol/L, and lactate 3 mmol/L. After 1 year at −18°C, the concentration of the labile coagulation factors V and VIII may have decreased, making some units inappropriate for therapy of patients in need of these coagulation factors. Stable clotting factors, however, are preserved.

FFP is prepared for administration by thawing at 30–37°C, with gentle agitation. Water baths are commonly used. It is recommended that the FFP be placed in a second heat-sealed bag for added protection when thawing in a water bath. More rapid thawing is possible with microwave ovens designed specifically for that purpose (2, 3).

The Standards of the American Association of Blood Banks (4) require that FFP once thawed may be stored at 1–6°C for no more than 24 hours before administration. However, thawed FFP is frequently not transfused and must be discarded. Several investigators have evaluated the stability of factors V and VIII in thawed FFP. Milam et al. (5) measured factor levels at various intervals up to 24 hours using plasma from 20 units of thawed FFP. Comparisons were made between units stored at 4 and 25°C. The mean factor V activity did not change significantly during the post-thaw period at either temperature. Mean factor VIII levels, which were 121% before freezing, dropped to 89% 4 hours after thawing and gradually declined to 67% at 24 hours. Refrigeration did not appear, to these investigators, to be necessary after thawing to preserve factor V and VIII activity. However, such cryophilic organisms as Pseudomonas and coliform bacteria may proliferate when FFP is thawed and stored at temperatures above 4°C. A pilot study by Smak Gregoor et al. (6) indicated that thawed FFP stored at 4°C for up to 28 days contained sufficient coagulation factors to support hemostasis.

Dzik et al. (1) examined the effects of refreezing previously thawed FFP. Experimental units were frozen, thawed, stored at 1–6°C for various periods up to 24 hours and then refrozen, stored at −65°C, rethawed, and stored again in the refrigerator for up to 24 hours. Aliquots of plasma were drawn periodically and batch-tested for prothrombin time (PT), activated partial thromboplastin time (APTT), and factor V and VIII:C activity. Although the results of coagulation testing in the twice-frozen plasma were always in the normal range, there was a slight but statistically significant prolongation of the PT and APTT and a decrease in the factor V and VIII:C levels as compared with controls. It was concluded that these altered values were not clinically significant and that refreezing may prove useful.

FFP may also be prepared from plasma obtained by apheresis. So-called "jumbo" plasma units contain 400–600 mL of plasma. The primary advantage of this preparation is in decreasing donor exposures. Ease of administration is another benefit, particularly in the operating room when multiple components are being administered.

LIQUID PLASMA

Liquid plasma, also referred to as single-donor plasma (SDP), is prepared by separation from RBCs at any time during storage, up to 5 days after expiration of the original unit. It may also be prepared from FFP that is outdated or has had cryoprecipitate removed. Liquid plasma differs from FFP only in its content of labile clotting factors. When cryoprecipitate has been removed, the component is deficient in factor VIII and fibrinogen and must be so labeled. Few blood centers make liquid plasma available for transfusion. It is usually used for the production of albumin, coagulation concentrates, and immune globulins.

USE OF FFP

The use of FFP increased 10-fold between 1974 and 1984 (7, 8). Use peaked at approximately 2.3 million units in 1984 and declined to approximately 2.1 million units in 1987 (9). Use in 1989, the most recent period for which data are available, was similar (10). The early increase in FFP use was attributed to multiple factors, not the least of which was the decreased availability of whole blood as the concept of component therapy became widespread. A significant proportion of this usage was for volume replacement in surgical patients. In addition, "reconstitution" of whole blood by concomitant transfusion of RBCs and FFP in fixed ratios accounted for a significant percentage of the FFP used. In an attempt to resolve some of the questions surrounding the increasing use of FFP, the National Heart, Lung, and Blood Institute, together with the Food and Drug Administration, convened a Consensus Development Conference in 1984. The Consensus Development Panel made very specific recommendations (7) that have been refined by others (11). Nevertheless, the use of FFP has remained relatively constant during the last decade.

Several investigators have examined the inappropriate use of FFP. Although many studies are flawed by the use of very liberal criteria, incomplete data on the indications for transfusion, and inclusion of patients with heterogeneous medical conditions, it is apparent that a significant percentage of FFP transfusions are not indicated. A problem of similar magnitude may be administration of inadequate volumes of FFP when therapy is indicated. Of the 135 patients studied by Blumberg et al. (12), 56% received 2 units of FFP or less. Approximately 38% of the FFP was used to reconstitute RBCs, primarily for surgical patients. In patients having open heart surgery at their institution in 1980, there was almost a 1:1 ratio between FFP and RBC use. Using the Consensus Conference recommendations as criteria for FFP administration, Stehling and Esposito (13) documented a 31% incidence of inappropriate FFP administration to noncardiac surgical patients during a 1-year period. Using similar criteria, Mozes et al. (14) found that 84% of FFP transfusions administered in a general teaching hospital in Israel were inappropriate.

The Sanguis Study group examined transfusion practices in a large number of hospitals in 10 European countries. They found that only 16% of surgical patients who received FFP had coagulation studies performed and in only 12% of the recipients was the result less than 60% of the normal control value (15). Despite instituting a program of mandatory pretransfusion approval by a hematologist, Hawkins and colleagues (16) in New Zealand documented a 33% inappropriate transfusion rate for FFP. Most cases involved administration of FFP after cardiac surgery. A recent study from Australia demonstrated inappropriate rates for transfusion episodes and numbers of units of FFP administered of 24% and 16%, respectively (17).

INDICATIONS FOR FFP

In the surgical population, FFP is most often administered to patients who are massively transfused and to those having cardiac surgery. An occasional patient on warfarin will require urgent surgery for which FFP may be indicated to reverse the effects of the drug. Patients with severe liver disease and documented coagulation abnormalities may require FFP administration preoperatively. In medical patients, large volumes of

FFP may be used during therapeutic plasma exchange procedures for thrombotic thrombocytopenic purpura (TTP) and other autoimmune, hematological, metabolic, and neurological conditions for which plasmapheresis is used (18).

The indications for FFP administration are actually quite limited. For convenience, clinical conditions are divided into those for which FFP is specifically recommended, those for which FFP may be indicated, and circumstances in which use of FFP is contraindicated.

CURRENTLY RECOMMENDED SPECIFIC INDICATIONS

Reversal of Warfarin Effect

Warfarin sodium (Coumadin) antagonizes vitamin K. In the absence of effective vitamin K, the protein precursors of factors II, VII, IX, and X and proteins C and S remain biologically inactive. Vitamin K acts as an essential cofactor for the hepatic microsomal enzyme system that, by carboxylating glutamic acid residues, enables the precursor protein to bind Ca^{++} and in turn be bound to phospholipid. Both steps are essential in the cascade of events that leads to clot formation. Vitamin K is oxidized during this reaction. Warfarin, by an unknown mechanism(s), blocks the regeneration of reduced vitamin K and produces a functional vitamin K deficiency. Reductases that act only at high concentrations of vitamin K and are less sensitive to warfarin are present in the hepatic microsomes. This may explain the ability of sufficient amounts of vitamin K to antagonize the effects of the anticoagulant (19).

Because anticoagulant reversal requires the completion of synthesis of active coagulation factors, 6–12 hours may be required for significant changes in clotting parameters to be observed after vitamin K administration. Maximum effects may not be seen for 24–36 hours (19). Immediate hemostasis can be achieved in anticoagulated patients who are actively bleeding or who require emergent surgery with FFP administration. Although a starting dose of 10–15 mL/kg is often recommended, a smaller volume may suffice. It should also be kept in mind that coagulation factor deficiencies that result in a prolongation of the PT and APTT of less than 1.5 times the mean control value may not be associated with increased bleeding.

In 1954, Müllertz and Storm (20) documented that anticoagulation with Dicumarol administered to prevent thromboembolism after major surgery was not associated with increased hemorrhage or other complications. However, they stressed the need for meticulous control of therapy with a standardized and sensitive method of determining the PT. Littman and Brodman (21), reporting their experience with patients who had a prolonged PT secondary to anticoagulation, concluded that the morbidity and mortality were no different than those observed in all other operations performed on the same surgical service during the same period of time.

Storm and Hansen (22) conducted a randomized study of patients having mitral commissurotomy who also received anticoagulant prophylaxis with Dicumarol. They concluded that no serious risk of bleeding is associated with such therapy when an accurate and sensitive method of estimating the prothrombin level is used in the control of treatment. Dietrich et al. (23) administered warfarin sodium to 125 patients before cardiac surgery. A control group of 115 patients had similar procedures. The International Normalized Ratio was 2.4 in the warfarin group and 1.1 in the control group. Approximately half the patients in each group received aprotinin intraoperatively. Neither the preoperative nor the postoperative PT correlated with blood loss or the need for allogeneic transfusion.

Recognizing the catastrophic potential of thromboembolic events in patients at risk, the reversal of anticoagulation with vitamin K or FFP should be seriously considered, especially when the PT and APTT are less than 1.5 times normal. Where feasible, delay of surgery to allow the effects of the anticoagulant to dissipate is preferable to FFP administration.

Replacement of Isolated Factor Deficiencies

Administration of FFP may be required when specific or combined factor concentrates are unavailable. Prothrombin complex containing factors II, VII, IX, and X is indicated in treating some patients with these deficiency states. Cryoprecipitate, which contains fibrinogen, fibronectin, and factor VIII, should be used as replacement therapy in patients who have a deficiency of fibrinogen. Desmopressin and some factor VIII preparations are alternatives to cryoprecipitate or FFP administration in the therapy of patients with von Willebrand disease. Factor VIII and IX concentrates are available for treating patients with hemophilia A and B (Christmas disease), respectively. Patients with factor XI deficiency are treated with FFP and those with factor XIII deficiency with FFP or cryoprecipitate. The dose depends on the specific factor being replaced because both the half-life and the concentration required vary for individual factors. This type of therapy is best managed by, or in consultation with, a physician conversant with these deficiency states.

Treatment of TTP

TTP is a relatively uncommon disease of unknown etiology that tends to occur between the second and fourth decades of life and is slightly more common in women. It is characterized by the pentad of severe microangiopathic hemolytic anemia, moderate to severe thrombocytopenia, fever, central nervous system dysfunction, and renal disease (24).

Although the management of TTP has been quite varied, the ultimate goal of therapy is the reversal of microvascular obstruction. Recent findings suggest that platelet-derived and/or endothelial ultralarge von Willebrand factor (vWF) multimers may play an important pathogenic role in development of the disease. Therapeutic plasma exchange with FFP is recognized by most hematologists as the most effective therapeutic modality in the management of TTP. Cryoprecipitate-poor plasma may be a better alternative because conventional FFP may replenish the vWF multimers (24). By the same token, platelet transfusion may aggravate TTP and should be avoided.

Antithrombin III Deficiency

Antithrombin III (ATIII), an alpha$_2$-glycoprotein, is the major circulating inactivator of thrombin. A serine protease inhibitor, it is also capable of inhibiting factors IXa, Xa, XIa, and XIIa, as well as plasmin. The inhibition of serine proteases by ATIII proceeds slowly in the absence of heparin but is greatly accelerated by its presence. Heparin, on the other hand, is devoid of anticoagulant action in the absence of ATIII.

ATIII deficiency can be inherited or acquired. The prevalence of the hereditary deficiency, transmitted as an autosomal dominant, is said to be 1:2000 to 1:5000 in the general population. In affected individuals, episodes of thrombosis and pulmonary embolism may be associated with ATIII levels of 40–60% of normal and usually occur after age 20. The incidence increases with increasing age and in association with surgery and pregnancy. The acquired form of the deficiency is associated with disseminated intravascular coagulation (DIC) during which ATIII is rapidly consumed. Whatever the cause of the DIC, the magnitude of the initial decrease in ATIII level is considered a reliable prognostic index of outcome.

Patients with hereditary ATIII deficiency should be treated before surgery, during pregnancy and delivery, and when they suffer a thromboembolic event. Therapy during DIC has shown some promise but requires further investigation before definitive recommendations can be made (25). Although FFP may be used to treat ATIII deficiency, serious consideration should be given to the use of ATIII concentrate (Thrombate III). This stable, lyophilized form of purified human ATIII is prepared from pooled plasma units obtained from normal donors by modification of Cohn's cold ethanol extraction method. It is heat treated at 60°C for not less than 10 hours to reduce the risk of transmitting viral infection. Because 5–10% of those infected with hepatitis B will persist as HBsAg carriers and HBsAg is carried in the fractions from which ATIII is derived, it is said to carry a risk of hepatitis B transmission.

CONDITIONAL USES: BLEEDING AND COAGULOPATHY

Massive Blood Transfusion

It has long been recognized that the transfusion of large volumes of stored blood over a short period of time can be associated with a bleeding diathesis. The etiology and treatment of such coagulopathies remained elusive until the late 1960s (26, 27). Two groups investigated coagulation disorders in combat casualties who had received massive blood transfusions. Thrombocytopenia proportional to the number of units transfused was observed in all massively transfused patients. Significant bleeding occurred after the administration of 20–25 units of acid citrate dextrose (ACD) bank blood when the platelet count approximated 65×10^9/L (26). Both groups of investigators observed prolongation of the PT and APTT, and, in one study, there was a moderate decrease in fibrinogen levels (27). Where bleeding was severe, transfusion with fresh whole blood proved an effective therapy. Although rarely used, FFP failed to reverse the observed coagulopathy. As a result of these studies conducted with casualties of the Vietnam conflict, an entire generation of anesthesiologists and surgeons was inculcated with the necessity to provide platelets to patients who received more than 20 units of whole blood in a 12-hour period.

Counts et al. (28) transfused traumatized patients who simultaneously received RBCs to provide oxygen-carrying capacity and plasma for volume replacement with whole blood from which platelets and cryoprecipitate had been removed (modified whole blood). They hypothesized that the transfusion of modified whole blood would lead to a primary hemostatic defect because of depletion of platelets rather than coagulation factors. Their results did indeed demonstrate that transfusion of large volumes of modified whole blood resulted in dilutional thrombocytopenia, but it did not cause clinically significant coagulation factor deficiencies. They recommended that when modified whole blood is used, a platelet count should be performed when a patient receives more then 15 units of blood and that the surgeon should be alert to signs of microvascular bleeding. Further, it was their belief that platelets are usually indicated if a patient receives over 20 units in a 12-hour period—a recommendation not too different from that made almost a decade earlier (26).

Because of the considerable evidence that dilutional thrombocytopenia is the major cause of the diffuse microvascular bleeding seen during massive transfusion, the same group undertook a prospective, randomized, double-blind clinical study to compare the effects of prophylactic administration of 6 units of platelets or 2 units of FFP with every 12 units of modified whole blood in patients receiving 12 or more units in 12 hours (29). Three patients in each group developed microvascular bleeding for an overall incidence of 18%, no different from that in the previous study where no prophylactic therapy was administered. The results of coagulation screening tests (PT, APTT, thrombin time, fibrinogen) were not significantly different between the two study groups at any point in time. Platelet counts were decreased significantly in both groups. There was a short-lived increase in platelet counts in the group that received this component. A progressive decline was seen for the remainder of the study. In the FFP group, the decline in platelet count was progressive. Thrombocytopenia developing as a result of rapid massive transfusion starts early; however, it appears to be counteracted by endogenous platelet release, resulting in platelet counts higher than predicted by standard washout curves. It was concluded that the prophylactic administration of platelets was not indicated, that it was almost impossible to predict which patients would develop microvascular bleeding, and that in the trauma patient, microvascular bleeding was, in all probability, secondary to a consumption coagulopathy.

Murray et al. (30) studied coagulation changes occurring during elective surgery when crystalloid solutions and RBCs were administered. They found coagulation factor levels to be correlated with the appearance of clinical bleeding. Prolongations of PT and APTT above control levels occurred in 9 of 12 patients before the replacement of one blood volume. None of the nine patients had a clinically detectable increase in bleeding. However, clinically evident increased bleeding was observed in four of seven patients who had greater than one blood volume replacement. Platelet counts were less than 100×10^9/L in all four patients. Bleeding decreased in two after the administration of platelets. Platelet counts increased in the two remaining patients, but bleeding persisted and was controlled by the administration of FFP. In both patients, PT and APTT were in excess of 1.5 times control values and fibrinogen levels were less than 75 mg/dL. If laboratory values alone were used as a guide to coagulation factor replacement, nine patients in this small series would have received FFP with its inherent dangers. It is evident from this study that clinical assessment of microvascular bleeding, along with laboratory confirmation of coagulation parameters, are the best indicators of the need for platelet transfusion or FFP administration.

A retrospective review of laboratory data, without clinical correlation, provided almost identical data. After transfusion of 20 or more units of RBCs, whole blood, or washed blood recovered intraoperatively, 75% of patients had platelet counts less than 50×10^9/L, whereas those who received fewer than 20 units had higher platelet counts. Transfusion with more than 12 units of RBCs or processed recovered blood along with crystalloid was consistently associated with PT and APTT values greater than 1.5 times the midrange of normal, values that have been associated with microvascular bleeding in massively transfused patients. In two patients who received fewer than 12 units, fibrinogen concentrations were 0.37 and 0.51 g/L (31).

Murray et al. (32), in an attempt to define the nature of coagulation abnormalities associated with clinically increased bleeding when RBCs and crystalloid were used to replace blood loss in excess of half a blood volume, prospectively studied 32 patients having elective posterior instrumentation of the vertebral column. A constant intravascular volume was maintained and estimates of blood loss were confirmed by appropriate invasive monitoring and serial hematocrit determinations. RBCs were administered when the hematocrit was less than 25%. Blood loss was assessed by observing the surgical field for signs of recurrent bleeding from the wound margins, increased bleeding in the absence of changes in arterial and venous pressure, and decreased clot formation. When a disorder of hemostasis was observed, coagulation studies were ordered. Before availability of the test results, however, FFP (10 mL/kg) was administered and the coagulation profile repeated after 20 minutes. If increased surgical bleeding persisted, platelets or additional FFP was administered on the basis of the laboratory results. In patients without evidence of increased bleeding, the coagulation profile was not sent to the laboratory until the completion of the surgical procedure. The PT and APTT were abnormal in 30 of 32 patients studied; however, bleeding was considered abnormal in only 17. Patients in whom increased bleeding was noted had smaller initial blood volumes and greater blood loss and replacement. The 17 patients who had increased bleeding had greater prolongations of PT and APTT than did those who did not bleed excessively. The decrease in platelet count and fibrinogen was similar in both groups. The decline in factor V, VII, and IX activity paralleled blood loss. It is evident from this study that PT and APTT increase above control values when more than 50% of the blood volume is replaced with crystalloid and RBCs. However, these abnormalities were not associated with increased bleeding until levels in excess of 1.5 times the mean control values were reached. At that time, surgical bleeding was successfully treated with FFP. Treatment of the coagulation factor deficiencies required therapy before the appearance of thrombocytopenia in this group of patients.

Hiippala et al. (33) reported a relatively similar study designed to determine changes in hemostatic factors and define the threshold for blood loss when RBCs and colloid were used to replace major blood loss. A critical fibrinogen deficiency (1 g/L) appeared when the blood loss approximated one and a half calculated blood volumes. Blood loss in excess of two calculated blood volumes caused a deficiency of factor II, factor V, platelets, and factor VII, in that order. The most significant result of this study was the demonstration of a rapid decay in fibrinogen. The critical level of factor II activity would be approached with a blood loss of two times the calculated blood volume, whereas the loss of an additional one-third of the calculated volume would result in compromise of factor VII activity. Levels of the labile factor V were most unpredictable, as was the platelet count. They concluded that fibrinogen deficiency develops earlier than any other deficiency when major blood loss is replaced with plasma-poor RBCs. It was their conclusion that administration of FFP should be the treatment of choice when coagulopathies are manifested under such clinical circumstances.

It is evident that abnormal laboratory values are not prognostic of microvascular bleeding after the rapid administration of large volumes of RBCs and crystalloid or colloid plasma substitutes. Prophylactic administration of neither FFP nor platelets is indicated. There may well be a difference in the etiology of microvascular bleeding in trauma patients and patients having elective surgery who receive comparable volumes of transfused blood. In the former case, the development of consumption coagulopathy may play a significant role, whereas in the latter instance, dilution of coagulation factors is probably most important.

Shock, independent of blood loss, may be associated with a consumptive coagulopathy and microvascular bleeding. Harke and Rahmen (34) studied 36 massively transfused patients and found that approximately 150 minutes of shock were required before significant prolongation of APTT or decreases in factor V activity were noted. A retrospective review of 64 massively transfused patients demonstrated that prolongation of APTT during the first 3–4 hours correlated with the volume of electrolyte solution administered. Thereafter, the prolongation of APTT was correlated with the duration of the preceding hypotension (35). Faringer et al. (36) also conducted a retrospective study of trauma patients and found that 33% with blunt trauma and brain injuries and 55% with penetrating trauma and no brain injuries had a PT greater than 18 seconds and an APTT greater than 55 seconds on arrival in the emergency department.

When determining whether administration of FFP (or other blood components) is indicated, laboratory values must be evaluated in relation to the patient's surgical condition and, most important, whether clinically significant microvascular bleeding is apparent. Microvascular bleeding, when it does occur, is most frequently associated with a PT and APTT in excess of 1.5 times normal. However, not all patients with coagulation profiles in this range exhibit microvascular bleeding. It is the rare laboratory that can provide PT and APTT results in less than an hour. On the other hand, the results of platelet counts should be available in a matter of minutes. If the platelet count is greater than 50×10^9/L, FFP (10–15 mL/kg) should be administered. It is important to note that platelet concentrates contain 50–70 mL plasma. If platelets are also administered, the volume of plasma administered with the platelets should be taken into account.

When the volume of blood transfused approaches 1–1.5 times the estimated blood volume, the anesthesiologist should, based on experience with both the surgeon and the procedure, anticipate the potential for continued blood loss. If it appears that hemostasis will not be achieved without further blood loss, the administration of FFP should be considered to prevent the almost inevitable onset of microvascular bleeding.

Liver Disease

Patients with liver disease may have multiple coagulation abnormalities. In addition to factor deficiencies, they may be thrombocytopenic and excessive fibrinolysis may occur. Bleeding, however, is seldom seen in the absence of such a precipitating factor as surgery or ruptured esophageal varices. Administration of FFP may be indicated if the patient is actively bleeding or if surgery is about to be undertaken and bleeding is anticipated. Large volumes of FFP are required to partially correct factor deficiencies and reduce the PT toward normal. Because there is a variable but rapid decay in factor levels, repeated transfusion of FFP is required to maintain any semblance of normalcy (37, 38).

The most significant question to be raised in patients with liver disease relates to the necessity to return the PT to normal before surgical intervention. It has been suggested that hemostasis in this group is more dependent on platelet function and vascular factors than on fibrin formation (39). In this regard, these patients may be no different from those treated with coumarin where major surgery can be performed without reversal of anticoagulation.

Percutaneous diagnostic and therapeutic procedures such as closed liver biopsy, paracentesis, and thoracentesis are frequently performed in this group of patients. The presence of a bleeding diathesis is often considered a contraindication to these procedures. Ewe (40) has pointed out that recommended acceptable limits of coagulation status before closed liver biopsy in this group vary widely. He performed needle biopsy of the liver during laparoscopy in 200 consecutive patients, regardless of abnormal clotting indices, and concluded that indices of coagulation in peripheral blood are unreliable guides to bleeding after liver biopsy and thus are of limited value in determining contraindications to the procedure. McVay and Toy (41) retrospectively examined data from 608 consecutive patients who had either thoracentesis or paracentesis where coagulation indices and preprocedure and postprocedure hemoglobin values were available. Almost half of the patients had significant hepatic disease. No increased bleeding was observed in patients with mild or moderate PT and APTT prolongation or mild thrombocytopenia. Because the incidence of clinically significant bleeding complications was so low (1/608 events), the investigators concluded that prophylactic blood component transfusion could not be recommended in patients with mild to moderate coagulopathy in the absence of clinical signs of active bleeding. It is worth noting that there was a sevenfold increase in bleeding in patients with a markedly elevated creatinine level.

Cardiac Surgery

Despite the lack of evidence indicating efficacy or necessity, many anesthesiologists and cardiothoracic surgeons administer FFP prophylactically after cardiopulmonary bypass to treat real or imagined coagulopathies. In a study designed to determine the reason for FFP transfusions at hospitals in southern Wisconsin, Snyder et al. (42) found that 45% of patients who had open heart surgery received FFP. That patient group accounted for 42% of the units of FFP transfused. In approximately 80% of the patients, FFP was given to replace coagulation factors. However, there is ample evidence that the reduction in coagulation factors as a result of hemodilution and exposure of blood to the trauma of roller pumps and plastic surfaces is not as significant as once believed.

Three decades ago, Trimble et al. (43) conducted a prospective randomized study designed to establish whether the routine use of FFP would measurably decrease bleeding after open heart surgery. Children received 1 unit of FFP and adults received 2 units. There was no reduction in bleeding in the patients who received FFP compared with control subjects. The authors concluded that the use of FFP to reduce bleeding after extracorporeal circulation is ineffective and not recommended. They advised hematological investigation followed by appropriate specific therapy when blood loss was excessive.

Milam et al. (44) studied alteration of coagulation and a number of clinical chemistry parameters in 75 patients who underwent open heart surgery without the transfusion of blood or blood components. One hour after surgery, the greatest reduction in coagulation factors was observed with factor V that decreased by 31%. Factor II was reduced by 12%, whereas factors VII and X fell by 16% and 14%, respectively. Fibrinogen declined by 16%. With the exception of factors VII and X, which remained at the 1-hour post-surgery level, other factors returned to or exceeded the preoperative level at 48 hours. Postoperative bleeding, then, could not be attributed to a deficiency in coagulation factors. There was a slight decrease in the platelet count at 1 hour postoperatively, with moderate recovery toward normal in 24–48 hours. Although there was wide variation in individual cases, decreases to 61×10^9/L did not result in excessive bleeding requiring transfusion.

A retrospective analysis of the records of 100 patients, 52 of whom received prophylactic FFP (2 units) after cardiopulmonary bypass revealed no difference between these patients and the 48 who did not receive FFP. The authors concluded that the prophylactic administration of FFP was not necessary for three reasons. First, although dilution of coagulation factors does occur, the postbypass levels are more than adequate to support hemostasis. Second, body stores and de novo synthesis by the liver create a sufficient pool of coagulation proteins. Finally, platelet dysfunction (not factor deficiency) is the major lesion causing bleeding after open heart surgery (45).

In an attempt to decrease bleeding associated with complex cardiac procedures, Swafford et al. (46) added FFP (30% of the patient's estimated plasma volume) to the cardiopulmonary bypass apparatus after rewarming of the patients. They found no significant improvement in coagulation profiles or clinical hemostasis. Blood component usage was slightly, but not statistically, higher in the plasma-treated group.

Assuming adequate heparin reversal and surgical hemostasis, bleeding in the postcardiopulmonary bypass period is, until proven otherwise, secondary to platelet dysfunction. The first line of therapy should be administration of platelets. There is no place for prophylactic FFP. Use of FFP should be reserved for those cases where a deficiency of clotting factors has been demonstrated by a prolongation of the PT or APTT.

UNJUSTIFIED USE OF FFP

"Formula Replacement"

The rapid rise in the use of FFP that accompanied the introduction of component therapy was no doubt due to predetermined replacement schedules. It was not uncommon to transfuse 1 unit of FFP for every 4 units of RBCs administered. There is no justification for such therapy because it is of no proven benefit and needlessly exposes the patient to unnecessary risk.

Hypovolemia

Volume deficits should be treated with crystalloid, synthetic plasma colloid substitutes, and, when necessary, human albumin solutions. These are cheaper, more readily available, and, above all, do not expose the patient to the risk, no matter how small, of transfusion-transmitted diseases.

Nutritional Support

The availability of parenteral and enteric hyperalimentation formulae have totally eliminated the need for FFP as nutritional support of the debilitated patient.

Immunodeficiency States

In the past, FFP was used to treat patients with inherited and acquired immunodeficiency states. The availability of purified intravenous immunoglobulin has replaced the need for FFP in these patients.

ADVERSE REACTIONS TO FRESH FROZEN PLASMA

The infusion of noncellular blood components is often considered to be a lesser cause of adverse reactions than is the transfusion of components containing the formed elements of blood. Although acute hemolytic transfusion reactions are not associated with FFP, a broad spectrum of adverse effects may accompany or follow the administration of FFP.

TRANSFUSION-TRANSMITTED DISEASE

A small but definable risk of viral transmission by FFP exists that is comparable with that of the whole blood from which it is prepared (47). Currently, "viral safety" depends solely on donor selection and donor blood screening methods. Two methods of viral chemical inactivation compatible with the preservation of the labile protein components of FFP are being investigated (48).

Solvent/detergent (S/D) treatment of FFP can inactivate most but not all viruses (49). The process involves the thawing and pooling of multiple liters of FFP of a single ABO group. The plasma is incubated with a mixture of the organic solvent tri-(n-butyl) phosphate (TNBP) and the detergent Triton X-100 for 4 hours at 30°C. Five percent soybean oil is added, and after centrifugation and filtration, the TNBP and Triton are removed by column-absorption chromatography. The plasma is then placed in plastic bags and refrozen.

The S/D FFP prepared by the pooling of plasma becomes a pharmaceutical product for which, in contrast to FFP, the potency of each component of the batch can be determined. When compared with the FFP from which it is prepared, the activity of the components of S/D FFP are reduced to a variable extent. Horowitz et al. (49) reported that all coagulation factors measured remained at or near normal levels when FFP was thawed and processed in 15- to 20-L pilot plant batches. Comparison of the start and end concentration of coagulation factors V, VIII, IX, and XI in four separate plasma pools showed recovery of 87%, 88%, 99%, and 108%, respectively. The PT and APTT were normal. At the 20-L scale, processing resulted in the loss of approximately 20% of the plasma volume. Others reported an overall reduction in the activity and concentration of coagulation factors, inhibitors, and immunoglobulins of 5–20% (50).

The S/D method is specific for viruses with a lipid envelope (e.g., human immunodeficiency virus types 1 and 2 and hepatitis B and C virus). Nonenveloped viruses such as hepatitis A or parvovirus B19 (PBV19) are unaffected. In contrast to the hepatitis A virus, PBV19 is rarely pathogenic and a rare infected unit will, in all probability, be neutralized by antibodies in the plasma pool. However, the effects of transfusion of FFP containing PBV19 to immunocompromised patients remain unclear.

Methylene blue can also be used for viral inactivation of plasma (51). In contrast to S/D treatment, this viral inactivation method is performed on single plasma units. Methylene blue is added and the unit is then exposed to visible light at room temperature for 1 hour. As is the case with S/D FFP, only lipid enveloped viruses are inactivated. Although the method has the distinct advantage of not requiring pooling of large batches of FFP, it has the disadvantage of a significant reduction in coagulation factor activity and a prolongation of the APTT (52).

A preliminary report by Highsmith et al. (53) indicated that it is possible to inactivate both lipid-enveloped and non-lipid-enveloped viruses in human plasma by treatment with cross-linked starch-iodine. This method has the advantage of retaining significant factor VIII and factor IX activity.

Both methylene blue- and S/D-treated FFP are available in Europe. Although S/D-treated plasma derivatives have been licensed for distribution in the United States, S/D FFP is not yet licensed. AuBuchon and Birkmeyer (54) examined the safety and cost-effectiveness of S/D FFP and concluded that from a public health prospective, the relatively high costs and small benefits do not appear to justify widespread implementation of this technology. Nevertheless, a plant for processing S/D FFP on a commercial scale is currently under construction. Once S/D FFP is made available, it is difficult to believe that clinicians would continue to use untreated FFP.

IMMUNOLOGICAL REACTIONS

A number of severe immunological reactions can result from the presence of antibodies in the plasma of either the donor or the recipient. Clinical severity varies from insignificant urticarial reactions or flushing to fulminant cardiorespiratory arrest. The most severe of these reactions probably represents true anaphylaxis. The less severe may well represent anaphylactoid reactions secondary to histamine release (55).

Immune Reactions Against Donor Plasma Protein Antigens

These reactions can usually be traced to the presence of class-specific anti-IgA formed as a result of previous transfusion in an IgA-deficient recipient. Small volumes of plasma will produce severe anaphylactic reactions in susceptible patients with IgA deficiency. Clinical manifestations that appear within seconds of transfusion include apprehension; chest, back, or abdominal pain; dyspnea; chills; and nausea. There is a rapid progression to circulatory collapse.

Anti-IgA antibodies of limited specificity against subclasses of IgA occur in low titer in subjects who usually have a normal serum IgA level. These reactions are milder and usually cutaneous in nature. Some allergic reactions of an IgE reaginic nature have been attributed to such exogenous antigens as drugs and food products to which the recipient is allergic and are present in donor plasma (56).

Reactions to Alloantibodies in Donor Plasma

The use of incompatible plasma or plasma components is usually tolerated if only small volumes are transfused and there is a low titer of anti-A or anti-B antibodies present. On the other hand, high titers of these proteins or infusion of large volumes of FFP with low titers of anti-A or anti-B may result in serious hemolytic reactions if ABO-incompatible plasma is transfused. For this reason, the Standards of the American Association of Blood Banks state that FFP should be ABO-compatible with the recipient's RBCs, especially when the component is to be transfused to infants (4). Cross matching is not required.

Transfusion-Related Acute Lung Injury

Noncardiogenic pulmonary edema resulting from the transfusion of blood components is a rare but life-threatening complication of hemotherapy. Indistinguishable from adult respiratory distress syndrome (ARDS), transfusion-related acute lung injury (TRALI) is said to have an incidence of 0.02% per unit transfused, or 0.16% per patient transfused (57). TRALI is characterized by acute respiratory distress, pulmonary edema, and hypoxemia. Fever and hypotension resistant to fluid challenges may be present. Signs and symptoms occur within 1–6 hours of transfusion of blood components. The diagnosis is usually one of exclusion after cardiogenic causes of pulmonary edema have been eliminated. Pulmonary capillary occlusion pressure is normal while the central venous pressure is in the normal or low range. Unlike ARDS, TRALI usually resolves in 48–96 hours provided there is prompt and vigorous intervention. However, death has been reported in up to 5% of reported cases.

Leukoagglutinating or specific human leukocyte antibodies (HLA) have been found in the plasma of patients with TRALI or of donors of the implicated components. In almost 90% of cases, the antibodies are found in the donor rather than the recipient plasma. This is not unexpected because the "target organs" are the white blood cells (WBCs). The pool of WBCs in the donor component is minimal when compared with the recipient's entire circulating and marginate pool of WBCs. Thus, in most cases, unlike most other immune reactions, TRALI begins with the passive transfer of antibodies from the donor's plasma to the recipient. HLA-A or -B antibodies of the donor correspond to one or more HLA antigenic determinants of the recipient, resulting in complement activation. In some instances, neutrophil-specific antibodies have been identified in the donor plasma. In a significant number of cases, the donors have been multiparous females or recipients of multiple transfusions. Unlike cardiogenic pulmonary edema where increased capillary hydrostatic pressure occurs, TRALI is the result of an increase in pulmonary capillary permeability, no doubt triggered by a sequence of events that follows the sequestration of leukocytes in the pulmonary microcirculation and activation of the complement cascade (57).

TRALI may be precipitated by transfusion of whole blood, RBCs, FFP, SDP, cryoprecipitate, or platelets. The volume of plasma and titer of antibody necessary to initiate the reaction remains unknown. Because FFP is the component containing the greatest volume of plasma, it is not unreasonable to expect that TRALI may be more common than it is after the administration of other components.

SUMMARY

Although there are few indications for the administration of FFP, it remains one of the most inappropriately transfused blood components. The principal reasons for this misuse relate to limited knowledge of its efficacy in specific situations, failure to recognize the risks associated with its administration, and its ready availability.

The administration of FFP is indicated for urgent reversal of warfarin therapy, correction of known coagulation factor deficiencies for which specific factor concentrates are unavailable, correction of microvascular bleeding in the presence of elevated (more than 1.5 times normal) PT or APTT, and correction of microvascular bleeding presumed to be secondary to coagulation factor deficiency in patients transfused with more than one blood volume when the PT and APTT cannot be obtained in a timely fashion.

When indicated, FFP should be administered in doses calculated to achieve a minimum of 30% of plasma factor concentrations. This is usually achieved with the administration of 10–15 mL/kg. When transfused for the reversal of warfarin, 5–8 mL/kg may suffice. It should be recalled that four to five platelet concentrates, 1 unit of single-donor apheresis platelets, or 1 unit of fresh whole blood provide a quantity of coagulation factors similar to those contained in 1 unit of FFP. The augmentation of blood volume or albumin concentration is not an indication for FFP administration.

REFERENCES

1. Dzik WH, Ribner MA, Linehan SK. Refreezing previously thawed fresh-frozen plasma. Stability of coagulation factors V and VIII:C. Transfusion 1989;29:600–604.
2. Rock G, Tackaberry ES, Dunn JG, Kashyp S. Rapid controlled thawing of fresh frozen plasma in a modified microwave oven. Transfusion 1984;24:60–65.
3. Churchill WH, Schmidt B, Lindsey J, Greenberg M, Boudrow S, Brugnara C. Thawing fresh frozen plasma in a microwave oven. A comparison with thawing in a 37°C waterbath. Am J Clin Pathol 1992;97: 227–232.
4. Standards for blood banks and transfusion services. Bethesda: AABB, 1994.
5. Milam JD, Buzzurro CJ, Austin SF, Stansberry SW. Stability of factors V and VIII in thawed fresh frozen plasma units. Transfusion 1980;20: 546–548.
6. Smak Gregoor PJH, Harvey MS, Briet E, Brand A. Coagulation parameters of CPD fresh frozen plasma and CPD cryoprecipitate-poor plasma after storage at 4°C for 28 days. Transfusion 1993;33:735–738.
7. Office of Medical Applications of Research. National Institutes of Health. Fresh frozen plasma: indications and risks. JAMA 1985;253: 551–553.
8. Silbert JA, Bove JR, Dulin S, Bush WS. Patterns of frozen plasma use. Conn Med 1981;45:507–511.
9. Surgenor DMN, Wallace EL, Hao SHS, Chapman RH. Collection and transfusion of blood in the United States, 1982–1988. N Engl J Med 1990;322:1646–1651.
10. Wallace EL, Surgenor DM, Hao HS, An J, Chapman RH, Churchill WH. Collection and transfusion of blood and blood components in the United States, 1989. Transfusion 1993;33:139–144.
11. Stehling L, Luban NLD, Anderson KC, et al. Guidelines for blood utilization review. Transfusion 1994;34:438–448.
12. Blumberg N, Laczin J, McMican A, Heal J, Arvan D. A critical survey of fresh-frozen plasma use. Transfusion 1986;26:511–513.
13. Stehling L, Esposito B. An analysis of the appropriateness of intraoperative transfusion. Anesth Analg 1989;68:S278.
14. Mozes B, Epstein M, Ben-Bassat I, Modan B, Halkin H. Evaluation of the appropriateness of blood and blood product transfusion using preset criteria. Transfusion 1989;29:473–476.
15. McClelland DBL. Red cell transfusion for elective surgery: a suitable case for treatment. Transfus Med 1994;4:247–249.
16. Hawkins TE, Carter JM, Hunter PM. Can mandatory pretransfusion approval programmes be improved? Transfus Med 1994;4:45–50.
17. Metz J, McGrath KM, Copperchini ML, et al. Appropriateness of transfusions of red cells, platelets and fresh frozen plasma. An audit in a tertiary care teaching hospital. Med J Aust 1995;162:572–577.
18. Strauss RG, Ciavarella D, Gilcher RO, et al. An overview of current management. J Clin Apheresis 1993;8:189–194.
19. Marcus R, Coulston AM. Fat-soluble vitamins. In: Gilman AG, Rall TW, Nies AS, Taylor P, eds. The pharmacologic basis of therapeutics. New York: Pergamon Press, 1990:1553–1571.
20. Müllertz S, Storm O. Anticoagulant therapy with dicumarol maintained during major surgery. Circulation 1954;10:213–220.
21. Littman JK, Brodman HR. Surgery in the presence of the therapeutic effect of dicumarol. Surg Gynecol Obstet 1955;100:709–714.
22. Storm O, Hansen AT. Mitral commissurotomy performed during anticoagulant prophylaxis with dicumarol. Circulation 1955;12: 981–985.
23. Dietrich W, Dilthey G, Spannagal M, Richter JA. Warfarin pretreatment does not lead to increased bleeding tendency during cardiac surgery. J Cardiothorac Vasc Anesth 1995;9:250–254.
24. Gilcher RO, Strauss RG, Ciavarella D, et al. Management of renal disorders. J Clin Apheresis 1993;8:258–269.
25. Fourrier F, Chopin C, Huart SS, Runge I, Caron C, Goudenand J. Double-blind, placebo-controlled trial of antithrombin III concentrates in septic shock with disseminated intravascular coagulation. Chest 1993;104:882–888.
26. Miller RD, Robbins TO, Tang MJ, Barton SL. Coagulation defects associated with massive blood transfusions. Ann Surg 1971;174: 799–801.
27. Simmons RL, Collins JA, Heisterkamp CA, Mills DE, Andren R, Phillips LL. Coagulation disorders in combat casualties. I. Acute changes after wounding. II. Effects of massive transfusion. III. Post-resuscitative changes. Ann Surg 1969;169:455–482.
28. Counts RB, Haisch C, Simon TL, Maxwell NG, Heimbach DM, Carrico CJ. Hemostasis in massively transfused trauma patients. Ann Surg 1979;190:91–99.
29. Reed RL, Ciavarella D, Heimbach DM, et al. Prophylactic platelet administration during massive transfusion. A prospective, randomized, double-blind clinical study. Ann Surg 1986;203:40–48.
30. Murray DJ, Olson J, Strauss R, Tinker JH. Coagulation changes during packed red cell replacement of major blood loss. Anesthesiology 1988; 69:839–845.
31. Leslie SD, Toy PTCY. Laboratory hemostatic abnormalities in massively transfused patients given red blood cells and crystalloid. Am J Clin Pathol 1991;96:770–773.
32. Murray DJ, Pennell BJ, Weinstein SL, Olson JD. Packed red cells in acute blood loss: dilutional coagulopathy as a cause of surgical bleeding. Anesth Analg 1995;80:336–342.
33. Hiippala ST, Myllylä GJ, Vahtera EM. Hemostatic factors and replacement of major blood loss with plasma-poor red cell concentrates. Anesth Analg 1995;81:360–365.
34. Harke H, Rahman S. Haemostatic disorders in massive transfusion. Bibl Haematol 1980;46:179–188.
35. Hewson JR, Neame PB, Kumar N, et al. Coagulopathy related to dilution and hypotension during massive transfusion. Crit Care Med 1985; 13:387–391.
36. Faringer PD, Mullins RJ, Johnson RL, Trunkey DD. Blood component supplementation during massive transfusion of AS-1 red cells in trauma patients. J Trauma 1993;34:481–487.
37. Spector I, Corn M, Ticktin HE. Effect of plasma transfusions on the prothrombin time and clotting factors in liver disease. N Engl J Med 1966;275;1032–1037.
38. Mannucci PM, Rranchi F, Dioguardi N. Correction of abnormal coagulation in chronic liver disease by combined use of fresh frozen plasma and prothrombin complex concentrates. Lancet 1976;2:542–545.

39. Stefanini M, Petrillo E. Relative importance of plasmic and vascular factors of hemostasis in pathogenesis of hemorrhagic diathesis of liver dysfunction. Acta Med Scand 1979;134:139–145.
40. Ewe K. Bleeding after liver biopsy does not correlate with indices of peripheral coagulation. Dig Dis Sci 1981;26:388–393.
41. McVay PA, Toy PTCY. Lack of increased bleeding after paracentesis and thoracentesis in patients with mild coagulation abnormalities. Transfusion 1991;31:164–171.
42. Snyder AJ, Gottschall JL, Menitove JE. Why is fresh-frozen plasma transfused? Transfusion 1986;26:107–112.
43. Trimble AS, Osborn JJ, Kerth WJ, Gerbode F. The prophylactic use of fresh frozen plasma after extracorporeal circulation. J Thorac Cardiovasc Surg 1964;48:314–316.
44. Milam JD, Austin SF, Martin RF, Keats AS, Cooley DA. Alteration of coagulation and selected clinical chemistry parameters in patients undergoing open heart surgery without transfusions. Am J Clin Pathol 1981;76:155–162.
45. Roy RC, Stafford MA, Hudspeth AS, Meredith JW. Failure of prophylaxis with fresh frozen plasma after cardiopulmonary bypass. Anesthesiology 1988;69:254–257.
46. Swafford MWG, Yawn D, Wenker O, Curling P. Effect of adding fresh frozen plasma to the cardiopulmonary bypass machine on blood component requirements in complex CV procedures. Anesth Analg 1995; 80:SCA128–SCA141.
47. Gerety RJ, Arouson DL. Plasma derivatives and viral hepatitis. Transfusion 1982;22:347–351.
48. Wieding JU, Hellstern P, Kohler M. Inactivation of viruses in fresh-frozen plasma. Ann Hematol 1993;67:259–266.
49. Horowitz B, Bonomo R, Prince AM, Chin SN, Brutman B, Shulman RE. Solvent/detergent-treated plasma: a virus-inactivated substitute for fresh frozen plasma. Blood 1992;79:826–831.
50. Hellstern P, Sachse H, Schwinn H, Oberfrank K. Manufacture and in-vitro characterization of solvent/detergent treated human plasma. Vox Sang 1992;63:178–185.
51. Mohr H, Lambrecht B, Knueuer-Hopf S. Virus inactivated single-donor fresh plasma preparations. Infusions Ther 1992;19:79–83.
52. Zeiler T, Riess H, Wittman G, et al. The effect of methylene blue photo treatment on plasma proteins and in vitro coagulation capability of single donor fresh-frozen plasma. Transfusion 1994;34:685–689.
53. Highsmith FA, Xue H, Caple M, Walthall B, Drohan WH, Shanbron E. Inactivation of lipid-enveloped and non-lipid-enveloped model viruses in normal human plasma by crosslinked starch-iodine. Transfusion 1994;34:322–327.
54. AuBuchon JP, Birkmeyer JD. Safety and cost-effectiveness of solvent-detergent-treated plasma. JAMA 1994;272:1210–1214.
55. Henderson RA, Pinder L. Acute transfusion reactions. N Z Med J 1990; 103:509–511.
56. Isbister JP. Adverse reactions to plasma and plasma components. Anaesth Intens Care 1993;21:31–38.
57. Popovsky MA, Chaplin HC, Moore SB. Transfusion-related acute lung injury: a neglected, serious complication of hemotherapy. Transfusion 1992;32:589–592.

Chapter 26

Pharmacological Approaches to Prevent or Decrease Bleeding in Surgical Patients

JERROLD H. LEVY
ANTONIO MORALES
JOHN H. LEMMER, JR.

INTRODUCTION

The pathophysiology of bleeding during cardiac surgery using cardiopulmonary bypass (CPB) is multifactorial and is predominantly due to the interaction among the patient's blood, the foreign surface of the extracorporeal circuit, and the complex array of humoral and cellular changes that ensue (see Chapter 28). Perturbation of the coagulation system and platelet function and activation of the fibrinolytic cascade contribute to the observed defect. Pharmacological approaches to reduce bleeding and transfusion requirements are based on either preventing or reversing the defects associated with the CPB-induced coagulopathy (1–3). Because in vivo coagulation depends on appropriate platelet-fibrinogen interactions, the ultimate goal is to preserve normal coagulation function but to avoid pathological effects of hypercoagulability. Different pharmacological agents have been reported to decrease perioperative bleeding, especially after cardiac surgery, as shown in Table 26.1. Because the normal homeostatic mechanisms are ultimately controlled by circulating serine protease inhibitors, including alpha$_2$-antiplasmin, C1 esterase inhibitors, and plasminogen activator inhibitor, most currently accepted pharmacological interventions are based on using a protease inhibitor, aprotinin, or the use of lysine analogues to inhibit fibrinolysis. Because platelet function plays an important role in perioperative hemostasis, studies evaluating desmopressin are also reviewed.

DESMOPRESSIN ACETATE

Desmopressin acetate (DDAVP) is a peptide with properties as shown in Table 26.2. It is a synthetic analogue of vasopressin created by substituting L-arginine for D-arginine, thus creating a drug with decreased vasopressor activity. DDAVP therapy causes a 2- to 20-fold increase in plasma levels of factor VIII and stimulates vascular endothelium to release the larger multimers of von Willebrand factor (vWF) (4). DDAVP also releases tissue plasminogen activator (tPA) and prostacyclin from vascular endothelium (4). Factor VIII is a plasma glycoprotein that accelerates activation of factor X by factor IXa in the presence of a phospholipid surface and calcium ions (5). Patients with hemophilia A have a variable decrease in plasma levels of factor VIII, and adequate levels of factor VIII also depend on the presence of adequate levels of vWF. vWF mediates platelet adherence to vascular subendothelium by functioning as a protein bridge between glycoprotein Ib receptors on platelets and subendothelial vascular basement membrane proteins. It also maintains plasma levels of factor VIII by protecting it from proteolytic enzymes and possibly by stimulating its synthesis (6). Patients who have von Willebrand disease have variable decreases in vWF levels, manifested by prolonged bleeding times (6).

TABLE 26.1. PHARMACOLOGICAL APPROACHES REPORTED TO DECREASE BLEEDING

Desmopressin (DDAVP)
Aprotinin
Fibrinolytic inhibitors: tranexamic acid, epsilon-aminocaproic acid
Nafamostat

TABLE 26.2. PHYSIOLOGICAL PROPERTIES OF DESMOPRESSIN

Synthetic analogue of vasopressin
Decreased vasopressor activity
Stimulates vascular endothelium to release multimers of vWF, but tPA and prostacyclin are also released
vWF mediates platelet adherence to vascular subendothelium

CLINICAL USES IN MEDICAL CONDITIONS

DDAVP shortens the bleeding time of patients with mild forms of hemophilia A or von Willebrand disease (7). However, patients with severe von Willebrand disease have little vWF to release and therefore do not respond to administration of desmopressin (5). In addition, patients with a rare form of von Willebrand disease, type IIb, have an exaggerated platelet response to release of vWF by DDAVP where platelets aggregate abnormally and are thus consumed, producing thrombocytopenia and worsening of hemostasis (8).

DDAVP has also been used to decrease bleeding and shorten bleeding times in various medical conditions (7, 9–15). Kobrinsky et al. (16) found that DDAVP was useful in shortening bleeding times of patients with aspirin-induced platelet dysfunction and patients with isolated platelet dysfunction. In addition, 18 of their patients treated with DDAVP and epsilon-aminocaproic acid underwent surgical procedures without requiring blood products. Other researchers have also shortened bleeding times of patients with acquired and inherited forms of platelet dysfunction with DDAVP treatment (17–19).

Uremic patients may have abnormal hemostasis caused by platelet dysfunction. Cryoprecipitate, which supplies factor VIII and vWF, is partially effective therapy for patients with uremia. Researchers have shortened bleeding times in these patients by using DDAVP. They were successful and temporarily shortened bleeding times by using intravenous or intranasal DDAVP (17, 19).

In patients with hepatic cirrhosis, Agnelli et al. (20) administered DDAVP to a group of patients and increased the levels of vWF and therapy, shortening their bleeding times.

CLINICAL USES DURING SURGICAL PROCEDURES

Kobrinsky et al. (16) were able to normalize bleeding times in 42 patients with various bleeding disorders by using DDAVP therapy. Eighteen of these patients underwent various surgical procedures ranging from dental extractions to repair of coarctation of the aorta without requiring the use of blood products. In 1987, Kobrinsky et al. (21) found decreased blood loss and decreased transfusion requirement in patients treated with DDAVP in a randomized double-blind trial of patients undergoing Harrington rod spine surgery. This group of patients should not have had preoperative platelet function abnormalities.

Salzman et al. (14) performed a randomized double-blind trial in which DDAVP or placebo was administered after protamine administration to 70 patients undergoing various cardiac operations requiring CPB. The group receiving DDAVP bled less (1317 ± 486 mL, mean ± SD) than the group receiving placebo (2210 ± 1415 mL) over the first 24 hours postoperatively. The DDAVP-treated group was also found to have higher plasma levels of vWF. However, because of the excessive amount of blood loss over 24 hours in both groups, there are important questions on the validity of the results of this study. In addition, the effects of DDAVP on transfusions are not reported in the study.

Efforts to confirm Salzman et al.'s original success with DDAVP therapy in open heart surgical patients have not been consistently positive. Czer and colleagues (22) administered DDAVP to patients bleeding more than 100 mL/hr at least 2 hours after termination of CPB. Control subjects were treated by transfusion therapy. Those treated with DDAVP required fewer blood products, especially platelets, while achieving similar reductions in bleeding. However, because this study was nonrandomized and unblinded, its results are also not accepted as proof that DDAVP is universally effective.

In 1988, Rocha et al. (13) reported a randomized double-blind trial of DDAVP in 100 patients at the conclusion of CPB after atrial septal defect repair or valvular replacement. There was no significant difference in overall blood loss between the DDAVP and the placebo group (131 versus 193 mL). Hackmann et al. (10) performed a double-blind randomized study comparing blood loss in patients undergoing primary coronary artery bypass grafting and/or valvular replacement with DDAVP or placebo. There was no difference in blood product transfusion rates or blood loss within the first 24 hours after operation. In addition, postoperative use of blood products did not differ between the groups. This finding led the authors to conclude that "the majority of patients who undergo elective cardiac surgery receive no hemostatic benefit from the use of desmopressin."

Which patients might benefit from use of DDAVP (23–26)? Patients with mild to moderate forms of hemophilia or von Willebrand disease undergoing surgery are likely to benefit from its use. In addition, patients with uremic platelet dysfunction and patients with chronic liver disease undergoing major surgery would benefit from DDAVP. It is yet to be seen if patients taking aspirin or other antiplatelet therapy would benefit from its use, but it may be worth trying in this type of patient who is bleeding excessively after surgery. Mongan and Hosking (23) reported that patients with a thromboelastogram (TEG) taken after protamine administration and with maximal amplitude less than 50 mm benefit from the effects of DDAVP (23). This study used a method to separate patients with platelet dysfunction from those with acceptable activity. Patients with reduced platelet function bled significantly more than those whose TEG was near normal. DDAVP was administered to patients with abnormal platelet function (TEG less than 50 mm) and the chest tube output was similar to that seen with those who had normal platelet function. This study brings into question the mechanism of DDAVP, and perhaps the elevation of factor VIII and vWF are effective only in the presence of abnormal platelet function. Universal application of DDAVP would not be expected to yield consistent efficacy if only certain subpopulations of patients were treatable. Perhaps Salzman et al.'s original patient population contained a relatively high number of patients with significant post-CPB platelet dysfunction. Some centers using TEG today do select patients with mild to moderate platelet dysfunction and target them for DDAVP therapy.

DDAVP is in some circumstances a profound releaser of tPA. It is well known that tPA rises during CPB and one has to wonder whether giving a tPA-releasing agent is counterproductive in some patients who are particularly susceptible to tPA release. Recent work so far has not shown an advantage to combining DDAVP with a lysine analogue fibrinolytic inhibitor (tranexamic acid) (26). This study, like many others, was done in "all covers" and not segregated as was Mongan and Hosking's work to those with demonstrated platelet dysfunction.

ADMINISTRATION

In the surgical patient, DDAVP should be administered intravenously. A dose of 0.3 mg/kg achieves maximal increases in levels of factor VIII and vWF in 30–60 minutes with no further increases achieved by higher doses. The drug, which is supplied in a 4-mg/mL preparation, should be diluted and administered over 15–30 minutes to avoid hypotension. Although the drug has a half-life of 2.5–4.4 hours, repeated administration results in tachyphylaxis (5).

UNDESIRABLE EFFECTS

Although few adverse effects are seen with the appropriate use of DDAVP, when given rapidly, it may cause flushing, hypotension, and increased heart rate, all attributable to vasodilatation due to release of prostacyclin from endothelial cells and direct effects on vascular smooth muscle (5, 24). These effects may be avoided by administering the drug over 15 minutes or more. Because DDAVP has a potent antidiuretic effect and is given in doses 15 times greater than those used to treat diabetes insipidus, there is a potential for free water retention and hyponatremia (5). However, few cases of fluid overload or hyponatremic seizures have been reported, and the drug appears to be safe even in patients with uremia (25). Of concern have been case reports of arterial thrombosis in patients receiving DDAVP (27). Several reports of myocardial infarction after DDAVP administration were of particular concern (28). These reports, however, were in patients not undergoing surgery. Reports of relatively large numbers of patients undergoing open heart surgery have failed to identify an increased incidence of thrombotic complications in DDAVP-treated patients, although it should be pointed out that a large prospective safety study has not been carried out. Studies in patients undergoing surgery have found no adverse thrombotic complications. The hemostatic defects associated with CPB may afford a certain level of protection from potential DDAVP-induced thrombotic complications observed in the nonsurgical patient. Until the safety of DDAVP is established, its use should be reserved for those patients who have a high likelihood of benefiting from this therapy.

APROTININ

Aprotinin (Trasylol) is one of a group of naturally occurring serine protease inhibitors. It is derived from bovine lung with properties as shown in Table 26.3 (29). Among the proteases it can inhibit are trypsin, chymotrypsin, plasmin, tPA, serum urokinase plasminogen activator, and both tissue and plasma kallikreins (29). Because of its inhibition of trypsin and chymotrypsin, it was originally used clinically for the treatment of acute pancreatitis. Although aprotinin was tried in the 1960s to diminish the effect of CPB on the hemostatic system, its use was mostly therapeutic and not prophylactic;

TABLE 26.3. CHEMICAL PROPERTIES OF APROTININ

Basic polypeptide (pKa 10)
Molecular mass 6512 Da
Derived from cow lung
Nonspecific protease inhibitor of trypsin, kallikrein, plasmin
Activity expressed as kallikrein inactivator units (KIU)

only evaluated low doses were used in an effort to treat bleeding after cardiac surgery rather than to prevent it. However, it was not until the late 1980s that a prophylactic high-dose technique was used (31).

In 1987, van Oeveren et al. (30) showed a 47% reduction in blood loss in patients receiving aprotinin during coronary bypass surgery. Royston et al. also published the results of three different groups of patient receiving either aprotinin or placebo during cardiac surgery. In 1987, they reported 22 patients with bubble oxygenators having repeat cardiac surgery (31). The original design of the study was to develop a pharmacological approach to inhibit inflammatory responses during extracorporeal circulation by administering a protease inhibitor in sufficient concentrations to inhibit pulmonary complications of bypass. They administered aprotinin as a loading dose of 2 million units after intubation and maintained therapeutic levels with a continuous infusion of 500,000 units/hr and a cardiopulmonary pump prime dose equal to the loading dose of 2 million units to compensate for the dilutional effects of extracorporeal circulation. Pulmonary dysfunction was not inhibited, but it was noted that the chest tube drainage from the aprotinin patients was minimal. The patients receiving aprotinin bled mean values of 286 mL compared with control subjects, who bled 1509 mL. There was an approximate 10-fold reduction of shed hemoglobin in the aprotinin versus placebo patients. In a subsequent study of 80 patients undergoing primary coronary bypass surgery, patients receiving aprotinin bled 46% less than control subjects, received fewer units of packed red blood cells (13 versus 75 units, aprotinin group versus placebo), and had no significant prolongation of their bleeding times, suggesting a platelet-preserving effect of aprotinin independent of its antifibrinolytic properties (32). A third group consisted of patients that required operations because of infective endocarditis. The mean chest tube drainage for these 15 patients was 388 mL, but there was no control group (29). These findings led to a number of studies investigating high-dose therapy in cardiac surgical patients (Table 26.4).

In 1990, Dietrich et al. (33) also found decreased blood loss in patients receiving aprotinin compared with those receiving placebo (738 versus 1431 mL) for primary coronary bypass surgery. They also found less formation of thrombin, fibrin split products, and D-dimers in patients receiving aprotinin and postulated that inhibition of contact activation of coagulation was the primary effect of the drug and that inhibition of fibrinolysis and platelet preservation was secondary.

Separate studies by Blauhut et al. (34), Havel et al. (35), Lemmer et al. (36), and Marx et al. (37) all confirmed decreased blood loss in patients receiving aprotinin at high doses based on the "Hammersmith regimen." Aprotinin also reduced blood loss 49–75% and allogeneic transfusion requirements 49–77% in three studies in patients receiving aspirin (38–40). Bertran et al. (41), using a 2 million unit loading dose before CPB and a 2 million unit loading dose in the CPB circuit in aspirin-pretreated patients, reported a reduction of blood loss of 370 versus 651 mL in the placebo-treated patients. Cosgrove et al. (42) reported in 171 patients significantly lower postoperative chest tube drainage in both full-dose and half-dose techniques compared with placebo-treated patients. The mean number of units transfused was similar for low-dose and placebo-treated patients. In 20 patients undergoing heart transplantation, Havel et al. (43) reported lower chest tube drainage and transfusion requirements in treated patients using a 2 million unit dose administered after intubation and 2 million units added to the CPB circuit; 70% of aprotinin-treated patients did not receive allogeneic blood compared with 30% of control subjects.

MECHANISMS OF ACTION

In the setting of cardiac surgery and CPB, aprotinin is thought to work by its inhibition of plasmin formation and activity and kallikrein. By inhibiting plasmin, the active proteolytic enzyme of the fibrinolytic system, aprotinin is able to inhibit fibrinolysis. In addition, by inhibiting kallikrein, which helps to amplify and accelerate contact activation of factor XII (Hageman factor) to XIIa, activation of the intrinsic pathway of coagulation is inhibited or attenuated. This contact activation, which occurs during CPB despite the use of heparin, leads to thrombin formation. Thrombin is the most important amplification agent for a wide range of coagulation factors and is a powerful platelet activator. By inhibiting kallikrein, aprotinin is suggested to decrease thrombin formation and potentially protect platelets from activation. Kallikrein in itself is also an activator of the fibrinolytic system, and therefore by inhibiting kallikrein, aprotinin inhibits fibrinolysis in a manner that is independent of its ability to inhibit plasmin. Van Oeveren (44) postulated that aprotinin inhibits the plasmin-related degradation of the platelet glycoprotein Ib receptor.

TABLE 26.4. SUMMARY OF TRIALS COMPARING TREATMENT WITH HIGH-DOSE[a] APROTININ WITH NO TREATMENT OR PLACEBO IN PATIENTS UNDERGOING CARDIAC SURGERY WITH CARDIOPULMONARY CONDITIONS

Reference	Study Design	Surgical procedure (no. patients)	Mean Total Postoperative Chest Tube Loss (mL)		Mean Total Allogeneic Transfusion Requirement (% of patients who did receive allogeneic products)	
			Aprotinin	Placebo	Aprotinin	Placebo
Repeat cardiac surgery						
Bidstrup et al.	p	HVR(15) or CABG (9) repeat surgery	245	1979	0.2 u (83)	
Lemmer et al.	mc, p, r, pl, db, pc	CABG repeat surgery (55)	1225	1700	0.3 u	10.7
Levy et al.	mc, p, r, pl, db, pc	CABG repeat surgery (126)	900	390	2.2 u	10.3
Orchard et al.[b]	p, r, pl, db, pc	Valve repeat surgery	288	1509	1435 mL[c]	1959 ml
Royston et al.	p, r, pl	Valve (18) or CABG (4) repeat surgery	286		0.5 u (64)	3.7
Primary cardiac surgery						
Alajmo et al.	p, r, pl	HVR (20) CABG (14)	486	830	213 mL	409
Baele et al.	p, r, pl, sb	CABG(75) valve (14) OTHER (26)[d]	699	1198	2.7 u	4.5u
Bidstrup et al.	p, r, pl, db, pc	CABG(77)	309	573	0.3 u	2.0
Bidstrup et al.	p, r, pl, db, pc	CABG(90)[e]	400	630	450 mL	795 ml
Dietrich et al.	p, r, pl, db, pc	CABG(39)	738	1431	0.6 u	2.3u
Dietrich et al.	p, r, pl	CABG(1085) valve CABG + valve[f]	678	1037	942 mL	1999 ml
Harder et al.	p, r, pl, db, pc	CABG(80)	559[g]	911[g]	2.4 u	
Havel et al.	p, r, pl	CABG(22)	610	1000		3.
Lemmer et al.	mc, p, r, pl, db, pc	CABG(141)	855	1053	2.2 u	5.7u
Swart et al.	p, r, pl, db, pc	CABG(50) valve	506	783	1.8 u	2.8u
van Oeveren et al.	p, r, pl	CABG(22)	357	674	700 mL	1400 ml

[a]The standard high-dose regimen consisted of 280 mg (2 million KIU) intravenous loading dose after anesthesia induction followed by 70 mg/hr (500,000 KIU/hr) continuous infusion for the duration of the operation and 280 mg.

[b]Patients received standard high-dose aprotinin regimen with 140 mg instead of the usual 280 mg added to the CPB pump prime fluid.

[c]Results include total homologous and autologous blood products transfused.

[d]Includes repeat surgery, combined HVR and CABG, combined cardiac and vascular surgery, bivalvular surgery and septal defect repairs.

[e]Results expressed as total median blood loss and transfusion requirements.

[f]Includes 201 patients who underwent repeat cardiac operations.

[g]Values expressed as milliliters of blood loss with a hemoglobin concentration of 7 mmol/L during the intraoperative and postoperative period.

p = prospective; mc = multicentered; r = randomized; db = double blind; pl = parallel; pc = placebo controlled; sb = single blind; u = units; CABG = coronary artery bypass.

The precise mechanism of action of aprotinin in reducing blood loss and transfusion requirement is not clear, and the optimal dose is not known. Further studies are needed to reveal how this drug decreases blood loss in patients undergoing CPB. However, it is apparent that whatever the mechanism is, the end result is a better functioning platelet possibly due to preservation of the glycoprotein Ib receptor, which mediates adhesion of platelets to vWF (44, 45). Lavee et al. (46) also postulated that aprotinin preserves platelet aggregation, possibly by preservation of the glycoprotein IIb/IIIa receptor, after studying platelets exposed to aprotinin during CPB under electron microscopy.

DOSAGE SCHEDULES

The biological activity of aprotinin is expressed in kallikrein inactivator units (KIU), where 1 inactivator unit is defined as that quantity that inhibits 1 unit of kallikrein. Royston developed the "Hammersmith regimen," which recommends giving a loading dose (for a 70-kg adult) of 280 mg (2,000,000 KIU) over 20 minutes, followed by an infusion of 70 mg/hr (500,000 KIU) and an additional 280 mg (2,000,000 KIU) in the CPB pump prime (31). Using this dosage regimen, Bidstrup and Royston were able to achieve plasma concentrations greater than 4 mmol/L, a concentration recommended by Fritz and Wunderer (47) to inhibit both plasmin and plasma kallikrein (31). Levy et al. (48) reported elimination half-lives to be approximately 5 hours, and based on their pharmacokinetic calculations, a full Hammersmith dose regimen would produce 200 KIU/mL. Different studies as listed in Table 26.4 have shown the full-dose technique to be effective.

Multiple modifications and dosing regimens have been tried to reduce drug costs and evaluate efficacy (Table 26.5). Studies using lower doses than those used in the Hammersmith regimen have reported variable results. However, more recent studies in repeat cardiac surgical patients using one half of the full Hammersmith dose have yielded favorable results as shown in Table 26.5. van Oeveren et al. (44) found similar results in perioperative chest tube drainage and blood loss in patients treated with either low-dose or high-dose aprotinin. Mean postoperative packed red blood cell transfusions were lower for low-dose and high-dose aprotinin versus placebo patients. Mohr et al. (49) reported similar results in patients undergoing primary coronary artery bypass graft (CABG) surgery. Schoenberger et al. (50, 51) reported that a single dose of aprotinin (2 million units added to the CPB prime) in primary CABG patients was also effective.

A study of 169 patients conducted by Cosgrove and associates (42) randomized patients to receive either high-dose aprotinin (Hammersmith dose), low-dose aprotinin (half Hammersmith dose), or placebo. They found that low-dose aprotinin was as effective as high-dose aprotinin in decreasing blood loss and blood transfusion requirements, but they did not study a pump prime dose.

Levy et al. (52) also reported the use of four different treatment groups in 287 patients undergoing repeat myocardial revascularization. The four groups were high-dose aprotinin, consisting of 2,000,000 KIU aprotinin loading dose, 2,000,000 KIU added to the CPB circuit prime, and a continuous infusion of 500,000 KIU during surgery; low-dose aprotinin, consisting of 1,000,000 KIU aprotinin loading dose, 1,000,000 KIU added to the CPB circuit prime, and a continuous infusion of 250,000 KIU/hr during surgery; pump prime aprotinin only, consisting of 2,000,000 KIU aprotinin added to CPB circuit prime; and placebo. The number of units of allogeneic packed red blood

TABLE 26.5. SUMMARY OF TRIALS COMPARING TREATMENT WITH LOW-DOSE (50% OF HIGH-DOSE REGIMEN) APROTININ (APR) WITH HIGH DOSE[a] OR PATIENTS UNDERGOING CARDIAC SURGERY WITH CPB

Reference	Study Design	Surgical Procedure (no. patients)	Treatment Regimen	Mean Total Postoperative Blood Loss (mL)
Cosgrove et al.	p, r, pl, db, pc	CABG repeat surgery (169)[b]	Apr1 high-dose regimen	720[c]
			Apr2 50% of high-dose regimen	866[c]
			PL	1121
Levy et al.	mc, p, r, pl, db, pc	CABG repeat surgery (254)	Apr1 high-dose regimen	900**
			Apr2 50% of high-dose regimen	1040**
			Apr3 280mg added to CPB pump prime fluid	1420
			PL	1700
Liu et al.	p, r, pl, db, pc	CABG (40)	Apr 50% of high-dose regimen	674**
			PL	1086

[a]The standard high-dose regimen consisted of 280 mg (2 million KIU) intravenous loading dose at induction followed by 70 mg/hr (500 000 KIU/hr) continuous infusion for the duration of the operation and 280 mg (2 million KIU) added to the CPB pump prime fluid.

[b]Twenty-one percent of patients received preoperative aspirin (acetylsalicylic acid).

[c]Statistically significant differences in blood loss ($P = .001$), transfusions requirements ($P = .006$), and patients transfused ($P = .001$) were reported between aprotinin recipients (results from high- and low-dose regimens combined) and placebo recipients.

cells was significantly less in the aprotinin-treated patients than in placebo patients (high dose, 1.6 units; low dose, 1.6 units; pump prime only, 2.5 units; placebo, 3.4 units). There were even greater reductions in total blood product exposure in high-dose and half-dose groups compared with placebo or pump prime. There were no differences in treatment groups for the incidence of perioperative myocardial infarction.

SAFETY PROFILE OF APROTININ

From the large number of patients that have received aprotinin in European studies, very few adverse effects have been reported. However, in the study performed by Cosgrove et al. (42) in patients undergoing repeat myocardial revascularization, they found only a trend toward a higher incidence of myocardial infarction and postoperative increases in serum creatinine levels in the aprotinin-treated groups, although these trends were not statistically significant. Other studies have not found any statistical differences in the incidence of these complications. van Oeveren (44) in almost 2000 patients noted no difference in intensive care unit stay time to extubation, congestive heart failure, or other surrogate markers for myocardial infarction in patients treated with aprotinin. Furthermore, several studies performed by the groups of Lemmer et al. (36), Bidstrup et al. (38), and Havel et al. (43) found no significant difference in patency of grafted vessels when examined postoperatively.

HEPARIN MANAGEMENT DURING USE OF APROTININ

After use of aprotinin became more common in Europe, it was apparent that the celite-activated activated clotting time (ACT) was prolonged by aprotinin (29). In 1990, after de Smet and associates (53) described this phenomenon, they suggested that the heparin dose administered to patients receiving aprotinin could be reduced. In 1992, Wang and associates (54) showed that the celite-activated ACT, but not the kaolin-activated ACT, was prolonged in the presence of aprotinin. Kaolin absorbs 98% or greater available aprotinin within seconds of contact. Therefore, any effect that aprotinin would have upon ACT is negated in kaolin-based ACT as long as the aprotinin dosage is not pushed far beyond a full Hammersmith dose. This led to speculations that the trend toward a higher incidence of myocardial infarction in Cosgrove et al.'s study was due to inadequate heparinization, because in that study the celite-activated ACT was maintained at only a minimum of 400 seconds even in the presence of aprotinin. If a kaolin-activated ACT had been used, the ACTs measured in that study would probably have been found to be significantly lower. In view of this, several recommendations have surfaced. Hunt et al. (55) and Royston recommended maintaining the ACT greater than 750 during CPB if the celite-activated ACT is used (31). Wang and associates (54) recommended that the celite-activated ACT should not be used at all in the presence of aprotinin. They recommend using only kaolin-activated ACTs. One appropriate method to maintain appropriate levels of anticoagulation is to administer additional doses of 100 U/kg heparin every hour in a fixed dosing scheme after the initial loading dose of heparin. Because of the controversy as to the appropriate heparin dose and ACT for patients undergoing CPB even without aprotinin, fixed doses of heparin every hour during bypass represent a clinically useful method for heparin administration if other monitors of heparin levels are not available. Certainly, kaolin-activated ACT is an acceptable method for monitoring even in the presence of aprotinin, and it appears that a controversy will rage for some time as to whether the celite-based ACT prolongation represents a problem or further anticoagulation due to aprotinin. Heparin dosing should not be reduced in the presence of aprotinin.

COSTS

Baele et al. (56) reported a 9% lower average hospital charge in high-dose aprotinin-treated patients due to complications in the control group and higher costs. Although the clinical studies in the United States are only now being designed to look at costs, the conserving of total blood products and operating room time suggest significant cost savings when compared with placebo-treated patients, especially from a half-dose perspective. More than one recent study does not suggest that aprotinin is more cost-effective than epsilon amino caproic acid in high-risk patients. If aprotinin's use allows for a reduction in surgical blood type and cross matching, further economic and other health care benefits may result (i.e., increased blood availability).

USE IN CHILDREN

Dietrich et al. (57) compared the clinical efficacy of high-dose and low-dose aprotinin for congenital heart surgery using a 4.2- or 2.1-mg/kg intravenous bolus dose administered after anesthesia induction and 4.2 or 2.1 mg/kg added to the CPB pump prime fluid in 60 children weighing less than 10 kg. Postoperative blood loss at 6 hours was lower in the high-dose group than in the low-dose and control groups, but no differences were observed in either the blood loss at 24 hours or in overall homologous transfusion requirements. Compared with 100 historical control patients, postoperative blood loss (154 versus 210 mL) and intraoperative (758 versus 1071 mL) and postoperative (53 versus 130 mL) transfusion requirements were significantly lower in 105 aprotinin-treated children. These children received

4.9–7.0 mg/kg intravenous loading dose after anesthesia induction followed by 2.8–4.2 mg/kg/hr continuous infusion and 4.9–7.0 mg/kg added to the CPB pump prime fluid.

Boldt et al. (58) reported lower aprotinin doses (3.5 mg/kg intravenous loading dose followed by 3.5 mg/kg/hr continuous infusion and 3.5 mg/kg added to the CPB pump prime fluid) in 48 children. No improvements in postoperative blood loss or transfusion requirements were reported among the children less than or more than 10 kg, with and without aprotinin. Higher homologous blood transfusion volumes in children weighing less than or more than 10 kg and postoperative blood loss in children weighing more than10 kg were observed in aprotinin-treated patients. Boldt et al. (59) also compared high-dose (4.9 mg/kg intravenous loading dose administered after induction followed by 1.4 mg/kg/min continuous infusion and 4.9 mg/kg added to the CPB pump prime fluid) and low-dose (2.8 mg/kg intravenous loading dose administered after anesthesia induction followed by 2.8 mg/kg/hr continuous infusion and 2.8 mg/kg added to the CPB pump prime fluid) regimens with those of control patients. Forty-two children weighing less than 20 kg undergoing cardiac surgery participated in the study, and similar postoperative blood losses and transfusion requirements were found in all three treatment groups. In an adult weighing 80 kg, equivalent dosages to those used in the last trial would largely exceed the clinically effective high-dose aprotinin regimen normally administered to adults. This demonstrates the difficulty in extrapolating drug doses in adults to infants and children. Although aprotinin has demonstrated clinical efficacy in some pediatric trials, the drug appears to be less effective in infants and small children in reducing allogeneic blood transfusions than in adults (57). Because of the severe dilutional changes that occur and obligate requirement of transfusion in small children and even adults, this may explain in part the difficulty in proving efficacy in this patient population. Therefore, more studies are needed to elucidate the role of aprotinin in pediatric cardiac surgery.

EFFECTS ON GRAFT PATENCY AND PERIOPERATIVE MYOCARDIAL INFARCTION

Potentially any drug that decreases bleeding and transfusion requirements has the potential to affect graft patency. The effects of aprotinin have been assessed in two randomized, double-blind, prospective, placebo-controlled studies in patients who underwent CABG surgery. Bidstrup et al. (38) reported vein graft patency 7–12 days postoperatively by magnetic resonance imaging in 90 patients who underwent primary CABG surgery. There were no differences between treatment and control groups and 46 evaluated internal mammary artery (IMA) grafts were patent. Lemmer et al. (36), using ultrafast computed tomography to assess vein and IMA graft patency 7–60 days after primary CABG surgery in 151 patients or repeat CABG surgery in 65 patients, found no statistically significant differences, although there was a trend toward lower vein and IMA graft patency rate in aprotinin recipient patients. Lemmer et al. also reported perioperative myocardial infarction and found no significant differences in patients between groups. Levy et al. (52) reported their results from a randomized prospective study of repeat coronary artery bypass surgical patients evaluating perioperative myocardial infarction in full-dose and half-dose aprotinin-treated patients using a blinded core laboratory to evaluate 24-hour serial creatine phospho-kinase myocardial band (CPK-MB) levels and electrocardiograms. The rate of myocardial infarction was not statistically different in high-dose, low-dose, pump-prime only, and placebo groups. The fact that not even a trend exists toward increased infarction largely negates the report by Cosgrove (42). With these three studies plus van Oeveren's experience from Germany, a large body of literature currently supports the claim that aprotinin does not independently increase the risk for graft thrombosis or perioperative myocardial infarction.

EFFECTS ON RENAL FUNCTION

Because aprotinin undergoes active reabsorption by the proximal tubules, aprotinin effect on renal function has been investigated. Bidstrup et al. (32) reported higher mean urine output in aprotinin compared with placebo treatment in 80 patients who underwent primary CABG surgery. Blauhut et al. (34) reported that osmolar clearance and fractional sodium excretion were higher in 13 aprotinin-treated patients compared with 13 control subjects after primary CABG. However, there were no differences in creatinine concentrations, electrolytes, or creatinine clearance between the two treatment groups. Lemmer et al. (60) also reported no differences in renal function in aprotinin- versus placebo-treated patients from recent U.S. studies. In patients undergoing thoracic or thoracoabdominal aortic surgery requiring CPB and hypothermic arrest, an increased risk of renal dysfunction was reported, described as an elevation of plasma creatinine greater than 1.5 preoperative values (61). The authors compared their data to 20 historical control subjects but found greater incidence of renal failure. However, the patients receiving aprotinin also received significantly lower doses of heparin compared with their historical control subjects (61).

HYPERSENSITIVITY REACTIONS

Aprotinin can produce allergic reactions associated with its administration. Because aprotinin is a protein of bovine origin, it is capable of causing anaphylactic reactions (62). In the literature, anaphylactic reactions have been reported in less than 0.5% of patients receiving it (63). However, these reactions will most likely become more common when aprotinin is given to patients who have received it previously. Aprotinin-specific IgG antibodies have been reported in 6 of 23 (26%) and 117 of 252 patients who underwent surgery 6 months previously (63). From European data, the incidence of hypersensitivity reactions ranges from 0.3 to 0.6% in patients receiving high-dose aprotinin who were not pretreated for prevention (63). Because anaphylaxis requires prior sensitization, the incidence of anaphylaxis to aprotinin is unclear; however, the incidence of anaphylactic reactions to another polypeptide with a similar molecular weight has been well-documented previously. The incidence of anaphylaxis to protamine is 0.6–2% in high-risk previously sensitized patients (64, 65). Therefore, the incidence of anaphylaxis to aprotinin may prove very similar upon reexposure. Therefore, patients who are to receive aprotinin should always get a small intravenous test dose at least 10 minutes before the loading dose. In addition, in cardiac surgical patients who are known to have received aprotinin in the past and are to undergo repeat exposure, the initial dose should be delayed until CPB can be instituted if cardiovascular collapse were to occur (i.e., with aortic or femoral artery exposure). The risk-to-benefit ratio for aprotinin in repeat exposure situations should be carefully weighed, and the efficacy of pretreatment with steroids and histamine blockers to prevent such complications is still not proven.

Aprotinin has also been studied for its ability to decrease bleeding and transfusion requirements after total hip replacement procedures. In these studies, aprotinin has decreased bleeding and transfusion requirements without an increased risk of postoperative thromboembolic complications (66, 67). After total hip replacement, patients are at a greater risk for postoperative thromboembolic complications. The lack of increased deep vein thrombosis in this patient population supports the lack of prothrombotic effects of aprotinin (66, 67).

LYSINE ANALOGUES AND ANTIFIBRINOLYTIC THERAPY

Epsilon-aminocaproic acid (EACA, Amicar) and its analogue, tranexamic acid (AMCA), are derivatives of the amino acid lysine (Fig. 26.1). Both drugs inhibit the proteolytic activity of plasmin and the conversion of plasminogen to plasmin by plasminogen activators as shown in Table 26.6. Their role in the pharmacological prevention of bleeding for cardiac surgery is reviewed.

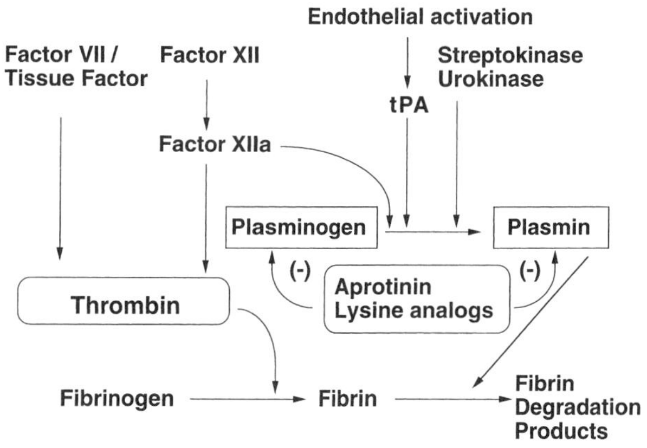

Figure 26.1. Coagulation and fibrinolytic pathways for initiation and inhibiting. Thrombin generation will convert fibrinogen to fibrin but also serves as an endothelial activator for tPA release. Contact activation via factor XIIa generation also converts plasminogen to plasmin. Aprotinin, a protease inhibitor, and lysine analogues epsilon-aminocaproic acid and tranexamic acid inhibit plasminogen and plasmin.

THE FIBRINOLYTIC SYSTEM

The fibrinolytic system inhibits the formation of intravascular fibrin, maintains fibrin localized to bleeding sites, and restores blood flow in obstructed vessels (Fig. 26.1). Plasminogen is the precursor of plasmin, the main proteolytic enzyme of the fibrinolytic system. It is a polypeptide consisting of 790 amino acids that has a unique conformation with five triple-loop regions called kringles, because of their resemblance to a Scandinavian biscuit of the same name (68). These kringles form binding sites for lysine and are responsible for binding fibrin, fibrinogen, factor V, factor VIII, platelet glycoprotein Ib, and complement. When activated by tPA, thrombin, kallikrein, urokinase, or streptokinase, plasminogen undergoes cleavage of two or more peptide bonds to become plasmin, a two-chain molecule linked by disulfide bonds. In the active form, plasmin is then able to lyse both fibrin and fibrinogen.

Fibrinogen is a dimer made of three polypeptide chains, synthesized in the liver, organized in mirror image, and bridged together by covalent disulfide bonds (69). Each side of this bond consists of three different polypeptide chains with distinct amino acid sequences. When thrombin is formed, it binds to the disulfide bonds, releasing fibrinopeptides A and B from the fibrinogen molecule, thus forming active fibrin, which then stacks together with other fibrin molecules that are then cross-linked at the alpha and gamma chains by factor XIII forming the fibrin mesh (69).

Plasmin cleaves fibrinogen by initially removing peptides from the A alpha chain and then from the B beta chains,

TABLE 26.6. CHEMICAL PROPERTIES OF FIBRINOLYTIC INHIBITORS

Low-molecular-weight molecules
Lysine analogues
Attach to the lysine binding site of plasmin(ogen)

leaving what is called fragment X. This fragment undergoes asymmetric cleavage of all three chains, releasing fragment D and leaving fragment Y (69). The three chains remaining in fragment Y undergo further cleavage, releasing one more fragment D, thus leaving a core called fragment E, a dimer that contains parts of all three fibrinogen chains (69).

Attack by plasmin or fibrin results in different end products because of the fact that the fibrin monomers are polymerized and cross-linked by the activated factor XIII (68). The major difference in the end products of fibrin digestion in contrast to fibrinogen digestion is the release of the cross-linked complex of two D fragments called the D-dimer. In addition, initial degradation of cross-linked fibrin results in X-oligomers that are X fragments bound together by polymerization and cross-linking (68).

Plasmin has also been shown to decrease the activity of factors V, VIII, and IX. Plasmin also can activate complement via the C1 esterase (62). However, the main clinical implications result from the breakdown of existing fibrin and fibrinogen. Plasmin is a potent platelet inhibitor at normothermia, but at hypothermia (less than 32°C), it is a platelet activator. The mechanism of this platelet effect is unclear, but this is thought to be important in the overall mechanism of CPB coagulopathy. Therefore, either the formed clot is broken down or formation of a further clot is inhibited. In addition, the breakdown products of the lysis of fibrinogen and fibrin have little or no clotting capacity, whereas they increase vascular permeability, inhibit platelet aggregation, and interfere with the formation of the fibrin mesh.

FIBRINOLYSIS DURING CARDIAC SURGERY

Fibrinolytic activity is initiated by incision and sternotomy, augmented by CPB, and peaks toward the end of extracorporeal circulation (70). Evidence for bypass-associated fibrinolysis has been shown by the presence of fibrin split products during and after CPB. Serum levels of tPA, an activator of plasmin released from endothelium, increase during CPB. In addition, plasminogen levels have been found to decrease at the same time that plasmin levels are increasing, indicating activation of plasminogen to plasmin.

THE LYSINE ANALOGUE ANTIFIBRINOLYTIC AGENTS

Drugs that inhibit activation of plasminogen to plasmin and interfere with the lysis of fibrinogen and fibrin are called antifibrinolytic or antiplasmin agents (Table 26.6). They are omega aminocarboxylic acid analogues of lysine that bind to the kringles on plasminogen and plasmin, occupying the binding site for fibrinogen and fibrin and therefore interfering with the fibrinolytic process (68). Both EACA (Amicar) and trans-p-amino methylcyclohexane-carboxylic acid (tranexamic acid) have been used to decrease fibrinolysis during cardiac surgery. Other analogues of lysine have been studied. Tranexamic acid is 6–10 times more potent than EACA (68).

Most early studies using antifibrinolytic agents showed decreased mediastinal drainage in patients treated with EACA. However, many of these studies lacked control subjects and were retrospective and unblinded. In 1967, Sterns and Lillehei (71) gave EACA to 240 patients at the end of CPB and again in the event of large amounts of blood loss. Compared with a historic group of 100 patients, the EACA-treated group had decreased blood loss.

In 1974, McClure and Izsac published a double-blind randomized study of 71 patients with cyanotic and noncyanotic cardiac defects requiring CPB (72). In this study, EACA was infused from the time of chest opening and then for 24 hours. Those receiving EACA showed less bleeding from the time of termination of CPB, until the end of surgery, and the difference in bleeding was more pronounced in patients with cyanotic cardiac defects and those requiring a prolonged period of CPB.

In 1988, Vander Salm et al. (73) administered either EACA or placebo to 60 patients undergoing first-time CABG before protamine administration and then they were given an infusion of the drug for 6 hours. Patients that received EACA bled less than the control subjects in the first 12 postoperative hours (273 versus 332 mL). In addition, those receiving EACA had higher platelet counts and shorter bleeding times than those receiving placebo. However, no data regarding blood product transfusions were reported.

In a large, randomized, blinded study of 350 patients undergoing routine CABG, Del Rossi et al. (74) reported a significant decrease in blood loss in the first 24 postoperative hours in those patients receiving a 5-g loading dose followed by a 1-g/hr infusion during the next 6–8 hours, starting before skin incision. Not only was blood loss reduced in the EACA versus placebo group (617 versus 883 mL), but transfusion of packed red blood cells was also reduced (2.8 versus 4.2). There were no differences in myocardial infarction, cerebrovascular accidents, or graft failures in those receiving EACA compared with those receiving placebo, although the overall complication rate was very low.

Horrow et al. (75–77) also studied the use of tranexamic acid given in a prophylactic manner before skin incision for primary CABG surgery. In one study, 12-hour postoperative blood loss was 496 mL in the tranexamic acid group compared with 750 mL in the placebo group (75). However, transfusion utilization was not different. Patients who received tranexamic acid had lower levels of fibrin split products and decreased plasminogen availability postoperatively. In a separate study, they again found decreased blood loss in patients receiving tranexamic acid compared with those receiving placebo but found no increased benefit by administering DDAVP concurrently (76). Efforts continue to determine the optimal dose using loading doses before incision of 2.5–40 mg/kg and one-tenth the loading dose hourly for 12 hours, as reported in 148 patients (77). Larger doses did not further decrease bleeding.

Rousou reported a clinical series of 415 consecutive patients undergoing primary CABG surgery where 209 received in the second 6 months of the study tranexamic acid as a 2-g bolus before the initiation of CPB and in 206, 8 g was given by slow infusion during bypass. In the patients who received tranexamic acid, there was a decrease in chest tube drainage from 1114 to 803 mL in the treated patients and small, but statistically significant, differences in allogeneic blood product use for red blood cells (1.7–0.69 units per patient), fresh-frozen plasma (0.23–0.024 units per patient), and platelets (1.06–0.3 units per patient). There were no differences in postoperative complications, although all data were collected by retrospective detailed chart reviews. The incidence of postoperative myocardial infarction was also low in both retrospective analysis (1% in controls versus 1.5% in the treated patients). One should note that the study was not blinded and no strict transfusion algorithm or guidelines were reported.

PHARMACOLOGY OF EACA AND TRANEXAMIC ACID

Because of their similarity to lysine, EACA and tranexamic acid attach to the lysine binding sites on plasminogen and plasmin to inhibit binding of lysine residues on fibrinogen and fibrin by plasminogen and plasmin. Because plasmin(ogen) is now unable to bind to fibrin(ogen), it is unable to lyse it. Tranexamic acid is 6–10 times more potent than EACA, probably because of subtle changes in the molecular structure that mimics lysine.

All antifibrinolytic drugs are water soluble and are therefore distributed through both the intravascular and extravascular compartments. Renal excretion accounts for most elimination of these drugs, with 80–90% of the drug recovered in the urine within 12 hours. Because of this method of elimination, urine levels of the drug can reach 50–100 times the plasma levels of the drugs.

Some studies reporting increased efficacy of the administration of antifibrinolytics have initiated therapy before skin incision. Recovered EACA loading doses of 5–10 g (approximately 75–150 mg/kg) should be given over 15–30 minutes, followed by an infusion of 10–15 mg/kg/hr. Tranexamic acid should be administered with loading doses of approximately 1 g (10–15 mg/kg) followed by an infusion of 1 mg/kg/hr. Even higher doses of tranexamic acid using 5–10 g have been reported in preliminary studies (29). These infusions are routinely continued until the end of CPB or surgery. Because tPA production is greatest during CPB and is rapidly cleared after weaning, lysine analogues should not be routinely continued into the intensive care unit unless there is bleeding or fibrinolysis is demonstrated.

UNDESIRABLE EFFECTS OF ANTIFIBRINOLYTIC DRUGS

When administered intravenously to patients undergoing cardiac surgery, the adverse effects of antifibrinolytic agents are relatively infrequent. The most common side effect is hypotension during rapid intravenous administration. It is therefore recommended that the intravenous loading doses be administered over 15–30 minutes with the patient in the supine position. Patients receiving these medications orally experience much more common side effects. Nausea, vomiting, diarrhea, and anorexia appear to be caused by a direct gastrointestinal irritation and are not related to plasma concentrations of the antifibrinolytic agents. Other side effects that have been reported after oral administration include nasal stuffiness, myalgias, muscle weakness, myoglobinuria, and skin rash.

Other undesirable effects seen after administration of antifibrinolytic agents are a direct result of inhibiting the fibrinolytic system. There is no definitive evidence that EACA, tranexamic acid, or any of the antifibrinolytic agents can actually produce thrombosis. However, fibrin formed intravascularly will be resistant to lysis by the fibrinolytic system, which normally inhibits formation of and removes intravascular fibrin. There are reports in the literature of glomerular capillary thrombosis, renal cortical necrosis, deep venous thrombosis, and pulmonary embolism, along with renal, carotid, and cerebral artery thrombosis (72). In addition, there is a report of widespread arterial and venous thrombosis in a patient with disseminated intravascular coagulation, a setting where use of antifibrinolytic therapy is particularly dangerous and may be contraindicated (72).

In the literature dealing with the use of antifibrinolytic therapy during cardiac surgery, there have been no reported differences in the incidence of thrombotic complications between patients receiving antifibrinolytic agents and those receiving placebo, although the design of these studies has not been prospective. The incidence of perioperative myocardial infarction and stroke has not been reported as different in the treatment group as compared with control subjects. However, because of the low incidence of these complications in routine CABG surgery and the small numbers of patients studied, one would be extremely surprised to find any difference with very small sample sizes. Prospective studies evaluating safety issues, including the risk of perioperative myocardial infarction, graft patency, and renal dysfunction, still need to be conducted, and although inhibiting fibrinolysis represents an effective way to reduce bleeding and transfusion requirements, other issues need to be addressed. Tranexamic acid is approved for use in the United States to prevent bleeding in patients with hereditary angioedema undergoing tooth extraction, but no U.S. Food and Drug Administration indication for use in CPB has been approved. Most work has focused on the use of lysine analogues in first-time CABG. Comparative research between aprotinin and these agents in complex cases, the case mix where hemorrhage is the greatest problem, is required. Such studies are underway today at multiple institutions.

NAFAMOSTAT MESILATE (FUT-175)

Nafamostat mesilate is a synthetic serine protease inhibitor that inhibits thrombin, factor XIIa, kallikrein, plasmin, and the C1 esterase. Nafamostat has been used in experimental models of acute pulmonary vasoconstriction to attenuate the complement-mediated pulmonary hypertension that can occur after protamine reactions. Murase et al. (78) reported their use of nafamostat during surgery in 20 patients in a randomized but nonblinded study in patients undergoing CABG surgery. Nafamostat inhibited fibrinolysis, preserved platelet counts, and decreased blood loss compared with the control group. In the nafamostat group, 33% of patients were transfused (1.4 units of red blood cells per patient) as compared with 53% of the control patients (7.7 units per patient) and no adverse effects of the pharmacological therapy were reported. Although the drug has been used as a protease inhibitor in Japan, there are currently little data supporting its application for clinical use.

COMPARISON STUDIES

There is a paucity of literature available to compare the efficacy and safety of pharmacological agents available for reducing allogeneic blood administration in cardiac surgical patients. Rocha et al. (79) compared aprotinin to DDAVP in 109 patients undergoing both CABG and valve operations. Aprotinin decreased blood loss and the need for transfusions, whereas DDAVP had no beneficial effect. Blauhut et al. (80) compared aprotinin to tranexamic acid in 43 patients undergoing CABG first-time surgery. Aprotinin reduced blood loss and transfusion requirements, but tranexamic acid failed to show a significant effect. In a retrospective study comparing aprotinin to EACA in high-risk cardiac surgery patients, Van Norman et al. (81) reported reductions in bleeding and transfusion requirements in the patients who received aprotinin, so aprotinin was a cost-effective strategy. Another trial compared dipyridamole, tranexamic acid, and aprotinin in 60 CABG patients (83). This study used a 2 million unit pump prime-only dose of aprotinin. Tranexamic acid and aprotinin both significantly reduced postoperative blood loss but did not affect the transfusion rates, although the investigators studied only 15 patients in each group. Another recent study compared tranexamic acid with a pump prime-only dose of aprotinin (84). Both drugs decreased blood losses compared with a control group, but the transfusion trigger was a hematocrit of 30% and only median transfused volumes were compared.

A meta-analysis study by Fremes and associates (85) reviewed 33 randomized placebo-controlled trials involving DDAVP, EACA, tranexamic acid, and aprotinin. All were published before June 1993 (therefore not including several large aprotinin trials published in 1994). The authors concluded that "the meta-analysis supports the prophylactic use of EACA, tranexamic acid, or preferably aprotinin rather than desmopressin for the reduction of postoperative bleeding associated with an open heart operation and the limitation of homologous blood use where indicated."

SUMMARY

The therapeutic approaches to decreasing the coagulation defect after CPB represent novel pharmacological approaches to preventing the coagulopathy that can ensue. DDAVP has not been consistently demonstrated to be effective in decreasing bleeding in cardiac surgical patients. However, with improved monitoring and targeting of platelet dysfunctional groups, perhaps DDAVP has an application.

The use of the lysine analogues (EACA or tranexamic acid) results in less chest tube drainage, but significant decreases in blood product transfusion requirements have not been consistently documented in blinded, placebo-controlled studies. Despite their widespread application in cardiac surgical patients, carefully controlled studies evaluating safety data regarding EACA and tranexamic acid are limited.

The serine protease inhibitors (in particular, aprotinin), by inhibiting both fibrinolysis and potentially other aspects of the inflammatory response to CPB, have theoretic advantages as compared with the lysine analogues. Aprotinin has been demonstrated to be highly effective in reducing bleeding and transfusion requirements in high-risk patients undergoing repeat median sternotomy or in patients who are taking aspirin. Results from multicenter studies of aprotinin show there is no greater risk of early graft thrombosis, perioperative myocardial infarction, or renal failure in aprotinin-treated patients. The incidence of stroke was actually significantly lower in aprotinin-treated patients compared with placebo in repeat CABG patients (52). Aprotinin use may produce occasional postoperative increases in serum creatinine that reverse postoperatively. Although additional pharmacological agents are on the horizon, prospective, well-designed, placebo-controlled studies are needed to determine the most effective modalities for decreasing bleeding and transfusion requirements in cardiac surgical patients.

REFERENCES

1. Harker LA. Bleeding after cardiopulmonary bypass. N Engl J Med 1986;314:1446–1448.
2. Woodman RC, Harker LA. Bleeding complications associated with cardiopulmonary bypass. Blood 1990;76:1680–1689.
3. Kestin AS, Valeri CR, Khuri SF, et al. The platelet function defect of cardiopulmonary bypass. Blood 1993;82:107–117.
4. Cash JD, Gader AMA, De Costa J. The release of plasminogen activator and factor VIII by LVP, AVP, DDAVP, AT III, and OT in man. Br J Haematol 1984;30:363–364.
5. Mannucci PM. Nontransfusional modalities. In: Loscalzo J, Schafer AI, eds. Thrombosis and hemorrhage. Boston: Blackwell Scientific Publications, 1994:1117–1135.
6. Cooney KA, Ginsburg D, Ruggeri ZM. von Willebrand disease. In: Loscalzo J, Schafer AI, eds. Thrombosis and hemorrhage. Boston: Blackwell Scientific Publications, 1994:657–682.
7. de la Fuente B, Kasper CK, Rickles FR, Hoyer LW. Response of patients with mild and moderate hemophilia A and von Willebrand disease to treatment with desmopressin. Ann Intern Med 1985;103:6–14.
8. Takahashi H, Nagayama R, Hattori A, Shibata A. Platelet aggregation induced by DDAVP in platelet-type von Willibrand's disease. N Engl J Med 1984;310:722–723.
9. Anderson TL, Solem JO, Tengborn L. Effects of desmopressin acetate on platelet aggregation, von Willebrand factor and blood loss after cardiac surgery with extracorporeal circulation. Circulation 1990;81:872–878.
10. Hackmann T, Gascoyne R, Naiman SC. A trial of desmopressin to reduce blood loss in uncomplicated cardiac surgery. N Engl J Med 1989;321:1437–1444.
11. Mannucci PM, Lusher JM. Desmopressin and thrombosis. Lancet 1989;2:675–676.
12. Reynolds LM, Nicolson SC, Jobes DR, et al. Desmopressin does not decrease bleeding after cardiac operation in young children. J Thorac Cardiovasc Surg 1994;106:954–958.
13. Rocha E, Llorens R, Paramo JA. Does desmopressin acetate reduce blood loss after surgery in patients on cardiopulmonary bypass? Circulation 1988;77:1319–1323.
14. Salzman EW, Weinstein MJ, Weintraub RM. Treatment with desmopressin acetate to reduce blood loss after cardiac surgery. N Engl J Med 1986;314:1402–1406.
15. Sean MD, Wadsworth LD, Rogers PC. The effect of desmopressin acetate (DDAVP) on postoperative blood loss after cardiac operations in children. J Thorac Cardiovasc Surg 1988;48:217–218.
16. Kobrinsky NL, Israel ED, Gerrard JM. Shortening of bleeding time by 1-deamino-8-D-arginine vasopressin in various bleeding disorders. Lancet 1984;1:1145–1148.
17. Mannucci PM, Remuzzi G, Pusineri F. Deamino-8-D-arginine vasopressin shortens the bleeding time in uremia. N Engl J Med 1983;308:8–12.
18. DiMichele DM, Hathaway WE. Use of DDAVP in inherited and acquired platelet dysfunction. Am J Hematol 1990;33:39–45.
19. Watson AJS, Koegh JAB. Effect of 1-deamino-8-D-arginine vasopressin on the prolonged bleeding time in chronic renal failure. Nephron 1982;32:49.
20. Agnelli G, Berrettini M, de Cunto M. Desmopressin-induced improvement of abnormal coagulation in chronic liver disease. Lancet 1983;1:645.
21. Kobrinsky NL, Letts RP, Patel R. DDAVP shortens the bleeding time and decreases blood loss in hemostatically normal subjects undergoing spinal fusion surgery. Ann Intern Med 1987;107:446–450.
22. Czer LSC, Bateman TM, Gray PJ. Treatment of severe platelet dysfunction and hemorrhage after cardiopulmonary bypass: reduction in blood product usage with desmopressin. J Am Coll Cardiol 1987;9:1139–1147.
23. Mongan PD, Hosking MP. The role of desmospressin acetate in patients undergoing coronary artery bypass surgery. A controlled clinical trial with thromboelastographic risk stratification. Anesthesiology 1992;77:38–46.
24. Bichet DG, Razi M, Lonergan M. Hemodynamic and coagulation responses to 1-desamino-8-D-arginine vasopressin in patients with congenital nephrogenic diabetes insipidus. N Engl J Med 1988;318:881.
25. Lowe J, Pettigrew A, Middleton S. DDAVP in hemophilia. Lancet 1977;2:614.
26. Horrow JC, van Ripper DF, Strong MD. The hemostatic effects of tranexamic acid and desmopressin during cardiac surgery. Circulation 1991; 84:2063–2070.
27. Byrnes JJ, Larcade A, Moake J. Thrombosis following desmospressin for uremic bleeding. Am J Hematol 1988;28:63–65.
28. Bond L, Bevan D. Desmopressin and myocardial infarction. Lancet 1988;1:664.
29. Davis R, Whittington R. Aprotinin: a review of its pharmacology and therapeutic efficacy in reducing blood loss associated with cardiac surgery. Drugs 1995;49:954–983.
30. van Oeveren W, Jansen NJG, Bidstrup BP. Effects of aprotinin on haemostatic mechanisms during cardiopulmonary bypass. Ann Thorac Surg 1987;44:640–645.
31. Royston D, Taylor KM, Bidstrup BP, Sapsfort RN. Effect of aprotinin on need for blood transfusion after repeat open-heart surgery. Lancet 1987;2:1289–1291.
32. Bidstrup BP, Royston D, Sapsfort RN, Taylor KM. Reduction in blood loss and blood use after cardiopulmonary bypass with high dose aprotinin (Trasylol). J Thorac Cardiovasc Surg 1989;97:364–372.
33. Dietrich W, Spannagl M, Jochum M, et al. Influence of high-dose aprotinin treatment on blood loss and coagulation patterns in patients

undergoing myocardial revascularization. Anesthesiology 1990; 73: 1119–1126.

34. Blauhut B, Gross C, Necek S. Effects of high-dose aprotinin on blood loss, platelet function, fibrinolysis, complement, and renal function after cardiopulmonary bypass. J Thorac Cardiovasc Surg 1991;101: 958–967.
35. Havel M, Teufelsbauer H, Knobl P, et al. Effect of intraoperative aprotinin administration on postoperative bleeding in patients undergoing cardiopulmonary bypass operation. J Thorac Cardiovasc Surg 1991; 101:968–972.
36. Lemmer JH, Stanford W, Bonney SL, et al. Aprotinin for coronary bypass surgery: efficacy, safety, and influence on early saphenous vein graft patency. J Thorac Cardiovasc Surg 1994;107:543–553.
37. Marx G, Pokar H, Reuter H, Doering V, Tilsner V. The effects of aprotinin on hemostatic function during cardiac surgery. J Cardiothorac Vasc Anesth 1991;5:467–474.
38. Bidstrup BP, Underwood SR, Sapsford RN, Streets EM. Effect of aprotinin (Trasylol) on aorta-coronary bypass graft patency. J Thorac Cardiovasc Surg 1993;105:147–153.
39. Dietrich W, Barankay A, Hahnel C, Meisner H, Richter JA. High dose aprotinin in cardiac surgery: three years experience in 1,784 patients. J Cardiothorac Vasc Anesth 1992;6:324–327.
40. Harder MP, Eijsman L, Roozendalal KJ. Aprotinin reduces intraoperative and postoperative blood loss in membrane oxygenator cardiopulmonary bypass. Ann Thorac Surg 1991;51:936–941.
41. Bertrand P, Mazzucotelli JP, Loisance D. L'aprotinine en chirurgie cardiaque chez les patients sous antiagregants plaquettaires. Arch Mal Coeur Vaiss 1993;86:1471–1474.
42. Cosgrove DM, Heric B, Lytle BW, et al. Aprotinin therapy for reoperative myocardial revascularization: a placebo-controlled study. Ann Thorac Surg 1992;54:1031–1038.
43. Havel M, Grabenwoger F, Schneider J. Aprotinin does not decrease early graft patency after coronary artery bypass grafting despite reducing postoperative bleeding and use of donated blood. J Thorac Cardiovasc Surg 1994;107:807–810.
44. van Oeveren W, Harder MP, Roozendaal KJ, Eijsman L, Wildevuur CRH. Aprotinin protects platelets against the initial effect of cardiopulmonary bypass. J Thorac Cardiovasc Surg 1990;99:788–797.
45. Rinder CS, Mathew JP, Rinder HM, Bonan J, Ault KA, Smith BR. Modulation of platelet surface adhesion receptors during cardiopulmonary bypass. Anesthesiology 1991;75:563–570.
46. Lavee J, Savion N, Smolinsky A, Goor DA, Mohr R. Platelet protection by aprotinin in cardiopulmonary bypass: electron microscopic study. Ann Thorac Surg 1992;53:477–481.
47. Fritz H, Wunderer G. Biochemistry and applications of aprotinin, the kallikrein inhibitor from bovine organs. Arzneimittelforshung 1983;33: 479–494.
48. Levy JH, Bailey JM, Salmenpera M. Pharmacokinetics of aprotinin in preoperative cardiac surgical patients. Anesthesiology 1994;80:1013–1018.
49. Mohr R, Goor DA, Lusky A. Aprotinin prevents cardiopulmonary bypass-induced platelet dysfunction. A scanning electron microscope study. Circulation 1992;86 (5 Suppl.):II405–II409.
50. Schoenberger JP, Everts PA, Ercan H. Low dose aprotinin in internal mammary artery bypass operations contributes to important blood saving. Ann Thorac Surg 1992;54:1172–1176.
51. Schoenberger JP, van Zundert A, Bredee JJ. Blood loss and use of blood in internal mammary artery and saphenous vein bypass grafting with and without adding a single, low dose of aprotinin (2 million units) to the pump prime. Acta Anaesthesiol Belg 1992;43:187–196.
52. Levy JH, Pifarre R, Schaff H, et al. A multicenter, placebo-controlled, double-blind trial of aprotinin undergoing repeat coronary artery bypass grafting. Circulation 1995;92:2236–2244.
53. de Smet AEA, Joen MCN, van Oeveren W. Increased anticoagulation during cardiopulmonary bypass by aprotinin. J Thorac Cardiovasc Surg 1990;100:520–527.
54. Wang JS, Lin CY, Hung WT, Karp RB. Monitoring of heparin-induced anticoagulation with kaolin activated clotting time in cardiac surgical patients treated with aprotinin. Anesthesiology 1992;77:1080–1084.
55. Hunt GJ, Segal H, Yacoub M. Guidelines for monitoring heparin by the activated clotting time when aprotinin is used during cardiopulmonary bypass. J Thorac Cardiovasc Surg 1992;104:211–212.
56. Baele PL, Ruiz-Gomez J, Londot C, Sauvage M, Van Dyck MJ, Robert A. Systematic use of aprotinin in cardiac surgery: influence on total homologous exposure and hospital cost. Acta Anaesth Belg 1992;43:103–112.
57. Dietrich W, Mossinger H, Spannagl M, et al. Hemostatic activation during cardiopulmonary bypass with different aprotinin dosages in pediatric patients having cardiac operations. J Thorac Cardiovasc Surg 1993;105:757–760.
58. Boldt J, Knothe C, Zickman B. Aprotinin in pediatric cardiac operations. Platelet function, blood loss, and homologous blood. Ann Thorac Surg 1993;55:1460–1466.
59. Boldt J, Knothe C, Zickman B. Comparison of two aprotinin dosage regimens in pediatric patients having cardiac operation. Influence on platelet function and blood loss. J Thorac Cardiovasc Surg 1993;105: 705–711.
60. Lemmer JH, Stanford W, Bonney SL. Aprotinin for coronary artery bypass grafting; effect on postoperative renal function. Ann Thorac Surg 1995;59:132–136.
61. Sundt TM, Kouchoukos NT, Saffitz JE, Murphy SF, Wareing TH, Stahl D. Renal dysfunction and intravascular coagulation with aprotinin and hypothermic circulatory arrest. Ann Thorac Surg 1993;55:1418–1424.
62. Levy JH. Anaphylactic reactions in anesthesia and intensive care. 2nd ed. Boston: Butterworth-Heinemann, 1992.
63. Leskiw U, Levy JH. Antigenicity of protamine and aprotinin in cardiac surgery. In: Pifarre R, ed. Blood conservation with aprotinin. Philadelphia: Hanely and Belfus, 1995:253–266.
64. Levy JH, Zaidan JR, Faraj BA. Prospective evaluation of risk of protamine reactions in NPH insulin-dependent diabetics. Anesth Analg 1986; 65:739–742.
65. Levy JH, Schwieger IM, Zaidan JR, Faraj BA, Weintraub WS. Evaluation of patients at risk for protamine reactions. J Thorac Cardiovasc Surg 1989;98:200–204.
66. Murkin JM, Lux J, Shannon NA, et al. Aprotinin significantly decreases bleeding and transfusion requirements in patients receiving aspirin and undergoing cardiac operations. J Thorac Cardiovasc Surg 1994;107: 554–561.
67. Janssens M, Joris J, David JL, Lemaire R, Lamy M. High-dose aprotinin reduces blood loss in patients undergoing total hip replacement surgery. Anesthesiology 1994;80:23–29.
68. Ouimet H, Loscalzo J. Fibrinolysis. In: Loscalzo J, Schafer AI, eds. Thrombosis and hemorrhage. Boston: Blackwell Scientific Publications, 1994:127–143.
69. Greenberg CS. Fibrin formation and stabilization. In: Loscalzo J, Schafer AI, eds. Thrombosis and hemorrhage. Boston: Blackwell Scientific Publications, 1994:107–126.
70. Tanaka K, Takao M, Yada I. Alterations in coagulation and fibrinolysis associated with cardiopulmonary bypass during open heart surgery. J Cardiothorac Anesth 1989;3:181–188.
71. Sterns LP, Lillehei CW. Effect of epsilon aminocaproic acid upon blood

loss following open heart surgery: an analysis of 340 patients. Can J Surg 1967;10:304–307.
72. McClure PD, Izsack J. The use of epsilon-amino-caproic acid to reduce bleeding during cardiac bypass in children with congenital heart disease. Anesthesiology 1974;40:604–608.
73. Vander Salm TJ, Ansell JE, Okike ON. The role of epsilon-aminocaproic acid in reducing bleeding after cardiac operation: a double-blind randomized study. J Thorac Cardiovasc Surg 1988;95:538–542.
74. DelRossi AJ, Cernaianu AC, Botros S. Prophylactic treatment of post-perfusion bleeding using EACA. Chest 1989;96:27–30.
75. Horrow J, Hlavacek J, Strong M, et al. Prophylactic tranexamic acid decreases bleeding after cardiac operations. J Thorac Cardiovasc Surg 1990;99:70–74.
76. Horrow JC, Wan Riper DF, Strong MD. The hemostatic effects of tranexamic acid and desmopressin during cardiac surgery. Circulation 1991;84:2063–2070.
77. Horrow JC, Van Riper DF, Strong MD, Grunewald KE, Parmet JL. The dose-response relationship of tranexamic acid. Anesthesiology 1995; 82:383–392.
78. Rousou JA, Engelmaan RM, Flack JE III, Deaton DW, Owen SG. Tranexamic acid significantly reduces blood loss associated with coronary revascularization. Ann Thorac Surg 1996;61:774–775.
79. Murase M, Usui A, Tomita Y. Nafamostat mesilate reduces blood loss during open heart surgery. Circulation 1993;88:432–436.
80. Rocha E, Hidalgo F, Llorens R. Randomized study of aprotinin and DDAVP to reduce postopertive bleeding after cardiopulmonary bypass surgery. Circulation 1994;90:921–927.
81. Blauhut B, Harringer W, Bettelheim P, Doran JE, Spath P, Lundsgaard-Hansen P. Comparison of the effects of aprotinin and tranexamic acid on blood loss and related variables after cardiopulmonary bypass. J thorac Cardiovasc Surg 1994;108:1083–1091.
82. Van Norman G, Ju J, Spiess B, Soltow L, Gillies G. Aprotinin versus aminocaproic acid in moderate-to-high-risk cardiac surgery; relative efficacy and costs. Anesth Analg 1995;80:SCA19.
83. Wong BI, McLean RF, Fermes SE, Harrington BA, Lee E. Aprotinin and tranexamic acid for complex open-heart surgery. Anesth Analg 1995;80:SCA–13.
84. Pugh SC, Wielogorski AK. A comparison of the effects of tranexamic acid and low-dose aprotinin on blood loss and homologous blood usage in patients undergoing cardiac surgery. J Cardiothorac Vasc Anesth 1995;9:240–244.
85. Fremes SE, Wong BI, Lee E, et al. Metaanalysis of prophylactic drug treatment in the prevention of postoperative bleeding. Ann Thorac Surg 1994;58:1580–1588.

Chapter 27

Fibrin Glue

ALEXANDER P. REINER

INTRODUCTION

Fibrin glue, also referred to as fibrin sealant, fibrin adhesive, biological glue, or tissue glue, is a topical hemostatic and adhesive agent used in a variety of surgical procedures. Although its use is more widespread in Europe, there has been a recent surge of interest in the use of fibrin glue in the United States (1–3). This chapter reviews the composition, mechanism of action, methods of application and clinical uses of fibrin glue and benefits and safety of fibrin glue in comparison with other available surgical hemostatic and adhesive agents.

HISTORICAL PERSPECTIVES

The central importance of fibrinogen and fibrin in hemostasis and wound healing has been recognized for many years. In the early 1900s, fibrin powder was used as a topical hemostatic agent (4), and fibrin patches or tampons were subsequently used to control bleeding during cerebral surgery (5) or from parenchymal organs (6). Fibrin glue was first used as a tissue adhesive during the 1940s. Fibrinogen in the form of autologous plasma was used for peripheral nerve repair (7), and plasma combined with bovine thrombin was used for skin graft attachment (8). These early attempts using "plasma glue" were largely unsuccessful, however, presumably because of the relatively low fibrinogen concentration of plasma.

The development of methods for isolating plasma coagulation proteins and improvements in microsurgical techniques led to the reemergence of fibrin glue as a topical surgical hemostatic and adhesive agent in Europe in the early 1970s. First in animal experiments (9) and later in humans (10), purified fibrinogen in the form of cryoprecipitate and bovine thrombin was used successfully for peripheral nerve reattachment. The subsequent development in Europe of commercial lyophilized fibrinogen concentrates manufactured from pooled human plasma led to the application of fibrin glue in a number of other surgical procedures. In the United States in 1978, however, the Food and Drug Administration banned the use of commercial fibrinogen concentrates derived from pooled human plasma because of the well-documented risk of viral hepatitis transmission (11). Despite the more recent addition of viral inactivation methods by European manufacturers and the well-documented viral safety record of these products, the commercial fibrinogen concentrates remain unlicensed in the United States.

Continued interest in the use of fibrin glue in this country led to the development of single-donor and autologous sources of fibrinogen. In 1983, a method using a small amount of patient autologous blood to make cryoprecipitate was introduced (12). Cryoprecipitation of single-donor plasma was later developed as a large-scale method for production of fibrinogen for use in fibrin glue (13). Because of the relatively inconsistent and low fibrinogen content of cryoprecipitate compared with commercial concentrates, various modifications of or alternatives to this procedure have been developed. These methods have been variably successful in increasing fibrinogen content. Because of the lack of a consistent and readily available source of fibrinogen, experimental and clinical use of fibrin glue in the Unites States has generally lagged behind use in other countries.

COMPOSITION AND MECHANISM OF ACTION

Fibrin glue is derived from two components. The first component contains human fibrinogen and coagulation factor XIII and varying amounts of other plasma proteins such as fibronectin and plasminogen. The second component contains thrombin (of either bovine or human origin) and calcium chloride. In Europe, both components are human derived and supplied in commercial fibrin glue "kits." In the United States, only the bovine thrombin component is commercially available, but commercially manufactured human thrombin and fibrinogen preparations are currently under investigation.

When mixed together, the two components of fibrin glue recapitulate the final stages of the coagulation cascade (Fig. 27.1). In the presence of calcium, thrombin, a coagulation enzyme, or serine protease catalyzes the conversion of fibrinogen to fibrin. Fibrinogen is a 340,000-Da plasma protein that consists of three pairs of Aα, Bβ, and γ polypeptide chains. After thrombin cleavage of fibrinopeptides A and B from the Aα and Bβ chains, fibrinogen begins to polymerize into a stable fibrin clot. Thrombin in the presence of calcium also catalyzes the conversion of factor XIII to activated factor XIII (factor XIIIa). Factor XIIIa, a transglutaminase, catalyzes the formation of cross-links between adjacent fibrin monomers, thus stabilizing and strengthening the insoluble fibrin clot. This imparts adhesive and tensile strength to the glue.

The fibrinogen and thrombin components of fibrin glue are usually applied in equal volumes, and maximal adhesive strength is generally achieved 3–5 minutes after application. The concentrations of the components are important for the desired hemostatic or adhesive effect. Fibrinogen concentration is directly proportional to the adhesive strength of fibrin glue (14, 15). Thrombin concentration, on the other hand, affects the rate of fibrin clot formation. A lower thrombin concentration (e.g., 4 units/mL) results in clot formation in 30 seconds to several minutes and is appropriate for procedures in which the glued surfaces may require some adjustment such as skin grafting or for presealing a porous vascular graft. A higher thrombin concentration (e.g., 500–1000 units/mL) results in clot formation within a few seconds and is used when immediate hemostasis is desired.

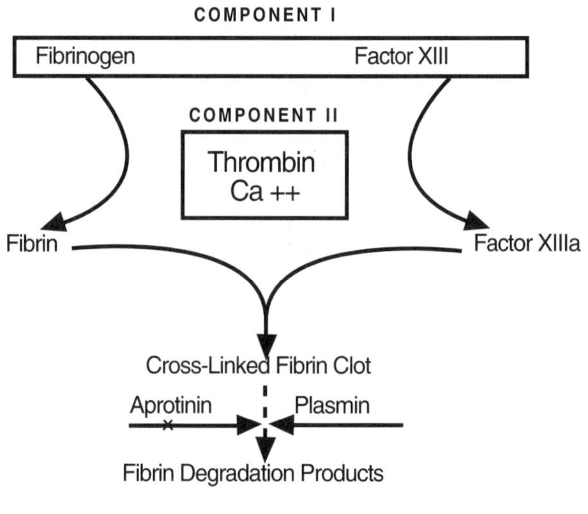

Figure 27.1. Mechanism of action of fibrin glue.

The fibrin clot or adhesive material eventually is completely resorbed by the fibrinolytic enzyme, plasmin (Fig. 27.1). The resorption process occurs within several days to weeks. An antifibrinolytic agent, aprotinin, is sometimes added to either the fibrinogen or thrombin component of fibrin glue to delay lysis of the adhesive material, particularly in areas containing high fibrinolytic activity, such as the lung, oral cavity, or urinary tract.

In addition to its hemostatic function, the components of fibrin glue are also involved in wound healing. Various components of fibrin glue, such as fibrin, thrombin, factor XIII, and fibrinonectin, have been implicated in fibroblast proliferation and granulation tissue formation (16, 17).

METHODS OF APPLICATION

Fibrin glue can be applied by a number of different techniques depending on the type of surgery. Most commonly, the two components of fibrin glue, fibrinogen and thrombin, are either premixed or injected simultaneously using a double-syringe applicator. This commercially available system consists of a holder for two syringes and allows a single plunger to inject equal volumes of the fibrinogen and thrombin solutions into a common "Y" joining piece to which a catheter or needle is attached (Fig. 27.2). This system allows accurate application of relatively small amounts of fibrin glue at the surgical site. For more delicate procedures such as middle ear reconstructive surgery, a microdrop delivery system is available (18). For large surfaces such as skin grafts, the heart, or mediastinum, spray application of fibrin glue is possible by attaching a multichannel catheter to a pressurized gas source (19–21). Finally, fibrin glue can be applied via a carrier such as gauze, collagen fleece, or Gelfoam.

METHODS OF FIBRINOGEN PREPARATION

In Europe, several commercial fibrinogen concentrates prepared from pooled human plasma are currently available (Table 27.1). These concentrates are manufactured using human plasma pooled from thousands of donors. Donors are carefully selected and screened for hepatitis viruses and human immunodeficiency virus (HIV). The fibrinogen is purified from plasma either by cryoprecipitation with or without glycine precipitation or by Cohn ethanol fractionation. These fibrinogen concentrates are either vapor heated, pasteurized,

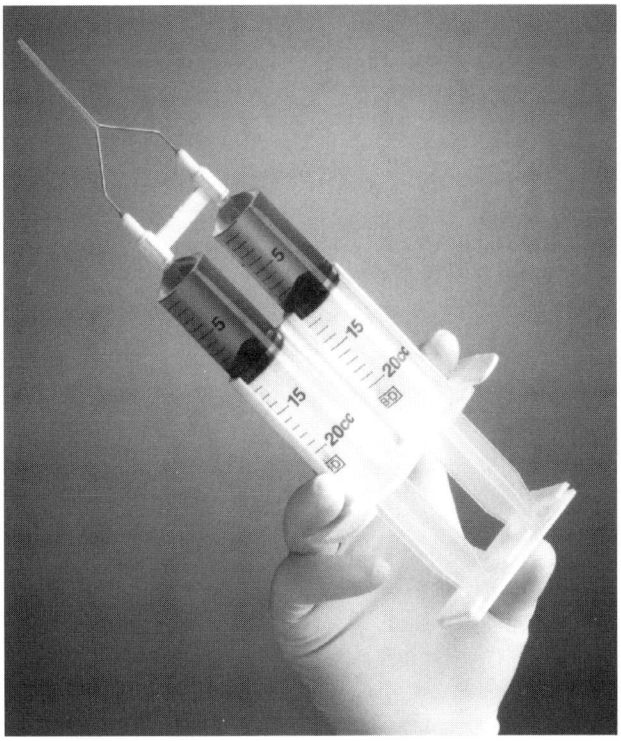

Figure 27.2. Dual-syringe delivery device for fibrin glue application (FibriJet, trademark of Micromedics, Eagan, MN). The two components of fibrin glue (fibrinogen and thrombin) are simultaneously injected into a common "Y: joining piece attached to a needle (shown here) or catheter. This allows mixing of equal volumes of the fibrinogen and thrombin components at the site of application. (Courtesy of Micromedics.)

or solvent/detergent treated to further reduce the risk of viral transmission. Because of the standardized manufacturing process, these products provide a relatively uniform and high concentration of fibrinogen in the range of 100 mg/mL. These concentrates also contain varying amounts of factor XIII, fibronectin, and plasminogen. The fibrinogen concentrates are lyophilized and supplied along with the thrombin component (approximately 500 U/mL) in two-component fibrin glue "kits." In some cases, the components are reconstituted with aprotinin, a fibrinolytic inhibitor.

In the United States, the fibrinogen component of fibrin glue is generally derived from standard blood bank single-donor (13, 22, 23) or autologous (12, 24, 25) cryoprecipitate (Table 27.2). In this sterile closed-system method, citrated plasma obtained by centrifugation of a unit of blood is frozen at −20°C or lower and then slowly thawed to 4°C over several hours. The insoluble cryoprecipitate containing the fibrinogen is separated from the serum supernatant and can be stored at −20°C for up to 1 year. Before use, the cryoprecipitate is resuspended in a small volume (1–10 mL) of plasma or saline. The advantage of autologous cryoprecipitate is the elimination of the risk of viral transmission, but this product requires at least 24 hours to produce and thus cannot be used in emergency settings.

Cryoprecipitation results in the recovery of approximately 50% of the original fibrinogen concentrated approximately 10-fold over normal plasma and can be performed using a variety of different blood volumes. The fibrinogen yield, however, varies widely from approximately 5–25 mg/mL and depends on the plasma fibrinogen concentration of the donor. Although the cryoprecipitation procedure is relatively simple and the closed system is easily adaptable to blood bank standard operating procedures, the yield of fibrinogen is relatively low compared with European commercial fibrinogen concentrates. As a result, various modifications of the standard cryoprecipitation procedure have been described (Table 27.2). The addition of an extra centrifugation step to further concentrate the precipitated fibrinogen can increase the final fibrinogen concentration to approximately 40 mg/mL (26).

TABLE 27.1. EUROPEAN FIBRINOGEN CONCENTRATES CONTAINED IN COMMERCIAL FIBRIN GLUE KITS[a]

Product Name	Manufacturer	Fibrinogen Concentration (mg/mL)	Factor XIII Concentration (U/mL)	Viral Inactivation Step
Tisseel	Immuno (Vienna, Austria)	70–110	10–50	Vapor heat
Beriplast P	Behringwerke AG (Marburg, Germany)	65–115	40–80	Pasteurization
Biocoll	CNTS (Lille, France)	116 ± 2.5	35 ± 2.88	Solvent-detergent

Reprinted with permission from Sierra DH. Fibrin sealant adhesive systems: A review of their chemistry; material properties and clinical applications. J Biomater Appl 1993;7:309–352. Byrne DJ, Hardy J, Wood RAB, McIntosh R, Cuschieri A. Effect of fibrin glues on the mechanical properties of healing wounds. Br J Surg 1991;78:841–843.

[a]These commercial fibrin glue kits also contain human thrombin (~500 units/mL) and varying amounts of the fibrinolytic inhibitor aprotinin.

TABLE 27.2. METHODS OF FIBRINOGEN PREPARATION USED IN THE UNITED STATES[a]

Method	System	Fibrinogen Concentration (mg/mL)	Reference
Standard cryoprecipitation	Closed	5–25	
Modified cryoprecipitation[b]			
1000 × *g*	Open	21.6	13
6500 × *g*	Closed	40 ± 5	26
Double cryoprecipitation[c]			
Whole Blood	Closed	39.8–58.5	14
Plasmapheresis	Closed	78.4 ± 18.3	28
Ammonium sulfate precipitation	Open	28 ± 12	29
Ethanol precipitation	Closed	26 ± 6	31
PEG precipitation	Closed	32.5 (27–39)	32
	Open	31.8 (13.4–47.5)	34
	Open	57–85	35

[a]Includes only references in which fibrinogen concentration is reported.
[b]Additional centrifugation step (centrifugation speed indicated).
[c]Additional freeze–thaw cycle.

The fibrinogen yield depends on the plasma anticoagulant and centrifugation speed used during the procedure (27). The addition of a second freeze–thaw cycle to the cryoprecipitation procedure can increase the fibrinogen yield to approximately 40–80 mg/mL (14, 28).

Various chemical precipitation methods using autologous plasma have been described. The precipitation of fibrinogen by the addition of ammonium sulfate to autologous plasma results in a mean fibrinogen concentration of 28 mg/mL (29). Bonding strength compares favorably with commercial fibrin glue (30). Ethanol precipitation of patient plasma has been used to prepare autologous fibrin glue containing fibrinogen concentration in the range of 25–40 mg/mL (31, 32). In addition, this procedure can be performed perioperatively using the patient's pericardial or mediastinal blood (33). The addition of 30% polyethylene glycol (PEG) to autologous or single-donor plasma absorbed with barium sulfate and magnesium sulfate (34) has resulted in final fibrinogen concentrations as high as 57–85 mg/mL (35).

Unlike standard cryoprecipitation, these modified cryoprecipitation or chemical precipitation procedures generally require the use of an open test tube system and thus are not applicable to blood banks. Exceptions include the modified cryoprecipitation procedure of Spotnitz et al. (26), the double cryoprecipitation methods (14, 28), and the ethanol precipitation method (31, 32), which can be performed in a closed system in which multiple bags or syringes are connected by sterile tubing.

Recently, an intraoperative method of preparing autologous fibrin glue has been described in patients undergoing open heart surgery. Patient plasma is procured from blood that is either withdrawn manually (36) or recovered from a cell-saver device (Haemonetics, Braintree, MA) (37, 38). The autologous plasma or platelet-rich plasma is directly mixed with bovine thrombin and a 10% calcium chloride solution at the operative site. Although fibrinogen content and adhesive strength of this fibrin glue preparation are reduced compared with standard cryoprecipitation procedures, hemostatic efficacy appears to be equivalent (37, 38).

CLINICAL APPLICATIONS

As described below, fibrin glue has been used in numerous surgical procedures that encompass virtually every surgical specialty. The precise role of fibrin glue in many instances, however, remains unclear. Many published reports of fibrin glue are preclinical studies performed in animal models. Furthermore, most human studies consist of uncontrolled observations involving relatively small numbers of patients and often using subjective evaluative criteria. Thus, in most surgical areas described next, there remains a need for prospective controlled clinical trials that compare fibrin glue with other surgical techniques with respect to object endpoints such as blood loss, hospital stay, and mortality. Another problem in interpreting the results of clinical studies of fibrin glue is the wide variation in fibrin glue preparation (particularly the fibrinogen concentration, which is significantly lower and less uniform in the United States). Thus, in comparing one study with another, it is important to keep in mind the particular fibrin glue preparation used.

CARDIOVASCULAR SURGERY

Commercially manufactured fibrin glue has been used extensively in Europe since the 1970s as a local hemostatic and adhesive agent in adults undergoing coronary artery bypass surgery or cardiac valve replacement (39–41) and in children undergoing repair of congenital heart defects (42, 43). More recently, fibrin glue derived either from cryoprecipitate or by ethanol precipitation of single-donor plasma has been used in patients undergoing open heart surgery in the United States (13, 15, 22–24). Fibrin glue is most efficacious in controlling low pressure venous bleeding from coronary grafts or vascular suture sites, anastomoses, and needle holes, especially during reoperative procedures in which bleeding is more difficult to control using conventional methods. Spray application of a uniform layer of fibrin glue can control hemorrhage from anterior mediastinal or cardiac surfaces (19, 39). Point application of fibrin glue is most effective when applied via a topical hemostatic carrier such as collagen.

The subjective utility of fibrin glue in controlling hemorrhage during open heart surgery has been documented in many studies (reviewed in ref. 15). Using more objective criteria, fibrin glue has been reported to reduce postoperative blood loss in patients undergoing open heart surgery. A multicenter, prospective, randomized study in the United States compared the efficacy of fibrin glue (Tisseel, Immuno AG, Vienna, Austria) to conventional methods for bleeding control in patients undergoing reoperative cardiac surgery or emergency resternotomy (44). The success rate for fibrin glue in controlling bleeding was 93% compared with 12% for conventional topical hemostatic agents ($P < .001$). In addition, fibrin glue successfully controlled hemorrhage in 82% of bleeding episodes in which conventional therapy had failed. Finally, the frequency of resternotomy was lower in the fibrin glue group compared with unmatched historical control subjects (6% versus 10%, $P > .0089$). Hospital stay and mortality rates, however, were not significantly different between the two groups. No study comparing fibrin glue to systemic aprotinin or lysis analogue antifibrinolytic has been carried out.

Fibrin glue is also effective in the pretreatment of woven and knitted double velour porous vascular grafts (39, 45–47). Compared with conventional sealing agents such as albumin or whole blood, pretreatment of porous vascular grafts with fibrin glue results in better handling characteristics of the graft and less blood leakage. Other studies indicate that fibrin glue is an optimal agent for the seeding of polytetrafluoroethylene vascular grafts with endothelial cells in vitro (48).

Although fibrin glue has generally been considered less effective in controlling high-pressure arterial bleeding, fibrin glue was used successfully instead of sutures to correct the acute aortic insufficiency associated with type A aortic dissection (49) and to reinforce the closure of an aortic stump after removal of an infected aortic graft (50). In patients with left ventricular free wall rupture, fibrin glue was used to reinforce a sutured autologous pericardial patch repair (51).

THORACIC SURGERY

Air leakage from lung parenchyma, pleurae, or bronchi not infrequently complicates pulmonary resection. Prolonged air leaks usually result from bronchopleural fistulae and are associated with prolonged length of hospitalization and increased mortality. In experimental studies of lung resection in animals, application of fibrin glue to pulmonary and bronchial suture lines is effective in reducing parenchymal air leaks and conserving pulmonary tissue without leading to an increase in postoperative intrapleural adhesions (52–54). In humans, however, the benefit of routine point and/or spray fibrin glue application during pulmonary resection to prevent air leaks is less clear. One randomized prospective study demonstrated a reduction in postoperative air leaks with the routine intraoperative use of fibrin glue in patients undergoing pulmonary resection (55). There was also a slight trend toward reduced hospitalization time in the fibrin glue-treated group. Other prospective studies, however, indicate that routine intraoperative spray application of fibrin glue during pulmonary resection does not have a significant effect on duration of pulmonary air leakage, chest tube drainage, or length of hospitalization in patients undergoing pulmonary resection compared with conventional stapling (56) or electrocautery (57).

Conventional postoperative management of prolonged air leaks due to thoracic fistulae generally consists of thoracostomy with closed drainage by suction. Administration of pleural adhesive agents through the chest tube is sometimes performed. Rarely, a second thoracotomy is required to close the leak, with either sutures or application of a pleural adhesive agent. Fibrin glue can be used as an alternative pleural adhesive agent for sealing postoperative air leaks. In 20 patients with persistent postoperative bronchopleural fistulae, Yasuda et al. (58) demonstrated that fibrin glue was 95% effective and compared favorably with other adhesive agents such as tetracycline. In addition, fibrin glue rarely resulted in the complications of pain and fever common with conventional pleural adhesive agents. Successful closure of bronchopleural fistulae can also be accomplished by rigid (59) or flexible (60–62) bronchoscopic application of fibrin glue. This method can avoid thoracotomy and thus reduce costs and length of hospitalization.

Fibrin glue has similarly been used to treat air leaks resulting from either spontaneous or traumatic pneumothoraces. A retrospective study indicated successful resolution of idiopathic spontaneous pneumothorax using thorascopic administration of fibrin glue in 94% of patients (63). In this setting fibrin glue appears to compare favorably with conventional pleural adhesive agents in terms of length of hospitalization, need for thoracotomy, and pneumothorax recurrence rate. Fibrin glue pleurodesis through a thoracostomy tube has also been used to successfully treat persistent air leakage due to traumatic pneumothorax (64).

Other possible uses of fibrin glue in thoracic surgery have been reported. Thorascopic application of fibrin glue was used to treat large emphysematous bullae (65). Postoperative chylothorax has been successfully managed by fibrin glue applied either thorascopically or via thoracotomy (66, 67). In a recent study of lung transplantation, fibrin glue was used to reduce postoperative air leaks from oversized donor lungs that had undergone staple pneumoreduction in preparation for transplantation into a smaller recipient (68). In a prospective randomized study, fibrin glue compared favorably with tetracycline pleurodesis in the treatment of malignant pleural effusion (69). Fibrin glue has also been effective in experimental studies of tracheal repair (70, 71).

NEUROSURGERY

In neurosurgery, fibrin glue has been used in the management of cerebrospinal fluid (CSF) leaks and in peripheral nerve repair. Neurosurgical procedures involving disruption of the dura can be complicated by CSF leakage. CSF leakage through a dural defect can result in several long-term sequelae such as pseudo-meningocele, arachnoiditis, meningitis, dural-cutaneous fistulae, reduced intracranial pressure, and neurological dysfunction. Conventional methods of dural closure include direct suturing; packing the defect with autologous muscle and fat tissue; and/or covering it with dural, fascial, or muscle homografts. Alternatively, fibrin glue can be applied directly to dural edges; fascia; or an overlying dural, skin or muscle graft. Experimental studies in animals indicate that fibrin glue compares favorably with sutures (72) and that reinforcement of muscle packing with fibrin glue is more effective in preventing CSF leakage during surgery than either agent alone (73). In several retrospective clinical studies of patients undergoing intracranial, craniofacial, or spinal operations, routine intraoperative adjunctive use of either autologous or single-donor cryoprecipitate-derived (74–76) or commercial (77) fibrin glue has been 93–100% successful in preventing postoperative CSF leakage. In a historical comparison of transsphenoidal resection of pituitary tumors, Van Velthoven et al. (77) noted an incidence of postoperative CSF rhinorrhea of 1.0–9.6% with conventional closure techniques versus 1.0–4.4% with conventional techniques supplemented with fibrin glue. Shaffrey et al. (74) reported a somewhat lower success rate of 67% for fibrin glue augmentation of dural closure of established CSF fistulae in 15 patients with posttraumatic, postsurgical, or spontaneous CSF fistulae. In those patients in whom the exact source of the leak could be identified intraoperatively, however, the success rate was higher (12 of 13 patients, or 92%).

Fibrin glue was first used during peripheral nerve repair in humans in 1942 (7). The development of a more consistent and concentrated form of fibrinogen led to the relatively widespread use of fibrin glue in Europe in the 1970s for peripheral nerve repair. The largest experience in Europe was reported by Narakas (78) in brachial plexus and nerve trunk repair. A retrospective review of 122 cases over a 7-year period indicated improved sensorimotor results and reduced operative duration with fibrin glue compared with conventional microsurgical suturing. Narakas' technique involved the application of fibrin glue as an adhesive cylinder around the repaired nerves or fascicles rather than between the transected ends of the nerves (78). The fibrin glue cylinder extends on either side of the apposed nerve ends, thus forming a "regeneration chamber" surrounding the anastomotic site that prevents ingrowth of epineural tissue. Other technical considerations that may be important include immobilization of the transected nerves, avoiding tension to prevent disruption of the apposed nerve ends, and application of only a small amount of fibrin glue to avoid scarring or adhesion to the surrounding tissues.

Despite the European experience, the role of fibrin glue in peripheral nerve repair compared with conventional microsurgical suturing remains controversial. Comparison of fibrin glue with sutures in animal models of nerve repair has yielded mixed results. Some studies suggest that fibrin glue may be superior to conventional suture repair (79, 80), whereas other studies have indicated the superiority of conventional microsuture techniques (81, 82). The potential advantages of fibrin glue over sutures include closer approximation of nerve ends, reduced nerve trauma, and the lack of foreign body reaction. Some problems associated with the use of fibrin glue in peripheral nerve repair may relate to the optimization of the various components of the adhesive. Elevated concentrations of the thrombin or fibrinogen components may lead to the development of nerve fibrosis after fibrin glue application (83). Nerve anastomotic dehiscence, on the other hand, may require the addition of antifibrinolytic agents such as aprotinin. More recent modifications of the fibrin adhesive technique may result in improved nerve repair. These modifications include applying fibrin glue mixed with nerve growth factors (84) or improving axonal alignment by freezing the nerve stumps before application of fibrin glue (85).

Other potential neurosurgical uses of fibrin glue include closure of carotid cavernous fistulae (86) and attachment of spinal cord-stimulating electrodes after limited laminectomy for treatment of pain syndromes and spasticity disorders (87).

OTORHINOLARYNGOLOGY

Middle ear reconstructive surgery may be required as a result of trauma, tumors, malformation, acute or chronic otitis, or cholesteatoma. Because of the disappointing results of synthetic glues such as cyanoacrylates in middle ear reconstructive surgery, commercial fibrin glue in Europe (88–90) and various preparations of autologous fibrin glue in the United States (25, 35, 91–93) have become widely used for myringoplasty and tympanoplasty. The methods of preparation of autologous or single-donor–derived fibrin glue have included cryoprecipitation (25, 92), ammonium sulfate precipitation (91, 93), or PEG precipitation (35). During tympanoplasty, fibrin glue can be used for fixation of fascial grafts, attachment of the graft to the malleus, and/or attachment of middle ear bony structures. Precise positioning of the tympanic graft or ossicular structures can be accomplished using fibrin glue itself or in combination with other tissues such as bone, cartilage, fascia, areolar tissue, biocompatible prostheses, or Gelfoam. Intraoperative application can be performed using either a standard dual-component syringe system or a microdrop delivery system (18). Although the reported success of fibrin glue in middle ear surgery in humans has been mainly subjective, experimental studies in animals have objectively documented the efficacy and long-term safety of fibrin glue (94–97).

Stapes surgery secondary to otosclerosis can sometimes be complicated by displacement of the stapes prosthesis. Marquet (90) reported successful stapedectomy without complications in 100 patients in which fibrin glue was applied after prosthesis placement. Nissen et al. (92) reported successful flap closure of the stapes using fibrin glue alone or by covering the prosthesis with fascia combined with fibrin glue. In chinchillas, Siedentop and Schobel (98) reported good results with the use of fascia grafting with fibrin glue to close the oval window after stapedectomy.

Perilymph fistulas due to rupture of the oval or round windows can occur secondary to surgery or trauma or spontaneously. Marquet (90) reported treatment of three cases of perilymph fistulas by implantation of allogeneic stapes covered with fibrin glue. Other investigators have repaired these defects using minced areolar tissue and/or fascia combined with fibrin glue (99, 100).

In reconstruction of the auditory canal, it is sometimes necessary to obliterate the mastoid cavity. A variety of materials such as autologous bone powder or paste, ceramics, or hydroxyapatite powder have been used. In some cases, fibrin glue has been combined with autologous bone powder before placement into the cavity (92, 101, 102).

Persistent CSF otorhinorrhea not infrequently complicates acoustic neurinoma surgery and may require surgical repair with mastoidectomy, translabyrinthine repair, or reexploration of the suboccipital craniectomy. Sierra et al. (103) reported four cases of acoustic neurinoma removal in which dural suture closure was augmented by fibrin glue combined with muscle and Gelfoam. No CSF leakage or adverse reactions to fibrin glue were noted. Symon and Pell (104) used bone dust combined with Surgicel and fibrin glue to seal mastoid air cells exposed during craniectomy for acoustic neurinoma removal. Compared with historical control subjects, there was a marked reduction in CSF leakage from 16% to 5%. Another recent retrospective study, on the other hand, found no improvement in CSF leakage with the use of fibrin glue during acoustic neuroma surgery (105).

Fibrin glue has been used in various other procedures in otorhinolaryngology. Successful control of postoperative hemorrhage in nasal septal surgery has been reported (106). This procedure avoids nasal packing, thus reducing patient discomfort and presumably length of hospitalization. Fibrin glue applied during endoscopic sinus surgery similarly results in improved hemostasis and mucosal healing and can eliminate the need for postoperative packing (107). Fibrin glue has also been effective in attachment of mucosal grafts during surgical treatment of laryngeal webs (108). A retrospective comparison of fibrin glue versus standard suture closure in thyroidectomy and parathyroidectomy indicated reduced postoperative drainage and length of hospitalization with a comparable complication rate (109).

PLASTIC SURGERY

A crude preparation of autologous fibrin glue was first used to adhere skin grafts in 1944 (8). Experimental models of skin grafting indicate that fibrin bonding of the elastin in skin grafts to the elastin in the recipient site is essential for initial graft adherence and graft survival (110). Numerous subsequent clinical studies have documented the utility of commercial, autologous, or single-donor fibrin glue in skin grafting. Fibrin glue is particularly useful as an adhesive agent in technically difficult areas that are either difficult to immobilize or contain contoured surfaces such as the face, neck, shoulders, axillae, eyelids, and buttocks (14, 111–116) and infected areas (116, 117). Graft success has been in the range of 90–100%. Fibrin glue is ineffective in parotidectomy, however, due to the high local fibrinolytic activity.

Compared with standard techniques, the advantages of fibrin glue in plastic surgery include improved hemostasis, improved graft adherence, reduced operative time, and reduced postoperative care and length of hospitalization. A retrospective study of aerosolized fibrin glue in patients undergoing facelifts demonstrated a statistically significant reduction in hematoma formation, decreased postoperative edema and ecchymoses, reduced postoperative care, and improved patient comfort (118). Similar results were reported by Flemming (119). In patients with dorsal hand burns, a retrospective comparison of fibrin glue in split-thickness skin grafting showed improved recovery of sensation and mobility compared with standard suturing (120). In a rat model, Brown et al. (121) demonstrated that fibrin glue reduced wound contraction in skin grafting. The mechanism may involve increased adherence of the skin grafts to wound beds or improved revascularization of the wound surface.

In patients with extensive burns, the transplantation of autologous epidermal cells or keratinocytes that have been grown in culture in vitro has been used as a supplement to conventional skin grafting. These cultured sheet grafts, however, are fragile, difficult to handle, and associated with variable rates of graft success. In an experimental model, fibrin glue was shown to enhance cultured epidermal graft stability and increase the rate of graft take (122). Recently, autologous keratinocytes cultured or suspended in fibrin glue have been used successfully in several patients with extensive burn wounds (123, 124). In some cases, the keratinocyte graft was covered with an allogeneic cadaver skin graft. Although further studies are required, this technique shows promise in the treatment of extensive burns.

Seromas are a common complication of mastectomy. Fibrin glue has been demonstrated to reduce postoperative seroma formation in rat mastectomy and modified radical neck dissection models (125–127). Recent prospective randomized studies in humans, however, show conflicting results. In one study, the use of fibrin glue was associated with a significant reduction in postoperative axillary lymphatic secretion in patients undergoing mastectomy for breast carcinoma (128). Other studies, however, failed to show an effect on postoperative drainage or hospital stay in patients undergoing radical mastectomy (129, 130). Fibrin glue has also been used in the postoperative management of rhinophyma (131) and for grafting of cartilage fragments during rhinoplasty (132).

ORTHOPEDIC SURGERY

In orthopedic surgery, fibrin glue has been used to attach periosteal and perichondral grafts, to repair cartilage and tendons, and to fill bony defects. Success has been variable, however, and there is a paucity of clinical studies. Furthermore, although earlier clinical and experimental studies indicated a favorable effect of fibrin glue on remodeling rates of homologous and heterologous bone grafts, the effects of fibrin glue on bone healing and osteoinduction are currently controversial (17, 133).

Articular cartilage defects heal spontaneously by formation of fibrocartilaginous tissue, which has relatively poor biomechanical properties. For this reason, chondral lesions are often covered with either an autologous (e.g., rib cartilage) or homologous perichondral graft. In the case of small chondral defects, transplanted chondrocytes are sometimes used. Fibrin glue has been used to attach perichondral grafts to subchondral bone (17, 134). In animal models, fibrin glue has been used as a delivery vehicle for transplanted chondrocytes (135, 136) or for chondrocyte allograft fixation (137), but the results have been variable. In other animal studies, fibrin glue has been used successfully for osteochrondral fracture repair, either alone (138, 139) or in combination with polytetrafluoroethylene patches (140).

Fibrin glue has been used in the arthroscopic repair of meniscal tears. A prospective analysis of 32 patients indicated a success rate of 80% by follow-up arthroscopy, and only 2 patients had recurrent meniscal symptoms with a follow-up up to 6 years (141). The authors indicate that fibrin glue is most useful in tears involving the posterior segment, which is difficult to suture without arthrotomy.

Excellent experimental and clinical results have been obtained using fibrin glue for Achilles tendon repair (17). When combined with absorbable sutures, fibrin glue reduces the need for sutures, thus reducing scar formation. In a rabbit model, compared with sutures, fibrin glue was shown to prevent adhesion formation in flexor tendon repair (142).

During orthopedic or craniofacial surgery, bony defects can be filled with either ceramic implants of calcium phosphate or hydroxyapatite or with autologous or homologous cancellous bone fragments. Filling bony defects with either bone grafts or ceramic implants can be complicated by early postoperative migration and displacement. In a study of 19 patients undergoing spine surgery, the adjunctive use of fibrin glue with autologous bone fragments was reported to prevent graft displacement and thus the complication of cord compression (143). Lack et al. (144) reported successful treatment of 29 bone defects caused by chronic osteomyelitis treated with radical excision followed by cancellous bone allografts fixed with fibrin glue. Fibrin glue combined with autologous bone powder has been applied as a paste to obliterate frontal sinuses during frontocranial remodeling (145).

ORAL AND MAXILLOFACIAL SURGERY

Fibrin glue has also been used as an adjunctive agent in the repair of bony defects in oral and maxillofacial surgery. Reconstruction of the anterior wall of the maxillary sinus has been accomplished without wire using homologous or autologous bone fragments combined with fibrin glue for filling bony defects (16). Tayapongsak et al. (146) reported 33 cases of mandibular reconstruction using autologous cancellous bone fragments in which the adjunctive use of fibrin glue prevented postoperative bone graft particle displacement and hastened the remodeling process by 50%. Fibrin glue has similarly been used to prevent postoperative dislocation of hydroxyapatite particles in patients undergoing maxillary alveolar ridge reconstructive surgery (147, 148). Fibrin glue has also been shown to be effective in the fixation of tissues and as a hemostatic agent compared with sutures in periodontal surgery (149).

In patients with congenital or acquired bleeding disorders, fibrin glue is an effective adjunctive local hemostatic agent during dental extractions (150, 151). Because of the high local concentration of fibrinolytic activators, a relatively high concentration of aprotinin (10,000 kallikrein inactivator units [KIU]/mL) should be included in the fibrin glue preparation.

TRAUMA AND GENERAL SURGERY

Blunt and penetrating abdominal trauma is frequently associated with injuries to the liver or spleen. Overall mortality is in the range of 10–15%, and hemorrhage is the most common cause of death (152). In the case of splenic injury, it is preferable to avoid splenectomy, because of the increased postoperative risk of early and late infection complications, particularly sepsis with encapsulated bacteria. Studies in trauma patients have demonstrated that commercial or single-donor fibrin glue is 90–100% effective in controlling hemorrhage from the liver and spleen (20, 153–157). In approximately 80% of cases, splenectomy could be avoided (153, 156). Because all the elements for formation of a hemostatic plug are contained within the fibrin glue, hemostasis can be achieved even in patients with underlying coagulopathy and/or thrombocytopenia (155, 157). In some cases, fibrin glue is effective only after larger arterial and venous bleeders are suture-ligated or clipped (157). Topical application of fibrin glue can control less severe sinusoidal bleeding, whereas intraparenchymal injection of fibrin glue may be required for more severe bleeding involving larger vessels (154, 157). Fibrin glue can also be applied with collagen fleece or by an aerosolized spray device. In relatively stable patients with parenchymal organ injury after abdominal trauma, laparoscopic injection of fibrin glue may be useful in controlling hemorrhage (158).

In a prospective randomized study, Kohno et al. (159) compared fibrin glue with collagen powder in 62 patients undergoing liver resection. Intraoperative hemostasis and morbidity and mortality were equivalent, but fibrin glue was associated with a reduction in postoperative complications such as rebleeding or bile leakage. A combination of fibrin glue and collagen has been described for controlling hemorrhage in patients undergoing partial hepatectomy (160). In living related liver transplantation, fibrin glue sprayed on the cut surface of the liver graft and remnant liver of the donor is hemostatically effective (161). Fibrin glue has also been effective in sealing the liver biopsy needle track in several high-risk patients (162, 163) and in radiological embolization of a large inferior mesenteric–caval shunt for treatment of portal hypertension (164).

Anastomotic dehiscence or leakage is a major complication of surgery involving the gastrointestinal tract. Anastomotic leakage is associated with significant morbidity and mortality, and the risk is particularly high in segments of the gastrointestinal tract that do not contain serosa, such as the esophagus and rectum. Adhesive materials such as cyanoacrylate glues have been studied to prevent postoperative bowel anastomotic leakage, but results have been poor. Fibrin glue has been used as an adjunctive agent in normal and high-risk bowel anastomoses to prevent leakage, but experimental studies have yielded conflicting results, and prospective clinical studies are lacking. Some experimental studies have suggested that fibrin glue reinforcement of high-risk intestinal anastomoses (165–168) or esophageal anastomoses (169, 170) has a beneficial effect in gastrointestinal tract surgery. Many of these earlier studies, however, suffer from poor experimental design and include small numbers of animals. Other animal studies indicate no benefit or even a detrimental effect of fibrin glue on colonic anastomosis healing in terms of adhesion formation, inflammatory reactions, anastomotic leakage, and abscess formation (171–174). Only two clinical studies have been reported. A retrospective analysis by Scheele et al. (165) indicated reduced anastomotic leakage and postoperative mortality in fibrin glue–treated patients. In contrast, a prospective clinical study of 100 patients demonstrated no beneficial effect of fibrin glue in the reinforcement of esophageal anastomoses (175).

There are several uncontrolled studies of the use of fibrin glue in sealing various fistulae and sinuses involving the gastrointestinal tract. Several reports describe successful closure of chronic perineal sinuses, rectovaginal, or anal fistulas in 70–80% of patients by blind injection of either commercial (176, 177) or autologous (178) fibrin glue. McCarthy et al. (179) successfully treated a patient with upper gastrointestinal bleeding due to a duodenal sinus secondary to Crohn's disease with endoscopic application of barium-impregnated fibrin glue. Surgical intervention could be avoided in this patient who had previously undergone numerous operative procedures for fistulae involving his gastrointestinal tract. Endoscopic application of fibrin glue was also successful in 11 of 17 patients with enterocutaneous fistulae and in 5 of 8 patients with intra-abdominal abscesses (180). Complications developed in four patients, however, including one patient who died of an air embolism as a result of the procedure.

Two recent randomized studies prospectively evaluated the use of fibrin glue in the surgical management of peptic ulcer disease. Berg et al. (181) found fibrin glue application at least as hemostatically effective as endoscopic sclerotherapy in the treatment of bleeding peptic ulcers. In a study of 100 patients with perforated peptic ulcers, laparoscopic application of fibrin glue was technically easier yet as effective as laparoscopic suture repair or patch repair laparotomy (182).

In a canine model, fibrin glue has been used successfully for sealing the common bile duct during biliary tract surgery (183). A retrospective clinical study indicated efficacy in preventing anastomotic leaks in pancreaticojejunostomy (184). In patients undergoing pancreatic surgery for traumatic and nontraumatic conditions, fibrin glue has been applied to pancreatic tissue and anastomoses. In one study, no postoperative pancreatic fistulas, abscesses, or pseudocysts developed in these patients (185). This was compared with a postoperative fistula rate of 29% in historical control subjects. Two recent prospective randomized studies were reported. A study of 56 patients undergoing distal pancreatectomy indicated a reduced incidence of pancreatic fistulae in patients treated with fibrin glue as compared with conventional surgical technique (186). A study of 97 patients, on the other hand, failed to show a benefit of fibrin glue in preventing postoperative pancreatic fistulas (187).

OPHTHALMIC SURGERY

Fibrin glue has been used in the repair of orbital defects. Härting et al. (188) used fibrin glue to attach a split-thickness skin graft to the bony orbit after exenteration. Compared with granulation techniques or pressure bandaging, this method was believed to shorten the time until an orbital prosthesis could be placed. In a patient with a traumatic nasal-orbital defect, fibrin glue was used to attach a fascial graft to repair a right medial orbital fistula (189). Fibrin glue was also used instead of sutures to attach a full-thickness mucosal graft during reconstruction of the lower fornix of an anophthalmic socket (190).

Fibrin glue has been used in various other types of ophthalmic surgery. Mori et al. (191) successfully repaired a spontaneous scleral perforation by attaching lyophilized homologous dura to the scleral defect using fibrin glue. In this case, the defect was in the posterior part of the eye and was too deep to suture. Zauberman and Hemo (192) reported the use of fibrin glue in 60 cases of ocular surgery, including 40 extracapsular cataract extractions, 10 retinal detachments, and 10 cases of strabismus. Fibrin glue was believed to be a good alternative to cauterization for hemostasis and to sutures for attachment of conjunctiva to the limbus. In the area of cataract surgery, Mester et al. (193) conducted a randomized prospective study of 385 patients undergoing phacoemulsification with posterior chamber lens implantation, comparing fibrin glue with single-stitch technique for wound closure. Results were comparable for the two techniques, and fibrin glue prevented the complication of postoperative against-the-rule astigmatism. Successful repair of perforated corneal ulcers has also been accomplished using fibrin glue (194). In some cases, keratoplasty could be postponed or avoided. In glaucoma surgery, Kajiwara (195) reported the use of fibrin glue to close a dehisced postoperative conjunctival wound in a patient who had undergone trabeculotomy that was complicated by a persistent aqueous leakage despite resuturing.

OBSTETRICS AND GYNECOLOGY

Reports of the use of fibrin glue in obstetrics and gynecologic surgery have been limited (196). Intracervical application of fibrin glue for sealing of premature ruptured amniotic membranes was first reported by Genz in 1979 (197). Over several years, Genz treated 20 cases of premature ruptured membranes with fibrin glue during the first or second trimester with a success rate of 60% (196). Baumgarten and Moser (198) achieved a similar success rate for intracervical application of fibrin glue in the treatment of premature ruptured membranes but found that the technique was most successful after the 32nd week of gestation. Perinatal mortality was 50% in patients treated before the 28th week of gestation. Thus, their results with fibrin glue were approximately the same as the results with patients receiving standard tocolytic treatment. At delivery, single-donor fibrin glue has been applied topically to control bleeding from the umbilical cannulation site when other hemostatic techniques have failed (199). Fibrin glue was used instead of serum or culture medium for uterine embryo transfer in 38 patients undergoing in vitro fertilization (200). It was proposed that the use of fibrin glue may decrease the complications of embryo expulsion and ectopic pregnancy. Pregnancy was established in 26% of 38 cases, compared with a pregnancy success rate of 19% in historical control subjects performed without fibrin glue.

In gynecological surgery, fibrin glue has been shown in clinical and experimental studies to be useful in the closure of vesicovaginal or rectovaginal fistulas (196). Fibrin glue has also been used successfully in vaginal reconstructive surgery (196). Experimental studies of the use of fibrin glue in microsurgical end-to-end anastomosis of fallopian tubes in animals have been summarized (196). It was concluded that compared with microsurgical techniques, the use of fibrin glue shortened operating time, reduced surgical trauma to oviduct stumps, reduced tissue ischemia, and decreased adhesion formation. In a clinical study, fibrin glue was used successfully in combination with a single-stitch technique for tubal anastomosis in women undergoing reversal of tubal ligation (201).

UROLOGY

In 1981, Fischer et al. (202) reported the use of fibrin glue in 61 cases of surgical removal of renal calculi (i.e., "coagulum pyelolithotomy"). Fibrin glue was injected into the renal pelvis via an angiocatheter; after 3 minutes, a pyelotomy was performed and the clot extracted. Calculus removal was successful in 90% of the cases in both dilated and nondilated pyelocaliceal systems. More recently, however, percutaneous nephrolithotomy and extracorporeal shock lithotripsy have replaced conventional kidney stone surgery. Percutaneous nephrolithotomy can be complicated by venous or arterial bleeding from the renal parenchyma. Fibrin glue was effective for the treatment of immediate and delayed renal parenchymal bleeding when applied via the nephrostomy tract in 26 patients undergoing percutaneous nephrolithotomy (203). In contrast, fibrin glue was no more effective than conventional sutures in reducing postoperative urinary leakage from the ureter in patients undergoing ureteral stone surgery (204).

Fibrin glue has been used in cases of renal and ureteral trauma and kidney surgery (205–207). Application of fibrin glue to the renal parenchyma can reduce venous oozing, and in some cases nephrectomy can be avoided. Ureteral anastomoses can be accomplished with less reliance on suture redundancy. Levinson et al. (208) reported the use of fibrin glue as an adjunctive agent for controlling venous bleeding from cut surfaces of the kidney in seven patients who underwent partial nephrectomy. Although there were no bleeding complications, urine leaks developed in two patients. Thus, fibrin glue may not be as effective in sealing or preventing urinary leaks because of the relatively high fibrinolytic activity of urine.

Other urological applications of fibrin glue have been reported. Fibrin glue has been used to seal peritoneal dialysis catheter leaks that have failed conventional management (209); catheter removal thus could be avoided. In 8 of 10 patients with severe hemophilia A undergoing circumcision, local fibrin glue application eliminated the need for factor VIII infusion (210). In animal studies, fibrin glue has been compared with conventional microsurgical techniques in animals undergoing vasovasostomy (211, 212). Vasovagal anastomosis with fibrin glue resulted in similar patency rates, reduced operative time, and greater postoperative tensile strength of the sutured anastomosis.

DELIVERY VEHICLE

Although studies have been limited, fibrin glue may be useful for localized delivery of antibiotics to prevent infection at surgical anastomotic or graft sites or treatment of preexisting infections (213–215). A potential advantage of localized delivery with fibrin glue is the relatively small dose of antibiotic required to produce an antibacterial effect; this may eliminate or reduce the side effects that can complicate systemic drug administration.

Fibrin glue has also shown potential for the localized delivery of growth factors or agents that promote wound healing to wounds, grafts, or tissues (84, 216, 217). Greisler et al. (218) demonstrated that perfusion of a combination of fibroblast growth factor type 1 and fibrin glue into polytetrafluoroethylene grafts that were transplanted into rabbit aortas resulted in graft endothelialization. This method may be an effective alternative to direct graft seeding with cultured endothelial cells.

BENEFITS AND RISKS OF FIBRIN GLUE

ADVANTAGES OF FIBRIN GLUE

Because it is derived from biological materials, fibrin glue has certain advantages over nonbiological hemostatic and adhesive agents such as sutures, staples, and synthetic glues. Compared with these nonbiological agents, fibrin glue is tissue-compatible and completely resorbed and thus less likely to induce inflammatory or foreign body reactions (72).

Fibrin and other components of fibrin glue (e.g., fibronectin, factor XIII, thrombin) are involved in the process of wound healing and tissue repair. Some, but not all, studies indicate a beneficial effect of fibrin glue on wound healing (17, 219, 220). These conflicting results may reflect the nonuniformity of fibrinogen concentration and other components within different fibrin glue formulations. For example, in animal models of wound healing, higher fibrinogen concentrations (as found in the commercial fibrin glue preparations) can actually *inhibit* wound healing (219, 220).

Although the use of fibrin glue might be expected to promote adhesion formation, paradoxically there is some experimental evidence of reduced intra-abdominal adhesion formation (221–223). This may be related to the formation of a physiochemical "barrier" to the influx of various inflammatory mediators at the wound site. This barrier phenomenon may also account for inhibition of both intra-abdominal abscess formation (224) and perianastomotic tumor cell migration (225) in animal models of fibrin glue application.

SAFETY OF FIBRIN GLUE

Despite earlier fears of viral transmission with the use of fibrinogen concentrates prepared from pooled human plasma, there has never been a single case reported of viral transmission with the use of these commercial concentrates in over 1 million applications in Europe (44). In addition to donor screening and testing for viral markers, the existing European commercial fibrinogen concentrates are treated with vapor heat, pasteurization, or solvent/detergent to inactivate viruses (Table 27.1). In the United States, although the safety of volunteer single-donor blood components continues to improve with more stringent donor screening criteria and the application of an increasing number of donor screening tests, a small but finite risk of disease transmission remains (see Chapter 7). In the United States, there has been one reported case of HIV transmission in a patient who received two homologous units of cryoprecipitate intraoperatively for fibrin glue (226). For this reason, autologous cryoprecipitate is preferred whenever possible, because the risk of infectious disease transmission is virtually eliminated.

The other major risk involved in the use of fibrin glue is the development of immune-mediated or hypersensitivity reactions. This is of particular concern with the exposure to bovine proteins (i.e., thrombin or aprotinin) contained within fibrin glue. An anaphylactic reaction to fibrin glue used to close a bronchopleural fistula was reported in a patient with hypogammaglobulinemia and elevated anti-IgA antibody titers (227). A patient undergoing pulmonary resection developed an anaphylactic reaction that was attributed to the aprotinin within a commercial fibrin glue preparation (228). Berguer et al. (229) reported two cases of severe hypotension after the injection of fibrin glue into deep hepatic wounds secondary to trauma. One patient died as a result, whereas the other survived with fluid resuscitation and vasopressors. The authors obtained a similar hypotensive effect upon injecting fibrin glue intravenously in an animal experiment. They also noted that the commercial manufacturer of bovine thrombin disclosed an additional 16 cases of hypotension or death associated with the use of its product. Although an anaphylactic reaction to bovine proteins is possible, a more likely explanation in this setting is activation of the coagulation system with resultant disseminated intravascular coagulation and hypotension caused by relatively large amounts of thrombin entering the circulation through the venous system of the liver.

Recently, it was noted that patients receiving fibrin glue, particularly during open heart surgery, can develop antibodies against bovine thrombin and/or factor V (230–233). The antibodies against bovine thrombin result in prolongation of the patient's thrombin time (because bovine thrombin is used for the in vitro assay) but are clinically insignificant. The factor V antibodies, on the other hand, occasionally cross-react with human factor V and can result in significant clinical bleeding complications postoperatively. Treatment with fresh-frozen plasma, intravenous gamma globulin, and plasmapheresis may be required. The recent development of human thrombin preparations in Europe and the United States should ultimately eliminate the problem of sensitization to bovine coagulation proteins.

REFERENCES

1. Gibble JW, Ness PM. Fibrin glue: the perfect operative sealant? Transfusion 1990;30:741–747.
2. Sierra DH. Fibrin sealant adhesive systems: a review of their chemistry, material properties and clinical applications. J Biomater Appl 1993;7: 309–352.
3. Spotnitz WD. Fibrin sealant in the United States: clinical use at the University of Virginia. Thromb Haemost 1995;74:482–485.
4. Bergel S. Uber Wirkugen des Fibrins. Dtsch Med Wochenschr 1909;35: 633–665.
5. Grey EG. Fibrin as a hemostatic in cerebral surgery. Surg Gynecol Obstet 1915;21:452–454.
6. Harvey SC. The use of fibrin papers and foams in surgery. Boston Med Surg J 1916;174:659–662.
7. Seddon HJ, Medawar PB. Fibrin suture of human nerves. Lancet 1942; 2:87–92.
8. Cronkite EP, Lozner EL, Deaver J. Use of thrombin and fibrinogen in skin grafting. JAMA 1944;124:976–978.
9. Matras H, Dinges HP, Lassmann H, Manoli B. Zur Nahtlosen Interfaszikularen Nerventransplantation im Tierexperiment [Suture-free interfascicular nerve transplantation in animal experiments]. Wien Med Wochenschr 1972;122:517–523.
10. Kuderna H, Matras H. Die Klinische Anwendung der Klebung von Nerveanatomosen bei der Rekonstruktion Verletzer Peripherer Nerven. Wien Klin Wochenschr 1975;87:495–501.

11. Bove JR. Fibrinogen—is the benefit worth the risk? Transfusion 1978; 18:129–136.
12. Gestring GF, Lerner R. Autologous fibrinogen for tissue-adhesion, hemostasis and embolization. Vasc Surg 1983;17:294–304.
13. Dresdale A, Rose EA, Jeevanandam V, Reemtsma K, Bowman FO, Malm JR. Preparation of fibrin glue from single-donor fresh-frozen plasma. Surgery 1985;97:750–754.
14. Saltz R, Sierra D, Feldman D, Saltz MB, Dimick A, Vasconez LO. Experimental and clinical applications of fibrin glue. Plast Reconstr Surg 1991;88:1005–1015.
15. McCarthy PM. Fibrin glue in cardiothoracic surgery. Transfus Med Rev 1993;7:173–179.
16. Matras H. Fibrin seal: the state of the art. J Oral Maxillofac Surg 1985;43:605–611.
17. Schlag G, Redl H. Fibrin sealant in orthopedic surgery. Clin Orthop 1988;227:268–285.
18. Arenberg IK, Altshuler JH. Autologous fibrin glue (AFG) and sealant: standard and microdrop delivery systems. Otolaryngol Head Neck Surg 1989;101:709–712.
19. Spotnitz WD, Dalton MS, Baker JW, Nolan SP. Reduction of perioperative hemorrhage by anterior mediastinal spray application of fibrin glue during cardiac operations. Ann Thorac Surg 1987;44:529–531.
20. Kram HB, Shoemaker WC, Clark SR, Macabee JR, Yamaguchi MA. Spraying of aerosolized fibrin glue in the treatment of nonsuturable hemorrhage. Am Surg 1991;57:381–384.
21. Ogawa J, Inoue H, Koide S, Shohtsu A. Newly devised instrument for spraying aerosolized fibrin glue in thoracoscopic operations. Ann Thorac Surg 1993;55:1595–1596.
22. Rousou JA, Engelman RM, Breyer RH. Fibrin glue: An effective hemostatic agent for nonsuturable intraoperative bleeding. Ann Thorac Surg 1984;38:409–410.
23. Lupinetti FM, Stoney WS, Alford WC Jr, et al. Cryoprecipitate—topical thrombin glue: initial experience in patients undergoing cardiac operations. J Thorac Cardiovasc Surg 1985;90:502–505.
24. Dresdale A, Bowman FO Jr, Malm JR, et al. Hemostatic effectiveness of fibrin glue derived from single-donor fresh frozen plasma. Ann Thorac Surg 1985;40:385–387.
25. Moretz WH Jr, Shea JJ Jr, Emmett JR, Shea JJ III. A simple autologous fibrinogen glue for otologic surgery. Otolaryngol Head Neck Surg 1986;95:122–124.
26. Spotnitz WD, Mintz PD, Avery N, Bithell TC, Kaul S, Nolan SP. Fibrin glue from stored human plasma: an inexpensive and efficient method for local blood bank preparation. Am Surg 1987;53:460–462.
27. DePalma L, Criss VR, Luban NLC. The preparation of fibrinogen concentrate for use as fibrin glue by four different methods. Transfusion 1993;33:717–720.
28. Casali B, Rodeghiero F, Tosetto A, et al. Fibrin glue from single-donation autologous plasmapheresis. Transfusion 1992;32:641–643.
29. Park MS, Cha CI. Biochemical aspects of autologous fibrin glue derived from ammonium sulfate precipitation. Laryngoscope 1993;103: 193–196.
30. Siedentop KH, Harris DM, Sanchez B. Autologous fibrin tissue adhesive. Laryngoscope 1985;95:1074–1076.
31. Kjaergard HK, Weis-Fogh US, Sørensen H, Thiis J, Rygg I. A simple method of preparation of autologous fibrin glue by means of ethanol. Surg Gynecol Obstet 1992;175:72–73.
32. Dahlstrøm KK, Weis-Fogh US, Medgyesi S, Rostgaard J, Sørensen H. The use of autologous fibrin adhesive in skin transplantation. Plast Reconstr Surg 1992;89:968–972.
33. Kjaergard HK, Weis-Fogh US, Thiis JJ. Preparation of autologous fibrin glue from pericardial blood. Ann Thorac Surg 1993;55:543–544.
34. Weisman RA, Torsiglieri AJ, Schreiber AD, Epstein GH. Biochemical characterization of autologous fibrinogen adhesive. Laryngoscope 1987; 97:1186–1190.
35. Silberstein LE, Williams LJ, Hughlett MA, Magee DA, Weisman RA. An autologous fibrinogen-based adhesive for use in otologic surgery. Transfusion 1988;28:319–321.
36. Hartman AR, Galanakis DK, Honig MP, Seifert FC, Anagnostopoulos CE. Autologous whole plasma fibrin gel: intraoperative procurement. Arch Surg 1992;127:357–359.
37. Oz MC, Jeevanandam V, Smith CR, et al. Autologous fibrin glue from intraoperatively collected platelet-rich plasma. Ann Thorac Surg 1992; 53:530–531.
38. Quigley RL, Perkins JA, Gottner RJ, et al. Intraoperative procurement of autologous fibrin glue. Ann Thorac Surg 1993;56:387–389.
39. Borst HG, Haverich A, Walterbusch G, Maatz W. Fibrin adhesive: an important hemostatic adjunct in cardiovascular operations. J Thorac Cardiovasc Surg 1982;84:548–553.
40. Köveker G. Clinical application of fibrin glue in cardiovascular surgery. Thorac Cardiovasc Surgeon 1982;30:228–229.
41. Wolner E. Fibrin gluing in cardiovascular surgery. Thorac Cardiovasc Surgeon 1982;30:236–237.
42. Huth C, Seybold-Epting W, Hoffmeister HE. Local hemostasis with fibrin glue after intracardiac repair of tetralogy of Fallot and transposition of the great arteries. Thorac Cardiovasc Surgeon 1983;31:142–146.
43. Stark J, de Leval M. Experience with fibrin seal (Tisseel) in operations for congenital heart defects. Ann Thorac Surg 1984;38:411–413.
44. Rousou J, Levitsky S, Gonzales-Lavin L, et al. Randomized clinical trial of fibrin sealant in patients undergoing resternotomy or reoperation after cardiac operations. J Thorac Cardiovasc Surg 1989;97:194–203.
45. Walterbusch G, Haverich A, Borst HG. Clinical experience with fibrin glue for local bleeding control and sealing of vascular prostheses. Thorac Cardiovasc Surgeon 1982;30:234–235.
46. Gundry SR, Behrendt DM. A quantitative and qualitative comparison of fibrin glue, albumin, and blood as agents to pretreat porous vascular grafts. J Surg Res 1987;43:75–77.
47. Kjaergard HK, Weis-Fogh US. Autologous fibrin glue for sealing vascular prostheses of high porosity. Cardiovasc Surg 1994;2:45–47.
48. Mazzucotelli JP, Klein-Soyer C, Beretz A, Brisson C, Archipoff G, Cazenave JP. Endothelial cell seeding: coating Dacron and expanded polytetrafluoroethylene vascular grafts with a biological glue allows adhesion and growth of human saphenous vein endothelial cells. Int J Artif Organs 1991;14:482–490.
49. Séguin JR, Picard E, Frapier JM, Chaptal PA. Aortic valve repair with fibrin glue for type A acute aortic dissection. Ann Thorac Surg 1994; 58:304–307.
50. Glimåker H, Björck CG, Hallstensson S, Ohlsén L, Westman B. Case report: avoiding blow-out of the aortic stump by reinforcement with fibrin glue. A report of two cases. Eur J Vasc Surg 1993;7:346–348.
51. Hvass U, Chatel D, Frikha I, Pansard Y, Depoix JP, Julliard JM. Left ventricular free wall rupture: long-term results with a pericardial patch and fibrin glue repair. Eur J Cardiothorac Surg 1995;9:75–76.
52. Türk RBM, Weidringer JW, Hartel W, Blümel G. Closure of lung leaks by fibrin gluing. Experimental investigations and clinical experience. Thorac Cardiovasc Surgeon 1983;31:185–186.
53. Bergsland J, Kalmbach T, Balu D, Feldman MJ, Caruana JA, Gage AA. Fibrin seal—an alternative to suture repair in experimental pulmonary surgery. J Surg Res 1986;40:340–345.

54. McCarthy PM, Trastek VF, Bell DG, et al. The effectiveness of fibrin glue sealant for reducing experimental pulmonary air leak. Ann Thorac Surg 1988;45:203–205.
55. Mouritzen C, Drömer M, Keinecke HO. The effect of fibrin glueing to seal bronchial and alveolar leakages after pulmonary resections and decortications. Eur J Cardiothorac Surg 1993;7:75–80.
56. Fleisher AG, Evans KG, Nelems B, Finley RJ. Effect of routine fibrin glue use on the duration of air leaks after lobectomy. Ann Thorac Surg 1990;49:133–134.
57. Wurtz A, Chambon JP, Sobecki L, Batrouni R, Huart JJ, Burnouf T. Utilisation d'une colle biologique en chirurgie d/exérèse pulmonaire partielle: résultats d'un essai contrôlé chez cinquante malades [Use of a fibrin glue in partial pulmonary excision surgery: results of a controlled trial in 50 patients]. Ann Chir 1991;45:719–723.
58. Yasuda Y, Mori A, Kato H, Fujino S, Asakura S. Intrathoracic fibrin glue for postoperative pleuropulmonary fistula. Ann Thorac Surg 1991; 51:242–244.
59. Jessen C, Sharma P. Use of fibrin glue in thoracic surgery. Ann Thorac Surg 1985;39:521–524.
60. Glover W, Chavis TV, Daniel TM, Kron IL, Spotnitz WD. Fibrin glue application through the flexible fiberoptic bronchoscope: closure of bronchopleural fistulas. J Thorac Cardiovasc Surg 1987;93:470–472.
61. Matar AF, Hill JG, Duncan W, Orfanakis N, Law I. Use of biological glue to control pulmonary air leaks. Thorax 1990;45:670–674.
62. Matthew TL, Spotnitz WD, Kron IL, Daniel TM, Tribble CG, Nolan SP. Four years' experience with fibrin sealant in thoracic and cardiovascular surgery. Ann Thorac Surg 1990;50:40–44.
63. Hansen MK, Kruse-Andersen S, Watt-Boolsen S, Andersen K. Spontaneous pneumothorax and fibrin glue sealant during thoracoscopy. Eur J Cardiothorac Surg 1989;3:512–514.
64. Nicholas JM, Dulchavsky SA. Successful use of autologous fibrin gel in traumatic bronchopleural fistula: case report. J Trauma 1992;32: 87–88.
65. Hillerdal G, Gustafsson G, Wegenius G, Englesson S, Hedenström, Hedenstierna G. Minimally invasive techniques: large emphysematous bullae. Successful treatment with thoracoscopic technique using fibrin glue in poor-risk patients. Chest 1995;107:1450–1453.
66. Akaogi E, Mitsui K, Sohara Y, Endo S, Ishikawa S, Hori M. Treatment of postoperative chylothorax with intrapleural fibrin glue. Ann Thorac Surg 1989;48:116–118.
67. Shirai T, Amano J, Takabe K. Thoracoscopic diagnosis and treatment of chylothorax after pneumonectomy. Ann Thorac Surg 1991;52: 306–307.
68. Shennib H, Adoumie R, Serrick C, Lulu H, Mulder D. Staple pneumoreduction with fibrin sealant application: A reliable method of transplanting oversized lungs. J Heart Lung Transplant 1994;13:43–47.
69. Gust R, Kleine P, Fabel H. Fibrinkleber- und Tetracyclinpleurodese bei rezidivierenden malignen Pleuraergüssen: Eine randomisierte Vergleichsuntersuchung [Intrapleural tetracycline and fibrin glue in the control of malignant pleural effusions]. Med Klin 1990;85:18–23.
70. Kram HB, Shoemaker WC, Hino ST, Chiang HS, Harley DP, Fleming AW. Tracheal repair with fibrin glue. J Thorac Cardiovasc Surg 1985; 90:771–775.
71. Hanawa T, Ikeda S, Funatsu T, et al. Development of a new surgical procedure for repairing tracheobronchomalacia. J Thorac Cardiovasc Surg 1990;100:587–594.
72. Cain JE Jr, Rosenthal HG, Broom MJ, Jauch EC, Borek DA, Jacobs RR. Quantification of leakage pressures after durotomy repairs in the canine. Spine 1990;15:969–970.
73. Nishihira S, McCaffrey TV. The use of fibrin glue for the repair of experimental CSF rhinorrhea. Laryngoscope 1988;98:625–627.
74. Shaffrey CI, Spotnitz WD, Shaffrey ME, Jane JA. Neurosurgical applications of fibrin glue: augmentation of dural closure in 134 patients. Neurosurgery 1990;26:207–210.
75. Stechison MT. Rapid polymerizing fibrin glue from autologous or single-donor blood: preparation and indications. J Neurosurg 1992;76: 626–628.
76. Toma AG, Fisher EW, Cheesman AD. Autologous fibrin glue in the repair of dural defects in craniofacial resections. J Laryngol Otol 1992; 106:356–357.
77. Van Velthoven V, Clarici G, Auer LM. Fibrin tissue adhesive sealant for the prevention of CSF leakage following transsphenoidal microsurgery. Acta Neurochir (Wien) 1991;109:26–29.
78. Narakas A. The use of fibrin glue in repair of peripheral nerves. Orthop Clin North Am 1988;19:187–199.
79. Feldman MD, Sataloff RT, Choi HY, Ballas SK. Compatibility of autologous fibrin adhesive with implant materials. Arch Otolaryngol Head Neck Surg 1988;114:182–185.
80. Bento RF, Miniti A. Comparison between fibrin tissue adhesive, epineural suture and natural union in intratemporal facial nerve in cats. Acta Otolaryngol [Stockh] 1989;105(Suppl. 465):1–36.
81. Nishihira S, McCaffrey TV. Repair of motor nerve defects: comparison of suture and fibrin adhesive techniques. Otolaryngol Head Neck Surg 1989;100:17–21.
82. Maragh H, Meyer BS, Davenport D, Gould JD, Terzis JK. Morphofunctional evaluation of fibrin glue versus microsuture nerve repairs. J Reconstr Microsurg 1990;6:331–337.
83. Herter T. Problems of fibrin adhesion of the nerves. Neurosurg Rev 1988;11:249–258.
84. Zeng L, Worseg A, Redl H, Schlag G. Peripheral nerve repair with nerve growth factor and fibrin matrix: An experimental study in rat model. Eur J Plast Surg 1994;17:228–232.
85. Bertelli JA, Mira JC. Nerve repair using freezing and fibrin glue: immediate histologic improvement of axonal coaptation. Microsurgery 1993;14:135–140.
86. Hasegawa H, Bitoh S, Obashi J, Maruno M. Closure of carotid-cavernous fistulae by use of a fibrin adhesive system. Surg Neurol 1985;24: 23–26.
87. Simpson RK Jr, Halter JA, Auzenne DG. Use of tissue adhesive to secure spinal epidural stimulating electrodes: technical note. Surg Neurol 1992;38:391–393.
88. Staindl O. Tissue adhesion with highly concentrated human fibrinogen in otolaryngology. Ann Otol 1979;88:413–418.
89. O'Connor AF, Shea JJ. A biologic adhesive for otologic practice. Otolaryngol Head Neck Surg 1982;90:347–348.
90. Marquet J. Fibrin glue in tympanoplasty. Am J Otol 1985;6:28–30.
91. Siedentop KH, Harris DM, Ham K, Sanchez B. Extended experimental and preliminary surgical findings with autologous fibrin tissue adhesive made from patient's own blood. Laryngoscope 1986;96:1062–1064.
92. Nissen AJ, Johnson AJ, Perkins RC, Welsh JE. Fibrin glue in otology and neurotology. Am J Otol 1993;14:147–150.
93. Park MS. Autologous fibrin glue for tympanoplasty. Am J Otol 1994; 15:687–689.
94. Siedentop KH, Harris DM, Loewy A. Experimental use of fibrin tissue adhesive in middle ear surgery. Laryngoscope 1983;93:1310–1313.
95. Mjøen S, Lindeman HH, Djupesland G, Schüler B, Sundby A, Skjørten F. Effect of human fibrin adhesive on the ear: an electrophysiological study of auditory function in the guinea pig correlated to light and

electron microscopy of middle ear mucosa and inner ear structures. Acta Otolaryngol [Stockh] 1986;102:257–265.
96. Wood AP, Harner SG. The effect of fibrin tissue adhesive on the middle and inner ears of chinchillas. Otolaryngol Head Neck Surg 1988; 98: 104–110.
97. Peters BR, Strunk CL, Fulmer RP. Autologous fibrin tissue adhesive for ossicular reconstruction in cats. Am J Otol 1992;13:540–543.
98. Siedentop KH, Schobel H. Stapedectomy modified by the application of fibrin tissue adhesive. Am J Otol 1991;12:443–445.
99. Palva T, Johnsson LG. Preservation of hearing after removal of the membranous canal with a cholesteatoma. Arch Otolaryngol Head Neck Surg 1986;112:982–985.
100. Gray RF, Bleach NR. Recurrent labyrinthine membrane rupture: Bioglue and five surgical repairs. J Laryngol Otol 1987;101:487–491.
101. Filipo R, Barbara M. Rehabilitation of radical mastoidectomy. Am J Otol 1986;7:248–251.
102. Portmann M. Results of middle ear reconstruction surgery. Ann Acad Med Singapore 1991;20:610–613.
103. Sierra DH, Nissen AJ, Welch J. The use of fibrin glue in intracranial procedures: preliminary results. Laryngoscope 1990;100:360–363.
104. Symon L, Pell MF. Cerebrospinal fluid rhinorrhea following acoustic neurinoma surgery: technical note. J Neurosurg 1991;74:152–153.
105. Lebowitz RA, Hoffman RA, Roland JT Jr, Cohen NL. Autologous fibrin glue in the prevention of cerebrospinal fluid leak following acoustic neuroma surgery. Am J Otol 1995;16:172–174.
106. Hayward PJ, Mackay IS. Fibrin glue in nasal septal surgery. J Laryngol Otol 1987;101:133–138.
107. Gleich LL, Rebeiz EE, Pankratov MM, Shapshay SM. Autologous fibrin tissue adhesive in endoscopic sinus surgery. Otolaryngol Head Neck Surg 1995;112:238–241.
108. Isshiki N, Taira T, Nose K, Kojima H. Surgical treatment of laryngeal web with mucosal graft. Ann Otol Rhinol Laryngol 1991;100:95–100.
109. Matthews TW, Briant TDR. The use of fibrin tissue glue in thyroid surgery: resource utilization implications. J Otolaryngol 1991;20: 276–278.
110. Burleson R, Eiseman B. Nature of the bond between partial-thickness skin and wound granulations. Surgery 1972;72:315–322.
111. Staindl O. The fibrin-adhesive-system in plastic surgery of head and neck. J Head Neck Pathol 1982;3:78–85.
112. Vibe P, Pless J. A new method of skin graft adhesion. Scand J Plast Reconstr Surg 1983;17:263–264.
113. Lilius P. Fibrin adhesive: its use in selected skin grafting. Practical note. Scand J Plast Reconstr Surg 1987;21:245–248.
114. Ellis DAF, Pelausa EO. Fibrin glue in facial plastic and reconstructive surgery. J Otolaryngol 1988;17:74–77.
115. Stuart JD, Morgan RF, Kenney JG. Single-donor fibrin glue for hand burns. Ann Plast Surg 1990;24:524–527.
116. Vedung S, Hedlund A. Fibrin glue: its use for skin grafting of contaminated burn wounds in areas difficult to immobilize. J Burn Care Rehabil 1993;14:356–358.
117. Jabs AD Jr, Wider TM, DeBellis J, Hugo NE. The effect of fibrin glue on skin grafts in infected sites. Plast Reconstr Surg 1992;89:268–271.
118. Marchac D, Sàndor GKB. Face lifts and sprayed fibrin glue: an outcome analysis of 200 patients. Br J Plast Surg 1994;47:306–309.
119. Flemming I. Fibrin glue in face lifts. Facial Plast Surg 1992;8:79–88.
120. Boeckx W, Vandevoort M, Blondeel P, Van Raemdonck D, Vandekerckhove E. Fibrin glue in the treatment of dorsal hand burns. Burns 1992;18:395–400.
121. Brown DM, Barton BR, Young VL, Pruitt BA. Decreased wound contraction with fibrin glue-treated skin grafts. Arch Surg 1992;127: 404–406.
122. Auger FA, Guignard R, López Valle CA, Germain L. Role and innocuity of Tisseel®, a tissue glue, in the grafting process and *in vivo* evolution of human cultured epidermis. Br J Plast Surg 1993;46: 136–142.
123. Ronfard V, Broly H, Mitchell V, et al. Use of human keratinocytes cultured on fibrin glue in the treatment of burn wounds. Burns 1991;17: 181–184.
124. Kaiser HW, Stark GB, Kopp J, Balcerkiewicz A, Spilker G, Kreysel HW. Cultured autologous keratinocytes in fibrin glue suspension, exclusively and combined with STS-allograft (preliminary clinical and histological report of a new technique). Burns 1994;20:23–29.
125. Lindsey WH, Masterson TM, Spotnitz WD, Wilhelm MC, Morgan RF. Seroma prevention using fibrin glue in a rat mastectomy model. Arch Surg 1990;125:305–307.
126. Harada RN, Pressler VM, McNamara JJ. Fibrin glue reduces seroma formation in the rat after mastectomy. Surgery 1992;175:450–454.
127. Lindsey WH, Masterson TM, Llaneras M, Spotnitz WD, Wanebo HJ, Morgan RF. Seroma prevention using fibrin glue during modified radical neck dissection in a rat model. Am J Surg 1988;156:310–313.
128. Gioffre-Florio MA, Mezzasalma F, Manganaro T, Pakravanan H, Cogliandolo A. The use of fibrin glue in the surgery of breast carcinoma. G Chir 1993;14:239–241.
129. Udén P, Aspegren K, Balldin G, Garne JP, Larsson SA. Fibrin adhesive in radical mastectomy. Eur J Surg 1993;159:263–265.
130. Vaxman F, Kolbe A, Stricher F, et al. Does fibrin glue improve drainage after axillary lymph node dissection? Prospective and randomized study in humans. Eur Surg Res 1995;27:346–352.
131. Staindl O. Surgical management of rhinophyma. Acta Otolaryngol [Stockh] 1981;92:137–140.
132. Fontana A, Muti E, Cicerale D, Rizzotti M. Cartilage chips synthesized with fibrin glue in rhinoplasty. Aesthetic Plast Surg 1991;15:237–240.
133. Schwarz N. The role of fibrin sealant in osteoinduction. Ann Chir Gynaecol 1993;82:63–68.
134. Homminga GN, Bulstra SK, Bouwmeester PSM, van der Linden AJ. Perichondral grafting for cartilage lesions of the knee. J Bone Joint Surg [Br] 1990;72:1003–1007.
135. Itay S, Abramovici A, Nevo Z. Use of cultured embryonal chick epiphyseal chondrocytes as grafts for defects in chick articular cartilage. Clin Orthop 1987;220:284–303.
136. Homminga GN, Buma P, Koot HWJ, van der Kraan PM, van den Berg WB. Chondrocyte behavior in fibrin glue in vitro. Acta Orthop Scand 1993;64:441–445.
137. Pitman MI, Menche D, Song EK, Ben-Yishay A, Gilbert D, Grande DA. The use of adhesives in chondrocyte transplantation surgery: invivo studies. Bull Hosp Jt Dis Orthop Inst 1989;49:213–220.
138. Meyers MH, Herron M. A fibrin adhesive seal for the repair of osteochondral fracture fragments. Clin Orthop 1984;182:258–263.
139. Keller J, Andreassen TT, Joyce F, Knudsen VE, Jørgensen PH, Lucht U. Fixation of osteochondral fractures: fibrin sealant tested in dogs. Acta Orthop Scand 1985;56:323–326.
140. Hanff G, Sollerman C, Abrahamsson SO, Lundborg G. Repair of osteochondral defects in the rabbit knee with Gore-Tex™ (expanded polytetrafluoroethylene): An experimental study. Scand J Plast Reconstr Hand Surg 1990;24:217–223.
141. Ishimura M, Tamai S, Fujisawa Y. Arthroscopic meniscal repair with fibrin glue. Arthroscopy 1991;7:177–181.
142. Frykman E, Jacobsson S, Widenfalk B. Fibrin sealant in prevention of

flexor tendon adhesions: an experimental study in the rabbit. J Hand Surg [Am] 1993;18:68–75.
143. Ono K, Shikata J, Shimizu K, Yamamuro T. Bone-fibrin mixture in spinal surgery. Clin Orthop 1992;275:133–139.
144. Lack W, Bösch P, Arbes H. Chronic osteomyelitis treated by cancellous homografts and fibrin adhesion. J Bone Joint Surg [Br] 1987;69:335–337.
145. Marchac D, Renier D. Fibrin glue in craniofacial surgery. J Craniofac Surg 1990;1:32–34.
146. Tayapongsak P, O'Brien DA, Monteiro CB, Arceo-Diaz LY. Autologous fibrin adhesive in mandibular reconstruction with particulate cancellous bone and marrow. J Oral Maxillofac Surg 1994;52:161–165.
147. Wittkampf ARM. Fibrin glue as cement for HA-granules. J Cranio Max Fac Surg 1989;17:179–181.
148. Hotz G. Alveolar ridge augmentation with hydroxyapatite using fibrin sealant for fixation. Part II. Clinical application. J Oral Maxillofac Surg 1991;20:208–213.
149. Pini Prato GP, Cortellini P, Agudio G, Clauser C. Human fibrin glue versus sutures in periodontal surgery. J Periodontol 1987;58:426–431.
150. Rakocz M, Mazar A, Varon D, Spierer S, Blinder D, Martinowitz U. Dental extractions in patients with bleeding disorders. Oral Surg Oral Med Oral Pathol 1993;75:280–282.
151. Martinowitz U, Schulman S. Fibrin sealant in surgery of patients with a hemorrhagic diathesis. Thromb Haemost 1995;74:486–492.
152. Stain S, Yellin A, Donovan A. Hepatic trauma. Arch Surg 1978;135:12–18.
153. Scheele J, Gentsch HH, Matteson E. Splenic repair by fibrin tissue adhesive and collagen fleece. Surgery 1984;95:6–13.
154. Hauser CJ. Hemostasis of solid viscus trauma by intraparenchymal injection of fibrin glue. Arch Surg 1989;124:291–293.
155. Kram HB, Nathan RC, Stafford FJ, Fleming AW, Shoemaker WC. Technique: fibrin glue achieves hemostasis in patients with coagulation disorders. Arch Surg 1989;124:385–387.
156. Kram HB, del Junco T, Clark SR, Ocampo HP, Shoemaker WC. Techniques of splenic preservation using fibrin glue. J Trauma 1990;30:97–101.
157. Ochsner MG, Maniscalco-Theberge ME, Champion HR. Fibrin glue as a hemostatic agent in hepatic and splenic trauma. J Trauma 1990;30:884–887.
158. Salvino CK, Esposito TJ, Smith DK, et al. Laparoscopic injection of fibrin glue to arrest intraparenchymal abdominal hemorrhage: an experimental study. J Trauma 1993;35:762–766.
159. Kohno H, Nagasue N, Chang YC, Taniura H, Yamanoi A, Nakamura T. Comparison of topical hemostatic agents in elective hepatic resection: a clinical prospective randomized trial. World J Surg 1992;16:966–970.
160. Sakon M, Monden M, Gotoh M, et al. Use of microcrystalline collagen powder and fibrinogen tissue adhesive for hemostasis and prevention of rebleeding in patients with hepatocellular carcinoma associated with cirrhosis of the liver. Surg Gynecol Obstet 1989;168:453–454.
161. Tokunaga Y, Tanaka K, Uemoto S, et al. Fibrin sealant of the cut surface of partial liver grafts from living donors. J Invest Surg 1995;8:243–251.
162. Rodriguez Fuchs CA, Bruno M. Plugging liver biopsy sites with coagulation factors. Lancet 1987;2:1087.
163. Chisholm RA, Jones SN, Lees WR. Fibrin sealant as a plug for the post liver biopsy needle track. Clin Radiol 1989;40:627–628.
164. Nagino M, Hayakawa N, Kitagawa S, et al. Interventional embolization with fibrin glue for a large inferior mesenteric-caval shunt. Surgery 1992;111:580–584.
165. Scheele J, Herzog J, Mühe E. Anastomosensicherung am Verdauungstrakt mit Fibrinkleber. Nahttechnische Grundlagen, experimentelle Befunde, klinische Erfahrungen [Fibrin glue protection of digestive anastomoses]. Zentralbl Chir 1978;103:1325–1336.
166. Petrelli NJ, Cohen H, DeRisi D, Ambrus JL, Williams P. The application of tissue adhesives in small bowel anastomoses. J Surg Oncol 1982;19:59–61.
167. Hjortrup A, Nordkild P, Christensen T, Sjøntoft E, Kjaergaard J. Rectal anastomosis with application of luminal fibrin adhesive in the rectum of dogs: An experimental study. Dis Colon Rectum 1989;32:422–425.
168. Saclarides TJ, Woodard DO, Bapna M, Economou SG. Fibrin glue improves the healing of irradiated bowel anastomoses. Dis Colon Rectum 1992;35:249–252.
169. Thorson GK, Perez-Brett R, Lillie DB, et al. The role of the tissue adhesive fibrin seal (FS) in esophageal anastomoses. J Surg Oncol 1983;24:221–223.
170. McCarthy PM, Trastek VF, Schaff HV, et al. Esophagogastric anastomoses: the value of fibrin glue in preventing leakage. J Thorac Cardiovasc Surg 1987;93:234–239.
171. Houston KA, Rotstein OD. Fibrin sealant in high-risk colonic anastomoses. Arch Surg 1988;123:230–234.
172. Byrne DJ, Hardy J, Wood RAB, McIntosh R, Hopwood D, Cuschieri A. Adverse influence of fibrin sealant on the healing of high-risk sutured colonic anastomoses. J R Coll Surg Edinb 1992;37:394–398.
173. van der Ham AC, Kort WJ, Weijma IM, van den Ingh HFGM, Jeekel H. Effect of fibrin sealant on the integrity of colonic anastomoses in rats with faecal peritonitis. Eur J Surg 1993;159:425–432.
174. van der Ham AC, Kort WJ, Weijma IM, Jeekel H. Transient protection of incomplete colonic anastomoses with fibrin sealant: An experimental study in the rat. J Surg Res 1993;55:256–260.
175. Fékété F, Gayet B, Panis Y. Apport de la colle de fibrine dans le renforcement des anastomoses œsophagiennes [Contribution of fibrin glue to the reinforcement of œsophageal anastomosis]. Presse Med 1992;21:157–159.
176. Kirkegaard P, Madsen PV. Perineal sinus after removal of the rectum: occlusion with fibrin adhesive. Am J Surg 1983;145:791–794.
177. Hjortrup A, Moesgaard F, Kjærgård J. Fibrin adhesive in the treatment of perineal fistulas. Dis Colon Rectum 1991;34:752–754.
178. Abel ME, Chiu YSY, Russell TR, Volpe PA. Autologous fibrin glue in the treatment of rectovaginal and complex fistulas. Dis Colon Rectum 1993;36:447–449.
179. McCarthy PM, Frazee RC, Hughes RW Jr, Beart RW Jr. Barium-impregnated fibrin glue: application to a bleeding duodenal sinus. Mayo Clin Proc 1987;62:317–319.
180. Lange V, Meyer G., Wenk H, Schildberg FW. Fistuloscopy—an adjuvant technique for sealing gastrointestinal fistulae. Surg Endosc 1990;4:212–216.
181. Berg PL, Barina W, Born P. Endoscopic injection of fibrin glue versus polidocanol in peptic ulcer hemorrhage: a pilot study. Endoscopy 1994;26:528–530.
182. Lau WY, Leung KL, Zhu XL, Lam YH, Chung SCS, Li AKC. Laparoscopic repair of perforated peptic ulcer. Br J Surg 1995;82:814–816.
183. Couto J, Kroczek B, Requena R, Lerner R. Autologous fibrin glue as a sealant of the common bile duct. Surgery 1987;101:354–356.

184. Tashiro S, Murata E, Hiraoka T, Nakakuma K, Watanabe E, Miyauchi Y. New technique for pancreaticojejunostomy using a biological adhesive. Br J Surg 1987;74:392–394.
185. Kram HB, Clark SR, Ocampo H, Yamaguchi MA, Shoemaker WC. Fibrin glue sealing of pancreatic injuries, resections, and anastomoses. Am J Surg 1991;161:479–481.
186. Suzuki Y, Kuroda Y, Morita A, et al. Fibrin glue sealing for the prevention of pancreatic fistulas following distal pancreatectomy. Arch Surg 1995;130:952–955.
187. d'Andrea AA, Costantino V, Sperti C, Pedrazzoli S. Human fibrin sealant in pancreatic surgery: is it useful in preventing fistulas? A prospective randomized study. Ital J Gastroenterol 1994;26:283–286.
188. Härting F, Koornneef L, Peeters HJF, Gillissen JPM. Glued fixation of split-skin graft to the bony orbit following exenteration. Plast Reconstr Surg 1985;76:633–635.
189. Bartley GB, McCaffrey TV. Cryoprecipitated fibrinogen (fibrin glue) in orbital surgery. Am J Ophthalmol 1990;109:227–228.
190. Watts MT, Collin R. The use of fibrin glue in mucous membrane grafting of the fornix. Ophthalmic Surg 1992;23:689–690.
191. Mori S, Komatsu H, Watari H. Spontaneous posterior bulbar perforation of congenital scleral coloboma and its surgical treatment: a case report. Ophthalmic Surg 1985;16:433–436.
192. Zauberman H, Hemo I. Use of fibrin glue in ocular surgery. Ophthalmic Surg 1988;19:132–133.
193. Mester U, Zuche M, Rauber M. Astigmatism after phacoemulsification with posterior chamber lens implantation: small incision technique with fibrin adhesive for wound closure. J Cataract Refract Surg 1993;19:616–619.
194. Lagoutte FM, Gauthier L, Comte PRM. A fibrin sealant for perforated and preperforated corneal ulcers. Br J Ophthalmol 1989;73:757–761.
195. Kajiwara K. Repair of a leaking bleb with fibrin glue. Am J Ophthalmol 1990;109:599–601.
196. Adamyan LV, Myinbayev OA, Kulakov VI. Use of fibrin glue in obstetrics and gynecology: a review of the literature. Int J Fertil 1991;36:76–88.
197. Genz HJ. Die Behandlung des vorzeitigen Blasensprungs durch Fibrinklebung [Treatment of premature rupture of the fetal membranes by means of fibrin adhesion]. Med Welt 1979;30:1557–1559.
198. Baumgarten K, Moser S. The technique of fibrin adhesion for premature rupture of the membranes during pregnancy. J Perinat Med 1986;14:43–49.
199. Moront MG, Katz NM, O'Connell J, Hoy GR. The use of topical fibrin glue at cannulation sites in neonates. Surg Gynecol Obstet 1988;166:358–359.
200. Feichtinger W, Barad D, Feinman M, Barg P. The use of two-component fibrin sealant for embryo transfer. Fertil Steril 1990;54:733–734.
201. Rücker K, Baumann R, Volk M, Taubert HD. Tubal anastomosis using a tissue adhesive. Hum Reprod 1988;3:185–186.
202. Fischer CP, Sonda LP III, Diokno AC. Further experience with cryoprecipitate coagulum in renal calculus surgery: a review of 60 cases. J Urol 1981;126:432–436.
203. Pfab R, Ascherl R, Blümel G, Hartung R. Local hemostasis of nephrostomy tract with fibrin adhesive sealing in percutaneous nephrolithotomy. Eur Urol 1987;13:118–121.
204. Schultz A, Christiansen LA. Fibrin adhesive sealing of ureter after ureteral stone surgery. Eur Urol 1985;11:267–268.
205. Urlesberger H, Rauchenwald K, Henning K. Fibrin adhesives in surgery of the renal parenchyma. Eur Urol 1979;5:260–261.
206. Brands W, Haselberger J, Mennicken C, Hoerst M. Treatment of ruptured kidney by gluing with highly concentrated human fibrinogen. J Pediatr Surg 1983;18:611–613.
207. Kram HB, Ocampo HP, Yamaguchi MP, Nathan RC, Shoemaker WC. Fibrin glue in renal and ureteral trauma. Urology 1989;33:215–218.
208. Levinson AK, Swanson DA, Johnson DE, Greskovich FJ III, Stephenson RA, Lichtiger B. Fibrin glue for partial nephrectomy. Urology 1991;38:314–316.
209. Joffe P. Peritoneal dialysis catheter leakage treated with fibrin glue. Nephrol Dial Transplant 1993;8:474–476.
210. Martinowitz U, Varon D, Bar-Maor A, Brenner B, Leibovitch I, Heim M. Circumcision in hemophilia: the use of fibrin glue for local hemostasis. J Urol 1992;148:855–857.
211. Silverstein JI, Mellinger BC. Fibrin glue vasal anastomosis compared to conventional sutured vasovasostomy in the rat. J Urol 1991;145:1288–1291.
212. Niederberger C, Ross LS, MacKenzie B Jr, Schacht MJ, Cho Y. Vasovasostomy in rabbits using fibrin adhesive prepared from a single human source. J Urol 1993;149:183–185.
213. Zilch H, Lambiris E. The sustained release of cefotaxim from a fibrin-cefotaxim compound in treatment of osteitis: pharmacokinetic study and clinical results. Arch Orthop Trauma Surg 1986;106:36–41.
214. Ney AL, Kelly PH, Tsukayama DT, Bubrick MP. Fibrin glue-antibiotic suspension in the prevention of prosthetic graft infection. J Trauma 1990;30:1000–1006.
215. Kram HB, Bansal M, Timberlake O, Shoemaker WC. Antibacterial effects of fibrin glue-antibiotic mixtures. J Surg Res 1991;50: 175–178.
216. Wadström J, Tengblad A. Fibrin glue reduces the dissolution rate of sodium hyaluronate. Ups J Med Sci 1993;98:159–167.
217. Fasol R, Schumacher B, Schlaudraff K, Hauenstein KH, Seitelberger R. Experimental use of a modified fibrin glue to induce site-directed angiogenesis from the aorta to the heart. J Thorac Cardiovasc Surg 1994;107:1432–1439.
218. Greisler HP, Cziperle DJ, Kim DU, et al. Enhanced endothelialization of expanded polytetrafluoroethylene grafts by fibroblast growth factor type 1 pretreatment. Surgery 1992;112:244–255.
219. Byrne DJ, Hardy J, Wood RAB, McIntosh R, Cuschieri A. Effect of fibrin glues on the mechanical properties of healing wounds. Br J Surg 1991;78:841–843.
220. Lasa CI, Kidd RR III, Nunez HA, Drohan WN. Effect of fibrin glue and Opsite on open wounds in db/db mice. J Surg Res 1993;54: 202–206.
221. Lindenberg S, Steentoft P, Sørensen SS, Olesen HP. Studies on prevention of intra-abdominal adhesion formation by fibrin sealant: an experimental study in rats. Acta Chir Scand 1985;151:525–527.
222. de Virgilio C, Dubrow T, Sheppard BB, et al. Fibrin glue inhibits intra-abdominal adhesion formation. Arch Surg 1990;125:1378–1382.
223. Sheppard BB, de Virgilio C, Bleiweis M, Milliken JC, Robertson JM. Inhibition of intra-abdominal adhesions: fibrin glue in a long term model. Am Surg 1993;59:786–790.
224. Dulchavsky SA, Geller ER, Maurer J, Kennedy PR, Tortora GT, Maitra SR. Autologous fibrin gel: bactericidal properties in contaminated hepatic injury. J Trauma 1991;31:991–995.
225. McGregor JR, Reinbach DH, Dahill SW, O'Dwyer PJ. Effect of fibrin sealant on perianastomotic tumor growth in an experimental model of colorectal cancer surgery. Dis Colon Rectum 1993;36:834–839.
226. Wilson SM, Pell P, Donegan EA. HIV-1 transmission following the use of cryoprecipitated fibrinogen as gel/adhesive [abstract]. Transfusion 1991;31(Suppl.):51S.

227. Milde LN. An anaphylactic reaction to fibrin glue. Anesth Analg 1989;69:684–686.
228. Mitsuhata H, Horiguchi Y, Saitoh J, et al. An anaphylactic reaction to topical fibrin glue. Anesthesiology 1994;81:1074–1077.
229. Berguer R, Staerkel RL, Moore EE, Moore FA, Galloway WB, Mockus MB. Warning: fatal reaction to the use of fibrin glue in deep hepatic wounds. Case reports. J Trauma 1991;31:108–111.
230. Zehnder JL, Leung LLK. Development of antibodies to thrombin and factor V with recurrent bleeding in a patient exposed to topical bovine thrombin. Blood 1990;76:2011–2016.
231. Rapaport SI, Zivelin A, Minow RA, Hunter CS, Donnelly K. Clinical significance of antibodies to bovine and human thrombin and factor V after surgical use of bovine thrombin. Am J Clin Pathol 1992;97:84–91.
232. Bänninger H, Hardegger T, Tobler A, et al. Fibrin glue in surgery: frequent development of inhibitors of bovine thrombin and human factor V. Br J Haematol 1993;85:528–532.
233. Nichols WL, Daniels TM, Fisher PK, Owen WG, Pineda AA, Mann KG. Antibodies to bovine thrombin and coagulation factor V associated with surgical use of topical bovine thrombin or fibrin "glue": a frequent finding [abstract]. Blood 1993;82:59a.

Section V
Transfusion Surgical Subspecialty Concerns

Chapter 28

Coagulation, Transfusion, and Cardiac Surgery

SIMON C. BODY
DAVID S. MORSE

INTRODUCTION

Nowhere in the practice of medicine do alterations in the coagulation state occur with such planned severity as during cardiac surgery. Indeed, they are vital. Preoperative antiplatelet agents (such as aspirin and dipyridamole) are effective in the prevention and treatment of myocardial ischemia and infarction; thrombolytics are used for therapy for myocardial infarction. Heparin and heparin alternatives are currently still essential for the practice of cardiopulmonary bypass (CPB). The management of perioperative coagulopathy and bleeding with blood products, heparin-reversal agents, and antifibrinolytics is a source of considerable investigation. The hypercoagulable state postoperatively remains a point of interest, probably worthy of greater study. Important areas of study and controversy surrounding cardiac surgery include the variability in allogeneic blood product transfusion, management of anticoagulation and coagulation during CPB, and management of specific patients with hematological disorders.

PREOPERATIVE ASSESSMENT

Most patients undergoing cardiac surgery have no congenital impairment of coagulation, yet a high percentage of patients exhibit an acquired deficit. The most common causes are drug induced, notably from aspirin, heparin, coumadin, and nitrosovasodilators. Preoperative impairments of fibrinolysis due to streptokinase, urokinase, and tissue plasminogen activator are also commonplace. Most coagulation defects occurring perioperatively are seen at the termination of CPB. Little information is available to the clinician except for that contained in the patient record. Accordingly, it is important to determine preoperatively all possible causes of perioperative coagulopathy. Patients should be queried preoperatively about any prior congenital or acquired coagulopathy, especially one associated with surgery. A history of spontaneous or excessive bleeding, purpura, or petechiae should be sought. Any medical conditions and current drug therapy should be recorded. A history of prior transfusions, pregnancy, and a family history must be established. In addition to routine physical examination, careful attention should be paid to the skin and nail beds, looking for evidence of prior bleeding. Routine laboratory testing before cardiac surgery is common. Most institutions require complete blood count, prothrombin time (PT), and activated partial thromboplastin time (APTT). Routine thrombin time (TT), template bleeding time, antithrombin III (ATIII) level, and coagulation protein levels are not warranted unless specifically indicated. In the heparinized patient, inappropriate intraoperative bleeding is assessed using platelet count and fibrinogen concentration. Additional tests of global coagulation can be performed. A useful example is thromboelastography upon blood where heparin has been metabolized by heparinase. In patients in whom heparin has been reversed using protamine, coagulation can be tested using platelet count, PT, APTT, TT, and fibrinogen level. Other tests such as the Sonoclot, thromboelastogram, activated clotting time (ACT), and Hepcon can be used. Measures of fibrinolysis such as fibrin degradation products can be measured.

Perioperative bleeding is frequently, but not always helpfully, defined as due to inadequate surgical techniques or due to alterations in hemostasis. This distinction is usually not clearcut, and both defects are often present concurrently. In the operating room, the distinction can be clearer. Oozing from the surgical wound, skin edges, grafts, suture lines, and catheter sites can be visualized. Postoperatively, there is a far greater reliance on total chest tube drainage, complete blood count, and measurements of coagulation status.

HEPARIN-INDUCED THROMBOCYTOPENIA AND ALTERNATIVES TO HEPARIN

Heparin-induced thrombocytopenia (HT) is a serious but uncommon complication of heparin therapy; its incidence varies from 1 to 10% (1–7). HT is more common with bovine-origin heparin than with porcine-origin heparin for unclear reasons (8). Paradoxically, HT is associated with thrombosis in approximately 50% of patients, of which approximately 10% is associated with organ injury, usually cerebral, myocardial, or mesenteric. HT most frequently occurs after a 4- to 10-day latent period but will usually abate 2–3 days after heparin cessation. Thromboembolic phenomena occur because of immune-mediated endothelial injury, complement activation, and platelet clumping.

HT is diagnosed by the presence of an anti-platelet IgG that can activate complement and cause platelet activation and aggregation. The IgG binds to heparin, at repeating epitopes, and to platelet receptors, probably Fc components (5, 9, 10). Additionally, serotonin release is pathognomic of HT, but no predictive test is available (11). Low-molecular-weight heparin may be associated with a lower incidence of HT (10, 11). Management of these patients for CPB is problematic. For elective CPB, it is recommended that heparin be completely avoided (12), yet the alternatives are limited and equally as challenging. Delay of CPB until measurable heparin-dependent IgG has disappeared has also been recommended (13). Suggested alternatives are listed in Table 28.1.

TABLE 28.1. ALTERNATIVES TO HEPARIN FOR ANTICOAGULATION FOR CARDIOPULMONARY BYPASS

Surgical delay
Plasmapheresis (15)
Warfarin (12)
Low-molecular-weight dextran (569)
Low-molecular-weight heparin (14, 47, 49, 57, 65, 570)
Heparinoids (571, 572)
Profound hemodilution (573)
Ancrod (25, 26, 34, 574, 575)
Hirudin (24)
Prostacyclins (64–67)

Delaying surgery until anti-platelet antibodies are unmeasurable and in vitro tests show the absence of heparin-induced aggregation has been undertaken without the recurrence of HT (14). Yet this strategy has not been shown to be protective for all individuals. Preoperative plasmapheresis to remove the anti-platelet IgG antibody has been described (15).

Thrombin inhibitors such as hirudin render heparin unnecessary. Hirudin is a heterogeneous polypeptide of 65–66 amino acids (molecular weight 7000) derived naturally from the salivary glands of the medicinal leech (*Hirudio medicinalis*). Recombinant forms of hirudin vary in form but preserve the structures responsible for binding of thrombin and inhibition of its catalytic site (Fig. 28.1). Hirudin is a specific thrombin inhibitor, with three to five times the potency of heparin. It requires no plasma cofactor such as ATIII and is not affected by inhibitors such as platelet factor 4. It appears to have no effect on platelets and is nonimmunogenic. It is cleared unchanged by the kidney with first-order kinetics, after initial redistribution with a half-life of 60 minutes (16–18). Hirudin effect is measured well at modest dose by assays of thrombin activity such as APTT and ACT (19, 20). TT is overly sensitive to hirudin activity and may be prolonged in the face of clinically normal coagulation. APTT seems to be best correlated with plasma hirudin levels and with clinical effect (Fig. 28.2) (16, 18, 21). At the high doses required for bypass, standard clotting tests may be prolonged beyond assay. As such, nontraditional tests such as amidolytic anti-IIa assays or thrombin-activated ACT may be required to provide meaningful data (20). Hirudin use has been described in angioplasty (22), in deep venous throm-

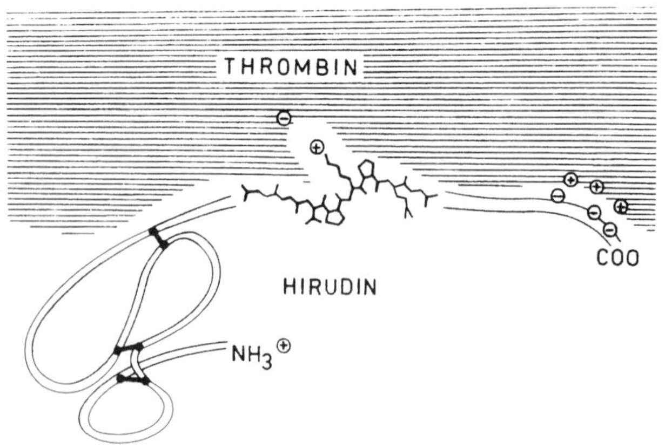

Figure 28.1. Hirudin interaction with thrombin. Secondary binding sites such as the polyanionic C-terminal region stabilize primary binding to and inhibition of the thrombin catalytic site. (Modified by permission from Markward TF. Pharmacology of selective thrombin inhibitors. Nouv Rev Fr Hematol 1988;30:161–165.)

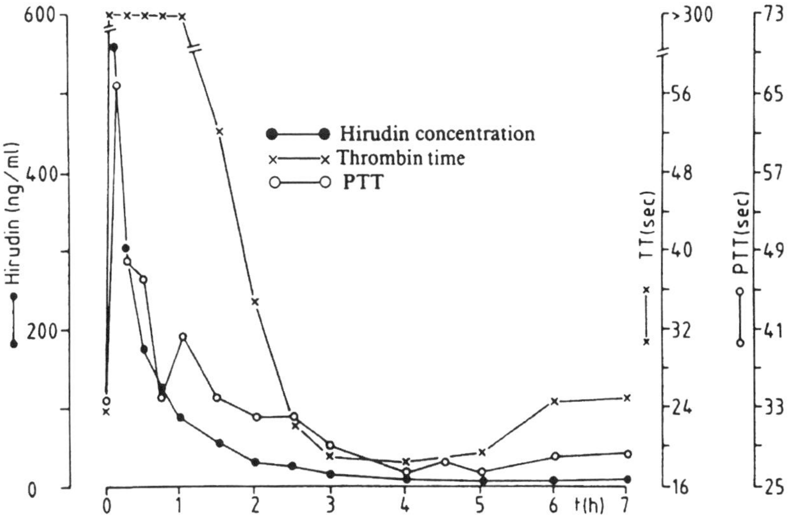

Figure 28.2. Hirudin plasma concentration correlates well to APTT but poorly to TT. (Modified by permission from Bichler J, Fichtl B, Siebeck M, Fritz H. Pharmacokinetics and pharmacodynamics of hirudin in man after single subcutaneous and intravenous bolus administration. Arzneim Forschung 1988;38:704–709.)

bosis (23), and in CPB surgery (24). Despite its many advantages, hirudin is likely an inferior anticoagulant to heparin, which promotes inhibition of many steps in the intrinsic (contact activated) pathway. In an in vitro model of CPB, hirudin resulted in higher levels of fibrinopeptide A and prothrombin fragment F1.2 compared with heparin. In canine bypass models, fibrin deposition in arterial line filters was significantly increased in those dogs receiving hirudin compared with heparin (18, 19). In reality, hirudin is rarely used for CPB.

Defibrinogenating agents such as Ancrod (Knoll Pharmaceutical Co., Whippary, NJ) also render heparin unnecessary. Ancrod, from the venom of the Malaya pit viper (*Agkistrodon rhodostoma*) (25, 26), selectively depletes blood of fibrinogen without effect on other clotting factors or platelets. Ancrod cleaves fibrinopeptide A from the α chain of fibrinogen but, unlike thrombin, does not cleave fibrinopeptide B and does not activate factor XIII (fibrin stabilizing factor). This results in an unstable water-soluble fibrin that is rapidly acted upon by the fibrinolytic system and cleared by the reticuloendothelial system (27, 28). Ancrod has been used in patients with deep venous thrombosis (29, 30), in major vascular surgery (31), and in dialysis (32). Ancrod has been used for anticoagulation in cardiac surgery (25, 26, 33–35) and in patients with HT (25, 26). In 20 patients undergoing cardiac surgery, adequate defibrinogenation (target fibrinogen concentration 0.2–0.7 g/L) required prolonged infusions lasting 10–15 hours (34). No thrombotic complications occurred, although postbypass coagulopathy was severe, requiring multiple transfusions of cryoprecipitate and other clotting factors. Other authors reported a mild postbypass coagulopathy easily treated with cryoprecipitate. An antidote for ancrod is available in the setting of overdose but is accompanied by a relatively high risk of allergy/anaphylaxis. Cryoprecipitate is the treatment of choice for overdose (26, 31).

Low-molecular-weight heparins present another alternative to unfractionated heparin in the patient with HT. These small heterogeneous oligosaccharides (4–6.5 kDa) possess the pentasaccharide ATIII binding region found in unfractionated heparin but are not large enough to bind ATIII and thrombin (factor IIa) simultaneously, as is required for thrombin inhibition (Fig. 28.3) (36). Platelet interaction is also minimal (37, 38). However, other activities of ATIII, such as inhibition of factors Xa and XIIa, are preserved (39, 40). This provides for a potent anticoagulant effect but with minimal platelet interaction and reduced risk for HT. Low-molecular-weight heparins are produced mainly via chemical or enzymatic digestion of unfractionated beef or pork heparin. This creates a heterogeneous array of low-molecular-weight oligosaccharides with varying bioavailability and antithrombin binding ability. As a result, the potency and relative anti-factor Xa and factor IIa activity of these products may vary considerably (41, 42).

Low-molecular-weight heparin may also precipitate HT, as has been reported (41, 43), and in vitro testing of platelets for low-molecular-weight heparin-induced platelet aggregation and serotonin release must be performed before clinical use in patients with a history of HT. Nevertheless, use of low-molecular-weight heparin has been reported in patients with deep venous thrombosis (44), with pulmonary embolism (45), for hemodialysis (46), and for CPB (47–49). A major obstacle to the use of low-molecular-weight heparin is in monitoring its anticoagulant effect. Assays such as TT, APTT, and ACT respond predominantly to thrombin inhibition and are likely to be unreliable. Amidolytic anti-factor Xa assays are the standard for low-molecular-weight heparin monitoring but require advanced expertise and are impractical in a clinical setting (37, 46, 50).

Low-molecular-weight heparin has less endothelial binding and cellular uptake and thus higher bioavailability and longer half-life than unfractionated heparin (51, 52). As such, it cannot be administered in doses normally used for unfractionated heparin. Given the abovementioned heterogeneity of different formulations, manufacturer's dosing recommendations must be adhered to carefully (46). Another difficulty with low-molecular-weight heparin is its resistance to inactivation by protamine. This is most pronounced in those formulations with high ratios of anti-factor Xa to anti-factor IIa activity. It is likely that protamine binds most avidly to large heparin oligosaccharides but with difficulty to smaller fragments. Anti-factor IIa activity is effectively reversed by protamine in milligram ratios of 1–1.5:1, as demonstrated by a return of TT and APTT to normal. However, anti-factor Xa activity, as measured by amidolytic assay, is incompletely reversed at best (48, 53, 54). The clinical implication of this residual anticoagulation is unclear, however. Animal studies demonstrate clinical hemostasis to be related to anti-factor IIa and not anti-factor Xa activity. Adequate reversal of anti-factor IIa activity results in adequate hemostasis (55, 56). Low-molecular-weight heparins have been used for CPB in patients with HT (47, 57); however, their anticoagulant effects are less reliable (49), and reversal by protamine is incomplete. Increased bleeding may be an accompaniment of the use of low-molecular-weight heparins (48, 49, 58).

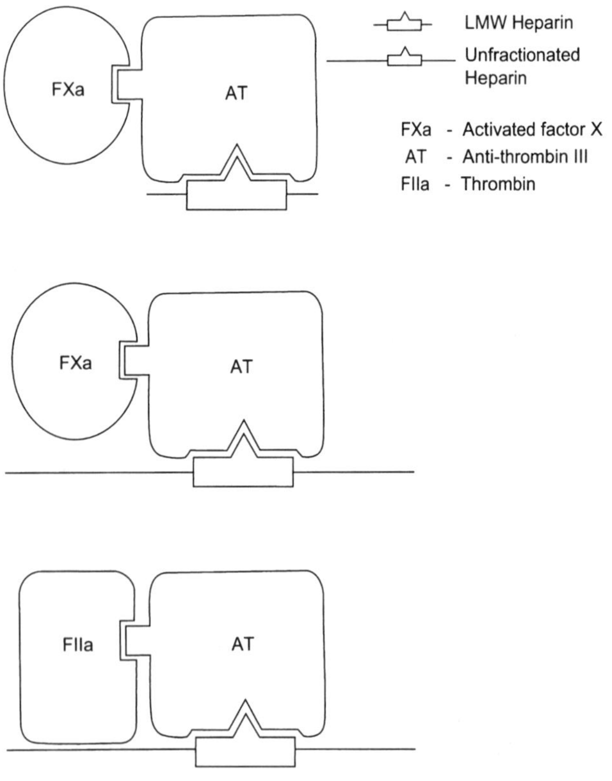

Figure 28.3. Low-molecular-weight heparin catalyzes ATIII mediated inhibition of factor Xa but not thrombin. (Modified by permission from Lane D, Denton J, Flynn A, Thunberg L, Lindhal U. Anticoagulant activities of heparin oligosaccharides and their neutralization by platelet factor 4. Biochem J 1984;218:725–732.)

Preoperative administration of anti-platelet agents has been described in patients with HT (59–62), although it has not been universally successful (62). Platelet inhibitors do not eliminate the need for heparin but prevent the platelet activation necessary for HT to occur. Use of aspirin and dipyridamole has been reported in two patients with known HT. Thrombotic and hemorrhagic complications were avoided (61). This technique cannot be recommended, however. In vitro study shows aspirin not to inhibit heparin-induced serotonin release, a sensitive assay of HT risk (63). In addition, the long duration of action of both aspirin and dipyridamole may increase the risk for postbypass bleeding.

Prostacyclin and its analogues have been used as inhibitors of platelet activation (64). Prostaglandins stimulate adenylate cyclase to produce cyclic AMP (cAMP), a potent inhibitor of platelet activation and aggregation. Unfortunately, both prostaglandin E_1 (PGE_1) and prostacyclin cause severe hypotension in clinical settings. In addition, prostacyclin is unstable at physiological pH. Iloprost is a stable prostacyclin analogue with a half-life of 15–30 minutes. This allows for administration by infusion with a rapid diminution of effect. Iloprost has been reported for use in CPB (63, 65, 66). In general, blood from patients with HT was tested preoperatively to ensure that iloprost would inhibit heparin-induced platelet aggregation and serotonin release. Iloprost was given by infusion before administration of heparin and continued until 15 minutes after protamine was given. Mild decreases in blood pressure were treated easily with infusion of phenylephrine or, rarely, norepinephrine. No abnormalities of bleeding were observed. Iloprost has been shown to prevent in vitro heparin-induced platelet aggregation in patients with HT (67), with PGE_2, and has also been used with aspirin to prevent platelet activation (68).

HEPARIN RESISTANCE

An occasional observation is the patient who receives a "usual" dose of heparin before CPB yet fails to adequately anticoagulate by laboratory estimation. Several etiologies have been offered and one clinical scenario aids our understanding. Numerous patients who have received heparin in the days and hours before CPB fail to anticoagulate adequately with usual doses of heparin (69–74). This phenomenon favors an etiology

TABLE 28.2. CAUSES OF HEPARIN RESISTANCE

Cogenital ATIII deficiency
Acquired ATIII deficiency
Thrombocytosis
Liver disease
Heparin therapy
Estrogen therapy
Pregnancy
Pregnancy
Sepsis
Hypercoaguable states
Coagulopathic processes

of either reduced ATIII levels (75–77), enhanced factor VIII activity (78, 79), or release of platelet factor 4 (73).

ATIII is an α_2-globulin that binds irreversibly to thrombin. Heparin binds to ATIII to increase its thrombin-binding activity manyfold (80). In the absence of ATIII, heparin has no anti-coagulant activity, and ATIII deficiency is associated with venous thrombosis (81). Administration of fresh-frozen plasma (as a source of ATIII) has been shown to attenuate heparin resistance (82). Although elevated factor VIII levels have been implicated as a cause of heparin resistance (78), others have not been able to confirm these results (83, 84). Other causes of heparin resistance are low-grade coagulopathic processes, severe thrombocytosis, pregnancy, and hypereosinophilia (85), which are outlined in Table 28.2.

COLD HEMAGGLUTININ DISEASE

Cold hemagglutinin disease (CHD) is mediated by several cold-reactive proteins. Cold-reactive proteins can occur without apparent etiology or in response to viral or mycoplasma infections and lymphoma. The overall incidence of cold-reactive proteins lies between 0.4 and 4% (86–88), with a higher incidence in human immunodeficiency virus-infected individuals (89) and males (86). Several classes of proteins are cold reactive, notably the cold agglutinins, cryoglobulins, cryofibrinogen, and Donath-Landsteiner antibodies.

Cold agglutinins are IgM autoantibodies usually directed against the red cell I antigen. Anti-I antibodies are present in low titers with low-temperature reactivity in normal individuals but in CHD are present in high titers and react at higher temperatures. After infections with organisms expressing I-like antigens, there is a higher titer of anti-I antibodies. Anti-I and other red-cell directed antibodies are not present in normal individuals but are occasionally identified in CHD. Clinical diagnosis of CHD by cold-provocation tests has been described (90). Coombs test, agglutinin titer, and thermal amplitude testing are usual laboratory tests (86). There is a wide thermal tolerance between individuals with CHD for laboratory-observable hemagglutination and hemolysis, occurring at temperatures between 25 and 34°C. At CPB, agglutination has been observed in the CPB circuit or coronary arteries or experimentally by placing a tube of heparinized blood on ice (88). Hemolysis in vitro and in vivo is rare because the activity of complement is temperature dependent but has been described during cardiac surgery (91).

Cryoglobulins are serum proteins that reversibly precipitate at low temperatures. Three types have been classified. Type I are monoclonal proteins such as in multiple myeloma, Waldenström's macroglobulinemia, and lymphoreticular disease. Types II and III are mixed immunoglobulins seen in autoimmune, infectious, and lymphoproliferative diseases. Few reports of CPB in patients with cryoglobulins are described.

Management of CPB depends on the severity of CHD. Although plasmapheresis, to reduce antibody titer, has been described, management is usually by avoidance of cold CPB and use of warm cardioplegia, depending on the thermal amplitude of the antibody. Where cold cardioplegia is believed to be necessary, anterograde or retrograde crystalloid cardioplegia is recommended (86). The efficacy of perioperative steroids in prevention of intraoperative CHD is unknown.

CONGENITAL COAGULATION FACTOR DISORDERS

HEMOPHILIA A (FACTOR VIII:C DEFICIENCY)

Hemophilia A (classic hemophilia) is inherited as a sex-linked recessive gene, and in 90% of individuals, both factor VIII:C and VIII:CAg are deficient, implying reduced production. Some individuals have missing factor VIII:C but VIII:CAg is present. Clinically, the diseases are identical, and factor VIII:C levels parallel the extent of disease.

Before the 1960s, fresh-frozen plasma was the only available therapy; however, cryoprecipitate and, lately, factor VIII concentrate have been mainstay therapy. Cryoprecipitate contains 75–100 units of factor VIII:C per unit, whereas factor VIII concentrate contains 1000 units in 30–100 mL. Before the early 1990s, viral transmission from multiple donors was problematic and heat treatment was used. Since then, recombinant DNA forms of factor VIII concentrate have become available. Clinically, patients present with spontaneous and excessive bleeding. Laboratory investigation reveals a prolonged APTT and normal PT, TT, and platelet count.

Desmopressin (DDAVP) has been shown to increase levels

of factor VIII by two- to fourfold, by causing release of endogenous factor VIII from peripheral stores (92–94). Accordingly, it is less effective as the severity of hemophilia A increases. Androgenic steroids have also been shown to increase factor VIII levels. Antifibrinolytics such as epsilon-aminocaproic acid and tranexamic acid have been used as adjuncts to treatment for hemophilia. Acute administration during dental procedures (95–97) and chronic administration for prevention of spontaneous bleeding (98) have been successful.

Before CPB, it is recommended that factor VIII:C levels be raised to 100% according to the following formula: units of factor VIII = weight (kg) × 40 (mL/kg) × % increase required. Because of the 8- to 12-hour half-life, repeated dosing with half the loading dose every 12 hours is required.

Antibodies to factor VIII:C develop in a significant proportion of patients and may make factor VIII concentrate requirements greater than usual. Accordingly, factor VIII activity must be measured preoperatively.

HEMOPHILIA B

Hemophilia B is a structural defect of factor IX that is inherited in a sex-linked manner. Two variants are categorized, albeit there are many structural defects described, based on whether the PT is normal with brain thromboplastin (hemophilia B) or abnormal (hemophilia B_M). Clinically, hemophilia B is indistinguishable from hemophilia A. Laboratory tests show a prolonged APTT with a normal TT and platelet count. Factor IX activity correlates with severity of the illness, although not as well as with hemophilia A. Unlike hemophilia A, inhibitors to factor IX rarely appear (1–5%).

Treatment is with prothrombin complex concentrations containing prothrombin and factors VII, IX, and X and factor IX concentrates (containing less than 5% of factors II, VII, and X). Because use of prothrombin complex concentrations has been associated with an incidence of thromboembolic disease (99) and disseminated intravascular coagulation, factor levels of 100% are not contemplated. Levels of 50–75% are usually adequate (100, 101).

Use of factor IX concentrates has been associated with fewer episodes of thromboembolism than occurs with prothrombin complex concentrations (102). In contrast to factor VIII dosing, factor IX requires twice the expected number of units to be given. The formula, units of factor IX = weight (kg) × 80 mL/kg × % increase required, is used. Because of the 18- to 24-hour half-life, only once daily dosing of half the loading dose is required.

VON WILLEBRAND DISEASE

von Willebrand disease (vWD) is a nonsex-linked document inheritance of a deficiency of von Willebrand factor (vWF). vWF is ionically bound to factor VIII complex and is an essential cofactor. This results in defective platelet adhesion and primary hemostasis at sites of vascular injury. Prevalence of the disease is approximately 1%. Unlike hemophilia, which presents with joint and soft-tissue hemorrhages and normal bleeding times, vWD is associated with mucocutaneous hemorrhages and prolonged bleeding times. Most patients with vWD have not had a significant bleeding episode and the diagnosis is made on the basis of an abnormal APTT. Subsequent laboratory testing to differentiate from hemophilia includes vWF antigen level, factor VIII:C level, ristocetin-induced platelet aggregation, ristocetin cofactor activity, and multimeric analysis. Diagnosis is based on a prolonged APTT, decreased vWF:Ag level, factor VIII:C level and vWF:RCoF activity, and a prolonged bleeding time.

The disease has been classified in five subtypes. Perioperative treatment of vWF depends upon the subtype of disease. The spectrum of therapies includes DDAVP, antifibrinolytics, factor VIII:C concentrates that contain vWF, cryoprecipitate, and platelets. Most patients (80%) have type I vWD and most of the remainder are type IIA. Therapy for these groups comprises DDAVP and antifibrinolytics (103). Type IIA patients also benefit from infusions of factor VIII:C concentrates containing vWF or cryoprecipitate. The rarer subtypes are not DDAVP-responsive and require blood products to replace higher molecular weight multimers (104).

ASPIRIN

A wide variety of drugs induce a functional defect in platelet function. These include the nitrosovasodilators, Ca^{++} channel blockers, β blockers, α blockers, antibiotics, local anesthetics, nonsteroidal anti-inflammatory agents, loop diuretics, hetastarch, and aspirin. These impairments occur by interference with intraplatelet cyclic adenine nucleotides, membrane receptors, prostaglandin synthesis, and other unknown mechanisms.

Aspirin is probably the most commonly prescribed antiplatelet drug in patients undergoing CPB. Aspirin irreversibly acetylates cyclooxygenase, inhibiting the production of thromboxane A_2. Termination of aspirin's action requires the production of new platelets because the aspirin-treated platelet is incapable of producing more cyclooxygenase. Aspirin inhibits the release of vitamin K-dependent coagulation factors. Aspirin, in clinical doses, prevents activation of platelets, thereby preventing platelet aggregation and binding to platelets adherent to the damaged vessel wall. Aspirin does not inhibit nonaggregatory platelet degranulation.

Aspirin has been shown to reduce the incidence of primary myocardial infarction, occlusion of coronary vessels, and grafts after coronary artery bypass graft (CABG) or coronary angioplasty (105) and the incidence of death and stroke in patients with transient ischemic attacks. Several studies have shown increased perioperative bleeding after CABG with preoperative aspirin (106–114). However, increased perioperative blood transfusion after aspirin ingestion has less frequently been demonstrated (108, 113, 115), and some have observed no differences (111, 114, 116). Some have observed an increased rate of reoperation for mediastinal bleeding (108, 112, 115), but others have not (111, 113, 114).

DDAVP may reduce the volume of chest tube drainage after CABG in patients who recently ingested aspirin (117–120), but this result is not universal (121). Aprotinin's ability to reduce fibrinolysis and blood loss after CABG is preserved after aspirin ingestion (122, 123).

MECHANICS OF CPB

During cardiac surgery, the CPB pump customarily replaces the function of the heart and lungs. The pump is usually "primed" with a crystalloid solution unless the patient is unusually small or anemic. Heparin is routinely added to the pump prime, in addition to direct administration to the patient. After placement of drainage (venous) and return (arterial) cannulae and assurance of adequate heparinization, CPB is commenced by allowing the blood to drain from the patient to the pump and is then returned to the patient. CPB is usually conducted with systemic flows of 1.0–2.2 L/min/m^{-2} and systemic pressures of 40–80 mm Hg at temperatures of 25–32°C. The path of blood within the bypass pump is as follows (Fig. 28.4). Venous blood from the right atrium of vena cavae is drained by gravity into an enclosed reservoir. The reservoir provides a buffer volume to account for variations in drainage of venous blood from the heart. In a so-called "bubble" oxygenator it also forms part of the oxygenator circuit. In addition, heparinized blood collected on the surgical field can also be suctioned back to the reservoir. The reservoir usually contains a "macro" filter (170 μm or similar) to filter foreign debris or particulate material before it is allowed to mix with the venous drainage blood from the patient.

From the reservoir, the blood is pumped, using either a roller pump or "centrifugal" pump, to the membrane oxygenator. The roller pump is comprised of two rollers, 180° apart, compressing a flexible plastic or rubber tubing contained within a metal "raceway." Each roller, as it rotates, compresses the tubing, almost completely, forcing blood along the tubing. As one roller disengages from the raceway, the other roller engages, giving a continuous flow with only minor flow and pressure fluctuations. Centrifugal pumps are cone-shaped pumps containing an impeller that spins at high

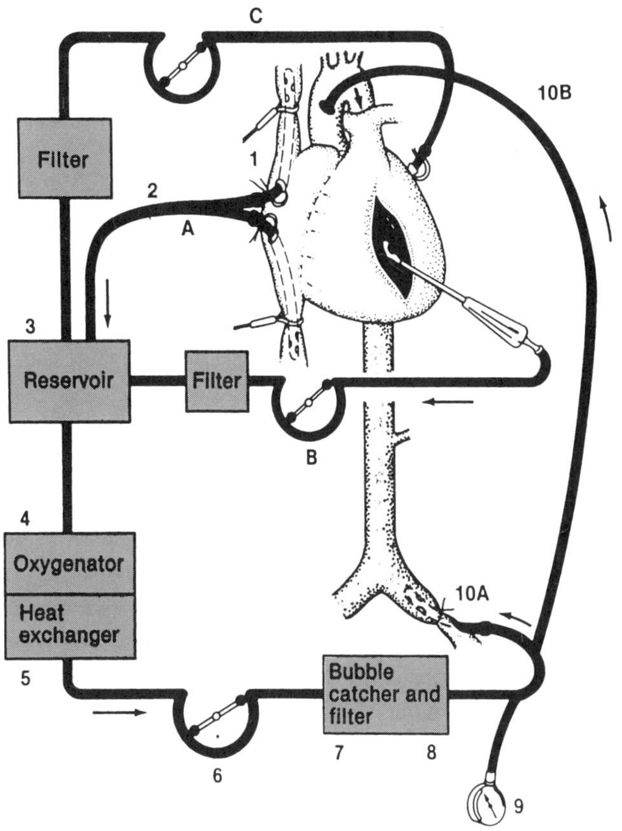

Figure 28.4. Schematic diagram of a cardiopulmonary bypass pump, bubble oxygenator, and circuit. Blood is drained by gravity from the vena cavae (1) through the venous cannula (2) into the venous reservoir (3). Heparinized blood from the surgical field and cardiotomy vent sites are pumped (B) to the venous reservoir (3). For circuits using bubble oxygenators, the blood is oxygenated (4) and then either heated or cooled (5), as appropriate, and pumped (6) back to the patient through a filter (7, 8) that can also act as a bubble trap. For membrane oxygenators, the order of the pump and oxygenator is reversed. The pressure in the arterial line is monitored (9). Blood can be returned to the patient via either the femoral artery (10A) or aorta (10B) or another arterial site. (Reprinted with permission from Antman E. Medical management of the patient undergoing cardiac surgery. In: Braunwald E, ed. Heart disease. A textbook of cardiovascular medicine. Philadelphia: WB Saunders, 1992:1670–1693.)

speed, forcing the blood outward, similar to water being thrown off an automobile tire. The pump is driven by an electric motor through a magnetic coupling. Bubble oxygenators have the pump placed downstream from the oxygenator; by contrast, membrane oxygenators have a high resistance and require the oxygenator to be downstream from the pump so that the pump can get blood through the oxygenator.

Membrane oxygenators separate the blood phase and gas phase using a thin (approximately 25 μm) membrane, through which oxygen and carbon dioxide diffuse. The membrane itself can be a thin sheet or, more usually, a hollow fiber composed of polypropylene. Other materials used are Teflon or polydimethylsiloxane. Most commonly, the gas is contained within the fiber and blood is allowed to circulate outside the wrapped fibers. The total surface area varies from 1 to 5 m^2, depending on the manufacturer and intended use of the pump (pediatric versus adult). The diffusion constant for oxygen through polypropylene is considerably less than that for carbon dioxide, hence the large surface area. Bubble oxygenators simply bubble a continuous stream of oxygen or an oxygen-air mixture throughout the blood contained in the hard-shell reservoir. Gas transfer is usually efficient and adequate for routine CPB. The gas-blood interface is a powerful stimulus to platelet and neutrophil activation along with complement activation.

Within the reservoir or oxygenator, the blood can be cooled or heated by the passage of water through stainless steel or aluminum alloy pipes, around which the blood flows. Most institutions place a 20- to 40-μm arterial filter in the outflow of the oxygenator. It is used to trap microemboli consisting of thrombus, fat, fibrin, foreign particles from the pump and circuit, and other debris. The blood is finally returned to the patient via an arterial cannula, usually placed in the ascending aorta.

VENTRICULAR DEVICES

Ventricular assist devices are designed to temporarily replace the function of either the right or left ventricle. Most commonly, they are placed on the left side of the heart and drain blood from the atrium or ventricle and pump it back into the ascending or descending aorta or the femoral artery. There is no oxygenator function to these devices. The pumping system can be either a roller or centrifugal pump or a valved, air-driven, bladder pump. Heparinization is required for their use, although their small foreign surface area usually means that lower doses are used than those required for CPB.

EXTRACORPOREAL MEMBRANE OXYGENATION

Extracorporeal membrane oxygenation is functionally identical to CPB but is used to provide long-term cardiac and pulmonary support, usually for pulmonary failure. Its efficacy is limited by the irreversibility of many diseases and the high rate of complications, usually hemorrhagic, renal, and cerebral. Structurally, the bypass system has many similarities to CPB, but the venous and arterial access points are often percutaneous. Systemic heparinization is required but usually at reduced levels compared with those for CPB. It appears to have most utility in the neonatal population, principally for respiratory distress of the newborn, meconium aspiration, and after cardiac or pulmonary surgery.

NORMAL PHYSIOLOGY OF THE COAGULATION SYSTEM

Hemostasis occurs along two, sometimes concurrent, phases. The first phase, primary hemostasis, occurs when platelets adhere to areas of intimal damage or loss to form a platelet plug. The second phase, secondary hemostasis, occurs when the platelet activates the coagulation cascade. These have been described in Chapters 5 and 6. Several components and products of normal vascular endothelium prevent platelet adherence and binding to endothelium. These include the heparins, nitric oxide, prostaglandins, thrombomodulin, prostacyclin, tissue plasminogen activator, and endonucleotidases. Loss or damage to the endothelium allows adherence of platelets to the damaged area. In the normal situation, platelets interact or roll along the vessel wall, exposing platelet receptors to the endothelium. When the endothelium is damaged or lost, these platelet receptors adhere to subendothelial matrix. Principally, platelet glycoprotein Ib binds to vWF of the matrix. Circulating vWF can also bind matrix collagen, acting as a bridge between the platelet and the matrix. Circulating vWF also acts as a platelet bridge. Collagen and other matrix adhesion (glyco) proteins vitronectin, fibronectin, and thrombospondin also bind to platelet membrane proteins to facilitate platelet adhesion.

The adhesion event causes several platelet changes; notably activation and degranulation. Dense and α-granules are fused with the platelet wall and release their contents, consisting of ADP, fibrinogen, vWF, fibronectin, vitronectin, thrombospondins, and other factors. Platelet ADP binds to its own platelet membrane receptors to induce a further sequence of events, including shape change (via actin filaments) and exteriorization of the glycoprotein IIb/IIIa receptor, which binds fibrinogen (Fig. 28.5) (124). Fibrinogen acts as the cross-link between platelets and is the primary mechanism of platelet aggregation and recruitment. Platelet phospholipases are also activated to manufacture and release thromboxanes. These cause vasoconstriction, altering shear stress, the washout or dilution of platelet products (ADP, etc.), and also directly recruit and activate platelets in the platelet plug.

PATHOPHYSIOLOGY OF CPB

The institution and maintenance of CPB require several components that alter coagulation and humoral function: heparinization, air and foreign surface exposure, hemodilution, hypothermia, nonpulsatile flow, and protamine administration. These changes induce a multitude of barely understood effects that have been described as an inflammatory response, involving the formed blood elements, coagulation, complement, and kallikrein/kinin systems.

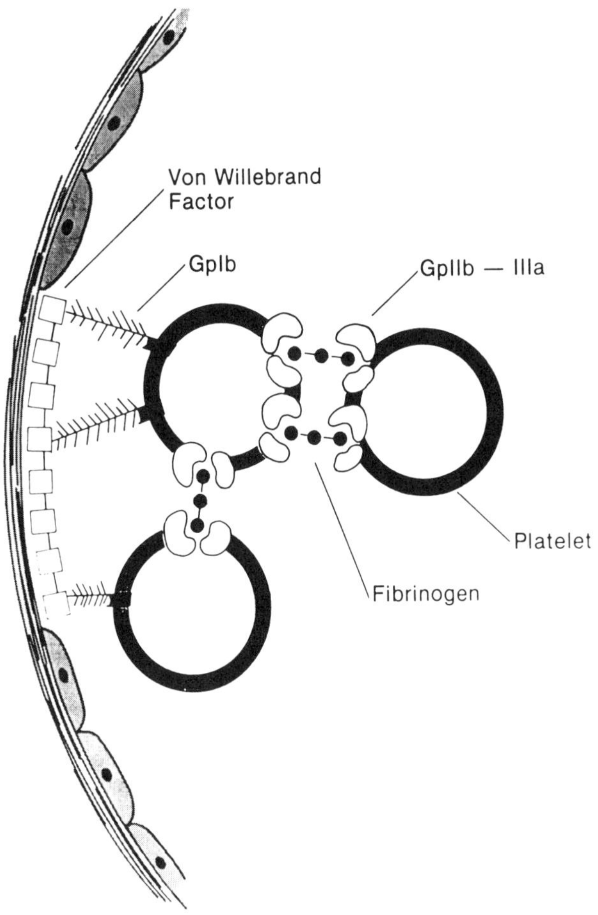

Figure 28.5. Molecular mechanism of platelet attachment to the vascular subendothelium (platelet adhesion) and of platelet-platelet adhesion. (Reprinted with permission from Handin R, Loscalzo J. Hemostasis, thrombosis fibrolysis and cardiovascular disease. In: Braunwald E, ed. Heart disease. A textbook of cardiovascular medicine. 4th ed. Philadelphia: WB Saunders, 1992:1767–1789.)

The most dramatic changes in the formed blood elements are induced by hemodilution. The CPB pump is primed with crystalloid solution, or rarely with colloids or blood. Depending on the blood volume and the volume of the priming solution, there is usually a reduction in hematocrit, white cell, and platelet count by approximately 40%. Further reductions in the platelet count are usually seen and depend on the volume of suctioned blood, degree of hypothermia, adherence of platelets to the bypass pump components, and destruction of platelets by the bypass pump.

HYPOTHERMIA

Local and/or systemic hypothermia increases bleeding in the surgical patient (125). It has long been noted by cardiac surgeons that rewarming the patient fully after systemic hypothermia reduces blood loss postoperatively. Animal studies have shown that hypothermia to 20°C causes thrombocytopenia because of hepatic platelet sequestration and increased fibrinolysis (126, 127). Local hypothermia causes an increase in the bleeding time and a decrease in the production of thromboxane B_2 in the bleeding time shed of blood. These changes are reversed by rewarming to 37°C (128).

The animal observations have been confirmed in humans. The bleeding time in humans undergoing systemic hypothermia on CPB to 25°C is prolonged (129). Furthermore, comparing the bleeding time in one arm of a patient with a systemic temperature of 25°C with the other arm (kept warm to 35°C by a local warming blanket), the "cold" arm has a prolonged bleeding time with lower shed thromboxane B_2 concentrations than the "warm" arm. Systemic hypothermia has also been shown to reduce the generation of C3a/C5a and neutrophil activation (87).

EFFECTS ON BLOOD CELLULAR ELEMENTS AND PROTEINS: COMPARISON OF MEMBRANE AND BUBBLE OXYGENATORS

The use of CPB during cardiac surgery inevitably results in humoral, hematological, and coagulation disturbances caused by blood contact and flow disturbances within the extracorporeal circuit. All types of oxygenators cause damage to the cellular and noncellular elements of the blood. The damage is greatest at the blood-gas and blood-surface interfaces but can occur without foreign-surface interaction because of shear rate injury to the blood. Protein denaturation is also caused by CPB. Within bubble oxygenators, there is circulation of these denatured proteins. In membrane oxygenators, the bound protein tends to adhere, perhaps reducing the systemic effect of denatured proteins. Bound proteins tend to reduce the adherence of platelets and white cells to the surface. In general, in vitro tests of oxygenators and the associated hardware easily demonstrate less injury with membrane oxygenators (130, 131). This is because the blood-surface (air or material) interface is larger with a bubble oxygenator. The continued blood-air interface with each passage through the oxygenator results in a greater injury than the reduced interaction with the proteinated solid surface of the membrane oxygenator. Comparisons of bubble and membrane oxygenators show that the reduced foreign-surface to blood interface in bubble oxygenators results in less initial binding of platelets than that in a membrane oxygenator. However, the air-blood interface in bubble oxygenators causes more platelet activation over time than the surface membrane to platelet interaction in a membrane oxygenator. It is well known that plasma proteins rapidly collect at blood-foreign surface interfaces (132). Fibrinogen, albumin, and, to a lesser extent, globulin bind to the surface. The rate and extent of binding are dependent on surface charge, surface chemistry, and the shear rate at the blood-surface interface. Bound, but not circulating, fibrinogen is a ligand for platelet receptors, thereby causing platelet adhesion and activation.

Platelets are very sensitive to damage during CPB. They are good intermediate outcome markers. Platelet quantitative, morphological, and receptor changes occur early in CPB with little evidence of other injury. Quantitative changes may occur as a result of dilution, sequestration, and subsequent release. Morphological and qualitative changes are variable and not well understood. Overall, membrane oxygenators are associated with less trauma and sequestration of the formed elements, less platelet activation, and better platelet preservation in vitro (131).

In vivo tests show less clear differences than in vitro tests. This is because the cellular and noncellular injury caused by the oxygenator and circuit is modified by the body. Variations in clinical techniques, especially suction from the field, are important. The reticulo-endothelial system, vascular endothelium, and solid organs act as filters and modifiers of the response. Many studies have examined the differences between bubble and membrane oxygenators. Most are flawed by the failure to exclude suctioned, and therefore traumatized, blood from the field and having too few patients. With CPB times of less than 2 hours, the difference between the two oxygenators is minimal (133, 134). Beyond 2 hours there is evidence to support less cellular damage with membrane oxygenators. However, markers of cellular and noncellular damage represent only intermediate outcomes. More appropriate outcomes to examine are blood product requirements, the incidence and severity of end-organ dysfunction and effect on duration, and cost of hospitalization. These are seldom well examined in most studies. When examined, the difference between the two oxygenators on blood loss is probably minimal because several studies have failed to demonstrate reductions in blood loss with membrane oxygenators (133, 135–137). Two studies have demonstrated advantages of membrane oxygenators for longer perfusion periods (138, 139).

COATED SURFACES AND ATTENUATION OF BYPASS-INDUCED INJURY

Blood contact with artificial surfaces leads to activation of the humoral inflammatory systems and cellular elements. The humoral systems involved include the complement, kallikrein, coagulation, and fibrinolytic pathways. The whole-body inflammatory response is responsible for considerable systemic organ dysfunction and coagulopathy (140–142). Several physical approaches to reduce this contact-activation have been adopted, the most common of which is heparin-coating of the exposed material. This approach mimics the endothelial adherence of the glycosaminoglycan heparin sulfate that binds ATIII, thereby inhibiting thrombin adherence to the vascular wall. Heparin is bound to the foreign surface by one of several mechanisms, leaving the ATIII-active portion, a pentasaccharide sequence, exposed (143). The surface-bound ATIII-heparin complex binds thrombin avidly. The stable ATIII-thrombin complex is subsequently released from the ATIII binding site on the surface-bound heparin, thereby allowing further circulating ATIII to bind to surface-bound heparin in a regenerative process (144). Initially, heparin was bound using quaternary ammonium salts (ionic binding) by using heparin's anionic charge to bind it to the cationic charge of the salt. The salt was then bound to the foreign surface. The ionic attachment of heparin to the salt is reversible and allows leaching of heparin; the rate of leaching depends on the salt used. Alternatively, heparin can be covalently bound to the foreign surface using a linking or "spacer" molecule. In general, covalent binding is more stable (145). Other considerations include heparin metabolism by circulating enzymes and achieving a structural configuration that exposes the ATIII binding site to the circulation. Early work demonstrated the importance of the length of the spacer chain between the surface and the active heparin site (144, 146) and the propensity of higher molecular weight heparins to activate platelets (144).

Heparin binding also reduces the area of foreign surface available for protein binding. As previously mentioned, fibrinogen and fibrin bind to the foreign surface and can subsequently bind and activate platelets. Heparin-coated surfaces reduce this process by reducing the thrombin-mediated conversion of fibrinogen to fibrin.

Two commercially available processes are available. An ionically bound surface is marketed by Bentley Laboratories (Duraflo II, Irvine, CA). Porcine mucosal heparin is bound to an alkylbenzyl dimethylammonium ligand attached to an 18-carbon alkyl chain (147). This salt-heparin complex is then washed through the circuit and binds to the surface of the circuit. A covalently bound surface is marketed by Medtronic (Carmeda Bioactive Surface, Anaheim, CA). Porcine mucosal heparin is degraded by nitrous acid and the fragments are then attached to a polyethylenimine spacer via a nitrous acid-created aldehyde group on each heparin fragment. The spacer is then bound to the foreign surface (143, 148).

Animal and ex vivo studies have shown reduced blood trauma with heparin-coated circuits and the ability to use markedly reduced levels of heparinization (147, 149–151). Studies have shown a reduced frequency of adherence of cellular elements to the surface, reduced blood trauma, reduced leukocyte, platelet and complement activation, and less blood loss with heparin-coated circuits (150, 152–157). However, its efficacy is debatable, and not all investigators have found reductions in blood loss or systemic inflammatory responses (158).

Human studies have found less consistent results. Comparing patients receiving conventional heparinization with and without heparin-coated bypass circuits, there is usually little difference noted (159, 160). This probably reflects the relative effectiveness of adequate heparinization in attenuation of bypass-induced hematological injury. Several studies and reports have examined the efficacy of using heparin-coated circuits in the presence of very low levels of heparinization (161–163). These have usually shown less bleeding and transfusion and have confirmed the utility of these devices. The most likely utility for these devices is in long-term extracorporeal support where heparinization entails increased likelihood or severity of bleeding (164). Clinical utility is still not well defined, in part because of the cost of the coatings. In situations where the risk of heparinization (usually of bleeding) is high, heparin-coated circuits will probably have the most utility.

COMPLEMENT ACTIVATION AND MODULATION

Complement constitutes a major part of the body's response to trauma, infection, or immunological stress. The classic pathway is most commonly initiated by antibody-antigen complexes. The alternative pathway is initiated by foreign bodies or surfaces and by various microbial organisms. Both classic and alternative pathways are initiated by circulating lipopolysaccharides/endotoxin and by tissue injury (165).

Complement activation is a ubiquitous aspect of CPB, with both the classic and alternative pathways involved (Fig. 28.6). The alternative pathway is activated by the surface of the circuit and oxygenator (166), although surface activation of factor XII may also activate C1 and initiate the classic pathway (167). Trauma to formed blood elements activates the alternative pathway, whereas denatured immunoglobulin aggregates, seen with blood-gas interfaces, activate the classic pathway (168–171).

Increases in the complement fragments C3a and the C5b-9 membrane attack complex are observed on bypass (130,

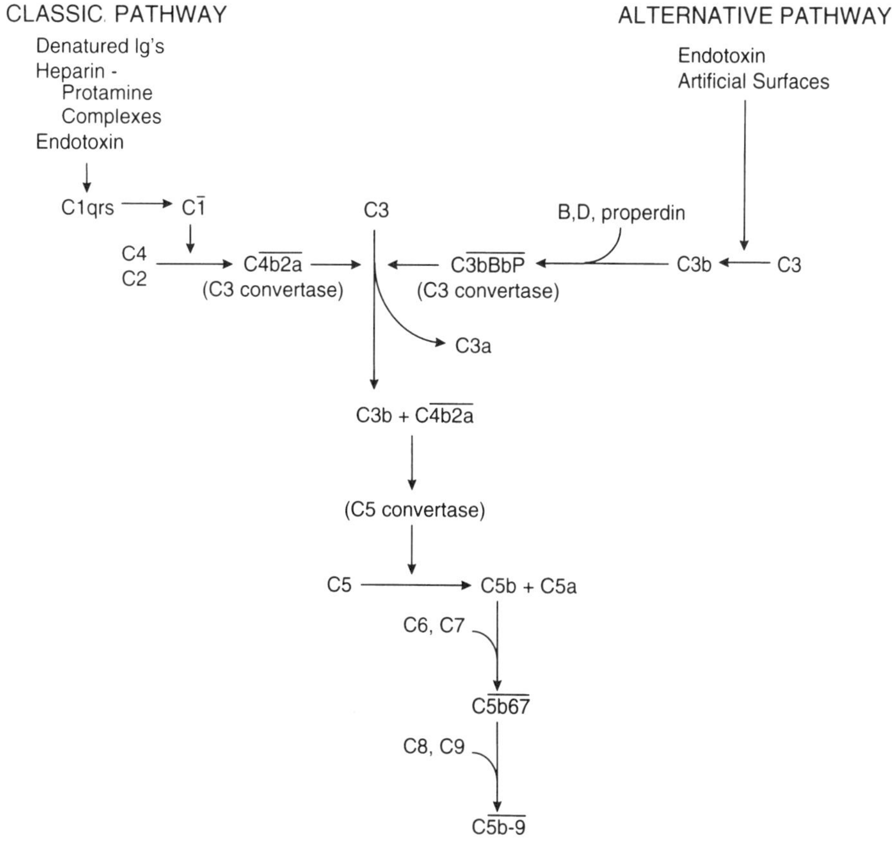

Figure 28.6. (A) Complement activation during CPB. (Modified by permission from Warren J, Ward P, Johnson K. The inflammatory response. In: Williams WJ, Beutler E, Erslev AJ, Lichman MA, eds. Hematology. New York: McGraw-Hall, 1990:63–70.)

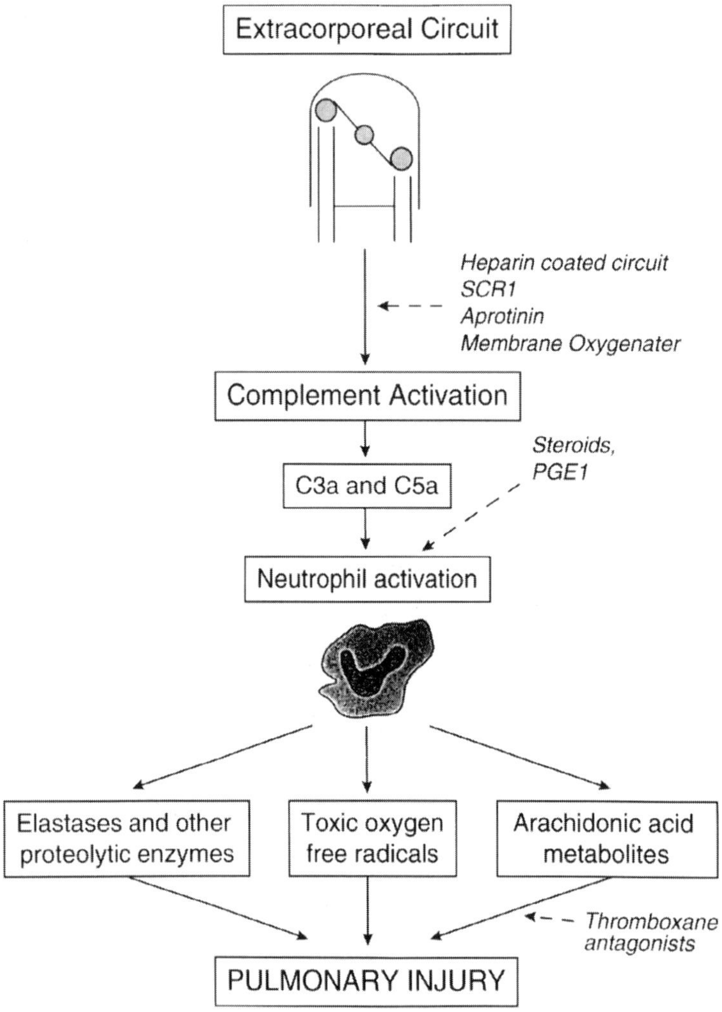

Figure 28.6. ***(continued)*** (**B**) Approaches to the prevention of complement-induced pulmonary injury during CPB. (Modified by permission from Sladen R, Berkowitz D. Cardiopulmonary bypass and the lung. In: Gravlee G, Davis R, Utley J, eds. Cardiopulmonary bypass: principles and practice. Baltimore: Williams & Wilkins, 1993:468–487.)

169, 172–174). Most but not all studies fail to detect an increase in C4a, indicating predominance of the alternative pathway in complement activation (169, 173, 175–178). C5a, although undoubtedly present on bypass, is difficult to detect because of rapid binding to neutrophils (172).

Protamine infusion causes complement activation in the postbypass period. Although protamine alone has no effect on complement, heparin-protamine complexes activate the classic pathway with production of C3a, C4a, and C5a (166, 176). The products of complement activation, particularly the anaphylatoxins C3a and C5a, result in pulmonary sequestration of neutrophils; increased capillary permeability; vasoconstriction; and cardiac, pulmonary, and renal dysfunction (175). The acute lung injury associated with bypass-induced complement activation is often referred to as the "post-pump" or "post-perfusion" lung syndrome. The pattern of injury involves an initial transient hypoxemia associated with an increase in pulmonary vascular resistance followed by a sustained increase in pulmonary capillary permeability and lung water, resulting in an adult respiratory distress-like syndrome (179, 180).

After release of the aortic cross-clamp and restoration of pulmonary blood flow, neutrophil counts decrease across the pulmonary vasculature. Peroxidation products and transvascular protein flux increase (176, 180, 181). These events are reduced (although not eliminated) in C3-deficient dogs (182) and in leukocyte-depleted sheep (183). This dysfunction is a result of complement activation of neutrophils, which adhere to endothelium and produce oxygen free radicals, peroxidase products, and arachidonic acid metabolites (176, 180, 184, 185). These activation products cause increased pulmonary vascular resistance and decreased arterial oxygenation that is ameliorated by cyclooxygenase inhibitors and/or free radical scavengers (179, 186).

Inhibition of complement activation involves direct inhibition of complement formation (e.g., membrane oxygenators, heparin-coated circuits, aprotinin, soluble complement inhibitors) or, alternatively, modulation of the effects of complement on leukocytes and leukocyte-based mediators of injury (e.g., steroids, prostaglandins, thromboxane antagonists) (Fig. 28.6).

The oxygenator (or any foreign surface) plays a primary role in the hematological and inflammatory changes of bypass. Vigorous bubbling of oxygen (i.e., the bubble oxygenator) through blood denatures and aggregates immunoglobulins, activating the classic complement pathway (133, 171). Membrane oxygenators may result in less complement activation. However, many membrane oxygenators also have a direct blood-gas interface (187). Moreover, membrane oxygenators with a high surface area may result in increased complement activation via the alternative pathway (188).

Studies comparing bubble to membrane oxygenators are hampered by variation in degree of hypothermia, hemodilution, heparin dosage, and priming solution (170, 171). These variables greatly affect complement activity. In addition, membrane oxygenators are quite heterogeneous, varying in materials, surface area, flow patterns, and porosity (130, 168, 187, 188). It is not surprising, therefore, that such comparisons are inconclusive (130, 133, 137, 168, 170, 171, 177, 189).

Heparin has been shown in vitro to inhibit complement activation by both classic and alternative pathways (190, 191). So-called biocompatible circuits seek to minimize activation of complement (and other inflammatory mediators) by coating the bypass circuit, oxygenator, or both with heparin. Studies comparing heparin-coated with noncoated surfaces have investigated complement activation, neutrophil activation, and pulmonary function with unclear results (192, 193). Some show heparin-coated circuits to decrease, but not eliminate, activation of C3 on bypass (191, 192). However, others show no change in C3 or a change that only occurs after bypass as a result of decreased protamine dose requirement (193–195). Similar confusion exists with regard to C5 activation. C5a binds rapidly to neutrophils and is thus difficult to assay (172, 173, 191). Studies that attempt to measure C5a or C5b-9 as a surrogate for C5 activation are equivocal with regard to heparin-coated circuits (191, 192, 194–196).

Aprotinin, the naturally occurring inhibitor of kallikrein and plasmin, has been proposed as an inhibitor of complement activation. In vitro, aprotinin reduces C1 activation at kallikrein-inhibiting doses and partially inhibits neutrophil elastase release (167). This is not likely to be a direct effect of aprotinin but a result of inhibition of kallikrein, plasmin, and factor XII. Aprotinin has no effect on generation of factors C3a or C4a in vivo (197).

Soluble complement receptor type 1 is a recombinant form of the membrane-bound complement inhibitor found on formed blood elements. An inhibitor of both the C3 and C5 convertases, it inhibits complement activation by both the classic and alternative pathways. In a porcine model of CPB, soluble complement receptor type 1 eliminated activation of C3 and C5. However, little effect was seen on neutrophil activation, pulmonary edema, or arterial oxygenation. This drug shows promise in future clinical use but also highlights the multiple systems (e.g., kallikrein, kinin, coagulation, fibrinolytic) at play in the inflammatory response to bypass (198).

Modulation of complement effect on neutrophils and the pulmonary vasculature without direct complement inhibition has been attempted with steroids, prostaglandins (specifically PGE_1), and thromboxane antagonists.

In general, steroids have not been shown to reduce complement activation on bypass (177, 199). In one study, methylprednisolone did reduce C3a activation by bubble oxygenators but not membrane oxygenators (133). However, steroids have been variously reported to reduce pulmonary sequestration of neutrophils, to reduce generation of tumor necrosis factor and leukotriene B_4, to reduce pulmonary vascular resistance and hypoxemia, and to reduce postoperative complications and intensive care unit duration (186, 189, 199, 200). Given the general lack of confirmation and a number of contradictory studies (201, 202), routine steroid use does not seem justified.

Prostaglandins, specifically PGE_1, inhibit pulmonary leukocyte activation and release of lysosomal enzymes. In a canine model of CPB, PGE_1 completely inhibited neutrophil aggregation in the lung (201).

Pulmonary vasoconstriction and hypoxemia are likely due to a complement and leukocyte-mediated release of thromboxane A_2 from the pulmonary vasculature. In a sheep model of complement activation, a selective thromboxane receptor antagonist completely ablated any change in pulmonary vascular resistance or arterial oxygenation (203).

KALLIKREIN

Kallikrein is activated from prekallikrein as part of the intrinsic or contact-activated coagulation pathway. It is a significant mediator of the "whole body inflammatory response" to CPB (167, 204–210). Polyanionic surfaces such as subendothelial collagen or foreign surfaces such as the bypass oxygenator and circuit bind prekallikrein and high-molecular-weight kininogen, bringing these two proenzymes into proximity with activated factor XII (210, 211). Factor XIIa converts prekallikrein to kallikrein, which correspondingly activates additional factor XII (Fig. 28.7). This positive feedback loop provides physiological amplification of the clotting cascade.

Kallikrein converts high-molecular-weight kininogen to bradykinin, which increases microvascular permeability and dilates arterioles, contributing to hypotension and pulmonary dysfunction in settings ranging from endotoxin shock to CPB (209, 212, 213). Bradykinin is metabolized by a converting enzyme associated with the pulmonary vascular endothelium. Consequently, exclusion of the pulmonary circuit during bypass leads to undiminished activity (206, 209). The degree of bradykinin generation appears to vary with time of bypass, depth of hypothermia, and composition of pump prime (209, 214).

More importantly, kallikrein leads to generation of plasmin from plasminogen, which in the setting of CPB quickly overwhelms its circulating inhibitors. Plasmin activates and aggregates platelets, rendering them susceptible to clearance from the circulation or, if uncleared, unable to participate in the release reaction (215–217). Plasmin cleaves platelet surface receptors for adhesion (glycoprotein Ib) (218–220) and aggregation (glycoprotein IIb/IIIa) (221, 222). Finally, it generates fibrinogen degradation products that interfere with platelet aggregation and fibrin cross-linking (223, 224). None of these effects taken alone are sufficient to produce abnormal clotting. However, taken together, these events, with plasmin as a common catalyst, contribute in a significant way to the multifaceted hemostatic defect seen after bypass.

Endogenous kallikrein modifiers include the C1 inhibitor, alpha$_2$-macroglobulin, alpha$_1$-antitrypsin and ATIII (225). C1 inhibitor is the most specific and most relevant inhibitor of kallikrein. It also has activity against the complement factor C1 and factor XIIa (226). Alpha$_2$-macroglobulin binds kallikrein with less specificity than C1 inhibitor but is an abundant, thus significant, plasma inhibitor. The kallikrein-macroglobulin complex retains enzymatic activity against some synthetic substrates, which makes some functional assays subject to confusion (227).

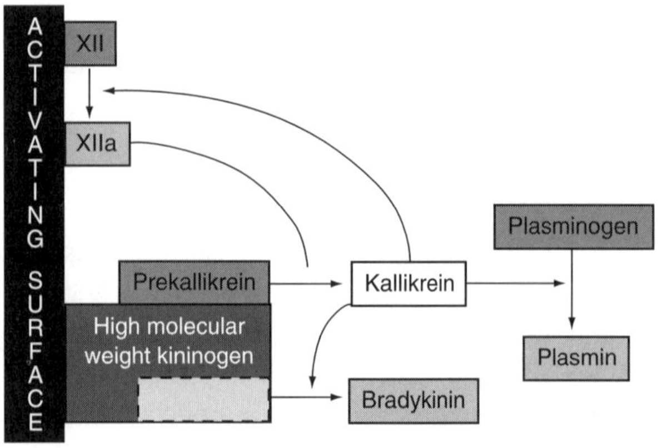

Figure 28.7. Role of kallikrein in surface activation.

ATIII inhibits kallikrein only in the presence of heparin, and its activity is the most controversial of the natural inhibitors. It is variously described as a slow inhibitor, with activity only in the absence of C1 inhibitor (226) or as a major inhibitor in the presence of high-molecular-weight kininogen (211). Heparin itself has been considered an activator of kallikrein. Reasons for this include contact activation via heparin's polyanionic structure (227), inhibition of the C1 inhibitor (228), or endotoxin contamination of the drug (204). This activation may also be simply an artifact of the assay (227).

Aprotinin is a bovine-derived, low-molecular-mass (6512 Da) polypeptide with multiple inhibitory activities (210). It is a potent inhibitor of serine proteases including trypsin and chymotrypsin but is required in large molecular excess (5–10 times) for inhibition of kallikrein to occur (213). Kallikrein inhibition occurs at 200–500 KIU/mL, whereas plasmin inhibition occurs at the much lower concentration of 75–125 KIU/mL (210, 213). The high dose "Hammersmith" protocol results in plasma aprotinin concentrations of 190–335 KIU/mL (229).

Aprotinin reduces kallikrein activity on bypass, reduces activation of the intrinsic pathway, and preserves ATIII (208, 230). C1 inhibitor is preserved in patients receiving high-dose aprotinin (205), whereas kallikrein-C1 inhibitor complexes are reduced in vitro (167, 197). Bradykinin production is reduced and high-molecular-weight kininogen is preserved (206). These findings remain in dispute, however (207, 212, 231), and the clinical benefits of kallikrein inhibition are not yet clear. It appears for now that aprotinin's most significant effect is to preserve hemostasis via direct inhibition of plasmin (210, 229, 232).

MONITORING HEPARIN ANTICOAGULATION

Individual patient response to heparin is variable. Blood heparin levels vary widely in response to a fixed dose as do assays of coagulation such as the ACT (233, 234). Empirical heparin therapy may result in excessive, or worse, inadequate anticoagulation depending on individual sensitivity to and metabolism of heparin (235). Because of this variability, monitoring of heparin anticoagulation is extremely important.

An ideal assay establishes an anticoagulant effect that is therapeutic without excessive anticoagulation. It is sensitive at high and low ranges of response, reproducible and easy to perform (236, 237). Other features of an ideal assay include: use of small amounts of whole blood, bedside availability, and reagents that are inexpensive, stable, and commercially available (238).

Assays of anticoagulation can be divided into functional and quantitative assays. Functional assays, such as the TT, PT, APTT, and ACT, demonstrate the response of the individual to anticoagulation but are also affected by factors unrelated to heparin anticoagulation. Quantitative assays, such as heparin concentration monitoring, verify and quantify the presence of anticoagulant but do not document its effect (239).

PT involves the addition of animal-derived tissue thromboplastin to recalcified, warmed, citrated plasma. PT prolongs predominantly in response to low (less than 50%) levels of factor V, VII, or X but is relatively insensitive to heparin (240, 241).

TT measures the effect of thrombin on fibrinogen. Thrombin is added to a warmed recalcified sample of plasma from citrated blood. Time to clot formation is recorded. TT is highly sensitive to the effect of low levels of heparin on thrombin but is unclottable at high heparin concentrations. TT is affected by levels of fibrinogen, ATIII, and fibrinogen/fibrin degradation products (240–242).

APTT involves this addition of phospholipid (partial thromboplastin reagent) plus a surface activator (kaolin, celite) to recalcified, warmed, citrated plasma (240, 241). APTT is sensitive to the effects of low-dose heparin on factor Xa and thrombin (239, 243–245), but reproducibility diminishes at higher doses (236). Like the TT, APTT is unclottable at concentrations of heparin seen during bypass (239, 243, 244). However, this sensitivity profile is advantageous when considering adequacy of protamine reversal of heparin (246).

APTT correlates poorly with heparin concentration and with other assays of anticoagulation such as ACT. Sources of variability in the APTT include levels of factor VIII and ATIII, type of activating reagent, and individual differences in response to a heparin dose. This variability results from differences in volume of distribution, metabolism, and clearance for the drug (236, 245–247).

A bedside APTT is also available. The Hemochron-APTT (International Technidyne, Edison, NJ) requires 1.5 mL of fresh whole blood to be added to a tube containing calcium, phospholipid, and diatomaceous earth. A normal clotting time is 45–65 seconds. This technique has been found to correlate well to both plasma APTT and heparin level at low heparin dose (237).

The ACT was originally introduced in 1966 (248). In 1975, Bull et al. (235, 249) suggested dosing heparin for bypass based on the response of the ACT to an initial heparin dose and continued monitoring of the ACT during bypass to predict additional heparin need. In doing so, heparin therapy was transformed from a collection of empirical protocols to that which included monitoring of anticoagulant effect. ACT is insensitive to low heparin levels but, unlike the TT or aPTT, gives meaningful results at the high levels of heparin required for bypass. ACT uses whole blood and is quick and easy to perform at the bedside (233, 248, 250).

Numerous problems, however, make the ACT a potentially inaccurate and imprecise assay. Individual response to heparin is variable, and the test is affected by factors unrelated to heparin. The relationship of ACT to heparin concentration is not always linear. Alterations in technique and test conditions affect precision (reproducibility). In addition, ACT endpoints are arbitrary and unrelated to clinical outcome.

The manually performed ACT is mainly of historical interest. Two milliliters of whole blood are withdrawn into a glass tube containing 12 mg of diatomaceous earth that serves as a contact activator. The tube is inverted vigorously and then rocked slowly at a constant temperature of 37°C. The tube is tilted or rolled at 15-second intervals until a clot is seen (248). Sources of error in this assay include variability in phlebotomy, mixing, temperature, and clot detection.

Automated ACT is easier to perform and accounts for less variability in technique and result. The Hemochron (International Technidyne) ACT device requires 2 mL of whole blood to be placed into a prewarmed glass tube containing celite (diatomaceous earth) or other contact activators and a magnet (Fig. 28.8). The tube is placed into a rotating well within a heat block. The magnet remains dependent until the formed clot displaces it toward the center of the tube. This displacement activates a proximity switch and stops the timer (233, 238, 244, 250–253).

The HemoTec (Medtronic/HemoTec Inc., Englewood, CO) device uses 0.4 mL of whole blood added into a prewarmed cartridge containing kaolin (Fig. 28.9). Mixing occurs by means of a plunger. As clotting blood impedes the action of the plunger, an optical detector is triggered and terminates the assay (250, 252).

In studies comparing the manual, Hemochron and HemoTec ACT vary greatly in their results, although the trend is for Hemochron ACT to be longer than the manual or HemoTec (250, 252–255). This difference is accentuated when ACT is prolonged (252). The variation may be a result of differences in concentration or quality of contact activator, mixing technique, and technique of clot detection (252, 255–257). The precision (reproducibility between identical samples) of the ACT varies up to 9% (233, 258).

Other factors contributing to variability in the ACT include hypothermia (234, 259), severe thrombocytopenia (260) or thrombocytosis (261), platelet activation (237, 262), and the antifibrinolytic, aprotinin (208, 229, 263, 264). Hypother-

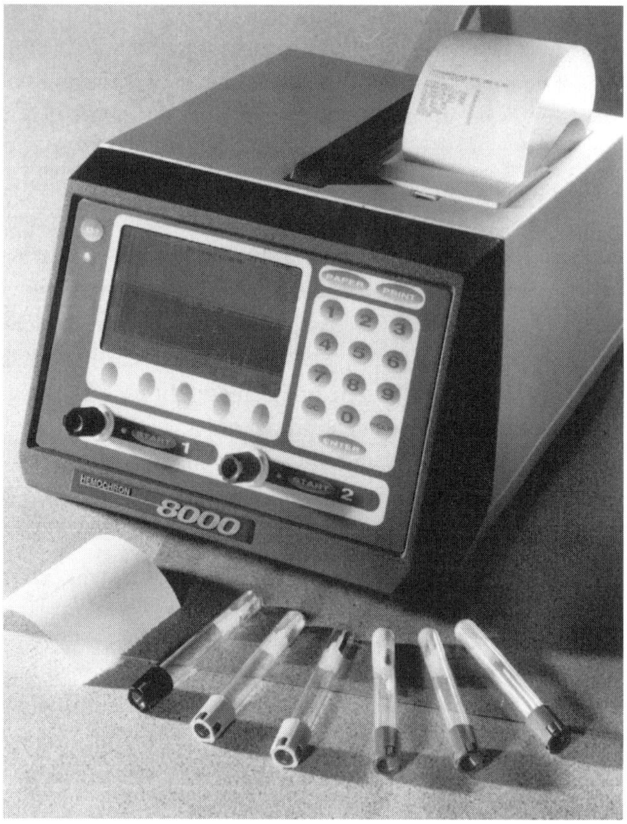

Figure 28.8. The Hemochron ACT monitor. (Courtesy of International Technidyne, Edison, NJ.)

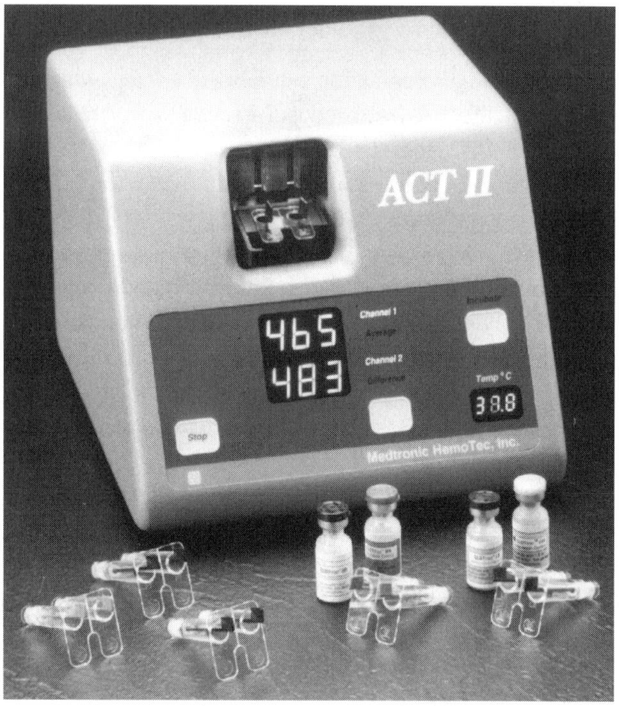

Figure 28.9. The HemoTec ACT monitor. (Courtesy of Medtronic/HemoTec Inc., Englewood, CO.)

mia impairs platelet activation and the rate of the coagulation cascade. Thrombocytopenia causes a deficiency of platelet phospholipid needed for clot organization, whereas thrombocytosis and/or platelet activation neutralizes heparin via release of platelet factor 4. Aprotinin delays contact activation through its inhibition of kallikrein.

Factors found not to contribute to ACT variability include age, weight, body surface area (249), platelet count (within the normal range), and ATIII (260). Hemodilution has been shown in vitro to prolong ACT (234), but other studies show no correlation between hematocrit (as a proxy for dilution) and ACT (259, 260).

Despite Bull et al.'s (235, 265) claims of a linear relationship between heparin dose and ACT, most studies find ACT to correlate weakly (244, 258, 266, 267) or not at all (234, 237, 245, 259, 268, 269) to heparin concentration during bypass. Lack of precision and large interpatient variability in response to heparin (up to 600%) are major factors in weakening the correlation (233, 234, 269, 270).

The optimal ACT for bypass is not clear. Bull et al. (249) based their optimal range of ACT of 300–600 seconds on their observation that a clot could appear in the surgical field if the ACT were beneath 300 seconds and that the ACT was unreliable if over 600 seconds.

Alternatively, fibrin monomer formation is inhibited at an ACT over 400, with preservation of ATIII, fibrinogen, and platelets (271). In addition, formation of fibrinopeptide A (a thrombin cleavage product of fibrinogen) is limited at an ACT exceeding 400 seconds (266, 272). As such, 400 seconds is the usual target range for anticoagulation. However, the clinical benefits of this target remain unproved. Many studies show no sequelae (based on fibrin monomer formation or absence of visible clot) of an ACT as low as 250–300 seconds (234, 273, 274).

Given the variability of the ACT, its imprecision, and its response to factors unrelated to heparin dose (e.g., hypothermia, platelet activation), heparin concentration monitoring is an alternative. Patients who undergo bypass with heparin concentration monitoring have significantly reduced fibrinopeptide A formation compared with those monitored by ACT alone (266). As such, monitoring adequacy of heparin concentration may result in decreased consumption of clotting factors on bypass and improved postbypass hemostasis.

Unfortunately, heparin concentration monitoring has never been shown to be superior to ACT in this regard. Heparin monitoring results in higher doses of heparin and protamine used (266, 275). Impaired postbypass hemostasis may occur in these patients as a result of excess anti-factor Xa activity that is not effectively neutralized by protamine (266). Worse yet, heparin concentration monitoring without a functional assay of anticoagulation may result in inadequate anticoagulation in the face of heparin resistance or ATIII deficiency (238, 276).

Ultimately, the combination of heparin concentration monitoring with functional monitoring (i.e., ACT) results in optimal anticoagulation on bypass and return to normal hemostasis in the postbypass period. Protocols using these two assays in concert compared with ACT alone (predominantly in historical control subjects) result in an up to 50% reduction in protamine dose, with reduced blood loss and blood product requirement (234, 269, 277, 278). Assays of heparin concentration can be functional, such as the protamine titration assay, or can involve chromogenic/fluorogenic substrates for thrombin or factor Xa. The protamine titration assay is based on the principle that a clot will form earliest in the presence of an optimal neutralizing ratio of protamine to heparin. Protamine in excess of heparin will paradoxically prolong clot formation (279–281) as will the predictable excess of heparin to protamine. Any functional assay of heparin activity (e.g., TT, APTT, ACT) can be subjected to protamine titration (282).

The Hepcon (Medtronic/HemoTec Inc.) is an automated protamine titration assay. It consists of a cartridge with glass wells, each containing an incrementally increasing dose of protamine to which whole blood is added (Fig. 28.10). Air is bubbled through the well, activating and mixing the protamine and blood. As a clot accumulates on a mesh filter at the top of each well, the level of blood in the well falls and a light detector is activated. The tube in which blood first clots contains the optimal ratio of heparin to protamine, approximately 10 μg protamine to 1 unit of heparin. From this ratio, the heparin concentration is calculated (277, 283). This technique of heparin monitoring is fast, is easy to perform, has good precision, and uses whole blood (234, 284).

A fluorogenic assay is available (Protopath, Miami, FL) using a fluorescent molecule (aminoisophthalic acid dimethyl ester) coupled by amide bond to a tripeptide sequence resembling the site of action of thrombin upon fibrinogen. Plasma from the patient is mixed with a pooled normal plasma containing an excess of ATIII and a fixed amount of thrombin. Thrombin uninhibited by heparin acts on the substrate and releases the fluorescent molecule (243, 282, 284, 285).

This assay is quick and has a high degree of accuracy and precision. It is not affected by patient levels of fibrinogen, fibrinogen/fibrin degradation products, or ATIII. It is sensitive to low concentrations of heparin and is more accurate than protamine titration (284). Drawbacks of the assay include the use of plasma rather than whole blood, the need for controls and standards for each assay, and the need for a highly skilled operator. Chromogenic assays are available using substrates for thrombin or factor Xa activity.

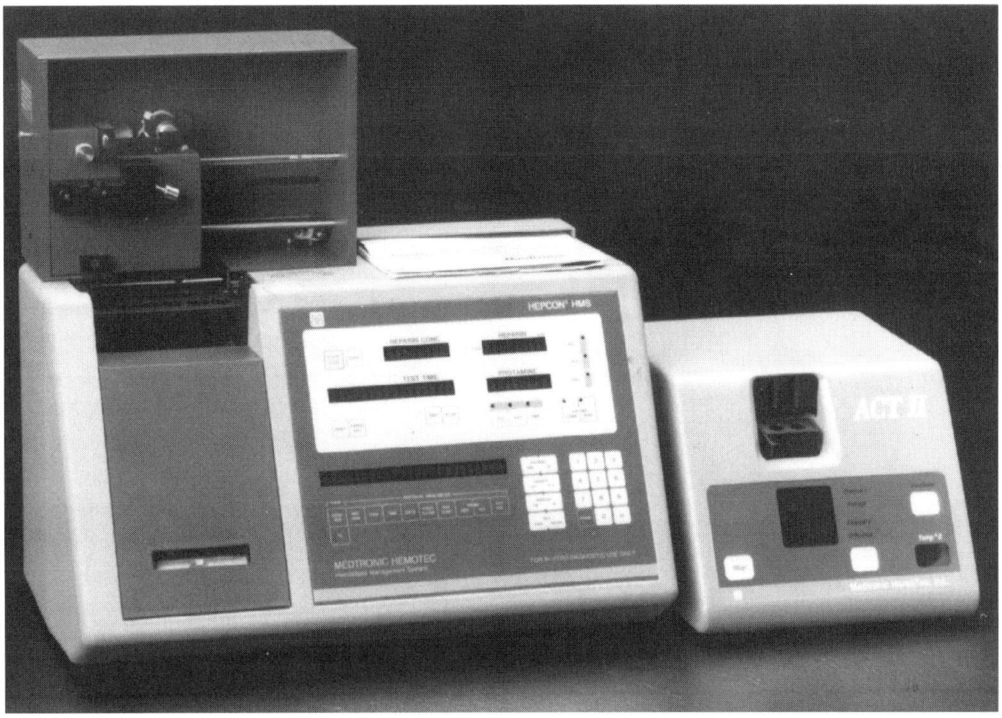

Figure 28.10. The Hepcon heparin concentration monitor (alongside the HemoTec ACT monitor). (Courtesy of Medtronic/HemoTec Inc., Englewood, CO.)

These assays are similar in technique to the fluorogenic assay and have similar drawbacks but have less precision (247).

PROTAMINE

Protamine, containing 67% arginine residues, is a densely positively charged substance derived from salmon sperm, although it is found in most other vertebrate species. It binds electrostatically to negatively charged heparin and effectively neutralizes heparin's anticoagulant effect. However, in large doses, protamine has anticoagulant activity and antiplatelet effects. Protamine inhibits the proteolytic activity of thrombin upon fibrinogen in a dose-dependent, reversible fashion (279). Excess protamine will prolong the ACT and other measures of coagulation in human and canine models (280, 281). This prolongation is reduced paradoxically by the presence of heparin.

Protamine reduces platelet count and impairs in vitro platelet response to agonists such as ADP, epinephrine, and thrombin (53, 281, 286–289). The mechanism for the reduction in platelet count is the electrostatic adherence of protamine to the platelet membrane. Protamine bridges platelets and causes microaggregates, resulting in decreased platelet number (288, 290–292). Protamine also causes release of tissue plasminogen activator from endothelium (53).

REVERSAL OF HEPARIN BY PROTAMINE

Calculation of the appropriate protamine dose at the termination of bypass presents difficulties resulting from interpatient variability in sensitivity to and metabolism of heparin. In addition, degree and duration of hypothermia on bypass affect heparin half-life and the resultant dose of protamine required (293). The result of such an inadequate calculation are obvious: inadequate reversal of heparin or protamine overdose.

Methods of protamine reversal include use of a fixed regimen, ACT titration, or determination of heparin concentration. Fixed, or empirical, regimens use a predetermined ratio of protamine to heparin that varies from less than 1 mg of protamine for every milligram of heparin to a 5:1 ratio. The amount of heparin to which this calculation is applied can be the initial dose of heparin or the total amount of heparin given before and during bypass (249). This technique is simple, requiring no additional equipment or operator training. However, the large variation in reversal protocols and the inability to respond to individual variability result in the problems discussed above (249, 293).

ACT titration uses the ACT before and during bypass to produce a heparin dose ACT dose-response curve. This curve is then used at the termination of bypass to predict the required protamine dose (235). This technique is simple, effective, and results in an average of 50–70% less protamine used than in the fixed regimen (249, 294).

Unfortunately, ACT titration presumes a linear heparin ACT-dose relationship that likely does not exist (234, 237, 245, 260, 268, 269). ACTs over 600 have virtually no relationship to heparin dose (249, 294). In addition, ACT is insensitive to low doses of heparin, so that inadequate reversal is unlikely to be detected (293).Measurement of heparin concentration by protamine titration has been described for 40 years (287) and has been shown to use less protamine than empirical therapy for almost as long (295). Methods of protamine titration have been described above (265, 282), although the most common in use is the automated Hepcon system (Medtronic/HemoTec Inc.) (234, 277, 283, 284). Heparin concentration monitoring results in an average 30% (up to 46%) reduction in protamine dose over the ACT dose-response curve (234).

PROTAMINE REACTIONS

Protamine reactions have been described since 1949. Jaques (296) described hypotension occurring on rapid injection, whereas Lowenstein in 1983 (297) described the idiosyncratic "catastrophic pulmonary vasoconstriction" response to protamine. Risk factors for protamine reactions are difficult to verify but may include valvular disease, preexisting pulmonary hypertension, use of protamine-containing insulin or other prior exposure, vasectomy, and fish allergy (298). Increased rate of administration might increase risk for systemic hypotension and/or pulmonary hypertension (297, 299). It has been theorized that left-sided administration of protamine (e.g., into the left atrium or the aorta) may reduce pulmonary exposure to heparin-protamine complexes with reduced risk of pulmonary histamine release and systemic hypotension (300), although this has not been borne out in most studies (313, 412, 434).

Protamine reactions have historically been classified into three categories (299, 301, 302): type I, transient systemic hypotension; type II, anaphylactic and anaphylactoid reactions; and type III, pulmonary vasoconstriction. Because type II-anaphylactoid and type III reactions do not occur in the presence of protamine alone but require the presence of both heparin and protamine, some authorities consider these reactions together (302).

Type I: Hypotension

Protamine acts like many other highly basic drugs (e.g., d-tubocurare, morphine) to induce histamine displacement from basophils and mast cells upon rapid injection (less than 3 minutes) and a reduction in arterial blood pressure (303,

304). Injection times of 5–10 minutes seem well tolerated (298). Interestingly, histamine receptor antagonists reduce but do not eliminate the response to rapid protamine infusion (305). Human lung tissue in vitro does not release histamine in response to protamine (306). Heparin is not necessary for this reaction to occur (304).

Hypotension is accompanied by reductions in filling pressure and systemic vascular resistance (SVR) and appears more severe in patients with impaired myocardial contractility. A role for a direct myocardial depressant effect of protamine has been proposed, but the evidence is inconclusive in this regard. In vitro, protamine alters the contractility of isolated porcine cardiac myocytes, with decreased response to beta-agonists and cardiac glycosides (307). This effect is also seen to a lesser extent in canine models (308). In humans, the effect is less clear. Canine models are known to be more sensitive to protamine than human (309). Patients with depressed ventricular function will often show a decrease in cardiac index in response to protamine that is not seen in patients with good function. However, this change is associated with decreased wedge pressure and likely does not reflect altered contractility (309–311).

Type II: Anaphylactic Reaction

Anaphylactic reactions are IgE-mediated. Again, heparin-protamine complexes are not required. IgE on the surface of mast cells interacts with protamine and cause mast cell degranulation (298). Clinical manifestations include all the potentially catastrophic events associated with anaphylaxis: urticaria, bronchospasm, stridor, edema, venodilation, arterial hypotension, and cardiac arrest (312).

Potential protamine allergy can be assessed in several ways. Intradermal skin testing can be used to confirm suspicion of an allergic reaction (298, 312). However, it subjects the patient to potentially dangerous reexposure. In addition, intraobserver variation may alter test results and interpretation. Whole blood leukocyte histamine release is an in vitro assay of response to protamine exposure. This test shows low specificity, however, and is poorly predictive of a clinical protamine reaction (313, 314). Radioallergosorbent testing identifies serum anti-protamine IgE (298, 314). Protamine saturated matrix is exposed to patient serum, washed, and then developed with radiolabeled anti-IgE. This test gives a semiquantitative result but is insensitive to low quantities of IgE. This is problematic in that protamine is a relatively weak antigen (315), and IgE levels are usually low (314). Moreover, a positive test does not predict a clinical protamine reaction (313).

Patients at an increased theoretical risk for anaphylactic reaction include diabetics with previous exposure to NPH or protamine-zinc insulin, patients with fish allergy, and vasectomized males.

Diabetics are noted to have increased titers of anti-protamine IgG and a large number also have anti-protamine IgE—as high as 53%—compared with the general population (316, 317). However, most reports indicate that diabetics do not have an increased rate of anaphylaxis to protamine (313, 314, 317, 318). Protamine-exposed diabetics have increased leukocyte histamine release to protamine in vitro, but as discussed previously, this test does not predict a clinical protamine reaction (314).

Many case reports exist of protamine reaction in diabetics, but most are not well documented as true type II-anaphylactic reactions. Moreover, these case reports must be compared with the relatively unreported or unknown rates of anaphylactic reaction in the nondiabetic community (298).

Conceivably, these reactions could be anaphylactoid in nature, mediated by anti-protamine IgG (313, 314, 317, 318). However, as mentioned above, protamine is a relatively weak antigen and documentation is lacking.

Understanding of anaphylactic reactions to protamine in patients with true fish allergy (as opposed to shellfish allergy) is based almost entirely on case reports (319–321) that suffer from the same problems of reporting bias discussed above with regard to diabetics. Protamine may serve as a cross-reacting antigen in the fish allergic patient (298). In addition, individual fish allergic patients have been reported to have increased IgE, leukocyte histamine release, and positive skin testing in response to protamine (313, 322). However, a retrospective study showed no increase in risk of anaphylactic reaction in fish allergic patients compared with the cardiac surgical population at large (313).

Vasectomized males also have a theoretical risk of anaphylaxis to protamine. A large number of men (22%) developed low titers of anti-protamine IgG within a year of vasectomy (315, 321). However, no increase in the risk of clinical anaphylactic or anaphylactoid reaction has been noted in this population (298, 311).

Type II: Anaphylactoid

Anaphylactoid reactions clinically resemble anaphylactic reactions except that IgE is not involved. In most, but not all, cases, heparin-protamine interaction is required. The heparin-protamine complex is an activator of the classic complement pathway (166, 323). Generation of the complement fragments C3a and C5a and other vasoactive mediators result in urticaria, bronchospasm, increased capillary permeability, and hemodynamic instability.

Nonheparin-requiring mechanisms have also been proposed. Protamine directly activates the classic complement pathway via C-reactive protein. Complexes of protamine and anti-protamine IgG can activate complement (323). Protamine inhibits plasma carboxypeptidase N, the enzyme responsible for metabolism of C3a, C5a, and bradykinin (324).

Case reports of noncardiogenic pulmonary edema occurring approximately 1 hour after bypass have implicated protamine as a causative agent. This delayed adult respiratory distress-like syndrome may be a variant of the type II-anaphylactoid reaction, with complement activation and subsequent vasodilation, neutrophil sequestration, and capillary leak in the pulmonary vasculature (325). However, no documentation of anti-protamine antibodies or of complement activation is presented in these reports. It remains unclear whether this is a complication of protamine or other factors such as bypass-induced complement activation, endotoxin, or transfusion reaction (298).

Alternatively, this syndrome may be a result of polycation-induced lung injury. Many types of polycations, protamine included, can cause damage to the pulmonary endothelium. Mechanisms include disruption of the normal endothelial anionic charge barrier, alteration of endothelial transport proteins, or release of mediators (e.g., leukotrienes, thromboxane) by pulmonary interstitial macrophages (297, 326, 327). Polycation-induced lung injury clinically resembles complement-mediated noncardiogenic pulmonary edema.

Type III: Catastrophic Pulmonary Vasoconstriction

Type III protamine reactions are associated with increased pulmonary vascular resistance, decreased left atrial pressure, right ventricular failure, and systemic hypotension (297, 298). Such episodes may be brief or may require reinstitution of bypass. Rechallenge may or may not result in repeat pulmonary hypertension. Heparin-protamine complexes are necessary (326, 328–331). It is unclear whether the rate of protamine infusion affects the likelihood and degree of the reaction (299, 332).

Animal studies strongly indicate that the type III reaction is similar to the type II-anaphylactoid reaction with heparin-protamine complexes causing activation of complement (via the classic pathway), mobilization of leukocytes, and generation of oxygen free radicals and thromboxane A_2 (318, 326, 330, 331). Type III reactions are not seen in animals given indomethacin or aspirin (326, 329–331). Similarly, thromboxane receptor antagonists eliminate the changes in pulmonary vascular resistance even in the presence of elevated thromboxane A_2 (287, 329, 333, 334). Thromboxane synthetase inhibitors reduce but do not eliminate the reaction in sheep, goats, and pigs (326, 329, 331, 335). Free radical scavengers partially block the reaction (326).

However, complement inhibition only partially inhibits thromboxane A_2 production (332). In addition, neither leukocytes nor platelets are necessary for the reaction to occur (336, 337). The source of thromboxane A_2 appears to be not platelets, but pulmonary interstitial macrophages, which respond to complement activation or to heparin-protamine complexes alone to produce thromboxane A_2 and other vasoactive mediators (332, 337, 338).

The idiosyncratic nature of the type III reaction is puzzling. Clearly, some individuals are at higher risk for the reaction than others. For example, it is well established that animal models, such as sheep, goats, pigs, and dogs, are far more prone to the reaction than humans, predictably responding to heparin-protamine complexes with pulmonary hypertension (330, 338). This difference may be in the degree of complement activation (318, 332) or, alternatively, the degree of response of leukocytes, platelets, and pulmonary interstitial macrophages (298, 338).

ALTERNATIVES TO PROTAMINE

Alternatives to protamine include hexadimethrine/polybrene, protamine filters, heparinase, and platelet factor 4. Hexadimethrine, also known as polybrene, is a synthetic quaternary ammonium salt with high positive charge. It effectively neutralizes heparin in a manner similar to protamine (339) but with reduced hemodynamic instability (340). Unfortunately, hexadimethrine also causes polycation-induced lung injury in a manner similar to protamine, with binding to endothelial anionic sites, an increase in capillary permeability, and a clinical picture of delayed noncardiogenic pulmonary edema (327, 328, 338). Hexadimethrine aggregates platelets via direct electrostatic interaction with resultant thrombocytopenia (291, 340, 341). It binds to anionic sites in the glomerular basement membrane (342), and in large doses (greater than 5 mg/kg) causes often fatal renal toxicity (338, 343, 344). For this reason, the drug is not available for clinical use.

A cellulose filter containing immobilized protamine can be placed on the arterial side of the bypass circuit at the termination of bypass. In vitro, the filter removes approximately 0.45 mg of heparin for every mg of protamine used. Several recirculations are required for optimal heparin neutralization, which in a dog model leads to increased resistance to flow and fibrin-platelet clot formation in the filter (345, 346). However, hemodynamic stability, stable platelet and leukocyte counts, and a 50% reduction in complement formation are noted in a species known to be highly sensitive to protamine (345, 347). This type of device might be best used in a partial bypass situation where large doses of heparin are not used (346).

Heparinase is produced from the microorganism flavobacterium heparinum. It cleaves the ATIII binding site of heparin, neutralizing its activity. Its half-life is 1 hour in vivo but can be expanded to 15 hours when covalently bound to a sepharose filter. The efficacy of heparinase has been shown in vitro in heparinized human blood from bypass patients (348). In canine studies, a heparinase-bonded filter has been shown to eliminate physiologically significant heparin concentrations at normal flow rates within two to three passes through the filter. Canine bypass models have shown complete elimination of heparin within 2 minutes (349).

Platelet factor 4 is a protein released from platelet alpha granules with highly specific heparin neutralizing properties (350–353). Platelet factor 4 is effective against low-molecular-weight heparin and may have more effective anti-factor Xa activity than protamine (352). It can be recombinantly produced and has a half-life of about 25 minutes.

In a phase I human trial, platelet factor 4 was found to effectively neutralize heparin in cardiac catheterization patients without significant hemodynamic side effects (354). In a rat model, platelet factor 4 did not affect platelet count, leukocyte count, or complement levels (350). However, in baboon models, leukopenia and increases in the complement fragment C3a are seen (352). Platelet factor 4 is an endogenous protein and does not evoke immune sensitization. However, it can contribute to HT in patients with such a predisposition (350, 352, 354). Platelet factor 4 has some homology with interleukin and may activate neutrophils and monocytes in theory, although this has not been observed in vitro or in vivo (353). Platelet factor 4, along with heparinase, present promising future alternatives to protamine for postbypass heparin reversal.

BLOOD PRODUCT ADMINISTRATION: CURRENT PRACTICE AND GUIDELINES

Over 300,000 cardiac surgical procedures are performed within the United States each year (355). These procedures consume approximately 18% of the 22 million blood bank products transfused every year within the United States, from approximately 14 million donations (356, 357). Accordingly, this represents a tremendous burden on an increasingly scarce resource. The use of allogeneic red cell transfusion for uncomplicated primary CABG surgery in a recent study remains high, at a median of 2 units. Yet there is considerable interinstitutional variability with institutional medians varying between 0 and 4 units (358). There remains considerable variability in transfusion practice that is unaccounted for by patient factors (359, 360). Both the Joint Commission in the Accreditation of Health Care Organizations and the American Association of Blood Banks require all institutions to maintain peer review of physicians' blood utilization patterns (361, 362). This peer review is the responsibility of the institution's Transfusion Committee. Two tasks of this committee include the establishment of transfusion guidelines and the monitoring of effectiveness of these guidelines. The effectiveness of guidelines in reducing transfusion rates at individual hospitals has been well established.

The estimated cost of a single red blood cell transfusion is approximately $150 (360, 363, 364), and there is evidence that programs to reduce unnecessary transfusion are cost-effective (365–368). In one institution, the introduction of new transfusion guidelines resulted in a reduction of transfusion costs by over $1,600,000 over 3 years with a reduction of transfusion rates by 20% (369). In one multi-institutional study, 15% of red cells, 32% of fresh-frozen plasma, and 47% of platelet transfusions were deemed to be inappropriately transfused. Total potential cost savings were estimated to be 24% (360). The efficacy of blood-conservation programs is well established for cardiac and other surgery (370).

PREOPERATIVE EVALUATION

All patients undergoing cardiac surgery require a review of their hematological and coagulation status. A history of congenital and acquired hematological disease should be sought, as well as a history of renal or hepatic disease. A history of easy bruising or bleeding should be sought. The most common preoperative cause of coagulation disorder is drug therapy. Although there are numerous drugs that can significantly impair platelet or serine protease function, the most common drugs in cardiac surgical patients are aspirin, heparin, persantin, thrombolytics, and the nitrosovasodilators. Others that are less likely to impair coagulation are nonsteroidal anti-inflammatory drugs, calcium antagonists, some β blockers, and antibiotics.

There is considerable variation in preoperative laboratory investigation between institutions. Every institution requests a complete blood count and most request a PT and APTT. A few order a more extensive screen, including a bleeding time, fibrinogen, TT, a qualitative platelet function assessment, and a cryoglobulin screen.

The value of the bleeding time before cardiac surgery has been extensively investigated. The bleeding time suffers from considerable operator dependence and is also local-site temperature dependent. It has been shown to be a poor predictor of postoperative bleeding and its use is condemned (371–373). The value of other preoperative tests is particularly limited, especially in predicting postoperative bleeding (371). The use of immediate postoperative tests is also limited because there are poor correlations between individual, or even multiple tests, in predicting postoperative bleeding

(371). However, recent work with whole blood clot strength tests does appear promising, but this test is not in wide use (see Chapter 16).

WHOLE BLOOD AND RED CELL ADMINISTRATION: TRANSFUSION TRIGGERS

The hemoglobin, hematocrit, or platelet count at which red cell or platelet transfusion is administered is often referred to as the transfusion "trigger" (Table 28.3). The origin and modifiers of these trigger values are probably more important than any single value. The etiology of the hemoglobin level or platelet count, the patient's disease state, operative procedure, ability to compensate, and the probable clinical course should have far greater impact on management than a single numeric value. Unfortunately, the implementation of transfusion guidelines places emphasis on numeric transfusion triggers. It is important to appreciate that transfusion guidelines are not indications for blood product administration, but they are laboratory values that are usually accepted as being reasonable indications for transfusion, below which no further justification for transfusion is necessary (270).

Surgeons and anesthesiologists have a long tradition of transfusion when the hemoglobin falls below 10 g/dL (or hematocrit below 30%). Originating in the 1940s, this practice has persisted, seemingly unchanged, until now (374). However, it is appropriate that this trigger be reevaluated. It is known that patients during and after cardiac surgery usually do well with hematocrits well below 30%. During CPB, hematocrits of 18% are usually tolerated. In several large series, the safety of a hemoglobin of greater than 8 g/dL has been demonstrated (375, 376). Patients with chronic renal failure usually tolerate anemia well, without adverse consequences attributable to the anemia. Experience with normovolemic hemodilution has shown that hemoglobin concentrations of 7 g/dL are well tolerated even in the elderly, provided euvolemia is maintained (377). In the young, hemoglobin concentrations of 5 g/dL are tolerated (378, 379).

The normal response to acute anemia in animals and humans is an increase in cardiac output, such that oxygen delivery is returned to normal or near normal. Oxygen extraction can also rise due to increased 2,3-DPG (diphosphoglycerate) levels. In patients who cannot increase their cardiac output, anemia may be unsafe and in the presence of hypovolemia may be lethal. Two studies have shown that the normal human heart does not produce lactate until the hematocrit is less than 18–20% (380, 381).

TABLE 28.3. PUTATIVE TRANSFUSION THRESHOLDS

Hemoglobin <7.0 g/dL
Hematocrit <21%
Platelets <50–100 × 10^9/dL
PT >20 sec
APTT >55 sec
Fibrinogen <200 mg/dL

Isovolemic hemodilution has the potential advantages of reduction in allogeneic blood transfusion requirements and improvements in organ blood flow. There is growing evidence that moderate hemodilution may be therapeutically useful in several disease states. In acute ischemic stroke, moderate hemodilution has been shown to improve moderate and long-term outcome (382–385). Yet not all studies have been able to reproduce these effects (386, 387). Alternative explanations for this, and perhaps other advantageous organ system effects, include increased cardiac output, reduced blood viscosity, reduced exposure of platelets and white cells to endothelium, and increased washout of ischemic byproducts (98, 388–392).

Several compensatory mechanisms occur in normovolemic hemodilution. The two primary events are reductions in oxygen-carrying capacity and viscosity. As hemoglobin concentration falls, oxygen-carrying capacity falls proportionately, yet whole-body oxygen supply remains constant (380, 393–405) or may even increase (406, 407) because of increased cardiac output. With progressive hemodilution, oxygen delivery will vary species-by-species, patient-by-patient, and also depend on other pathophysiological states (e.g., CPB, sepsis, and arterial disease). Despite the reduction in oxygen delivery, the oxygen extraction is able to be adjusted to maintain O_2 consumption, as oxygen extraction is rarely maximized at the baseline state (Fig. 28.11) (393, 408).

The compensatory increase in cardiac output occurs by three mechanisms: a decrease in blood viscosity, an increase in cardiac sympathetic stimulation, and a reduction in SVR (409–412).

The reduction in SVR that occurs (413, 414) is not primarily caused by a reduction in viscosity (415, 416). Yet the reduction in viscosity is a vital component of the increase in cardiac output seen in hemodilution (417–421). When the oxygen-carrying capacity of blood is reduced equivalently by anemia or methemoglobinemia in dogs, there is a greater increase in cardiac output in anemic dogs (417). Increased cardiac sympathetic stimulation has been shown to be a further mechanism of increased cardiac output. Plasma norepinephrine but not epinephrine levels are raised in euvolemic hemodilution (422–424), and denervation or cardiac β blockade reduces the compensatory cardiac output response by only a small fraction (425, 426). These responses are not attenuated

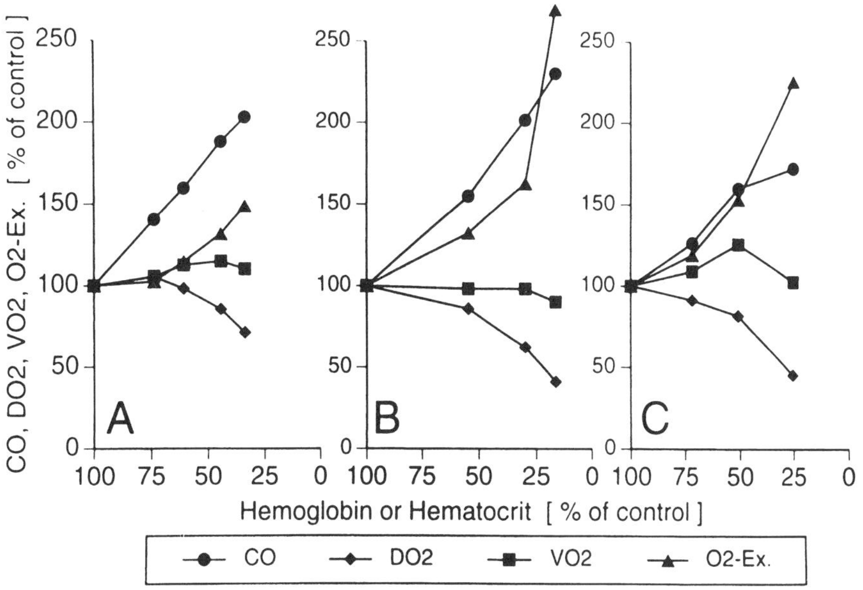

Figure 28.11. Relative changes in cardiac output (CO), oxygen delivery (Do_2), oxygen consumption (Vo_2), and oxygen extraction (O_2-Ex.) during progressive hemodilution: (**A**) in pigs (redrawn by permission according to van Woerkens E, Trouwborst A, Duncker D, Koning M, Boomsma F, Verdouw P. Catecholamines and regional hemodynamics during isovolemic hemodilution in anesthetized pigs. J Appl Physiol 1992;72:760–769); (**B**) in baboons [redrawn by permission according to Moss G, DeWoskin R, Rosen A, Levine H. Palani C. Transport of oxygen and carbon dioxide by hemoglobin-saline solution in the red-cell free primate. Surg Gynecol Obstet 1976;142:357–362); (**C**) in dogs [redrawn by permission according to Messmer K, Sunder-Plassmann L, Klovenkorn W, Holper K. Circulatory significance of hemodilution: rheological changes and limitations. Adv Microcirc 1972;4:1–77). Note that during initial hemodilution, the increase in cardiac output is the most important compensatory mechanism to maintain oxygen delivery at prehemodilution values. In more advanced hemodilution stages, the increase in cardiac output cannot fully compensate for the decrease in arterial oxygen-carrying capacity any more and oxygen delivery decreases. Oxygen consumption is then maintained via an increase in oxygen extraction. Redistribution in favor of heart and brain is observed only during extreme hemodilution. (Reprinted with permission from Spahn D, Leone B, Reves J, Pasch T. Cardiovascular and coronary physiology of acute isovolemic hemodilution: a review of non-oxygen carrying and oxygen-carrying solutions. Anesth Analg 1994;78:1000–1021.)

during long periods of hemodilution such as in anemia of chronic duration. Concomitant to the increase in cardiac output, there are increases in organ blood flow, specifically of the coronary bed (422). The type of hemodiluting solution is relatively unimportant provided the blood volume and degree of anemia are maintained. Stable euvolemia is, however, more difficult to obtain with crystalloid solutions (406, 427).

Coronary blood flow is increased during hemodilution in individuals without coronary artery disease (CAD) (380, 393, 400, 403, 419, 428–432) due to decreased myocardial vascular resistance and decreased viscosity. Oxygen extraction is maintained during moderate hemodilution (380, 393, 400, 403, 419, 429–433), and oxygen consumption is maintained or increased (428). With extreme hemodilution, oxygen extraction is unchanged in primates (405), indicating the reliance on increased cerebral blood flow. Epicardial predominance of blood flow in extreme hemodilution is observed (393, 429), indicating the relative susceptibility of the endocardium to ischemia.

In patients with CAD, moderate hemodilution does not appear to be deleterious, and routine use of postbypass moderate hemodilution appears to be safe (395, 434–437). Animal experimental evidence supports the clinical data (438, 439). The reserves of coronary blood flow and oxygen extraction are exceeded by extreme hemodilution to levels of 6 g/dL in animals (438, 440, 441). In addition to compensatory reserves of myocardial oxygen consumption, there are significant reserves in myocardial mechanical function. Accordingly, the impairment in mechanical function in ischemic areas of the heart can be compensated for by normally contractile and perfused myocardium (438, 440).

Importantly, the hospital course and postoperative exercise tolerance were not different between patients transfused to hematocrits of 0.32 and those transfused to 0.25 (442).

There is no evidence regarding the safety of normovolemic hemodilution in β-blocked patients with CAD. The normal compensatory increase in cardiac output is diminished by β-blockade in animals (413, 426). Yet the additional workload, and therefore oxygen demand, is also decreased. A "safe" hematocrit level probably depends on the extent of stenotic CAD, ventricular function and reserve, myocardial workload, and other as yet undetermined factors. It would be unwise to state a single safe hematocrit for patients with CAD. It is likely that a hemoglobin of at least 7.5 g/dL is not a cause of ischemia or impaired contractile function in most patients with CAD.

PLATELET ADMINISTRATION

Thrombocytopenia is routinely associated with CPB. Hemodilution accounts for a significant proportion of this process. Sequestration, adhesion, and destruction within a CPB pump oxygenator and tubing account for the remainder (443). There is considerable controversy regarding platelet transfusion. In the patient with excessive bleeding after CPB, there are usually coexisting etiologies: thrombocytopenia, factor deficiency, fibrinolysis, and activation of inflammatory processes. Treatment of excessive bleeding necessitates an algorithmic approach of which platelet transfusion is only one methodology.

The CPB-induced reduction in platelet count depends on patient blood volumes and pump prime volume; a reduction of platelet count of approximately 30% is usual. Within minutes after the initiation of CPB, there is a further reduction in platelet count. Sequestration of platelets (usually intrahepatic) as a consequence of hypothermia accounts for some of this thrombocytopenia. Platelet adhesion to the foreign surface of the pump and oxygenator undoubtedly accounts for a significant proportion. Platelets adhere to fibrinogen and other proteins that are bound to the tubing. Activation and aggregation are inevitable consequences of adhesion. An often overlooked etiology of thrombocytopenia is activation and destruction by surgical suction. In addition, platelets aggregate and are activated by protamine and heparin-protamine complexes. Platelet counts usually rise by about 50% over the first 2 days after CPB and are normal within 1 week. The delayed return to normal probably reflects the ongoing inflammatory and procoagulant response to CPB.

Not only are platelet numbers reduced by CPB, but platelet function is also reduced. Less qualitative emphasis has been placed on this aspect because it is more difficult to measure. Although we can confidently say that CPB induces a platelet function deficit and that this deficit is due to platelet aggregation and activation, the exact mechanisms of this process are less clear. Hypothermia is a causal etiology. Factors associated with impaired platelet function are duration of CPB, type of CPB apparatus, volume of surgical suction, degree of hypothermia, heparin, protamine, and endogenous circulation platelet inhibitors.

Clinical practice across institution, with regard to platelet transfusion rates, varies considerably (358). These variations cannot be accounted for by patient factors. Part, but not all, of the explanation for the variability is due to inability to qualify the platelet contribution to bleeding. Platelet count, by automated counters, may be artificially high due to red cell and platelet fragments being counted as platelets. Platelet function is difficult to measure in the clinical environment. An estimate of platelet function can be obtained by thromboelastography, sonoclot, and other semiautomated methods. All of these methodologies are time-consuming and sporadically used. Systematic laboratory approaches in concert with systematic clinical protocols are the best implementation of this technology. Because of the time required to obtain results and subsequently obtain blood products, it is necessary to obtain heparinized blood while on bypass. One approach is to use heparinase to obtain a coagulable sample.

The use of platelet count as a transfusion trigger for prophylactic platelet administration is to be condemned. There is no evidence of clinical benefit from prophylactic platelet transfusion (444, 445). There is, however, a place for platelet transfusion in the bleeding thrombocytopenic patient. Both the extent of bleeding and level of thrombocytopenia that indicate platelet transfusion are open to debate and clinical interpretation. Many different arbitrary volumes of chest tube drainage and platelet counts have been proposed as being triggers for platelet transfusion.

Platelets are available in single-donor platelet pheresis or multiple-donor pooled platelet products. Single-donor platelets have the advantages of reduced possibility of infection and alloimmunization but are more expensive and difficult to harvest. Between five and eight single-platelet pack equivalents are contained in a single-donor pheresis pack. Pooled platelet bags contain platelets from five to eight donors, with greater than 55×10^9 platelets per donor in 50–75 mL of plasma. Once pooled, platelets should be transfused within 6 hours. Platelets can be transfused without regard to ABO or Rh grouping under most circumstances.

COAGULATION FACTOR ADMINISTRATION

Plasma products, obtained from the fractionation of donor whole blood, have undergone a meteoric rise in use over the last 20 years. Like all other blood products, their use is variable across institutions, unexplained by patient parameters. The largest use of blood products during surgery is seen with CABG surgery.

Fresh-frozen plasma is separated from whole blood and frozen within 6 hours of collection at −18°C. Some loss of the labile factors V and VIII occurs (approximately 50%), but the remaining factors are close to 100% preserved. Because only 25–40% of normal circulating factor levels are required for normal hemostasis, most coagulation factor deficiencies are corrected by transfusion of 4 units of fresh-frozen plasma. Larger requirements will be seen in ongoing losses and fibrinolysis.

It is highly likely that a significant portion of fresh-frozen plasma transfusions in cardiac surgery are unnecessary and do not contribute to preventing postoperative bleeding, especially those for "prophylactic indications."

BLOOD CONSERVATION TECHNIQUES FOR CPB

In the early days of CPB technology, the need for large pump-priming volumes and extensive pump-induced destruction of the formed elements of blood resulted in a requirement for very large allogeneic blood requirements. Fresh whole blood was a routine requirement and use of platelets and fresh-frozen plasma was also routine. This requirement has been largely reduced by technological advances; however, practitioners have also learned to appreciate the safety of hemodilution.

Because of the financial and social cost of allogeneic transfusion and the limited blood supply, it is incumbent upon the physician to use all opportunities to reduce the use of allogeneic blood products. Several techniques are used for prevention of transfusion during cardiac surgery (Table 28.4). Avoidance of allogeneic transfusion has many advantages, notably reduction in viral and bacterial transmission (446–453), isoimmunization, incidence of wound and other infections, cancer recurrence, and graft-versus-host reactions (454–465). The need for blood conservation is crucial given the increasing demand for blood products and the still residual possibility of transfusion of an antibody-negative virus-containing allogeneic unit.

Several studies have demonstrated an increased incidence of wound or other infections in patients receiving allogeneic red cell or factor products (see Chapters 7 and 8). Frequently, these studies have not been well controlled for confounding variables or effect modifiers and are criticized on the basis of sicker patients or those with more advanced disease receiving higher rates of blood transfusion and also being more likely to have an infection. Despite these criticisms, blood transfusion has been identified as an independent risk factor in several studies (460, 463, 465), yet not all studies have confirmed these results (466, 467).

TABLE 28.4. AVAILABLE MEANS OF REDUCING ALLOGENEIC BLOOD TRANSFUSION WITH CARDIAC SURGERY

Preoperative
Autologous predonation of whole blood, red blood cells, FFP, platelets
Pheresis of platelets and FFP
Erythropoietin
Intraoperative
Institutional program of guidelines for allogeneic blood product administration
Rigorous surgical technique
Pre-CPB isovolemic hemodilution
Pheresis of FFP and platelets
Nonsanguinous prime
Whole blood collection at CPB onset
Retransfusion of pump blood
Cell saver or ultrafiltration of pump blood
Drug therapy
Antifibrinolytic agents
DDAVP
Postoperative
Institutional program of guidelines for allogeneic blood product administration
Shed mediastinal blood transfusion

FFP, fresh-frozen plasma.

AUTOLOGOUS RED CELL DONATION

Preoperative autologous donation represents a theoretically ideal mechanism of blood conservation. Unfortunately, it is perceived to be feasible only in a relatively small subgroup of patients, because of short waiting times and other factors that are perceived to prevent donation (468–470), and its cost-effectiveness has been questioned (471). However, some practitioners have used this as an excuse for complete failure to practice this technique. Others have failed to pursue the full potential of autologous donation. Some reasons for this failure are because patients do not always have the requisite 1–3 weeks available to them before their surgery, come from distant locations, are anemic, or are correctly or incorrectly perceived to be too unstable to donate blood. In addition, the costs of autologous blood donation are higher than those for allogeneic blood transfusion (363). Yet the practice of autologous donation is increasing, primarily because of patient perceptions of disease risk (357). Several large studies have investigated the use of autologous predonation (468, 472–475) and all have shown the efficacy of collection and transfusion of an average of 3 units of autologous blood. Collections of less than 3 units have conventionally been less efficacious because the rate of allogeneic transfusion in this group has been high. Transfusion of 3 or more units of autologous blood has been associated with reduced rates of allogeneic transfusion and higher discharge hematocrits.

Predonation of autologous blood has been shown to reduce preoperative hemoglobin by approximately 2 g/dL when an average of 2 units are harvested over 2–3 weeks (468). Donation is very rarely associated with morbidity, usually minor, and overall appears to be well tolerated even in relatively sick patients (468, 472–474, 476, 477). A proportion of patients require operation during the harvest period. This fraction does not appear to be higher than the natural course of disease (473), although this is open to debate (478).

Because of concerns over the time taken to achieve an adequate harvest of autologous blood, erythropoietin has been used to increase red cell mass for harvest. Administration of erythropoietin with or without concurrent iron administration enables greater harvest of red cells before surgery (see Chapter 10) (479–484). Erythropoietin has also been shown to improve hematocrit in anemic patients before CABG surgery (485). It may also have a role in improvements in cell-mediated immunity after CPB (486). Its physiology and efficacy have been recently reviewed (487).

AUTOLOGOUS PLATELET DONATION

The most common clinical use for plasmapheresis is to remove pathogenic antibodies. Examples of this use are HT with thrombosis, cold agglutinin disease, and hyperviscosity syndrome. Approximately 10% of patients treated with heparin develop thrombocytopenia, primarily due to heparin-induced anti-platelet antibodies. Only a very small percentage develop thrombosis, and only some of those fail to respond to cessation of heparin alone. Cold agglutinin disease is an occasional cause of autoimmune hemolytic anemia. Several temperature-dependent autoantibodies bind to erythrocyte antigens, causing intravascular agglutination. Complement is usually activated. Conduct of hypothermic bypass can trigger antibody-induced agglutination with resultant thrombosis and hemolysis. The degree of agglutination depends on the temperature dependence and titer of cold agglutinins. Plasmapheresis in the 24 hours before surgery, due to the short half-life of the IgM autoantibody, has been shown to be useful. Rarely, hyperviscosity syndrome secondary to hematological malignancy is reported. Hyperviscosity and the frequently concurrent platelet defect are attenuated by plasmapheresis.

Preoperative harvest of platelet-rich plasma (PRP) must be performed in the 24–72 hours before surgery or during surgery because of the relatively short half-life of stored platelets (5 days). Practically, because of shorter preoperative admissions, PRP collection is usually performed in the operating room, before CPB. Patients with preexisting thrombocytopenia, coagulation disorders, and hemodynamic instability, but not those with moderately low left ventricular ejection fractions, are usually excluded. Platelets are collected by discontinuous flow centrifugation using a Haemonetics Plasma Collecting System. PRP is collected by draining whole blood into a centrifuge bowl. The centrifuge is run at 3400–3800 rpm, and PRP is separated from red cells, white cells, and plasma. These are then returned to the patient and a new aliquot of whole blood is drawn from the patient. The process is repeated until sufficient PRP is obtained. The volume of platelets obtained by this method is between 9 and 30% of the circulating platelet pool (488–491). Unfortunately, this may frequently be an inadequate number of platelets to be effective in reduction of blood loss after surgery. An effective platelet pheresis product requires 3×10^{11} platelets (492), yet this is frequently not achieved with smaller volumes of platelet pheresis (491). It has been recommended that at least 2.4×10^{11} platelets are withdrawn for use after cardiac surgery (493). The failure or inability to withdraw adequate numbers of platelets probably represents the single greatest obstacle to the efficacy of platelet pheresis. The use of one to two blood volumes of pheresis does not produce the number of platelets needed for treatment of a severe bleeding diathesis. Accordingly, when most needed, platelet pheresis is ineffective, but it is most commonly used when there is little bleeding or coagulopathy, a situation that rarely requires platelet transfusion. Technical advances may improve the harvest of platelets (494). Platelets that are harvested are unaffected by harvest and storage for 2–3 hours (495).

The use of intraoperative autologous PRP transfusion has been associated with (489–491, 495–501) and without a reduction in transfusion requirement (488, 502–505). Most of these studies are flawed by difficulties with blinding and failure to define transfusion triggers. Nevertheless, most studies have found an effect of platelet pheresis. The two largest studies of PRP (498, 500) totaling 577 patients receiving PRP found reductions in blood loss and allogeneic red cell replacement. Some studies have failed to show a reduction in allogeneic blood product transfusion but have demonstrated improvements in intermediate markers of coagulation status. Boldt et al. (495) were able to show differences in intermediate outcomes such as a blood loss reduction and higher ATIII and fibrinogen concentrations in the pheresis group but were unable to show reductions in transfusion. In a similar study that also examined the use of cell-saver techniques, Boldt et al. (496) were able to demonstrate that platelet count 45 minutes after termination of CPB was higher in the PRP group. There were no differences in blood loss or transfusion in the PRP group. Del Rossi et al. (491) were able to demonstrate in a small population that PRP transfusion was associated with an increased platelet count 15 minutes after transfusion (but not on postoperative day 1), reduced chest drainage on the day of surgery, and less transfusion of fresh-frozen plasma, but not of red cells. Giordano et al. (490) and Noon et al. (506) were able to show a reduction in red cell and platelet transfusion volumes with platelet pheresis. In addition, PRP contains an excess of smaller platelets (507) that appear to have attenuated hemostatic function compared with larger platelets (508–511). Accordingly, some have argued that unprocessed autologous whole blood is as effective as PRP (512). Autologous whole blood, however, is impracticable to harvest in anemic and smaller patients. Improvements in technical expertise may result in improved results for platelet pheresis because of better platelet yields.

ACUTE NORMOVOLEMIC HEMODILUTION

Acute normovolemic hemodilution (ANH) entails the simultaneous removal of whole blood from the patient and transfusion of crystalloid or colloid volume replacement before CPB. ANH has been both associated with (368, 513–520) and without (515, 521–523) decreases in allogeneic transfusion requirement. Supporters of ANH have observed higher platelet counts (515–518, 524, 525). These platelet count increases are probably not sufficient to prevent bleeding.

ANH has not been associated with an increase in cardiovascular or other morbidity or in pulmonary extravascular water (436, 526). Its safety appears to be well established, but its efficacy is open to debate (527, 528).

The rationale for this debate revolves around the volume of red cells (and platelets) that can be safely harvested in the immediate pre-bypass period. Two techniques are used. The most common is the removal of blood from the central or arterial line into citrated bags before heparinization. It is rare with this technique to be able to harvest more than 1000 mL of blood given the time constraint. The second technique is the removal of blood from the venous line to the pump, after heparinization, at the onset of bypass. Similarly, it is rare to be able to withdraw more than 1000 mL of blood.

The aims of ANH are the transfusion of red cells and normal platelets. Removal and transfusion of 1000 mL of blood rarely improves platelet count or function by a clinically significant amount, because the number of retransfused platelets is low compared with the circulating platelet pool (515, 524). The number of red cells is less important because red cells are consumed less than platelets during bypass. Accordingly, their number and function are little affected by ANH, provided the contents of the oxygenator and all suctioned blood are transfused at the end of CPB.

CELL SAVERS AND ULTRAFILTRATION OF PUMP BLOOD

Three methods of processing the remaining pump blood volume at the end of CPB are possible. These are centrifugation using a cell saver, ultrafiltration using a hollow-fiber ultrafilter, and retransfusion of unprocessed blood. The latter two techniques have the advantage of retaining platelets, plasma proteins, and coagulation factors but the infusate is heparinized, therefore requiring additional protamine for reversal (529, 530). In addition, ultrafiltration exposes the infusate to high transmembrane pressures that can potentially worsen hemolysis. Cell-saver technology produces a red cell-only infusate with negligible circulating heparin, platelet plasma protein, and coagulation factor levels. Comparing the use of cell savers with ultrafiltration, upon discarded surgical suction and the remainder of the CPB pump volume, the ultrafiltered blood is a more red-cell concentrated and less platelet and coagulation factor-depleted product than the cell-saver blood (531). Infusion of centrifuged blood has been associated with longer PT, APTT, and TT than direct infusion or ultrafiltration; infusion of ultrafiltered blood is associated with higher fibrinogen levels and colloid oncotic pressures (532). These changes do not persist beyond 6 hours. Some studies have been unable to differentiate between the coagulation states after infusion of ultrafiltered and "cell-saved" infusate (533).

SHED MEDIASTINAL BLOOD TRANSFUSION

In 1978, Schaff et al. (534) demonstrated a 50% reduction in allogeneic red cell transfusion requirement with transfusion of the shed blood from chest drainage tubes. The same authors and others have demonstrated the efficacy of shed mediastinal blood transfusion after CABG surgery in reducing allogeneic red blood cell transfusion (368, 535–541). However, the safety and efficacy of shed mediastinal blood is currently being debated (542, 543). Other studies have failed to demonstrate significant reduction in red blood cell transfusion (544–551). In addition, in several studies that showed an effect of shed mediastinal blood transfusion, the reduction in allogeneic red cell transfusion seen was greater than the volume of red cells transfused in the shed mediastinal blood transfusion. Complicating several studies has been the stated or implied rationale for the study, being a justification for a change in institutional practice or the introduction of shed mediastinal blood to the institution. Additionally, it is also difficult to blind investigators and providers to the use of shed mediastinal blood.

Transfusion of shed mediastinal blood has been shown to affect measurements of coagulation, both with (552) and without (534, 549, 553) an increase in postoperative bleeding. Shed mediastinal blood is a defibrinogenated thrombocytopenic admixture that does not usually clot in the collection system. Several studies have examined the composition of shed mediastinal blood. The hematocrit of shed mediastinal blood is approximately 20% but varies considerably, depending on the rate of active bleeding, time after surgery, and volume of surgical wash remaining in the pleural cavity and pericardium at the end of surgery (554). Additionally, considerable red cell hemolysis occurs. Plasma hemoglobin levels of 4g/L in the infusate are common (555). Transfusion of shed mediastinal blood has not been associated with hemoglobin-induced renal failure (550, 556, 557) because the total free hemoglobin load is low (approximately 3 g for an infusate of 700 mL). Although some studies have found automated platelet counts to be normal, or elevated above the patient's circulating platelet count (534, 550, 556), manual counting of shed mediastinal blood shows severe thrombocytopenia. The apparent discrepancy is explained by platelet and other cellular fragments being counted as platelets by automatic counters (558).

Fibrinolysis occurs in shed mediastinal blood, as expected (368, 551, 553, 559). Tissue plasminogen activator is elevated after shed mediastinal blood transfusion (430, 552). When shed mediastinal blood is transfused, circulating fibrin degradation products are elevated (547, 553, 559), and although some investigators have believed this to be evidence of a circulating whole-body response, this elevation of fibrin degradation products most likely merely indicates infusion of a completed fibrinolytic process (545). It is unlikely that routine volumes of shed mediastinal blood transfusion can overwhelm the body's mechanisms for "mopping up" products of fibrinolysis. Studies, with few exceptions, have not been able to demonstrate increased bleeding in patients who received shed mediastinal blood transfusion. Only one group has shown an increased chest tube drainage (552, 560). No study has demonstrated an increased rate of reoperation for bleeding (554, 561).

Some studies have demonstrated bacterial contamination of shed mediastinal blood, predominantly by diphtheroids and coagulase-negative staphylococci, albeit without clinical evidence of sepsis (562–565).

Cardiac enzymes, notably creatine kinase and lactate dehydrogenase, are elevated in shed mediastinal blood fluid. Transfusion of shed mediastinal blood elevates circulating creatine kinase and lactate dehydrogenase levels (566–568). Some have argued that shed mediastinal blood should not be transfused because it may confuse the diagnosis of myocardial infarction. This is rarely of importance, and avoidance of potential difficulty in a laboratory diagnosis is not justification for reduction in the therapeutic benefit of shed mediastinal blood transfusion.

REFERENCES

1. Ansell J, Slepchuk N Jr, Kumar R, Lopez A, Southard L, Deykin D. Heparin-induced thrombocytopenia: a prospective study. Thromb Haemost 1980;43:61–65.
2. Bell WR, Tomasulo PA, Alving BM, Duffy TP. Thrombocytopenia occurring during the administration of heparin: a prospective study in 52 patients. Ann Intern Med 1976;85:155–160.
3. Gollub S, Ulin A. Heparin-induced thrombocytopenia in man. J Lab Clin Med 1962;59:430–435.
4. Hackett T, Kelton J, Powers P. Drug induced platelet destruction. Semin Thromb Haemost 1982;8:116–137.
5. King D, Kelton J. Heparin associated thrombocytopenia. Ann Intern Med 1984;100:535–540.
6. Warkentin T, Kelton J. Heparin-induced thrombocytopenia. Prog Hemost Thromb 1991;10:1–34.
7. Zalcberg JR, McGrath K, Dauer R, Wiley JS. Heparin-induced thrombocytopenia with associated disseminated intravascular coagulation. Br J Haematol 1983;54:655–657.
8. Stead RB, Schafer AI, Rosenberg RD, Handin RI, Josa M, Khuri SF. Heterogeneity of heparin lots associated with thrombocytopenia and thromboembolisn. Am J Med 1984;77:185–188.
9. Lynch D, Howe S. Heparin-associated thrombocytopenia: antibody binding specificity to platelet antigens. Blood 1985;66:1176–1187.
10. Chong B, Castaldi P, Berndt M. Heparin-induced thrombocytopenia: effects of rabbit IgG and its FAB and Fc fragments on antibody-heparin-platelet interaction. Thromb Res 1989;55:292–295.
11. Kelton J, Sheridan D, Santos A, et al. Heparin-induced thrombocytopenia: laboratory studies. Blood 1988;72:925–930.
12. Hines R, Rinder C. Perioperative coagulopathy: Cardiac surgery. In: Lake C, Moore R, eds. Blood: hemostasis, transfusion, and alternatives in the perioperative period. New York: Raven Press, 1985:476.
13. Woodman R, Harker L. Bleeding complications associated with cardiopulmonary bypass. Blood 1990;76:1680–1697.
14. Olinger G, Hussey C, Olive J. Cardiopulmonary bypass for patients with previously documented heparin-induced platelet aggregation. J Thorac Cardiovasc Surg 1984;87:673–677.
15. Vender J, Matthew E, Silverman I, Konowitz H, Dau P. Heparin-associated thrombocytopenia: alternative managements. Anesth Analg 1986; 65:520–522.
16. Bichler J, Fichtl B, Siebeck M, Fritz H. Pharmacokinetics and pharmacodynamics of hirudin in man after single subcutaneous and intravenous bolus administration. Arzneim Forschung 1988;38:704–709.
17. Markwardt F. Pharmacology of selective thrombin inhibitors. Nouv Rev Fr Hematol 1988;30:161–165.
18. Walenga J, Bakhos M, Messmore H, Fareed J, Pifarre R. Potential use of recombinant hirudin as an anticoagulant in a cardiopulmonary bypass model. Ann Thorac Surg 1991;51:271–277.
19. Walenga J, Bakhos M, Messmore H, Fareed J, Pifarre R. Comparison of recombinant hirudin and heparin as an anticoagulant in a cardiopulmonary bypass model. Blood Coag Fibrinol 1991;2:105–111.
20. Koza M, Walenga J, Fareed J, Pifarre R. A new approach in monitoring recombinant hirudin during cardiopulmonary bypass. Semin Thromb Hemost 1993;19:90–96.
21. Zoldhelyi P, Webster M, Fuster V, et al. Recombinant hirudin in pa-

tients with chronic stable coronary artery disease. Circulation 1993;88: 2015–2022.

22. Topol E, Bonan R, Jewitt D, et al. Use of a direct antithrombin, hirulog, in place of heparin during angioplasty. Circulation 1993;87:1622–1629.
23. Nand S. Hirudin therapy for heparin-associated thrombocytopenia and deep venous thrombosis. Am J Hematol 1993;43:310–311.
24. Riess F, Lower C, Seelig C, et al. Recombinant hirudin as a new anticoagulant during cardiac operations instead of heparin successful for aortic valve replacement in man. J Thorac Cardiovasc Surg 1995;110: 265–267.
25. O-Yurvati A, Laub G, Southgate T, McGrath L. Heparinless cardiopulmonary bypass with ancrod. Ann Thorac Surg 1994;57:1656–1658.
26. Teasdale S, Zulys V, Mycyk T, Baird R, Glynee M. Ancrod anticoagulation for cardiopulmonary bypass in heparin-induced thrombocytopenia and thrombus. Ann Thorac Surg 1989;48:712–713.
27. Reid H, Chan K, Thean P. Prolonged coagulation defect (defibrination syndrome) in Malayan viper bite. Lancet 1963;3:621–626.
28. Ewart M, Hatton M, Basford J, Dodgson K. The proteolytic action of Arvin on human fibrinogen. Biochem J 1970;118:603–609.
29. Barrie W, Wood E, Crumlish P, Forbes C, Prentice C. Low-dosage ancrod for prevention of thrombotic complications after surgery for fractured neck of femur. Br Med J 1974;4:130–133.
30. Davies J, Merrick M, Sharp A, Holt J. Controlled trial of ancrod and heparin in treatment of deep-vein thrombosis of lower limb. Lancet 1972;1:113–115.
31. Cole C, Bormanis J, Luna G, et al. Ancrod versus heparin for anticoagulation during vascular surgical procedures. J Vasc Surg 1993;17: 288–293.
32. Hall G, Holman H, Webster A. Anticoagulation by ancrod for haemodialysis. Br Med J 1970;4:591–593.
33. Spiekermann B, Lake C, Rich G, Humphries J. Normal activated clotting time despite adequate anticoagulation with Ancrod in a patient with heparin-associated thrombocytopenia and thrombosis undergoing cardiopulmonary bypass. Anesthesiology 1994;80:686–688.
34. Zulys V, Teasdale S, Michel E, et al. Ancrod (Arvin®) as an alternative to heparin anticoagulation for cardiopulmonary bypass. Anesthesiology 1989;71:870–877.
35. Kiers L, Grigg L, Cade J, Street P, Chong B. Use of ORG 10,172 in the treatment of heparin-induced thrombocytopenia and thrombosis. Aust NZ J Med 1986;16:719.
36. Danielsson A, Raub E, Lindahl U, Bjork I. Role of ternary complexes, in which heparin binds both antithrombin and proteinase, in the acceleration of the reactions between antithrombin and thrombin or factor Xa. J Biol Chem 1986;261:15467–15473.
37. Mannen E. Why low molecular weight heparin? Semin Thromb Hemost 1990;16:1–4.
38. Salzman E. Low-molecular-weight heparin: is small beautiful? N Engl J Med 1986;315:957–959.
39. Lane D, Denton J, Flynn A, Thunberg L, Lindahl U. Anticoagulant activities of heparin oligosaccharides and their neutralization by platelet factor 4. Biochem J 1984;218:725–732.
40. Holmer E, Kurachi K, Soderstrom G. The molecular-weight dependence of the rate enhancing effect of heparin on the inhibition of thrombin, factor Xa, factor IXa, factor XIIa and kallikrein by antithrombin. Biochem J 1981;193:395–400.
41. Hirsh J, Levine M. Low molecular weight heparin. Blood 1992;79: 1–17.
42. Fareed J. Development of heparin fractions: some overlooked considerations. Semin Thromb Hemost 1985;11:227–236.
43. Horellou MH, Conard J, Lecrubier C, et al. Persistent heparin induced thrombocytopenia despite therapy with low molecular weight heparin. Thromb Haemost 1984;51:134.
44. Vitoux J, Mathieu J, Roncato M, Fiessinger J, Aiach M. Heparin-associated thrombocytopenia treatment with low molecular weight heparin. Thromb Haemost 1986;55:37–39.
45. Roussi J, Houbouyan L, Goguel A. Use of low-molecular-weight heparin in heparin-induced thrombocytopenia with thrombotic complications. Lancet 1984;1:1183.
46. Rowlings P, Mansberg R, Rozenberg M, Evans S, Murray B. The use of a low molecular weight heparinoid (Org 10172) for extracorporeal procedures in patients with heparin dependent thrombocytopenia and thrombosis. Aust NZ J Med 1991;21:52–54.
47. Gouault-Heilmann M, Huet Y, Contant G, Payen D, Bloch G, Rapin M. Cardiopulmonary bypass with a low-molecular-weight heparin fraction. Lancet 1983;2:1374.
48. Massonnet-Castel S, Pelissier E, Bara L, et al. Partial reversal of low molecular weight heparin (PK 10169) anti-Xa activity by protamine sulfate: in vitro and in vivo study during cardiac surgery with extracorporeal circulation. Haemostasis 1986;16:139–146.
49. Robitaille D, Leclerc J, Laberge R, Sahab P, Atkinson S, Cartier R. Cardiopulmonary bypass with a low-molecular-weight heparin fraction (enoxaparin) in a patient with a history of heparin-associated thrombocytopenia. J Thorac Cardiovasc Surg 1992;103:597–599.
50. Abildgaard U, Norrheim L, Larsen A, Nesvold A, Sandset P, Odegarrd O. Monitoring therapy with LMW heparin: a comparison of three chromogenic substrate assays and the heptest clotting assay. Haemostasis 1990;20:193–203.
51. Bara L, Billaud E, Kher A, Samama M. Increased anti-Xa bioavailability for a low molecular weight heparin (POK10169) compared with unfractionated heparin. Semin Thromb Hemost 1985;11:316–317.
52. Boneu B, Caranobe C, Cadroy Y, et al. Pharmacokinetic studies of standard unfractionated heparin, and low molecular weight heparins in the rabbit. Semin Thromb Hemost 1988;14:18–27.
53. Racanelli A, Fareed J, Walenga J, Coyne E. Biochemical and pharmacologic studies on the protamine interactions with heparin, its fractions and fragments. Semin Thromb Haemost 1985;11:176–189.
54. Harenberg J, Wurzner B, Zimmermann R, Schettler G. Bioavailability and antagonizaton of the low molecular weight heparin CY 216 in man. Thromb Res 1986;44:549–554.
55. Doutremepuich C, Bonini F, Toulemonde F, Bertrand H, Bayrou B, Quilichini R. In vivo neutralization of low-molecular weight heparin fraction CY216 by protamine. Semin Thromb Hemost 1985;11: 318–322.
56. Van Ryn-McKenna J, Ofosu F, Hirsh J, Buchanan M. Neutralization of enoxaparine-induced bleeding by protamine sulfate. Thromb Haemost 1990;63:271–274.
57. Altes A, Martino R, Gari M, et al. Heparin-induced thrombocytopenia and heart operation: management with tedelparin. Ann Thorac Surg 1995;59:508–509.
58. Massonnet-Castel S, Pelissier E, Dreyfus G, et al. Low-molecular-weight heparin in extracorporeal circulation. Lancet 1984;1:1182–1183.
59. Long R. Management of patients with heparin-induced thrombocytopenia requiring cardiopulmonary bypass [letter]. J Thorac Cardiovasc Surg 1985;89:950–951.
60. Kappa JR, Fisher CA, Berkowitz HD, Cottrell ED, Addonizio VP Jr. Heparin-induced platelet activation in sixteen surgical patients: diagnosis and management. J Vasc Surg 1987;5:101–109.

61. Makhoul R, McCann R, Austin E, Greenberg C, Lowe J. Management of patients with heparin-associated thrombocytopenia and thrombosis requiring cardiac surgery. Ann Thorac Surg 1987;43:617–621.
62. Smith JP, Walls JT, Muscato MS, et al. Extracorporeal circulation in a patient with heparin-induced thrombocytopenia and thrombosis requiring cardiac surgery. Anesthesiology 1985;62:363–365.
63. Kappa J, Fisher C, Todd B, et al. Intraoperative management of patients with heparin-induced thrombocytopenia. Ann Thorac Surg 1990;49: 714–723.
64. Gorman R, Blunting S, Miller O. Modulation of human adenylate cyclase by prostacyclin (PGX). Prostaglandins 1977;13:377–388.
65. Addonizio V, Fisher C, Kappa J, Ellison N. Prevention of heparin-induced thrombocytopenia during open heart surgery with iloprost (ZK36374). Surgery 1987;102:796–807.
66. Kraenzler E, Starr N. Heparin-associated thrombocytopenia: management of patients for open heart surgery. Case reports describing the use of iloprost. Anesthesiology 1988;69:964–967.
67. Kappa R, Horn D, McIntosh C, Fisher C, Ellison N, Addonizio PJ. Iloprost (IZK36374), a new prostacyclin analogue, permits open cardiac operation in patients with heparin-induced thrombocytopenia. Surg Forum 1985;36:285–286.
68. Shorten G, Communale M, Johnson R. Management of cardiopulmonary bypass in a patient with heparin-induced thrombocytopenia using prostaglandin E, and aspirin. J Cardiothorac Vasc Anesth 1994;8: 556–558.
69. Carreras L. Thrombosis and thrombocytopenia induced by heparin. Scand J Haematol 1981;25:64–80.
70. Esposito R, Culliford A, Colvin S, Thomas S, Lackner H, Spencer F. Heparin resistance during cardiopulmonary bypass. J Thorac Cardiovasc Surg 1983;85:346–353.
71. Esposito R, Culliford A, Colvin S, Thomas S, Lackner H, Spencer F. The role of the activated clotting time in heparin administration and neutralization for cardiopulmonary bypass. J Thorac Cardiovasc Surg 1983;85:174–185.
72. Michalski R, Lane D, Pepper D, Kakkar V. Neutralization of heparin in plasma by platelet factor 4 and protamine. Br J Haematol 1978;38: 561–571.
73. Thaler E, Lechner K. Antithrombin III deficiency and thromboembolism. Clin Haematol 1981;10:369–390.
74. White P, Sadd J, Nonsel R. Thrombotic complications of heparin therapy. Ann Surg 1979;190:595–601.
75. Conrad J, LeCompte T, Horellou M, Cazenave B, Samama M. AT III in patients treated with subcutaneous or intravenous heparin. Thromb Res 1981;22:507–511.
76. Miciniak E, Gockerman J. Heparin induced decrease in circulating AT III. Lancet 1980;2:581–584.
77. O'Brien J, Etherington M. Effect of heparin and warfarin on antithrombin III. Lancet 1977;2:1231.
78. Denson K. Ratio of factor VIII-related antigen and factor VIII biological activity as an index of hypercoagulability and intravascular clotting. Thromb Res 1977;10:107–119.
79. Denson K, Redman C. Heparin induced decrease in circulating AT III. Lancet 1977;2:1028–1029.
80. Jordan R, Oosta G, Gardener W, Rosenberg R. The kinetics of the hemostatic enzyme-antithrombin interactions in the presence of low molecular weight heparin. J Biol Chem 1980;255:10081–11090.
81. Hyers T, Hull R, Weg J. Antithrombotic therapy for venous thromboembolic disease. Chest 1989;95:37S–51S.
82. Sabbagh AH, Chung GK, Shuttleworth P, Applegate BJ, Gabrhel W. Fresh frozen plasma: a solution to heparin resistance during cardiopulmonary bypass. Ann Thorac Surg 1984;37:466–468.
83. Pusineri F, Bini A, Mussoni L, Remuzzi G, Donati M. Intermittent heparin treatment does not induce hypercoagulopathy in hemodialyzed patients. J Clin Pathol 1980;33:631–634.
84. Milan J, Austin S, Martin R, Keats A, Cooley D. Alternation of coagulation and selected clinical chemistry parameters in patients undergoing open heart surgery without transfusions. Am J Clin Pathol 1981;76: 155–162.
85. Anderson E. Heparin resistance prior to cardiopulmonary bypass. Anesthesiology 1986;64:504–507.
86. Agarwal S, Ghosh P, Gupta D. Cardiac surgery and cold-reactive proteins. Ann Thorac Surg 1995;60:1143–1150.
87. Moore FJ, Warner K, Assousa S, Valeri C, Khuri S. The effect of complement activation during cardiopulmonary bypass. Attenuation by hypothermia, heparin and hemodilation. Ann Surg 1988;208:95–103.
88. Bracken C, Gurkowski M, Naples J. Cardiopulmonary bypass in two patients with previously undetected cold agglutinins. J Cardiothorac Vasc Anesth 1993;7:743–749.
89. Pruzanski W, Roelcke D, Donnelly E, Lui L. Persistent cold agglutinins in AIDS and related disorders. Acta Hematol 1986;75:171–173.
90. Foerster J. Autoimmune hemolytic anemias. In: Lee G, Bithell T, Foerster J, Athens J, Lukens J, eds. Wintrobe's clinical hematology. Philadelphia: Lea & Febiger, 1993:1170–1196.
91. Wertlake P, McGinniss M, Schmidt P. Cold antibody and persistent intravascular hemolysis after surgery under hypothermia. Transfusion 1969;9:70–73.
92. Kobrinsky NL, Israels ED, Gerrard JM, et al. Shortening of bleeding time by 1-deamino-8-D-arginine vasopressin in various bleeding disorders. Lancet 1984;1:1145–1148.
93. Mannucci P, Ruggeri Z, Pareti F, Capitanio A. 1-Deamino-8-D-arginine vasopressin: a new pharmacologic approach to the management of haemophilia and von Willebrand's disease. Lancet 1977;1:869–872.
94. Warrier A, Lusher J. DDAVP: a useful alternative to blood components in moderate hemophilia A and von Willebrand disease. J Pediatr 1983;102:228–233.
95. Osterud B, Rapaport S. Activation of factor IX by the reaction product of tissue factor and factor VII: additional pathway for initiating blood coagulation. Proc Natl Acad Sci USA 1977;74:5260–5264.
96. Eisenberg J, Clarke J, Sussman S. Prothrombin and partial thromboplastin times as preoperative screening tests. Arch Surg 1982;117: 48–51.
97. Simon T, Akl B, Murphy W. Controlled trial of routine administration of platelet concentrates in cardiopulmonary bypass surgery. Ann Thorac Surg 1984;37:359–364.
98. Vorstrup S, Anderson A, Juhler M, Brun B, Boysen G. Hemodilution increases cerebral blood flow in acute ischemic stroke. Stroke 1989;20: 884–889.
99. Blatt P, Lundblad R, Kingdon H, McLean G, Roberts H. Thrombogenic materials in prothrombin complex concentrates. Ann Intern Med 1974; 81:766–770.
100. Kasper C. Surgical operation in hemophilia B: use of factor IX concentrate. Cald Med 1970;113:4–8.
101. Levine P. Clinical manifestations and therapy of hemophilia A and B. In: Colman R, Hirsch J, Marder V, Salzman E, eds. Hemostasis and thrombosis. Philadelphia: J.B. Lippincott, 1987:97–111.
102. Menache D. New concentrates of factors VII, IX and X. In: Kasper C, ed. Recent advances in hemophilia care. New York: Alan R. Liss, 1990:177–187.

103. Ruggeri Z, Mannucci P, Lombardi R, Frederici A, Zimmerman T. Multimeric composition of factor VIII/von Willebrand factor following administration of DDAVP: implications for pathophysiology and therapy of von Willebrand's disease subtypes. Blood 1982;59: 1272–1278.
104. Holmberg L, Nilsson I, Borge L, Gunnarsson M, Sjorin E. Platelet aggregation induced by 1-desamino-8-D-arginine vasopressin (DDAVP) in type IIB von Willebrand's disease. N Engl J Med 1983;309: 816–821.
105. Gavaghan TP, Gebski V, Baron DW. Immediate postoperative aspirin improves vein graft patency early and late after coronary artery bypass graft surgery. A placebo-controlled, randomized study. Circulation 1991;83:1526–1533.
106. Goldman S, Copeland J, Moritz T, et al. Improvement in early saphenous vein graft patency after coronary artery bypass surgery with antiplatelet therapy: results of a Veterans cooperative study. Circulation 1988;77:1324–1332.
107. Kallis P, Tooze JA, Talbot S, Cowans D, Bevan DH, Treasure T. Preoperative aspirin decreases platelet aggregation and increases postoperative blood loss—a prospective, randomized, placebo controlled, double-blind clinical trial in 100 patients with chronic stable angina. Eur J Cardiothorac Surg 1994;8:404–409.
108. Ferraris VA, Ferraris SP, Lough FC, Berry WR. Preoperative aspirin ingestion increases operative blood loss after coronary artery bypass grafting. Ann Thorac Surg 1988;45:71–74.
109. Ferraris VA, Ferraris SP. 1988: Preoperative aspirin ingestion increases operative blood loss after coronary artery bypass grafting. Updated in 1995. Ann Thorac Surg 1995;59:1036–1037.
110. Michelson E, Morganroth J, Torosian M, MacVaugh H. Relation of preoperative use of aspirin to increased mediastinal blood loss after coronary artery bypass graft surgery. J Thorac Cardiovasc Surg 1978; 76:694–697.
111. Reich DL, Patel GC, Vela-Cantos F, Bodian C, Lansman S. Aspirin does not increase homologous blood requirements in elective coronary bypass surgery [see comments]. Anesth Analg 1994;79:4–8.
112. Sethi GK, Copeland JG, Goldman S, Moritz T, Zadina K, Henderson WG. Implications of preoperative administration of aspirin in patients undergoing coronary artery bypass grafting. Department of Veterans Affairs Cooperative Study on Antiplatelet Therapy. J Am Coll Cardiol 1990;15:15–20.
113. Taggart DP, Siddiqui A, Wheatley DJ. Low-dose preoperative aspirin therapy, postoperative blood loss, and transfusion requirements [see comments]. Ann Thorac Surg 1990;50:424–428.
114. Torosian M, Michelson E, Morganroth J, MacVaugh H. Aspirin- and coumadin-related bleeding after coronary-artery bypass graft surgery. Ann Intern Med 1978;89:325–328.
115. Bashein G, Nessly ML, Rice AL, Counts RB, Misbach GA. Preoperative aspirin therapy and reoperation for bleeding after coronary artery bypass surgery. Arch Intern Med 1991;151:89–93.
116. Rawitscher RE, Jones JW, McCoy TA, Lindsley DA. A prospective study of aspirin's effect on red blood cell loss in cardiac surgery. J Cardiovasc Surg (Torino) 1991;32:1–7.
117. Sheridan DP, Card RT, Pinilla JC, et al. Use of desmopressin acetate to reduce blood transfusion requirements during cardiac surgery in patients with acetylsalicylic-acid-induced platelet dysfunction. Can J Surg 1994;37:33–36.
118. Gratz I, Koehler J, Olsen D, et al. The effect of desmopressin acetate on postoperative hemorrhage in patients receiving aspirin therapy before coronary artery bypass operations. J Thorac Cardiovasc Surg 1992;104:1417–1422.
119. Kam PC. Use of desmopressin (DDAVP) in controlling aspirin-induced coagulopathy after cardiac surgery. Heart Lung 1994;23: 333–336.
120. Chard RB, Kam CA, Nunn GR, Johnson DC, Meldrum-Hanna W. Use of desmopressin in the management of aspirin-related and intractable haemorrhage after cardiopulmonary bypass. Aust NZ J Surg 1990;60: 125–128.
121. Lazenby WD, Russo I, Zadeh BJ, et al. Treatment with desmopressin acetate in routine coronary artery bypass surgery to improve postoperative hemostasis. Circulation 1990;82:IV413–IV419.
122. Murkin JM, Lux J, Shannon NA, et al. Aprotinin significantly decreases bleeding and transfusion requirements in patients receiving aspirin and undergoing cardiac operations. J Thorac Cardiovasc Surg 1994;107:554–561.
123. Tabuchi N, Huet RC, Sturk A, Eijsman L, Wildevuur CR. Aprotinin preserves hemostasis in aspirin-treated patients undergoing cardiopulmonary bypass. Ann Thorac Surg 1994;58:1036–1039.
124. Handin R, Loscalzo J. Hemostasis, thrombosis, fibrolysis and cardiovascular disease. In: Braunwald E, ed. Heart disease. A textbook of cardiovascular medicine. 4th ed. Philadelphia: WB Saunders, 1992:1767–1789.
125. Khuri S, Wolfe J, Jsa M, et al. Hematologic changes during and after cardiopulmonary bypass and their relationship to the bleeding time and nonsurgical blood loss. J Thorac Cardiovasc Surg 1992;104:94–107.
126. Pina-Cabral J, Ribeiro-da-Silva A, Almeida-Diaz A. Platelet sequestration during hypothermia in dogs treated with sulphinpyrazone and ticlopidine—reversability accelerated after intra-abdominal rewarming. Thromb Haemost 1985;43:838–841.
127. Yoshihara H, Yamanmoto T, Mihara H. Changes in coagulation and fibrinolysis occurring in dogs during hypothermia. Thromb Res 1985; 37:503–512.
128. Valeri C, Feingold H, Cassidy G, Ragno G, Khuri S, Altschule M. Hypothermia-induced platelet dysfunction. Ann Surg 1987;205:175–181.
129. Valeri C, Khabbaz K, Khuri S, et al. Effect of skin temperature on platelet function in extracorporeal bypass patients. J Thorac Cardiovasc Surg 1992;7:108–116.
130. Videm V, Fosse E, Mollnes T, Ellingsen O, Pedersen T, Karlsen H. Different oxygenators for cardiopulmonary bypass lead to varying degrees of human complement activation in vitro. J Thorac Cardiovasc Surg 1989;97:764–770.
131. Voorhees CJ, Grover RW, Voorhees ME. Evaluation of platelet damage in extracorporeal circuits using a visual platelet morphology method. ASAIO Trans 1990;36:M664-M667.
132. Baier R. The organization of blood components near interfaces. Ann NY Acad Sci 1977;283:17–36.
133. van Oeveren W, Kazatchkine M, Descamps-Latscha B, et al. Deleterious effects of cardiopulmonary bypass: a prospective study of bubble versus membrane oxygenation. J Thorac Cardiovasc Surg 1985;89: 888–889.
134. Bick R. Hemostasis defects associated with cardiac surgery, prosthetic devices and other extracorporeal circuits. Semin Thromb Haemost 1985;11:249–280.
135. Hessel E, Johnson D, Ivey T, Miller D. Membrane versus bubble oxygenator for cardiac operations. J Thorac Cardiovasc Surg 1980;80: 111–112.
136. Sade R, Bartles D, Dearing J, Campbell L, Loadholt C. A prospective randomized study of membrane versus bubble oxygenators in children. Ann Thorac Surg 1980;29:502–511.
137. Nilsson L, Bagge L, Nystrom S-O. Blood cell trauma and postoperative bleeding: comparison of bubble and membrane oxygenators and

observations on coronary suction. Scand J Thorac Cardiovasc Surg 1990;24:65–69.
138. Clark R, Beauchamps R, Magrath R, Brooks J, Ferguson T, Weldon C. Comparison of bubble and membrane oxygenators in short and long perfusions. J Thorac Cardiovasc Surg 1979;78:655–666.
139. van den Dungen J, Karliczek G, Brenken U, Homan van der Hiede J, Wildevuur C. Clinical study of blood trauma during perfusion with membrane and bubble oxygenators. J Cardiothorac Vasc Surg 1982; 83:108–116.
140. Royston D. Blood cell activation. Semin Thorac Cardiovasc 1990;2: 341–357.
141. Butler J, Rocker G, Westaby S. Inflammatory response to cardiopulmonary bypass. Ann Thorac Surg 1993;55:552–559.
142. Downing S, Edmunds LJ. Release of vasoactive substances during cardiopulmonary bypass. Ann Thorac Surg 1992;54:1236–1243.
143. Larm O, Larsson R, Olsson P. A new non-thrombogenic surface prepared by selective covalent binding of heparin via a modified reducing terminal residue. Biomater Med Devices Artif Organs 1983;11:161–173.
144. Ito Y. Antithrombogenic heparin-bound polyurethanes. J Biomater Appl 1987;2:235–265.
145. Liu L, Ito Y, Imanishi Y. Synthesis and antithrombogenicity of heparinized polyurethanes with intervening spacer chains of various kinds. Biomaterials 1991;12:390–396.
146. Park K, Okano T, Nojiri C, Kim S. Heparin immobilization onto segmented polyurethaneurea surfaces—effect of hydrophilic spacers. J Biomed Mater Res 1988;22:977–992.
147. von Segesser L, Turina M. Cardiopulmonary bypass without systemic heparinization for 24 hours. Proceedings of AmSECT Annual Meeting, Atlanta, GA, 1989.
148. Hsu L. Principles of heparin-coating techniques. Perfusion 1991;6: 209–219.
149. Bagge L, Thelin S, Hultman J, Nilsson L, Thorelius J, Hillstrom P. Heparin-coated CPB-sets increase biocompatibility and reduce endothelial cell damage in pigs. J Cardiothorac Anesth 1989;3 (Suppl. 1):84.
150. Thelin S, Bagge L, Hultman J, Borowiec J, Nilsson L, Thorelius J. Heparin-coated cardiopulmonary bypass circuits reduce blood cell trauma. Experiments in the pig. Eur J Cardiothorac Surg 1991;5:486–491.
151. von Segesser L, Weiss B, Pasic M, et al. Experimental evaluation of heparin-coated cardiopulmonary bypass equipment with low systemic heparinization and high-dose aprotinin. Thorac Cardiovasc Surg 1991; 39:251–256.
152. Borowiec J, Thelin S, Bagge L, Nilsson L, Venge P, Hansson H. Heparin coated circuits reduce activation of granulocytes during cardiopulmonary bypass—a clinical study. J Thorac Cardiovasc Surg 1992;104:642–647.
153. Borowiec J, Thelin S, Bagge L, van der Linden J, Thörnö E, Hansson H. Heparin-coated cardiopulmonary bypass circuits and 25% reduction of heparin dose in coronary artery surgery—a clinical study. Ups J Med Sci 1992;97:55–66.
154. Borowiec J, Bylock A, van der Linden J, Thelin S. Heparin coating reduces blood cell adhesion to arterial filters during coronary bypass: a clinical study. Ann Thorac Surg 1993;55:1540–1545.
155. Pasche B, Kodama K, Larm O, Olsson P, Swedenborg J. Thrombin inactivation on surfaces with covalently bonded heparin. Thromb Res 1986;44:739–748.
156. Arnander C, Dryjski M, Larrson R, Olsson P, Swedenborg J. Thrombin uptake and inhibition on endothelium and surfaces with a stable heparin coating. A comparative in vitro study. J Biomed Mater Res 1986;20:235–246.
157. Videm V, Mollnes T, Garred P, Svennevig J. Biocompatibility of extracorporeal circulation. In vitro comparison heparin-coated and uncoated circuits. J Thorac Cardiovasc Surg 1991;101:654–660.
158. Wagner W, Johnson P, Thompson K, Marrone G. Heparin-coated cardiopulmonary bypass circuits: Hemostatic alterations and post-operative blood loss. Ann Thorac Surg 1994;58:734–741.
159. Gravlee G, Phipps J, Mills S, Stump D, ATR. Hematologic evaluation of a heparin-coated circuit for cardiopulmonary bypass. Anesthesiology 1992;77:A99.
160. Gu Y, van Oeveren W, van der Kamp K. Heparin-coating of extracorporeal circuits reduces thrombin formation in patients undergoing cardiopulmonary bypass. Perfusion 1991;6:221–225.
161. von Segesser L, Weiss B, Garcia E, von Felten A, Turina M. Reduction and elimination of systemic heparinization during cardiopulmonary bypass. J Thorac Cardiovasc Surg 1992;103:790–799.
162. von Segesser L, Weiss B, Garcia E, Gallino A, Turina M. Reduced blood loss and transfusion requirements with low systemic heparinization: preliminary clinical results in coronary artery revascularization. Eur J Cardiothorac Surg 1990;4:639–643.
163. von Segesser L, Weiss B, Garcia E, Turina M. Clinical application of heparin-coated perfusion equipment with special emphasis on patients refusing homologous transfusions. Perfusion 1991;6:227–233.
164. Roissant R, Slama K, Lewandowski K, et al. Extracorporeal lung assist with heparin-coated systems. Int J Artif Organs 1992;15:29–34.
165. Knudsen F, Andersen L. Immunological aspects of cardiopulmonary bypass. J Cardiothorac Vasc Anesth 1990;4:245–258.
166. Kirklin J, Chenoweth D, Naftel D, et al. Effects of protamine administration after cardiopulmonary bypass on complement, blood elements, and the hemodynamic state. Ann Thorac Surg 1986;41:193–199.
167. Wachtfogel Y, Kucich U, Hack C, et al. Aprotinin inhibits the contact, neutrophil, and platelet activation systems during simulated extracorporeal perfusion. J Thorac Cardiovasc Surg 1993;106:1–10.
168. Gillinov A, Bator J, Zehr K, et al. Neutrophil adhesion molecule expression during cardiopulmonary bypass with bubble and membrane oxygenators. Ann Thorac Surg 1993;56:847–853.
169. Collett B, Alhaq A, Abdullah A, et al. Pathways of complement activation during CPB. Br Med J 1984;289:1251–1254.
170. Tamiya T, Yamasaki M, Maeo Y, Yamashiro T, Ogoshi S, Fujimoto S. Complement activation in cardiopulmonary bypass, with special reference to anaphylaxotoxin production in membrane and bubble oxygenators. Ann Thorac Surg 1988;46:47–57.
171. Videm V, Fosse E, Mollnes T, Garred P, Svennevig J. Complement activation with bubble and membrane oxygenators in aortocoronary bypass grafting. Ann Thorac Surg 1990;50:387–391.
172. Chenoweth D, Cooper S, Hughli T, Stewart R, Blackstone E, Kirklin J. Complement activation during cardiopulmonary bypass. N Engl J Med 1981;304:497–503.
173. Howard R, Crain C, Franzini D, Hood C, Hugli T. Effects of cardiopulmonary bypass on pulmonary leukostasis and complement activation. Arch Surg 1988;123:1496–1501.
174. Salama A, Hugo F, Heinrich D, et al. Deposition of terminal C5b-9 complement complexes on erythrocytes and leukocytes during cardiopulmonary bypass. N Engl J Med 1988;318:408–414.
175. Kirklin J, Westaby S, Blackstone E, Kirklin J, Chenowth D, Pacifico A. Complement and the damaging effects of cardiopulmonary bypass. J Thorac Cardiovasc Surg 1983;86:845–857.
176. Cavarocchi N, England M, Schaff H, et al. Oxygen free radical generation during cardiopulmonary bypass: correlation with complement activation. Circulation 1986;74:130–133.

177. Jones H, Matthews N, Vaughan R, Stark J. Cardiopulmonary bypass and complement activation. Involvement of classical and alternative pathways. Anaesthesia 1982;37:629–633.
178. Kirklin J, Blackstone E, Kirklin J. Cardiopulmonary bypass: studies on its damaging effects. Blood Purif 1987;5:168–178.
179. Perkowski S, Havill A, Flynn J, Gee M. Role of intrapulmonary release of eicosanoids and superoxide anion as mediators of pulmonary dysfunction and endothelial injury in sheep with intermittent complement activation. Circ Res 1983;53:574–583.
180. Royston D, Fleming J, Desai J, Westaby S, Taylor K. Increased production of peroxidation products associated with cardiac operations. J Thorac Cardiovasc Surg 1986;91:759–766.
181. Braude S, Nolop K, Fleming J, Krausz T, Taylor K, Royston D. Increased pulmonary transvascular protein flux after canine cardiopulmonary bypass. Am Rev Respir Dis 1986;134:857–872.
182. Gillinov A, Redmond J, Winkelstein J, et al. Complement and neutrophil activation during cardiopulmonary bypass: a study in the complement-deficient dog. Ann Thorac Surg 1994;57:345–352.
183. Flick M, Perel A, Staub N. Leukocytes are required for increased lung microvasculature permeability after microembolization in sheep. Circ Res 1981;49:344–351.
184. Sacks T, Moldow C, Craddock P, Bowers T, Jacob H. Oxygen radicals mediate endothelial cell damage by complement stimulated granulocytes. J Clin Invest 1978;21:1161–1167.
185. Rinder C, Rinder H, Smith B, et al. Blockade of C5a and C5b-9 generation inhibits leukocyte and platelet activation during extracorporeal circulation. J Clin Invest 1995;96:1564–1572.
186. Borg T, Gerdin B, Hallgren R, Modig J. The role of polymorphonuclear leucocytes in the pulmonary dysfunction induced by complement activation. Acta Anaesthesiol Scand 1985;29:231–240.
187. Nilsson L, Nilsson U, Venge P, et al. Inflammatory system activation during cardiopulmonary bypass as an indicator of biocompatibility: a randomized comparison of bubble and membrane oxygenators. Scand J Thorac Cardiovasc Surg 1990;24:53–58.
188. Gu Y, Boonstra P, Akkerman C, Mungroop H, Tigchelaar I, Van Oeveren W. Blood compatibility of two different types of membrane oxygenator during cardiopulmonary bypass in infants. Int J Artif Organs 1994;17:543–548.
189. Cavarocchi N, Pluth J, Schaff H, et al. Complement activation during cardiopulmonary bypass. Comparison of bubble and membrane oxygenators. J Thorac Cardiovasc Surg 1986;91:252–258.
190. Ekre H, Naparstek Y, Lider O, et al. Anti-inflammatory effects of heparin and its derivatives: inhibition of complement and of lymphocyte migration. Adv Exp Med Biol 1992;313:329–340.
191. Videm V, Svennevig J, Fosse E, Semb G, Osterud A, Mollnes T. Reduced complement activation with heparin-coated oxygenator and tubing in coronary bypass operations. J Thorac Cardiovasc Surg 1992;103:808–813.
192. Fosse E, Moen O, Johnson E, et al. Reduced complement and granulocyte activation with heparin-coated cardiopulmonary bypass. Ann Thorac Surg 1994;58:472–477.
193. Redmond J, Gillinov A, Stuart R, et al. Heparin-coated bypass circuits reduce pulmonary injury. Ann Thorac Surg 1993;56: 474–479.
194. Pekna M, Hagman L, Halden E, Nilsson U, Nilsson B, Thelin S. Complement activation during cardiopulmonary bypass: effects of immobilized heparin. Ann Thorac Surg 1994;58:421–424.
195. Svennevig J, Geiran O, Karlsen H, et al. Complement activation during extracorporeal circulation. In vitro comparison of Duraflo II heparin-coated and uncoated oxygenator circuits. J Thorac Cardiovasc Surg 1993;106:466–472.
196. Mollnes T, Videm V, Gotze O, Harboe M, Oppermann M. Formation of C5a during cardiopulmonary bypass inhibition by precoating with heparin. Ann Thorac Surg 1991;52:92–97.
197. Blauhut B, Gross C, Necek S, Doran J, Spath P, Lundsgaard-Hansen P. Effects of high-dose aprotinin on blood loss, platelet function, fibrinolysis, complement, and renal function after cardiopulmonary bypass. J Thorac Cardiovasc Surg 1991;101:957–967.
198. Gillinov A, DeValeria P, Winkelstein J, et al. Complement inhibition with soluble complement receptor type 1 in cardiopulmonary bypass. Ann Thorac Surg 1993;55:619–624.
199. Jansen N, van Oeveren W, van den Broek L, et al. Inhibition by dexamethasone of the reperfusion phenomena in cardiopulmonary bypass. J Thorac Cardiovasc Surg 1991;102:515–525.
200. Teoh K, Bradley C, Gauldie J, Burrows H. Steroid inhibition of cytokine-mediated vasodilation after warm heart surgery. Circulation 1995;92:347–353.
201. Bolanowski P, Bauer J, Machiedo G, Neville W. Prostaglandin influence on pulmonary intravascular leukocytic aggregation during cardiopulmonary bypass. J Thorac Cardiovasc Surg 1977;73:221–224.
202. Coffin L, Shinozaki T, DeMeules J, Browdie D, Deane R, Morgan JG. Ineffectiveness of methylprednisolone in the treatment of pulmonary dysfunction after cardiopulmonary bypass. Am J Surg 1975; 130:555–559.
203. Smith W, Murphy M, Appleyard R, et al. Prevention of complement-induced pulmonary hypertension and improvement of right ventricular function by selective thromboxane receptor antagonism. J Thorac Cardiovasc Surg 1994;107:800–806.
204. Kongsgaard U, Smith-Erichsen N, Geiran O, Amundsen E, Mollnes T, Garred P. Different activation patterns in the plasma kallikrein-kinin and complement systems during coronary bypass surgery. Acta Anaesthesiol Scand 1989;33:343–347.
205. Fuhrer G, Gallimore M, Heller W, Hoffmeister H. Aprotinin in cardiopulmonary bypass—effects on the Hageman factor (FXII)-Kallikrein system and blood loss. Blood Coagul Fibrinol 1992;3:99–104.
206. Nagaoka H, Yamado T, Hatano R, Tsukuura T, Sakamoto T. Clinical significance of bradykinin liberation during cardiopulmonary bypass and its prevention by a kallikrein inhibitor. Jpn J Surg 1975;5: 222–233.
207. Heller W, Fuhrer G, Gallimore M, Michel J, Hoffmeister H. Changes in the kallikrein-kinin system after different dose regimen of aprotinin during cardiopulmonary bypass operation. Adv Exp Med Biol 1989; 247B:43–48.
208. de Smet A, Joen M, van Oeveren W, et al. Increased anticoagulation during cardiopulmonary bypass by aprotinin. J Thorac Cardiovasc Surg 1990;100:520–527.
209. Pang L, Stalcup S, Lipset J, Hayes C, Bowman FJ, Mellins R. Increased circulating bradykinin during hypothermia and cardiopulmonary bypass in children. Circulation 1979;60:1503–1507.
210. Westaby S. Aprotinin in perspective. Ann Thorac Surg 1993;55: 1033–1041.
211. Olson S, Sheffer R, Francis A. High molecular weight kininogen potentiates the heparin-accelerated inhibition of plasma kallikrein by antithrombin: role for antithrombin in the regulation of kallikrein. Biochemistry 1993;32:12136–12147.
212. Siebeck M, Fink E, Weipert J, et al. Inhibition of plasma kallikrein with aprotinin in porcine endotoxin shock. J Trauma 1993;34: 193–198.

213. Fritz H, Wunderer G. Biochemistry and applications of aprotinin, the kallikrein inhibitor from bovine organs. Drug Res 1983;33:479–494.
214. Ellison N, Behar M, HD M, Marshall B. Bradykinin, plasma protein fraction and hypotension. Ann Thorac Surg 1980;29:15–19.
215. Niewiarowski S, Senyi A, Gillies P. Plasmin-induced platelet aggregation and platelet release reaction: effects on hemostasis. J Clin Invest 1973;52:1647–1659.
216. Fitzgerald D, Catella F, Roy L, FitzGerald G. Marked platelet activation in vivo after intravenous streptokinase in patients with acute myocardial infarction. Circulation 1988;77:142–150.
217. Penny W, Ware J. Platelet activation and subsequent inhibition by plasmin and recombinant tissue-type plasminogen activator. Blood 1992;79:91–98.
218. Adelman B, Michelson A, Loscalzo J, Greenberg J, Handin R. Plasmin effect on platelet glycoprotein Ib-von Willebrand factor interactions. Blood 1985;65:32–40.
219. Adelman B, Michelson A, Greenberg J, Handin R. Proteolysis of platelet glycoprotein Ib by plasmin is facilitated by plasmin lysine-binding regions. Blood 1986;68:1280–1284.
220. Michelson A, Barnard M. Plasmin-induced redistribution of platelet glycoprotein Ib. Blood 1990;76:2005–2010.
221. Beer J, Coller B. Evidence that platelet glycoprotein IIIa has a large disulfide-bonded loop that is susceptible to proteolytic cleavage. J Biol Chem 1989;264:17564–17573.
222. Pasche B, Ouimet H, Francis S, Loscalzo J. Structural changes in platelet glycoprotein IIb/IIIa by plasmin: determinants and functional consequences. Blood 1994;83:404–414.
223. Bick R, Arbegast N, Crawford L, Holterman M, Adams T, Schmalhorst W. Hemostatic defects induced by cardiopulmonary bypass. Vasc Surg 1975;9:228–243.
224. McKenna R, Bachmann F, Whittaker B, Gilson J, Weinberg M. The hemostatic mechanism after open-heart surgery. II. Frequency of abnormal platelet functions during and after extracorporeal circulation. J Thorac Cardiovasc Surg 1975;70:298–308.
225. Schachter M. Kallikreins (kininogenases)—a group of serine proteases with bioregulatory actions. Pharmacol Rev 1979;31:1–17.
226. Fritz H, Fink E, Truscheit E. Kallikrein inhibitors. Fed Proc 1979;38: 2753–2759.
227. Kongsgaard U, Aasen A, Simth-Erichsen N, Bjornskau L. Effects of heparin on proteolytic activities in human plasma. Eur Surg Res 1992;24:119–128.
228. Fuhrer G, Gallimore M, Heller W, Hoffmeister H. Studies on components of the plasma kallikrein-kinin system in patients undergoing cardiopulmonary bypass. Adv Exp Med Biol 1986;198B:385–391.
229. Dietrich W, Spannagl M, Jochum M, et al. Influence of high-dose aprotinin treatment on blood loss and coagulation patterns in patients undergoing myocardial revascularization. Anesthesiology 1990;73: 1119–1126.
230. Gallimore M, Fuhrer G, Heller W, Hoffmeister H. Augmentation of kallikrein and plasmin inhibition capacity by aprotinin using a new assay to monitor therapy. Adv Exp Med Biol 1989;247B:55–60.
231. Hoffman H, Stebeck M, Thetter O, Jochum M, Fritz H. Aprotinin concentrations effective for the inhibition of tissue kallikrein and plasma kallikrein in vitro and in vivo. Adv Exp Med Biol 1989;247B:35–42.
232. Royston D, Bidstrup B, Taylor K, Sapsford R. Effect of aprotinin on the need for blood transfusion after repeat open heart surgery. Lancet 1987;2:1289–1291.
233. Gravlee G, Case L, Angert K, Rogers A, Miller G. Variability of the activated coagulation time. Anesth Analg 1988;67:469–472.
234. Culliford A, Gitel S, Starr N, et al. Lack of correlation between activated clotting time and plasma heparin during cardiopulmonary bypass. Ann Surg 1981;193:105–111.
235. Bull B, Huse W, Brauer F, Korpman R. Heparin therapy during extracorporeal circulation. II. The use of a dose-response curve to individualize heparin and protamine dosage. J Thorac Cardiovasc Surg 1975; 69:685–689.
236. Brandt J, Triplett D. Laboratory monitoring of heparin. Effect of reagents and instruments on the activated partial thromboplastin time. Am J Clin Pathol 1981;76:530–537.
237. O'Neill A, McAllister C, Corke C, Parkin J. A comparison of five devices for the bedside monitoring of heparin therapy. Anaesth Intens Care 1991;19:592–601.
238. Jobes D, Schwartz A, Ellison N, Andrews R, Ruffini R, Ruffini J. Monitoring heparin anticoagulation and its neutralization. Ann Thorac Surg 1981;31:161–166.
239. Gompets E, Bethlehem B, Hockley J. The monitoring of heparin activity during extracorporeal circulation. S Afr Med J 1977;51: 973–976.
240. Bithell T. The diagnostic approach to the bleeding disorders. In: Lee G, Bithell T, Foerster J, et al., eds. Wintrobe's clinical hematology. Philadelphia: Lea & Febiger, 1993:1301–1324.
241. White GI, Marder V, Colman R, et al. Approach to bleeding patient. In: Colman R, Hirsh J, Marder V, Salzman E, eds. Hemostasis and thrombosis. Philadelphia: J.B. Lippincott, 1994:1134–1147.
242. Delorme M, Inwood M, O'Keefe B. Sensitivity of the thrombin clotting time and activated partial thromboplastin time to low level of antithrombin III during heparin therapy. J Clin Lab Haematol 1990;12: 433–436.
243. Choo I, Didisheim P, Doerge M, et al. Evaluation of a heparin assay method using a fluorogenic synthetic peptide substrate for thrombin. Thromb Res 1982;25:115–123.
244. Kurec A, Morris M, Davey F. Clotting activated partial thromboplastin and coagulation times in monitoring heparin therapy. Ann Clin Lab Sci 1979;9:494–500.
245. Reiner J, Coyne K, Lundergan C, AM R. Bedside monitoring of heparin therapy: comparison of activated clotting time to activated partial thromboplastin time. Cathet Cardiovasc Diagn 1994;32:49–52.
246. Dauchot P, Berzina-Moettus L, Rabinovitch A, Ankeney J. Activated coagulation and activated partial thromboplastin times in assessment and reversal of heparin-induced anticoagulation for cardiopulmonary bypass. Anesth Analg 1983;62:710–719.
247. van Putten J, van de Ruit M, Beunis M, Hemker H. Automated spectrophotometric heparin assays. Comparison of methods. Haemostasis 1984;14:195–204.
248. Hattersley P. Activated coagulation time of whole blood. JAMA 1966;196:150–154.
249. Bull B, Korpman R, Huse W, Briggs B. Heparin therapy during extracorporeal circulation. I. Problems inherent in existing heparin protocols. J Thorac Cardiovasc Surg 1975;69:674–684.
250. Ferguson J. All ACTs are not created equal. Tex Heart Inst J 1992; 19:1–3.
251. Mabry C, Thompson B, Read R, Campbell G. Activated clotting time monitoring of intraoperative heparinization: our experience and comparison of two techniques. Surgery 1981;90:889–895.
252. Avendano A, Ferguson J. Comparison of Hemochron and HemoTec activated coagulation time target values during percutaneous transluminal coronary angioplasty. J Am Coll Cardiol 1994;23:907–910.
253. Hill J, Dontigny L, de Leval M, Mielke CJ. A simple method of hep-

arin management during prolonged extracorporeal circulation. Ann Thorac Surg 1974;17:129–134.
254. Reich D, Zahl K, Perucho H, Thys D. An evaluation of two activated clotting time monitors during cardiac surgery. Proceedings of the Society of Cardiovascular Anesthesiologists 12th Annual Meeting, 1990.
255. Varga Z, Papp L, Andrassy G. Hemochron versus HemoTec activated coagulation time target values during percutaneous transluminal coronary angioplasty. J Am Coll Cardiol 1995;25:803–804.
256. Jobes D, Ellison N, Campbell F. Limit(ation)s for ACT. Anesth Analg 1989;69:142–144.
257. Uden D, Seay R, Kriesmer P, Cipolle R, Payne N. The effect of heparin on three whole blood activated clotting tests and thrombin time. ASAIO Trans 1991;37:88–91.
258. Green T, Isham-Schopf B, Steinhorn R, Smith C, Irmiter R. Whole blood activated clotting time in infants during extracorporeal membrane oxygenation. Crit Care Med 1990;18:494–498.
259. Kase P, Dearing J. Factors affecting the activated clotting time. J Extracorp Technol 1985;17:27–30.
260. Kesteven P, Pasaoglu I, Williams B, Savidge G. Significance of the whole blood activated clotting time in cardiopulmonary bypass. J Cardiovasc Surg 1986;27:85–89.
261. Gravlee G, Brauer S, Roy R, et al. Predicting the pharmacodynamics of heparin: a clinical evaluation of the Hepcon System 4. J Cardiothorac Anesth 1987;1:379–387.
262. Moorehead M, Westengard J, Bull B. Platelet involvement in the activated coagulation time of heparinized blood. Anesth Analg 1984;198: 394–398.
263. Despotis G, Joist J, Joiner-Maier D, et al. Effect of aprotinin on activated clotting time, whole blood and plasma heparin measurements. Ann Thorac Surg 1995;59:106–111.
264. Wang J, Lin C, Hung W, Thisted R, Karp R. In vitro effects of aprotinin on activated clotting time measured with different activators. J Thorac Cardiovasc Surg 1992;104:1135–1140.
265. Bull M, Huse W, Bull B. Evaluation of tests used to monitor heparin therapy during extracorporeal circulation. Anesthesiology 1975;43: 346–353.
266. Gravlee G, Haddon W, Rothberger H, et al. Heparin dosing and monitoring for cardiopulmonary bypass. J Thorac Cardiovasc Surg 1990; 99:518–527.
267. Stenbjerg S, Berg E, Albrechtsen O. Heparin levels and activated clotting time (ACT) during open heart surgery. Scand J Haematol 1981; 216:281–284.
268. Cohen J. Activated coagulation time method for control of heparin is reliable during cardiopulmonary bypass. Anesthesiology 1984;60: 121–124.
269. Esposito R, Culliford A, Colvin S, Thomas S, Lackner H, Spencer F. The role of activated clotting time in heparin administration and neutralization for cardiopulmonary bypass. J Thorac Cardiovasc Surg 1983;85:174–185.
270. Stehling L, Simon T. The red blood cell transfusion trigger. Arch Pathol Lab Med 1994;1118:429–434.
271. Young J, Kisker C, Doty D. Adequate anticoagulation during cardiopulmonary bypass determined by activated clotting time and the appearance of fibrin monomer. Ann Thorac Surg 1978;26:231–240.
272. Davies G, Sobel M, Salzman E. Elevated plasma fibrinopeptide A and thromboxane B_2 levels during cardiopulmonary bypass. Circulation 1980;61:808–814.
273. Cardoso P, Yamazaki F, Keshavjee S, et al. A reevaluation of heparin requirements for cardiopulmonary bypass. J Thorac Cardiovasc Surg 1991;101:153–160.
274. Metz S, Keats A. Low activated coagulation time during cardiopulmonary bypass does not increase postoperative bleeding. Ann Thorac Surg 1990;49:440–444.
275. Gravlee G, Rogers A, Dudas L, et al. Heparin management protocol for cardiopulmonary bypass influences postoperative heparin rebound but not bleeding. Anesthesiology 1992;76:393–401.
276. Nielsen L, Bell W, Borkon A, Neill C. Extensive thrombus formation with heparin resistance during extracorporeal circulation. A new presentation of familial antithrombin III deficiency. Arch Intern Med 1987;147:149–152.
277. Bowie J, Kemna G. Automated management of heparin anticoagulation in cardiovascular surgery. Proc Am Acad Cardiovasc Perfusion 1985;6:1–10.
278. Despotis G, Joist J, Hogue CJ, et al. The impact of heparin concentration and activated clotting time monitoring on blood conservation. A prospective, randomized evaluation in patients undergoing cardiac operation. J Thorac Cardiovasc Surg 1995;110:46–54.
279. Cobel-Geard R, Hassouna H. Interaction of protamine sulfate with thrombin. Am J Hematol 1983;14:227–233.
280. Ellison N, Ominsky A, Wollman H. Is protamine a clinically important anticoagulant? A negative answer. Anesthesiology 1971;35:621–629.
281. Kresowik T, Wakefield T, Fessler R, Stanley J. Anticoagulant effects of protamine sulfate in a canine model. J Surg Res 1988;45:8–14.
282. Anido G, Freeman D. Heparin assay and protamine titration. Am J Clin Pathol 1981;76:410–415.
283. Verska J. Control of heparinization by activated clotting time during bypass with improved postoperative hemostasis. Ann Thorac Surg 1977;24:170–173.
284. Saleem A, Shenaq S, Yawn D, Harshberger K, Diemunsch P, Mohindra P. Heparin monitoring during cardiopulmonary bypass. Ann Clin Lab Sci 1984;14:474–479.
285. Gauvin G, Umlas J, Chin N. Measurement of plasma heparin levels using a fluorometric assay. Med Instrum 1983;17:165–168.
286. Ellison N, Edmunds L, Colman R. Platelet aggregation following heparin and protamine administration. Anesthesiology 1978;48:65–68.
287. Hurt R, Perkins H, Osborn J, Gerbode F. The neutralization of heparin by protamine in extracorporeal circulation. J Thorac Surg 1856;32: 612–619.
288. Horrow J. Thrombocytopenia accompanying a reaction to protamine sulfate. Can Anaesth Soc J 1985;32:49–52.
289. Lindblad B, Wakefield TW, Whitehouse WM Jr, Stanley JC. The effect of protamine sulfate on platelet function. Scand J Thorac Cardiovasc Surg 1988;22:55–59.
290. Bjoraker D, Ketcham T. In vivo platelet response to clinical protamine sulfate infusion. Anesthesiology 1982;57:A7.
291. Eika C. On the mechanism of platelet aggregation induced by heparin, protamine and polybrene. Scand J Haematol 1972;9:248–254.
292. Rådegran K, McAshlan C. Circulatory and ventilatory effects of induced platelet aggregation and their inhibition by acetylsalicylic acid. Acta Anaesthesiol Scand 1972;16:76.
293. Arén C. Heparin and protamine therapy. Semin Thorac Cardiovasc Surg 1990;2:364–372.
294. Akl B, Vargas G, Neal J, Robillard J, Kelly P. Clinical experience with the activated clotting time for the control of heparin and protamine therapy during cardiopulmonary bypass. Thorac Cardiovasc Surg 1980;79:98–102.

295. Hawksley M. De-heparinisation of blood after a cardiopulmonary bypass. Lancet 1966;1:563–565.
296. Jaques L. A study of the toxicity of the protamine, salmine. Br J Pharmacol 1949;4:135.
297. Lowenstein E, Johnston W, Lappas D, et al. Catastrophic pulmonary vasoconstriction associated with protamine reversal of heparin. Anesthesiology 1983;59:470–473.
298. Horrow J. Protamine allergy. J Cardiothorac Vasc Anesth 1988;2: 225–228.
299. Morel D, Mo Costabeela P, JF P. Adverse cardiopulmonary effects and increased thromboxane concentrations following the neutralization of heparin with protamine in awake sheep are infusion rate-dependent. Anesthesiology 1990;73:415–424.
300. Frater R, Oka Y, Hong Y, Tsubo T, Loubser P, Masone R. Protamine-induced circulatory changes. J Thorac Cardiovasc Surg 1984;87: 687–692.
301. Horrow J. Management of coagulation and bleeding disorders. In: Kaplan JA, ed. Cardiac anesthesia. Philadelphia: WB Saunders, 1983: 951–994.
302. Moorman R, Zapol W, Lowenstein E. Neutralization of heparin anticoagulation. In: Gravlee GP, Davis RF, Utley JR, eds. Cardiopulmonary bypass. Principles and practice. Baltimore: Williams & Wilkins, 1993:381–406.
303. Keller R. Interrelation between different types of cells. II. Histamine release for the mast cells of various species by cationic polypeptides of polymorphonuclear leukocytes, lysosomes and other cationic compounds. Int Arch Allergy Appl Immunol 1968;34:139–144.
304. Stoelting R, Henry D, Verbur K, McCammon R, King R, Brown J. Haemodynamic changes and circulating histamine concentrations following protamine administration to patients and dogs. Can Anaesth Soc J 1984;31:534–540.
305. Parsons R, Mohandas K. The effect of histamine-receptor blockade on the hemodynamic responses to protamine. J Cardiothorac Anesth 1989;3:37–43.
306. Levy J, Faraj B, Zaidan J, Camp V. Effects of protamine on histamine release from human lung. Agents Actions 1989;28:70.
307. Hird R, Wakefield T, Mukherjee R, et al. Direct effects of protamine sulfate on myocyte contractile processes: cellular and molecular mechanisms. Circulation 1995;92II:443–446.
308. Iwatsuki N, Matsukawa S, Iwatsuky K. A weak negative inotropic effect of protamine sulfate upon the isolated canine heart muscle. Anesth Analg 1980;59:100–102.
309. Michaels I, Barash P. Hemodynamic changes during protamine administration. Anesth Analg 1983;62:831–835.
310. Sethna D, Gray R, Bussell J, Raymond M, Matloff J, Moffitt E. Further studies on the myocardial metabolic effect of protamine sulfate following cardiopulmonary bypass. Anesth Analg 1982;61:476–677.
311. Sethna D, Moffitt E, Gray R, et al. Effects of protamine sulfate on myocardial oxygen supply and demand in patients following cardiopulmonary bypass. Anesth Analg 1982;61:247–251.
312. Doolan L, McKenzie I, Kratchek J, Parsons B, Buxton B. Protamine sulfate hypersensitivity. Anaesth Intens Care 1981;9:1–47.
313. Levy J, Schwieger I, Zaidan J, Faraj B, Weintraub W. Evaluation of patients at risk for protamine reactions. J Thorac Cardiovasc Surg 1989;98:200–204.
314. Levy J, Zaidan J, Faraj B. Prospective evaluation of risk protamine reactions in patients with NPH insulin-dependent diabetes. Anesth Analg 1986;65:739–742.
315. Samuel T, Kolk A, Rumke P, Van Lis J. Autoimmunity to sperm antigens in vasectomized men. Clin Exp Immunol 1975;21:65–74.
316. Sharath M, Metzger W, Richerson H, et al. Protamine-induced fatal anaphylaxis, prevalence of antiprotamine immunoglobin E antibody. J Thorac Cardiovasc Surg 1985;90:86–90.
317. Weiss M, Nyhan D, Peng Z, et al. Association of protamine IgE and IgG antibodies with life-threatening reactions to intravenous protamine. N Engl J Med 1989;320:886–892.
318. Morel D, Zapol W, Thomas S, et al. C5a and thromboxane generation associated with pulmonary vaso- and broncho-constriction protamine reversal of heparin. Anesthesiology 1987;66:597–604.
319. Stewart W, McSweeney S, Kellett M, Faxon D, Tyan T. Increased risk of severe protamine reactions in NPH insulin-dependent diabetes undergoing cardiac catheterization. Circulation 1984;70:788–792.
320. Caplan S, Berkman E. Letter: Protamine sulfate and fish allergy. N Engl J Med 1976;295:172.
321. Knape J, Schuller J, De Haan P, De Jong A, Bovill JG. An anaphylactic reaction to protamine in a patient allergic to fish. Anesthesiology 1981; 55:324–325.
322. Casthely P, Goodman K, Fryman P, Abrams L, Aaron D. Hemodynamic changes after the administration of protamine. Anesth Analg 1986;65:78–80.
323. Lakin J, Blocker T, Strong D, Yocum M. Anaphylaxis to protamine sulfate mediated by a complement-dependent IgG antibody. J Allergy Clin Immunol 1978;61:102–107.
324. Lock R, Hessel E. Probable reversal of protamine reactions by heparin administration. J Cardiothorac Vasc Anesth 1990;4:604–608.
325. Olinger G, Becker R, Bonchek L. Noncardiogenic pulmonary edema and peripheral vascular collapse following cardiopulmonary bypass: rare protamine reaction? Ann Thorac Surg 1980;29:20–25.
326. Horiguchi T, Enzan K, Mitsuhata H, Murata M, Suzuki M. Heparin-protamine complexes cause pulmonary hypertension in goats. Anesthesiology 1995;83:786–791.
327. Toyofuku T, Koyama S, Kobayashi T, Dusama S, Ueda G. Effects of polycations on pulmonary vascular permeability in conscious sheep. J Clin Invest 1989;83:2063.
328. Horrow J. Heparin reversal of protamine toxicity: have we come full circle? J Cardiothorac Vasc Anesth 1990;4:539.
329. Conzen P, Habazettl H, Gutmann R, et al. Thromboxane mediation of pulmonary hemodynamic responses after neutralization of heparin by protamine in pigs. Anesth Analg 1989;68:25–31.
330. Hobbhahn J, Conzen P, Zenker B, Goetz A, Peter K, Brendel W. Beneficial effect of cyclooxygenase inhibition on adverse hemodynamic responses after protamine. Anesth Analg 1988;67:253.
331. Morel D, Lowenstein E, Nguyenduy T, et al. Acute pulmonary vasoconstriction and thromboxane release during protamine reversal of heparin anticoagulation in awake sheep. Circ Res 1988;62: 905–915.
332. Lowenstein E, Zapol W. Protamine reactions, explosive mediator release, and pulmonary vasoconstriction [editorial]. Anesthesiology 1990;73:373–374.
333. Nuttall G, Murray M, Bowie J. Protamine-heparin-induced pulmonary hypertension in pigs; effects of treatment with a thromboxane receptor antagonist on hemodynamics and coagulation. Anesthesiology 1991; 74:138–145.
334. Schumacher W, Heran C, Ogletree M. Effect of thromboxane receptor antagonism on pulmonary hypertension caused by protamine-heparin interaction in pigs. Circulation 1988;78:207.

335. Colman R. Humoral mediators of catastrophic reactions associated with protamine neutralization. Anesthesiology 1987;66:595–596.
336. Degges R, Foster M, Dan A, Read R. Pulmonary hypertensive effect of heparin and protamine interaction: evidence for thromboxane B2 release from the lung. Am J Surg 1987;154:696–699.
337. Montalescot G, Lowenstein E, Ogletree M, et al. Thromboxane receptor blockade prevents pulmonary hypertension induced by heparin-protamine reactions in awake sheep. Circulation 1990;82:1765–1777.
338. Schapira M, Christman B. Neutralization of heparin by protamine: time for a change? Circulation 1990;82:1877–1879.
339. Godal H. A comparison of two heparin-neutralizing agents: protamine and polybrene. Scand J Clin Lab Invest 1960;12:446.
340. Weiss W, Gilman J, Catenacci A, Osterberg A. Heparin neutralization with polybrene administered intravenously. JAMA 1958;166: 630–637.
341. Egerton W, Robinson C. The anti-heparin, anticoagulant and hypotensive properties of hexadimethrine and protamine. Lancet 1961;2: 635–637.
342. Bertolatus J, Hunsicker L. Polycation binding to glomerular basement membrane. Effect of biochemical modification. Lab Invest 1987;56: 170–179.
343. Haller J, Ransdell H, Stowens D, Rubel W. Renal toxicity of polybrene in open heart surgery. J Thorac Cardiovasc Surg 1962;44:486–491.
344. Ransdell H, Haller J, Stowens D, Barton P. Renal toxicity of polybrene (hexadimethrine bromide). J Surg Res 1965;5:195.
345. Yang V, Port F, Kim G, Teng C, Till G, Wakefield T. The use of immobilized protamine in removing heparin and preventing protamine-induced complications during extracorporeal blood circulation. Anesthesiology 1991;75:288–297.
346. Teng C, Kim J, Port F, Wakefield T, Till G, Yang V. A protamine filter for extracorporeal blood heparin removal. ASAIO Trans 1988;34: 743–746.
347. Kim J-S, Vincent C, Teng C, Wakefield T, Yang V. A novel approach to anticoagulation control. ASAIO Trans 1989;35:644–646.
348. Despotis G, Summerfield A, Joist J, et al. In vitro reversal of heparin effect with heparinase: evaluation with whole blood prothrombin time and activated partial thromboplastin time in cardiac surgical patients. Anesth Analg 1994;79:670–674.
349. Langer R, Linhardt RJ, Hoffberg S, et al. An enzymatic system for removing heparin in extracorporeal therapy. Science 1982;217:261–263.
350. Cook J, Niewiarowski S, Yan Z, et al. Platelet factor 4 efficiently reverses heparin anticoagulation in the rat without adverse effects of the heparin-protamine complexes. Circulation 1992;85:1102–1105.
351. Levy J, Cormack J, Morales A. Heparin neutralization by recombinant platelet factor 4 and protamine. Anesth Analg 1995;81:35–37.
352. Bernabei A, Gikakis N, Maione T, et al. Reversal of heparin anticoagulation by recombinant platelet factor 4 and protamine sulfate in baboons during cardiopulmonary bypass. J Thorac Cardiovasc Surg 1995;109:765–771.
353. Williams R, D'Ambra M, Maione T, Lynch K, Keene D. Recombinant platelet factor 4 reversal of heparin in human cardiopulmonary bypass blood. J Thorac Cardiovasc Surg 1994;108:975–983.
354. Dehmer G, Fisher M, Tate D, Teo S, Bonnem E. Reversal of heparin anticoagulation by recombinant platelet factor 4 in humans. Circulation 1995;91:2188–2194.
355. Andet A, Goodnough L. Practice strategies for elective red blood cell transfusion. Ann Intern Med 1992;116:403–408.
356. Goodnough L, Honston M, Ramsey G, et al. Guidelines for transfusion support in patients undergoing coronary artery bypass grafting. Ann Thorac Surg 1990;50:675–683.
357. Wallace E, Surgenor D, Hao HAJ, Chapman R, Churchill W. Collection and transfusion of blood and blood components in the United States, 1989. Transfusion 1993;33:139–144.
358. Stover E, Siegel L, Parks R, et al. Variability in transfusion practice for coronary artery bypass surgery persists despite national consensus guidelines: a 24-institution study. Anesthesiology 1994;81:A1124.
359. Goodnough LT, Johnston MFM, Toy PTCY, Transfusion Medicine Academic Award Group. The variability of transfusion practice in coronary artery bypass surgery. JAMA 1991;265:86–90.
360. Goodnough L, Soegiarso R, Birkmeyer J, Welch H. Economic impact of inappropriate blood transfusions in coronary artery bypass graft surgery. Am J Med 1993;94:509–514.
361. Organizations JCoAoHC.Accreditation Manual for Hospitals, 1994.
362. Widman F. Standards for blood banks and transfusion services. American Association of Blood Banks, 1993.
363. Forbes J, Anderson M, Anderson G, Bleecher G, Rossi E, Moss G. Blood transfusion costs: a multicenter study. Transfusion 1991;31: 318–323.
364. Lubarsky DA, Hahn C, Bennett DH, et al. The hospital cost (fiscal year 1991/1992) of a simple perioperative allogeneic red blood cell transfusion during elective surgery at Duke University. Anesth Analg 1994;79:629–637.
365. Tyson G, Sladen R, Spainhour V, Savitt M, Ferguson T, Wolfe W. Blood conservation in cardiac surgery. Preliminary results with an institutional commitment. Ann Surg 1989;209:736–742.
366. Jones J, Rawitscher R, McLean T, Beal A, Thornby J. Benefit from combining blood conservation measures in cardiac operations. Ann Thorac Surg 1991;51:541–546.
367. Scott W, Rode R, Castlemain B, et al. Efficacy, complications, and cost of a comprehensive blood conservation program for cardiac operations. J Thorac Cardiovasc Surg 1992;103:1001–1007.
368. Dietrich W, Barankay A, Dilthey G, Mitto H, Richter J. Reduction of blood utilization during myocardial revascularization. J Thorac Cardiovasc Surg 1989;97:213–219.
369. Rosen N, Bates L, Herod G. Transfusion therapy: improved patient care and resource utilization. Transfusion 1993;33:341–347.
370. Spiess B, Gillies B, Chandler W, Verrier E. Changes in transfusion therapy and reexploration rate after institution of a blood management program in cardiac surgical patients. J Cardiothorac Vasc Anesth 1995;9:168–173.
371. Gravlee G, Arora S, Lavender S, et al. Predictive value of blood clotting tests in cardiac surgical patients. Ann Thorac Surg 1994;58: 216–221.
372. Rogers R, Levin J. A critical reappraisal of the bleeding time. Semin Thromb Haemost 1990;16:1–20.
373. Lind S. The bleeding time does not predict surgical bleeding. Blood 1991;77:2547–2552.
374. Zander H. Preoperative hemoglobin requirement. Anesth Clin North Am 1990;8:471–480.
375. Carson J, Spence R, Poses R, Bonavita G. Severity of anemia and operative mortality and morbidity. Lancet 1988;1:727–729.
376. Spence R, Costabule J, Young G, et al. Is hemoglobin level alone a reliable predictor of outcome in the severely anemic surgical patient. Ann Surg 1992;2:92–95.
377. Stehling L, Zander H. Acute normovolemic hemodilution. Transfusion 1991;31:857–868.

378. Martin E, Ott E. Extreme hemodilution in the Harrington procedure. Bibl Hematol 1981;47:322–327.
379. Haberkerin M, Dangel P. Normovolemic hemodilution and intraoperative autotransfusion in children: experience with 30 cases of spinal fusion. Eur J Pediatr Surg 1991;1:30–55.
380. Jan K, Chien S. Effect of hematocrit variations on coronary hemodynamics and oxygen utilization. Am J Physiol 1977;233:H106–H113.
381. Delano BG, Nacht R, Friedman EA, Krasow N. Myocardial anaerobiosis in anemia in uremic man. Am J Cardiol 1972;29:39–46.
382. Koller M, Haenny P, Hess K, Weniger D, Zangger P. Adjusted hypervolemic hemodilution in acute ischemic stroke. Stroke 1990;21: 1429–1434.
383. Group THiSS. Hypervolemic hemodilution treatment of acute shock. Results of a randomized multicenter trial using pentastarch. Stroke 1989;20:317–320.
384. Strand T. Evaluation of long-term outcome and safety after hemodilution therapy in acute ischemic stroke. Stroke 1992;23:657–662.
385. Goslinga H, Eijzenbach V, Heuvelmans J, et al. Custom tailored hemodilution with albumin and crystalloids in acute ischemic stroke. Stroke 1992;213:181–188.
386. Group SSS. Multicenter trial of hemodilution in acute ischemic stroke. Results of subgroup analyses. Stroke 1988;19:464–471.
387. Mast H, Marx P. Neurological deterioration under isovolemic hemodilution with hydroxyethyl starch in acute cerebral ischemia. Stroke 1991;22:680–683.
388. Heros R, Korosue K. Hemodilution for cerebral ischemia. Stroke 1989;20:423–427.
389. Korosue K, Heros R, Ogilvy C, Hyodo A, Tu Y, Graichen R. Comparison of crystalloids and colloids for hemodilution in a model of focal cerebral ischemia. J Neurosurg 1990;73:576–584.
390. Hyodo A, Heros R, Tu Y, et al. Acute effects of isovolemic hemodilution with crystalloids in a canine model of focal cerebral ischemia. Stroke 1989;20:534–540.
391. Korosue K, Heros R. Mechanism of cerebral blood flow augmentation by hemodilution in rabbits. Stroke 1992;23:1487–1492.
392. Cole D, Schell R, Drummond J, Reynolds L. Focal cerebral ischemia in rats. Effect of hypervolemic hemodilution with diaspirin crosslinked hemoglobin versus albumin on brain injury and edema. Anesthesiology 1993;78:335–342.
393. van Woerkens E, Trouwborst A, Duncker D, Koning M, Boomsma F, Verdouw P. Catecholamines and regional hemodynamics during isovolemic hemodilution in anesthetized pigs. J Appl Physiol 1992;72: 760–769.
394. Crystal G, Rooney M, Salem M. Regional hemodynamics and oxygen supply during isovolemic hemodilution alone and in combination with adenosine-induced controlled hypotension. Anesth Analg 1988;67: 211–218.
395. Catoire P, Saada M, Liu N, Delauney L, Rauss A, Bonnet F. Effect of preoperative normovolemic hemodilution on left ventricular segmental wall motion during abdominal aortic surgery. Anesth Analg 1992; 75:654–659.
396. Noldge G, Priebe H, Bohle W, Buttler K, Geiger K. Effects of acute normovolemic hemodilution on splanchnic oxygenation and on hepatic histology and metabolism in anesthetized pigs. Anesthesiology 1991;74:908–918.
397. Trouwborst A, Tenvrinck R, van Woerkens E. Blood gas analysis of mixed venous blood during normoxic acute isovolemic hemodilution in pigs. Anesth Analg 1990;70:523–529.
398. Tarnow J, Eberlein H, Hess W, Schneider E, Schwiechel E, Zimmermann G. Hemodynamic interactions of hemodilution, anaesthesia, propranolol pretreatment and hypovolaemia. II. Coronary circulation. Basic Res Cardiol 1979;74:123–130.
399. Wright C. The effects of severe progressive hemodilution on regional blood flow and oxygen consumption. Surgery 1976;79:299–305.
400. Holtz J, Bassenge E, von Restoriff W, Mayer E. Transmural differences in myocardial blood flow and in coronary dilatory capacity in hemodiluted conscious dogs. Basic Res Cardiol 1976;71:36–46.
401. Escobar E, Jones N, Rapaport E, Murray J. Ventricular performance in acute normovolemic anemia and effects of beta blockade. Am J Physiol 1966;211:877–884.
402. Chapter C, Cain S. Blood flow and O_2 uptake in dog hindlimb with anemia, norepinephrine, and propranolol. J Appl Physiol 1981;51: 565–570.
403. von Restorff W, Hofling B, Bassenge E. Effect of increased blood fluidity through hemodilution on general circulation at rest and during exercise in dogs. Pflugers Arch 1975;357:25–34.
404. Cain S, Chapler C. O_2 extraction by hind limb versus whole dog during anemic hypoxia. J Appl Physiol 1978;45:966–970.
405. Wilkerson D, Rosen A, Sehgal L, Gould S, Sehgal H, Moss G. Limits of cardiac compensation in anemic baboons. Surgery 1988;103: 665–670.
406. Messmer K, Sunder-Plassmann L, Klovenkorn W, Holper K. Circulatory significance of hemodilution: rheological changes and limitations. Adv Microcirc 1972;4:1–77.
407. Messmer K, Sunder-Plassmann L, Jesch F, Gornandt L, Sinagowitz E, Kessler M. Oxygen supply to the tissues during limited normovolemic hemodilution. Res Exp Med (Berl) 1973;159:152–166.
408. Spahn D, Leone B, Reves J, Pasch T. Cardiovascular and coronary physiology of acute isovolemic hemodilution: a review of non-oxygen carrying and oxygen-carrying solutions. Anesth Analg 1994;78: 1000–1021.
409. Rand P, Lacombe E, Hunt H, Austin W. Viscosity of normal human blood under normothermic and hypothermic conditions. J Appl Physiol 1964;19:117–122.
410. Replogle R, Meiselman H, Merrill E. Clinical implications of blood rheology studies. Circulation 1967;36:148–160.
411. Flowler N, Holmes J. Blood viscosity and cardiac output in acute experimental anemia. J Appl Physiol 1973;39:453–456.
412. Guyton A, Richardson T. Effect of hematocrit on venous return. Circ Res 1961;9:157–164.
413. Clarke T, Foex P, Roberts J, Saner C, Bennett M. Circulatory responses of the dog to acute isovolumic anaemia in the presence of high-grade adrenergic beta-receptor blockade. Br J Anaesth 1980;52: 337–341.
414. Crystal G, Salem M. Myocardial and systemic hemodynamics during isovolemic hemodilution alone and combined with nitroprusside-induced controlled hypotension. Anesth Analg 1991;72:227–237.
415. Fan F, Chen R, Schuessler G, Chien S. Effects of hematocrit variations on regional hemodynamics and oxygen transport in the dog. Am J Physiol 1980;238:H545–H552.
416. Rooney M, Hirsch L, Mathru M. Hemodilution with oxyhemoglobin. Mechanism of oxygen delivery and its superaugmentation with a nitric oxide donor (sodium nitroprusside). Anesthesiology 1979;79:60–72.
417. Murray J, Escobar E. Circulatory effects of blood viscosity: comparison of methemoglobinemia and anemia. J Appl Physiol 1968; 25:594–599.
418. Dedichen H, Race D, Schenk W. Hemodilution and concomitant hyperbaric oxygenation. J Thorac Cardiovasc Surg 1967;53:341–348.

419. Biro G. Comparison of acute cardiovascular effects and oxygen-supply following haemodilution with dextran, stromafree haemoglobin solution and fluorocarbon suspension. Cardiovasc Res 1982;16: 163–168.
420. Biro G. Fluorocarbon and dextran hemodilution in myocardial ischemia. Can J Surg 1983;26:163–168.
421. Gelin L, Bergentz S, Helander C, et al. Hemodynamic consequences from increased viscosity of blood. In: Copley A, ed. Hemorheology. Oxford: Pergamon Press, 1968:722–728.
422. Bowens C, Spahn D, Smith L, McRae R, Leone B. Hemodynamic effects of acute, extended isovolemic hemodilution. Anesth Analg 1993; 76:1027–1032.
423. Berman W, Lister G, Alverson D, Olsen S. Ouabain effect on oxygen physiology in anemic lambs. Pediatr Res 1987;21:447–452.
424. Adams H, Ratthey K, Rupp D, Hemplemann G. Endokrine Reaktionen bei akuter normovolamischer Hamodilution. Anaesthetist 1990;39: 269–274.
425. Glick G, Plauth W, Brauwald E. Role of the autonomic nervous system in the circulatory response to acutely induced anemia in unanesthetized dogs. J Clin Invest 1964;43:2112–2124.
426. Shinoda T, Smith C, Khairallah P, Fouad-Tarazi F, Estafanous F. Effects of propranolol on myocardial performance during acute normovolemic hemodilution. J Cardiothorac Vasc Anesth 1991;5:15–22.
427. Michalski A, Lowenstein E, Austen W, Buckley M, Laver M. Patterns of oxygenation and cardiovascular adjustment of acute, transient normovolemic anemia. Ann Surg 1968;168:946–956.
428. Fisselsson L, Rosberg B, Ericsson M. Myocardial blood flow, oxygen uptake and carbon dioxide release of the human heart during hemodilution. Acta Anaesthesiol Scand 1982;26:589–591.
429. Buckberg G, Brazier J. Coronary blood flow and cardiac function during hemodilution. Bibl Haematol 1975:173–189.
430. Brazier J, Cooper N, Maloney J, Buckberg G. The adequacy of myocardial oxygen delivery in acute normovolemic anemia. Surgery 1974;75:508–516.
431. Tarnow J, Eberlein H, Hess E, Schneider E, Schweichel E, Zimmermann G. Hemodynamic interactions of hemodilution, anaesthesia, propranolol pretreatment and hypovolaemia. I. Systemic circulation. Basic Res Cardiol 1979;74:109–122.
432. Crystal G. Coronary hemodynamic responses during local hemodilution in canine hearts. Am J Physiol 1988;254:H525–H531.
433. Most A, Ruocco N, Gewirtz H. Effect of a reduction in blood viscosity on maximal myocardial oxygen delivery distal to a moderate coronary stenosis. Circulation 1986;74:1085–1092.
434. Laxenaire M, Aug F, Voisin C, Chevreaud C, Bauer P, Bertrand A. Effects of hemodilution on the ventricular function of the coronary patient. Ann Fr Anesth 1986;5:218–222.
435. Singbartl G, Becker M, Frankenberg C, Maleszka H, Schleinzer W. Intraoperative online ST-segment analysis with extreme normovolemic hemodilution. Anesth Analg 1992;74:S295.
436. Boldt J, Bormann B, Kling D, Scheld H, Hempelmann G. Influence of acute normovolemic hemodilution on extravascular lung water in cardiac surgery. Crit Care Med 1988;16:336–339.
437. Cosgrove D, Loop F, Lytle B, et al. Determinants of blood utilization during myocardial revascularization. Ann Thorac Surg 1985;40: 380–384.
438. Spahn D, Smith L, McRae R, Leone B. Effects of acute isovolemic hemodilution and anesthesia on regional function in left ventricular myocardium with compromised coronary blood flow. Acta Anaesthesiol Scand 1992;36:628–636.
439. Gould K, Lipscomb K, Hamilton G. Physiologic basis for assessing critcial coronary stenosis. Instantaneous flow response and regional distribution-during coronary hyperemia as measures of coronary flow reserve. Am J Cardiol 1974;33:87–94.
440. Spahn D, Smith R, Veronee C, et al. Acute normovolemic hemodilution and blood transfusion: effects on regional function and metabolism in myocardium with compromised coronary blood flow. J Thorac Cardiovasc Surg 1993;105:694–704.
441. Spahn D, Frasco P, White W, Smith L, McRae R, Leone B. Is esmolol cardioprotective? Tolerance of pacing tachycardia, acute afterloading and hemodilution in dogs with coronary stenosis. J Am Coll Cardiol 1993;21:809–821.
442. Johnson RG, Thurer RL, Kruskall MS, et al. Comparison of two transfusion strategies after elective operations for myocardial revascularization. J Thorac Cardiovasc Surg 1992;104:307–314.
443. Hope A, Heyns A, Lotter M, et al. Kinetics and site of sequestration of Indium III-labeled human platelets during cardiopulmonary bypass. J Thorac Cardiovasc Surg 1981;81:880.
444. Conference C. Platelet transfusion therapy. JAMA 1987;257: 177–1780.
445. Harding S, Skakoor M, Grindon A. Platelet support for cardiopulmonary bypass. J Thorac Cardiovasc Surg 1975;70:350–353.
446. Cohen N, Munoz A, Reitz B, et al. Transmission of retrovirus by transfusion of screened blood in patients undergoing cardiac surgery. N Engl J Med 1989;320:1172–1176.
447. Ward J, Holmber S, Allen J, et al. Transmission of human immunodeficiency virus (HIV) by blood transfusion screened as negative for HIV antibody. N Engl J Med 1988;318:473–478.
448. Bove J. Transfusion-associated hepatitis and AIDS. What is the risk? N Engl J Med 1987;317:242–245.
449. Peterman T, Jaffe H, Feorino P, et al. Transfusion associated acquired immunodeficiency syndrome in the United States. JAMA 1985;254: 2913–2917.
450. Jaffe H, Sarngadharan M, DeVico A. Infection with HTLV-III/LAV and transfusion-associated acquired immunodeficiency syndrome. Serologic evidence of an association. JAMA 1985;254:770–773.
451. Cumming P, Wallace E, Schoor J, Dodd R. Exposure of patients to human immunodeficiency virus through the transfusion of blood components that test antibody-negative. N Engl J Med 1989;321:941–946.
452. Gaines H, von Sydow M, Sonnerborg A, et al. Antibody response in primary human immunodeficiency virus infection. Lancet 1987;1: 1249–1253.
453. Ranki A, Valle S, Krohn M, et al. Long latency precedes overt seroconversion in sexually transmitted human-immunodeficiency-virus infection. Lancet 1987;2:589–593.
454. Waymack J, Warden C, Alexander J, Miskell P, Gonce S. Effect of blood transfusion and anesthesia on resistance to bacterial peritonitis. J Surg Res 1987;42:528–535.
455. Triulzi D, Blumberg N, Heal J. Association of transfusion with postoperative bacterial infection. Crit Rev Clin Lab 1990;28:95–107.
456. Tartter P, Driefuss R, Malon A, Heimann T, Aufses A. Relationship of postoperative septic complications and blood transfusion in patients with Crohn's disease. Am J Surg 1988;155:43–48.
457. Rosemurgy A, Hart M, Murphy C, et al. Infection after injury: association with blood transfusion. Am Surg 1992;58:104–107.
458. Simchen E, Raz R, Stein H, Danon Y. Risk factors for infection in fracture war wounds (1973 and 1982 wars, Israel). Milit Med 1991;156: 520–527.
459. Galandiuk S, George C, Pietsch J, Byck D, DeWeese R, Polk HJ. An

experimental assessment of the effect of blood transfusion on susceptibility to bacterial infection. Surgery 1990;108:567–571.

460. Tartter P, Quintero S, Barron D. Perioperative blood transfusion associated with infectious complications after colorectal cancer operations. Am J Surg 1986;152:479–482.
461. Tartter P. Blood transfusion and infectious complications following colorectal cancer surgery. Br J Surg 1988;75:789–792.
462. Nichols R, Smith J, Klein D, et al. Risk of infection after penetrating abdominal trauma. N Engl J Med 1984;311:1065–1070.
463. Dawes L, Aprahamian C, Condon R, Malangoni M. The risk of infection after colon injury. Surgery 1986;100:796–803.
464. Mezrow C, Bergstein I, Tartter P. Postoperative infections following autologous and homologous blood transfusions. Transfusion 1992;32:27–30.
465. Murphy P, Heal J, Blumberg N. Infection or suspected infection after hip replacement surgery with autologous or homologous blood transfusions. Transfusion 1991;31:212–217.
466. Bock M, Grevers G, Koblitz M, Heim M, Mempel W. Influence of blood transfusion on recurrence, survival and postoperative infections of laryngeal cancer. Acta Otolaryngol (Stockh) 1990;110:155–160.
467. Fernandez M, Gottlieb M, Menitove J. Blood transfusion and postoperative infection in orthopedic patients. Transfusion 1992;32:318–322.
468. Love T, Hendren W, O'Keefe D, Daggett W. Transfusion of predonated autologous blood in elective cardiac surgery. Ann Thorac Surg 1987;43:508–512.
469. Gluck D, Kubanek B, Ahnefeld F. Autologous transfusion. Objectives and benefits, limits and risks shown in a practical clinical concept. Anaesthesia 1988;37:565–571.
470. Anderson B, Tomasulo P. Current autologous transfusion practices. Implications for the future. Transfusion 1988;28:394–396.
471. Birkmeyer JD, AuBuchon JP, Littenberg B, et al. Cost-effectiveness of preoperative autologous donation in coronary artery bypass grafting. Ann Thorac Surg 1994;57:161–169.
472. Britton L, Eastlund T, Dziuban S, et al. Predonated autologous blood use in elective cardiac surgery. Ann Thorac Surg 1989;47:529–532.
473. Owings D, Kruskall M, Thurer R, Donovan L. Autologous blood donations prior to elective cardiac surgery. JAMA 1989;262:1963–1968.
474. Cove H, Matlotf J, Sacks H, Sherbecoe R, Goldfinger D. Autologous blood transfusion in coronary artery bypass surgery. Transfusion 1976;16:245–246.
475. Dzik W, Fleischer A, Ciavarella D, Karlsson K, Reed G, Berger R. Safety and efficacy of autologous blood donation before elective aortic valve operation. Ann Thorac Surg 1992;54:1177–1181.
476. Goldfinger D, Capon S, Czer L, et al. Safety and efficacy of preoperative donation of blood for autologous use by patients with end-stage heart or lung disease who are awaiting organ transplantation. Transfusion 1993;33:336–340.
477. Spiess B, Sassetti R, McCarthy R, Narbone R, Tuman K, Ivankovich A. Autologous blood donation: hemodynamics in a high-risk population. Transfusion 1992;32:17–22.
478. Gravlee G. Con: autologous blood collection is not useful for elective coronary artery bypass graft surgery. J Cardiothorac Vasc Anesth 1994;8:238–241.
479. Goodnough L, Price T, Rudnick S, Soegiarso R. Preoperative and red cell production in patients undergoing aggressive autologous phlebotomy with and without erythropoietin therapy. Transfusion 1992;32.
480. Kulier A, Gombotz H, Fuchs G, Vuckovic U, Metzler H. Subcutaneous recombinant human erythropoietin and autologous blood donation before coronary artery bypass surgery. Anesth Analg 1993;76:102–106.
481. Kyo S, Omoto R, Hirashima K, Eguchi S, Fujita T. Effect of human recombinant erythropoietin on reduction of homologous blood transfusion in open-heart surgery. A Japanese multicenter study. Circulation 1992;86:413–418.
482. Hayashi J, Shinonaga M, Nakazawa S, Miyamura H, Eguchi S, Shinada S. Does recombinant human erythropoietin accelerate erythropoiesis for predonation before cardiac surgery. Jpn Circ J 1993;57:475–479.
483. Hayashi J, Kumon K, Takanashi S, et al. Subcutaneous administration of recombinant human erythropoietin before cardiac surgery: a double blind, multicenter trial in Japan. Transfusion 1994;34:142–146.
484. Schmoekel M, Nollert G, Mempel M, Mempel W, Reichart B. Effects of recombinant human erythropoietin on autologous blood donation before open heart surgery. Thorac Cardiovasc Surg 1993;41:364–368.
485. Konishi T, Ohbayashi T, Kaneko T, Ohki T, Saitou Y, Yamato Y. Preoperative use of erythropoietin for cardiovascular operations in anemia. Ann Thorac Surg 1993;56:101–103.
486. Hisatomi K, Isomura T, Galli SJ, Yasunaga H, Hayashida N, Ohishi K. Augmentation of interleukin-2 production after cardiac operations in patients treated with erythropoietin. J Thorac Cardiovasc Surg 1992;104:278–283.
487. Helm RE, Gold JP, Rosengart TK, Zelano JA, Isom OW, Krieger KH. Erythropoietin in cardiac surgery. J Card Surg 1993;8:579–606.
488. Wong C, Franklin M, Wade L. Coagulation tests, blood loss, and transfusion requirements in platelet rich plasmapheresed versus nonpheresed cardiac surgery patients. Anesth Analg 1994;78:29–36.
489. Jones J, McCoy T, Rawitscher R, Lindsley P. Effects of intraoperative plasmapheresis on blood loss in cardiac surgery. Ann Thorac Surg 1990;49:585–590.
490. Giordano G, Rivers S, Chung G, et al. Autologous platelet-rich plasma in cardiac surgery: effect on intraoperative and postoperative transfusion requirements. Ann Thorac Surg 1988;46:416–419.
491. Del Rossi A, Cernaianu A, Vertrees R, et al. Platelet-rich plasma reduces postoperative blood loss after cardiopulmonary bypass. J Thorac Cardiovasc Surg 1990;100:281–286.
492. Holland P, Schmidt PE. Standards for blood banks and transfusion services. 12th ed. Washington, DC: American Association of Blood Banks, 1987.
493. Davies G, Wells D, Mabee T, Sadler R, Melling N. Platelet-leukocyte plasmapheresis attenuates the deleterious effects of cardiopulmonary bypass. Ann Thorac Surg 1992;53:274–277.
494. Boldt J. Acute platelet-rich plasmapheresis for cardiac surgery. J Cardiothorac Vasc Anesth 1995;9:79–88.
495. Boldt J, Von Bormann B, Kling D, Jacobi M, Moosdorf R, Hempelmann G. Preoperative plasmapheresis in patients undergoing cardiac surgery procedures. Anesthesiology 1990;72:282–288.
496. Boldt J, Kling D, Zickmann B, Jacobi M, Dapper F, Hempelmann G. Acute preoperative plasmapheresis and established blood conservation techniques. Ann Thorac Surg 1990;50:62–68.
497. Ferrari M, Zia S, Valbonesi M, et al. A new technique for hemodilution, preparation of autologous platelet-rich plasma and intraoperative blood salvage in cardiac surgery. Int J Artif Org 1987;10:47–50.
498. Giordano GS, Giordano GJ, Rivers S, et al. Determinants of homologous blood usage, utilizing autologous platelet rich plasma in cardiac operations. Ann Thorac Surg 1989;47:897–902.
499. Harke H, Tanger D, Fürst-Denzer S, Paochrysnathou C, Bernhard A. Effects of a preoperative separation of platelets on the postoperative

blood loss subsequent to extracorporeal circulation in open heart surgery. Anaesthetist 1977;26:64–71.
500. Tawes R, Sydorak G, Duvall T, et al. The plasma collection system: a new concept in autotransfusion. Ann Vasc Surg 1989;3:304–306.
501. Wells D, Davies G. Platelet salvage in cardiac surgery. J Cardiothorac Vasc Anesth 1993;7:448–451.
502. Calandra D, Lanser R. Blood utilization and the role of the transfusion medicine specialist in cardiac surgery. In: DiFarre R, ed. Anticoagulation, hemostasis, and blood preservation in cardiovascular surgery. Philadelphia: Hanely and Belfus, 1989.
503. Boey S, Ong B, Dhara S. Preoperative plateletpheresis does not reduce blood loss during cardiac surgery. Can J Anaesth 1993;40:844–850.
504. Ereth M, Oliver WJ, Beynen F, et al. Autologous platelet-rich plasma does not reduce transfusion of homologous blood products in patients undergoing repeat valvular surgery. Anesthesiology 1993;79: 540–547.
505. Tobe C, Vocelka C, Sepulvada R, et al. Infusion of autologous platelet rich plasma does not reduce blood loss and products use after coronary artery bypass. J Thorac Cardiovasc Surg 1993;105:1007–1014.
506. Noon G, Jones J, Fehir K, Yawn D. Use of preoperatively obtained platelets and plasma in patients undergoing cardiopulmonary bypass. J Clin Apheresis 1990;5:91–96.
507. Mohr R, Goor D, Yellin A, Moshkovitz Y, Shinfeld A, Martinowitz U. Fresh blood units contain large potent platelets that improve hemostasis after open heart surgery. Ann Thorac Surg 1992;53:650–654.
508. Hirsh J, Glynn M, Mustard F. The effect of platelet age on platelet adherence to collagen. J Clin Invest 1968;47:466–473.
509. Kaufman M. Platelet size in thrombocytopenias and thrombosis of various origin. Blood 1973;41:587–598.
510. Karpatkin S, Charmatz A. Heterogeneity of human platelets. I. Metabolic and kinetic evidence suggestive of young and old platelets. J Clin Invest 1969;48:1073–1082.
511. Whitten C, Allison P. Why is acute preoperative plasmapheresis not uniformly effective at decreasing bleeding following cardiac surgery. J Cardiothorac Vasc Anesth 1993;7:766.
512. Mohr R, Sagi B, Lavee J, Goor D. The hemostatic effect of autologous platelet-rich plasma versus autologous whole blood after cardiac operations: is platelet separation really necessary? J Thorac Cardiovasc Surg 1993;105:371–373.
513. Hallowell P, Bland J, Buckley M, Lowenstein E. Transfusion of fresh autologous whole blood in open-heart surgery. A method for reducing blood bank requirements. J Cardiothorac Vasc Surg 1972;64:941–948.
514. Newland P, Pastoriza-Pinol J, McMillan J, Smith B, Stirling G. Maximal conservation and minimal usage of blood products in open-heart surgery. Anaesth Intens Care 1980;8:178–182.
515. Kaplan J, Cannarella C, Jones E, Kurter M, Hatcher C, Dunbar R. Autologous blood transfusion during cardiac surgery. J Thorac Cardiovasc Surg 1977;74:4–10.
516. Lilleaasen P, Frysaker T. Fresh autologous blood in open heart surgery: influence on blood requirements, bleeding, and platelet counts. Scand J Thorac Cardiovasc Surg 1979;13:41–46.
517. Ochsner J, Mills N, Leonard G, Lawson N. Fresh autologous blood transfusions with extracorporeal circulation. Ann Surg 1973;77: 811–817.
518. Lawson L, Ochsner J, Mills N, Leonard G. The use of hemodilution and fresh autologous blood in open heart surgery. Anesth Analg 1974;53:672–683.
519. Petry AF, Jost J, Sievers H. Reduction of homologous blood requirements by blood-pooling at the onset of cardiopulmonary bypass. J Thorac Cardiovasc Surg 1994;107:1210–1214.
520. Schonberger JP, Bredee JJ, Tjian D, Everts PA, Wildevuur CR. Intraoperative predonation contributes to blood saving. Ann Thorac Surg 1993;56:893–898.
521. Pliam M, McGoon D, Tarhan S. Failure of transfusion of autologous whole blood to reduce banked-blood requirements in open-heart surgical patients. J Thorac Cardiovasc Surg 1975;70:338–343.
522. Sherman M, Dobnik D, Dennis R, Berger R. Autologous blood transfusion during cardiopulmonary bypass. Chest 1976;70:592–595.
523. Cohn L, Fosberg A, Anderson W, Collins JJ. The effect of phlebotomy, hemodilution and autologous transfusion on systemic oxygenation and whole blood utilization in open heart surgery. Chest 1975;68:283–287.
524. Wagstaffe J, Clarke A, Jackson P. Reduction of blood loss by restoration of platelet levels using fresh autologous blood after cardiopulmonary bypass. Thorax 1972;27:410–416.
525. Hardesty R, Bayer W, Bahnson H. A technique for the use of autologous fresh blood during open heart surgery. J Thorac Cardiovasc Surg 1968;56:683–688.
526. Niinikoski J, Laato V, Laaksonen V, et al. Effects of extreme haemodilution on the immediate post-operative course of coronary artery bypass patients. Eur Surg Res 1983;15:1–10.
527. Robblee J. Pro: blood should be harvested immediately before cardiopulmonary bypass and infused after protamine reversal to decrease blood loss following cardiopulmonary bypass. J Cardiothorac Anesth 1990;4:519–521.
528. Starr N. Con: blood should not be harvested immediately before cardiopulmonary bypass and infused after protamine reversal to decrease blood loss following cardiopulmonary bypass. J Cardiothorac Anesth 1990;4:522–525.
529. Henderson L, Besarab A, Michaels A, Bluemle LJ. Blood purification by ultrafiltration and fluid replacement (diafiltration). Trans Am Soc Artif Intern Organs 1967;13:216–226.
530. Magilligan D, Oyama C. Ultrafiltration during cardiopulmonary bypass: laboratory evaluation and initial clinical experience. Ann Thorac Surg 1984;37:33–39.
531. Boldt J, Kling D, von Bormann B, Züge M, Scheld H, Hempelmann G. Blood conservation in cardiac operations: cell separation versus hemofiltration. J Thorac Cardiovasc Surg 1989;97:832–840.
532. Sutton R, Kratz J, Spinale F, Crawford F. Comparison of three blood-processing techniques during and after cardiopulmonary bypass. Ann Thorac Surg 1993;56:938–943.
533. Solem J, Tengborn L, Steen S, Lührs C. Cell saver versus hemofilter for concentration of oxygenator blood after cardiopulmonary bypass. Thorac Cardiovasc Surg 1987;35:42–47.
534. Schaff HV, Hauer JM, Bell WR, et al. Autotransfusion of shed mediastinal blood after cardiac surgery: a prospective study. J Thorac Cardiovasc Surg 1978;75:632–641.
535. Schaff HV, Hauer J, Gardner TJ, et al. Routine use of autotransfusion following cardiac surgery: experience in 700 patients. Ann Thorac Surg 1979;27:493–499.
536. Breyer RH, Engelman RM, Rousou JA, Lemeshow S. Blood conservation for myocardial revascularization. Is it cost effective? J Thorac Cardiovasc Surg 1987;93:512–522.
537. Eng J, Kay PH, Murday AJ, et al. Postoperative autologous transfusion in cardiac surgery. A prospective, randomized study. Eur J Cardiothorac Surg 1990;4:595–600.
538. Johnson RG, Rosenkrantz KR, Preston RA, Hopkins C, Daggett WM. The efficacy of postoperative autotransfusion in patients undergoing cardiac operations. Ann Thorac Surg 1983;36:173–179.

539. Page R, Russell GN, Fox MA, Fabri BM, Lewis I, Williets T. Hard-shell cardiotomy reservoir for reinfusion of shed mediastinal blood. Ann Thorac Surg 1989;48:514–517.
540. Parrot D, Lancon J, Merle J, et al. Blood salvage in cardiac surgery. J Cardiothorac Vasc Anesth 1991;5:454–456.
541. Weniger J, Shanahan R. Reduction of blood requirements in cardiac surgery. Thorac Cardiovasc Surg 1982;30:142–146.
542. Dietrich W. Pro: shed mediastinal blood retransfusion should be used routinely in cardiac surgery. J Cardiothorac Vasc Anesth 1995;9: 95–99.
543. Mazer CD. Con: shed mediastinal blood retransfusion should be used routinely in cardiac surgery. J Cardiothorac Vasc Anesth 1995;9: 100–102.
544. Adan A, Riviere A, Haas F, Zalk A, deNooij E. Autotransfusion of drained mediastinal blood after cardiac surgery: a reappraisal. Thorac Cardiovasc Surg 1988;36:10–14.
545. Axford TC, Dearani JA, Ragno G, et al. Safety and therapeutic effectiveness of reinfused shed blood after open heart surgery. Ann Thorac Surg 1994;57:615–622.
546. Bennett JG. Autotransfusion of drained mediastinal blood. Thorac Cardiovasc Surg 1982;30:28–30.
547. Bouboulis N, Kardara M, Kesteven P, Jayakrishnan AG. Autotransfusion after coronary artery bypass surgery: is there any benefit? J Card Surg 1994;9:314–321.
548. Ikeda S, Johnston MF, Yagi K, Gillespie KN, Schweiss JF, Homan SM. Intraoperative autologous blood salvage with cardiac surgery: an analysis of five years' experience in more than 3,000 patients. J Clin Anesth 1992;4:359–366.
549. Roberts SR, Early GL, Brown B, Hannah HD, McDonald HL. Autotransfusion of unwashed mediastinal shed blood fails to decrease banked blood requirements in patients undergoing aortocoronary bypass surgery. Am J Surg 1991;162:477–480.
550. Thurer RL, Lytle BW, Cosgrove DM, Loop FD. Autotransfusion following cardiac operations: a randomized, prospective study. Ann Thorac Surg 1979;27:500–507.
551. Ward HB, Smith RR, Landis KP, Nemzek TG, Dalmasso AP, Swaim WR. Prospective, randomized trial of autotransfusion after routine cardiac operations. Ann Thorac Surg 1993;56:137–141.
552. de Haan J, Schonberger J, Haan J, van Oeveren W. Tissue-type plasminogen activator and fibrin monomers synergistically cause platelet dysfunction during retransfusion of shed blood after cardiopulmonary bypass. J Thorac Cardiovasc Surg 1993;106:1017–1023.
553. Griffith LD, Billman GF, Daily PO, Lane TA. Apparent coagulopathy caused by infusion of shed mediastinal blood and its prevention by washing of the infusate. Ann Thorac Surg 1989;47:400–406.
554. Adoumie R, Lockananthan R, Yen A, Chiu R-J. Character of shed blood in cardiac and thoracic surgery patients: implications for reinfusion. Can J Surg 1994;37:203–207.
555. Kongsgaard UE, Tollofsrud S, Brosstad F, Ovrum E, Bjornskau L. Autotransfusion after open heart surgery: characteristics of shed mediastinal blood and its influence on the plasma proteases in circulating blood. Acta Anaesthesiol Scand 1991;35:71–76.
556. Hartz RS, Smith JA, Green D. Autotransfusion after cardiac operation. J Thorac Cardiovasc Surg 1988;96:178–182.
557. Body S, Parks R, Ley C, et al. for the McSPI Research Group. Safety and efficacy of autotransfusion Efficacy of re-transfusion of shed mediastinal blood after CABG surgery: a multi-institutional analysis. Anesthesiology 1994;81:A1245.
558. Kongsgaard UE, Hovig T, Brosstad F, Geiran O. Platelets in shed mediastinal blood used for postoperative autotransfusion. Acta Anaesthesiol Scand 1993;37:265–268.
559. Markovitz M, Smith P, Brown M, Bloom R, Mammen E. Hemostasis markers in cardiac surgery patients following postoperative autotransfusion. Anesth Analg 1988;67:S140.
560. de Haan J, Boonstra P, Monnink S, Ebels T, van Oeveren W. Retransfusion of suctioned blood during cardiopulmonary bypass impairs hemostasis. Ann Thorac Surg 1995;59:901–907.
561. Salas J, Munoz M, Peran S, Negri S, de Vega N. Autotransfusion of shed mediastinal blood after cardiac operations. Ann Thorac Surg 1995;59:257–258.
562. Bland LA, Villarino ME, Ardunino MJ, et al. Bacteriologic and endotoxin analysis of salvaged blood used in autologous transfusions during cardiac operations. J Thorac Cardiovasc Surg 1992;103:582–588.
563. Schwieger IM, Gallagher CJ, Finlayson DC, Daly WL, Maher KL. Incidence of cell-saver contamination during cardiopulmonary bypass. Ann Thorac Surg 1989;48:51–53.
564. Solem JO, Steen S, Tengborn L, Lindgren S, Olin C. Mediastinal drainage blood. Potentialities for autotransfusion after cardiac surgery. Scand J Thorac Cardiovasc Surg 1987;21:149–152.
565. Thurer RL, Popovski MA, Johnson RG. Shed mediastinal blood transfusion in open heart surgery [letter]. Lancet 1991;338:1078–1079.
566. De Paulis R, Bassano C, Ricci A, Actis DG. Enzyme levels in shed blood after cardiac operations. Ann Thorac Surg 1993;56:1001–1003.
567. Hannes W, Keilich M, Koster W, Seitelberger R, Fasol R. Shed blood autotransfusion influences ischemia-sensitive laboratory parameters after coronary operations. Ann Thorac Surg 1994;57:1289–1294.
568. Wahl GW, Feins RH, Alfieres G, Bixby K. Reinfusion of shed blood after coronary operation causes elevation of cardiac enzyme levels. Ann Thorac Surg 1992;53:625–627.
569. Schwartz A, Howie M. Case conference. J Cardiothorac Anesth 1987; 1:577–583.
570. Malik M, Collins J, Ludorf M, et al. Laboratory confirmation of heparin-associated thrombocytopenia (HAT) [abstract]. Blood 1989; 74:11a.
571. Ortel T, Gockermann J, Califf R, McCann R, Greenberg C. Anticoagulant therapy with heparinoid (ORG 10172) in patients with heparin associated thrombocytopenia (HAT) and thrombosis (HATT) [abstract]. Blood 1989;74:136a.
572. Harenberg J, Zimmermann R, Schwarz R, Kubler W. Treatment of heparin-induced thrombocytopenia with thrombosis by new heparinoid. Lancet 1983;1:986–987.
573. Palmer Smith J, Walls J, Muscato M, et al. Extracorporeal circulation in a patient with heparin induced thrombocytopenia. Anesthesiology 1985;62:363–365.
574. Zulys V, Teadale S, Michel E, Skala R, Glynn M. Ancrod anticoagulation for cardiopulmonary bypass [abstract]. Clin Invest Med 1987; 10:C44a.
575. Cole C, Bormanis J. Ancrod: a practical alternative to heparin. J Vasc Surg 1988;8:59–63.
576. Antman E. Medical management of the patient undergoing cardiac surgery. In: Braunwald E, ed. Heart disease. A textbook of cardiovascular medicine. Philadelphia: WB Saunders, 1992:1670–1693.
577. Warren J, Ward P, Johnson K. The inflammatory response. In: Williams WJ, Beutler E, Erslev AJ, Lichtman MA, eds. Hematology. New York: McGraw-Hall, 1990:63–70.
578. Sladen R, Berkowitz D. Cardiopulmonary bypass and the lung. In: Gravlee G, Davis R, Utley J, eds. Cardiopulmonary bypass: principles and practice. Baltimore: Williams & Wilkins, 1993:468–487.
579. Moss G, DeWoskin R, Rosen A, Levine H, Palani C. Transport of oxygen and carbon dioxide by hemoglobin-saline solution in the red-cell free primate. Surg Gynecol Obstet 1976;142:357–362.

Chapter 29

Blood Utilization in Major Peripheral Vascular Surgery

KAJ JOHANSEN

INTRODUCTION

Most surgical operations risk blood loss and therefore warrant consideration of prudent blood utilization. In a majority of such settings, however, unexpected or excessive blood loss results from an accident or a technical maneuver gone awry. Only in cardiovascular surgery—reconstructive procedures of the heart and the great vessels—are the pump and the conduits for the body's circulating blood deliberately opened, bypassed, sutured, ligated, patched, or otherwise manipulated. In such cases, the potential for substantial blood loss is always understood, anticipated, and, upon occasion, even accepted.

Blood resource management during cardiac surgery is specifically discussed in Chapter 30: numerous pre-, intra-, and postoperative tools and tactics for appropriate blood management are detailed there and in other chapters. This chapter describes safe, prudent, and cost-effective strategies for blood management in patients undergoing major peripheral vascular surgery. The interested reader is referred to several recent publications relevant to blood utilization strategies in the vascular surgical setting (1–3).

THE VASCULAR SURGICAL PATIENT

Most vascular surgical patients are elderly. Aged chronologically or at least physiologically (or both), they are commonly also debilitated and harbor advanced generalized atherosclerosis. Because such "vasculopaths" are presumed to be at high risk for coronary artery disease and its attendant complications (e.g., myocardial infarction, cardiac arrhythmias, sudden death, congestive heart failure), usual physiological compensatory mechanisms and "margins of error" may be less available or even absent. Such patients may be less likely to tolerate many exigencies of major vascular surgery such as significant and persistent blood loss, massive transfusion, acidosis, tissue ischemia, hypothermia, and prolonged administration of anesthetics and various vasoactive medications. Such patients may also have other significant comorbidities, such as chronic obstructive pulmonary disease, cancer, malnutrition, diabetes, and hypertension. Their capacity to tolerate hypotension, hypovolemia, or a reduced oxygen-carrying capacity is accordingly diminished.

Most elderly patients today receive multiple medications that may have a direct impact on elements of the blood or on cardiovascular compensatory mechanisms. Commonly administered, for example, is aspirin, which has demonstrable beneficial effects for the prevention (or treatment) of cardiac disease, transient ischemic cerebrovascular ischemic attacks, or arthritis (4). However, virtually all such patients will also consequently have diminished platelet function, prolonged bleeding times, and increased risks of perioperative bleeding and wound hematomas.

TYPES OF VASCULAR OPERATIONS

Although the scope of vascular reconstructive surgery sometimes seems bound only by the patient's anatomy, the surgeon's imagination, and the limits of optical magnification, in reality, elective peripheral vascular surgery can be divided, for the purposes of a discussion about blood utilization, into three types: reconstruction of the aorta and its primary branches, either for aneurysm or for atherosclerosis; arterial reconstruction in the neck and upper and lower extremities, almost always for atherosclerotic arterial occlusive disease; and thromboembolectomy, the management of vascular trauma, and other miscellaneous vascular procedures performed primarily in nonatherosclerotic patients. As is demonstrated, such a division of vascular reconstructive procedures by anatomic site and, in part, by the general status of the patients undergoing a given operation permits accurate and cost-effective blood utilization planning. It will distinguish between patients at substantial risk of major blood loss (or of suffering the physiological consequences of major hemorrhage) and those whose risk is less significant or negligible.

SURGERY OF THE AORTA AND ITS MAJOR BRANCH VESSELS

Surgical reconstruction of the aorta or its major brachycephalic or visceral branches is associated with the greatest blood utilization implications among the various forms of vascular surgery. This is not only because of the obvious risk of profuse and difficult-to-control hemorrhage typified by such operative procedures, but also because many of these patients' coronary and myocardial comorbidity makes them intolerant of even moderate hemorrhage. Accordingly, preoperative blood planning in such patients must be liberal, and the transfusion threshold may be met at higher hemoglobin or hematocrit levels or lesser amounts of blood lost.

Two major types of aortic reconstruction occur: those directed toward the management of *aneurysms* and those designed to reconstruct *atherosclerotic aortic occlusive disease*. Liberal blood utilization planning is prudent in these two types of patients, but for different reasons.

Elective aortic aneurysm repair has become relatively predictable and safe, primarily because these patients' anesthetic and surgical risks are relatively low. A burgeoning recognition has developed that such patients' advanced age (mean 70 years) notwithstanding, they are frequently quite healthy. For example, although aortic aneurysm patients, because of their age and other risk factors, might be presumed to be at risk for the presence of significant atherosclerotic coronary artery disease (5), operative mortality for elective abdominal aortic aneurysm repair is well under 5% (6), even in octogenarians (7). Aneurysm patients are unlikely to have a prior or subsequent history of symptomatic coronary artery disease (8–10). On an actuarial basis, an aortic aneurysm is the leading mortality risk for the patient who has one, and successful repair of an aneurysm returns such patients to the survival curve of an age-matched nonaneurysmal population (6). These facts underscore the basically favorable physiological status of abdominal aortic aneurysm patients, their relatively well-preserved compensatory hemodynamic mechanisms, and their ability to withstand moderately significant hemorrhagic insults.

On the other hand, patients with atherosclerotic aortic occlusive disease, although much younger (mean age 50–60 years), have a significant likelihood of concurrent accelerated coronary atherosclerosis: more than 90% will have a prior or subsequent history of myocardial infarction or a cardiac intervention (9). Accordingly, patients undergoing operation for aortoiliac atherosclerosis are at highest risk for intraoperative complications; their elevated risk of major bleeding and their diminished ability to tolerate sudden hypotension, hypovolemia, or anemia makes their margin for error less and thoughtful blood planning crucial.

Patients undergoing reconstructive procedures on primary branches of the aorta—the brachycephalic arteries, the celiac, mesenteric, and renal vessels or the common iliac arteries—require equivalently close attention to blood planning, because of their combined risks of sudden major hemorrhage and their diminished physiological tolerance to hypotension, hypovolemia, and diminished oxygen-carrying capacity. These patients' intolerance to blood loss is made more significant by the fact that such patients are usually about 10 years older than those undergoing operation for aortoiliac atherosclerosis.

ARTERIAL RECONSTRUCTIVE PROCEDURES OF THE NECK AND EXTREMITIES

Most peripheral arterial reconstructive procedures involve endarterectomy of the extracranial carotid artery or the insertion of bypass grafts, using vein or synthetic material, from the femoral artery at the groin to the popliteal or the tibial arteries. Blood planning should generally be more straightforward and parsimonious for elective reconstruction at these sites. This results from the fact that although such patients are generally elderly and have a high risk of harboring significant coronary atherosclerosis (11), nonetheless their operative wounds are smaller, the major body cavities are not entered, and the likelihood of significant blood loss is low. For example, I have not had to perform an intraoperative or early postoperative transfusion for blood loss in a patient undergoing infrainguinal bypass or carotid artery reconstruction for more than a decade.

MISCELLANEOUS VASCULAR PROCEDURES

A variety of surgical patients undergoing elective or emergency vascular procedures may incur a substantial risk from unexpectedly profuse blood loss. For example, significant hemorrhage may ensue during thrombectomy procedures intended to relieve acute occlusion of dialysis access grafts. Such operations are unfortunately not uncommonly performed as relatively unplanned procedures at the end of the day, often by junior trainees, and their risk for significant blood loss is too often minimized. Because these patients are by definition significantly physiologically comprised, their tolerance for such blood loss may be low, and an early "transfusion trigger" (12) may be involved.

At even greater risk from unexpected blood loss are patients undergoing operation for arterial embolus, usually to an extremity artery. More than 90% of these emboli arise from the heart, predominantly due to prior myocardial infarctions with resulting areas of left ventricular mural thrombosis. Because such patients often have active ongoing cardiac failure or arrhythmias, even relatively minor thromboembolectomy operations accompanied by only moderate blood loss are fraught with risk, with operative mortality rates in some series approaching 20% (13). Nonoperative therapies such as systemic heparinization (14) or transcatheter infusion of thrombolytic agents (15) have been proposed as safer and equivalently effective alternative approaches to the acutely ischemic extremity.

Trauma victims requiring vascular repair are generally young and healthy and have a substantial capacity to withstand even prodigious blood loss and shock. However, the cumulative effects of massive transfusion and crystalloid infusion, prolonged anesthetic administration, and hypothermia can ultimately nullify this physiological advantage (see Chapters 23 and 24).

The blood use implications of operations for patients with cirrhosis and portal hypertension, usually portal decompressive shunts, hepatic resection, or orthotopic liver transplantation (see Chapter 30), are legendary. Not only do such patients have a significant risk of intraoperative blood loss due to the nature of the operations themselves, but bleeding frequently continues inexorably because of cirrhotic patients' low platelet counts and hypoprothrombinemia.

BLOOD UTILIZATION STRATEGIES IN MAJOR VASCULAR SURGERY

As noted elsewhere, blood utilization strategies are properly directed toward the goals of patient safety and conservation of a scarce medical and societal resource. In addition, conservative blood use will reserve administration of particular components of blood to those specific clinical scenarios for which they are most appropriate, thereby limiting the risks of blood exposure assumed by both those receiving blood and those administering it.

Blood should be drawn preoperatively for typing and cross matching in a fashion appropriate to the surgeon's expectation of a rapid need for blood intraoperatively. This decision relates not only to the nature of the operation itself (as noted above, an aortic operation is much more likely to require blood than a carotid endarterectomy or a femoral-popliteal bypass graft), but also, importantly, should be based on the surgeon's assessment of this particular patient. Factors such as whether the procedure is reoperative or the patient has a known coagulopathy and how important it may be to maintain an adequate oxygen-carrying capacity all play a role in this judgment.

Further, just as every vascular surgeon should know his or her outcomes for commonly performed procedures (e.g., stroke and death rate with carotid endarterectomy or mortality after abdominal aneurysm repair), so too should he or she be able to accurately predict the likelihood of blood loss associated with various common procedures. For example, among my carotid surgery patients, none has required transfusion in 15 years, but every other aortic reconstruction patient has required 2 units of transfused blood in the perioperative period in the past 5 years. Such knowledge permits simultaneously safe and cost-effective blood-ordering strategies in the perioperative period.

PREOPERATIVE SURGICAL PLANNING

Most reconstructive vascular operations can be performed electively, which means that an effective assessment of bleeding risk and the need for perioperative blood replacement can be accomplished (Fig. 29.1). History can be very useful, if sought. A recent patient scheduled for aortic aneurysm repair revealed that two different hip operations 20 years previously had required multiple transfusions, a history that resulted in the diagnosis of his previously undocumented von Willebrand disease.

Most vascular patients will have been chronically treated with aspirin (4), and the antiplatelet effect of this agent may have an impact on blood loss at the time of vascular reconstruction. Some such patients may be anticoagulated chronically, for example, for atrial arrhythmias, whereas others may receive nonsteroidal anti-inflammatory agents for arthritis or other chronic conditions and thus be at increased risk of perioperative bleeding (16).

In the absence of a well-documented bleeding history, diagnostic tests can be relatively limited. Assessment of a hemogram is appropriate; hospital charges are relatively low ($36 inpatient charges at my institution), and documentation of the hematocrit (sometimes elevated because of some vascular patients' chronic obstructive pulmonary disease) and

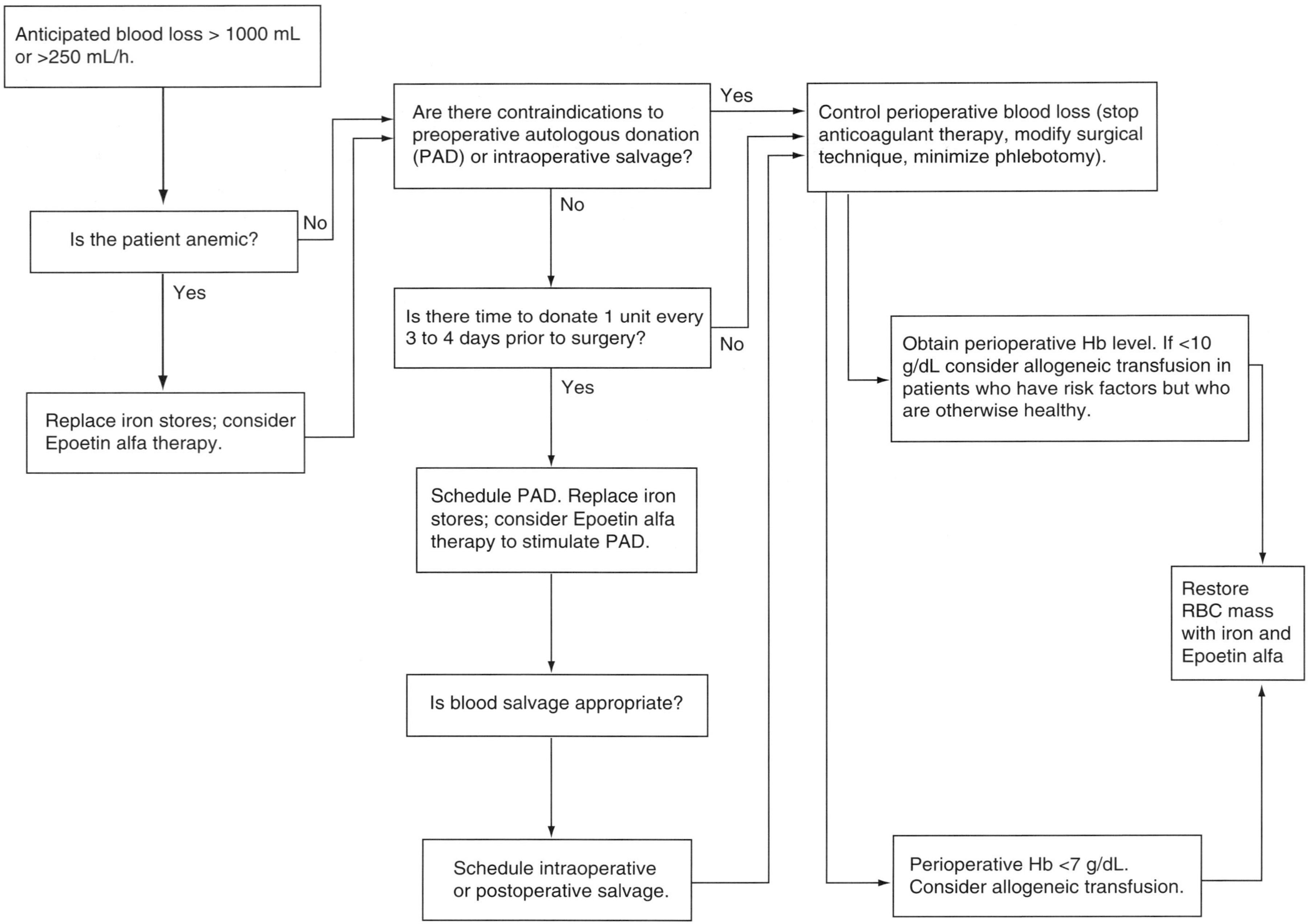

Figure 29.1. A blood utilization algorithm. (Reprinted with permission from Spence RK. Blood Management Practice Guidelines Conference. Surgical red blood cell transfusion policies. Am J Surg 1995;170 (Suppl.):3S–15S, copyright 1995 by Excerpta Medica Inc.

the platelet count can be useful baseline values. The assessment of the coagulation status—measurement of the prothrombin time or International Normalized Ratio and the partial thromboplastin time—is probably *not* warranted in the absence of a history of easy bleeding or unusually extensive blood loss at the time of prior operations (17). Assessment of bleeding time as a test of platelet function is not cost-effective in the absence of clinical indications (18).

For elective vascular procedures in those circumstances where preoperative autologous donation (19,20) seems warranted, either because of patient request, difficulty with cross matching, or concerns about alloimmunization, time is generally available for this to be carried out. As noted later, attractive though the concept of preoperative autologous donation seems, decision analysis has raised significant questions about its actual cost-effectiveness (21).

A history of reconstructive procedures *is* crucial; a decision regarding reoperative surgery, with its risk of excessive blood loss, versus an alternative reconstructive approach involves solution of an important equation relating the implications of reoperative surgery against the comparative long-term efficacies of the alternative operation. For example, after failure of an aortofemoral bypass graft, the surgeon must weigh the relative risks and benefits of a "redo" aortic reconstruction versus the technical ease but lesser patency of an extra-anatomic axillofemoral bypass graft.

ANESTHETIC PLANNING

Numerous variables govern the choice of anesthetic technique for major vascular procedures, including the nature of the operation, the patient's underlying cardiopulmonary and metabolic status, available expertise, and physician and patient preference. Regarding blood utilization, anesthetic planning will be affected by the patient's apparent tolerance for significant hemorrhage and the likelihood that major bleeding will occur (certain operations, and certain surgeons, are known to be associated with a higher risk of blood loss).

It has become clear that anesthetic technique may affect amount and rate of intraoperative hemorrhage. For example, several different types of operations involving hip reconstruction or other operations related to the lower torso or pelvis performed under regional anesthesia are associated with a significantly lower blood loss than the same operations performed under a general anesthetic (22–24). The physiological basis for this blood-conserving effect of spinal or epidural anesthesia is not precisely clear but may relate to the lower mean arterial pressure and greater venous compartmentalization of blood that results from conduction anesthetic techniques.

Although the blood-conserving effect of spinal and epidural anesthesia has been noted for radical prostatectomy (22), total hip replacement (23), and major scoliosis surgery (24), comparative studies in patients undergoing aortic reconstruction have shown at best only trends toward less blood loss in patients whose operations are performed under continuous spinal or epidural anesthesia (25). On the other hand, conduction anesthesia appears to be associated with a significantly reduced likelihood of early peripheral bypass graft occlusion when compared with general anesthesia (26).

Theoretically, an increased risk of epidural or subarachnoid bleeding with potentially catastrophic spinal or peripheral neurological complications might accompany conduction anesthetic techniques in vascular patients who will virtually always be anticoagulated intraoperatively. However, retrospective and prospective series have been reassuring; no increased risk of epidural hematoma, intradural bleeding, or neurological complication has been demonstrated in vascular surgical patients undergoing spinal or epidural anesthesia (27), even when fully anticoagulated preoperatively (28).

As intimated previously, preoperative autologous blood donation may be neither cost-effective nor safe in peripheral vascular surgical patients, most of whom must be presumed to have significant underlying coronary artery disease (4, 11). In certain settings, however, where a planned large and potentially complex vascular reconstructive procedure is contemplated, careful preoperative donation of 1–2 units of blood, combined with administration of iron (29) or erythropoietin (30, 31), may be useful (19, 20, 31). Alternatively, in patients in whom an acute reduction in hematocrit to 20–22 can be tolerated, immediate preoperative isovolumic hemodilution via rapid withdrawal of 2–3 units of blood, maintaining normal volume by simultaneous administration of crystalloid, fresh-frozen plasma, or hetastarch, may provide a highly useful source of fresh autologous blood available later in the operation (32, 33). This technique has not commonly been used in peripheral vascular surgical patients.

INTRAOPERATIVE BLOOD CONSERVATION AND UTILIZATION

By far the most important aspect of prudent blood utilization is proper surgical planning, that is, maximizing the chances of avoiding unanticipated bleeding by minimizing the risk of technical misadventure. Attendant important issues include assurance of the availability of adequate surgical and anesthetic expertise and availability of appropriate equipment (e.g., autotransfusion devices and personnel knowledgeable in their function) and adequate blood bank capabilities. Although intraoperative accidents by definition cannot be anticipated, the likelihood of their occurrence can be minimized by thoughtful conservative preoperative planning. Repetitive consideration of solutions to the question, "what is the worst possible thing that could happen in this setting?" can be lifesaving by permitting establishment of effective and redundant safety systems to be used during the perioperative period.

Appropriate large-bore venous access catheters should be inserted using the "n + 1" principe (n is the minimum safe number of sites of venous access). Appropriate cardiovascular monitoring lines (arterial pressure measuring catheters, central venous pressure, or pulmonary artery catheters) should be placed, keeping in mind the implications of the proposed operation (e.g., avoiding placement of an arterial pressure-monitoring catheter in the radial artery ipsilateral to the axillary artery anastomosis for an axillofemoral bypass graft).

Patient positioning may be relevant to planning for blood loss. Neck operations (e.g., carotid endarterectomy) should be performed in a reverse Trendelenburg position because venous bleeding is less in this position. Similarly, operations on lower extremity veins (which may result in a substantial blood loss) are most safely performed with the legs elevated 30 degrees from the horizontal, once again diminishing venous pressure at the operative site(s).

Although data are conflicting (26, 34–36) as to whether blood loss is mitigated with extraperitoneal compared with transperitoneal exposure of the abdominal aorta, I am strongly convinced by the published evidence for the general physiological benefit of the former approach (25, 34–36) and perform almost all aortic reconstructions through a left retroperitoneal incision. Most studies have suggested less blood loss (although somewhat greater crystalloid replacement) in patients undergoing a retroperitoneal approach for aortic reconstruction. This form of exposure appears to result in a more rapid resumption of gastrointestinal function, fewer postoperative pulmonary complications, and a shorter length of stay than equivalent operations performed through a transperitoneal approach (34–36).

A number of other technical strategies can have a major impact on intraoperative blood loss. For example, failure to obtain adequate exposure for clamp placement proximal to an arteriotomy site threatens uncontrollable hemorrhage if a technical accident occurs. On the other hand, injudicious dissection in anatomically remote sites may risk disruption of nearby large veins (e.g., around the common iliac arteries or in the "tunnel" beneath the inguinal ligament proximal to a femoral artery exposure). Failure to recall that knitted Dacron grafts must be preclotted before systemic heparinization may result in massive bleeding through the interstices of the graft and require emergency replacement with a woven Dacron or expanded Teflon graft.

Hemostatic techniques during and at the end of a vascular reconstructive procedure are a crucial aspect of blood conservation; in addition, they play a major role in the outcome of the early postoperative course. As noted, strategies for obtaining proximal and distal vascular control should be neither too miserly nor overly aggressive; the principle that "the enemy of good is perfect" should be kept in mind. On occasion, the use of balloon catheters (e.g., placed antegrade into the iliac artery orifices during aortic aneurysm repair) may completely eliminate the need for dissection and clamp placement. In certain clinical settings, in the extremities, the use of a sterile proximal tourniquet or Esmarch bandage may obviate the proximal and distal dissection for vascular control (37).

Hemostasis after completion of vascular anastomoses is predominantly technique and material dependent. For example, large vascular suture needles result in more anastomotic bleeding than small ones; suture holes in expanded Teflon bleed more than those in an autogenous artery or vein patch or in Dacron. Clearing an arteriotomy of adherent adventitia or of underlying atherosclerotic plaque may permit better apposition of graft and native vessel. Taking a few minutes to remove adherent atheromatous intima from the inner surface of an aortic aneurysm permits a more accurate suturing of back-bleeding lumbar arteries.

The vascular surgeon straddles the "knife edge" between thrombosis of the native vessel during clamping and vascular reconstruction and uncontrolled bleeding after restoration of flow. Virtually all vascular patients are anticoagulated with heparin during the period of vessel reconstruction or graft insertion, usually at doses between 50 and 100 mg/kg body weight. Bleeding tendency does not appear to be correlated with residual heparin, and although cardiac surgeons routinely use protamine to reverse heparin's effect, I (and numerous other peripheral vascular surgeons [38]) only infrequently administer this agent. This is due not only to the thrombogenic nature of the protamine-heparin complex (use of protamine results in a significantly higher risk of stroke after carotid endarterectomy [39]) but also to the rare but unpredictable (and occasionally catastrophic) hypotension that can accompany protamine administration (38, 40).

Instead, vascular hemostasis can generally be obtained by topical and local techniques. Gelfoam soaked in thrombin is placed liberally over fresh vascular suture lines; fine hemostatic sutures coapt adventitia only at bleeding sites, and diffuse bleeding is controlled by tamponade pressure with gauze pads or with surrounding soft tissues. Large bleeding surfaces are problematic, and devices such as the argon laser coagulator are demonstrably useful in such settings (41). Fibrin glue is touted as a safe and useful topical hemostatic agent (42); it is not currently commercially available in the United States (although it can be produced de novo at the operating table by combining thrombin and albumin [43]).

Drains are mandatory in most cardiothoracic operations, primarily to provide a monitor of early postoperative bleeding; because mediastinal bleeding persists in part due to defibrination of shed blood, chest tube drainage can be an accurate indicator of blood loss (and even a source of postoperative autologous blood [44]). In contrast, drains are virtually never helpful in peripheral vascular operations; they do not prevent hematoma formation, rarely provide an accurate assessment of blood loss, and theoretically act as an entrée for exogenous bacterial contamination of prosthetic grafts or the wound itself.

Autotransfusion devices have become routine in the performance of aortoiliac reconstruction; they clearly have diminished the need for allogeneic blood administration in these patients, with a concomitant reduction in patient risk and cost (44–46). In my practice, the Cell-Saver autotransfuser (Haemonetics, Braintree MA) is used in all aortic reconstructive cases (see Chapter 23), initially as a suction device; calculations have demonstrated that actual processing and reinfusion of shed blood with the autotransfusion device is cost-effective once total blood volume aspirated into the reservoir exceeds 1000 mL. Blood is not automatically returned to the patient as soon as it is processed; it may be processed, stored, and reinfused postoperatively if the patient's volume status and oxygen-carrying capacity remains adequate intraoperatively (44).

Several more specialized strategies for diminishing perioperative blood loss may be contemplated, although they have only occasionally been used in peripheral vascular surgery. These include the administration of agents such as epsilon-aminocaproic acid (47), desmopressin (48), tranexamic acid (49), or aprotinin (50, 51), discussed in detail in other chapters. Concerns that the use of such agents might diminish early patency of peripheral or coronary artery bypass grafts are controversial (51, 52).

Perhaps the most straightforward hemostatic maneuver is the readministration of fresh autologous blood (and the platelets and clotting factors contained therein) drawn and stored preoperatively (19, 20) or at the time of isovolumic hemodilution (32, 33) at the beginning of the procedure (see above). Administration of platelet-rich plasma made available by use of devices such as the Plasma-Saver (Haemonetics) plasmapheresis device may be indicated (53), although it may not always significantly assist in hemostasis (54).

Intraoperative transfusion strategies are similar to those in cardiac surgical patients, with replacement of blood (usually by transfusion of packed red blood cells) in patients with known or suspected cardiac disease whose serum hemoglobin level has fallen below 10 mg% (12). On the other hand, hemoglobin levels in healthy younger patients have frequently been permitted to fall to as low as 5 mg% in the absence of hypotension or hypoxemia, a practice demonstrated to be safe in the "natural experiment" provided by observations of the physiological consequences of major blood loss in Jehovah's Witness patients (55).

Persistent intraoperative bleeding for nontechnical reasons (i.e., due to intrinsic or acutely acquired coagulopathies) thankfully are rare in major vascular surgical patients. Frequently exacerbated by hypothermia (56, 57) and acidosis (57), such coagulopathies are difficult to reverse. Techniques found useful in trauma surgery—packing, temporary wound closure, and transfer to the intensive care unit for warming and metabolic resuscitation—may be life-saving (58). The most common acquired cause of persistent nontechnical bleeding is dilutional thrombocytopenia after multiple blood transfusions to treat major intraoperative blood loss (59). Other more rare causes of intraoperative coagulopathy include major transfusion reactions (60), heparin-induced thrombosis and thrombocytopenia (61), and true disseminated intravascular coagulation (62), usually confined to critically ill patients with massive tissue infarction or sepsis.

EARLY POSTOPERATIVE BLOOD ADMINISTRATION

RESPONDING TO MASSIVE BLOOD LOSS

For reasons previously mentioned, vascular patients may suffer sudden massive hemorrhage, usually because of a technical misadventure. In other circumstances, rupture of an abdominal aortic aneurysm or major vascular trauma confronts the surgeon with the need simultaneously to halt bleeding, repair the vascular defect, and restore blood volume. The implications of massive transfusion are discussed in Chapters 23, 24, and 30, and need not be repeated in detail. Suffice it to say that especially in elderly ruptured aneurysm patients, or even in the younger trauma victim who has already incurred a substantial blood volume replacement, issues of dilution, tissue ischemia, hypothermia, red-cell damage, and acidosis may result in a refractory coagulopathy that renders both homeostasis and hemostasis impossible. In an extensive experience with ruptured abdominal aortic aneurysm (63), my surgical and anesthesiological colleagues and I have aggressively promoted trauma center blood utilization techniques—administration of type-specific blood and use of the autotransfuser (64), the rapid-infusion device (65), and the in-line intravenous fluid warmer (66)—in the management of massive bleeding in this complex patient population. By so doing, survival in hypotensive ruptured aortic aneurysm patients, generally less than 10%, has been trebled (63).

Certain strategies used to make vascular reconstruction optimal may have an impact on perioperative blood utilization. For example, perioperative administration of dextran-40 has been demonstrated to provide a statistically significant improvement in early infrainguinal graft patency (67), presumably by virtue of its antiplatelet effect (although aspirin does not appear to confer a similar patency advantage [68]). An interesting consequence of the routine use of dextran in patients undergoing femoral-popliteal or femoral-distal bypass is that many such patients will postoperatively demonstrate a significant reduction in hematocrit, even though intraoperative blood loss has been negligible. This postoperative anemia is caused, of course, by another effect of dextran, the volume-expanding properties that were the basis for its original development (69). (It is this temporary postoperative anemia that leads to occasional postoperative packed red cell transfusion in my infrainguinal bypass patients, as noted above.)

Similarly, recent evidence suggests that the use of low-molecular-weight heparin (70) or warfarin (71) may provide a similar patency advantage to infrainguinal bypass grafts; in each setting, of course, a somewhat increased risk of postoperative bleeding might be anticipated.

WHEN TO TRANSFUSE THE VASCULAR SURGICAL PATIENT

Perhaps no population exemplifies the implications, both positive and negative, of attention to sagacious blood utilization planning than the peripheral vascular surgical patient. Because virtually all must be presumed to have significant coronary artery disease and therefore to be intolerant of significant reductions in oxygen-carrying capacity, the "transfusion trigger" is frequently invoked earlier or at higher hematocrits than in other patient populations (12). Similarly, by virtue of this same anticipated myocardial and coronary insufficiency, such patients may be significantly less able to withstand the sometimes major metabolic consequences and shifts in oxygen-carrying capacity that may result from major transfusion.

Sensible practice guidelines for prudent blood and blood product utilization have resulted from a recent National Institutes of Health Consensus Conference (72). The value of these guidelines arises from the fact that they have been derived from seminal basic physiological studies (73–75). These studies, and others, demonstrate that the previous generally held transfusion threshold of a serum hemoglobin concentration equaling 10 mg% may be appropriate for patients with active cardiac disease (angina pectoris, recent myocardial infarction, congestive heart failure) undergoing most surgical procedures (other than cardiopulmonary bypass). On the other hand, data and clinical experience have clearly demonstrated that patients without active coronary artery disease need not be transfused until hemoglobin levels fall below 8 or even 7; iron replacement, the administration of erythropoietin, and assurance of adequate nutrition may be an appropriate substitute for homologous blood transfusion in many such cases.

A useful algorithm has been developed for blood utilization in peripheral arterial surgery patients (76) (Fig. 29.1). The algorithm uses the three major alternatives to allogeneic blood transfusion—preoperative autologous donation, immediate preoperative isovolumic hemodilution, and intraoperative autotransfusion—and introduces the concept of the maximum surgical blood-ordering schedule (MSBOS). The MSBOS, itself an algorithm used by blood bank personnel to facilitate cross match and storage efficiency, is based on serial institutional reviews of ratios of cross matched to transfused units for given procedures and surgeons (76–78).

Although each surgeon, in concert with his or her colleagues and institution(s), should modify this protocol to fit local circumstances, attention to such a plan should maximize patient safety and institutional cost-effectiveness by reducing to a minimum homologous blood transfused and autologous predonated blood wasted. A randomized trial has suggested that a directed continuing medical education approach to parsimonious blood utilization can significantly improve physician behavior regarding this important medical and societal resource (79).

REFERENCES

1. Spence RK. Transfusion practices in vascular surgery. Perspec Vasc Surg 1993;6:14–48.
2. Tawes RL, Spence RK. Blood transfusion and the vascular surgeon. Semin Vasc Surg 1994;7:65–130.
3. Spence RK. Consensus conference. Blood management: surgical practice guidelines. Am J Surg 1995;178(Suppl. 6A):1S–73S.
4. Stein B, Fuster V, Israel DH, et al. Platelet inhibitor agents in cardiovascular disease: an update. J Am Coll Cardiol 1989;14:813–836.
5. Hertzer NR, Young JR, Beven EG, et al. Late results of coronary bypass in patients with infrarenal aortic aneurysms. Am Surg 1987;205: 360–368.
6. Rutherford RB. Infrarenal abdominal aortic aneurysms. In: Rutherford RB, ed. Vascular surgery. 4th ed. Philadelphia: WB Saunders, 1995.
7. Harris KA, Ameli FM, Lally M, et al. Abdominal aortic aneurysm resection in patients more than 80-years old. Surg Gynecol Obstet 1986;162: 536–542.
8. Roger VL, Ballard DJ, Hallett JW, et al. Influence of coronary artery disease on morbidity and mortality after abdominal aortic aneurysmectomy: a population-based study 1971–1987. J Am Coll Cardiol 1989;14: 1245–1250.

9. Tilson DM, Stansel HC. Differences in results for aneurysms vs. occlusive disease after bifurcation grafts: the results of a hundred elective grafts. Arch Surg 1980;107:1173–1180.
10. Golden MA, Whittemore AD, Donaldson MC, et al. Selective evaluation and management of coronary artery disease in patients undergoing repair of abdominal aortic aneurysm. Ann Surg 1990;212:415–421.
11. Hertzer NR, Beven EG, Young JR, et al. Coronary artery disease in peripheral vascular patients: a classification of 1,000 coronary angiograms and results of surgical management. Ann Surg 1984;199:223–233.
12. Spence RK, Carson JA. Transfusion decision-making in vascular surgery: blood ordering schedules and the transfusion trigger. Semin Vasc Surg 1994;7:76–81.
13. Tawes RL, Harris EJ, Brown WH. Arterial thromboembolism: a twenty year perspective. Arch Surg 1985;120:595–599.
14. Blaisdell FW, Steele M, Allen RE. Management of acute lower extremity arterial ischemia due to embolism and thrombosis. Surgery 1978;84:822–834.
15. MacNamara TO, Bomberger RA, Merchant RF. Intraarterial urokinase as the initial therapy for acutely ischemic lower limbs. Circulation 1991;83(Suppl. 1):I106-I119.
16. Schafer AI. Effects of non-steroidal inflammatory drugs on platelet function and systemic hemostasis [review]. J Clin Pharmacol 1995;35: 209–219.
17. Erban S, Kinman J, Schwartz J. Routine use of the prothrombin and partial thromboplastin times. JAMA 1989;263:2428–2432.
18. Rodgers RPC. A critical reappraisal of the bleeding time. Semin Thromb Hemost 1990;16:1–20.
19. Chambers LA, Kruskall MS. Preoperative autologous blood donation. Transfus Med Rev 1990;4:35–46.
20. Spiess BD, Sassetti R, McCarthy RJ, et al. Autologous blood donation: hemodynamics in a high-risk population. Transfusion 1992;32:17–22.
21. Etchason J, Petz L, Keeler E, et al. The cost effectiveness of postoperative autologous blood donation. N Engl J Med 1995;32:719–724.
22. Shir Y, Raja SN, Frank SM, Brendler CB. Intraoperative blood loss during radical retropubic prostatectomy: epidural versus general anesthesia. Urology 1995;45:993–999.
23. Sharrock NE, Mineo R, Urquhart B, Salvati EA. The effect of two levels of hypotension on intraoperative blood loss during total hip arthroplasty performed under lumbar epidural anesthesia. Anesth Analg 1993;76:580–584.
24. Brodsky JW, Dickson JH, Erwin WD, Rossic D. Hypotensive anesthesia for scoliosis surgery in Jehovah's Witnesses. Spine 1991;16: 3044–3306.
25. Cambria RP, Brewster DC, Abbott WM, et al. Transperitoneal versus retroperitoneal approach for aortic reconstruction: a randomized prospective study. J Vasc Surg 1990;11:314–320.
26. Christopherson R, Beattie C, Frank SM, et al. Perioperative morbidity in patients randomized to epidural or general anesthesia for lower extremity vascular surgery. Anesthesiology 1993;79:422–434.
27. Baron HC, LaRaja RD, Rossi G, Atkinson D. Continuous epidural analgesia in the heparinized vascular surgical patient: a retrospective review of 912 patients. J Vasc Surg 1987;6:144–146.
28. Odoom JA, Sih IL. Epidural analgesia and anticoagulant therapy. Anesthesia 1983;38:254–259.
29. Burns DL, Mascioli EA, Bistrian BR. Parenteral iron-dextran therapy: a review. Nutrition 1995;11:163–168.
30. Goldberg MA. Erythropoiesis, erythropoietin, and iron metabolism in elective surgery: preoperative strategies for avoiding allogeneic blood exposure. Am J Surg 1995;170(Suppl.):37S-43S.
31. Graff H, Watzinger U, Ludvik B, et al. Recombinant human erythropoietin as adjuvant treatment for autologous blood donation. Br Med J 1990;300:1627–1630.
32. Stehling L, Zauder HL. Acute normovolemic hemodilution. Transfusion 1991;31:857–868.
33. D'Ambra MN, Kaplan DK. Alternatives to allogeneic blood use in surgery. Acute normovolemic hemodilution and preoperative autologous donation. Am J Surg 1995;170(Suppl.):49S-52S.
34. Leather RP, Shaw CM, Kaufman JL, et al. A comparative analysis of retroperitoneal versus transperitoneal aortic replacement for aneurysm. Surg Gynecol Obstet 1989;168:337–345.
35. Sicard GA, Reilly JM, Rubin BG, et al. Transabdominal versus retroperitoneal incision for abdominal aortic surgery: report of a prospective randomized trial. J Vasc Surg 1995;21:174–183.
36. Johnson JN, McLaughlin GA, Wake PN, Helsby CR. Comparison of extraperitoneal and transperitoneal methods of aortoiliac reconstruction. J Cardiovasc Surg 1986;27:561–564.
37. Shindo S, Tada Y, Sato O, et al. Esmarch's bandage technique in distal bypass surgery. J Cardiovasc Surg 1992;33:609–612.
38. Wakefield TW, Lindblad B, Stanley TJ, et al. Heparin and protamine use in peripheral vascular surgery: a comparison between surgeons of the Society for Vascular Surgery and the European Society for Vascular Surgery. Eur J Vasc Surg 1994;8:193–198.
39. Mauney MC, Buchanan SA, Lawrence WA, et al. Stroke rate is markedly reduced after carotid endarterectomy by avoidance of protamine. J Vasc Surg 1995;22:264–269.
40. Kirklin JW, Chenoweth DE, Naftel DC, et al. Effects of protamine administration after cardiopulmonary bypass on complement, blood elements and the hemodynamic state. Ann Thorac Surg 1986;41:193–199.
41. Ward PH, Castro DJ, Ward S. A significant new contribution to radical head and neck surgery. The argon beam coagulator is an effective means of limiting blood loss. Arch Otolaryngol Head Neck Surg 1989; 115:921–923.
42. Dresdale A, Rose EA, Jeevanandam V, et al. Preparation of fibrin glue from single-donor fresh frozen plasma. Surgery 1985;97:750–753.
43. Hartman AR, Galanakis DK, Honig MP, et al. Autologous whole plasma fibrin gel. Intraoperative procurement. Arch Surg 1992;127: 357–359.
44. Schaff HV, Hauer JM, Beall WR, et al. Autotransfusion of shed mediastinal blood after cardiac surgery: a prospective study. J Thorac Cardiovasc Surg 1978;75:632–640.
45. Tawes RL, Scribner RG, DuVall TB, et al. The cell-saver and autotransfusion: an under-utilized resource in vascular surgery. Am J Surg 1986;152:105–109.
46. Tawes RL. Blood replacement and autotransfusion in major vascular surgery. In: Rutherford RB, ed. Vascular surgery. Philadelphia: WB Saunders, 1995:433–447.
47. VanderSalm TJ, Ansell JE, Okike ON, et al. The role of epsilon aminocaproic acid in reducing bleeding after cardiac operation: a double-blind, randomized study. J Thorac Cardiovasc Surg 1988;95: 538–540.
48. Hackmann T, Gascoyne RD, Naiman SC, et al. A trial of desmopressin to reduce blood loss in uncomplicated cardiac surgery. N Engl J Med 1989;321:1437–1440.
49. Teasdale S, Norman P, Carroll J, et al. Prevention of post bypass bleeding with tranexamic acid and epsilon-aminocaproic acid. J Cardiothorac Vasc Anesth 1993;7:431–435.
50. Dietrich W, Barankay A, Hahnel C, et al. High-dose aprotinin in cardiac surgery: three years experience in 1,784 patients. J Cardio Thorac Anesth 1992;7:324–327.

51. Lemmer GH, Stanford W, Bonney SL, et al. Aprotinin for coronary bypass operations: efficacy, safety, and influence on early saphenous vein graft patency—a multicenter, randomized, double-blind, placebo controlled study. J Thorac Cardiovasc Surg 1994;107:543–553.
52. Samama CM, Mazoyer E, Bruneval P, et al. Aprotinin could promote arterial thrombosis in pigs. A prospect of randomized blinded study. Thromb Haemost 1991;71:663–669.
53. Giordano GF, Rivers SL, Chung GKT, et al. Autologous platelet-rich plasma in cardiac surgery: effect on intraoperative and postoperative transfusion requirements. Ann Thorac Surg 1988;46:416–422.
54. Tobe CE, Vocelka C, Sepulvada R, et al. Infusion of autologous platelet-rich plasma does not reduce blood product use after coronary bypass: a prospective randomized blinded study. J Thorac Cardiovasc Surg 1993;105:1007–1014.
55. Viele M, Weiskopf R. What can we learn about the need for transfusion from patients who refuse blood? The experience with Jehovah's Witnesses. Tranfusion 1994;34:396–401.
56. Valeri CR, Feingold H, Cassidy G, et al. Hypothermia-induced reversible platelet dysfunction. Ann Surg 1987;205:175–182.
57. Ferrara A, MacArthur JD, Wright HK, et al. Hypothermia and acidosis worsen coagulopathy in the patient requiring massive transfusion. Am J Surg 1990;160:515–518.
58. Rotondo MF, Schwab CW, McGonigal MD, et al. "Damage control": an approach for improved survival in exsanguinating penetrating abdominal injury. J Trauma 1993;35:375–382.
59. Reid RI, Ciaverella D, Heimbach D, et al. Prophylactic platelet administration during massive transfusion. N Surg 1986;203:40–50.
60. Davenport RD, Kunkel SL. Cytokine roles in hemolytic and nonhemolytic transfusion reactions. Transf Med Rev 1994;8:157–163.
61. Chong BH. Heparin-induced thrombocytopenia. Br J Haematol 1995; 89:431–439.
62. Capson SM, Goldfinger D. Acute hemolytic trransfusion reaction a paradigm of the systemic inflammatory response: new insights into pathophysiology and treatment. Transfusion 1995;35:513–520.
63. Johansen K, Kohler TR, Nicholls SC, et al. Ruptured abdominal aortic aneurysm: the Harborview experience. J Vasc Surg 1991;13:240–248.
64. McKenzie FN, Heimbecher RO, Wall W, et al. Intraoperative autotransfusion in elective and emergency vascular surgery. Surgery 1978; 83:470–478.
65. Towes RL, DuVall TB. The rapid-infusion system. In: Braverman M, Tawes RL, eds. Surgical technology international. London: Century Press, 1991:112–113.
66. Satiani B, Fried SJ, Zeeb P, et al. Normothermic rapid volume replacement in traumatic hypovolemia. Arch Surg 1987;122:1044–1051.
67. Rutherford RB, Jones DN, Bergentz SE, et al. The efficacy of Dextran 40 in preventing early postoperative thrombosis following difficult lower extremity bypass. J Vasc Surg 1984;1:765–773.
68. Kohler TR, Kaufman JL, Kacoyannis G., et al. The effect of aspirin and dipyridamole on the patency of lower extremity bypass grafts. Surgery 1984;96:462–466.
69. Gong R, Lindberg J, Abrams J, et al. Comparison of hypertonic saline solutions and dextran in dialysis-induced hypotension. J Am Soc Nephrol 1993;3:1808–1812.
70. Edmondson RA, Cohen AT, Dass K, et al. Low molecular weight heparin vs. aspirin and dipyridamole after femoral popliteal bypass grafting. Lancet 1994;344:914–918.
71. Kretschmer G, Herbst F, Prager M, et al. A decade of oral anticoagulant treatment to main autologous vein grafts for femoral popliteal atherosclerosis. Arch Surg 1992;127:1112–1115.
72. National Institutes of Health Consensus Conference. Perioperative red cell transfusion. JAMA 1988;260:2700–2714.
73. Leone BJ, Spahn DSR. Anemia, hemodilution and oxygen delivery. Anesth Analg 1992;75:651–653.
74. Greenburg AG. A physiologic basis for red blood cell transfusion in incisions. Am J Surg 1995;170(Suppl.):44S–48S.
75. Schlichtig R, Kramer DJ, Pinsky MR. Flow redistribution during progressive hemorrhage is a determinant of critical oxygen (O_2) delivery. J Appl Physiol 1991;70:169–178.
76. Spence RK. Blood management practice guidelines conference. Surgical red blood cell transfusion practice policies. Am J Surg 1995; 170(Suppl.):3S–15S.
77. Kuriyan M, Kim D. Implications of utilization of a maximum surgical blood order schedule. Vox Sang 1989;57:152–154.
78. Goodnough LT, Despotis GJ. Establishing practice guidelines for surgical blood management. Am J Surg 1995;170(Suppl.):16S–20S.
79. Soumerai SB, Salem-Schatz S, Avorn J, et al. A controlled trial of educational outreach to improve blood transfusion practice. JAMA 1993; 270:961–966.

Chapter 30

Blood Coagulation During Liver, Kidney, Pancreas, and Lung Transplantation

YOOGOO KANG
THOMAS A. GASIOR

LIVER TRANSPLANTATION

Intraoperative bleeding is common during orthotopic liver transplantation. On average, 10–15 units each of packed red blood cells (RBC) and fresh-frozen plasma (FFP) are lost, and massive blood loss (more than 50 units) may occur when the surgical procedure is complicated (1). Bleeding may result from surgical or medical causes, and it is often difficult to distinguish between these causes. Surgical bleeding is caused by difficulties in the removal of the diseased liver in the presence of portal hypertension, numerous collateral vessels, adhesions from previous abdominal surgery and fragile tissues, and complexity of reconstruction of the major vessels (the inferior vena cava, portal vein, and hepatic artery). Surgical bleeding is compounded by abnormal coagulation associated with the hepatic dysfunction and dynamic intraoperative dilutional and pathological coagulopathy. Anemia and a major fluid shift may also complicate the intraoperative management of recipients.

Intraoperative transfusion therapy is complex and difficult. Two of the first seven liver transplant patients in the 1960s and six of the first 43 patients in Pittsburgh in the early 1980s died of uncontrollable intraoperative bleeding (2, 3). Therefore, an understanding of the principles of transfusion in patients undergoing liver transplantation requires a thorough knowledge of the pathophysiology of coagulation, fluid balance, hematopoiesis, and proper selection of monitoring and treatment mode.

COAGULATION IN PATIENTS WITH END-STAGE LIVER DISEASE

Normal hepatic function is essential for homeostasis in all five steps of the coagulation process. The role of liver disease in the vascular phase of coagulation is unclear, but liver disease may impair the elasticity and contraction of blood vessels and the interaction between the vessel walls and platelets (4). Quantitative and qualitative impairment in the platelet phase is common in patients with liver disease. Thrombocytopenia has been observed in up to 70% of patients (5), although the production of platelets may have been normal or increased (6). Thrombocytopenia is caused by splenomegaly (7), shortened platelet survival (8), platelet consumption (6), sequestration of platelets in the regenerating liver (6), folic acid deficiency in alcoholic liver disease (9), and toxic effects of ethanol on megakaryocytes (10). Platelet dysfunction is frequently observed in these patients with end-stage liver disease: platelet count does not correlate with bleeding time (4), clot retraction is diminished, and platelet aggregation is impaired (11, 12). Platelet dysfunction may be caused in part by decreases in arachidonic acid, which is required for production of thromboxane A_2, and decreases in platelet content of adenine nucleotides (13). The impaired aggregation of platelets appears to be caused by an increase in small hypofunctional platelets (14). Abnormal platelet function in patients with the hepatorenal syndrome is caused by dialyzable or nondialyzable plasma factors.

The coagulation cascade is adversely affected by low levels of procoagulants and inhibitors produced by the liver. These include most coagulation factors (I, II, V, VII, VIII, IX, X, XI, XII, XIII, prekallikrein, and high-molecular-weight kininogen), inhibitors (antithrombin III and α_1-antitrypsin), and regulatory proteins (C_1 inhibitor and α_2-macroglobulin). The deficiency of coagulation factors is more severe with factors VII, IX, X, and II; however, the fibrinogen level is normal or increased, although dysfibrinogenemia caused by excessive sialic acid in the fibrinogen molecule affects the polymerization of fibrin monomers, resulting in prolonged thrombin time (15, 16). It is interesting to note that enzymatic removal of sialic acid residue from the fibrinogen of these patients restores thrombin time (17). The level of factor VIII is frequently increased because of increases in the von Willebrand factor antigen and its activity (18). A generalized deficiency in coagulation factors prolongs prothrombin time (PT) and decreases in levels of factors IX and XII prolong activated partial thromboplastin time (APTT). In addition, the low level of proteinases with antithrombin activity (antithrombin III and α_1-antitrypsin) and regulatory proteins (C_1 inhibitor and α_2-macroglobulin) may theoretically result in thrombosis (19).

Fibrin polymerization is impaired by the low level of factor XIII and dysfibrinogenemia. Fibrinolysis is also affected because the levels of inhibitors of lysis (α_2-antiplasmin and plasminogen activator inhibitor) are low and the tissue plasminogen activator (TPA) level is high because of the enlarged endothelial area (20). In addition, impairment of hepatic clearance of activated factors involved in coagulation and fibrinolysis may cause intravascular coagulation or fibrinolysis (21).

In another view, homeostasis of coagulation is maintained through an optimal balance between coagulation and fibrinolysis, which are activated simultaneously on vascular injury. An imbalance in defective coagulation and fibrinolysis, which is common in patients with liver disease, results in all types of coagulopathy. Hypocoagulation is caused by quantitative and qualitative defects in clotting factors and platelets. Insufficient hepatic clearance of activated coagulation factors may result in a hypercoagulable state (disseminated or localized intravascular coagulation). Fibrinolysis is prone to develop when levels of fibrinolysis inhibitors (α_2-antiplasmin and histidine glycoprotein) are low or the hepatic clearance of TPA is decreased (22–25). Impaired fibrinolysis caused by deficiency of protein C or protein S may result in a hypercoagulable state.

The degree of abnormality of coagulation may vary depending on the cause and severity of liver disease. Severe coagulopathy is seen in patients with hepatocellular disease such as viral or alcoholic postnecrotic cirrhosis or fulminant hepatic failure. Coagulation disturbances are less severe in patients with cholestatic disease than those with hepatocellular diseases, although similar changes may be seen in the terminal stage of cholestatic liver disease. The coagulation profile may be normal in patients with uncomplicated neoplasms, although necrosis of a tumor may trigger disseminated intravascular coagulation (DIC). Patients with congenital metabolic disorders such as Dubin-Johnson, Gilbert, or Rotor's syndrome have low titers of factor VII (26, 27), and patients with familial antithrombin deficiency, an autosomal-dominant genetic disease, are prone to developing thromboembolism.

PERIOPERATIVE CHANGES IN COAGULATION

Perioperative changes in coagulation in liver transplantation have been described since the development of the procedure (28–30) and confirmed in more recent reports (Table 30.1) (5, 31, 32). Preoperative coagulation profiles were abnormal in most patients undergoing liver transplantation: PT in 65%, APTT in 71%, fibrinogen in 14%, factor V in 59%, factor VII in 56%, factor VIII in 3%, and platelet count in 70% of patients. The euglobulin lysis time (ELT) was less than 2 hours in 27% of patients, and fibrin degradation products (FDP) were positive in 24% of patients (5).

During the preanhepatic stage, preexisting coagulopathy is compounded by dilutional coagulopathy caused by surgical bleeding, resulting in a generalized decrease in the levels of coagulation factors and thrombocytopenia (Fig. 30.1). In patients with a severe hepatocellular disease, fibrinolysis may begin to develop during this stage. In addition, ionized hypocalcemia and acidosis, complications of massive blood transfusion, may impair coagulation.

Coagulopathy is more severe during the anhepatic stage. When venovenous bypass is used, prolonged APTT and reaction time as measured by thromboelastography (TEG) are observed at the onset of the bypass. This heparin effect is caused by a small dose of heparin (2000–5000 units) added to the priming solution and dissipates gradually within 1 hour without treatment. Dilutional coagulopathy becomes more pronounced during this period because of difficulty in dissection of the retrohepatic area in the presence of portal hypertension, particularly in patients without venovenous bypass. In addition, absence of hepatic synthetic function results in further decreases in coagulation factor levels. Fibrinolytic activity demonstrated by shortened ELT and fibrinolysis time (f) of TEG becomes more evident during this period and occurs in about 20% of patients. Fibrinolysis appears to be caused by the absence of the hepatic clearance of TPA based on a progressive increase in the TPA level (Fig. 30.2) (33, 34). The loss of hepatic clearance of activated coagulation factors may lead to

TABLE 30.1. COAGULOPATHY DURING ORTHOTOPIC LIVER TRANSPLANTATION

Preanhepatic stage
Preexisting coagulopathy
Dilution
Fibrinolysis (mild)
Ionized hypocalcemia
Acidosis
Anhepatic stage
Dilution
Heparin effect (mild, with venovenous bypass)
Fibrinolysis (moderate)
Activation of coagulation
Hypothermia
Ionized hypocalcemia
Acidosis
Neohepatic stage (early)
Fibrinolysis (severe)
Heparin effect (moderate)
Intravascular coagulation (localized)
Dilution
Hypothermia
Ionized hypocalcemia
Acidosis
Neohepatic stage (late)
Gradual recovery

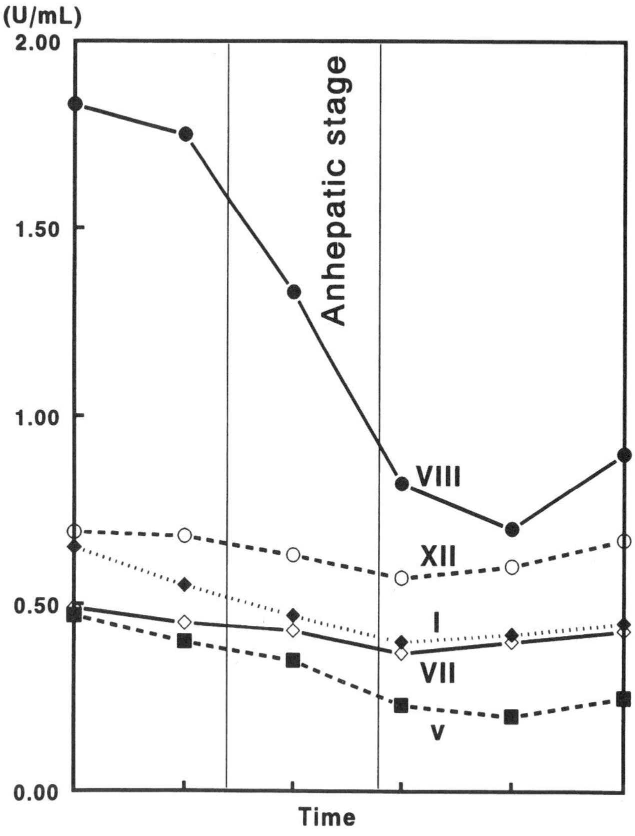

Figure 30.1. Coagulation profile during liver transplantation. (Modified by permission from Lewis JH, Bontempo FA, Awad SA, et al. Liver transplantation: intraoperative changes in coagulation factors in 100 first transplants. Hepatology 1989;9:710–714.)

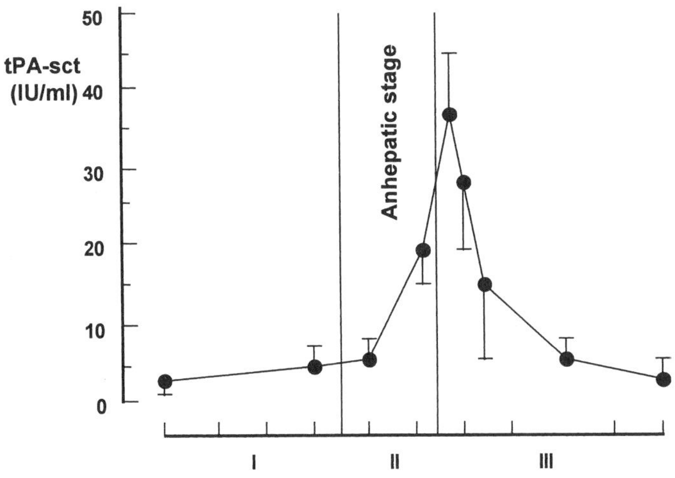

Figure 30.2. TPA level during liver transplantation. (Reprinted with permission from Porte RJ, Bontempo FA, Knot EA, et al. Systemic effects of tissue plasminogen activator-associated fibrinolysis and its relation to thrombin generation in orthotopic liver transplantation. Transplantation 1989;47:978–984.)

activation of coagulation or a tendency to develop intravascular coagulation, evidenced by gradual increases in TAT complex and FDP (Fig. 30.3) (35). Clinically significant DIC or thromboembolic phenomena are rare, however.

A severe coagulopathy, the postreperfusion syndrome of coagulation, develops on reperfusion of the grafted liver. Changes are prolonged PT, APTT, reptilase time, and thrombin time; a generalized decrease in coagulation factor levels including factors I, V, VII, and VIII; a sudden increase in TPA; thrombocytopenia; a shortened ELT; a moderate increase in FDP; and a very high level of TAT complex (5, 28, 31). The cause of the postreperfusion coagulopathy is believed to be multifactorial. A sudden influx of heparin that is leaked from the donor hepatocytes causes a moderate to severe heparin effect in about one-third of patients. The heparin effect is seen as a prolongation of APTT and reaction time of TEG and is reversed by the administration of protamine sulfate (Fig. 30.4). Other coagulation inhibitors or heparin-like substances have been suggested to play a role in the development of the postreperfusion syndrome (28). Severe fibrinolysis, seen as generalized oozing in the previously dry surgical field, occurs in about half of patients on reperfusion (36). Laboratory findings include shortened ELT (as low as 0–15 min), an abrupt increase in TPA level, a very low level of plasminogen activator inhibitor (PAI), and a reduction in fibrinolysis time and maximum amplitude, and prolonged reaction time of TEG. Fibrinolysis is caused by a massive release of TPA from the grafted liver, congested viscera, and lower extremities together with insufficient hepatic clearance of TPA and a reduction of PAI (33, 34). Other potential causes of fibrinolysis include contact activation of fibrinolysis and activation of protein C or urokinase-type plasminogen activator (37). Postreperfusion fibrinolysis is believed to be primary in origin based on several factors: a relatively steady level of antithrombin III (38); only moderate levels of fibrin(ogen) degradation products and D-dimers (5); an association between fibrinolysis and a selective decrease in factors I, V, and VIII (31); no known microembolization; and the effectiveness of epsilon-aminocaproic acid (EACA) in treating fibrinolysis without complications (36).

Intravascular coagulation with secondary fibrinolysis has been suggested to occur on reperfusion because the levels of TAT complex, FDP, and fibrin monomers increase gradually during the anhepatic stage and reach their peak immediately after reperfusion (35). Intravascular coagulation appears to be caused either by TPA-induced activation of platelet aggregation or by extracellular release of lysosomal proteinases from macrophages (cathepsin B) and granulocytes (elastase) (39, 40). The role of intravascular coagulation in postreperfusion coagulopathy does not appear to be clinically significant, however, because administration of antithrombin III to inhibit thrombin activity neither improves the coagulation profile nor reduces blood loss and fibrinolytic activity (41).

Quantitative and qualitative defects in platelets may cause reperfusion coagulopathy. Thrombocytopenia occurs in most patients on reperfusion (42), and the transhepatic decrease in platelet count has been shown to be as much as 55% (43, 44). Although unclear, reperfusion thrombocytopenia may be caused by extravasation of platelets into Disse's spaces or phagocytosis by Kupffer cells. Platelet function can be impaired by the loss of granulation (45) and decreased platelet aggregation (46).

Reperfusion hypothermia (by 1–2°C), dilutional coagulopathy caused by an influx of preservation solution, and bleeding and ionic hypocalcemia may also interfere with coagulation (47).

Postreperfusion coagulopathy dissipates gradually and the levels of coagulation factors and platelet count increase toward

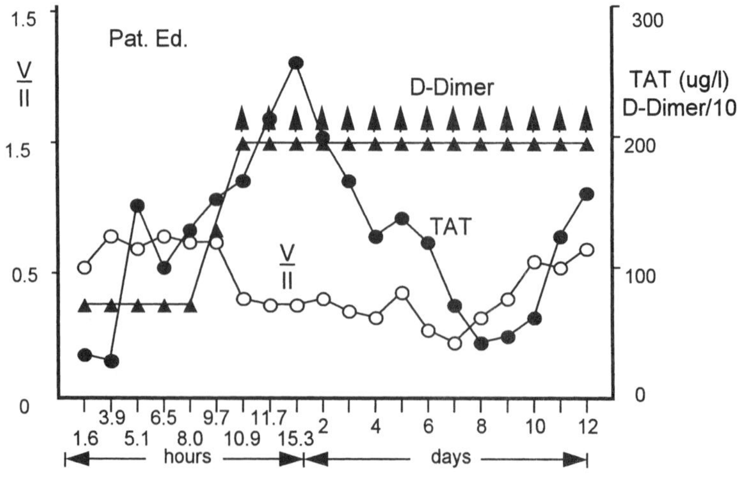

Figure 30.3. Intraoperative changes in coagulation factors, D-dimers, and TAT. (Reprinted with permission from Kratzer MAA, Dieterich J, Denecke H, Knedel M. Hemostatic variables and blood loss during orthotopic human liver transplantation. Transplantation Proc 1991;23:1906–1911. Reprinted by permission of Appleton & Lange, Inc.)

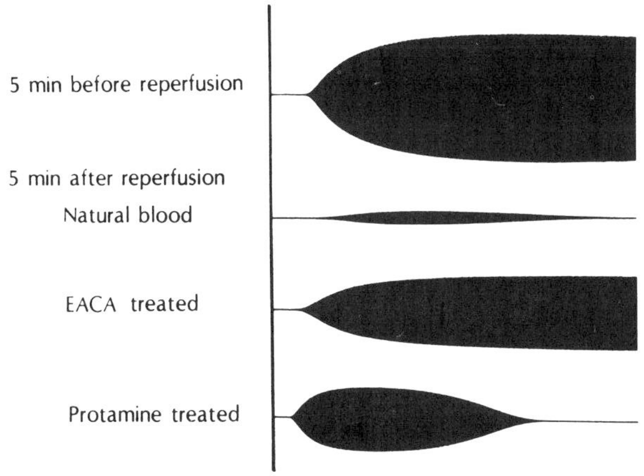

Figure 30.4. Thromboelastography of reperfusion coagulopathy.

baseline levels as the grafted liver begins to function. Bleeding or oozing, however, may persist in some patients. Oozing in the presence of an abnormal coagulation profile and TEG may indicate insufficient administration of coagulation factors and platelets; insufficient production of clotting factors from the poorly functioning grafted liver; inadequate hepatic clearance of activated clotting factors; complication of untreated fibrinolysis as plasminogen selectively destroys factors I, V, and VIII (31); or localized intravascular coagulation in the graft liver as a result of ischemic insult or immunological reaction (28). In patients with an acceptable coagulation profile and TEG, oozing may result from inadequate or delayed treatment of fibrinolysis because a certain lag time exists between the activation of fibrinolysis and lysis of the preformed clots or oozing in the surgical field. Systemic or local intravascular coagulation by a poorly functioning liver graft or graft with ischemic injury may also contribute to coagulopathy.

The postoperative evolution of coagulation depends on the graft function. In general, with adequate graft function, the coagulation factor level increases steadily toward a normal value, and PT, APTT, and platelet count return to normal values within 2 weeks (Fig. 30.5).

MONITORING OF COAGULATION

Coagulation is commonly monitored using a traditional coagulation profile including PT, APTT, fibrinogen level, platelet count, ELT, and FDP level. If more information is needed, factor assays (I, V, VII, XII), reptilase time, and thrombin time can be determined. However, a coagulation profile has limitations for clinical monitoring, namely the lack of availability and difficulty in assessing blood coagulability in patients with dynamic and multiple coagulation defects.

Recently, TEG was introduced to monitor whole-blood coagulation (48, 49). TEG determines the shear elasticity of fibrins formed in real-time fashion, and its advantages are its capability to assess the interaction of all cellular and noncellular elements involved in coagulation and the ease of accessibility. More importantly, TEG assists in making differential diagnosis of coagulopathy and guides selective replacement and pharmacological therapy.

Commonly determined TEG variables are shown in Figure 30.6. Reaction time is the interval from the start of the TEG recording to the point where amplitude reaches 2 mm. It is the time taken to generate initial fibrin strands, a primary function of the coagulation cascade. Maximum amplitude, the largest amplitude reached, is a function of the platelets. Clot formation rate, the speed with which a solid clot forms, is a primary function of fibrinogen and a secondary function of platelet. The time interval between the maximum amplitude and subsequent zero amplitude is the fibrinolysis time.

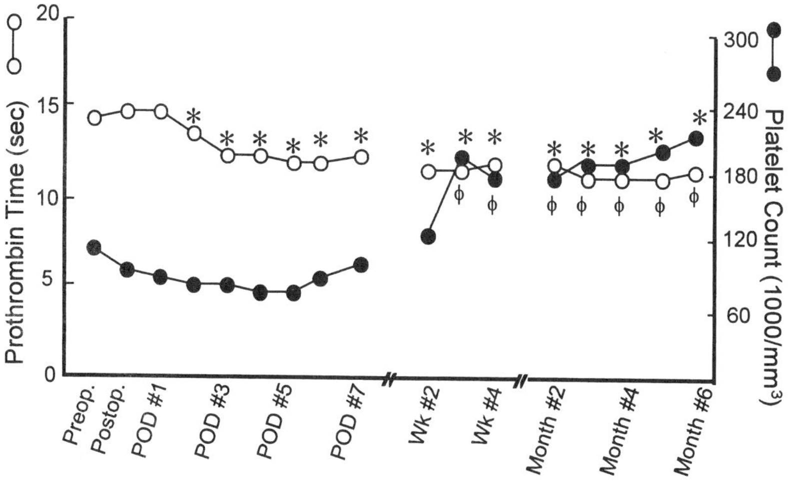

Figure 30.5. Postoperative evolution of the coagulation profile. (Courtesy of Dr. Mahmood Tabatabai of University of Pittsburgh School of Medicine.)

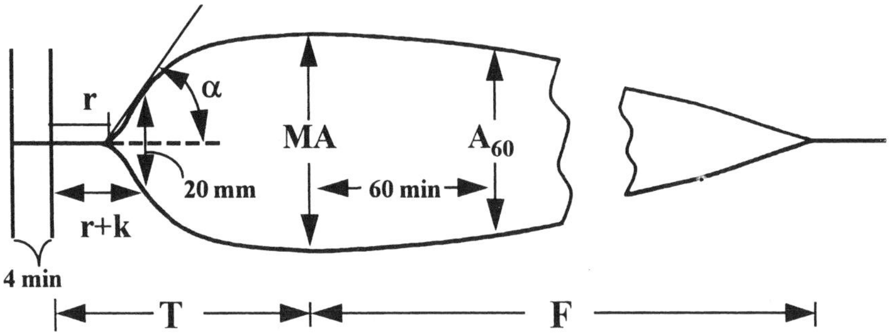

Figure 30.6. Variables and normal values measured by thromboelastography. r, reaction time, 6–8 min; r + k, coagulation time, 10–12 min; α, clot formation rate, >50°; MA, maximum amplitude, 50–70 mm; A_{60}, amplitude at 60 min after MA; A_{60}/MA × 100, fibrinolysis index, >85%; F, fibrinolysis time, >300 min. (Reprinted with permission from Kang YG, Martin DJ, Marquez J, et al. Intraoperative changes in blood coagulation and thromboelastographic monitoring in liver transplantation. Anesth Analg 1985;64:888–896.)

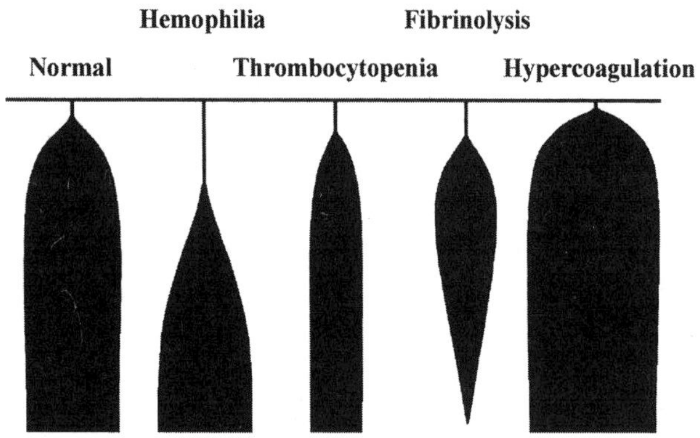

Figure 30.7. Thromboelastographic patterns of normal and disease states. (Reprinted with permission from Kang YG. Monitoring and treatment of coagulation. In: Winter PM, Kang YG, eds. Hepatic transplantation: anesthetic and perioperative management. New York: Praeger, 1986:151–173, With permisison of Greenwood Publishing Group Inc, Westport, CT.)

The amplitude 60 minutes after maximum amplitude (A_{60}) is used to determine the fibrinolysis index (A_{60}/MA × 100). A fibrinolysis index less than 85% indicates fibrinolysis. The relationship between TEG variables and activity of blood components, however, is not precise because TEG is a summary of interactions of cellular and noncellular components of coagulation.

A normal TEG pattern is characterized by an initial fluid state, followed by a gradual increase in fibrin shear elasticity that reaches maximum amplitude in 30–60 minutes (Fig. 30.7). The fibrinolysis index remains above 85%. Coagulation in a patient with hemophilia is characterized by a prolonged reaction time and reduced clot formation rate because of the delayed formation of thrombin caused by insufficient activity of factor VIII; however, maximum amplitude (platelet function) is normal. A similar TEG pattern is observed in patients with ionized hypocalcemia (less than 0.6 mmol/L) or hypothermia (less than 34°C). In thrombocytopenia, the maximum amplitude is decreased. In addition, a prolonged reaction time and a reduced clot formation rate are observed in thrombocytopenia because aggregation and activation of platelets are essential to the activation of the coagulation cascade. In fibrinolysis, a rapid decrease in amplitude is accompanied by a prolonged reaction time and decreased maximum amplitude. The deterioration of reaction time and maximum amplitude is caused by a net decrease in the amount of fibrin as the number of fibrin fibers decreases by fibrinolysis. Hypercoagulation is characterized by a short reaction time and an increased clot formation rate and maximum amplitude.

For the differential diagnosis, TEG of untreated blood (0.36 mL) is compared with that of blood (0.33 mL) treated with blood components (0.03 mL of FFP, cryoprecipitate, and platelets) or pharmacological agents (0.03 mL of 1% EACA and 0.01% protamine sulfate). Differential diagnosis of postreperfusion coagulopathy is shown in Figure 30.4 (49). Relatively normal prereperfusion TEG changed abruptly to a hypocoagulable state with a prolonged reaction time, reduced clot formation rate and maximum amplitude, and a demonstrable fibrinolysis. Improvement in reaction time, maximum amplitude, and clot formation rate in blood treated with protamine sulfate suggests the presence of the heparin effect, and improvement in all variables in blood treated with EACA demonstrates fibrinolysis.

PERIOPERATIVE MANAGEMENT OF COAGULATION

Preoperative Management

Preoperative optimization of coagulation, although ideal, is difficult because replacement therapy may not sustain satisfactory levels of coagulation factors and transfusion of a large volume of FFP may cause fluid overloading. Preoperative management of coagulation should be tailored to the specific clinical circumstances such as the degree and type of coagulation defects, the type of invasive procedure planned, and the nature or location of bleeding. Treatment of coagulation includes administration of vitamin K, FFP, platelets, cryoprecipitate, and antifibrinolytic agents and plasmapheresis.

Vitamin K

Hepatic synthesis of coagulation factors (II, VII, IX, and X) depends on vitamin K, a cofactor for posttranslational carboxylation. Vitamin K, a lipid-soluble vitamin, is either obtained directly from dietary intake or produced from a precursor by the action of intestinal flora. Intestinal absorption of vitamin K requires bile salts. Consequently, deficiencies of vitamin K-dependent coagulation factors result from a poor dietary intake, inadequate production or excretion of bile salts, or suppression of normal intestinal flora by antibiotics. Drugs such as cholestyramine resin bind to bile salts and thus inhibit the absorption of vitamin K.

For a mild vitamin K deficiency, oral administration of vitamin K and bile salts is a sufficient treatment and intramuscular or intravenous administration of vitamin K1 (5 mg/day) is effective in correcting PT within 24–48 hours. Repeated administration of vitamin K1 and coagulation factors may be necessary to treat bleeding tendency. Vitamin K is not effective in patients with severe hepatocellular disease because of either an inadequate amount of coagulation factor precursors or incomplete carboxylation (50); however, it may be given to evaluate the effectiveness of the therapy in these patients (10 mg for 3 days).

Fresh-Frozen Plasma

FFP is the most suitable agent for the correction of multiple coagulation defects in patients with liver disease because it contains all coagulation factors and inhibitors present in the blood. It is generally accepted that FFP is given to patients with a prolonged PT (more than 15 seconds) before the needle biopsy of the liver. FFP administration, however, only improves coagulation temporarily in cirrhotic patients with hemorrhagic symptoms, and the large volume required to treat coagulopathy may cause fluid overloading. Therefore, overzealous FFP administration is not recommended in the immediate preoperative period.

Platelets

Platelet transfusion is required for severe thrombocytopenia. Platelet transfusion is only temporarily effective in patients with liver disease, however, because transfused platelets are removed rapidly from circulation by the spleen and liver. Clinically, a bleeding tendency is not seen when the platelet count is greater than 75,000/mm^3, but satisfactory hemostasis can be obtained with lesser platelet counts (more than 30,000/mm^3).

Cryoprecipitate

Cryoprecipitate contains fibrinogen and factors VIII and XIII. Because of a high level of factor VIII in patients with liver disease, transfusion of cryoprecipitate is indicated only when hypofibrinogenemia is documented. One unit of cryoprecipitate contains 300 mg of fibrinogen, and transfusion of 1 unit of cryoprecipitate increases the fibrinogen level about 10 mg/dL in a patient weighing 60 kg. The half-life of the fibrinogen is about 3–4 days, and repeated transfusion of cryoprecipitate is necessary to supplement the loss.

Anticoagulation Therapy

Anticoagulation therapy is rarely used in cirrhotic patients. Heparin is rarely used to avoid heparin-induced thrombocytopenia, although a subcutaneous injection of a small dose appears to be acceptable. Oral anticoagulants are also not recommended because of the unpredictable response.

Antifibrinolytic Agents

Antifibrinolytic agents stabilize fragile hemostatic plugs in localized bleeding such as a gastric mucosal ulcer or bleeding esophageal varices and may decrease the bleeding tendency in patients without signs of fibrinolysis. EACA has been shown to be ineffective in improving coagulopathy in patients with liver disease, however (51). Antifibrinolytic therapy should be reserved for patients with demonstrable fibrinolysis to avoid thrombotic complications.

Plasmapheresis

Plasmapheresis (30–40 mL/kg) in combination with replacement therapy may improve coagulation by removing filterable humoral elements and coagulation inhibitors, particularly in patients with fulminant hepatic failure. Plasmapheresis of 36.8 mL/kg of blood has reportedly decreased PT from 28.3 to 17.7 seconds and APTT from 64.8 to 43.3 seconds in patients awaiting liver transplantation (52).

Intraoperative Management

Physiological Therapy

Hypothermia, ionized hypocalcemia, and acidosis are common during liver transplantation and are known to impair the coagulation process (47). Hypothermia impairs coagulation by inhibiting the activity of proteases involved in the coagulation cascade; this phenomenon is seen as a prolonged reaction time and reduced clot formation rate of TEG. Ionized hypocalcemia delays coagulation because calcium ions are cofactors of coagulation. Therefore, physiological variables including body temperature, tissue perfusion, gas exchange, acid-base state, and fluid-electrolyte balance should be normalized to maintain normal blood coagulability.

Replacement Therapy

Replacement therapy is guided by conventional coagulation profile or TEG variables. Replacement guidelines based on conventional coagulation vary widely from institution to institution, ranging from specific guidelines (PT greater than 50% International Normalized Ratio; hematocrit, 30%; platelet count greater than 30,000/mm^3; and antithrombin III level greater than 70%) to more ambiguous guidelines (hemoglobin greater than 9 g%, FFP to correct coagulopathy, and platelet count greater than 100,000/mm^3) (53, 54).

At the University of Pittsburgh Medical Center, coagulation therapy is guided by TEG variables because maintenance of blood coagulability with administration of minimal blood products is the clinical goal. In general, continuous replacement of FFP is required to compensate for a progressive decrease in coagulation factor levels. This is achieved by administration of a mixture of blood products (RBC:FFP:PlasmaLyte-A = 300:200:250 mL) containing 20–50% of normal levels of coagulation factors. Additional blood products may be administered according to TEG variables and platelet count: platelets (10 units) when maximum amplitude is less than 40 mm, cryoprecipitate (6 units) when clot formation rate is less than 40° even after platelet administration, and additional FFP (2 units) when reaction time is persistently longer than 15 minutes even after the administration of platelets and cryoprecipitate (55). Administration of cryoprecipitate is rarely necessary, however, unless the patient develops fibrinolysis.

During the anhepatic stage with venovenous bypass, aggressive administration of platelets and cryoprecipitate is avoided to prevent potential thromboembolism. More aggressive replacement therapy may be needed during the neohepatic stage when surgical bleeding persists or treatment of fibrinolysis or the heparin effect is delayed. Untreated fibrinolysis may require replacement of factors I, V, and VIII by administration of cryoprecipitate containing factors I and VIII and FFP containing factor V. Patients with poorly functioning graft livers or patients who are highly sensitized to class 1 human lymphocyte antigens may require transfusion of a large volume of platelets (56, 57).

Administration of antithrombin III was recommended because its level can be low during the anhepatic and early neohepatic stages. The antithrombin III level remains stable when FFP is adequately administered (38), however, and its use is reserved only for patients with excessively low antithrombin III levels.

The TEG patterns and coagulation profile of a patient with fulminant hepatic failure, who received TEG-guided replacement therapy, are shown in Figures 30.8 and 30.9 (5). The baseline TEG pattern showed a prolonged reaction time, decreased maximum amplitude, and decreased clot formation rate, indicating a generalized decrease in coagulation factor levels and platelets. Administration of 2 units of FFP improved reaction time. The administration of 10 units of platelets brought maximum amplitude to close to normal range, but mild fibrinolysis began to develop. Transfusion of 6 units of cryoprecipitate did not improve clot formation rate due to continuous deterioration of coagulation. The anhepatic stage was characterized by pronounced fibrinolysis. On reperfusion, a severe coagulopathy was noted with prolonged reaction time, decreased clot formation rate, decreased maximum amplitude, and signs of fibrinolysis. Reperfusion co-

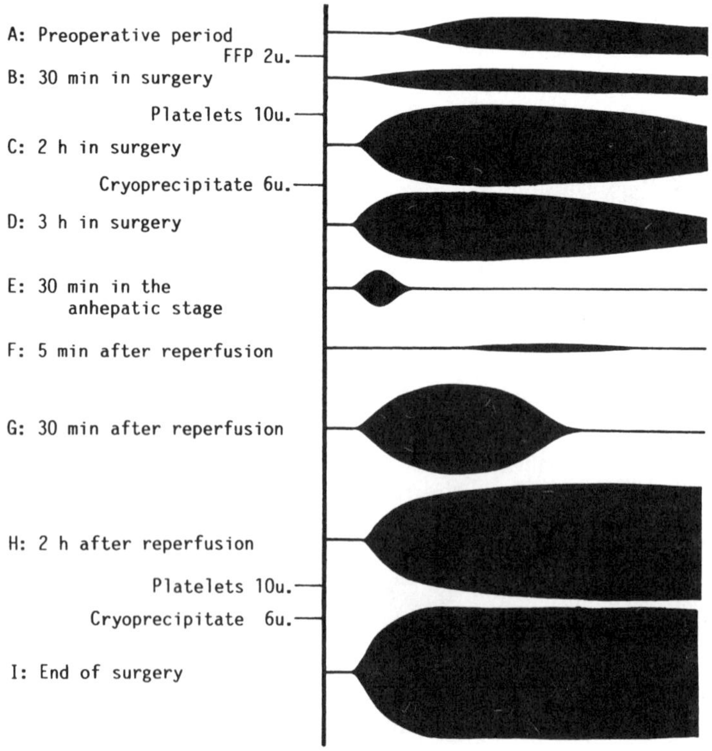

Figure 30.8. TEG-guided replacement therapy during liver transplantation. (Reprinted with permission from Kang YG, Martin DJ, Marquez J, et al. Intraoperative changes in blood coagulation and thromboelastographic monitoring in liver transplantation. Anesth Analg 1985;64:888–896.)

Coagulation profile (LW)

	Preanhepatic Stage		Anhepatic Stage		Neohepatic Stage		End
Platelet (K/mm3)	28	109	92	85	107	110	125
PT (sec)	27.7	18.5	19.1	15.3	14.6	14	13.5
aPTT (sec)	47.1	43.4	72.9	41.3	40.9	39.3	33.3
Thrombin time (sec)	28.2	21.4	34.2	21.7	20.3	18.8	20.9
Reptilase time (sec)	33.5	24.1	24.6	24.4	23.4	21.6	23.1
Fibrinogen (mg/mL)	95	130	130	175	225	230	250
Factor II (U/mL)	0.17	0.24	0.24	0.31	0.33	0.35	0.43
Factor V (U/mL)	0.12	0.18	0.16	0.25	0.29	0.29	0.41
Factor VII (U/mL)	0.04	0.09	0.09	0.22	0.29	0.34	0.44
Factor VIII (U/mL)	2.75	1.95	1.75	1.9	0.15	1.25	1.4
Factor IX (U/mL)	0.31	0.36	0.33	0.52	0.62	0.58	1.15
Factor X (U/mL)	0.17	0.22	0.25	0.23	0.33	0.38	0.49
Factor XI (U/mL)	0.44	0.52	0.78	0.58	0.66	0.6	0.84
Factor XII (U/mL)	0.52	0.52	0.52	0.6	0.6	0.33	0.4
FDP (ug/mL)	0	0	0	0	0	0	20
ELT (h)	2	1	1	1	2.5	2.75	4

Figure 30.9. Complete coagulation profile of the patient presented in Figure 30.8. Shaded cells indicate mild abnormality and dark cells, severe abnormality.

agulopathy gradually improved 2 hours after reperfusion. The administration of platelets and cryoprecipitate normalized TEG by the end of surgery, even in the presence of a mild abnormality in the coagulation profile.

PHARMACOLOGICAL THERAPY

The synthetic antifibrinolytic agents (EACA and tranexamic acid) accelerate the conversion of plasminogen to plasmin but inhibit the formation of plasmin-fibrin(ogen) complex. In the first clinical trial of EACA, three patients undergoing liver transplantation were given the agent (5 g loading dose followed by 1 g/hr) to treat bleeding presumably caused by fibrinolysis. All three patients died of continuous bleeding or pulmonary embolism (29). Based on this negative experience with EACA, it was concluded that no antifibrinolytic therapy should be given because reperfusion coagulopathy reverses itself with a functioning graft liver.

Oozing induced by fibrinolysis is a clinical concern, however, because patients with a short ELT (15 min) have been found to require more blood transfusions (31). In a subsequent study using a low dose of EACA (1 g), 82.5% of the 79 patients studied developed some degree of fibrinolysis (36). EACA administered to 20 patients who developed severe fibrinolysis (fibrinolysis time less than 120 min or fibrinolysis index less than 80%) demonstrated complete inhibition of fibrinolysis with improved maximum amplitude, fibrinolysis time, and fibrinolysis index without thrombotic or hemorrhagic complications. The reduction in EACA dose was an important finding of this study. The conventional EACA dosage schedule is based on the recommendation of McNicol et al. (58) for complete inhibition of fibrinolysis in vitro and includes a priming dose of 4–5 g followed by 1 g/hr to achieve a plasma level of 13 mg/dL. In patients undergoing liver transplantation, fibrinolysis is transient, although severe, and inhibition of plasmin in the early stage of fibrinolysis is sufficient to stop fibrinolysis. Furthermore, EACA is almost completely eliminated in urine within 6 hours, and no residual effect of EACA is anticipated at the end of or after surgery. Recently, even a smaller dose of EACA (250–500 mg) was found to be effective in treating most types of fibrinolysis (59), although its short half-life may necessitate a second dose when an extremely high TPA level persists over a prolonged period. The prophylactic use of EACA is not recommended, however, to avoid any potential thrombotic complications (60). Recently, importance of early diagnosis and treatment of fibrinolysis is recognized because it reduces bleeding; prevents selective destruction of factors I, V, and VIII to minimize the need for FFP and cryoprecipitate; and reduces warm ischemia of the liver by reducing the surgical hemostasis time. Fibrinolysis can be diagnosed in its early stage by observing a significant improvement in TEG variables (reaction time and clot formation rate) in blood treated with EACA compared with untreated blood in the first 10–15 minutes of recordings. A typical replacement and pharmacological therapy guided by TEG differential diagnosis is shown in Figure 30.10.

Tranexamic acid appears to have similar beneficial effects without noticeable complications in pediatric patients (61) and in adults (62).

Protamine sulfate (25–50 mg) has been used to treat the heparin effect (59), a common phenomenon at the onset of venovenous bypass and immediately after reperfusion. The heparin effect is readily detected by prolonged APTT and by comparing the TEG of untreated blood and blood treated with protamine sulfate as described above.

Aprotinin, a nonspecific inhibitor of serine protease, has been shown to decrease blood loss in patients undergoing liver transplantation (63–65) by decreasing the TPA level and fibrinolysis (66). A generalized inhibition of coagulation and fibrinolysis in vitro (67) together with reduction of blood loss suggests that the beneficial role of aprotinin may be associated with reduced activation of coagulation. Further investigation on the mechanism of action of aprotinin may serve to decrease blood loss and to increase our understanding of coagulation during liver transplantation.

Desmopressin acetate (DDAVP), a synthetic analogue of 8-arginine vasopressin, increases the levels of factor VIII, von Willebrand factor, and plasminogen. It has been used in patients undergoing cardiac surgery (68) and in uremic patients (69) with platelet dysfunction to improve coagulation by increasing von Willebrand factor and by promoting the endothelial release of factor VIII (70). DDAVP appears to improve blood coagulability of patients undergoing liver transplantation in vitro, possibly by activating coagulation factors and platelets (71); however, further clinical investigation is needed.

The treatment of DIC is controversial because clinically significant DIC is rare, although localized intravascular coagulation is known to occur. Moreover, diagnosis is difficult. Generally, replacement therapy using FFP and platelets, with or without heparin (less than 5000 units), is accepted by most clinicians while the underlying cause is corrected. Administration of antithrombin III has been reported to be beneficial in modifying DIC (72).

Postoperative Management

Postoperative management of coagulation is similar to that during the intraoperative period.

Coagulation in Specific Conditions

Pediatric patients undergoing liver transplantation have been shown to have a less severe degree of coagulopathy be-

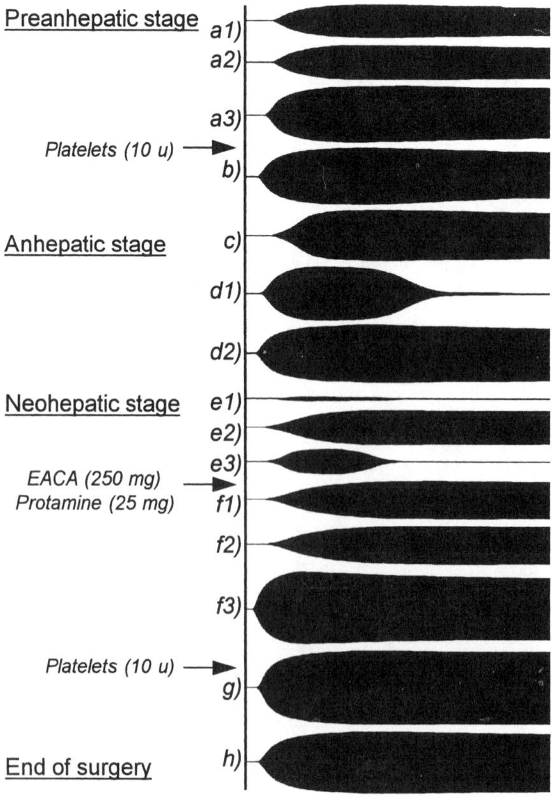

Figure 30.10. Replacement and pharmacologic therapy guided by thromboelastographic differential diagnosis. A patient with postnecrotic cirrhosis caused by hepatitis C received a fluid mixture (RBC:FFP:PlasmaLyte-A = 300:200:250 mL) throughout surgery to maintain acceptable levels of hematocrit (26–28 vol%) and coagulation factors (>30% of normal). The patient received 32 units of RBCs, 32 units of FFP, and 20 units of platelets. a1, baseline TEG showed some degree of coagulopathy with platelet count of 32,000/mm^3; comparison of a1, a2 (FFP-treated blood in vitro), and a3 (platelet-treated blood in vitro) demonstrated platelet deficiency without significant improvement with additional FFP; b, coagulation improved after transfusion of 10 units of platelets, which increased platelet count to 65,000/mm^3; c, reaction time was prolonged 10 minutes after the onset of venovenous bypass indicating the heparin effect. The heparin effect was not treated to avoid thrombosis during venovenous bypass. d1, fibrinolysis occurred 30 minutes before reperfusion; d2, inhibition of fibrinolysis is seen in blood treated with EACA in vitro. The moderate fibrinolysis was not treated to avoid thromboembolism in the presence of activation of coagulation at the end of the anhepatic stage; e1, severe coagulopathy is seen 5 minutes after reperfusion. A comparison of e1, e2 (EACA-treated blood in vitro), and e3 (protamine sulfate-treated blood in vitro) suggests the presence of severe fibrinolysis and heparin effect, and they were treated with administration of EACA (250 mg) and protamine sulfate (25 mg). f1, TEG of 30 min after reperfusion showed less than optimal recovery of coagulation. A comparison of f1, f2 (FFP-treated blood in vitro), and f3 (platelet-treated blood in vitro) indicated platelet deficiency (platelet count 40,000/mm^3). g, transfusion of 10 units of platelets improved TEG dramatically; h, coagulation deteriorated somewhat at the end of surgery because of continuous loss of clotting factors, insufficient recovery of hepatic function, and localized intravascular coagulation.

cause cholestatic disease is more common, the duration of disease is shorter, and donor organs may have better function (73). Some centers prefer minimal replacement and pharmacological therapy because overtransfusion of clotting factors has been suggested as a contributing factor for hepatic arterial thrombosis in children (74, 75).

Coagulopathy is also less severe during heterotopic liver transplantation because the surgical technique avoids the anhepatic state. The hypercoagulable state seen in patients with the Budd-Chiari syndrome may not require treatment because dilutional and pathological coagulopathy are common. Administration of a small dose of heparin (1000–2000 units), however, may be necessary postoperatively. Patients with hemophilia A or B require specific coagulation factors to increase levels to greater than 30% of the normal values during the preanhepatic and anhepatic stages. Additional treatment is unnecessary once the graft liver begins to function (76). Patients with protein C deficiency are prone to developing thromboembolism, and heparin may be given until the grafted liver begins to produce protein C. Patients with familial antithrombin III deficiency may also develop thromboembolism. They are resistant to heparin, and the administration of FFP and/or antithrombin III is required until the grafted liver begins to produce antithrombin III.

BLOOD TRANSFUSION

Hematopoiesis and Fluid Balance in Patients with End-Stage Liver Disease

Anemia (hematocrit, 25–30 vol%) is commonly observed in patients with end-stage liver disease. It is caused by a combination of iron and folic acid deficiency, impaired iron reuptake secondary to inflammatory changes in the liver, sequestration and destruction of RBC in the presence of portal hypertension and hypersplenism, and blood loss from variceal and gastrointestinal bleeding (77). Further, chronic hepatocellular disease is associated with the lack of normal hematopoietic response to anemia, and the erythroid marrow may fail to compensate for the increased destruction of RBC. In its severe form, irreversible marrow failure may occur, in which most or all RBC precursors are lost.

Ascites develop when an imbalance of Starling's forces in the hepatic sinusoids and splanchnic capillaries causes excessive lymph formation, exceeding the capacity of the thoracic duct. Consequently, excess lymph accumulates in the peritoneal space as ascites. Fluid imbalance is also complicated by hypoalbuminemia because albumin is the major determinant of colloid osmotic pressure. Normally, albumin is the most abundant protein in human serum (approximately 60% of the total protein) and 99.95% of newly formed albumin in the liver (11 mg/day/g of liver) is secreted through the hepatic sinusoidal wall into the plasma or directly into the ascitic fluid (78, 79). As a result, development of ascites causes progressive redistribution of plasma volume and contraction of circulating plasma volume. Subsequently, the diminished effective plasma volume signals the renal tubule to retain sodium and water, resulting in massive ascites and peripheral edema. Plasma volume can be increased when water retention is excessive, but patients who receive diuretics to promote urinary excretion of water and sodium may develop hypovolemia.

Hence, the goals of transfusion therapy include maintenance of normal intravascular blood volume, oxygen-carrying capacity, colloid osmotic pressure, and blood coagulability and avoidance of complications associated with massive blood transfusion.

Guideline and Mode of Blood Transfusion

In general, RBCs are transfused to maintain a hematocrit of 26–28% intraoperatively. This relatively low hematocrit was chosen to reduce RBC requirements, improve circulation in potentially hypothermic patients, and avoid thrombosis of the reconstructed vessels. A large volume of colloid and crystalloid is required to compensate for the continuous formation of ascites and third space fluid loss and to maintain colloid osmotic pressure. This goal is met by administration of a fluid mixture of RBC:FFP:PlasmaLyte-A = 300:200:250 mL (5). Administration of this fluid mixture provides relatively constant hematocrit, colloid osmotic pressure, coagulation factor level, and hydration in patients with more than 5 L of blood loss. When blood loss is less than 5 L, additional colloids (FFP or 5% albumin) or crystalloids are necessary.

Conventional pressurized transfusion devices with blood warmers have several major drawbacks when massive bleeding (more than 300 mL/min) occurs (80). Transfusion speed is limited by the low flow rate (maximum flow rate approximately equal to 130 mL/min) and time required to prepare devices and spike blood bags. Hypothermia may result from the limited blood-warming capacity of these devices (less than 25°C at a high flow rate). More importantly, operation of several devices by multiple personnel may make fine adjustments in intravascular blood volume and composition difficult, resulting in inadvertent hypovolemia or hypervolemia and variable levels of hemoglobin and coagulation factors.

Therefore, a device that delivers a large volume of premixed, prewarmed blood on demand with minimal human resources is necessary to maintain homeostasis. This goal is achieved by the use of some type of massive transfusion device or the Rapid Infusion System (Fig. 30.11) (81). The Rapid Infusion System includes a 2.5-L cardiotomy reservoir lined with a 170-μm filter, a countercurrent heat exchanger, a roller pump, a 40-μm micropore filter, two air detectors, a

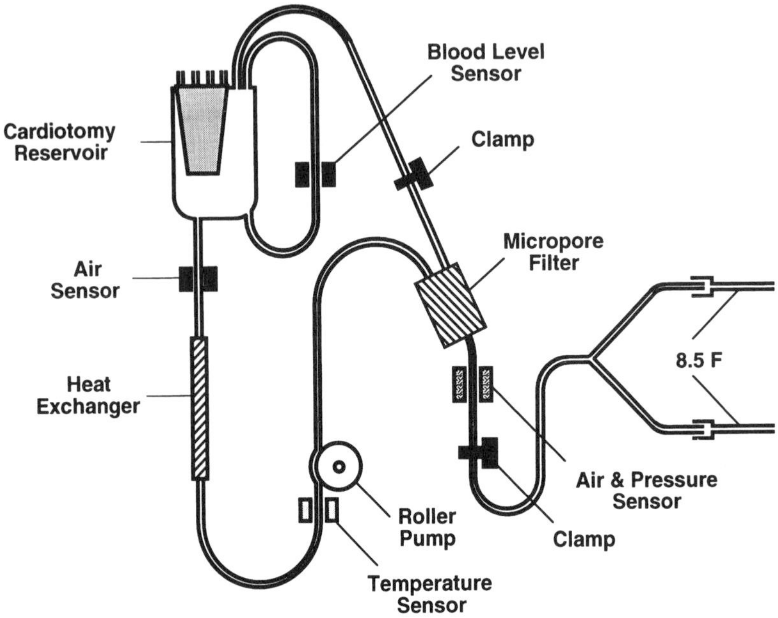

Figure 30.11. A schematic diagram of the Rapid Infusion System (Haemonetics, Inc., Braintree, MA.) (Reprinted with permission from Kang Y. The diagnosis and management of massive blood loss during liver transplantation. In: Abouna GM, Kumar MSA, White AG, eds. Organ transplantation 1990. Kluwer Academic Publishers, 1990:314, with kind permission from Kluwer Academic Publishers.)

temperature sensor, a pressure sensor, recirculation tubing, two large-bore transfusion tubes, and a control panel.

The cardiotomy reservoir has four large spikes to facilitate the rapid transfer of blood from the blood bags and removes large particles from the RBCs. RBC, FFP, and glucose-free isotonic solution (normal saline or PlasmaLyte-A) are added to the reservoir in a desirable ratio. The addition of a calcium-containing solution, which forms clots in the reservoir, should be avoided. The heat exchanger column efficiently warms the blood flowing outside the spirally grooved heat exchanger element in a countercurrent fashion. In one pass, cold blood (less than 10°C) can be warmed to greater than 33°C and warmer blood (20°C) can be warmed to greater than 36°C. The roller pump delivers blood at a rate of between 1 mL/hr and 1.5 L/min. The fluid-challenge mode delivers either 100 or 500 mL at a flow rate of 400 mL/min. The recirculation tubing returns warmed blood to the reservoir (400 mL/min) where it is mixed evenly and kept warm. The online micropore filter (40 μm) removes most of the aggregates. Two large-caliber tubes (0.188 inch, ID) are attached to two 8.5-French intravenous catheters for rapid delivery of the blood. Activation of the fluid-level sensor (fluid level less than 200 mL) and air sensor stops the roller pump, and low blood temperature (less than 36°C) and too high pressure of the system (more than 100, 200, or 300 mm Hg) slows the infusion speed. The control panel has several touch-sensitive buttons for transfusion control and displays system function and transfusion mode including total infusion volume. A rechargeable battery is installed as a backup power source and for transfusion during transportation.

The Rapid Infusion System is a safe and convenient mode of massive blood transfusion. A large volume of warmed fluid may be infused in a predetermined composition to prevent hypovolemia, hypothermia, and the fluctuation of levels of hemoglobin and coagulation factors. The system also allows precise titration of intravascular volume by evaluating the relation of pressure volume in the circulation. There have been few scientific studies on the system, however, because of the difficulty in conducting a double-blind clinical trial. Dunham et al. (82) reported the results of a randomized clinical trial of the Rapid Infusion System in 36 hypovolemic trauma patients who received approximately one blood volume of RBCs. The results of the study showed that the Rapid Infusion System group patients maintained greater body temperature and urine output and lower serum lactate level and base deficit compared with control group patients (Fig. 30.12). The authors concluded that the device is safe, preserves normothermia, improves cellular perfusion, reduces coagulopathy, and delivers fluids more rapidly to hypovolemic patients.

Potential complications of any massive transfusion device are direct complications associated with operator error and indirect complications associated with massive blood transfusion. The blood in the reservoir forms a clot when any calcium-containing solution is added, thereby losing the function of the reservoir. The filter lining the reservoir may be blocked by RBC debris and aggregates when more than 50 units of RBCs are added to the system. Hypervolemia may occur if the operator does not pay attention to the speed of blood transfusion, particularly with the continuous infusion mode. Collection of air released from the cold blood in the

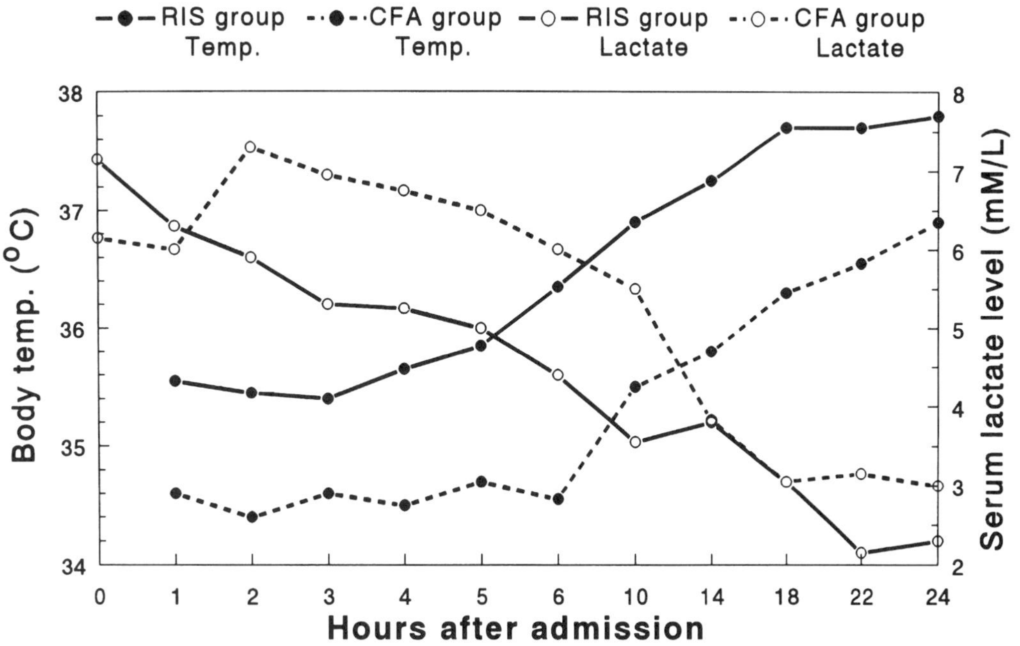

Figure 30.12. Metabolic effects of the RIS Rapid Infusion System on hypovolemic trauma patients. RIS group (n = 18) patients received blood products using the rapid infusion system and CFA group (n = 18) patients using the conventional fluid administration techniques. Reprinted with permission from Dunham CM, Belzberg H, Lyles R, et al. The rapid infusion system: a superior method for the resuscitation of hypovolemic trauma patients. Resuscitation 1991;21:207–227. With kind permission from Elsevier Science Ltd.

distal micropore filter may trigger the air sensor to make the system inoperable.

Complications of Massive Blood Transfusion

Complications are common with massive blood transfusion during liver transplantation because the volume of transfusion is greater than in traditional massive blood transfusion (one blood volume within a 24-hour period) (83), and hepatic function is negligible or absent during surgery.

Ionic hypocalcemia or citrate intoxication is a serious concern during liver transplantation because ionic hypocalcemia invariably occurs in patients with hepatic dysfunction. Inadequate hepatic clearance of citrate-calcium complex results in severe ionized hypocalcemia during liver transplantation; the serum citrate level reaches the level in the homologous RBC and has an inverse relationship to the serum ionized calcium level. Ionic hypocalcemia (0.56 mmol/L) is associated with myocardial dysfunction with decreased blood pressure, cardiac index, and stroke-work index; however, these negative hemodynamic changes have been reversed by the administration of calcium preparation (84). A prolonged Q-T interval may be seen on the electrocardiogram, but it is an unreliable indicator for ionic hypocalcemia. The ionic calcium level should be monitored hourly or more frequently and should be normalized to prevent serious hemodynamic and coagulation complications. For the treatment of hypocalcemia, $CaCl_2$ and equimolar doses of calcium gluconate are equally effective (85).

Ionic hypomagnesemia is observed during liver transplantation because citrate also binds with magnesium (86). Ionic hypomagnesemia may lead to tachycardia, hypotension, seizures, a prolonged Q-T interval, myocardial depression, or sudden death (87). Although the clinical significance of ionic hypomagnesemia during liver transplantation is unclear, $MgCl_2$ may be given if a magnesium deficiency is considered to be the cause of hemodynamic instability.

Progressive hyperkalemia (up to 7–8 mmol/L) inevitably occurs when a large volume of homologous RBCs with a high potassium content is transfused rapidly, particularly in patients with renal dysfunction (88). The degree of hyperkalemia is associated with the rate of transfusion, age of RBC, and degree of renal dysfunction. Hyperkalemia manifests as a tall peaked T wave on the electrocardiogram and bradycardia progressing to sinus arrest. Untreated hyperkalemia (more than 6 mmol/L) reduces conduction velocity and myocardial contractility by decreasing the resting membrane potential and the number of open calcium channels during depolarization (89). Hyperkalemia is treated effectively with the infusion of insulin (5–10 units) and glucose (12.5 g) within 15–30 minutes, even in the absence of hepatic function (90). The transfusion of potassium-free blood should be considered when the serum potassium level increases progressively (greater than 5.5 mmol/L) even after the administration of insulin. Blood with low potassium content is available as washed RBCs at the blood bank or it can be prepared by washing RBCs with saline solution using an autotransfusion system on site (91, 92).

Progressive metabolic acidosis is caused by acid load from the transfused blood and inadequate hepatic clearance of acidic substances. It should be treated aggressively (base deficit less than 5 mmol/L) to preserve myocardial function, tissue perfusion, and cellular respiration. The acute side effects of $NaHCO_3$ are transient myocardial depression and hypotension caused by the hyperosmolar solution. Therefore, incremental administration of $NaHCO_3$ is recommended instead of bolus (50 mmol) administration. If hypernatremia and hyperosmolality, which contribute to the development of central pontine myelinolysis, are a concern, administration of tromethamine is preferred (93); 150 mL of 0.3 molar tromethamine solution is equivalent to 50 mmol of $NaHCO_3$.

Intraoperative Autotransfusion

Intraoperative autotransfusion has been used during liver transplantation as in other major surgical procedures (94–96), and the potential complications of autotransfusion during liver transplantation such as the effects of residual anticoagulants, contamination of tissue thromboplastin, dissemination of infection, electrolyte imbalance, and renal dysfunction caused by hemoglobinuria have been addressed (97). In a recent two-phase study, the biochemical, hematological, coagulatory, and bacteriological characteristics of autotransfusion were investigated (98).

In this study, acid-citrate-dextrose solution was used to anticoagulate collected blood because of the ease of monitoring citrate level and treatment of hypocalcemia, and the blood was washed with 1 L of PlasmaLyte-A solution. The washing cycle of the system removed most of the contaminants, including bilirubin, citrate, potassium, fragments of RBCs, coagulation factors (I, II, and VIII), platelets, FDP, and fibrin monomers. Plasma-free hemoglobin decreased after washing (from 678 ± 332 to 264 ± 127 mg/dL), and infusion of the washed blood (500 mL) increased plasma-free hemoglobin to an insignificant level (from 32.4 ± 12.0 to 40.4 ± 17.2 mg/dL). The effects of autotransfusion on patients undergoing liver transplantation appear to be negligible; the levels of coagulation factors and FDP, platelet count, ELT, FDP, fibrin monomers, and TEG variables remained unchanged, and postoperative renal function was not affected.

In a qualitative bacteriological study, rare coagulase (−)*Staphylococcus epidermidis* was found in 6 of 30 washed blood samples, and the blood cultures of all patients were negative. The results of a quantitative bacteriological study in 15 patients showed skin culture positive for coagulase (−)*Staphylococci* in two patients, washed blood positive for coagulase (−)*Staphylococci* in three patients, and air positive for coagulase (−)*Staphylococci* or *Bacillus* sp. in three patients. One of three patients whose washed blood contained coagulase (−)*Staphylococci* had the same bacteria on the skin and the other two had the same bacteria in the culture of air from the mock reservoir. Therefore, the source of contamination was most likely environmental. The bacterial count was rare (less than two colonies) in all washed blood samples. Two of three positive air cultures each contained two colonies of coagulase (−)*S. epidermidis,* and the third contained three. The culture containing *Bacillus* sp. had 12 colonies. This bacterial contamination is not surprising, because blood collected during cardiac surgery contained similar types of bacteria (99, 100), and about 5% of bacteria remained even after washing the blood with 10 L of fluid (101). Bacterial contamination associated with autotransfusion does not appear to pose a significant threat for postoperative infection in patients who receive prophylactic broad-spectrum antibiotics as supported by sterile blood cultures for 1 week postoperatively. Autotransfusion should be avoided in patients with a source of malignancy and infection, however, such as peritonitis, abscess, or recent abdominal surgery. Additionally, it is recommended that autotransfusion begin after ascites are drained to avoid contamination of thromboplastin and end before biliary reconstruction to avoid contamination of gastrointestinal contents.

KIDNEY AND PANCREAS TRANSPLANTATION

Blood transfusion issues relevant to kidney and pancreas transplantation are combined in this section. Most pancreas recipients have diabetic nephropathy, and increased capillary permeability may be the only additional observation in these patients (102).

COAGULATION IN PATIENTS WITH END-STAGE RENAL DISEASE

Bleeding from mucous membranes is the most common hemorrhagic complication in patients with end-stage renal disease. Other complications include gastrointestinal bleeding, hemorrhagic pericardial effusions, or intracranial hemorrhage (103, 104). In general, the levels of coagulation factors are well maintained, and platelet count and survival are within the normal range.

The most characteristic change in coagulation is prolonged bleeding time, which can be reversed by dialysis (105). Prolonged bleeding time appears to be associated with platelet dysfunction, and several mechanisms have been proposed. It is known that the availability of platelet factor 3 and platelet retention to glass bead columns are reduced (106). Certain dialyzable plasma factors may impair platelet-endothelium interaction; guanidinosuccinic acid, phenol, and phenolic acid from the serum of uremic patients have been found to inhibit platelet aggregation (107, 108) and middle molecules (500–3000 Da) purified from the serum of uremic patients to inhibit the release of serotonin from platelets by inhibiting glucose utilization (109). The increased calcium ions in platelets resulting from increased parathyroid hormonal activity may adversely affect platelet function (110). In addition, an imbalance between the reduced production of procoagulants (thromboxane A_2) by platelets and enhanced formation of antiaggregatory endoperoxides (prostacyclin, prostaglandin E_2, and prostaglandin I_2) by vessel walls has been shown to contribute to the bleeding (111, 112). Other contributing factors may include modified platelet membrane receptors for von Willebrand factor binding and altered platelet production of β-thromboglobulin, platelet factor 4 (antiheparin), and platelet growth factor (113).

Hemodialysis affects coagulation because the residual heparin effect can increase the bleeding tendency. The heparin effect is a lesser concern with regional heparinization, however, in which heparin is administered as blood leaves the patient and neutralized as blood is returned. Repeated hemodialysis may cause thrombosis and the activation of fibrinolysis (114). The thrombotic tendency appears to be caused by recurrent platelet activation, imbalance between platelets and vascular prostaglandin, activation of fibrinolysis by the release of TPA from endothelial cells, and consumption of PAI (115). The release of TPA has been shown to be caused by complement activation (116), platelet activation (117), heparin administration (118), and tissue hypoxia (119). Fibrinolysis does not appear to be caused by the dialyzer, because the cross-linked FDP level is unaffected by hemodialysis and the coagulation profile of arterial blood is similar to that of venous blood.

MANAGEMENT OF COAGULATION

Bleeding time is considered to be the best screening test, because it correlates with clinical bleeding (105, 112). Dialysis is the treatment of choice for a prolonged bleeding time. Additionally, platelets may be administered to patients with a markedly prolonged bleeding time, and cryoprecipitate may reduce bleeding time in certain patients (120). The administration of DDAVP may also shorten bleeding time, possibly by improving the binding of von Willebrand factor with platelet membranes (121). The residual heparin effect from hemodialysis can be detected by determination of the activated clotting time (ACT), APTT, or TEG and reversed by protamine sulfate (25–50 mg), although rebound heparinization can occur in some patients (122). Antiplatelet agents (prostacyclin and sulfinpyrazone) may be used for patients with long-term dialysis to prevent activation of platelets and to maintain patency of the shunts (123, 124), although the therapy may result in bleeding when platelet dysfunction is present (125).

Bleeding is not a clinical concern during transplantation because the patient received dialysis before surgery and surgical bleeding is limited. Thrombocytopenia is the most common coagulation defect during and after surgery and is caused by hyperacute or acute rejection. Antiplatelet agents (prostacyclin) and immunosuppressants may be effective in treating rejection-related thrombocytopenia (126). In severe cases of thrombocytopenia with rejection, allograft nephrectomy improves thrombocytopenia. Platelet dysfunction may also occur from depletion of serotonin from platelets (127), activation of platelets by the circulating immune complex, and development of microvascular thrombosis (128).

BLOOD TRANSFUSION

End-stage renal disease is complicated by significant anemia (hematocrit less than 25 vol%). Anemia develops when creatinine exceeds 3 mg/dL and is caused by decreased erythropoietin production with the loss of renal mass, bone marrow depression, shortened RBC survival secondary to hemolysis from oxidizing drugs and microangiopathic lesions, iron deficiency with blood loss, decreased iron absorption due to phosphate binding antacids, deficiency of folic acid and vitamin B_{12} and B_6 and other proteins, secondary hyperparathyroidism, and hemodialysis-induced platelet dysfunction (129). Generally, hematocrit 24–28 vol% is considered satisfactory, because kidney transplantation patients tolerate anemia quite well by increasing the level of 2,3-diphosphoglycerate and cardiac output and by decreasing oxygen-hemoglobin affinity. In addition, blood transfusion may induce the formation of alloantibodies to leukocyte antigens (130), which may lead to febrile nonhemolytic reaction and hyperacute rejection or poor survival of the graft kidney (131). Therefore, blood transfusion is minimized in these patients, and frozen-deglycerolized RBCs containing a minimal volume of white blood cells is administered to reduce the development of alloantibodies.

It was shown, however, that graft survival in patients who received frozen-deglycerolized RBCs was better than in patients who did not receive RBC transfusion (134). This observation has been confirmed by other investigators, and it appears that maximal benefit is achieved when 2–5 units of RBCs are transfused approximately 3 weeks to 6 months before transplantation (135). The mechanism for this protective effect is still unclear, although it may be associated with patient selection or modulation of immune response (136). The patient selection theory proposes that a patient who develops multiple cytotoxic antibodies after homologous blood transfusion is likely to receive a better matching graft and to have improved graft survival. On the other hand, blood transfusion-induced changes in T-cell mediated regulatory and effector mechanisms may modulate immune response by nonspecific suppression of major histocompatibility complex (MHC) reactivity and lymphocyte proliferative response to antigens (137), proliferation of cells directed against antigens expressed by transfused cells (138), overloading of the reticuloendothelial system (139), and induction of anti-idiotypic antibodies against T lymphocytes (140).

LUNG TRANSPLANTATION

Lung transplantation has become a viable therapy for patients with irreversible pulmonary disease of various etiologies. Initially, combined heart and lung transplantation was the only option for such patients, but with improved surgical technique, scarcity of suitable heart-lung donors, and the ability to benefit several recipients from one donor, there has been a decrease in the number of combined heart and lung transplants performed and a concomitant increase in the number of single and double lung transplants. As of December 1993, the Registry of the International Society for Heart and Lung Transplantation has recorded 1567 combined heart and lung transplants, 1943 single lung transplants, and 943 bilateral or double lung transplants (141).

BLEEDING AND COAGULATION IN PATIENTS FOR HEART-LUNG OR LUNG TRANSPLANTATION

Perioperative bleeding can be a major complication of either combined heart and lung transplantation or isolated lung transplantation, and the frequency and severity of bleeding depend on a combination of factors (Table 30.2).

TABLE 30.2. FACTORS AFFECTING THE FREQUENCY AND SEVERITY OF PERIOPERATIVE BLEEDING

1. Type of intrathoracic transplantation
2. Underlying disease state
3. Requirement for cardiopulmonary bypass
4. Preoperative medications
5. Preoperative hepatic function
6. Previous intrathoracic surgery

Combined heart and lung transplantation is commonly performed for patients with end-stage cardiopulmonary disease, particularly those with complex congenital heart disease and Eisenmenger's syndrome and those with primary pulmonary hypertension with right heart failure. It was not uncommon to experience extensive perioperative bleeding, multiple blood product transfusion, compromised function of the transplanted lung, the development of multiorgan failure, and ultimate death (142). Perioperative bleeding was a major cause of early postoperative morbidity and mortality in early series (143–145) and accounted for 36% of intraoperative deaths and for 8% of total deaths in one large series (146). Therefore, control of hemostasis during either combined heart and lung transplantation or isolated lung transplantation requiring cardiopulmonary bypass (CPB) represents another challenge in these already demanding procedures.

Causes for bleeding during combined heart and lung transplantation are several. These patients are prone to developing pulmonary thromboembolic events because of their disease state, and concomitant polycythemia and preoperative medications might include aspirin, dipyridamole, and oral anticoagulants such as warfarin. In the past, because of the emergent nature of the transplant procedure, these drugs would often have been ingested just before the operation. Presently, anticoagulants are being administered more selectively. Right ventricular dysfunction or failure caused by long-standing pulmonary arterial hypertension may result in hepatic congestion leading to diminished synthetic function and decreased coagulant levels. Because of chronic hypoxemia, there are large posterior mediastinal and pleural collateral blood vessels, and prolonged CPB was often required for dissection and control of these vessels.

Modifications of the surgical technique used during combined heart and lung transplantation include limited dissection of the posterior mediastinum, increased surgical stapling, use of the argon beam coagulator, and use of fibrin glue. These have all led to better posterior mediastinal hemostasis and a significant reduction in bleeding and subsequent transfusion requirements (142, 147). The recent introduction of the "clamshell" incision, a bilateral thoracosternotomy (148), further facilitates exposure and takedown of adhesions. Although a previous sternotomy or thoracotomy was once thought to be an absolute contraindication, presently, patients with previous intrathoracic surgery are considered on a case by case basis. With the improved surgical technique and pharmacological drugs to be mentioned below, exsanguinating hemorrhage during combined heart and lung transplantation is becoming less of a problem at experienced centers (149).

Patients with either primary pulmonary hypertension or Eisenmenger's syndrome with a correctable intracardiac defect such as an atrial septal defect or patent ductus arteriosus may receive only a single lung transplant. They require CPB for correction of the intracardiac defect and subsequent lung transplantation. They resemble the patients for combined heart and lung transplantation but likely have less severe right heart dysfunction that could contribute to a perioperative coagulopathy. Patients with septic pulmonary disease such as cystic fibrosis or bronchiectasis may undergo bilateral sequential lung transplants, in most cases without the need for CPB. Because of repeated infections, these patients are likely to have pleural adhesions that may bleed. The greatest number of patients awaiting lung transplantation are the chronic obstructive pulmonary disease patients, and they are likely to receive only a single lung transplant. CPB is not necessary in most of these patients. Bleeding is not often an issue, but repeated chest tube insertions for pneumothoraces and the recent introduction of thorascopic pulmonary reduction procedures for bullous disease can lead to pleural adhesions. Therefore, the degree of bleeding is greatest in combined heart and lung transplantation, next in single lung transplantation and double lung transplantation requiring CPB, and least in single lung transplantation done without CPB.

Effects of CPB on the hemostatic mechanisms are numerous and complicated and include but are not limited to contact activation through factor XII, activation of the complement cascade, leukocyte activation, quantitative and qualitative platelet defects, fibrinolysis, hemodilution, hypothermia, and the effects of heparin and its reversal with protamine. Discussion of these effects is beyond the scope of this chapter and is dealt with elsewhere. The effect of CPB on pulmonary function after any cardiothoracic procedure remains unclear but clinically ranges from frank pulmonary edema or "pump lung," to pulmonary infiltrates, to experimentally measured increased interstitial lung water. Although the incidence of severe pulmonary dysfunction has fortunately decreased in recent years because of improvements in CPB materials and techniques, subtle changes in the microvascular permeability of the pulmonary endothelium still occur. Proposed mechanisms have included complement activation with subsequent leukocyte and platelet activation (150).

Ischemia and subsequent reperfusion are known to damage the endothelium of all organs. The pulmonary endothelial permeability in several transplanted lungs was demonstrated to be greater than that of healthy volunteers, but not uniformly (151). The effects of CPB on early allograft dysfunction in a large series were recently reported. Patients undergoing lung transplantation requiring CPB had lower arterial/alveolar oxygen tension ratios, more severe pulmonary infiltrates on chest roentgenograms, prolonged intubation, and a slightly worse graft survival and patient survival compared with patients who did not require CPB for their lung transplantation (152). Not surprisingly, there was a significant difference in the amount of transfused blood products between the two groups. The use of a heparin-coated CPB circuit combined with reduced systemic heparinization did not improve early graft function in a canine model of single lung transplantation (153).

MONITORING OF COAGULATION

Preoperative evaluation of patients undergoing intrathoracic transplantation is typically extensive and includes evaluation of right heart function; assessment of hepatic congestion and renal dysfunction, both of which could compromise hemostatic mechanisms (154); and a baseline coagulation profile consisting of platelet count, PT, and APTT. Bleeding time, fibrinogen, and fibrin/fibrinogen degradation products are not normally obtained. However, the value of these blood clotting tests in predicting postoperative mediastinal drainage in 897 patients undergoing cardiac surgical procedures (coronary operations, valve replacement, and reoperative procedures) requiring CPB was shown to be low (155). The value of these clotting tests in predicting perioperative hemorrhage during lung transplantation remains unstudied.

TRANSFUSION AND MANAGEMENT OF COAGULATION

Preoperative Management

Because of the emergent nature of lung transplantation, autologous predonation by the patient is of limited value. The different patient groups will also vary in their baseline hemoglobin levels. Typically, patients scheduled for combined heart and lung transplantation are polycythemic, patients with chronic obstructive pulmonary disease have normal or slightly elevated hemoglobin, whereas septic patients (i.e., cystic fibrosis and bronchiectasis) are often chronically anemic. Although erythropoietin has been used safely in other cardiac patients (156), its use in patients undergoing lung transplantation has yet to be tested. The administration of vitamin K to antagonize a warfarin effect will be of limited immediate value but may be of benefit in the postoperative period.

Intraoperative Management

The complications and risks involved with blood product transfusion are outlined elsewhere and include possible fluid overload, nonallergic reactions, hemolytic transfusion reactions, and transmission of infectious agents such as viral hepatitis, human immunodeficiency virus, and cytomegalovirus (CMV). Although these are concerns in any patient, the perioperative management of lung transplant patients requires judicious fluid administration (157) and the avoidance of CMV infection.

The preoperative collection of autologous blood is often possible in the patients with complex congenital heart disease because of their marked polycythemia associated with chronic hypoxemia. Several units of blood can be collected with normovolemic hemodilution, bringing the hemoglobin down to a relatively "normal" level before initiation of CPB. Another option is to sequester blood while on CPB. In either case, the autologous blood is reinfused after heparin neutralization with protamine. The intraoperative collection of autologous blood is often not possible in the chronically anemic patients and of limited value in the uncomplicated single lung transplants where bleeding is not an issue.

The efficacy of autologous platelet plasmapheresis during routine cardiac surgical procedures has yet to be established, likely because of the inability to obtain large platelet volumes in a timely fashion (158, 159). Because of the emergent nature of lung transplantation, autologous platelet plasmapheresis is presently of limited value. One of the mainstays of blood conservation methods remains the use of intraoperative salvage by means of a cell-saving device with reinfusion of the washed RBCs.

After discontinuation of CPB, protamine is administered to neutralize the heparin. Various methods to determine the protamine dosage are used, including a dose matched to the total heparin administered or a dose determined by a measurement of residual heparin concentration. Whatever method is used, a return to baseline ACT is the goal. Surgical hemostasis should be attempted, and if bleeding persists, clotting tests including platelet count, PT, APTT, fibrinogen, and fibrin/fibrinogen degradation products can be obtained to help guide blood product therapy. The use of TEG with algorithms for interpretation has been effective in guiding therapy during liver transplantation and has been advocated to guide replacement therapy during cardiac procedures (160), but it is not uniformly accepted (161, 162).

Replacement therapy is usually with blood components. Modified whole blood is sometimes available and would be indicated when the combination of red cells and plasma is expected. Transfusion of packed RBCs is used to improve oxygen delivery and would typically be indicated to maintain the hemoglobin level between 7 and 10 g/dL in the operative lung transplant patient. The lowest acceptable hemoglobin is determined by patient need and the operative team. Lung transplant patients receive leukocyte-depleted blood to attenuate human leukocyte antigen alloimmunization and possible leukocyte-mediated lung injury and CMV seronegative blood to minimize the occurrence of CMV pneumonitis. Platelets are administered for persistent bleeding, typically after a prolonged CPB run with a normal or near-normal ACT. A measured platelet count may not indicate a qualitative platelet defect. Platelets can be administered as pooled random-donor platelets or as a single-donor apheresis product. Transfusion of FFP is ideally dictated by a measured PT with administration of FFP if the PT is 1.5 times the laboratory's normal value, in the presence of clinical bleeding. In the case of massive bleeding with unavailability of laboratory data, FFP is sometimes transfused in combination with RBC. Transfusion of cryoprecipitate is limited to patients with massive bleeding and is governed by a fibrinogen concentration, typically less than 100 mg/dL.

Pharmacological agents are sometimes used as prophylaxis to reduce perioperative bleeding. These include the antifibrinolytics, EACA and tranexamic acid, and platelet agents such as dipyridamole, DDAVP, and aprotinin. Most studies of these agents have been on more routine cardiac patients at increased risk for bleeding. These include patients undergoing "redo" cardiac procedures, patients with preexisting coagulopathy, and patients on antiplatelet or anticoagulant drugs. The results of studies are often conflicting because patient populations are often dissimilar between studies and no uniform method is available to assess efficacy (163). The antifibrinolytic drugs, EACA and tranexamic acid, clearly influence coagulation and the hemostatic mechanisms during cardiac procedures using CPB, typically with a decrease in postoperative chest tube drainage and sometimes transfusion requirements (164, 165). Aprotinin has been shown to be efficacious in decreasing chest tube drainage and transfused blood products (166, 167). A meta-analysis of prophylactic drug treatment in the prevention of postoperative bleeding found that DDAVP, antifibrinolytic drugs, and aprotinin were all effective in decreasing postoperative chest tube drainage; aprotinin and the antifibrinolytics were effective in decreasing the amount of transfused blood products. However, only aprotinin was effective in increasing the percentage of patients that did not receive any transfused blood products. None of the prophylactic drug therapies had an effect on mortality (168). A small series of patients undergoing combined heart and lung transplantation and double lung transplantation appeared to benefit from the administration of aprotinin by decreased transfused blood products and decreased chest tube drainage (169). A large, randomized, placebo-controlled study needs to be done to confirm these results.

REFERENCES

1. Kang Y, Aggarwal S, Freeman JA. Update on anesthesia for adult liver transplantation. Transplant Proc 1987;19(Suppl. 3):7–12.
2. Starzl TE, Groth CG, Makowka L. Clio chirurgica: liver transplantation. Austin: Silvergirl, 1988.
3. Kang Y, Aggarwal S, Freeman JA. Intraoperative mortality during liver transplantation. Transplant Proc 1988;20(Suppl. 1):600.

4. Ballard HS, Marcus AJ. Platelet aggregation in portal cirrhosis. Arch Intern Med 1976;136:316–319.
5. Kang YG, Martin DJ, Marquez J, et al. Intraoperative changes in blood coagulation and thrombelastographic monitoring in liver transplantation. Anesth Analg 1985;64:888–896.
6. Stein SF, Harker LA. Kinetic and functional studies of platelets, fibrinogen, and plasminogen in patients with hepatic cirrhosis. J Lab Clin Med 1982;99:217–230.
7. Aster RH. Pooling of platelets in the spleen: Role in the pathogenesis of "hypersplenic" thrombocytopenia. J Clin Invest 1966;45:645–657.
8. Canoso RT, Hutton RA, Deykin D. The hemostatic defect of chronic liver disease. Gastroenterology 1979;76:540–547.
9. Lindenbaum J. Folate and vitamin B12 deficiencies in alcoholism. Semin Hematol 1980;17:119–129.
10. Cowan DH. Effect of alcoholism on hemostasis. Semin Hematol 1980; 17:137–147.
11. Thomas DP, Ream VJ, Stuart RK. Platelet aggregation in patients with Laennec's cirrhosis of the liver. N Engl J Med 1967;276:1344–1348.
12. Rubin MH, Weston MJ, Bullock G, et al. Abnormal platelet function and ultrastructure in fulminant hepatic failure. Q J Med 1977;46:339–352.
13. Owen JS, Hutton RA, Day RC, Bruckdorfer KR, McIntyre N. Platelet lipid composition and platelet aggregation in human liver disease. J Lipid Res 1981;22:423–430.
14. Karpatkin KS, Freedman ML. Hypersplenic thrombocytopenia differentiated from increased peripheral destruction by platelet volume. Ann Intern Med 1978;89:200–203.
15. Martinez J, Palascak JE, Kwasniak D. Abnormal sialic acid content of the dysfibrinogenemia associated with liver disease. J Clin Invest 1978;61:535–538.
16. Green G, Thomson JM, Dymock IW, Poller L. Abnormal fibrin polymerization in liver disease. Br J Haematol 1976;34:425–439.
17. Narvaiza JM, Fernàndez J, Cuesta B, Pàramo JA, Rocha E. Role of sialic acid in acquired dysfibrinogenemia associated with liver cirrhosis. Ricerca Clin Lab 1986;16:563–568.
18. Green AJ, Ratnoff OD. Elevated antihemophilic factor (AHF, factor VIII) procoagulant activity and AHF-like antigen in alcoholic cirrhosis of the liver. J Lab Clin Med 1974;83:189–197.
19. Colman RW, Rubin RN. Blood coagulation. In: The liver: biology and pathobiology. Arias IM, Jakoby WB, Popper H, et al. eds. New York: Raven Press, 1988:1033–1042.
20. Grossi CE, Rousselot LM, Panke WF. Coagulation defects in patients with cirrhosis of the liver undergoing porta-systemic shunts. Am J Surg 1962;104:512–517.
21. Straub PW. Diffuse intravascular coagulation in liver disease. Semin Thromb Hemost 1977;4:29–39.
22. Knot EAR, Drijfhout HR, ten Cate JW, et al. α_2-Antiplasmin inhibitor metabolism in patients with liver cirrhosis. J Lab Clin Med 1985;105: 353–358.
23. Saito H, Goodnough LT, Boyle JM, Heimburger N. Reduced histidine-rich glycoprotein levels in plasmas of patients with advanced liver cirrhosis: possible implications for enhanced fibrinolysis. Am J Med 1982;73:179–182.
24. Fletcher AP, Biederman O, Moore D, Alkjaersig N, Sherry S. Abnormal plasminogen-plasmin system activity (fibrinolysis) in patients with hepatic cirrhosis: its cause and consequences. J Clin Invest 1964;43: 681–695.
25. Tytgat G, Collen D, De Vreker R, Verstraete M. Investigators on the fibrinolytic system in liver cirrhosis. Acta Haematol (Basel) 1968; 40:265–274.
26. Seligsohn U, Shani M, Ramot B, Adam A, Sheba C. Dubin-Johnson syndrome in Israel. II. Association with factor-VII deficiency. Q J Med 1970;39:569–584.
27. Seligsohn U, Shani M, Ramot B. Gilbert syndrome and factor VII deficiency [letter]. Lancet 1970;1:1398.
28. Groth CG, Pechet L, Starzl TE. Coagulation during and after orthotopic transplantation of the human liver. Arch Surg 1969;98:31–34.
29. Von Kaulla KN, Kaye H, Von Kaulla E, Marchioro TL, Starzl TE. Changes blood coagulation, before and after hepatectomy or transplantation in dogs and man. Arch Surg 1966;92:71–79.
30. Flute PT, Rake MO, Williams R, Seaman MJ, Calne RY. Liver transplantation in man. IV. Haemorrhage and thrombosis. Br Med J 1969;3: 20–23.
31. Lewis JH, Bontempo FA, Awad SA, et al. Liver transplantation: intraoperative changes in coagulation factors in 100 first transplants. Hepatology 1989;9:710–714.
32. Owen CA Jr, Rettke SR, Bowie EJW, et al. Hemostatic evaluation of patients undergoing liver transplantation. Mayo Clin Proc 1987;62:761–772.
33. Porte RJ, Bontempo FA, Knot EA, Lewis JH, Kang YG, Starzl TE. Systemic effects of tissue plasminogen activator-associated fibrinolysis and its relation to thrombin generation in orthotopic liver transplantation. Transplantation 1989;47:978–984.
34. Virji MA, Aggarwal S, Kang Y. Alterations in plasminogen activator and plasminogen activator inhibitor levels during liver transplantation. Transplant Proc 1989;21(Suppl. 3):3540–3541.
35. Kratzer MAA, Dieterich J, Denecke H, Knedel M. Hemostatic variables and blood loss during orthotopic human liver transplantation. Transplant Proc 1991;23:1906–1911.
36. Kang Y, Lewis JH, Navalgund A, et al. Epsilon-aminocaproic acid for treatment of fibrinolysis during liver transplantation. Anesthesiology 1987;66:766–773.
37. Himmelreich G, Dooijewaard G, Breinl P, et al. Changes in urokinase-type plasminogen activator in orthotopic liver transplantation. Semin Thromb Hemost 1993;19:311–314.
38. Lewis JH, Bontempo FA, Ragni MV, Starzl TE. Antithrombin III during liver transplantation. Transplant Proc 1989;21:3543–3544.
39. Böhgmig HJ. The coagulation disorder of orthotopic hepatic transplantation. Semin Thromb Hemost 1977;4:57–82.
40. Riess H, Jochum M, Machliedt W, et al. Possible role of extracellular released phagocyte proteinase in the coagulation disorder during liver transplantation. Transplantation 1991;52:482–490.
41. Palareti G, Legagni C, Maccaferri M, et al. Coagulation and fibrinolysis in liver transplantation: the role of the recipient's disease and the use of antithrombin III concentrates. Haemostasis 1991;21:68–76.
42. Hutchinson DE, Genton E, Porter KA, et al. Platelet changes following clinical and experimental hepatic homotransplantation. Arch Surg 1968; 97:27–33.
43. Homatas J, Wasantapruek S, von Kaulla E, von Kaulla KN, Eisenman B. Clotting abnormalities following orthotopic and heterotopic transplantation of marginally preserved pig livers. Acta Hepato Splenol 1969;2:14–27.
44. Porte RJ. Coagulation and fibrinolysis in orthotopic liver transplantation: current views and insights. Semin Thromb Hemost 1993;19: 191–196.
45. Schlam SW, Terpstra JL, Achterberg JR, et al. Orthotopic liver transplantation: an experimental study on mechanisms of hemorrhagic diathesis and thrombosis. Surgery 1975;78:400–507.
46. Himmelreich GK, Hundt K, Neuhaus P, Roissant R, Riess H. Decreased platelet aggregation after reperfusion in orthotopic liver transplantation. Transplantation 1992;53:582–586.

47. Ferrara A, MacArthur JD, Wright HK, Modlin IM, McMillen MA. Hypothermia and acidosis worsen coagulopathy in the patient requiring massive transfusion. Am J Surg 1990;160:515–518.
48. Zuckerman L, Cohen L, Vagher JP, Woodward E, Caprini JA. Comparison of thrombelastography with common coagulation tests. Thromb Haemost 1981;46:752–756.
49. Kang YG. Monitoring and treatment of coagulation. In: Winter PM, Kang YG, eds. Hepatic transplantation. Anesthetic and perioperative management. New York: Praeger, 1986:151–173.
50. Blanchard RA, Furie BC, Jorgensen M, Kruger, BA, Furie B. Acquired vitamin K-dependent carboxylation deficiency in liver disease. N Engl J Med 1981;305:242–248.
51. Lewis JH, Doyle AP. Effect of epsilon aminocaproic acid on coagulation and fibrinolytic mechanism. JAMA 1964;188:56–63.
52. Munoz SJ, Ballas BE, Moritz MM, et al. Perioperative management of fulminant and subfulminant hepatic failure with therapeutic plasmapheresis. Transplant Proc 1989;21:3535–3536.
53. Azad SC, Kratzer MAA, Groh J, Welte M, Haller M, Pratschke E. Intraoperative monitoring and postoperative reevaluation of hemostasis in orthotopic liver transplantation. Semin Thromb Hemost 1993;19: 233–237.
54. Ickz B, Pradier O, Degroote F, et al. Effect of two different dosages of aprotinin on perioperative blood loss during liver transplantation. Semin Thromb Hemost 1993;19:300–301.
55. Kang Y, Gelman S. Liver transplantation. In: Gelman S, ed. Anesthesia and organ transplantation. Philadelphia: WB Saunders, 1986:139–186.
56. Weber T, Marino IR, Kang YG, Esquivel CD, Starzl TE, Duquesnoy J. Intraoperative blood transfusions in highly immunized patients undergoing orthotopic liver transplantation. Transplantation 1989;47: 797–801.
57. Dutcher JP, Schiffer CA, Aisner J, Wiernik. Alloimmunization following platelet transfusion: the absence of dose-response relationship. Blood 1981;57:395–398.
58. McNicol GP, Fletcher AP, Alkjaersig N, Sherry S. The absorption, distribution, and excretion of e-aminocaproic acid following oral or intravenous administration to man. J Lab Clin Med 1962;59:15–24.
59. Kang Y. Coagulation and liver transplantation. Transplant Proc 1993; 25:2001–2005.
60. Rake MO, Flute PT, Parnell G, Williams R. Intravascular coagulation in acute hepatic necrosis. Lancet 1970;1:533–537.
61. Carlier M, Veyckemans F, Scholtes JL, et al. JB. Anesthesia for pediatric hepatic transplantation: experience of 33 cases. Transplant Proc 1987;19:3333–3337.
62. Klinck JR, Boylan JF, Sandler AN, et al. Tranexamic acid prophylaxis during liver transplantation: a randomized controlled study [abstract]. Hepatology 1993;18:728.
63. Neuhaus P, Bechstein WO, Lefebre B, Blumhardt G, Slama K. Effect of aprotinin on intraoperative bleeding and fibrinolysis in liver transplantation. Lancet 1989;2:924–925.
64. Mallett SV, Cox D, Burroughs AK, Rolles K. Aprotinin and reduction of blood loss and transfusion requirements in orthotopic liver transplantation [letter]. Lancet 1990;336:886–887.
65. Grosse H, Lobbes W, Frambach M, von Broen O, Ringe B, Barthels M. The use of high dose of aprotinin in liver transplantation: the influence of fibrinolysis and blood loss. Thromb Res 1991;63:287–297.
66. Himmlreich G, Kierzek B, Neuhaus P, Slamer KJ, Riess H. Fibrinolytic changes and the influence of the early perfusate in orthotopic liver transplantation with intraoperative aprotinin treatment. Transplant Proc 1991;23:1936–1937.
67. Kang Y, De Wolf AM, Aggarwal S. In vitro study of the effects of aprotinin on coagulation during orthotopic liver transplantation. Transplant Proc 1991;23:1934–1935.
68. Anderson TLG, Solem JO, Tengborn L, Vinge E. Effects of desmopressin acetate on platelet aggregation, von Willebrand factor, and blood loss after cardiac surgery with extracorporeal circulation. Circulation 1990;81:872–878.
69. Mannuccio PM, Vicente V, Vianello L, et al. Controlled trial of desmopressin in liver cirrhosis and other conditions associated with a prolonged bleeding time. Blood 1986;67:1148–1153.
70. Mannucci PM. Desmopressin: a nontransfusional form of treatment for congenital and acquired bleeding disorders. Blood 1988;72:1449–1455.
71. Kang Y, Scott V, De Wolf A, Roskoph J, Aggarwal S. In vitro effects of DDAVP during liver transplantation. Transplant Proc 1993;25: 1821–1822.
72. Rake MO, Shilkin KB, Winch J, Lewis LM, Williams R. Early and intensive therapy of intravascular coagulation in acute liver failure. Lancet 1971;2:1215–1218.
73. Kang Y, Borland LM, Picone J, Martin LK. Intraoperative coagulation changes in children undergoing liver transplantation. Anesthesiology 1989;71:44–47.
74. Massaferro V, Esquivel CO, Makowka L, et al. Hepatic artery thrombosis after pediatric liver transplantation: medical or surgical event? Transplantation 1989;47:971–977.
75. Esquivel CO, Koneru B, Karrer F, et al. Liver transplantation before one year of age. J Pediatr 1987;110:545–548.
76. Bontempo FA, Lewis JH, Gorenc TJ, et al. Liver transplantation in hemophilia A. Blood 1987;69:1721–1724.
77. Douglas SE, Adamson JW. The anemia of chronic disorders: studies of marrow regulation and iron metabolism. Blood 1975;45:55.
78. Kelman, L, Saunders SJ, Frith L, Wicht S, Corrigal A. Effects of dietary protein restriction on albumin synthesis, albumin catabolism, and the plasma aminogram. Am J Clin Nutr 1972;25:1174.
79. Zimmon DS, Oratz M, Kessler R, Schreiber SS, Rothschild MA. Albumin to ascites: demonstration of a direct pathway bypassing the systemic circulation. J Clin Invest 1967;48:2074.
80. Dula DJ, Muller HA, Donovan JW. Flow rate variance of commonly used IV infusion techniques. J Trauma 1981;21:480–482.
81. Sassano JJ. The rapid infusion system. In: Winter PM, Kang YG, eds. Hepatic transplantation: anesthetic and perioperative management. New York: Praeger, 1986:120–134.
82. Dunham CM, Belzberg H, Lyles R, et al. The rapid infusion system: a superior method for the resuscitation of hypovolemic trauma patients. Resuscitation 1991;21:207–227.
83. Holland, PV. The diagnosis and management of transfusion reactions and other adverse effects of transfusion. In: Petz LD, Swisher SN, eds. Clinical practice of transfusion medicine. 2nd ed. New York: Churchill Livingstone, 1989:713–736.
84. Marquez J, Martin D, Kang YG, et al. Cardiovascular depression secondary to citrate intoxication during hepatic transplantation in man. Anesthesiology 1986;65:457–461.
85. Martin TJ, Kang Y, Robertson KM, Virji MA, Marquez JM. Ionization and hemodynamic effects of calcium chloride and calcium gluconate in the absence of hepatic function. Anesthesiology 199;3:62–650.
86. Scott V, Kang Y, De Wolf A, et al. Altered ionized magnesium level in plasma during orthotopic liver transplantation [abstract]. Hepatology 199;8:7253.
87. Altura BM, Altura BT. Mg, Na, and K interactions and coronary heart disease. Magnesium 1982;1:241–265.

88. Young LE. Complications of blood transfusion. Ann Intern Med 1964;61: 136–146.
89. Leight L, Roush G, Rafi E, McGaff CJ. The effect of intravenous potassium on myocardial contractility and cardiac dynamics. Am J Cardiol 1962;12:686–691.
90. De Wolf A, Frenette L, Kang Y, Tang C. Insulin decreases the serum potassium concentration during the anhepatic stage of liver transplantation. Anesthesiology 1993;78:677–682.
91. Belani KG, Estrin JA. Biochemical and hematologic effects of intraoperative processing of CPDA-1 and AS-1 packed red cells [abstract]. Anesthesiology 1985;7:A1567.
92. Brown MR, Ramsay MA, Swygert TH. Exchange autotransfusion using the cell saver during liver transplantation. Anesthesiology 1989;70: 168–169.
93. Videira R, Kang YG, Martinez J, De Wolf AM, Aggarwal S, Gasior T. A rapid increase in sodium is associated with CPM after liver transplantation [abstract]. Anesthesiology 1991;75(3A):A222.
94. Lindop MJ, Farman JV, Smith MF. Anaesthesia. Assessment and intraoperative management. In: Calne RY, ed. Liver transplantation. London: Grune & Stratton, 1983:128–129.
95. Dzik WH, Jenkins R: Use of intraoperative blood salvage during orthotopic liver transplantation. Arch Surg 1985;120:946–948.
96. Van Voorst SJ, Peters TG, Williams JW, Vera SR, Britt LG. Autotransfusion in hepatic transplantation. Am Surg 1985;51:623–626.
97. Hauer JM, Thurer RL. Controversies in autotransfusion. Vox Sang 1984;46:8–12.
98. Kang Y, Aggarwal S, Virji M, et al. Clinical evaluation of autotransfusion during transplantation. Anesth Analg 1991;72:94–100.
99. Thurer RL, Lytle BW, Cosgrove DM, Loop FD. Autotransfusion following cardiac operations: a randomized, prospective study. Ann Thorac Surg 1979;27:500–507.
100. Cosgrove DM, Amiot DM, Meserko JJ. An improved technique for autotransfusion of shed mediastinal blood. Ann Thorac Surg 1985;40: 519–520.
101. Boudreaux JP, Bornside GH, Cohn I Jr. Emergency autotransfusion: partial cleansing of bacteria-laden blood by cell washing. J Trauma 1983;23:31–35.
102. Lowe GD, Lowe JM, Drummond MM, et al. Blood viscosity in young mild diabetics with and without retinopathy. Diabetologia 1980;18: 359–363.
103. Kazatchkine M, Sultan YU, Caen JP, Bariety J. Bleeding in renal failure: a possible cause. Br Med J 1976;2:612–615.
104. Carvalho A. Editorial: Bleeding in uremia-a clinical challenge. N Engl J Med 1983;308:38–39.
105. Stewardt JH, Castaldi PA. Uraemic bleeding: a reversible platelet defect corrected by dialysis. Q J Med 1967;36:409–423.
106. Rabiner SF, Hrodek O. Platelet factor 3 in normal subjects and patients with renal failure. J Clin Invest 1968;47:901–912.
107. Horowitz HI, Stein IM, Cohen BD, White JG. Further studies on the platelet inhibitory effect of guanidinosuccinic acid: its role in uremic bleeding. Am J Med 1970;49:336–345.
108. Rabiner SF, Molinas F. The role of phenol and phenolic acids on the thrombocytopathy and defective platelet aggregation of patients with renal failure. Am J Med 1970;49:346–351.
109. Castaldi PA, Rosenberg MC, Stewart JH. Bleeding disorder of uraemia. Lancet 1966;2:66–69.
110. Gura V, Creter D, Levi J. Elevated thrombocyte calcium content in uremia and its correction by a 1 alpha (OH) vitamin D treatment. Nephron 1982;30:237–239.
111. Rao AK, Walsh PN. Acquired qualitative platelet disorders. Clin Haematol 1983;12:201–238.
112. DiMinno G, Martinez J, McKeann M, DeLaRosa J, Burke JF, Murphy S. Platelet dysfunction in uremia: multifaceted defect partially corrected by dialysis. Am J Med 1985;79:552–559.
113. Green D, Santhanam S, Krumlovsky FA, del Greco F. Elevated betathromboglobulin in patients with chronic renal failure: effect of hemodialysis. J Lab Clin Med 1980;95:679–685.
114. Jorgensen KA, Ingeberg S. Platelets and platelet function in patients with chronic uremia on maintenance hemodialysis. Nephron 1979;23: 233–236.
115. Nakamura Y, Tomura S, Tachibana K, Chida Y, Marumo F. Enhanced fibrinolytic activity during the course of hemodialysis. Clin Nephrol 1992;38:90–96.
116. Hakim RM, Breillatt J, Lazarus JM, Port FK. Complement activation and hypersensitivity reactions to dialyser membranes. N Engl J Med 1984;311:878–882.
117. Hakim RM, Schafer AI. Hemodialysis-associated platelet activation and thrombocytopenia. Am J Med 1985;78:57–80.
118. Speiser W, Wojta J, Korninger C, Kirchheimer JC, Zazgornik J, Binder BR. Enhanced fibrinolysis caused by tissue plasminogen activator release in hemodialysis. Kidney Int 1987;32:280–283.
119. Tappy L, Hauert J, Bachmann F. Effects of hypoxia and acidosis on vascular plasminogen activator release in the pig ear perfusion system. Thromb Res 1984;33:117–124.
120. Janson PA, Jubelirer SJ, Weinstein MS, Beykin D. Treatment of bleeding tendency in uremia with cryoprecipitate. N Engl J Med 1980;303: 1318–1322.
121. Mannucci PM, Remuzzi G, Pusineri F, et al. Deamino-8-D-arginine vasopressin shortens the bleeding time in uremia. N Engl J Med 1983;308:8–12.
122. Hampers CL, Blanfox MD, Merrill JP. Anticoagulant rebound after hemodialysis. N Engl J Med 1988;275:776–778.
123. Turney JH, Williams LC, Fewell MR, Parsons V, Weston MJ. Platelet protection and heparin sparing with prostacyclin during regular dialysis therapy. Lancet 1980;2:224–226.
124. Woods, HF, Ash G, Weston MJ. Sulfinpyrazone reduced deposition of fibrin on dialyser membranes [abstract]. Thromb Haemost 1979;42: 401.
125. Lindsay RM, Prentice CRM, Davidson JF, Burton JA, McNicol GP. Hemostatic changes during dialysis, associated with thrombus formation on dialysis membrane. Br Med J 1972;4:454–458.
126. Mundy AR, Bewick M, Moncada S, Vane JR. Short term suppression of hyperacute renal allograft rejection in presensitized dogs with prostacyclin. Prostaglandins 1980;19:595–603.
127. Capitanio A, Mannucci PM, Ponticelli C, Pareti F. Detection of circulating released platelets after renal transplantation. Transplantation 1982;33:298–301.
128. Moncada S, Vane JR. Arachidonic acid metabolites and the interactions between platelets and blood vessel walls. N Engl J Med 1979; 300:1142–1147.
129. Fried W. Hematological abnormalities in chronic renal failure. Semin Nephrol 1981;1:176.
130. Dausset J. Leuko-agglutinins. IV. Leuko-agglutinins and blood transfusion. Vox Sang 1957;4:190.
131. Kissmeyer-Nielsen F, Olsen S, Petersen VP, Fjeldborg O. Hyperacute rejection of kidney allografts associated with pre-existing humoral antibodies against donor cells. Lancet 1966;1:662.
132. Patel R, Terasaki PI. Significance of the positive crossmatch test in kidney transplantation. N Engl J Med 1969;280:735.

133. Terasaki PI, Kreisler M, Michey RM. Presensitization and kidney transplant failures. Postgrad Med J 1971;47:89.
134. Opelz G, Terasaki PI. Poor kidney-transplant survival in recipients with frozen-blood transfusions or no transfusions. Lancet 1974;2:696.
135. Feduska NJ, Amend WJ, Vincenti F, Duca R, Salvatierra O. Blood transfusions before and on the day of transplantation: effects on cadaver graft survival. Transplant Proc 1982;13:175.
136. Joysey VC. Some effects of blood transfusion. In: Calne RY, eds. Transplantation immunology. Oxford: Oxford University Press, 1984: 278.
137. Maki T, Monaco AP. Impaired T-cell function after allogeneic blood transfusion in mice. Transplant Proc 1985:9973.
138. Terasaki PI. The beneficial transfusion effect on kidney graft survival attributed to clonal deletion. Transplantation 1984;37:119–125.
139. Keown PA, Descamps B. Hypothesis: improved renal allograft survival after blood transfusion: a nonspecific, erythrocyte-mediated immunoregulatory process? Lancet 1979;1:20–22.
140. Singal DP, Joseph S. Role of blood transfusions on the induction of antibodies against recognition sites on T lymphocytes in renal transplant patients. Hum Immunol 198;:93–1082.
141. Hosenpud JD, Novick RJ, Breen TJ, Daily OP. The Registry of the International Society for Heart and Lung Transplantation: Eleventh Official Report—1994. J Heart Lung Transplant 1994;13:561–70.
142. Novick RJ, Menkis AH, McKenzie FN, et al. Reduction in bleeding after heart-lung transplantation: the importance of posterior mediastinal hemostasis. Chest 1990;98:1383–1387.
143. Dawkins KD, Jamieson SW, Hunt SA, et al. Long-term results, haemodynamics and complications after combined heart-lung transplantation. Circulation 1985;71:919–926.
144. McCarthy PM, Starnes VA, Theodore J, Stinson EB, Oyer PE, Shumway NE. Improved survival after heart-lung transplantation. J Thorac Cardiovasc Surg 1990;99:54–60.
145. Griffith BP, Hardesty RL, Trento A, et al. Heart-lung transplantation: lessons learned and future hopes. Ann Thorac Surg 1987;43:6–16.
146. Sarris GE, Smith JA, Shumway NE, et al. Long-term results of combined heart-lung transplantation: the Stanford experience. J Heart Lung Transplant 1994;13:940–949.
147. Vouhe PR, Dartevelle PG. Heart-lung transplantation: technical modifications that may improve the early outcome. J Thorac Cardiovasc Surg 1989;97:906–910.
148. Pasque MK, Cooper JD, Kaiser LR, Haydock DA, Triantafillou A, Trulock EP. Improved technique for bilateral lung transplantation: rationale and initial clinical experience. Ann Thorac Surg 1990;49: 785–791.
149. Hunt BJ, Sack D, Amin S, Yacoub MH. The perioperative use of blood components during heart and heart-lung transplantation. Transfusion 1992;32:57–62.
150. Kirklin JK. The postperfusion syndrome: inflammation and the damaging effects of cardiopulmonary bypass. In: Tinker J, ed. Cardiopulmonary bypass: current concepts and controversies. Philadelphia: WB Saunders, 1989:131–146.
151. Hunter DN, Morgan CJ, Yacoub M, Evans TW. Pulmonary endothelial permeability following lung transplantation. Chest 1992;102: 417–421.
152. Aeba R, Griffith BP, Kormos RL, et al. Effect of cardiopulmonary bypass on early graft dysfunction in clinical lung transplantation. Ann Thorac Surg 1994;57:15–22.
153. Francalancia NA, Aeba R, Yousem SA, Griffith BP, Marrone GC. Deleterious effects of cardiopulmonary bypass on early graft function after single lung allotransplantation: evaluation of a heparin-coated bypass circuit. J Heart Lung Transplant 1994;13:498–507.
154. Taylor KM. Perioperative approaches to coagulation defects. Ann Thorac Surg 1993;56:S78–S82.
155. Gravlee GP, Arora S, Lavender SW, et al.: Predictive value of blood clotting tests in cardiac surgical patients. Ann Thorac Surg 1994;58: 216–221.
156. Rosengart TK, Helm RE, Klemperer J, Krieger KH, Isom OW. Combined aprotinin and erythropoietin use for blood conservation: results with Jehovah's Witnesses. Ann Thorac Surg 1994;58:1397–1403.
157. Cheng DC, Demajo W, Sandler AN. Lung transplantation. Anesthesiol Clin North Am 1994;12:749–767.
158. Tobe CE, Vocelka C, Sepulvada R, et al. Infusion of autologous platelet rich plasma does not reduce blood loss and product use after coronary artery bypass. J Thorac Cardiovasc Surg 1993;105: 1007–1014.
159. Stover EP, Siegel LC.: Plateletpheresis before cardiopulmonary bypass [letter; comment]. Anesthesiology 1990:715–7174.
160. Spiess BD, Ivankovich AD. Thromboelastography: a coagulation-monitoring technique applied to cardiopulmonary bypass. In: Ellison N, Jobes DR, eds. Effective hemostasis in cardiac surgery. Philadelphia: WB Saunders, 1988:163–181.
161. Wang JS, Lin CY, Hung WT, et al. Thromboelastogram fails to predict postoperative hemorrhage in cardiac patients. Ann Thorac Surg 1992; 53:435–439.
162. Spiess BD,Tuman KJ, McCarthy RJ, et al. Thromboelastogram and postoperative hemorrhage [letters and reply]. Ann Thorac Surg 1992; 54:810–813.
163. Lemmer JH. Reporting the results of blood conservation studies: the need for uniform and comprehensive methods. Ann Thorac Surg 1994; 58:1305–1306.
164. Blauhut B, Harringer W, Bettelheim P, Doran JE, Spath P, Lundsgarard-Hansen P. Comparison of the effects of aprotinin and tranexamic acid on blood loss and related variable after cardiopulmonary bypass. J Thorac Cardiovasc Surg 1994;108:1083–1091.
165. Horrow JC, Van Riper DF, Strong MD, Grunewald KE, Parmet JL. The dose response relationship of tranexamic acid. Anesthesiology 1995;82:383–392.
166. Lemmer JH, Stanford W, Bonney SL, et al. Aprotinin for coronary bypass operations: efficacy, safety, and the influence on early saphenous vein graft patency. J Thorac Cardiovasc Surg 1994;107:543–553.
167. Royston D. High-dose aprotinin therapy: a review of the first five years' experience. J Cardiothor Vasc Surg 1992;6:76–100.
168. Fremes SE, Wong BI, Lee E, et al. Metaanalysis of prophylactic drug treatment in the prevention of postoperative bleeding. Ann Thorac Surg 1994;58:1580–1588.
169. Royston D. Aprotinin therapy in heart and heart-lung transplantation. J Heart Lung Transplant 1993;12:S19–S25.

Chapter 31

Blood Conservation in Orthopedic Surgery

JOSEPH C. MCCARTHY
RODERICK H. TURNER
AGNES KIM
PATRICIA O'DONNELL
ROBERT G. VALERI
BRUCE D. SPIESS

INTRODUCTION

Blood loss during reconstructive orthopedic surgery can be extensive. Improvements in anesthetic techniques and agents coupled with dramatic improvements in technology and surgical expertise have resulted in the ability to tackle increasingly complex and lengthy reconstructive problems. The first total hip replacement was performed in the United States in the mid-1960s. Now in this country there are nearly 300,000 total hip and knee replacement procedures performed annually. Concomitant with the increase in frequency of these primary arthroplasties is the number of revision joint replacements necessary. In 1992, there were 17,192 such operations performed. It is during these repeat arthroplasty procedures that the most dramatic blood loss occurs (up to 35 units). Routine total hip replacement usually causes approximately 1000 mL of blood loss, and although tourniquets are used for total knee surgery, the postoperative period (when the tourniquet is released) may account for 500–700 mL of blood loss. In addition to total joint reconstruction, surgery for multiple trauma and spinal fusion also incur substantial blood loss. In spinal surgery, the number of segments being operated has a direct impact on the amount of blood loss. The extent, and on occasion the rapidity, of this loss can tax the availability of homologous blood.

To add to this dilemma, the need for blood transfusion has increased 100% over the past 10 years, whereas the amount of blood collected has increased only 30%. It is for this reason that the Red Cross has imported blood from Europe since 1986. This shortfall has also propelled efforts toward alternatives to homologous transfusion. Orthopedic surgery, because of its large number of cases and the potential for major blood loss, as a specialty is of particular interest to transfusion medicine. A number of studies have looked at the transfusion behavior and utilization within orthopedics and compared with other specialties. Because of the nature of a number of these high demand (for blood) surgeries, the orthopedic specialty is uniquely poised to take advantage of certain programs that may be much less effective in other specialties. Particularly, predeposit autologous donation is useful in elective orthopedic surgery. It is discussed in a separate chapter on autologous blood and is also covered here, but the fact that orthopedic surgery can be planned in advance for many large blood loss cases makes autologous predonation possible and widely studied for its cost effectiveness. Along with predonation is the utilization of erythropoietin, again uniquely able to be studied in large series of patients that have similar operations, blood requirements, and planned surgeries.

Because much of orthopedics' large blood demand surgeries are elective with several weeks to months of advance notice, autologous blood donation is now a mainstay of most orthopedic programs. Some might suggest that it is less than the standard of care to not offer autologous donation to elective orthopedic surgery patients. Agreement appears to be very broad on the usefulness of predeposit programs. However, the use of the blood harvested may have considerable disagreement when the point of reinfusion is encountered. Clearly, orthopedic surgeons have listened loud and clear to the public's demands for autologous blood donation. The concerns regarding virus transmission and costs have been imparted to the practitioners.

Reinfusion of predonated blood is an area of considerable controversy. A number of consensus conferences at the National Institutes of Health and practice guidelines for transfusion therapy have occurred or have been published by specialties. The American College of Physicians' guidelines for transfusion therapy was the basis for one study examining the appropriateness of transfusions. The use of blood in internal medicine and general surgery showed that 52.8 and 56.4% of red cell transfusions did not fit prescribed criteria as described by these guidelines. However, 73.5% of red cell transfusions for orthopedic surgery could not be justified (1). The most common events leading to unjustified transfusions were ordering 2 units at a time and using red cells in hemodynamically stable, normovolemic anemic patients without ongoing blood loss. This relays a philosophy of a defined transfusion trigger clearly in the mind of those practicing in the specialty. This study subjected autologous blood units to the same scrutiny as allogeneic units.

Although it appears that autologous blood has less potential "risk" than allogeneic blood, that may be limited to viral transmission alone. One added risk is that if a patient has donated autologous blood, he or she may develop severe dissatisfaction with the care team if allogeneic blood is transfused either before autologous blood is used or in lieu of existing predonated supplies. This happens in almost 10% of patients studied at one institution. There appears to be as of yet no fail-safe mechanism for informing practitioners that autologous blood is available and should be used first (2). The study just quoted focused on the "mistakes" of giving allogeneic blood when autologous was available, but it also looked at the appropriateness of transfusion and found that 40% of interoperative transfusion did not meet criteria and 38% of postoperative failed as well. If one views the use of allogeneic blood when autologous was available as a human error (perhaps multiple human errors in a system), then a 10% error rate is very high. One argument for having the same criteria for transfusion triggers in allogeneic and autologous is that human error can occur, leading to ABO-Rh incompatibility problems. This most disastrous complication of transfusion appears to happen at a rate of 1–2000 to 1–20,000 units transfused. However, a patient transfused with allogeneic blood when autologous blood was available may become extremely unhappy with the medical care system, and if a viral transmission occurs, then the legal liabilities would be tremendous. That 10% error rate in orthopedic surgery would suggest that we as a health care system are failing in our management of autologous blood.

Another study has tried to find the appropriateness of transfusions via a medical chart review (3). As one can imagine, this technique may be quite ineffective in understanding the decision-making in practitioners. Symptoms requiring transfusion were recorded in only 10% of charts. An indication for transfusion was indicated in the chart in only 27% of cases postoperatively but 95% of cases intraoperatively. Interestingly, the documentation of criteria for transfusion was not different between autologous and allogeneic blood. The documentation in charts may be so poor that using them for appropriateness of transfusion is wrong, which is what the authors of this study concluded. Discharge hematocrit has been suggested as a way to decide whether transfusion therapy by either autologous or allogeneic blood was appropriate. However, a study examining the use of discharge hematocrit has found similar blood utilization in orthopedic patients in three different discharge groups. The appropriateness of transfusion was similar between groups with only about 6.5–13% of transfusions being deemed excessive (4).

So what is the appropriateness of transfusion in orthopedic surgery? Inappropriate transfusion ranges from 6.5% to as high as 73.5%. The vast range of these numbers can be explained not only in the way in which they are assessed, but also in the philosophy prevalent in orthopedic surgery that autologous blood is transfused more liberally than allogeneic. That practice has been documented (5). One can debate the point, and perhaps it should be debated in light of the data of a 10% error rate in having autologous blood available and transfusing allogeneic blood. But if the specialty views autologous blood differently, and clearly it does, then can it be judged by outside criteria based on allogeneic blood? That is a question that cannot be answered in this text.

RISKS OF HOMOLOGOUS TRANSFUSION

Efforts to avoid homologous blood transfusion during reconstructive orthopedic surgery have taken on increasing importance in the era of the acquired immunodeficiency syndrome (AIDS) (6). Although the risk of human immunodeficiency virus (HIV) seroconversion from homologous blood is quite small, estimated at 1 in 40,000 to 1 in 300,000, patient perception deems this likelihood unacceptably high. Although the threat of AIDS remains firmly rooted at the forefront of one's conscience, other diseases are much more likely to be transmitted. The risk of developing hepatitis B after transfusion is 1 in 200,000, whereas that of hepatitis C virus is 1 in 3300. It has been shown that up to 5% of blood donors tested in the United States have a positive infectious disease serotest. Other potentially transmissible diseases include cytomegalovirus, human T-lymphotropic virus types 1 and 2, yersinia, malaria, leishmania, and other parasites and viruses (7) (Valeri RC, personal communication.)

ABO incompatibility may result in an acute hemolytic reaction. Symptoms may range from mild to catastrophic. In one New York study, 58% of errors were caused by personnel outside the blood bank (8). Of these errors, 43% resulted from failure to identify either the patient or the unit of homologous blood correctly before transfusion. Personnel errors have also resulted in antigen-antibody incompatibility reactions. Febrile reactions are the most common transfusion reaction and occur in up to 1 in 100 cases. Although these are usually mild and self-limited, acute lung injury has been reported and may result in pulmonary edema (9). These allergic reactions and the development of coagulopathies such as disseminated intravascular coagulation have caused patients concern and physicians to avoid homologous transfusion whenever possible (10–14) (Keith J, Dishoneh L, Bunfein L, et al., unpublished data).

In addition to the above complications, homologous transfusion may have an immunosuppressive effect. This effect is mediated by both humeral and cellular factors. Several animal studies corroborate this immunosuppressive effect (15–19) (Sistino JJ, Owitz D, Monero LB, unpublished data). More recently, human clinical studies have demonstrated decreases in T lymphocytes (20) and in killer cell formation (21). This dysfunction persisted up to 30 days. The potential consequences for orthopedic patients with implants are of considerable concern. Triulzi et al. (22) showed a fourfold decrease in killer cell function in patients after homologous transfusion but not after autologous transfusion. This resulted in an increased postoperative spinal infection rate. In a small series, Murphy et al. (23) demonstrated a 26% increase in prosthetic infections in those patients who had received homologous blood. Triulzi et al. (24) reviewed 11 clinical studies; in 10, homologous blood transfusion increased the risk for postoperative infection.

Many strategies have been developed to avoid homologous transfusion, including lowering the transfusion trigger, hemodilution, hypotensive anesthesia, predeposit autodonation, erythropoietin, and cell-saving techniques (7, 16, 25–35). This last method involves red cell recovery, washing, and readministration intraoperatively. More recently, filtration of shed blood and portable cell-washing techniques have become available for postoperative use (27, 28) (Semkin LB, Schurman DJ, Goodman SB, et al., unpublished data). In addition, the surgeon can have an impact on transfusion requirements by shortening operative time, obtaining thorough hemostasis, and using hemostatic agents on exposed bony beds (25, 36). Recently, autologous fibrin glue has become available for use as a hemostatic agent in vascular surgery and orthopedics.

By far the most common techniques to conserve blood used in major reconstructive orthopedic surgery are autologous predonation, operative cell washing, postoperative reinfusion, and erythropoietin to increase autologous donation. There are limitations to preoperative autodonation, including anemia, a 35-day limit on liquid preservation, operative postponement, and geographical access to an autodonation facility. For these reasons, all the techniques have been used at our institution and they are viewed as complementary.

PREOPERATIVE AUTOLOGOUS BLOOD DONATION PROGRAM

The autologous blood donation program has proved highly successful in managing blood loss in primary total hip arthoplasty (THA). All orthopedic patients scheduled for elective surgery in which blood replacement is anticipated are encouraged to participate in the autologous blood donation program, which began in 1983 (Table 31.1). Patients may donate up to 1 unit of their own blood per week before surgery. Blood is stored in a liquid state for up to 35 days and may be frozen for a period of 3 years. Although freezing blood is a widely accepted technique, a small number of red cells are lost in the freezing process. In addition, blood freezing incurs added cost, technician time, and storage space problems. Patients under the age of 18 and over 65 years are required to have medical clearance before donation. Chronic respiratory disorders, cardiac conditions, and any illness that may be worsened by decreasing the patient's oxygen-carrying capacity are contraindications to predonation. Patients with hematocrit less than 34% are not phlebotomized. However, this may change in the future. Autologous blood harvest is efficacious in orthopedic surgery (5, 37). In total hip and total knee surgery, predeposit of blood is very effective in decreasing the need for allogeneic blood (38). However, autologous blood harvest has been criticized as quite cost ineffective (39). If one examines the literature on a cost-effectiveness model for

TABLE 31.1. NUMBER OF AUTOLOGOUS DONATIONS AT NEBH AND ELSEWHERE

	1984	1987	1990	1993
Total no. of units	241	2135	2690	3399
No. of units donated at NEBH	241	1416	1960	2200
No. of units donated elsewhere	0	719	336	602
No. of patients	97	837	1536	2113

quality added life years saved by using autologous blood donation, then it seems to be very costly (40). The added cost to society for saving one human life might be well in excess of hundreds of thousands of dollars. The authors of this one study asked if it is worth the cost and if there are less expensive ways to decrease blood utilization (39).

Those questions are appropriate, but the analysis may have some built-in bias. The computer model that shows autologous predeposit as extremely costly for society in orthopedic surgery has a rather myopic view of the problem. They examine only the potential risks of viral transmission and therefore the avoided costs by using autologous blood. Clearly, the risks of allogeneic transfusion go beyond just viral transmission. Immunosuppression has recently been investigated in orthopedic surgery, and if autologous blood is used as compared with allogeneic, the risk of postoperative infection is significantly reduced. The cost of a major infection in a total joint arthroplasty patient must be tremendous and calculable; however, the literature examining the "high cost" of autologous predonation does not even consider this in its model. It deems that as controversial and any data that are controversial are just not computed. Other risks such as sepsis, minor transfusion reaction including allergic reaction, and graft-versus-host disease (a substantial killer in Japan) were not even considered. The data on viral transmission were taken from the best data ever reported and are present in only one very important paper. However, one should realize that the cost of autologous predonation is far from established in orthopedic surgery and that although an article exists saying that it is cost ineffective, some major inadequacies of that analysis do exist.

Autologous predonation does cost more than allogeneic blood, however, and therefore it is worthwhile targeting the collection of blood to the operation planned (40). Studies have shown that most of the surgeries will be serviced effectively by harvesting 3 units of autologous blood for total hip surgery and 2 units for total knee surgery. Indeed, if one increases these numbers by 1 unit more for each surgery, only an additional 5% of patients will benefit. That would be quite cost ineffective. Spinal surgery with 3 units harvested shows that some 66% of autologous blood is not used and perhaps that harvest should be reduced. Of course, those patients having "redo" operations or large extensive spine surgeries could be candidates for even more blood harvested before surgery. These data should be taken with some element of introspection when one looks at the appropriateness of transfusion previously discussed. If 3 units are harvested for total hip surgery but significant numbers of them are being transfused against the clinical guidelines of a number of societies, then one has to wonder if it would not be even more cost effective to harvest less and transfuse with different guidelines.

The use of autologous blood predonated in orthopedic surgery has allowed the study of not only cost effectiveness and appropriateness of transfusion, but also the risks of immunosuppression and infection. These areas of research have contributed a great deal of knowledge to the transfusion literature. Interestingly, not examined in the analysis of cost effectiveness is an effect of autologous blood transfusion on the relative risk of perioperative hypercoagulability. It is well known that many different types of surgical patients develop a propensity for postoperative thrombosis, deep venous thrombosis, and pulmonary emboli. Total hip surgery patients appear particularly prone to this problem, and some have thought this might be due to bed rest, immobilization, blockage of venous drainage from the limb operated on, and welling. Today, it appears that changes in the fibrinolytic coagulation system may predispose patients to an increased risk for thrombosis. In one orthopedic study using autologous or allogeneic blood transfusions in total hip surgery, there were significant differences in the risks for deep venous thrombosis (38).

This study looked not only at the use of autologous blood versus allogeneic blood, but also at some of the pro- and anticoagulant proteins (38). Interestingly, plasminogen activator inhibitor-1 (PAI-1) was elevated postoperatively much higher in the group that only received homologous blood. That protein, by blocking the local action of tissue plasminogen activator, is quite prothrombotic. It essentially blocks the early disaggregation of platelet microthrombi. It is elevated in acute myocardial infarction, vascular disease, pulmonary emboli, and acutely postoperatively. The mechanism of its release is unclear, but this finding from the orthopedic literature that PAI-1 is different in matched groups receiving allogeneic and autologous blood may shed more light on the mechanism of its release. Perhaps there are inflammatory or immunological mechanisms involved.

The data on infectious and tumor recurrence from allogeneic versus autologous blood transfusions have been widely investigated. Data from orthopedics have been some of the best in terms of being well controlled and randomized (37). Several studies have investigated the incidence of postoperative infection: pulmonary, urinary, wound, and joint (37, 41). In studies where patients were randomized to receive either autologous or allogeneic blood, those who received autologous blood had a major reduction of overall infections (2.6 times less) (37). That supports the contention that allogeneic blood has immunosuppressive properties. Again, when discussions of cost effectiveness of autologous blood transfusion are written, they do not take into account the immunosuppressive effects of allogeneic transfusion. All patients are placed on ferrous sulfate supplementation. Referral patients unable to donate blood at the hospital bank may have their blood processed at local facilities (33). A recent prospective, randomized trial of blood salvage techniques by Rothman showed that predonation was the single most important factor to avoid homologous transfusion in primary total hip patients (Rothman R, unpublished data). If the hematocrit is borderline or low, then patients may not be able to donate their full complement of autologous blood. The use of erythropoietin can increase the amount of autologous blood donated. Paiement et al. (42) demonstrated a 450% increase in reticulocyte count and a 1 unit decrease in the amount of blood transfused in patients receiving erythropoietin compared with placebo. Studies from orthopedics have laid the ground work for how effective erythropoietin therapy can be. A large multicentered study with 204 patients having baseline hematocrits at 39% or below was undertaken (43). Autologous blood was harvested every 3–4 days if the hematocrit was above 33%, and patients were randomized to receive recombinant human erythropoietin (600 U/kg) or a placebo. More blood was collected from patients taking erythropoietin (4.5 ± 1.0 units) than from placebo patients (3.0 ± 1.0 units) ($P < .001$). The use of allogeneic blood transfusion was greater in the placebo group (31%) than the erythropoietin group (20%). This study is often quoted to show the usefulness of erythropoietin in assisting harvest of autologous blood from patients with low hematocrit. It should be applied to those patient groups with expected limited abilities to donate. Once again, cost effectiveness is important, and one should keep in mind the target number of units to be donated. If one is trying to harvest more than 3 units and prolonged erythropoietin therapy is planned, unless a truly complex operation is expected to require such large amounts of blood, it may be very cost ineffective to do this technique.

EXPERIENCE WITH THE CELL SAVER AT THE NEW ENGLAND BAPTIST HOSPITAL

The introduction of the Cell Saver (Haemonetics Corp., Braintree, MA) at the New England Baptist Hospital (NEBH) in 1978 has been a major factor in reducing the number of homologous blood transfusions needed in major orthopedic cases at our institution. The initial application of the use of Cell Saver in orthopedic surgery was discussed in Turner et al. (33). The Cell Saver, during the first year of operation, was used in 76 orthopedic cases and has reached approximately 600 orthopedic cases per year. The orthopedic applications have been total hip replacements, total knee replacements, spinal fusions, revision total hip replacements, and revision total knee replacements. Table 31.2 displays the types of surgeries and numbers of cases that have used the Cell Saver. In total, the NEBH has used the Cell Saver in 4656 operative cases from 1978 to 1994. The Cell Saver is used on all revision THAs in which blood loss is estimated to be greater than 1500 mL. At this volume of blood loss, the Cell Saver should be able to salvage at least 2 units of packed red blood cells from the operative field. Data from 1992 showed that 73% of all revision THAs were able to salvage 2 or more units of blood. These cases now account for more than 40% of the Cell Saver case load at the NEBH. Data from the use of the Cell Saver in 1992 showed 70% of the revision THAs did not require homologous blood transfusions. They received their own predonated blood and/or the intraopera-

TABLE 31.2. CELL SAVER CASES VS. TYPE OF SURGERY AT NEBH (1984 TO JUNE 1994)

	THR	Rev. Hip	Spinal	Vascular	Miscellaneous	Total
1984	68	151	79	11		312
1985	47	172	73	13		310
1986	20	174	53	8		255
1987	77	199	73	16	12	377
1988	80	202	63	11	8	364
1989	120	210	137	13	15	495
1990	114	236	151	18	20	539
1991	92	238	215	25	41	611
1992	101	192	246	13	28	580
1993	103	203	234	12	7	559
1994	52	88	99	9	6	254

THR, Total hip replacement; Rev. Hip, revision of prior hip replacement tive autotransfused blood replacement via the Cell Saver. The Cell Saver is currently not used in routine primary THA because of a dramatic decrease in blood loss from decreased operative time and improved surgical technique (26, 33). However, the reinfusion machine continues to be used for those primary hip arthroplasties that are complex congenital deformities of the hip (CDH), protrusio, etc.) or where blood loss is expected to be greater than 2 units (bilateral total hip replacement (THR), blood dyscrasia, etc.).

CELL SAVER SAFETY

The Cell Saver cases performed at the NEBH from 1978 through its present use have proved that intraoperative autologous blood transfusion is a safe method of blood replacement. In our review of cases from 1978 to 1986, no complications were reported. During the same period of time, more than 6000 patients received more than 33,000 units of homologous blood at NEBH. In these patients, there were 22 known transfusion-related cases of hepatitis, 81 allergic reactions, 164 episodes of posttransfusion chills and fever, and 2 known cases of exposure of HIV (AIDS).

The advantages of using the Cell Saver for autotransfusion are prevention of transmission of disease such as hepatitis and AIDS; no risk of allergic or graft-versus-host reactions; no risk of isoimmunization; ready availability; systemic anticoagulation is not required and regional anticoagulant is removed by cell washing; and the finished product is devoid of activated clotting factors, platelets, plasma free hemoglobin, bone particles, fat, air, and cellular debris.

COST

With cost as a sole consideration, the findings at NEBH demonstrate that the Cell Saver has been effective if 2 or more units of blood are salvaged from the operative site. Presently, a single unit of homologous blood costs approximately \$250. This charge effects red blood cell processing, cross matching, and blood administration. The charge for the Cell Saver during a surgical procedure is approximately \$500. This charge includes the disposable set for collecting and reinfusing blood, technician time, heparin, saline, and machine maintenance. The patient will use only one set of disposables, no matter how many units of blood are processed. When comparing prices, one must also consider the financial burden associated with the risks of homologous transfusions. The cost evaluation of transfusion reactions can range from \$125 for a mild reaction to \$3000 for a mild case to \$24,000 for a severe case. The cost of treatment for AIDS is expensive and can be estimated at an excess of \$180,000 in addition to indirect costs of lost earnings from recovery time (44). Although red cell washing is widely accepted as part of major surgical procedures, its use postoperatively has only recently become available. To date, most orthopedic surgeons have resorted to filtration methods to return shed blood after total joint replacement surgery (27). Despite the ease of application and successful use of the filtration devices, concern continues to be raised about deleterious side effects, both chemical and clinical (7, 10, 11, 14–16, 26).

Unlike cardiac surgery, shed blood during the perioperative period of a reconstructive orthopedic procedure often contains additional contaminants, such as fat particles, bone chips, bone cement, and fibrin degradation products (7, 27, 28). Because of concern about these orthopedic byproducts, we critically analyzed representative constituent elements of shed blood during and after major reconstructive orthopedic surgery. Blood was analyzed before and after cell washing, and clinical parameters were monitored during the first 24 hours postoperatively.

PORTABLE CELL WASHING TECHNIQUES

Recently, cell-saving machines have become available that are smaller, lighter, more portable, and automated. The Haemolite II cell saver (Haemonetics) was used in our study (Fig. 31.1). The unit is lightweight (less than 45 lb), small ($12 \times 20 \times 10$ inches), and can be transported on the patient's bed after total hip or knee surgery. The same machine can be used intra- and postoperatively. Should postoperative blood loss exceed 1 unit, the software tubing, unlike the filtered units, does not have to be changed. This automated machine processed shed blood within 6 minutes for return to the patient.

Using the Haemolite II portable machine, we attempted to determine the ability of the cell-washing process to remove byproduct material from orthopedic reconstructive procedures. We tested shed blood collected intraoperatively and postoperatively for supernatant hemoglobin, fat particles, D-dimer, complement C3a, and heparin. In addition, we studied the effect of transfusing washed intraoperatively and postoperatively collected shed blood into patients on their hematocrit value, platelet count, D-dimer, fat, plasma, hemoglobin, C3a, and heparin level after transfusion. Finally, we monitored the impact of transfusing cell-washed shed blood on patients' clinical parameters, including blood pressure, pulse and respiratory rate, and temperature.

METHODS

A prospective series of 37 patients had their shed blood collected intraoperatively and postoperatively during major orthopedic reconstructive surgery. The shed blood was washed using the Haemolite II cell washer. Samples of the shed

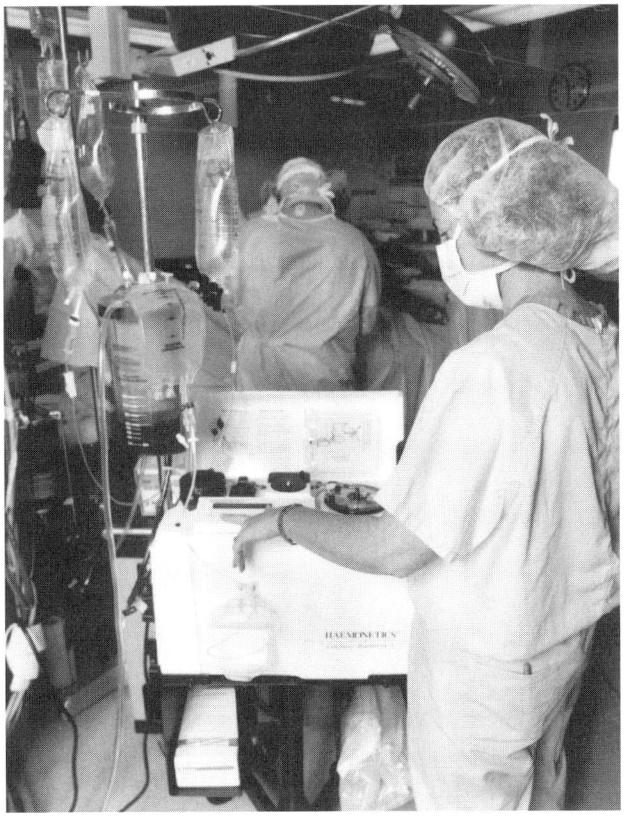

Figure 31.1. Haemolite II cell saver.

blood were drawn before washing, after washing, and from the waste solution. Those patients receiving postoperative reinfusion had their shed blood washed and transfused within 6 hours of collection.

The following measurements were made. The hematocrit value was determined using a microhematocrit centrifuge. Hemoglobin was obtained using a hemoglobinometer. The white blood cell count was measured using an electronic particle counter (Coulter Model ZBI). Supernatant hemoglobin was analyzed using the cyanomethemoglobin method. D-dimer was measured using a monoclonal antibody. C3a (complement) was determined using a radioimmune assay. Fat particles were measured and stratified using a nile red dye and fluorescent microscopy. Heparin was analyzed using an automated chemistry system (Cobras).

Each patient had vital signs (blood pressure, heart rate, respiratory rate, and core temperature) measured before, during, and 1 hour after transfusion of *each* unit of washed shed blood. The vital signs were then repeated 24 hours after transfusion.

Hematocrit value, hemoglobin concentration, white blood cell count, and platelet count were determined using an electronic particle counter; plasma hemoglobin was measured using a dual-beam spectrophotometer (Perkin-Elmer). D-dimer, C3a, fat particles, and heparin levels were measured as described above. Blood samples were drawn from each patient before each transfusion, 1 hour after transfusion, and 24 hours after transfusion of each unit of washed shed blood.

RESULTS

Table 31.3 reports data obtained on units of intraoperatively collected shed blood. Table 31.4 summarizes the data on units on postoperatively collected shed blood. Table 31.5 reports data on patients before and after transfusion of intraoperatively shed blood. Table 31.6 reports information from patients before and after transfusion of postoperatively shed blood. Table 31.7 shows the correlation between red blood cell volume washed and supernatant hemoglobin washout in intraoperatively shed blood. The red blood cell volume washed was determined by the post-wash volume and hematocrit values. Table 31.8 shows the correlation between red blood cell volume washed and supernatant hemoglobin washout in postoperatively shed blood. The red blood cell volume washed was determined by the post-wash volume and hematocrit values.

The Haemolite cell washer was more efficient in removing supernatant hemoglobin, D-dimer, C3a, and fat particles from intraoperatively shed blood than from postoperatively shed blood. Intraoperatively shed blood does contain more supernatant volume than postoperatively shed blood, which allows greater concentration of the red blood cells, and this is probably responsible for the increased washout values.

Patients receiving intraoperatively shed blood showed no changes in vital signs or hematological measurements after transfusion of up to 3 units of washed shed blood. A slight increase in the D-dimer level was observed after transfusion; however, this returned to baseline levels by 24 hours after transfusion. Patients receiving postoperatively shed blood showed no changes in vital signs during and after transfusion. Increases in fat particles, C3a, and D-dimer were observed 1 hour after transfusion; however, they returned to near baseline levels 24 hours after transfusion.

CONCLUSIONS

After major reconstructive orthopedic surgery, there are clearly advantages to reinfusing shed blood. Intraoperatively, cell washing is a safe, effective, and efficient technique of returning more than half of the shed red cells in surgery. Our study has demonstrated that red cell washing can be effectively accomplished postoperatively as well. Although red cells can be returned to the patient via a filtration method after surgery (27), cell washing provides additional aggregated

TABLE 31.3. INTRAOPERATIVE DATA

	Hct (v%)	Hgb (g/dL)	WBC ($\times 10^3$/mL)	SHC (mg/dL)	Volume (mL)	FAT PARTICLES <9µm (#/mL)	FAT PARTICLES 9–40 µm (#/mL)	FAT PARTICLES >40µm (#/mL)	D-Dimer (ng/mL)	C3a (ng/mL)	Heparin (U/mL)	Waste Hgb Spillage (%)	Cell Recovered (%)	Hgb Account (%)
Pre-Wash														
Mean	10.8	4.8	2.8	921	1405	21,374	500	37	21,175	3492	1.5			
SD	5.4	2.4	2	352	626	20,566	673	103	5615	1778	1.5			
Post-Wash														
Mean	40.4	14	3	534	199.6	4390	267	5	5544	1000	0.21	3.4	52	57
SD	6.5	2.4	3.3	208		8134	750	16	4615	1099	0.02	3.6	16	18

Hct, hematocrit; Hgb, hemoglobin; WBC, white blood cell; SHC, supernatant hemoglobin content.

TABLE 31.4. POSTOPERATIVE DATA

	Hct (v%)	Hgb (g/dL)	WBC ($\times 10^3$/mL)	SHC (mg/dL)	Volume (mL)	FAT PARTICLES <9µm (#/mL)	FAT PARTICLES 9–40 µm (#/mL)	FAT PARTICLES >40µm (#/mL)	D-Dimer (ng/mL)	C3a (ng/mL)	Heparin (U/mL)	Waste Hgb Spillage (%)	Cell Recovered (%)	Hgb Account (%)
Pre-Wash														
Mean	23.6	8.2	23.6	406	634	2004	148	2	22,907	5490	1.9			
SD	12.7	4.2	2.1	374	227	2423	225	6	5127	2196	2.6			
Post-Wash														
Mean	34.7	11.7	4.2	408	202	1269	71	0	20,080	779	0.4	1.7	55	54
SD	11.2	3.9	3.1	235		1863	170	0	4477	280	0.3	2.4	18	16

Hct, hematocrit; Hgb, hemoglobin; WBC, white blood cell; SHC, supernatant hemoglobin content.

TABLE 31.5. INTRAOPERATIVE PATIENT DATA

	Hct (v%)	Hgb (g/dL)	WBC (×10³/mL)	PL Hgb (mg/dL)	PLT CT (×10⁶/mL)	MPV (u3)	FAT PARTICLES <9μm (#/mL)	FAT PARTICLES 9–40μm (#/mL)	FAT PARTICLES >40μm (#/mL)	D-Dimer (ng/mL)	C3a (ng/mL)	Heparin (U/mL)	Blood Pressure Systolic (Torr)	Blood Pressure Diastolic (Torr)	Heart Rate (bpm)	Re-spira-tory Rate (/min)	Tem-pera-ture (°C)
Pre-transfusion																	
Mean	30	10	6.6	36	221	9.4	597	145	4	1119	1147	0.2	105	64	67	8	34.9
SD	5	1.7	2.4	36	89	1.7	1665	623	23	1327	1949	0	14	12	13	2	0.8
During Transfusion 1																	
Mean	—	—	—	—	—	—	—	—	—	—	—	—	113	68	68	9	34.5
SD	—	—	—	—	—	—	—	—	—	—	—	—	9	11	16	3	0.7
During Transfusion 2																	
Mean	—	—	—	—	—	—	—	—	—	—	—	—	110	65	69	8	34.5
SD	—	—	—	—	—	—	—	—	—	—	—	—	16	9	13	2	0.8
During Transfusion 3																	
Mean	—	—	—	—	—	—	—	—	—	—	—	—	110	65	69	10	34.4
SD	—	—	—	—	—	—	—	—	—	—	—	—	13	19	13	4	0.7
1 Hour Posttransfusion 1																	
Mean	31.2	10.4	13.7	40	212	9.2	233	57	5	3478	723	0.2	122	70	76	13	34.8
SD	4	1.3	5.7	55	84	1.4	478	184	25	4655	467	0	23	13	20	6	1.2
1 Hour Posttransfusion 2																	
Mean	31.3	10.4	13.5	66	222	8.6	148	115	7	1974	683	0.2	120	71	77	12	34.3
SD	4.7	1.5	5.8	56	57	1.4	448	422	27	1216	315	0	19	14	19	6	1.2
1 Hour Posttransfusion 3																	
Mean	32.2	10.8	14.9	38	192	9.4	23	13	13	4906	534	0.2	125	69	73	12	34.4
SD	3	1	9.9	22	63	1.5	73	37	45	3946	360	0	37	17	17	5	1.2
24 Hour Posttransfusion																	
Mean	27	9	10.3	15	187	9	34	17	0	1702	625	0.2	123	67	87	20	37.4
SD	5.6	1.9	3.1	10	68	1.7	93	73	0	1369	389	0.1	18	8	13	2	0.6

Hct, hematocrit; Hgb, hemoglobin; WBC, white blood cell; SHC, supernatant hemoglobin content; PL, plasma hemoglobin; PLT CT, platelet count; MPV, mean platelet volume.

TABLE 31.6. POSTOPERATIVE PATIENT DATA

	Hct (v%)	Hgb (g/dL)	WBC (×10³/mL)	PL Hgb (mg/dL)	PLT CT (×10⁶/mL)	MPV (u3)	FAT PARTICLES <9μm (#/mL)	FAT PARTICLES 9–40μm (#/mL)	FAT PARTICLES >40μm (#/mL)	D-Dimer (ng/mL)	C3a (ng/mL)	Heparin (U/mL)	Blood Pressure Systolic (Torr)	Blood Pressure Diastolic (Torr)	Heart Rate (bpm)	Re-spira-tory Rate (/min)	Tem-pera-ture (°C)
Pre-transfusion																	
Mean	31.1	10.5	11.9	29.2	164	8.6	59	9	0	2262	581	0.2	131	64	85	17	35.6
SD	7.6	2.5	5.7	14.3	68	1.8	116	22	0	2759	143	0	27	22	18	4	0.8
During Transfusion 1																	
Mean	—	—	—	—	—	—	—	—	—	—	—	—	136	65	90	17	36.7
SD	—	—	—	—	—	—	—	—	—	—	—	—	25	16	14	4	0.6
1 Hour Posttransfusion 1																	
Mean	30.5	10.1	13.1	18.8	180	8.5	54	0	0	6920	731	0.3	130	67	90	17	36.6
SD	4.1	1	7.4	13.2	53	0.8	336	0	0	6777	571	0.2	23	14	14	3	0.7
24 Hour Posttransfusion																	
Mean	27.7	9.2	9.1	15.4	170	8.6	6	0	0	3234	621	0.2	117	69	84	17	37.3
SD	5.4	2.3	3.3	15.4	62	0.7	12	0	0	2127	306	0	16	9	11	3	0.6

Hct, hematocrit; Hgb, hemoglobin; WBC, white blood cell; SHC, supernatant hemoglobin content.

TABLE 31.7. Correlation Between Red Cell Volume Washed and Supernatant Hemoglobin

	Supernatant Hemoglobin		Fat Particles <9μm		Fat 9–40μm		Fat >40μm		D-Dimer		C3a		Heparin		WBC
	Washout (%)	Account (%)	Washout (%)	Account (%)	Washout (%)	Account (%)	Washout (%)	Account (%)	Washout (%)	Account (%)	Washout (%)	Account (%)	Washout (%)	Account (%)	Washout (%)
Post-wash															
Mean	94.9	74.7	96.4	112	95.3	70	84.3	107	98.3	108	97.5	115.9	96.6	87.1	84.2
SD	2.5	31.5	12.7	198	14.8	253	33.4	416	2.7	55	2.7	50.4	4.1	58.1	12.2

Hct, hematocrit; Hgb, hemoglobin; WBC, white blood cell; SHC, supernatant hemoglobin content.

TABLE 31.8. Correlation Between Red Blood Cell Volume Washed and Supranatant Hemoglobin

	Supranatant Hemoglobin		Fat Particles <9μm		Fat 9–40μm		Fat >40μm		D-Dimer		C3a		Heparin		WBC
	Washout (%)	Account (%)	Washout (%)	Account (%)	Washout (%)	Account (%)	Washout (%)	Account (%)	Washout (%)	Account (%)	Washout (%)	Account (%)	Washout (%)	Account (%)	Washout (%)
Post-wash															
Mean	69.2	101.3	84.2	582	93.7	336	100		61.2	484	95.9	100	80.4	168	51.6
SD	22.6	38	13.9	664	10.2	378	0		18.1	138	2.7	63	23.7	145	27.5

features. Potentially deleterious materials such as plasma free hemoglobin, D-dimer, C3a (complement), and fat can be confidently removed. In our study, washing shed blood intraoperatively reduced the total amount of supernatant hemoglobin by 95% and the total amount of complement C3a and D-dimer by 98%. Fat particles less than 9 μm and 9–40 μm in size were also reduced by 98%, whereas fat particles of greater than 40 μm were reduced by 92%. Washing postoperatively shed blood reduced supernatant hemoglobin by 78% and fat particles of less than 9 μm by 85%, 9–40 μm by 98%, and greater than 40 μm by 100%. The cell washer is slightly less effective postoperatively because of the smaller amount of red cells and a washing bowl that was, at times, less than full. Because each of these materials is potentially toxic, the process of cell washing provides a higher quality red cell product. The smallest filter currently available on filtered units is 40 μm, so none of the smaller fat particles would be removed. The accumulation of these materials in the aggregate may be associated with increased morbidity, particularly in those cases with higher blood loss. In addition, the hematocrit of the washed product averages 45%, whereas that of a filtered unit averages 20%. The effectiveness of the Haemolite cell washer is such that one could reliably reinfuse 9 units of shed blood perioperatively for every unit of filtered blood returned to the patient (3). Recently, it has been published that the use of antibiotics in the surgical wound, such as Tobramycin, should be used with caution in a filtered system (45). No such concern for reinfusion exists if cell washing occurs. There were no adverse clinical effects in patients after reinfusion of up to 2 units postoperatively or 9 units intraoperatively. Postoperative reinfusion can now be accomplished in a continuous fashion through use of a portable cell washer. The technique is safe, effective, and dramatically reduces the potential for the morbidity associated with conventional blood administration.

SUMMARY

Blood conservation in orthopedic surgery is safe, cost effective, and efficient with the use of the Cell Saver for intraoperative autotransfusion. The use of the Cell Saver at NEBH has dramatically reduced the requirement for homologous transfusions in reconstructive surgery. The more recent addition of postoperative reinfusion techniques will yet further reduce the morbidity associated with homologous transfusion.

REFERENCES

1. Ghali WA, Palepu A, Paterson WG. Evaluation of red blood cell transfusion practices with the use of preset criteria. Can Med Assoc J 1994; 150:1449–1454.
2. Simpson MB, Georgopoulos G, Orsini E, Eilert RE. Autologous transfusions for orthopaedic procedures at a children's hospital. J Bone Joint Surg [Am] 1992;74:652–658.
3. Audet AM, Goodnough LT, Parvin CA. Evaluating the appropriateness of red blood cell transfusions: the limitations of retrospective medical record reviews. Int J Qual Health Care 1996;8:41–49.
4. Goodnough LT, Vizmeg K, Riddell J, Soegiarso RW. Discharge haematocrit as clinical indicator for blood transfusion audit in surgery patients. Transfus Med 1994;4:35–44.
5. Pinkerton PH. Use of autologous blood in support of orthopaedic surgery using a hospital-based autologous donor programme. Transfus Med 1995;5:139–144.
6. Peterman TA, Jaffe HW, Feorino PM, et al. Transfusion-associated acquired immunodeficiency syndrome in the United States. JAMA 1985; 254:2913–2917.
7. Keeling MM, Gray LA, Brink MA, Hillerich VK. Intraoperative autotransfusion. Experience in 725 consecutive cases. Am Surg 1983;197: 536–541.
8. Linden JV, Paul B, Dressler KP. A report of 104 transfusion errors in New York State. Transfusion 1992;32:601–606.
9. Popovsky MA, Chaplin HC Jr, Moore SB. Transfusion-related acute lung injury: a neglected, serious complication of hemotherapy. Transfusion 1992;32:589–592.
10. Hohn DC, Meyers AJ, Gherini ST, et al. Production of acute pulmonary injury by leukocytes and activated complement. Surgery 1980;88: 48–58.
11. Luscher EF. Activated leukocytes and the hemostatic system. Rev Infect Dis 1987;9:S546–552.
12. Myhre BA. Fatalities from blood transfusion. JAMA 1980;244: 1333–1335.
13. Thomas L. Possible role of leukocyte granules in the Schwartzmann and Arthus reaction. Proc Soc Exp Biol Med 1964:115:235.
14. Woda R, Tetzzaff JE. Upper airway edema following autologous blood transfusions from a wound drainage system. Can J Anesth 1922; 39:290–292.
15. Sieunarine K, Langton S, Lawrence-Brown M, et al. Elastase levels in salvaged blood and the effect of cell washing. Aust NZ J Surg 1990; 60:613–616.
16. Tawes RL Jr, Scribner RG, Duval TB, et al. The cell saver and autologous transfusion: an underutilized resource in vascular surgery. Am J Surg 1986;152:105–109.
17. Waymack JP, Yurt RW. The effect of blood transfusions on immune function. V. The effect on the inflammatory response to bacterial infections. J Surg Res 1990;48:147–153.
18. Bradley JA. The blood transfusion effect: experimental aspects. Immunol Lett 1991;29:127–132.
19. Perkins HA. Transfusion-induced immunologic unresponsiveness. Transfus Med Rev 1988;2:196–203.
20. Kaplan J, Sarnaik S, Gitlin J, Lusher J. Diminished helper/suppressor lymphocyte ratios and natural killer activity in recipients of repeated blood transfusions. Blood 1984;64:308–310.
21. Gascon P, Zoumbos NC, Young NS. Immunologic abnormalities in patients receiving multiple blood transfusions. Ann Intern Med 1984; 100:173–177.
22. Triulzi DJ, Vanek K, Ryan DH, et al. A clinical and immunologic study of blood transfusion and postoperative bacterial infection in spinal surgery. Transfusion 1992;32:517–524.
23. Murphy P, Heal JM, Blumberg N. Bacterial infection after hip replacement surgery. Transfusion 1989;29:S90.

24. Triulzi DJ, Blumberg N, Heal JM. Association of transfusion with post-operative bacterial infection. Crit Rev Clin Lab Sci 1990;28:95–107.
25. Culter BS. Avoidance of homologous transfusion in aortic operations: the role of autotransfusion, hemodilution and surgical technique. Surgery 1984;95:717–723.
26. Eckardt JJ, Gossett TC, Amstutz HC. Autologous transfusion and total hip arthroplasty. Clin Orthop 1978;132:39–45.
27. Faris PM, Ritter MA, Keating EM, et al. Unwashed filtered shed blood collected after knee and hip arthroplasties. A source of autologous red blood cells. J Bone Joint Surg [Am] 1991:73:1169–1178.
28. Keeling MM, Schmidt-Clay P, Kotcamp WW. Autotransfusion in the postoperative orthopedic patient. Clin Orthop 1993:291:251–258.
29. Mattox KL. Comparison of techniques of autotransfusion. Surgery 1978;84:700–702.
30. Kristensen PW, Sorensen LS, Thyregod HC. Autotransfusion of drainage blood in arthroplasty. A prospective, controlled study of 31 operations. Acta Orthop Scand 1992;63:377–380.
31. Popovsky MA, Devine PA, Taswell HF. Intraoperative autologous transfusion. Mayo Clin Proc 1985;60:125–134.
32. Thompson JD, Callaghan JJ, Savory G, et al. Prior deposition of autologous blood in elective surgery. J Bone Joint Surg [Am] 1987:69: 320–324.
33. Turner RH, Capozzi JD, Kim A, Anas PP, Hardman E. Blood conservation in major orthopedic surgery. Clin Orthop 1990;256:299–305.
34. Woolson ST, Marsh JS, Tanner JB. Transfusion of previously deposited autologous blood for patients undergoing hip replacement surgery. J Bone Joint Surg [Am] 1987;69:325.
35. Young JN, Ecker RR, Moretti RL, et al. Autologous blood retrieval in thoracic, cardiovascular, and orthopedic surgery. Am J Surg 1982;144: 48–52.
36. Clements DH, Sculco TP, Burke SW, et al. Salvage and reinfusion of postoperative sanguineous wound drainage. J Bone Joint Surg [Am] 1992:74:646–651.
37. Healy JC, Frankforter SA, Graves BK, et al. Preoperative autologous blood donation in total-hip arthroplasty. A cost-effectiveness analysis. Arch Pathol Lab Med 1994;118:465–470.
38. Hedstrom M, Flordal PA, Ahl T, Svensson J, Dalén N. Autologous blood transfusion in hip replacement. No effect on blood loss but less increase of plasminogen activator inhibitor in a randomized series of 80 patients. Acta Orthop Scand 1996;67:317–320.
39. Berman AT, Levenberg RJ, Tropiano MT, Parks B, Bosacco SJ. Post-operative autotransfusion after total knee arthroplasty. Orthopedics 1996;19:15–22.
40. Blumberg N, Kirkley SA, Heal JM. A cost analysis of autologous and allogeneic transfusions in hip-replacement surgery. Am J Surg 1996; 171:324–330.
41. Fernandez MC, Gottlieb M, Menitove JE. Blood transfusion and post-operative infection in orthopedic patients. Transfusion 1992;32: 318–322.
42. Canadian Orthopedic Perioperative Erythropoietin Study Group. The effectiveness of perioperative recombinant human erythropoietin in elective hip replacement. Lancet 1993;341:1227–1232.
43. Price TH, Goodnough LT, Vogler WR, et al. The effect of recombinant human erythropoietin on the efficacy of autologous blood donation in patients with low hematocrits: a multicenter, randomized, double-blind, controlled trial. Transfusion 1996;36:29–36.
44. Nelson CL, Nelson RL, Cone J. Blood conservation techniques in orthopedic surgery. Review articles. 21 REFS Instr Course Lect 1990; 39:425–429.
45. Lux PS, Martin JW, Whiteside LA. Reinfusion of whole blood following addition of Tobramycin powder to the wound during total knee arthroplasty. J Arthroplasty 1993;8:269–271.

Chapter 32

Obstetrical and Gynecological Transfusion Practice

J. A. COHEN
M. E. BRECHER

INTRODUCTION

The practice of transfusion owes much to the 19th century work of the pioneering and innovative English obstetrician James Blundell. Dr. Blundell, concerned with the loss of blood in puerperal hemorrhage, successfully reintroduced blood transfusion to medical practice after 150 years of mandated prohibition in Europe. His studies laid the groundwork for the rational use of blood transfusion for years to come.

The practice of both obstetrics and gynecology and transfusion medicine has advanced greatly since the time of Dr. Blundell. This chapter focuses on the unique aspects of current transfusion practice in obstetrics and gynecology.

BLOOD USE IN OBSTETRICS AND GYNECOLOGY

Blood use by obstetrical and gynecological patients is infrequent. In a typical tertiary care hospital, only 2.3% of these patients are transfused, consuming just 1.6% of all transfused units (1). These percentages reflect a dramatic decreasing trend in blood use. In a retrospective review of 30,621 deliveries between 1976 and 1986, Klapholz (2) found that in 1976, 4.6% of women received blood transfusions. This percentage fell to 1.9% in 1986. Similarly, over the interval from 1989 to 1991, Morrison et al. (3) documented a 60% decrease in the number of obstetrical and gynecological patients receiving transfusions and a 75% decrease in the number of units used. Finally, Maxwell (4) reported that 13.7% of women undergoing cesarean sections in 1971–1974 were transfused, whereas only 5.7% were transfused during 1984–1986. These marked decreases in blood use were seen not only in obstetrics and gynecology, but in all medical and surgical specialties, and likely reflect the recognition that human immunodeficiency virus (HIV) could be transmitted by transfusion. In addition, transfusion practice is now more closely audited by quality assurance committees, which use recently published consensus guidelines to evaluate blood use. Specifically, these guidelines recommend adoption of a lower transfusion trigger, which has certainly contributed to a decline in blood use.

Because of this decline, older reviews overestimate current practice. Representative "current" published maximum surgical blood ordering schedules (MSBOS) for obstetrical and gynecological procedures are summarized in Table 32.1 and serve as a useful guide in preparing blood for surgery. The MSBOS provides for the transfusion requirements of most patients undergoing the stated procedure.

GYNECOLOGICAL TRANSFUSION PRACTICE

As with other surgical disciplines, blood use in gynecology is determined by specific operative procedure, although in some cases, published data are limited. For many procedures, such as dilatation and curettage, cone cervical excision, tubal ligation, abdominal hysterectomy (nontumor), and vaginal hysterectomy, blood use is uncommon (less than 10% of cases). Thus, for these procedures, most MSBOS require only a preoperative blood type and antibody screen. This is supported by the finding that only 2 of 88 patients

TABLE 32.1 REPRESENTATIVE MODELS OF MSBOS OF OBSTETRICS AND GYNECOLOGICAL PROCEDURES

Procedure	University of North Carolina	University of Michigan[5]	University of Cincinnati[6]
C-section			
Elective	Type and screen	Type and screen	Type and screen
Emergency			As ordered
Hysterectomy			
Vaginal or abdominal	Type and screen	Type and screen	Type and screen
Radical with pelvic node dissection	2	4	4
Total pelvic exenteration	4		6
Vulvectomy			
Simple			Type and screen
Radical with/without nodes	2	1 (with) 2 (without)	2
Debulking procedure			2
Cervical conization	Type and screen	Type and screen	Type and screen
Ectopic pregnancy	2		Type and screen
Oophorectomy		Type and screen	Type and screen
Tubuloplasty/ligation		Type and screen	Type and screen
Pelvic lymph node dissection		3	4
Ovarian wedge resection		Type and screen	Type and screen
Hysterotomy (other than C-section)			2
Abortion, therapeutic		Type and screen	
Cervical circlage		Type and screen	
Dilatation and curettage		Type and screen	No cross match, no type and screen
Salpingo-oophorectomy		Type and screen	

Such schedules are based primarily on local blood utilization, regional and national practice, and consensus between the transfusion service and the surgery services.

(2.3%) undergoing vaginal hysterectomy in a community hospital were transfused (1–2 units each) (7). In the same study, 20 of 233 patients (8.6%) undergoing abdominal hysterectomy were transfused a total of 42 units of blood (2.1 units per patients; range 1–4 units). On retrospective review, only 15 of 20 cases were found to be appropriately transfused. More complicated cancer operations require transfusion of 3–4 units of red blood cells (Table 32.1).

Gynecological patients, in general, receive less blood than other surgical patients. They have a lower transfusion trigger and receive fewer units of blood (Table 32.2). In one study, an average of 2.4 units of red blood cells were transfused to gynecological patients; however, 81% of these patients received only 1–2 units (7). For the most part, the transfusion issues facing the gynecological patient are similar to those faced by the general surgical patient. These issues are covered extensively elsewhere in this book. Special situations do arise in the transfusion of obstetrical patients, and for this reason, the remainder of this chapter is devoted to these patients.

BLOOD USE IN PREGNANCY

Approximately 0.5–2.5% of pregnant women are transfused at or near the time of delivery. This percentage is low compared with that of the average adult surgical patient; obstetrical patients are generally young, healthy, and have volume expansion and are thus better able to tolerate blood loss.

The transfusion needs of most pregnant women can be met by 2 units of blood. In a review of 16,462 deliveries, Sherman et al. (8) found that 3.5% suffered from obstetrical hemorrhage; of these, only 4.7% received more than 2 units.

TABLE 32.2. TRANSFUSION PRACTICE AT CEDARS-SINAI MEDICAL CENTER IN LOS ANGELES IN 1987 WITH 4365 CONSECUTIVE RED CELL TRANSFUSIONS

	Mean Red Blood Cells Per Patient (units)	Mean Hemoglobin Pretransfusion (g/L)	Percent of Patients Using			
			1–2 units	3–4 units	5–8 units	>8 units
Obstetrics	2.5	76	81	15	0	4
Gynecology	2.4	82	81	9	7	3
Hematology/oncology	4.7	82	43	24	20	13
Orthopedics	2.6	88	61	28	10	1
Urology	2.3	95	71	21	8	0
Cardiovascular Surgery	3.9	85	47	29	16	8
General Surgery	3.9	90	57	23	12	8

From Pepkowitz HS. Autologous blood donation and obstetric transfusion practice. In: Sacher RA, Bucher ME, eds. Obstetric transfusion practice. Bethesda, MD: American Association of Blood Banks, 1993.

At other institutions, 19% (1) and 29% (2) of transfused women received more than 2 units (Table 32.2). These latter results are tempered by the fact that they included some data obtained before the acquired immunodeficiency syndrome epidemic, when blood use was more liberal.

Despite the fact that obstetrical transfusion is infrequent and typically uses only 1–2 units of blood, obstetrical hemorrhage remains the major cause of maternal mortality (overall mortality of 9.1 per 100,000 live births) (8). In one study, peripartum hemorrhage accounted for 799 of 2666 (30.2%) maternal deaths; other major causes of death included pulmonary embolism (23.4%) and pregnancy-induced hypertension (18.1%) (8). Of the 799 hemorrhage-related deaths, ruptured ectopic pregnancies alone accounted for 37%; other major causes included abruptio placentae (16%) and uterine bleeding (10%). Because maternal blood volume, cardiac output, and uterine blood flow are massively increased by the third trimester of gestation, uterine bleeding during this time can rapidly become a serious event. For example, uterine blood flow at 10 weeks gestation is only 50 mL/min; by term, blood flow has accelerated to 500 mL/min (9).

Although the overall risk of peripartum transfusion is low, there are subpopulations of women for whom this risk is increased. Factors associated with increased risk of transfusion include previous abortion (2.6%), bleeding during pregnancy (2.6%), oligohydramnios (3.9%), polyhydramnios (7.1%), operative/instrumental delivery (4.8–29%), breech extraction (12.5%), multiple pregnancy (8.3% for twins, 12.5% for triplets/quadruplets), abnormal placentation (9.1% for marginal to 41.7% for accreta), cesarean section (5.2%), drug induction/augmentation (oxytocin 5.5–45.4%, prostaglandin 4.8%), magnesium sulfate therapy for preeclampsia (21.8%) or for tocolysis for preterm labor (10.9%), and HELLP syndrome (hemolytic anemia, elevated liver enzymes, and a low platelet count) (100%) (2, 8, 10).

A number of studies have implicated abnormal placentation as the most frequently transfused diagnosis. Nearly one-third of patients with placenta previa sustain peripartum blood loss warranting transfusion. These patients also required the largest transfusions; in 12 patients, a mean of 5.0 units of red blood cells (range 1–28 units) were used. Transfused patients with abruptio placentae ($n = 4$) received an average of 4.0 units of red blood cells (range 2–7 units) (8). Sherman et al. (8) found that the need for transfusion could only be anticipated on the basis of antepartum causes in 23.7% of patients ultimately receiving blood products.

AUTOLOGOUS BLOOD DONATION IN PREGNANCY

Autologous blood donation is widely used in elective surgery and is discussed in detail in Chapter 8. Briefly, autologous blood is collected to protect the patient from blood-borne infections, most importantly HIV, hepatitis B and C, and human T-lymphotropic virus (HTLV). Other adverse effects of transfusion, such as sensitization to cellular antigens, febrile reactions, and anaphylaxis, are also eliminated. Risks of blood collection and storage include reduction in blood volume and hematocrit, bacterial contamination and loss of red blood cell viability during prolonged storage, and clerical error. When autologous blood collection is clinically indicated, these risks are minimal (1).

SAFETY AND TIMING OF AUTOLOGOUS BLOOD DONATION IN PREGNANCY

Although blood may be collected at any point during a pregnancy, the third trimester is usually recommended. Pronounced maternal autonomic instability and a high incidence of spontaneous abortion have discouraged blood collection during the first trimester (1); thus, the safety of donation during this time has not been evaluated. In addition, blood collected during the first and the second trimesters must be stored frozen and then deglycerolized before use, which not only provides additional potential for error and increases cost but also limits availability on an emergency basis.

Autologous donation is optimal during the third trimester of pregnancy in terms of both blood storage issues and maternal and fetal safety. A number of studies have demonstrated, through continuous fetal heart tracings during blood donation and through correlation with fetal outcome, that third trimester donation causes no apparent harm to the fetus (11–14). More recent work by Droste et al. (15) used Doppler ultrasound techniques to sensitively analyze maternal and fetal hemodynamic parameters (cardiac output, total peripheral vascular resistance, and fetal umbilical artery systolic:diastolic ratio) during autologous blood donation in the third trimester of uncomplicated pregnancies. Significant differences in maternal variables were not observed during donation or afterward when the patients were subjected to orthostatic stress. In fact, hemodynamic responses of the pregnant women were similar to those observed in the nongravid age-matched control group. Fetal hemodynamic parameters were also without change, and fetal heart tracings and uterine activity remained normal. Thus, the collection of blood in the third trimester of pregnancy is supported both by its clinical safety record and by prospective studies documenting hemodynamic stability.

Despite these data, there are still concerns regarding the safety of blood donation during pregnancy. The data thus far are limited; Droste et al. (15) studied only 16 completely normal women with routine singleton pregnancies, and other authors report small numbers as well. Adverse reactions such as fainting and seizures occur in 1–2.9% of nonpregnant women who donate blood (1, 16, 17). Because the sample size of pregnant autologous donors is relatively small, significant numbers of low frequency reactions have not been encountered, and their impact on maternal and fetal outcome is unknown. In addition, the data do not adequately address the effects of blood donation in more complicated pregnancies (e.g., multiple gestations) or those in which there is underlying maternal disease.

RECOMMENDATIONS FOR AUTOLOGOUS BLOOD DONATION DURING PREGNANCY

Predelivery autologous blood collection is an absolute indication for women who have developed antibodies to very common ("high frequency") red blood cell antigens, such as k (18,19). These antigens are present on nearly all donor cells, making it extremely difficult if not impossible to provide allogeneic blood for such patients. These women should donate as much blood as possible, beginning early in, or preferably before, pregnancy.

Autologous blood collection is strongly indicated for women with placental abnormalities, particularly placenta previa, because they have a higher incidence of peripartum bleeding and blood use (20). Relative indications for autologous blood collection include any other situations in which there is an increased incidence of transfusion, such as cesarean section. Because there are many situations in which blood is required but in which this need cannot be anticipated antepartum (8) and because of the risk of transfusion-transmitted viral diseases, many women with routine pregnancies now elect to donate autologous blood. Although the safety of blood donation in the third trimester has been demonstrated, physicians should still proceed cautiously, because there are risks inherent to blood collection and administration that are best avoided if these procedures are unnecessary.

In terms of cost effectiveness, a review of 424 red cell transfusions in 15,000 full-term gestations (without placenta previa) estimated that prevention of a single case of post-transfusion HIV by the use of autologous blood would cost between \$26 million and \$300 million dollars (21).

The safety of blood collection during pregnancy has been studied most thoroughly in healthy women during the third trimester and thus can only be recommended for these patients during this interval. Most authors collect blood after 32–36 weeks of gestation (1, 11–14); blood collected 6 weeks before delivery can be stored in liquid (as opposed to frozen) form. One 450-mL unit of blood can be collected each week, with a goal of 2 units (more in a high-risk diagnosis such as placenta previa), as long as the patient's predonation hematocrit exceeds 34%. While donating, the patient should assume the left lateral decubitus position to maintain blood flow through the inferior vena cava. Women should receive daily iron supplementation ($FeSO_4$, 325 mg orally tid) as replacement for iron lost in the donated units (1, 11–14).

As with all transfusion, to minimize complications of transfusion, we recommend that autologous blood be administered only when a predetermined hematocrit (e.g., 25% in a healthy woman) is reached or if the patient develops symptomatic anemia.

RED BLOOD CELL PROBLEMS UNIQUE TO PREGNANCY

HEMOLYTIC DISEASE OF THE NEWBORN

Hemolytic disease of the newborn (HDN) represents a wide spectrum of disease, the most severe manifestations of which are the life-threatening syndromes erythroblastosis fetalis and kernicterus. Erythroblastosis fetalis is an immune hemolytic anemia that develops as a consequence of transplacental passage of maternal antibodies directed against paternal antigens present on fetal erythrocytes. Fetal red blood cell destruction results in anemia, heart failure, generalized edema, portal hypertension, liver failure, and hepatosplenomegaly. Ongoing hemolysis leads to excessive production of unconjugated bilirubin, which in utero is cleared by the maternal liver. The metabolic capacity of the newborn liver cannot keep up with bilirubin production, and the bilirubin is deposited in the basal ganglia of the brain. This deposition is known as kernicterus, which in severe untreated cases can result in 90% mortality. The remaining 10% will be left with chronic neurological sequelae, including neurosensory deafness, spastic choreoathetosis, and mental retardation (22).

RH-RELATED HDN

HDN is most commonly due to production of anti-Rh-D antibodies by a mother who is Rh negative. This disease is thus most frequent in the white population, in which 16% of mothers are Rh negative. Approximately 7.8% of blacks, 3.6% of Native Americans, and 0.3% of Asians are Rh negative (23).

Rh-negative mothers become immunized (i.e., produce anti-Rh-D antibody) when Rh-positive fetal red blood cells enter into the maternal circulation. Fetal erythrocytes have been identified within maternal blood in 0.4–5.8% of pregnant women at 28–30 weeks gestation and in 3.5–7% during the third trimester; however, transfer of fetal cells most commonly occurs at the time of delivery (24, 25). After one pregnancy with an Rh-positive, ABO-compatible infant, approximately 4.9% of Rh-negative mothers become immunized; this percentage rises to 17% after the second such pregnancy and to 50% after the fifth such pregnancy (26–28). ABO incompatibility between the fetus and the mother offers considerable protection, because fetal cells entering the maternal circulation are rapidly destroyed by preformed ABO antibodies before Rh immunization can be initiated. In whites, for example, group A incompatibility between infant and mother provides 90% protection from Rh immunization, whereas B incompatibility provides 55% protection (29).

Rh-immune globulin (RhIg) may be administered to at-risk mothers at times of suspected fetal-maternal blood exchange (i.e., with delivery or trauma). RhIg consists of anti-Rh-D antibodies that bind Rh-D epitopes on fetal red blood cells, thereby preventing them from inciting a maternal immune response. After RhIg administration at the time of delivery became commonplace, the incidence of Rh sensitization decreased to 1.8% (28). After the routine administration of RhIg at 28 weeks gestation, this rate fell to 0.1% (28). Although the incidence of Rh-D mediated HDN has declined from 45.1% per 10,000 total births in 1970 to 15.6 per 10,000 total births in 1983, Rh-D-related disease still accounts for 85–90% of the most severe cases of HDN. Inadvertent omission of RhIg, inadequate dosing, or lack of prenatal care likely account for many of these residual cases.

HDN DUE TO ANTIBODIES OTHER THAN ANTI-RH-D

ABO incompatibility between mother and fetus accounts for most cases of HDN, although most cases are mild. The incidence of jaundice in ABO-incompatible live births is less than 1% (30); in comparison, nearly 50% of Rh-incompatible pregnancies result in moderate or severe disease. Maternal antibodies to other fetal red cell antigens, such as Rh-c, Kell (K), Duffy A (Fya), and Kidd (Jka and Jkb), may also cause severe disease. In Australia, women of reproductive age routinely receive Kell-negative blood. Antibodies to Rh-C and Rh-E, usually in conjunction with Rh-D antibody, can also cause severe disease.

DIAGNOSIS AND MANAGEMENT

Antibody Detection

Routine antibody screening should be performed at the first prenatal visit. If an alloantibody with a specificity known to be associated with HDN is identified, a titer should be performed. A titer (using anti-human globulin) greater than 8 (positive reaction at a 1:8 dilution) is a critical value, requiring additional testing. If the father's erythrocytes are shown to lack the antigen in question and there is no doubt as to paternity, no further investigation is necessary.

Amniocentesis

Amniocentesis (percutaneous transabdominal aspiration of fluid from the amniotic sac) was the primary method of fetal surveillance for many years. In 1961, Liley (31) analyzed amniotic fluid from 101 Rh-D-sensitized pregnancies at 27–41 weeks gestational age. Using the optical density at 450 nm subtracted from a point on a line drawn from the OD at 375 and 525 nm, he identified three zones related to gestational age that were predictive of the severity of hemolytic disease and of the need for clinical intervention. Unfortunately, extrapolation of these curves to earlier gestational ages led to underdiagnosis of anemic infants (32). Newer modified curves more accurately address OD_{450} values between 14 and 40 weeks gestation and provide four different management zones (Fig. 32.1) (33). Amniocentesis can be performed as early as 13–14 weeks; ultrasound guidance should be used to minimize damage to the fetus, placenta, or umbilical cord. Amniotic fluid samples must be protected from light to prevent oxidation of bile pigments and should be free of meconium or blood, which can artifactually increase the optical density at 450 nm. Centrifugation before analysis can clear a specimen of red blood cells.

Recently, polymerase chain reaction- (PCR) based techniques have been used to demonstrate the presence of the Rh-D gene in amniotic fluid and chorionic villi in a research setting (34). This procedure would facilitate earlier diagnosis of the at-risk fetus. In utero PCR-based identification of other red blood cell antigens is currently under investigation.

Periumbilical Blood Sampling

Periumbilical blood sampling (PUBS) or "cordocentesis" provides more information than amniocentesis (Fig. 32.2). Through direct sampling of the fetal circulation, rapid fetal blood typing is performed to determine whether the fetus is at risk. In addition, antibody coating of fetal cells (Coombs test) can be identified, and fetal hematocrit, reticulocyte count, and bilirubin can be quantitated (35–37). Like amniocentesis, this procedure requires ultrasound guidance and is not without risk. In particular, when the placenta is located on the anterior uterine wall, sampling must occur transplacentally. This can lead to leakage of fetal cells into the maternal circulation with subsequent stimulation of the maternal immune system, increase in antibody titer, and worsening of fetal hemolysis (38, 39). This approach is therefore contraindicated. In any PUBS, there is always the risk of umbilical hematoma, fetal bradycardia (typically transient), and fetal loss (1.2%) (39).

INTRAUTERINE TRANSFUSION

Intraperitoneal transfusion (IPT), first described by Liley in 1963, involves the introduction of red cells into the peritoneal cavity; these cells then enter the fetal circulation via the peritoneal lymphatic system. Repeated transfusions were performed and the fetuses delivered at 32 weeks gestation. In the early 1980s, direct transfusion of fetal vessels, using either chorionic plate vessels under direct fetoscopic guidance or umbilical venous puncture under ultrasound guidance, were described (intravascular transfusion [IVT]). These techniques offered more rapid and efficient delivery of red cells to the fetal circulation and rapidly supplanted IPT (40, 41). More recently, Moise et al. (42) have used a combined IVT and IPT approach to minimize the wide swings in hematocrits that occur between transfusions. When IVT alone is used, the fetus is serially transfused to a hematocrit of 50–65%. With the combined IVT/IPT approach, IVT transfusions are given until a fetal hematocrit of 35–40% is achieved. For severely anemic and hydropic infants, a more gradual rise in hematocrit has been advocated; posttransfuion

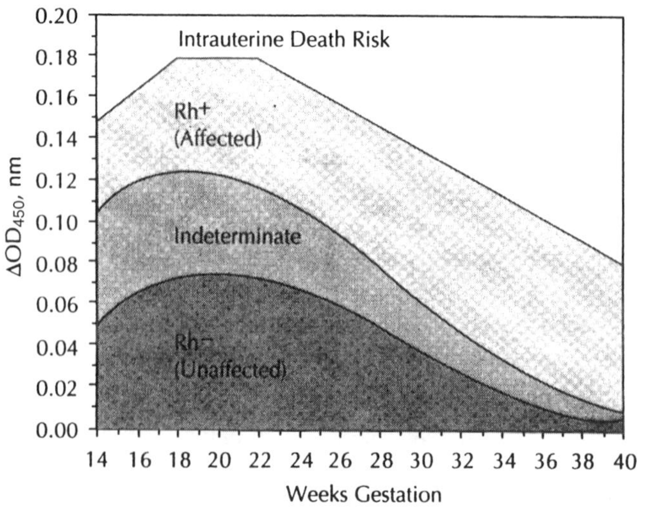

Figure 32.1. ΔOD_{450} amniotic fluid management zones as a function of gestional age. (Reprinted with permission from Queenan JT, Tomai TP, Ural SH, King JC. Deviation in the amniotic fluid optical density at a wavelength of 450 nm in Rh-immunized pregnancies from 14–40 weeks' gestation: a proposal for clinical management. Am J Gynecol 1993:168:1370–1376.)

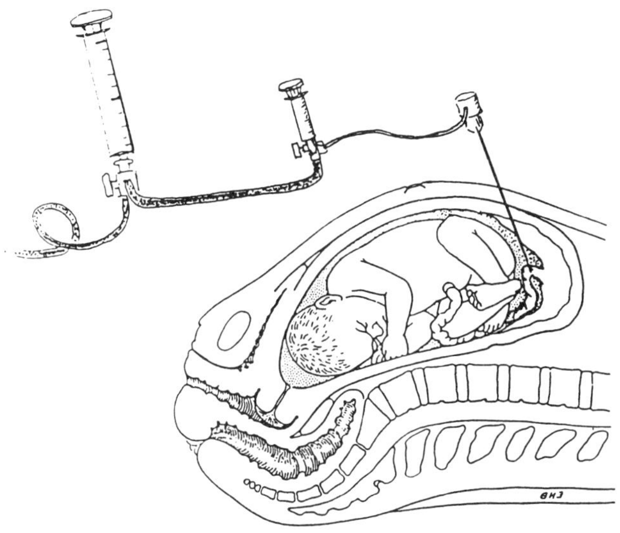

Figure 32.2. Diagrammatic representation of intravascular intrauterine transfusion or cordocentesis. (Reproduced with permission from King JC, Sacher RS. Percutaneous umbilical blood sampling. In: Sacher RA, Strauss R, eds. Contemporary issues in pediatric transfusion medicine. Arlington, VA: American Association of Blood Banks, 1989:33–53.)

hematocrit should not exceed 25% or a fourfold increase from the pretransfusion value (43). In both the IVT and IVT/IPT procedures, the last transfusion is given at 35 weeks and the fetus is delivered at 38 weeks gestation. In general, a fetal hematocrit of less than 30% is considered an indication for intrauterine transfusion.

CHOICE OF BLOOD FOR TRANSFUSION

Historically, type O-negative, Rh-D- or specific antigen-negative, cytomegalovirus-(CMV) negative, "fresh" (less than 7 days old) irradiated red cells were used for intrauterine transfusion. However, recent interest in autologous blood has led to the use of washed maternal blood. Such blood offers the advantage of readily available fresh antigen-negative red cells. Before transfusion, these red cells are leukocyte depleted to minimize the possible transmission of CMV, washed to rid the blood of the offending antibody, packed to a hematocrit of approximately 80%, and irradiated to prevent in utero graft-versus-host disease (44). ABO-incompatible maternal red cells have been used successfully, because ABO antibodies are not formed by the fetus before delivery. As is the case for all other donors, the mother must undergo routine screening for HIV, hepatitis B and C, HTLV-1, and syphilis. Because viruses with poor or partial vertical transmission, such as hepatitis C virus or HIV, may be transmitted by maternal blood, mothers who test positive for these viruses should not donate.

EFFICACY OF INTRAUTERINE TRANSFUSION

A recent study of 1087 IVTs (389 fetuses) performed at 16 centers in the United States and Canada revealed a survival rate of 90% for nonhydropic fetuses and 82% for hydropic fetuses (44). In a follow-up study of children who received IVT, 35 of 38 children had normal neurological development at 2 years of age; in the remaining 3, abnormal development was not believed to be a direct complication of IVT (45).

ALTERNATIVE THERAPIES

In patients with a history of early fetal loss due to HDN and a high titer antibody, serial plasmapheresis may be successful in lowering the maternal antibody titer until intrauterine transfusion becomes feasible (minimum 16 weeks gestational age for IVT and 22 weeks for IPT). Maternal antibody has been detected within the fetus by 6 weeks gestational age; thus, early intervention is recommended in these cases. Plasmapheresis may also be useful when intravascular or IPT is not available or not technically possible (i.e., anterior placental placement).

Administration of intravenous immunoglobulin (IVIG) to the mother before 38 weeks gestation has been reported to be effective in the prevention of hydrops. If confirmed, this modality may significantly reduce the need for invasive therapies (46).

PLATELET PROBLEMS UNIQUE TO PREGNANCY

NEONATAL ALLOIMMUNE THROMBOCYTOPENIC PURPURA

Neonatal alloimmune thrombocytopenia (NAIT) is a rare condition (1 in 3000 to 1 in 5000 births) that occurs when maternal antibodies are formed against paternally derived antigens on fetal platelets (47, 48). These IgG antibodies are capable of crossing the placenta and binding to antigens on the fetal platelets, resulting in their destruction by the fetal reticuloendothelial system. Fetal thrombocytopenia may ensue and, in some cases, may be quite severe. Clinically, the most important consequence of thrombocytopenia is intracranial hemorrhage (and associated neurological sequelae) sustained by up to 30% of affected neonates (48).

Human platelets have five groups of surface glycoproteins; antibodies may be synthesized against a variety of epitopes on these molecules. Antibodies against HPA-I (formerly known as PLA-1) are most frequent, comprising more than 75% of cases of NAIT (47–50). Even though fetal platelets may possess paternally derived antigens that the mother lacks, antibodies are produced in only 4–10% of cases (47–50). The ability to respond (i.e., produce antibodies) in cases of platelet antigen mismatch appears to be linked to the maternal HLA-types DRw52 and Dqw2 (47) The second most common antiplatelet antibody, anti-HPA5b, accounts for about 20% of cases of NAIT; ability to produce this antibody is also associated with maternal human leukocyte antigen- (HLA) types DRw52 and DQw1. Other varieties of anti-platelet antibody are rarely seen. Antibodies directed against the HLA system and the ABO system are of negligible importance in NAIT (47, 49).

Initial Diagnosis and Management (First Pregnancy)

In contrast to the situation in HDN, the first pregnancy is affected in 60% of cases (48). In addition, rapid prenatal platelet typing and antibody screening is not routinely available. Thus, there is no real method by which to predict the first at-risk pregnancy. The diagnosis is suggested by the presence of intracranial hemorrhage on prenatal ultrasound. This is detectable by 20 weeks (47), but the actual hemorrhagic event may theoretically occur as early as 14 weeks, because fetal platelet antigens are already expressed by this gestational age (49). Approximately 10% of intracranial hemorrhages occur in utero; the remainder are due to trauma incurred during vaginal delivery. At birth, petechiae and purpura (present in 85% of HPA-1a mediated cases) in an otherwise healthy neonate are signs of a platelet-mediated hemostatic defect (48). A complete blood count will typically reveal an isolated thrombocytopenia, although there may be some component of anemia due to bleeding. Thrombocytopenia may be quite severe; in one study, the platelet count was less than 10,000 in 27% and 10,000–30,000 in 26% of affected neonates with anti-HPA-1a disease (48). Underlying maternal causes, such as medications and autoimmune diseases, should be ruled out. The maternal platelet count is usually normal. Laboratory confirmation of clinically suspected NAIT is time consuming. Because the consequences of not treating symptomatic NAIT may be grave and the treatment is low risk, clinically suspicious cases should be treated immediately while diagnostic evaluation is in progress (47).

The treatment of choice is transfusion of maternally matched platelets, which may be obtained from the mother by platelet pheresis or from a large regional blood bank. Maternal platelets must be washed to remove ABO-related antibodies and irradiated to destroy contaminating lymphocytes that are capable of causing graft-versus-host disease. Unrelated donor platelets should be CMV seronegative or leukocyte depleted. After platelet transfusion, platelet counts should be repeated daily, because the transfused platelets have a limited life span (3–4 days) and neonatal platelet counts may continue to decline, necessitating repeat transfusion. If platelets are not available, high-dose IVIG (1.0–1.5 g/day) and steroids may be administered; however, 12–24 hours are necessary for response to these medications, so platelet transfusion is preferable if at all possible (47).

To confirm the diagnosis of NAIT, maternal and paternal platelets should be phenotyped to determine if a mismatch exists. Assays for anti-platelet antibodies, such as the platelet immunofluorescence test and glycoprotein-specific immunoassays, will determine whether the mother has produced relevant antibodies. However, it may not be possible to identify antibodies with currently available techniques (26% of cases are antibody negative). Moreover, the presence or titer of antibodies does not always predict clinical disease (48). These specialized tests are usually performed by large reference laboratories and may take several days to complete.

Management of Subsequent Pregnancies

Once an immunized mother has been identified, subsequent pregnancies should be followed carefully for evidence of recurrent NAIT (recurs in 85% of at-risk infants), with the ultimate goal of preventing in utero and perinatal intracranial hemorrhage (48). PUBS may be performed to determine the fetal platelet count at 16–21 weeks. The treatment of fetal thrombocytopenia thus discovered is controversial, and the data are limited. Some authors report successful prevention of intracranial hemorrhage in this population using maternal IVIG therapy. However, there are also several contradictory reports (47). Another option for these pregnancies is serial intrauterine platelet transfusion. This approach is limited by the short life span of transfused platelets, necessitating weekly transfusions and invasive procedures. Regardless of approach, PUBS should be repeated at 38 weeks gestation, and platelets administered as necessary. Some authors suggest cesarean delivery to minimize birth-related trauma. Appropriately prepared maternal or donor platelets should be immediately available at the time of delivery. As noted above, platelet counts should be checked daily after birth because of the short life span of transfused platelets and postnatal decreases in platelet count (49).

The data are limited regarding the prevention of intracranial hemorrhage before 16 weeks gestation. Treatment options under investigation include maternal or fetal administration of IVIG and/or corticosteroids (49).

Future Technologies

With advances in current technology, it may soon be possible to screen all pregnant women to identify those that are negative for common platelet antigens and are thus at risk for NAIT. Development of a medication to prevent maternal sensitization, analogous to Rh-immune globulin used in HDN, would also prove useful.

GESTATIONAL THROMBOCYTOPENIA AND IDIOPATHIC THROMBOCYTOPENIC PURPURA

Gestational Thrombocytopenia

In 1986, Freedman et al. (51) observed that 5% of healthy women developed isolated thrombocytopenia during pregnancy (platelet count less than 136 $\times$ 10^9/L); subsequent prospective studies reported percentages as a high as 8.3% (52). In each case, the workers carefully excluded other causes of thrombocytopenia, notably hypertension and preeclampsia, and other underlying maternal disease and drugs. Thrombocytopenia in these normal women was usually discovered during routine peripartum laboratory determinations. This finding has come to be known as thrombocytopenia of pregnancy or gestational thrombocytopenia (GT) (51, 52).

In 95% of women with GT, thrombocytopenia was mild; only 5% had platelet counts less than 100,000/L (53). Platelet-mediated bleeding diathesis did not occur during pregnancy, delivery (vaginal or cesarean), with administration of spinal or epidural anesthesia, or in the postpartum period. In one study, excessive bleeding during these events was not observed even with platelet counts less than 50,000 (54). In almost all cases of GT, the maternal platelet count returned to normal by the seventh postpartum day (53). Of note, many affected women had experienced GT in earlier pregnancies; thus, this is a recurrent phenomenon. In summary, the maternal effects of GT are minimal; the women are asymptomatic and their platelet counts recover rapidly after delivery.

GT also appears to have little effect on fetal platelet count or outcome. In 756 mothers with GT, Burrows and Kelton (55) found only one neonate with a platelet count of less than 20,000. Neonatal platelet counts were normal even when mothers had marked thrombocytopenia (less than 50,000) at delivery (54).

Thus, GT appears to be a benign phenomenon in terms of both maternal and fetal outcome. However, the differential diagnosis of isolated maternal thrombocytopenia includes idiopathic thrombocytopenic purpura (ITP).

Idiopathic Thrombocytopenic Purpura

ITP occurs most commonly in young women of childbearing age and can present during pregnancy (56). In this disease, the mother produces autoantibodies directed against her own platelet antigens. These antibodies can cross the placenta and recognize shared antigens on fetal platelets, leading to destruction of these platelets and subsequent fetal thrombocytopenia. Fetal thrombocytopenia has potentially dangerous consequences, the most important being intracranial hemorrhage sustained during the trauma of vaginal delivery (55–58). For this reason, many experts have recommended cesarean section for women with ITP. However, the incidence of severe fetal thrombocytopenia is low, and intracranial hemorrhage is rare. In their 1993 study, Burrows and Kelton (55) documented cord blood platelet counts less than 20,000 in only 4 of 46 neonates born to women with known ITP. Moreover, there was no associated fetal morbidity or mortality.

Women with ITP are often treated with steroids and IVIG during their pregnancies, and their fetuses may undergo prenatal blood sampling. These therapies all have associated morbidity and mortality, and if applied to all pregnant women with isolated thrombocytopenia, large numbers of women with GT (up to 8.3% of all pregnant women) would be exposed to unnecessary risk. Because a new presentation of ITP is much less frequent than GT and the incidence of a poor outcome is low in ITP, prenatal manipulations and cesarean section are not warranted, except in cases of known ITP and when there is strong clinical suspicion of ITP (57).

Management of Pregnant Patients with Isolated Thrombocytopenia

Healthy women who present with isolated thrombocytopenia during pregnancy should be managed conservatively, because the risk of a poor outcome is low. A detailed medical history should be obtained, and use of medications should be ruled out. A history of thrombocytopenia or of symptoms consistent with a platelet-related hemostatic defect should suggest a diagnosis of ITP. History of a pregnancy complicated by thrombocytopenia in an otherwise healthy woman most likely represents recurrent GT.

Physical examination of the mother should be performed, with particular attention to evidence of submucosal (gingival, gastrointestinal) and subcutaneous hemorrhage. A complete blood count and peripheral blood smear will help to exclude other hematological disorders or artifactual thrombocytopenia. Maternal platelet counts should be repeated periodically and followed monthly for several months after delivery to ensure that adequate recovery has occurred (54). Failure of the platelet count to return to normal after several months suggests an etiology other than GT and merits further hematological evaluation (54).

If the clinical suspicion of maternal ITP is low, prenatal fetal platelet counts are not indicated. A platelet count should be obtained from the cord blood upon delivery. The count should be repeated within the first few days of life, because this value usually decreases after delivery (55, 57).

The maternal platelet count should be measured before delivery; it typically increases at this time and was generally found to exceed 50,000, thus ensuring adequate maternal hemostasis for vaginal delivery or cesarean section, as well as spinal or epidural anesthesia (52, 53, 55, 57, 58).

OTHER IMMUNE PHENOMENA THAT COMPLICATE PREGNANCY

THE ANTIPHOSPHOLIPID-ANTIBODY (APL) SYNDROME

Antiphospholipid-antibody syndrome is a recently recognized syndrome in which antibodies to negatively charged phospholipids (such as cardiolipin, phosphatidyl serine, or phosphatidylinositol) are associated with a thrombotic diathesis, fetal wastage, and thrombocytopenia. Laboratory findings can include a prolonged activated partial thromboplastin time (APTT) or, less frequently, a prolonged prothrombin time (PT), a falsely positive screening test for sero diagnosis of syphilis, and a positive lupus anticoagulant (59). Patients may have clinical manifestations of connective tissue disease or may be asymptomatic. Theoretically, fetal wastage occurs as a result of antibody-induced placental vascular thrombosis; however, the data do not support this theory (60). Alternatively, these antibodies could bind placental phospholipid antigens, possibly inhibiting placental growth or the passage of nutrients (60). Untreated, over 90% of pregnancies in women with a significant anti-phospholipid antibody who have previously experienced fetal wastage fail to produce a viable infant (61).

Recent reports of three patients suggest that plasma exchange or immunoabsorbent plasmapheresis in conjunction with steroids and aspirin may reduce the risk of recurrent abortion (62a–64). Similarly, anecdotal reports suggest a beneficial role for combination therapy with IVIG, steroids, and anticoagulants (61). The use of subcutaneous heparin has been more extensively studied and appears to offer the most promise. In a study of 15 patients receiving subcutaneous heparin every 12 hours, at a dose sufficient to prolong the mid-interval APTT to 1.5–2.0 times normal, a pregnancy success rate of 93% was observed (62). Similarly, in a multicenter study in which all women received 80 mg of aspirin daily but were randomized to receive either prednisone (40 mg orally each day) or subcutaneous heparin (every 12 hours), the fetal survival was 75% in both groups (63). These data are encouraging; however, there was significantly increased prematurity and maternal morbidity in those women receiving steroids.

ANTI-P

Women with the rare red cell phenotypes p or Pk lack the high incidence P antigen and can form either the antibody complex anti-P, anti-P1, anti-Pk (in p individuals, formerly known as anti-Tja), or anti-P (in Pk individuals). These antibodies have been associated with an increased risk of first trimester spontaneous abortions (64–66); in contrast, fetal wastage associated with HDN and other red cell antibodies such as anti-D or anti-K typically manifest in the third trimester. Plasma exchange or plasma exchange with antibody absorption was successfully used in six pregnancies of four patients (two Pk phenotype and two p phenotype) who all had repeated abortions (64–68). These reports suggest that plasmapheresis be initiated early (as soon as conception is confirmed) because a delay of even 9 weeks in one case was associated with failure (64, 65). It is not known whether plasma exchange should be continued past the 20th week of gestation because fetal loss due to these antibodies is uncommon after this time.

COMPLETE CONGENITAL HEART BLOCK

The development of complete congenital heart block (CCHB) in the fetus is strongly associated with the presence of antibodies to soluble ribonucleoproteins, principally SSA (Ro) and SSB (La) (69–71). This antibody-mediated myocarditis and inflammation with subsequent fibrosis of the cardiac conducting system has been described as CCHB type I to distinguish it from CCHB resulting from major cardiac malformations (type II) or from mass lesions (type III) (69). By the time CCHB is detected, the damage is irreversible.

Most cases occur in women with subclinical connective tissue disease (70). In 41% of cases there was at least one other affected sibling (71). Although the risk of CCHB is 1 in 20 for the first pregnancy in women who produce anti-Ro, the risk in subsequent pregnancies rises to 1 in 3 (71–73). Other risk factors include high titer antibodies, the presence of anti-La in addition to anti-Ro, and the presence of HLA DR3 in the mother (70, 73).

As yet, there is no optimal management for pregnant patients with anti-Ro or anti-La. It has been suggested that for high-risk patients, plasma exchange (three times per week) in addition to steroids should be started as early as possible in the pregnancy.

Plasma exchange was used in four pregnancies with mixed results (71, 74–76). However, in the two cases resulting in healthy infants, therapy was initiated before 20 weeks gestation. Because the data are so limited, it is not possible to accurately assess the efficacy of plasma exchange on outcome.

MYASTHENIA GRAVIS

Myasthenia gravis (MG) is an autoimmune disorder in which specific IgG autoantibodies bind to and inactivate acetylcholine receptors on skeletal muscle. This leads to a spectrum of disease, from mild, transient fatigue to severe weakness requiring ventilator assistance. Pregnancy increases the risk of exacerbation, and MG increases the risk of adverse reactions to anesthesia (77). Fetal risks include prematurity, neonatal myasthenia, or, rarely, arthrogryposis (77, 78). In a summary of 16 reports, 36.5% (19 of 52 pregnancies) of myasthenic mothers delivered premature infants (77).

Plauche (77) reviewed 322 pregnancies in 225 myasthenic mothers and identified acute exacerbations of MG in 41% of patients during gestation and in 29.8% of patients in the puerperium. There was no change in the status of the disease in 31.7% of patients. Twenty-nine percent showed at least a partial remission during pregnancy. Four patients (1%) had remissions during pregnancy followed by significant puerperal exacerbation.

Because uterine contraction is not dependent on acetylcholine receptors, MG does not affect the first stage of labor. However, in the second and third stages of labor, the striated abdominal muscles are required for expulsion. These muscles may be weakened by MG or the patient may fatigue, thus necessitating forceps or vacuum-assisted delivery (77).

Plauche (77) reported that 52 of 276 newborns (18.8%) developed neonatal myasthenia. Neonatal myasthenia is transient and is due to the passive transfer of anti-acetylcholine receptor antibodies from the mother. Symptoms of neonatal myasthenia can occur within hours of birth or up to 3 days after delivery. Severity of symptoms varies from mild generalized weakness to respiratory distress. Unfortunately, the maternal antibody titer does not correlate with the severity of symptoms in the mother or the baby; thus, the occurrence or severity of neonatal myasthenia cannot be predicted (77, 78).

RISKS OF PLASMA EXCHANGE AND PREGNANCY

A major concern in pregnant patients is the precipitation of labor. Because plasma exchange removes plasma proteins nonspecifically, removal of certain as yet uncharacterized "circulating factors" may involve some risk. Although the mechanisms leading to the onset of parturition are poorly understood, there is mounting evidence suggesting that an immune modulating system turns off the mother's ability to recognize and mount an effective cell-mediated or humoral cytotoxic attack against the fetus (79). The onset of labor may thus be due to relaxation of this suppression of graft (the fetus) rejection. Further, it has been suggested that maternal immunotolerance may be mediated by a soluble factor that could be removed by plasma exchange. In goats, ultrafiltration of extracorporeally circulated blood predictively precipitated the onset of labor in all three trimesters of pregnancy (79). In controlled experiments, only the removal of a low-molecular-weight fraction predictably induced labor. Although worrisome, such has not been the experience reported in the numerous studies of pregnant women in which pregnancies were sustained (typically against high odds) until term.

A second possible risk would be a decrease in the mother's and in the infant's immune response to infection because of the removal of maternal immunoglobulin. Infections are uncommon in most nonpregnant patients undergoing plasma exchange; however, they have been documented in patients with renal disease (80). If the IgG level falls to less than 200 mg/dL during a series of exchanges, an infusion of IVIG should be considered (81, 82). This may be relevant in pregnant patients due to the immunomodulation of pregnancy.

A third concern in the pregnant patient is the removal of plasma cholinesterase. Plasma cholinesterase is important in the metabolism of drugs such as succinylcholine, which may be used during anesthesia. If these medications are used shortly after plasma exchange with albumin or crystalloid replacement, the patient may be predisposed to apnea as a result of excessive blockade of acetylcholine receptors by the unexpectedly high levels of succinylcholine (83).

Plasma exchange using fluids other than plasma for replacement can result in transient (less than 4 hours) prolongation of PT, partial thromboplastin time (PTT), and thrombin time; the concentrations of specific clotting factors may not normalize until 24 hours after the procedure (84). However, whether a patient is predisposed to hemorrhage due to depletion of coagulation factors such as fibrinogen or to a thrombotic event as a result of decreased antithrombin III (ATIII) and elevated factor VIII levels (due to stress) is unpredictable. Fortunately, few thrombotic or hemorrhagic complications have been reported, and in those reports, it is not clear whether they were related to apheresis procedures or the underlying disease. In a study of seven alloimmunized pregnant patients undergoing plasma exchange five times per week, coagulation factor concentrations stayed within normal limits with the exception of one patient with decreasing ATIII levels (85). This study suggests most otherwise healthy pregnant patients will be able to compensate for loss of coagulation factors by increasing their synthesis.

COAGULOPATHIES AND PREGNANCY

THROMBOTIC

Obstetrical patients, because of increased lower extremity stasis associated with a gravid uterus and their decreased mobility, are at increased risk of thrombosis. It has been estimated that 0.09% of women without a history of a thrombotic tendency experience thrombosis during pregnancy (86). This rate increases to 0.2–0.4% in the postpartum period. Women with a personal or family history of venous thromboembolism should be evaluated for a possible hypercoagulable state. Such entities include ATIII deficiency, protein C deficiency, protein S deficiency, and the newly described protein C resistance. Diagnosis and treatment of these entities is complex and exceeds the scope of this chapter. Readers are referred to Chapter 20 on preexisting problems of hypercoagulability and other extensive reviews (87). In such cases, consultation with coagulation experts is highly recommended. In general, subcutaneous heparin is the anticoagulant of choice during pregnancy, although in certain circumstances, specific factor replacement may be warranted (87). Warfarin is known to be teratogenic during the first trimester (88–90), being associating with nasal malformations, epiphyseal stippling, central nervous system alterations, and optic atrophy. However, the use of oral anticoagulants does not appear to be teratogenic during the first 6 weeks of gestation (89). If oral anticoagulation is used later in pregnancy and premature labor occurs, the fetus may be at risk of bleeding because warfarin is known to cross the placenta (91). Low-molecular-weight heparin does not cross the placenta (92).

CONGENITAL BLEEDING DISORDERS AND PREGNANCY

Autosomal dominant inherited bleeding disorders such as factor IX deficiency or von Willebrand disease can complicate a pregnancy. Other factor deficiencies are quite rare. In general, factor levels hemostatic for surgery are adequate for parturition (87). If factor replacement is administered, it should probably be administered for at least 48 hours after delivery to ensure adequate hemostasis (87).

DISSEMINATED INTRAVASCULAR COAGULATION

Disseminated intravascular coagulation (DIC) during pregnancy has been associated with abruptio placentae, amniotic fluid embolism, septic or hypertonic abortion, intrauterine infections, retained dead fetus or necrotic placental tissue, and acute fatty liver of pregnancy (93). DIC is characterized by elevated PT and APTT (which help distinguish it from thrombotic thrombocytopenic purpura [TTP]/hemolytic uremic syndrome [HUS] or HELLP syndrome), decreased platelets and fibrinogen with increases in fibrin degradation products, and a microangiopathic hemolytic anemia (MHA). Thromboplastin (tissue factor) released from a dead fetus or necrotic placental tissue initiates DIC. As in other causes of DIC, the removal of the source of the DIC is of major importance in controlling it. Until the source of DIC is controlled, it is crucial that the patient's blood volume is maintained through the administration of red blood cells and other blood components. Heparin in obstetrical DIC is generally indicated only in the rare case of two or more fetuses in which one or more has died, leaving a remaining viable fetus. In such cases, heparin has been used to control ongoing DIC, allowing successful maturation and delivery of the remaining viable infant (94, 95). Use of heparin in obstetrical DIC in which there is preexisting placental bleeding such as in an abruptio placentae or after an abortion or delivery may exacerbate and prolong hemorrhage.

Abruptio placentae, the premature separation of a normally located placenta from the uterine wall, is the most frequent cause of obstetrical DIC. Such separation may be associated with vaginal bleeding; however, in some cases, an abruption may not produce vaginal bleeding and can conceal up to 5 L of blood, resulting in hypovolemic shock (93). Examination of placentas has shown evidence of abruption in 4.5% of pregnancies, most (65%) of which are not clinically apparent before delivery (96). If more than 30–40% of the maternal surface is involved, it will result in fetal hypoxia and death (96).

Amniotic fluid embolism is a very rare (approximately 1 in 87,000 pregnancies) but catastrophic complication of pregnancy (93). Shortly after the entry of amniotic fluid into the maternal circulation, symptoms of respiratory distress (51%), cardiovascular collapse (27%), convulsions (10%), and hemorrhage (12%) manifest. If the patient survives 1 hour, pulmonary edema and DIC (seen in as many as 37% of cases) further complicate the course of the patient. Maintenance of adequate tissue oxygenation is crucial, and patients should be managed in an intensive care setting. As in a pulmonary embolism from a venous thrombus, too rigorous attempts at fluid resuscitation can lead to fluid overload. Therefore, central vascular pressure monitoring is recommended. The goal is to sustain the patient until the thrombi are cleared from the pulmonary circulation. In some cases, red cell transfusions and maintenance of intravascular volume have been sufficient to allow reversal of the coagulopathy (97, 98). Overall, mortality is estimated to be 86% (95).

Fatty liver of pregnancy is a rare third trimester complication of pregnancy that is often associated with variable degrees of DIC. Initial presentations frequently include severe nausea, intractable vomiting, malaise, right upper quadrant abdominal pain, headache, fever, jaundice, and easy bruising. Histologically, hepatocellular swelling is present (resulting from the presence of fat-filled microvesicles). These histological changes are most prominent in the pericentral regions of the hepatic lobules. Elevation in liver transaminases (typically less than 500 IU/L), hyperbilirubinemia (usually less than 10 mg/dL), elevated blood ammonia, decreased blood glucose, and rising blood urea nitrogen and creatinine all are suggestive of liver failure (99). These findings help to distinguish this etiology from other causes of DIC or MHAs. Aggressive stabilization of the patient with fluids, red cells, fresh-frozen plasma, platelets, and cryoprecipitate and aggressive treatment of hypoglycemia with glucose infusions should be undertaken as needed. Infusion of ATIII concentrates has been used with apparent benefit in these patients because ATIII levels in this condition are extremely low (100–102). The etiology of this condition is not understood. However, if immediate delivery is undertaken, the condition is potentially reversible. The maternal mortality rate for this disorder is 75–85% with a fetal mortality of around 85%; more recently, with earlier recognition and prompt supportive therapy, the maternal and fetal mortality rates have decreased to 7–18% and 14–32%, respectively (99, 103).

OTHER CAUSES OF MHA

Three other rare syndromes characterized by MHA but not DIC that are seen in pregnancy are TTP, HELLP syndrome, and HUS. TTP is characterized by MHA, severe thrombocytopenia, mild renal failure, fever, and fluctuating neurological symptoms (104). TTP can be either acute or chronic and relapsing. HELLP syndrome is a complication of preeclampsia/eclampsia (105). HUS presents with MHA, mild thrombocytopenia, mild to severe renal failure, fever, and, infrequently, neurological symptoms (104). Although frequently considered separately, TTP and HUS may represent a spectrum of disease.

Clinically, these syndromes are very similar, and it may be impossible to distinguish one from another and may in fact represent a spectrum of disease. Schwartz (106) makes a case for grouping all patients with MHA and thrombocytopenia as preeclamptic/eclamptic.

However, it is important to differentiate among these syndromes because plasma therapy is the primary treatment for TTP and HUS, but termination of the pregnancy is required in HELLP syndrome. TTP/HUS is not usually ameliorated by delivery; plasma therapy before delivery has no therapeutic benefit in HELLP syndrome (104, 107, 108).

It has been suggested that coagulation studies may help in differentiating among the syndromes (108). In HELLP syndrome, the PT/PTT are prolonged and ATIII activity is reduced. In TTP/HUS, the ATIII levels are normal. Clinically, acute upper abdominal pain (thought to be due to stretching of the liver capsule) is a major symptom and can aid in the differential diagnosis.

Unexplained fever strongly favors the diagnosis of TTP, and the gestational age at onset may aid in arriving at the correct diagnosis. TTP is more commonly reported during the first two trimesters (108–111). In one series of 65 women with TTP, 38 (58%) of the patients were less than 24 weeks gestation at the time of diagnosis (108). HELLP syndrome usually occurs in the third trimester of pregnancy (104, 107). HUS is most frequently reported in the postpartum period after a normal delivery. Weiner's review (108) of reports totaling 62 patients shows that 58 (98%) HUS was diagnosed 0–180 days postpartum (26.6 ± 35 days). In retrospect, nine patients had symptoms antepartum.

Patient management depends on the severity of the patient's symptoms and the status of the fetus. Owen and Brecher (112) suggested management based on categorizing patient presentations into one of four groups:

1. If the gestational age is less than 28 weeks, the fetus is viable and the mother is stable, TTP is the most likely diagnosis. Plasma therapy should be started immediately.
2. When the gestational age is between 28 and 34 weeks, the course of action is more problematic. If the diagnosis is HELLP, failure to terminate the pregnancy could result in maternal and fetal death. However, if the patient has TTP, terminating the pregnancy may result in severe prematurity for the infant without maternal benefit. If the patient has normal ATIII levels and clinical status allows, a trial of plasma therapy should be tried. If the patient does not respond within 1 week or the mother's condition worsens (falling platelet count, increasing lactate dehydrogenase), the pregnancy should be terminated while continuing plasma therapy until a response is achieved.
3. If the clinical picture is that of preeclampsia/eclampsia or DIC or the gestational age is at least 34 weeks, the patient should be treated for HELLP syndrome; the pregnancy should be terminated immediately. If the patient presents when symptoms first develop and treatment is prompt, maternal recovery is usually seen within 72 hours of delivery. If maternal recovery does not occur (relief of maternal symptoms, elevated platelet count, reduced lactate dehydrogenase) within 72 hours or she relapses, plasma therapy should be started immediately.
4. Patients with postpartum HUS syndrome make up the fourth group. HUS is very similar to TTP and the primary treatment is plasma exchange.

A recent study by the Canadian Apheresis Study Group shows that plasma exchange is more effective than plasma infusion in the treatment of TTP (109). This is of special significance in the pregnant patient when a few days or weeks could make the difference in fetal survival.

Currently, there is no consensus on the volume of plasma to be exchanged or the optimal frequency of exchange. Typically, 1–1.5 plasma volumes are exchanged daily. The efficiency of exchange decreases beyond this point, whereas the risks of exposure to fresh-frozen plasma continue to mount as the patient is exposed to more donors. Usually, fresh-frozen plasma is used for replacement, but "cryo-poor" plasma (the supernatant plasma remaining after cryoprecipitate has been removed) to reduce the infusion of high-molecular-weight von Willebrand multimers has also been used. Therapy should not be discontinued until the platelet count is greater than 150 $\times$ 10^9/L on 2 consecutive days, the hematocrit is stable or rising, and the lactate dehydrogenase is within or approaching the normal range. Patients with chronic relapsing TTP or prepartum TTP may require a long course of therapy and/or repeat courses of plasma exchange until delivery (18).

RED CELL EXCHANGE FOR SICKLE CELL DISEASE

The ideal management of a pregnancy in a mother with a major sickling hemoglobinopathy (hemoglobin SS or hemoglobin SC disease) is both difficult and controversial. Maternal complications include a propensity for infection (particularly urinary or pulmonary), vaso-occlusive crisis, and pregnancy-induced hypertension (110, 111, 113). Fetal complications include a high incidence of premature infants (17–39%), miscarriage (5–25%), and intrauterine growth retardation (14–18%) (110, 111, 113). Red cell transfusion therapy is used either for prophylactic red cell exchange (to maintain hemoglobin A at the 40–60% level, with a hematocrit of 30–35%) or only when severe complications arise. Transfusion is frequently accomplished by erythrocytapheresis because it is rapid, minimizes fluid fluxes, and avoids the iron overload associated with simple transfusion. Unfortunately, different clinical trials have arrived at different conclusions, and there remains no consensus regarding the approach to red cell transfusion for the pregnant sickle cell patient.

CONCLUSIONS

Two of the most remarkable success stories of modern medicine include the implementation of blood transfusion therapy (due in large part to Dr. Blundell and his desire to treat postpartum hemorrhage) and the prophylaxis of Rh-mediated HDN. If the past is any predictor of the future, we can expect great and exciting innovations to occur when the specialties of transfusion medicine and obstetrics and gynecology unite.

REFERENCES

1. Pepkowitz HS. Autologous blood donation and obstetric transfusion practice. In: Sacher RA, Brecher ME, eds. Obstetric transfusion practice. Bethesda, MD: American Association of Blood Banks, 1993.
2. Klapholz H. Blood transfusion in contemporary obstetric practice. Obstet Gynecol 1990;75:940–943.
3. Morrison JC, Sumrall D, Chevalier SP, Robinson SV, Morrison FS, Wiser WL. The effect of provider education on blood utilization practices. Am J Obstet Gynecol 1993;169:1240–1245.
4. Maxwell CN. Blood transfusion and caesarean section. Aust NZ J Obstet Gynaecol 1989;29:121–123.
5. Oberman HA. Surgical blood ordering, blood shortage situations, and emergency transfusion. In: Petz LD, Swisher SN, eds. Clinical practice of transfusion medicine. New York: Churchill Livingstone, 1989.
6. Greenwalt TJ. Human blood groups and compatibility testing. In: Rossi EC, Simon TL, Moss GS, eds. Principles of transfusion medicine. Baltimore: Williams & Wilkins, 1991.
7. Hill ST, Lavin JP. Blood ordering in obstetrics and gynecology: recommendations for the type and screen. Obstet Gynecol 1983;62: 236–240.
8. Sherman SJ, Greenspoon JS, Nelson JM, Paul RH. Obstetric hemorrhage and blood utilization. J Reprod Med 1993;38:929–934.
9. Mattison D. Anatomical, physiologic and biochemical adaptations to pregnancy. In: Sacher RA, Brecher ME, eds. Obstetric transfusion practice. Bethesda, MD: American Association of Blood Banks, 1993.
10. Klapholz H. In reply [letter]. Obstet Gynecol 1990;76:890–891.
11. Druzin ML, Wolf CFW, Edersheim TG, Hutson JM, Kogut JM, Salamon JLN. Donation of blood by the pregnant patient for autologous transfusion. Am J Obstet Gynecol 1988;159:1023–1027.
12. Herbert WNP, Owen HG, Collins ML. Autologous blood storage in obstetrics. Obstet Gynecol 1988; 72:166–170.
13. Kruskall MS, Leonard S, Klapholz H. Autologous blood donation during pregnancy: analysis of safety and blood use. Obstet Gynecol 1987;70: 938–941.
14. Lindenbaum CR, Schwartz IR, Chibber G, Teplick FB, Cohen AW. Safety of predeposit autologous blood donation in the third trimester of pregnancy. J Reprod Med 1990;35:537–540.
15. Droste S, Sorensen T, Price T, et al. Maternal and fetal hemodynamic effects of autologous blood donation during pregnancy. Am J Obstet Gynecol 1992;167:89–93.
16. Sayers MH. Autologous blood donation in pregnancy: Con. Transfusion 1990;30:172–174.
17. Tomasulo PA, Anderson AJ, Paluso MB, Gutschrenritter MA, Aster RA. A study of criteria for blood donor deferral. Transfusion 1980; 20:511–518.
18. Kruskall MS. The safety and utility of autologous donations by pregnant patients: Pro. Transfusion 1990;30:168–171.
19. Sandler SG, Beyth Y, Laufer N, Levene C. Autologous blood transfusions and pregnancy. Obstet Gynecol 1979;53(Suppl.):62S-66S.
20. McShane PM, Heyl PS, Epstein MF. Maternal and perinatal mortality resulting from placenta previa. Obstet Gynecol 1985;65:176.
21. Combs CA, Murphy EL, Laros RK. Cost-benefit analysis of autologous blood donation in obstetrics. Obstet Gynecol 1992;80:621–625.
22. Bowman JM. Treatment options for the fetus with alloimmune hemolytic disease. Trans Med Rev 1990;4:191–207.
23. Vengelen-Tyler V, ed. Technical manual. 12th ed. Bethesda, MD: American Association of Blood Banks, 1996.
24. Bowman JM, Pollock JM. Failures of intravenous RH immune globulin prophylaxis: an analysis of the reasons for such failures. Transfus Med Rev 1987;1:101–112.
25. Huchet J, Defossez Y, Brossard Y. Detection of transplacental haemorrhage during the last trimester of pregnancy [letter]. Transfusion 1988;28:506.
26. Eklund J, Nevanlinna HR. Rh prevention—a report and analysis of a national programme. J Med Genet 1973;10:1.

27. Mollison PL, Engelfriet CP, Contreras M. Blood transfusion in clinical medicine. 9th ed. Boston: Blackwell Scientific Publications, 1993.
28. Bowman J. The prevention of Rh immunization. Trans Med Rev 1988;2:129–150.
29. Murray S, Knox EG, Walker W. Rhesus haemolytic disease of the newborn and the ABO groups. Vox Sang 1965;10:6–31.
30. Hsia DY-Y, Gellis SS. Studies on erythroblastosis due to ABO incompatibility. Pediatrics 1954;13:503.
31. Liley AW. Intrauterine transfusion of foetus in haemolytic disease. Br Med J 1963;2:1107–1109.
32. Nicolaides KH, Rodeck CH, Mibashan RS, Kemp JR. Have Liley charts outlived their usefulness? Am J Obstet Gynecol 1991;165: 546–553.
33. Queenan JT, Tomai TP, Ural SH, King JC. Deviation in the amniotic fluid optical density at a wavelength of 450 nm in Rh-immunized pregnancies from 14–40 weeks' gestation: a proposal for clinical management. Am J Obstet Gynecol 1993:168:1370–1376.
34. Bennett PR, Kim CL, Colin Y, et al. Prenatal determination of fetal RhD type by DNA amplification following chorion villus biopsy or amniocentesis. N Engl J Med 1993;329:607–610.
35. Leduc L, Moise KJ, Carpenter RJ, Cano LE. Fetoplacental blood volume estimation in pregnancies with Rh alloimmunization. Fetal Diagn Ther 1990;5:138–146.
36. Nicolaides KH, Thilaganathan B, Mibashan RS. Cordocentesis in the investigation of fetal erythropoiesis. Am J Obstet Gynecol. 1989;161: 1197–2000.
37. Weiner CP. Human fetal bilirubin levels and fetal hemolytic disease. Am J Obstet Gynecol 1992;166:1449–1454.
38. Nicolini U, Kochenour NK, Greco P, et al. Consequences of fetomaternal haemorrhage after intrauterine transfusion. BMJ 1988;297:1379–1381.
39. Ludomirsky A. Intrauterine fetal blood sampling-a multicenter registry, evaluation of 7462 procedures between 1987–1991. Am J Obstet Gynecol 1993;168:318.
40. Rodeck CH, Kemp JR, Holman CA, et al. Direct intravascular fetal blood transfusion by fetoscopy in severe Rhesus isoimmunization. Lancet 1981;1:625–627.
41. Bang J, Bock JE, Trolle D. Ultrasound-guided fetal intravenous transfusion for severe Rhesus haemolytic disease. BMJ 1982;284:373–374.
42. Moise KJ, Carpenter RJ, Kirshon B, Deter RL, Sala JD, Cano LE. Comparison of four types of intrauterine transfusion: effect on fetal hematocrit. Fetal Ther 1989;4:126–137.
43. Radunovic N, Lockwood CJ, Alvarez M, Plecas D, Chitkara U, Berkowitz RL. The severely anemic and hydropic isoimmune fetus: changes in fetal hematocrit associated with intrauterine death. Obstet Gynecol 1992;79:390–393.
44. Moise KJ. Changing trends in the management of red blood cell alloimmunization in pregnancy. Arch Pathol Lab Med 1994;118:421–428.
45. Doyle LW, Kelly EA, Rickards AL, Ford GW, Callanan RJ. Sensorineural outcomes at 2 years for survivors of erythroblastosis treatment with fetal intravascular transfusions. Obstet Gynecol 1993;81: 931–935.
46. Marguiles M, Voto LS, Mathet E, Marguiles M. High dose intravenous IgG for the treatment of severe Rhesus alloimmunization. Vox Sang 1991;61:181–189.
47. Goldman M, Filiion M, Proulx C, Chartrand P, Decary F. Neonatal alloimmune thrombocytopenia. Transfus Med Rev 1994;8:123–131.
48. Muellar-Eckhardt C, Kiefel V, Grubert A, et al. 348 cases of suspected neonatal alloimmune thrombocytopenia. Lancet 1989; 1:363–366.
49. Waters A, Murphy M, Hambley H, Nicolaides K. Management of alloimmune thrombocytopenia in the fetus and neonate. In: Nance SJ, ed. Clinical and basic science aspects of immunohematology. Arlington, VA: American Association of Blood Banks, 1991.
50. Muellar-Eckhardt C, Kiefel V, Santoso S. Review and update of platelet alloantigen systems. Transfus Med Rev 1990;4:98–109.
51. Freedman J, Musclow E, Garvey B, Abbott D. Unexplained peripartunient thrombocytopenia. Am J Hematol 1986;21:397–407.
52. Burrows RF, Kelton JG. Incidentally detected thrombocytopenia in healthy mothers and their infants. N Engl J Med 1988;319: 142–145.
53. Burrows RF, Kelton JG. Thrombocytopenia at delivery: a prospective survey of 6715 deliveries. Am J Obstet Gynecol 1990;162:731–734.
54. Anteby E, Shalev O. Clinical relevance of gestational thrombocytopenia of $<$100,000/μl. Am J Hematol 1994;47:118–122.
55. Burrows RF, Kelton JG. Fetal thrombocytopenia and its relation to maternal thrombocytopenia. N Engl J Med 1993; 329:1463–1466.
56. George JN, El-Harake MA, Raskob GE. Chronic idiopathic thrombocytopenic purpura. N Engl J Med 1994;331:1207–1211.
57. Aster RH. "Gestational" thrombocytopenia. A plea for conservative management. N Engl J Med 1990; 323:264–266.
58. Nagey DA, Alger LS, Edelman BB, Heyman MR, Pupkin MJ, Crenshaw C. Reacting appropriately to thrombocytopenia in pregnancy. South Med J 1986; 79:1385–1388.
59. Sontheimer RD. The anticardiolipin syndrome: a new way to slice an old pie, or a new pie to slice? Arch Dermatol 1987;123:590–595.
60. Lockshin MD, Druzin ML, Goei S, et al. Antibody to cardiolipin is a predictor of fetal distress or death in pregnant patients with systemic lupus erthematosus. N Engl J Med 1985;313:152–156.
62A.Fulcher D, Stewart G, Exner T, et al. Plasma exchange and the anticardiolipin syndrome in pregnancy [letter]. Lancet 1989;2:171.
63A.Kobayashi S, Tamura N, Tsuda H, et al. Immunoadsorbent plasmapheresis for a patient with antiphospholipid syndrome during pregnancy. Ann Rheum Dis 1992;51:399–401.
64A.Frampton G, Cameron JS, Thorn M, et al. Successful removal of antiphospholipid antibody during pregnancy using plasma exchange and low dose prednisolone [letter]. Lancet 1987;2:1023–1024.
61. Parke A. The role of IVIG in the management of patients with antiphospholipid antibodies and recurrent pregnancy losses. In: Ballow M, ed. IVIG therapy today.Totowa, NJ: The Humana Press Inc., 1992: 105–118.
62. Rosove MH, Tabsh K, Wasserstrum N, et al. Heparin therapy for pregnant women with lupus anticoagulant or anticardiolipin antibodies. Obstet Gynecol 1990;75:630–634.
63. Cowchock FS, Reece EA, Balaban D. Repeated fetal losses associated with antiphospholipid antibodies: a collaborative randomized trial comparing prednisone with low-dose heparin treatment. Am J Obstet Gynecol 1992;166:1318–1323.
64. Shechter Y, Timor-Tritsch IE, Lewit N, Sela R, Levene C. Early treatment by plasmapheresis in a woman with multiple abortions and the rare blood group p. Vox Sang 1987;53:135–138.
65. Shirey RS, Ness PM, Kickler TS, et al. The association of anti-P and early abortion. Transfusion 1987;27:189–119.
66. Rock JA, Rosetta SS, Braine HG, et al. Plasmapheresis for the treatment of repeated early pregnancy wastage associated with anti-P. Obstet Gynecol 1985;66(Suppl.):57–60.
67. Yoshida H, Ito K, Emi N, Kanzaki H, Matsuura S. A new therapeutic antibody removal method using antigen-positive red cells: application to a P-incompatible pregnant woman. Vox Sang 1984;47:216–223.
68. Yoshida H, Ito K, Kusakari T, et al. Removal of maternal antibodies from a woman with repeated fetal loss due to P blood group incompatibility. Transfusion 1994;34:702–705.

69. Buyon J, Szer I. Passively acquired autoimmunity and the maternal fetal dyad in systemic lupus erythematosus. Semin Immunopathol 1986; 9:283–304.
70. Olah KS, Gee H. Fetal heart block associated with maternal anti-Ro (SS-A) antibody—current management. A review. Br J Obstet Gynaecol 1991;98:751–755.
71. Buyon J, Roubey R, Swersky S, Pompeo L, Parke A, Baxi L, Winchester R. Complete congenital heart block: risk of occurrence and therapeutic approach to prevention. J Rheumatol 1988;15:1104–1108.
72. Ramsey-Goldman R, Hom D, Deng JS, et al. Anti-SS-A antibodies and fetal outcome in maternal systemic lupus erythematosus. Arthritis Rheum 1986;29:1269–1273.
73. McCune AB, Weston WL, Lee LA. Maternal and fetal outcome in neonatal lupus erythematosus. Ann Intern Med 1987;106:518–523.
74. Barclay CS, French MAH, Ross LD, Sokol RJ. Successful pregnancy following steroid therapy and plasma exchange in a woman with anti-Ro (SS-A) antibodies. Case report. Br J Obstet Gynaecol 1987;94:369–371.
75. Venning MC, Burn DJ, Ward RM, et al. Neonatal lupus syndrome: optimism justified [letter]? Lancet 1988;2:640.
76. Buyon J, Swersky SH, Fox HE, et al. Intrauterine therapy for presumptive fetal myocarditis with acquired heart block due to systemic lupus erythematosus. Experience in a mother with a predominance of SS-B (La) antibodies. Arthritis Rheum 1987;30:44–49.
77. Plauche WC. Myasthenia gravis in mothers and their newborns. Clin Obstet Gynecol 1991;34:82–99.
78. Fennell DF, Ringel SP. Myasthenia gravis and pregnancy. Obstet Gynecol Surv 1987;41:414–421.
79. Lentz MR, Saltonstahl WP. Apheresis of low molecular weight protein fraction and the onset of labor. J Clin Apher 1990;5:62–70.
80. Wing EJ, Bruns FJ, Fraley DS, et al. Infectious complications with plasmapheresis in rapidly progressive glomerulonephritis. JAMA 1980; 244:2423–2426.
81. Huestis DW, Bove JR, Case J. Therapeutic hemapheresis. In: Huestis DW, Bove JR, Case J, eds. Practical blood transfusion. 4th ed. Boston: Little, Brown, 1988:367–386.
82. Huestis DW. Complications of therapeutic apheresis. In: Valbonesis M, Pineda A, Biggs JC, eds. Therapeutic hemapheresis. Milano, Italy: Wichtig Editore Milano, 1986:179–186.
83. Evans RT, Robinson A. The combined efects of pregnancy and repeated plasma exchange on serum cholinesterase activity. ACTA Anaesthesiol Scand 1984;28:44–46.
84. Flaum MA, Cuneo RA, Applebaum FR, Deisseroth AB, Engel WK, Gralnick HR. The hemostatic imbalance of plasma-exchange transfusion. Blood 1979;54:694–702.
85. Nilsson T, Rudolphi O, Cedergren B. Effects of intensive plasmapheresis on the hemostatic system. Scand J Haemat 1983;30:201–206.
86. Conrad J, Horellou MH, Van Dreden P, et al. Thrombosis and pregnancy in congenital deficiencies in AT III, protein C or protein S: study of 78 women. Thromb Haemost 1990:63:319–320.
87. Alving BM. Management of congenital and acquired hemostatic disorders during pregnancy. In: Sacher RA, Brecher ME, eds. Obstetric transfusion practice. Bethesda, MD: American Association of Blood Banks, 1993.
88. Hall JG, Pauli RM, Wilson KM. Maternal and fetal sequelae of anticoagulation during pregnancy. Am J Med 1980;68:122–140.
89. Iturbe-Alessio I, de Carmen FM, Mutchinik O, et al. Risks of anticoagulant therapy in pregnant women with artificial heart valves. N Engl J Med 1986;315:1390–1393.
90. Ginsberg JS, Hirsh J. Use of anticoagulants during pregnancy. Chest 1989;95(Suppl.):156s–160s.
91. Hirsh J, Ginsberg J, Turner C, Levine MN. Management of thromboembolism during pregnancy: risks to the fetus. In: Bern MM, Frigoletto FD Jr, eds. Hematologic disorders in maternal-fetal medicine. New York: Wiley-Liss, Inc., 1990:523–543.
92. Hirsh J, Levine MN. Low molecular weight heparin. Blood 1992;79: 1–17.
93. Boulton FE, Letsky E. Obstetric haemorrhage: causes and management. Clin Haematol 1985;14:683–728.
94. Romero R, Duffy TP, Berkowitz RL et al. Prolongation of a preterm pregnancy complicated by death of a single twin in utero and disseminated intravascular coagulation. Effects of treatment with heparin. N Engl J Med 1984;310:772–774.
95. Skelly H, Marivate M, Norman R, et al. Consumptive coagulopathy following fetal death in a triplet pregnancy. Am J Obstet Gynecol 1982;142:595–596.
96. Howell RJS. Haemorrhage from the placental site. Clin Obstet Gynecol 1986;13:633–658.
97. Morgan M. Amniotic fluid embolism. Anesthesia 1979;34:20–32.
98. Killam A. Amniotic fluid embolism. Clin Obstet Gynecol 1985;28: 32–36.
99. Fisher J. Acute fatty liver of pregnancy. Biomed Prog 1994;7:17–21.
100. Liebman HA, McGhee WG, Patch MJ, Feinstein DI. Severe depression of antithrombin III associated with disseminated intravascular coagulation in women with fatty liver of pregnancy. Ann Intern Med 1983;98:330–333.
101. Laursen B, Mortensen JZ, Frost L, Hansen KB. Disseminated intravascular coagulation in hepatic failure treated with antithrombin III. Thromb Res 1981;22:701–704.
102. Owen J. Antithrombin III replacement therapy in pregnancy. Semin Hematol 1987;24:82–100.
103. Burroughs AK, Seong NG, Dojcinoov DM, Scheuer PJ, Sherlock SVP. Idiopathic acute fatty liver of pregnancy in 12 patients. Q J Med 1982;51:481–497.
104. Watson WJ, Katz VL, Bowes WA. Plasmapheresis during pregnancy. Obstet Gynecol 1990;76:451–457.
105. Weinstein L. Syndrome of hemolysis, elevated liver enzymes, and low platelet count: a severe consequence of hypertension in pregnancy. Am J Obstet Gynecol 1982;142:159–167.
106. Schwartz ML. Possible role for exchange plasmapheresis with fresh frozen plasma for maternal indications in selected cases of preeclampsia and eclampsia. Obstet Gynecol 1986;68:136–139.
107. Martin JN, Blake PG, Perry KG, et.al. The natural history of HELLP syndrome: patterns of disease progression and regression. Am J Obstet Gynecol 1991;164:1500–1513.
108. Weiner CL. Thrombotic microangiopathy in pregnancy and the postpartum period. Semin Hematol 1987;24:119–129.
109. Rock GA, Shumak KH, Buskard NA, et al. Comparison of plasma exchange with plasma infusion in the treatment of thrombotic thrombocytopenic purpura. N Engl J Med 1991;325:393–403.
110. Koshy M, Burd L, Wallace D, et al. Prophylactic red cell transfusions in pregnant patients with sickle cell disease. N Engl J Med 1988;319: 1447–1452.
111. Powars DR, Sandhu M, Niland-Weiss J, et al. Pregnancy in sickle cell disease. Obstet Gynecol 1986;67:217–222.
112. Owen HG, Brecher ME. Therapeutic apheresis of the pregnant patient. In: Sacher RA, Brecher ME, eds. Obstetric transfusion practice. Bethesda, MA: American Association of Blood Banks, 1993.
113. Morrison JC, Morrison FS, Floyd RS, et al. Use of continuous flow erythroctyapheresis in pregnant patients with sickle cell disease. J Clin Apher 1991;6:224–229.

Chapter 33

Transfusion in the Trauma and Burn Patient

KEITH D. CLANCY
RICHARD L. GAMELLI

INTRODUCTION

The use of blood transfusion as a treatment for hemorrhage began in the early 19th century when James Blundell, a London physician, reinfused 8 ounces of shed blood into a woman suffering from postpartum hemorrhage (1). Transfusion therapy did not gain widespread acceptance, however, until Landsteiner described the major blood groups (ABO) (2, 3). Experience during World War I and the Spanish Civil War led to technologies to collect, store, and transfuse blood in emergencies. By 1937, the first blood bank in the United States was opened at Cook County Hospital by Bernard Fantus (1). The use of acid-citrate-dextrose blood was practiced by the end of World War II and expanded our ability to store blood for emergency use. During this same time period, the use of crystalloid fluids for the resuscitation of injured patients was begun and the importance of preventing hypotension and hypovolemia documented.

The ability to store blood in large quantities for use in emergency situations and in remote locations was an important advance for the field of trauma surgery (3). The availability of low-titer type O blood at division clearing stations during the Vietnam War reduced mortality significantly (4). The nearly unlimited supply of blood during that war was demonstrated by the average amount of blood transfused for injuries to various anatomic regions: head and neck, 4.1 units; thorax, 8.1 units; abdomen, 11.3 units; upper extremity, 4.4 units; and lower extremity, 6.3 units (4).

During the Vietnam War, the increased use of transfusion therapy was accompanied by reduced resuscitation times and earlier operative intervention in patients not responding to resuscitative measures compared with management in previous wars. The time from admission to operation during the Vietnam War was often 30 minutes or less, significantly less than World War II times of 4 hours (4). The wartime experience with the resuscitation of the injured patient and the use of blood transfusion has been incorporated into the management of civilian injuries. The late 1960s brought the development of organized prehospital emergency medical services resulting in the rapid transport of injured patients to trauma centers that were capable of treating the critically injured. Patients who would have succumbed to massive hemorrhage could now be salvaged with transfusion in combination with early therapeutic interventions and aggressive intensive care management.

The use of blood for the resuscitation and treatment of the thermally injured patient was advocated as early as the 1920s and 1930s by various groups (5, 6). Whole blood, packed cells, and plasma have been components of various treatment regimens and "burn formula" for the initial resuscitation of the burn patient (7). The availability of blood and blood products during the perioperative phase of treatment has resulted in decreased mortality of elderly burn patients and those with associated medical problems who would not have tolerated low hemoglobin levels. Intraoperative transfusion therapy has permitted a more extensive area of débridement and grafting, reducing the required number of operations.

The current indications for blood transfusion in the trauma or burn patient have evolved with the recognition of the relative merits of this form of treatment and practical considerations. The limitations of the blood supply became apparent as increasing demand outpaced availability. In addition, the incidence of transfusion reactions and the transmission of hepatitis was well documented by the mid 1970s. The incidence of posttransfusion associated non-A, non-B hepatitis in the United States was estimated to be between 5% and 18% during the 1970s and early 1980s (8). A more recent study evaluated the risk of the hepatitis C virus (HCV), now known to cause approximately 90% of posttransfusion hepatitis. Since May 1990, blood banks have been able to test for the HCV antibody and the risk of posttransfusion hepatitis C was 0.57% per patient and 0.03% per unit transfused (8). The first case of transfusion-related transmission of the human immunodeficiency virus (HIV) was documented in 1982 (9). The transmission of this universally fatal disease by transfused blood caused a reevaluation of the use of blood transfusion in the injured patient because the risk-to-benefit considerations had now changed.

Beyond disease transmission, several recent studies have demonstrated the immunosuppressive effect of blood transfusions. One such study in burn patients identified the number of transfusions as an independent variable for an increased incidence of infectious complications (10). In another study of patients receiving perioperative transfusion for resection of colorectal cancer, the only independent variables found correlating with tumor recurrence were Dukes' stage and the administration of a blood transfusion (11). These studies demonstrate that in the absence of hepatitis and HIV risk, the immunosuppressive effects of blood transfusion can have an adverse impact on patient outcome.

The use of a specific hemoglobin level as a "transfusion trigger" has been criticized, and recent evidence suggests that patients can tolerate lower hemoglobin levels under various circumstances without untoward effects. Although still a lifesaving therapy in appropriate circumstances, these recent events have led to a more judicious use of erythrocytes and other blood products (2). The current blood use in trauma and burn patients is the result of best practice, availability, and risk assessment.

ASSESSING THE PHYSIOLOGICAL NEED FOR TRANSFUSION

Hypovolemic shock is defined as the state in which oxygen availability at the tissue level is inadequate to meet the metabolic needs of the tissue, resulting in anaerobic tissue metabolism (12). A critical management principle for the trauma or burn patient is the optimization of oxygen delivery and the correction of tissue hypoxia. Ideally, a single laboratory value would identify those whose oxygen delivery requires the administration of red blood cells. Unfortunately, this is not the case; therefore, the decision to transfuse must be based on an understanding of the role of red blood cells in the scheme of oxygen delivery.

Oxygen delivery (DO_2) is a measure of oxygen transport to tissues and is the product of arterial oxygen content (CaO_2) and cardiac output (CO) (2, 13–15):

$$DO_2 = CaO_2 \times CO \text{ (mL } O_2\text{/min)}$$

In the healthy patient, the DO_2 index (DO_2 normalized for body surface area) is 500–800 mL of O_2/min/m^2 or 10–12 mL of O_2/min/kg (13, 16).

Arterial oxygen content (CaO_2) reflects both the hemoglobin-bound oxygen and the oxygen dissolved in the plasma and is represented by the equation

$$CaO_2 = SaO_2 \times 1.34 \times \text{Hemoglobin} \times 10 + (0.003 \times PaO_2)$$

where 1.34 is an estimate of the mean volume of O_2 that can be bound to 1 g of fully saturated normal hemoglobin (17). SaO_2 is the oxygen saturation and PaO_2 is the partial pressure of oxygen. Ten is a correction factor that converts the hemoglobin concentration from g/dL to g/L. From this equation, it is evident that the dissolved oxygen in plasma contributes minimally to the total CaO_2 at atmospheric pressure. This contribution increases under hyperbaric conditions.

Oxygen consumption ($\dot{V}O_2$) is a measure of the total oxidative metabolism and is a product of the arterial-venous oxygen difference ($CaO_2 - CvO_2$) and the CO (2, 13):

$$\dot{V}O_2 = [CaO_2 - CvO_2] \times CO \text{ (mL } O_2\text{/min)}$$

The $\dot{V}O_2$ index ranges from 130 to 160 mL of O_2/min/m^2 or 3–4 mL of O_2/min/kg.

In most cases, oxygen consumption is relatively independent of hemoglobin level over a wide range of oxygen delivery values because of compensation made in CO and oxygen uptake by the tissue. The oxygen extraction ratio (OER) is a measure of the oxygen extracted by the tissues in a single pass through the circulatory system.

$$OER = \dot{V}O_2/DO_2$$

Under normal conditions, the OER is approximately 25–30% (13, 18), but this varies in different tissues, from 7% to 10% for the skin and kidneys to 55% in the heart at rest (16, 19). Different tissues have a variable ability to increase oxygen extraction, further increasing tissue oxygen availability to those tissues. However, the heart, which is at near maximal oxygen extraction, depends on increased oxygen delivery to meet increased cellular O_2 requirements. The physiological impact of acute normovolemic anemia on the trauma and burn patient is therefore dependent on the compensatory ability of the myocardium.

In the acutely injured patient, the prevention of tissue ischemia is of utmost importance. The compensatory mechanisms for acute tissue hypoxia include increased CO, increased oxygen extraction, and redistribution of blood flow to those tissues whose oxygen consumption is supply dependent, namely the heart and brain (15, 16). It should be noted that oxygen delivery is decreased in the hypovolemic patient regardless of hematocrit level (15, 20–22). Therefore, the initial emphasis during the resuscitation of the trauma patient in hemorrhagic shock should be asanguineous volume expansion to restore normovolemia and support CO.

Numerous studies have demonstrated that with normovolemia, CO progressively increases with reductions from baseline hematocrits down to hematocrits of approximately 8.6% in dogs (18) and 6% in primates (23). Compensatory mechanisms supporting the increased CO with normovolemic anemia were largely due to reductions in blood viscosity (Fig. 33.1) (16, 24). Decreases in viscosity were most prominent in the postcapillary venules, which accounted in part for the increased venous return noted (19, 25). Additionally, decreases in blood viscosity resulted in reduced total peripheral resistance that in turn yielded afterload reduction and preload augmentation (24). In addition to these increases in CO, which are largely passive, the aortic chemoreceptors are believed to contribute to increased CO by affecting the venomotor tone, which further improves venous return and decreases venous pooling of blood (16, 19, 26). Finally, altered cardiac sympathetic nerve activity maintains and increases CO via augmented cardiac contractility (19, 27, 28).

Under normal conditions, oxygen delivery exceeds oxygen requirement two- to threefold. This "margin of safety" provides sufficient oxygen to meet alterations in metabolic demands without increasing blood flow to the tissue (19). DO_2 increases to approximately 110% of baseline levels as the hematocrit declines from normal values to 30% (16). This is predominantly due to increased CO. These compensatory responses allow oxygen uptake to be maintained until the hematocrit has been lowered to about 10% (19). At hematocrit levels below 10%, the oxygen delivery demonstrates a significant decline in primates (23).

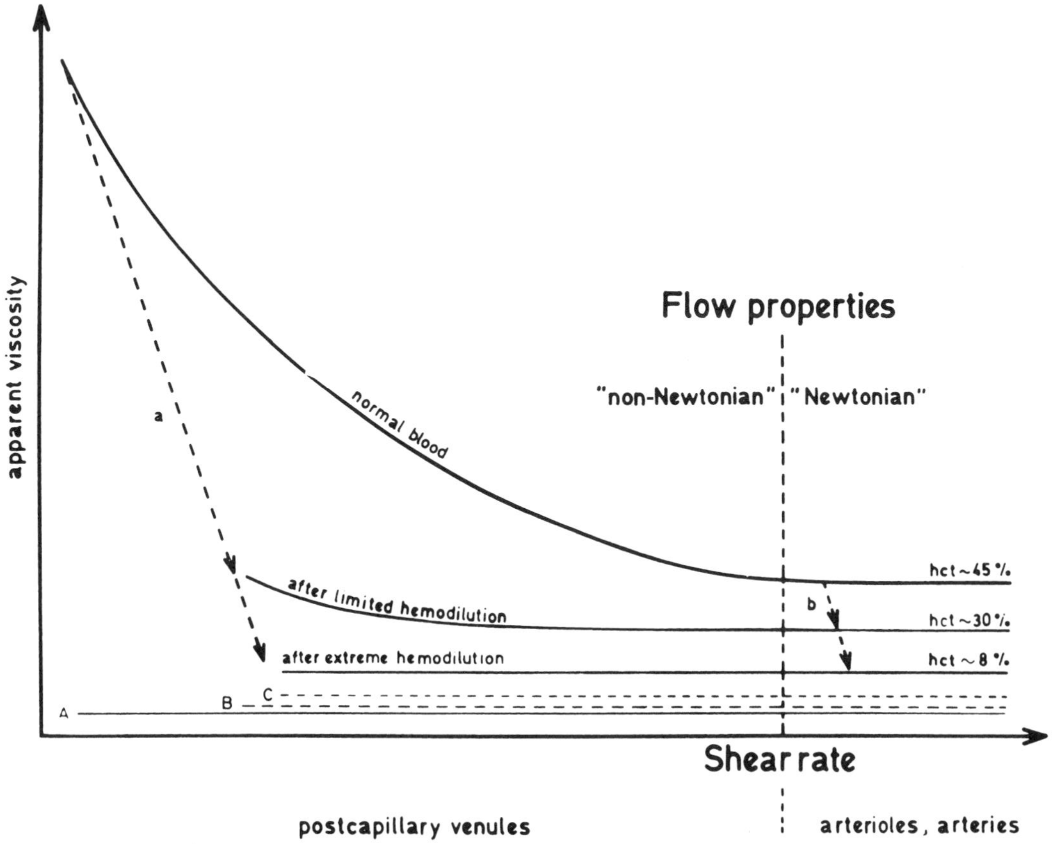

Figure 33.1. Schematic representation of the effect of hemodilution on changes in viscosity at various hematocrits in different vascular compartments. (Reprinted with permission from Messmer K. Hemodilution. Surg Clin North Am 1975;55:662.)

The relationship between DO_2 and $\dot{V}O_2$ demonstrates a biphasic response (Fig. 33.2). Below a critical level of DO_2, the $\dot{V}O_2$ is related to the DO_2 in a linear relationship. Above the critical DO_2, the $\dot{V}O_2$ is independent of delivery (16, 29). An analysis of patients undergoing coronary artery bypass surgery demonstrated that in the anesthetized prebypass period, the critical value of DO_2 was 330 mL/min/m^2. Above this level, the $\dot{V}O_2$ was independent of delivery (109 $\pm$ 16 mL/min/m^2) (29). Lactate levels obtained in these patients revealed that those patients with DO_2 levels below the critical level had lactate values significantly above baseline. This suggests that below the critical oxygen delivery value, some tissues undergo anaerobic metabolism. The applicability of these data to other classes of patients is unclear because the $\dot{V}O_2$ plateau in this study was 22% below that of other studies (30). This likely reflects the decreased oxygen requirements due to the effects of anesthesia and mechanical ventilation on the body's metabolic requirements.

In addition to increasing CO as a means of improving tissue oxygen delivery, different tissues have a variable ability to increase oxygen extraction (OER). To improve the oxygen extraction from the blood, the body redistributes flow to tissues with greater oxygen requirements. The heart extracts about 55% of the delivered oxygen at rest and has limited ability to increase further O_2 extraction. The increase in myocardial oxygen demand is compensated by increased coronary blood flow through autoregulatory mechanisms. A study of isovolemic anemia in primates demonstrated that oxygen consumption was maintained by increased CO until a hematocrit of 6% and an improved OER was reached, which increased in a linear fashion as the hematocrit decreased to 10% and the OER reached 50% (23). Below this hematocrit value, oxygen consumption progressively declined. A change in the myocardium from lactate consumption to lactate production was noted to have occurred at these hematocrit values.

These findings imply that the myocardial metabolism was anaerobic, which would correspond clinically to myocardial failure. Because this change of the myocardium from a lactate consumer to lactate producer occurred at an OER of 50%, the authors offered the OER, which is easily derived from hemodynamic monitoring devices, as a sensitive indicator of marginal oxygen reserve. These investigators performed additional canine studies in which a critical left anterior descending (LAD) coronary artery stenosis was experimentally created (18). Cardiac failure occurred in the control animals at a hematocrit of 8.6% and in the LAD stenosed animals at hematocrit of 17.0%. The maintenance of oxygen delivery in the stenosed animals was achieved primarily from increased oxygen extraction and not by increased CO. This confirmed that cardiac compensatory mechanisms in the anemic animal are limited, requiring a higher hematocrit to support oxygen delivery. However, in both animal groups, the myocardial lactate production occurred at OER of 50%. In both groups, myocardial lactate production preceded the onset of hemodynamic instability and cardiac failure, whereas oxygen consumption remained normal even after the onset of cardiac failure. These data in aggregate clearly call into question traditional approaches advocating hematocrit values of 30% or higher in injured persons.

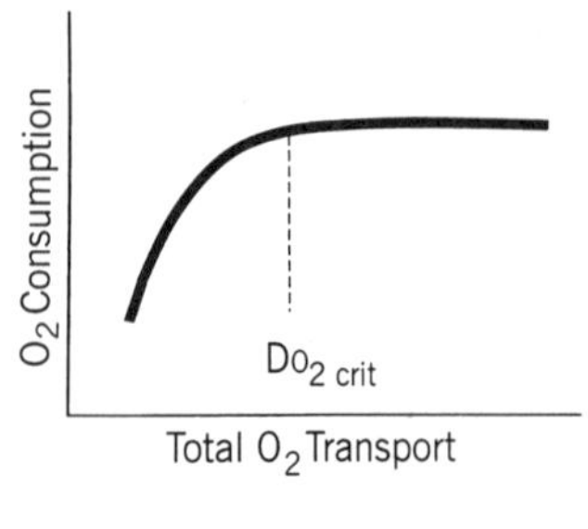

Figure 33.2. Schematic representation of biphasic relationships of oxygen consumption to oxygen delivery. Above the critical DO_2, the $\dot{V}O_2$ is dependent on DO_2. (Reprinted with permission from Tuman KJ. Tissue oxygen delivery: the physiology of anemia. Anesthesiol Clin North Am 1990;8:453.)

IMPACT OF THE CLINICAL STATE ON THE NEED FOR TRANSFUSION

When assessing the need for transfusion in the trauma or burn patient, it is clear that these patients do not comprise a homogenous group but rather form several separate groups for consideration. It may be more appropriate to consider the trauma patient's transfusion needs at four different stages: the acute resuscitative phase, the intraoperative phase, the nonoperative management of ruptured solid organs, and the recovery phase. The burn patient is considered separately.

ACUTE TRAUMA: RESUSCITATIVE PHASE

The initial management of the acute hypotensive trauma patient includes maintenance of the airway and ventilation, stabilization of the cervical spine as appropriate, and fluid resuscitation. The administered fluid is usually crystalloid and is initiated as a 2-L bolus of lactated Ringer's solution or normal saline for adults and a 20-mL/kg bolus for the pediatric patient. The hemodynamic response to this initial bolus determines the amount of additional fluid required and the nature of the fluid. Table 33.1 defines the four classes of shock according to the American College of Surgeons Committee on Trauma (31). The patient who remains hemodynamically stable after the initial fluid bolus usually continues to be supported with crystalloid at a maintenance rate with careful

TABLE 33.1. THE FOUR CLASSES OF SHOCK BASED ON BLOOD LOSS WITH ASSOCIATED CLINICAL SIGNS

	Class I	Class II	Class III	Class IV
Blood loss (mL)	up to 750	750–1500	1500–2000	2000 or more
Blood loss (%BV)	up to 15%	15–30%	30–40%	40% or more
Pulse rate	<100	>100	>120	140 or higher
Blood pressure	Normal	Normal	Decreased	Decreased
Pulse pressure (mm Hg)	Normal or increased	Decreased	Decreased	Decreased
Capillary refill test	Normal	Positive	Positive	Positive
Respiratory rate	14–20	20–30	30–40	>35
Urine output (mL/hr)	30 or more	20–30	5–15	Negligible
CNS–mental status	Slightly anxious	Mildly anxious	Anxious and confused	Confused-lethargic
Fluid replacement (3:1 rule)	Crystalloid	Crystalloid	Crystalloid + blood	Crystalloid + blood

Values based on a 70-kg male.

Reprinted with permission from American College of Surgeons Committee on Trauma. Advanced Trauma Life Support Course. Chicago: American College of Surgeons, 1989:72.

monitoring of hemodynamic parameters and urine output. In the patient who becomes hemodynamically unstable or remains unstable despite the initial bolus, continued crystalloid administration is recommended. Transfusion of erythrocytes is appropriate for those who remain hypotensive or are experiencing obvious massive hemorrhage. Patients who manifest ongoing volume loss require expeditious evaluation and definitive intervention to arrest ongoing hemorrhage.

The administration of erythrocytes in the trauma room should be reserved for those patients who demonstrate a transient response to initial fluid resuscitation or those who present in severe shock refractory to the initial crystalloid bolus. These two groups represent patients who have lost greater than 30% of their blood volume and who are still actively bleeding. The transfusion of blood in the trauma room must not delay definitive surgical intervention, and these patients should be transported to the operating room without delay.

An interesting correlation between low initial hemoglobin levels and mortality in trauma patients has been documented by Knottenbelt (32). In a retrospective study of 1000 patients with an age range of 15–85 years, those patients who died of moderate shock (systolic blood pressure 60–79) and severe shock (systolic blood pressure < 60) had significantly lower hemoglobin levels when compared with the group of patients who did not present in shock. In addition, the mean hemoglobin levels of the patients who died of hypovolemic causes were significantly lower regardless of the initial blood pressure (32). It is notable that 48% of the patients in this study arrived by private conveyance and therefore received no prehospital fluids, and of those patients who arrived by ambulance, the average prehospital fluid volume infused was 148 mL with no patient having received more than 600 mL of fluid. This suggests that the decreases in hemoglobin level were largely due to blood loss and were not due to the dilutional effects of fluid infusion before laboratory confirmation of the hemoglobin level. Although it is generally believed that 24 hours is required for hemoglobin levels to stabilize after acute blood loss (while fluid shifts from the interstitial space into the vascular space), these data suggest this may be true only for limited amounts of blood loss. Patients who present with low initial hemoglobin levels may have suffered blood loss that exceeds the compensatory mechanism. Knottenbelt concluded that the finding of a low hemoglobin on presentation after injury indicates severe and ongoing blood loss.

Once the decision to transfuse blood has been made, there are several options for the type of blood used. Ideally, typed and cross-matched blood should be used. However, it may take up to 1 hour for the laboratory to perform the appropriate testing and transport the specimen and blood between the blood bank and trauma unit, which is an unacceptably long delay for the patient in class III or IV shock. Alternatively, the use of type-specific uncross-matched blood may be used. This is usually available within 20–30 minutes. Finally, O-negative blood, which should be immediately available in an institution treating victims of trauma, may be used. Multiple studies have documented that the administration of O-negative blood is a safe means by which to restore red blood cell volume for the patient in severe shock.

ACUTE TRAUMA: INTRAOPERATIVE PHASE

The initial operative management of the acute trauma patient includes hemostatic control of the injured organs. In the case of abdominal trauma, this includes packing the abdomen while allowing the anesthesia team to administer intravenous fluids. The use of fluid warmers and a heated ventilatory circuit reduces hypothermia and the coagulopathy associated with decreased body temperature.

The rationale to transfuse the patient intraoperatively can be problematic. Traditionally, a hemoglobin of 10 g/dL has been considered the lowest safe level in elective surgical patients. More recently, numerous studies have demonstrated the safety of lower hemoglobin levels in elective surgical patients (33–35) and nonsurgical patients (36). In a study of 54 Jehovah's Witness patients with severe anemia (hemoglobin less than 7.0 g/dL, mean 4.6) who had refused blood transfusion on religious grounds, Spence et al. (33) found that hemoglobin values as an isolated variable were not reliable predictors of outcome. Sepsis was noted to be the only independent predictor of mortality, with a probability of survival of less than 10%. Active bleeding was an independent predictor of survival with hemoglobin levels below 4.0 g/dL with a probability of survival of less than 10%. Despite a trend for increased mortality with decreasing hemoglobin, the hemoglobin level became an independent predictor of mortality only at hemoglobin levels below 3.0 g/dL. In a similar study by the same authors, the primary predictor of mortality in 107 Jehovah's Witness patients with preoperative hemoglobin values as low as 6.0 g/dL was an intraoperative blood loss of greater than 500 mL (34).

How these data might be used in the trauma patient must be tempered by the recognition that hemoglobin levels obtained for the acutely hemorrhaging trauma patient may be falsely elevated because the blood has not had time to completely equilibrate with the interstitial space and infused volume expanders. In addition, there is no way to rapidly and reliably estimate the extent of blood loss in the acutely hemorrhaging trauma patient preoperatively. Finally, the physiological adaptations that typically occur with chronic anemia require more time than transpires with acute hemorrhage. These studies do support the concept that the use of a specific hematocrit level as a transfusion trigger is inappropriate, and the decision to transfuse should be based on an assessment of the patient's overall condition and an estimate of ongoing blood loss once the surgical exploration has begun.

The autotransfusion of the patient's own blood has become a widely used practice in elective surgery. It has been successfully used in elective vascular, gynecological, general, thoracic, and neurosurgical cases. The major advantages include conservation of the blood supply, the avoidance of complications related to transfusion reactions, the ready availability of autologous blood in the intraoperative setting, and the absence of infectious risk of viral pathogens from banked blood (22). The use of intraoperative blood salvage has been successfully used in cases of thoracic trauma. Blood from the chest cavity may be reinfused after simple filtration. As the shed blood is defibrinogenated, it does not require further anticoagulation. This blood has a hematocrit of approximately one-half the patient's and contains few platelets.

The use of intraoperative blood salvage with abdominal injuries has not been universally accepted. Particular concerns include the potential transfusion of contaminated blood secondary to hollow viscus injuries and the potential that intraoperative blood salvage from the peritoneal cavity may contribute to coagulopathy or abnormalities in the clotting mechanism (22, 37). Conversely, such devices have been used in which known contaminated blood has been reinfused with no untoward effects (38). It would seem prudent, however, to refrain from the use of autotransfused blood from the abdominal cavity in the presence of enteric injuries.

ACUTE TRAUMA: NONOPERATIVE MANAGEMENT OF SOLID ORGANS

Historically, the treatment of splenic trauma has been splenectomy. During the early part of the 20th century, the mortality from splenic rupture approached 90% (39). With the introduction of splenectomy, the mortality decreased to approximately 27% (40). Because of the significant reduction of mortality with splenectomy, this practice was unquestioned until King and Schumaker (41) reported overwhelming postsplenectomy infection (OPSI) in children who had splenectomies in infancy. Surgeons did not change their treatment, however, until a report from Toronto established the safety of nonoperative management in the stable pediatric population (42). The success of nonoperative management of splenic injury in the pediatric patient has been confirmed in numerous studies (43–46). In the 1980s, as the use of computed tomography for the evaluation of abdominal trauma gained acceptance, trauma surgeons began to advocate the nonoperative management of certain splenic and liver injuries in carefully selected adult patients with success rates for splenic salvage ranging between 30% and 100% (39, 47). The benefits of splenic salvage include prevention of postsplenectomy sepsis and sparing the patient from a laparotomy. Critics of nonoperative management of splenic injury cite the potential of continued hemorrhage with the subsequent decreased ability to achieve splenic repair and the increased transfusion requirements in nonoperative patients as reasons to proceed with immediate laparotomy.

Flaherty and Jurkovich (48) reported on the safety of the

nonoperative management of minor splenic injuries in the hemodynamically stable patient with limited transfusion requirements. In a retrospective review of 182 minor blunt splenic injuries, they compared the transfusion requirements of those patients managed nonoperatively, including those who failed nonoperative management, with those patients operated for hemoperitoneum. The median transfusion requirement in the group initially managed nonoperatively was not significantly different from the group who underwent immediate exploration (2.0 versus 2.5 units). The authors concluded that transfusion requirements in the stable patient with minor splenic injury would not be reduced by immediate exploration.

The findings of Feliciano et al. (39), using decision analysis, were somewhat different. They determined that the nonoperative management of splenic injuries was associated with an increased mortality from transfusion-related deaths. Their work supports the findings of Luna and Dellinger (49). After an extensive review of the literature, they noted that 35–40% of patients who are successfully managed nonoperatively require blood transfusion approximating 40–50% of their blood volume. They determined that the risk of OPSI is overestimated and that death from OPSI is 0.026% for at-risk adults and 0.052% for children. Based on an incidence of posttransfusion hepatitis of 3% per unit, the authors estimate the posttransfusion mortality to be approximately 0.14% per unit. It is worth noting that studies estimating the incidence of posttransfusion hepatitis are based on data before May 1990, when the HCV antibody screening became a standard part of blood screening (8). As the incidence of posttransfusion hepatitis and its associated mortality and morbidity decline from these improved screening tests, the safety of blood transfusion in the nonoperative management of splenic injuries may allow the transfusion of several units before the need to operate. Finally, there appears to be no data on the incidence of OPSI in splenectomized patients who have received the polyvalent pneumococcal vaccine currently in use. As these data become available, it may indicate a decreased mortality from OPSI that might sufficiently reduce the infectious risk for the asplenic patient. In the present environment, the relative risk of a 1- or 2-unit transfusion in the otherwise stable patient seems a reasonable alternative to splenectomy.

ACUTE TRAUMA: RECOVERY PHASE

The period of time after the trauma patient has been operated on or has been successfully managed nonoperatively until discharge may be the period where the greatest reduction of transfusion may occur without compromising the patient. During this period, there is no ongoing blood loss, and the intravascular volume has equilibrated with the interstitial space so dramatic that changes in the hematocrit should not be expected. The decision to transfuse during this period should not be based on maintaining the hematocrit above a certain level but rather based on evidence of symptomatic anemia. In the absence of chest pain, dyspnea, fatigue, or significant tachycardia, transfusion should not be necessary. Maintaining adequate nutrition and iron supplementation are important. The progressive anemia from routine daily blood draws must be carefully considered. If the patient is tolerating an enteral diet, remains afebrile, and has no other symptoms, there may be no need for routine blood testing.

BURN PATIENT

Similar to severely injured trauma patients, thermally injured patients may demonstrate anemia throughout their hospital course. Unlike trauma patients, however, the etiological factors responsible for the anemia of thermal injury are quite different (50–54). As such, these patients present a different challenge when evaluating their need for transfusion. The particular factors that predominate as the cause of anemia in the burn patient vary with respect to the time of evaluation during their hospital course (51, 52).

In the early hours after thermal injury, the most important factors accounting for anemia include direct thermal injury to erythrocytes within the cutaneous circulation and hemorrhage from the burn wounds. In the days after the injury, the predominant factors accounting for the anemia of thermal injury include ongoing blood loss during dressing changes and further hemolysis of erythrocytes that were damaged but not destroyed at the time of thermal injury. Further hemolysis occurs as erythrocytes pass through burn eschar and other tissue damaged as a result of thermal injury. Additional contributing factors in the anemia of thermal injury include blood loss at the time of surgery, from continued dressing changes, and occasionally blood loss from the gastrointestinal tract (51, 52). The amount of blood withdrawn for laboratory testing, which is not inconsequential and is routinely underestimated, serves to exacerbate further the resultant postburn anemia.

The thermally injured patient demonstrates an altered response to the anemia of thermal injury (51–54). Several studies have documented an increase in erythropoietin in response to anemia of thermal injury (53, 54). This increase has not been documented in all studies, and these differences may be related to the specific method used to measure the erythropoietin levels (54). When reticulocyte counts were measured in response to thermal injury, the results again were variable. A study of 27 patients by Vasko et al. (54) showed that although erythropoietin levels were inversely correlated with hemoglobin, these patients developed a reticulocytopenia that was present early in the hospital course and persisted throughout the hospitalization. This study suggested that the bone marrow response to the elevated level of erythropoietin was not associated with the expected increase in erythrocyte production.

Several studies have evaluated the effect of recombinant human erythropoietin (rEPO) on burn patients. In one study of pediatric burn patients and healthy volunteers receiving 150 units/kg/day of rEPO for 7 days, the authors documented increased erythrocyte formation based on increased reticulocyte counts (50). The hematocrit failed to show a statistically significant increase in either the burn patients or healthy volunteers. The authors suggested that the failure of the hematocrit level to increase in burn patients may have been related to the short duration of treatment, whereas the failure to respond in the healthy volunteers was due to the induction of an iron-deficiency anemia.

Studies of the erythropoietic response to thermal injury have documented an increase in erythropoietic levels that correlated with the size of the burn (53). Although a reticulocytosis was also documented in the burned patients, it did not appear to reach the levels anticipated for a normal bone marrow response. This may be the result of an inhibitory factor in the sera of burn patients. In a study using the sera from burn patients with greater than 20% full-thickness burn cocultured in vitro with target mouse bone marrow, a decrease in erythroid colonies was noted when erythropoietin was added to the culture system. Whereas erythropoiesis was inhibited, however, granulocytopoiesis was not affected. Furthermore, when the erythropoietin was subsequently assayed in vivo, there was no decrease in activity documented, suggesting that the mechanism of erythroid colony inhibition was not at the level of erythropoietin (52). In another experimental animal study, the erythroid colony forming cells were noted to return to normal as the animals healed. This study also noted that contrary to the inhibition of erythropoiesis, granulocytopoiesis and thrombopoiesis proceeded at an accelerated rate (51). The authors postulated that the redirection of the pluripotent stem cells away from erythroid formation to the granulocyte, macrophage, and platelet progenitor cell compartment may yield a survival advantage in the burned patient because infection and sepsis are major causes of morbidity and mortality in this patient population.

The safety of hemoglobin and hematocrit levels lower than previously thought advisable for burn patients has recently been reported (55, 56). Mann et al. (56) retrospectively compared transfusion practices in 1980 versus 1990 for patients with a greater than 10% total body surface area (TBSA) burn who required at least one operation. In 1980, patients received an average of 133 ± 24 mL% TBSA compared with 20 ± 6 mL% TBSA in 1990. None of the patients treated in 1990 suffered increased morbidity such as cardiac complications as a result of this more restricted use of blood transfusion. Based on these findings, the authors suggested that healthy patients do not need to be transfused if the hematocrit is greater than 15% and they are expected to undergo only one operation, or 25% if multiple surgeries are anticipated. For those patients with limited cardiovascular reserve or with critical burn injury, a hematocrit of 30% should be maintained. The findings of Sittig and Deitch (55) support the work of Mann et al. A policy of withholding transfusion for patients until hemoglobin levels were below 6.0–6.5 g/dL was initiated, and the results were compared with a cohort of patients treated when patients were transfused under a policy of routine transfusion to maintain hemoglobin levels above 9.5–10.0 g/dL. The adequacy of hemoglobin was determined by the patients' clinical stability. The routinely transfused patients received 7.4 ± 7.6 units, whereas the selectively transfused patients received only 2.1 ± 1.7 units. None of the patients treated under the policy of selective transfusion developed anemia associated with cardiac failure. In addition, 86% of the transfusions received in the selectively managed group of patients were given during the operative period (Figs. 33.3 and 33.4) (55). These studies support the safety

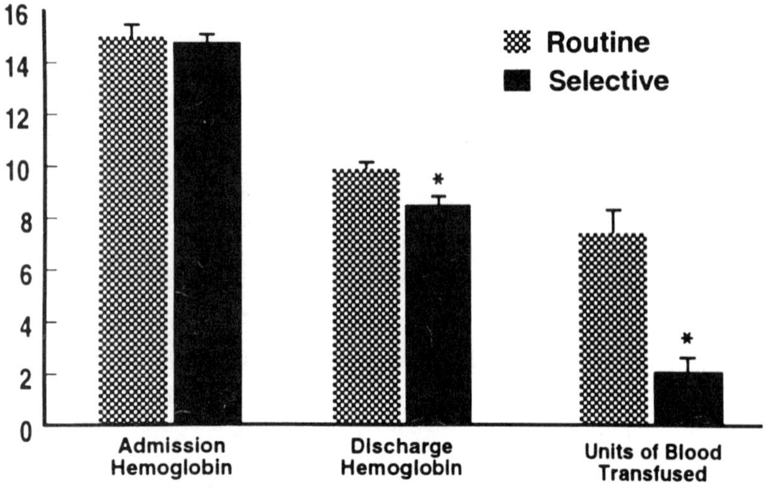

Figure 33.3. Comparison of admission and discharge hemoglobin levels for patients treated under a routine vs. selective transfusion policy. Data expressed as mean ± SEM; *P* < .01. (Reprinted with permission from Sittig KM, Deitch EA. Blood transfusions: for the thermally injured or for the doctor? J Trauma 1994;36:370.)

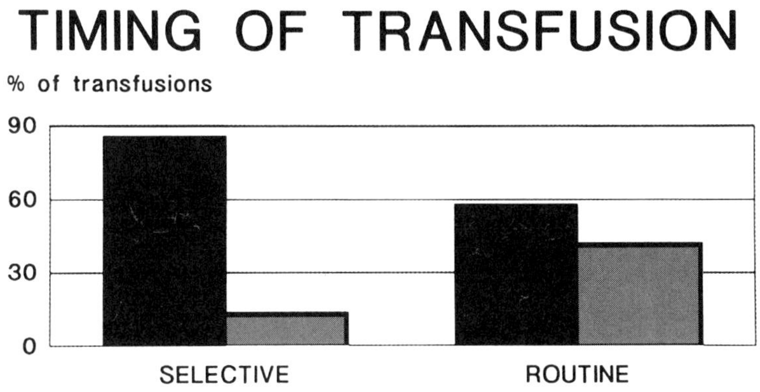

Figure 33.4. The timing of transfusion was different between the two groups, with the selective transfusion group receiving most transfusions during the operative period. $P < .004$ by chi-square analysis. ■, operative; ■, nonoperative. (Reprinted with permission from Sittig KM, Deitch EA. Blood transfusions: for the thermally injured or for the doctor? J Trauma 1994;36:371.)

of selective transfusion in the previously healthy burn patient. In addition, the reduction of infectious risk and the considerable cost savings from reduced utilization of blood services represent additional advantages with this approach.

The use of hemostatic agents in the operative phase of burn management can provide further reductions in the need for transfusion. Because the amount of intraoperative blood loss becomes one of the factors limiting the extent of excision, the control of hemorrhage either from the donor sites or from tangentially excised burn tissue is beneficial. Thrombin spray and laparotomy pads soaked with thrombin and epinephrine are commonly used (55, 57). In addition, tourniquets can be used for hemorrhage control when grafting extremities (58). Given the functional coagulopathy that can occur with normal coagulation factors in the presence of hypothermia, the importance of maintaining normothermia cannot be overlooked. This includes infusing warmed intravenous solutions and maintaining the operating room at a higher temperature than may be comfortable for the operative team but will limit heat loss from the patient.

MASSIVE TRANSFUSION

Massive transfusion has been defined as the administration of the patient's entire blood volume within a 24-hour time period (59). Others define this as the transfusion of greater than 10 units of packed red blood cells within 24 hours (60). The necessity for massive transfusion in the trauma patient, although potentially life-saving to the exsanguinating trauma patient, has a number of complications associated with it. The coagulopathy of massive transfusion is perhaps the most commonly cited complicating factor associated with massive transfusion. Recommended treatment of the massively transfused patient follows a proscribed protocol in some institutions. However, most recommend only treating documented factor and platelet deficiencies as opposed to replacement of these components based on the number of units of blood transfused.

TRANSFUSION OF OTHER BLOOD PRODUCTS

One problem associated with severe trauma and resuscitation with crystalloid solutions and massive transfusion of packed red blood cells is microvascular bleeding. Sometimes called "medical bleeding," this is differentiated from surgical bleeding by the presence of mucous membrane bleeding, oozing from surgical wounds and raw tissue surfaces, oozing from catheter sites after the application of direct pressure, and generalized petechiae or increase in the size of ecchymoses (61). This has resulted in the recommendation that platelet transfusion and fresh frozen plasma (FFP) should be prophylactically administered to correct platelet and coagulation deficiencies. A variety of formulas are used to guide the administration of these products, including the transfusion of 1 unit of FFP for every 3–6 units of packed red blood cells (62–64). In addition, the administration of 1 unit of platelet concentrate for every 10–12 units of packed red blood cells has been widely practiced (61). Recent studies indicate that the transfusion-associated risk of HCV is 0.03% per unit since May 1990 when the HCV antibody screening of the blood supply was initiated (8). Therefore, the inappropriate use of these blood products may not decrease the incidence of microvascular bleeding but may increase the patient's risk of HCV exposure.

Several studies have evaluated the changes in coagulation factors and platelet counts and their role in microvascular bleeding after trauma and massive transfusion (30, 61–66). These studies document a decrease in both coagulation factors and platelet count. Several explanations for these decreases have been suggested. First, a dilutional coagulopathy and thrombocytopenia has been documented. This has been called the "washout phenomenon" that occurs from the use of crystalloid fluid in the initial resuscitation and the transfusion of "old" bank blood that is deficient in both platelets and coagulation factors. In a study of 98 patients by Lucas and Ledgerwood (64), patients were resuscitated with a balanced

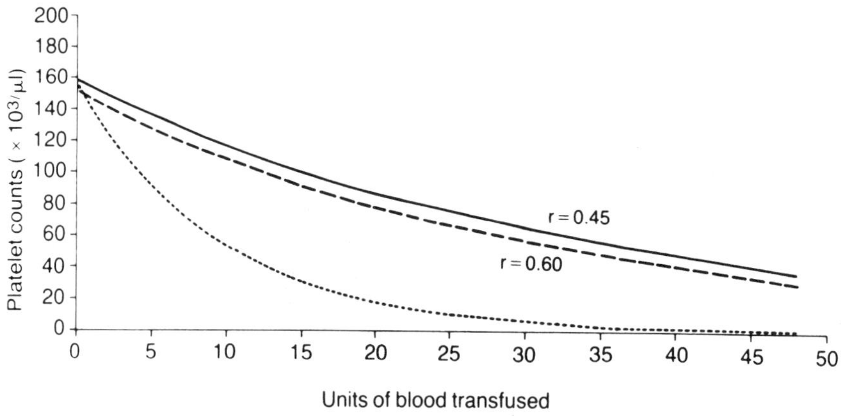

Figure 33.5. Exponential regressions of lines representing the change in platelet counts with number of units transfused for both treatment groups (platelet vs. FFP). Note that both groups have higher platelet counts than would be predicted if counts were solely dependent on dilutional factors. —, platelet group; ---, FFP group; ···, predicted levels. (Reprinted with permission from Reed RL, Ciavarella D, Heimbach DM, et al. Prophylactic platelet administration during massive transfusion. Ann Surg 1986;203:46.)

electrolyte solution and whole blood when it became available. This approach included administering 1 unit of FFP and one ampule of calcium chloride for each 5 units of whole blood transfused. They found that the washout phenomenon was not the only cause of coagulation factor depletion and that the duration of shock during the resuscitation period and the amount of stored blood transfused during the shock phase had a substantial impact on factor depletion.

A study by Reed et al. (61) supported the role of dilution as a contributing factor in thrombocytopenia but found that other factors were also involved. Approximately 35% of the decrease in platelet count could be attributable to dilutional factors by regression analysis (Fig. 33.5). In addition, 50% of the patients exhibiting microvascular bleeding required multiple platelet transfusions after the period of massive fluid and erythrocyte transfusion, suggesting that dilutional factors did not play a role in persistent thrombocytopenia during this period. In another study by the same group, dilutional factors accounted for only 43% of the platelet count variability, whereas other causes of platelet consumption were believed to account for the thrombocytopenia. The etiologies of the consumptive thrombocytopenia are believed to be related to the pathophysiological response accompanying lung, brain and massive tissue injury, shock, sepsis, and endothelial damage (65).

The Lucas and Ledgerwood group subsequently performed work in a canine model of hemorrhagic shock where the animals received a balanced electrolyte solution and packed red blood cell transfusion alone or with FFP (30). They found that although the coagulation factors decreased significantly at the end of the shock insult, the levels were still above those considered adequate for normal hemostasis. Furthermore, only factor II and antithrombin III were significantly higher in the group resuscitated with FFP versus the group resuscitated without FFP. Based on this study, the use of FFP to replace coagulation factors in the absence of microvascular bleeding could not be supported.

Recent prospective studies by Reed and colleagues (61, 63) evaluated the clotting factor abnormalities and platelet levels in 36 massively transfused patients (mean 21 units, ratio of whole blood to packed red blood cells, 4) and its relationship with microvascular bleeding. In addition, they evaluated the benefit of prophylactic platelet concentrate transfusion versus prophylactic FFP transfusion in the prevention of microvascular bleeding. These two comparison groups were chosen because 6 units of platelets contain approximately 1.5–2 units of FFP. These two study groups were able to evaluate the effects of platelet transfusion alone by comparing them with a group of patients treated with approximately the same FFP content as would be found in the platelet transfusion. They found that mild to moderate prolongations of the prothrombin time (PT) and partial thromboplastin time (PTT) were common in this patient population but did not predict microvascular bleeding. Regression analysis revealed that approximately 15–35% of the elevation of the PT and PTT could not be attributable to coagulation factor deficiencies. This suggests that other unidentified factors play a role in the elevation of the PT and PTT.

Although no laboratory test alone can identify those patients who would benefit from the transfusion of platelets, FFP, or cryoprecipitate, certain tests are more valuable than others in the decision process (63). A PT of no more than 1.3 times the control value has a 94% predictive value of indicating the absence of microvascular bleeding. Although the sensitivity of the PT or PTT to identify microvascular bleeding is only about 50%, PT or PTT values of at least 1.8 times the control value are 96% specific for microvascular bleeding. The bleeding time is not a helpful predictor of microvascular bleeding. In one study of 22 hypotensive trauma patients, 86% were noted to have a significantly elevated bleeding time, none of whom exhibited any evidence of microvascular bleeding (66).

The most sensitive laboratory predictors of microvascular bleeding are a platelet count of no more than 50×10^9/L

(50,000/mm³) and a fibrinogen of no more than 0.5 g/L. The combination of these two had a sensitivity of 89% and a negative predictive value of 96%; that is to say, if both values were above these levels, there was only a 4% chance of developing microvascular bleeding. The authors recommend that platelet transfusion be the initial response to microvascular bleeding with platelet counts less than 100×10^9/L (100,000/mm³) because platelet counts above this level may be required to control bleeding in patients with platelet dysfunction. Prophylactic transfusion with platelets is advocated for platelet counts of no more than 50×10^9/L (50,000/mm³), because this level correlates highly with microvascular bleeding in the trauma patient. Supplemental FFP or cryoprecipitate is recommended with fibrinogen less than 0.8 g/L. Fibrinogen levels less than 0.6–0.8 g/L can elevate PT and PTT even when middle level coagulation factors are appropriate. When the fibrinogen level is adequate but the PT or PTT ratio is at least 1.8, FFP should be administered (63).

Several studies of the effects of hypothermia on platelet counts and coagulation function have produced interesting results. Villalobos et al. (67) studied the mechanisms for the thrombocytopenia that occurs with cooling. Twenty-two dogs were cooled to 17°C and platelet counts, bone marrow aspirations, and tissue biopsies were obtained. The decrease of [^{32}P]-labeled platelets with hypothermia was secondary to sequestration by the liver, spleen, and other sites in the portal circulation rather than platelet destruction. Bone marrow aspiration revealed no difference in the megakaryocytes during hypothermia or rewarming, suggesting that platelet production was unchanged during the study.

Reed and others (68–70) established the coagulation factor dysfunction due to hypothermia. Standard coagulation testing in the laboratory is typically performed at 37°C. This method indicates coagulation abnormalities only if specific factor levels are decreased. The function of the coagulation cascade is dependent on enzymatic activity; thus, coagulation times may be prolonged with hypothermia in the presence of normal coagulation factor levels. They found that the PT was prolonged at all temperatures less than 33°C, whereas the PTT was prolonged at all temperatures less than 35°C despite normal coagulation factor levels (69). The study concluded that if clinical oozing exists in a hypothermic patient and coagulation tests performed at 37°C are within the normal range, rewarming the patient is more appropriate than empiric transfusion of FFP. Another study by the same group indicated that hypothermia exhibits a greater effect on the kinetic function of the coagulation factors than on the factor levels (70).

Finally, in a study that compared the equivalent clotting time prolongation that would be produced by a specific factor deficiency, hypothermia caused coagulation factors to behave as if there was a deficiency of factors (68). The findings represented in Table 33.2 and Figure 33.6 demonstrate that at temperatures of 29°C and below, all factors function as if the factor levels were less than 10%, levels that would cause severe bleeding abnormalities. At temperatures above 35°C, the factors functioned at levels equivalent to greater than 50% for all factors, which are sufficient for normal hemostasis. Clinically, there is rarely a coagulopathy above 35°C that can be related to the reduced temperature. Between 29 and 35°C there exist variable decreases in factor function that are

TABLE 33.2. THE FUNCTIONAL EQUIVALENCE OF CLOTTING FACTOR ACTIVITY

Temperature (°C)	Percentage of Factor							
	II	V	VII	VIII	IX	X	XI	XII
25°	5	3	5	0	0	4	2	1
27°	7	5	7	0	0	6	2	1
29°	10	8	12	3	3	10	4	1
31°	17	22	34	16	7	20	16	10
33°	24	50	60	59	32	44	60	17
35°	82	75	82	79	66	81	85	65
37°	100	100	100	100	100	100	100	100

At various temperatures, normal levels of clotting factor function as if there were a factor deficiency which is inversely related to temperature.
(Reprinted with permission from Johnston TD, et al. Trauma. Baltimore: Williams & Wilkins, 1994;37:415.)

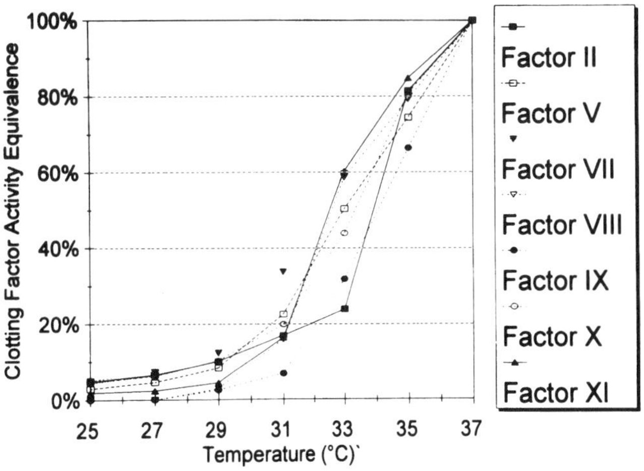

Figure 33.6. A graphical representation of the data from Table 33.2. (Reprinted with permission from Johnston TD, Chen Y, Reed RL II. Functional equivalence of hypothermia to specific clotting factor deficiencies. J Trauma 1994;37:415.)

not likely to cause clinical coagulopathy due to hypothermia alone, but may in combination with factor deficiencies from consumptive processes cause clinical evidence of microvascular bleeding. These studies support the importance of correcting hypothermia that may be more important than the administration of FFP in correcting coagulopathy.

SUMMARY

Massive hemorrhage continues to be the leading cause of death during the resuscitation phase of the severely injured trauma patient. The early use of blood transfusion combined with an aggressive approach to therapeutic intervention has significantly decreased mortality. However, the potential for disease transmission has increased the relative risk of blood transfusions and caused trauma and burn surgeons to reevaluate their transfusion practices. The lower limit of safe hemoglobin level for the trauma and burn patient is not yet entirely known. Although data from general surgical patient populations have helped us to realize that previously adhered to transfusion triggers are not appropriate, the acute nature of traumatic hemorrhage with the scenario of the unknown extent of injury means that these data are not universally transferrable to the trauma population. Recognizing that the care of the trauma and burn patient follows several distinct clinical phases, it is possible to optimize transfusion practices. Patients needing blood products for improved oxygen delivery or for the correction of coagulation abnormalities will be transfused in a timely fashion while avoiding transfusions in those instances where there is little benefit realized physiologically. Although blood transfusion continues to be a lifesaving therapy, the judicious use of blood can provide maximal benefit while limiting the potential risks to the patient.

REFERENCES

1. Bordley J III, Harvey AM. Two centuries of American medicine. Philadelphia: WB Saunders, 1976:303–314.
2. Spence RK, Cernaianu AC, Carson J, DelRossi AJ. Current problems in surgery: transfusions and surgery. 30th ed. St. Louis: Mosby-Year Book, 1993:1101–1192.
3. Hamilton SM. The use of blood in resuscitation of the trauma patient. Can J Surg 1993;36:21–27.
4. Whelan TJ Jr, Burkhalter WE, Gomez A. Management of war wounds. In: Welch CE, ed. Advances in surgery. Chicago: Year Book Medical Publishers, 1968:227–350.
5. Artz CP. Historical aspects of burn management. Surg Clin North Am 1970;50:1193–1200.
6. Talbott JH. A biographical history of medicine: excerpts and essays on the men and their work. New York: Grune and Stratton, 1970:1104–1105.
7. Moore FD. The body-weight burn budget: basic fluid therapy for the early burn. Surg Clin North Am 1970;50:1249–1265.
8. Donahue JG, Munoz A, Ness PM, et al. The declining risk of post-transfusion hepatitis C virus infection. N Engl J Med 1992;27:369–373.
9. Faust RJ, Warner MA. Transfusion risks. Int Anesthesiol Clin 1990;28: 184–189.
10. Graves TA, Cioffi WG, Mason AD Jr, McManus WF, Pruitt BA Jr. Relationship of transfusion and infection in a burn population. J Trauma 1989;29:948–954.
11. Tartter PI. The association of perioperative blood transfusion with colorectal cancer recurrence. Ann Surg 1992;216:633–638.
12. Abramson D, Scalea TM, Hitchcock R, Trooskin SZ, Henry SM, Greenspan J. Lactate clearance and survival following injury. J Trauma 1993;35:584–589.
13. Greenburg AG, Renzi RM, Kaye W. Oxygen delivery concepts in critically ill patients. In: Najarian JS, Delaney JP, eds. Progress in trauma and critical care surgery. St. Louis: Mosby-Year Book, 1992:297–302.
14. Reed RL II. Monitoring of circulatory oxygen delivery. Trauma Quart 1994;11:18–30.
15. Robertie PG, Gravlee GP. Safe limits of isovolemic hemodilution and recommendations for erythrocyte transfusion. Int Anesthesiol Clin 1990;4:197–204.
16. Tuman KJ. Tissue oxygen delivery: the physiology of anemia. Anesthesiol Clin North Am 1990;8:451–469.
17. Stehling L, Zauder HL. Acute normovolemic hemodilution. Transfusion 1991;31:857–868.
18. Levy PS, Chavez RP, Crystal GJ, et al. Oxygen extraction ratio: a valid indicator of transfusion need in limited coronary vascular reserve? J Trauma 1992;32:769–774.
19. Chapler CK, Cain SM. The physiologic reserve in oxygen carrying capacity: studies in experimental hemodilution. Can J Physiol Pharmacol 1986;64:7–12.
20. Domsky MF Wilson RF. Hemodynamic resuscitation. In: Milzman DP, Boulanger BR, Rodriguez A, eds. Critical care clinics. Philadelphia: WB Saunders, 1993:715–726.
21. Weigelt JA. Resuscitation and initial management. In: Rodriguez A, Boulanger BR, Milzman DP, eds. Critical care clinics. Philadelphia: WB Saunders, 1993:657–671.
22. Somers J Greenburg AG. Transfusion therapy in surgical emergencies. In: Najarian JS, Delaney JP, eds. Progress in trauma and critical care surgery. St. Louis: Mosby-Year Book, 1992:25–39.
23. Wilkerson DK, Rosen AL, Gould SA, Sehgal LR, Sehgal HL, Moss GS. Oxygen extraction ratio: a valid indicator of myocardial metabolism in anemia. J Surg Res 1987;42:629–634.
24. Fowler NO, Holmes JC. Blood viscosity and cardiac output in acute experimental anemia. J Appl Physiol 1975;39:453–456.
25. Messmer K. Hemodilution. Surg Clin North Am 1975;55:659–668.
26. Szlyk PC, King C, Jennings DB, Cain SM, Chapler CK. The role of aortic chemoreceptors during anemia. Can J Physiol Pharmacol 1984;62: 519–523.
27. Chapler CK, Cain SM. Blood flow and O_2 uptake in dog hindlimb with anemia, norepinephrine, and propranolol. J Appl Physiol 1981;51:565–570.
28. Glick G Jr, Plauth WH, Braunwald E. Role of the autonomic nervous system in the circulatory response to acutely induced anemia in unanesthetized dogs. J Clin Invest 1964;43:2112–2124.
29. Shibutani K, Komatsu T, Kubal K, Sanchala V, Kumar V, Bizzarri DV. Critical level of oxygen delivery in anesthetized man. Crit Care Med 1983;11:640–643.
30. Martin DJ, Lucas CE, Ledgerwood AM, Hoschner J, McGonigal MD, Grabow D. Fresh frozen plasma supplement to massive red blood cell transfusion. Ann Surg 1985;202:505–511.

31. Committee on Trauma. A.C.S. Advanced Trauma Life Support Course, Chicago: American College of Surgeons, 1989.
32. Knottenbelt JD. Low initial hemoglobin levels in trauma patients: an important indicator of ongoing hemorrhage. J Trauma 1991;31: 1396–1399.
33. Spence RK, Costabile JP, Young GS, et al. Is hemoglobin level alone a reliable predictor of outcome in the severely anemic surgical patient? Am Surg 1992;58:92–95.
34. Spence RK, Carson JA, Poses R, et al. Elective surgery without transfusion: influence of preoperative hemoglobin level and blood loss on mortality. Am J Surg 1990;159:302–324.
35. Czer LSC, Shoemaker WC. Optimal hematocrit value in critically ill postoperative patients. Surg Gynecol Obstet 1978;147:363–368.
36. Dietrich KA. Cardiovascular and metabolic response to blood cell transfusion in critically ill volume-resuscitated non-surgical patients. Crit Care Med 1990;18:940–944.
37. Horst HM, Dlugos S, Fath JJ, Sorensen VJ, Obeid FN, Bivins BA. Coagulopathy and intraoperative blood salvage (IBS). J Trauma 1992;32: 646–653.
38. Ozmen V, McSwain NE, Nichols RL, Smith J, Flint LM. Autotransfusion of potentially culture—positive blood (CPB) in abdominal trauma: preliminary data from a prospective study. J Trauma 1992;32:36–39.
39. Feliciano PD, Mullins RJ, Trunkey DD, Crass RA, Beck JR, Helfand M. A decision analysis of traumatic splenic injuries. J Trauma 1992;33: 340–348.
40. Beal SL, Spisso JM. The risk of splenorrhaphy. Arch Surg 1988;123: 1158–1163.
41. King H, Schumaker HB Jr. Splenic studies. I. Susceptibility to infection after splenectomy performed in infancy. Ann Surg 1952;136:239–242.
42. Upadhyaya P, Simpson JS. Splenic trauma in children. Surg Gynecol Obstet 1968;126:781–790.
43. Consentino CM, Luck SR, Barthel MJ, Reynolds M, Raffensperger JG. Transfusion requirements in conservative nonoperative management of blunt splenic and hepatic injuries during childhood. J Pediatr Surg 1990;25:950–954.
44. Delius RE, Frankel W, Coran AG. A comparison between operative and nonoperative management of blunt injuries to the liver and spleen in adult and pediatric patients. Surgery 1989;106:788–793.
45. Umali E, Andrews HG, White JJ. A critical analysis of blood transfusion requirements in children with blunt abdominal trauma. Am Surg 1992;58:736–739.
46. Molin MR, Shackford SR. The management of splenic trauma in a trauma system. Arch Surg 1990;125:840–843.
47. Smith JS Jr, Wengrovitz MA, DeLong BS. Prospective validation of criteria, including age, for safe, nonsurgical management of the ruptured spleen. J Trauma 1992;33:363–369.
48. Flaherty L, Jurkovich GJ. Minor splenic injuries: associated injuries and transfusion requirements. J Trauma 1991;31:1618–1621.
49. Luna GK, Dellinger EP. Nonoperative observation therapy for splenic injuries: a safe therapeutic option? Am J Surg 1987;153:462–468.
50. Fleming RYD, Herndon DN, Vaidya S, et al. The effect of erythropoietin in normal healthy volunteers and pediatric patients with burn injuries. Surgery 1992;112:424–432.
51. Wallner S, Vautrin R, Murphy J, Anderson S, Peterson V. The haematopoietic response to burning: studies in an animal model. Burns 1984;10:236–251.
52. Wallner SF, Vautrin R. The anemia of thermal injury: mechanism of inhibition of erythropoiesis. Proc Soc Exp Biol Med 1986;181:144–150.
53. Deitch EA, Sittig KM. A serial study of the erythropoietic response to thermal injury. Ann Surg 1993;217:293–299.
54. Vasko SD, Burdge JJ, Ruberg RL, Verghese AS. Evaluation of erythropoietin levels in the anemia of thermal injury. J Burn Care Rehabil 1991;12:437–441.
55. Sittig KM, Deitch EA. Blood transfusions: for the thermally injured or for the doctor? J Trauma 1994;36:369–372.
56. Mann R, Heimbach DM, Engrav LH, Foy H. Changes in transfusion practices in burn patients. J Trauma 1994;37:220–222.
57. Prasad JK, Taddonio TE, Thomson PD. Prospective comparison of a bovine collagen dressing to bovine spray thrombin for control of haemorrhage of skin graft donor sites. Burns 1991;17:70–71.
58. Housinger TA, Lang D, Warden GD. A prospective study of blood loss with excisional therapy in pediatric burn patients. J Trauma 1993;34: 262–263.
59. Johnson RL Campbell JA. Blood transfusion therapy in the surgical intensive care unit. In: Maull KI, Cleveland HC, Feliciano DV, Rice CL, Trunkey DD, Wolferth CC, eds. Advances in trauma and critical care. St. Louis: Mosby-Year Book, 1993:51–84.
60. Ferrara A, MacArthur JD, Wright HK, Modlin IM, McMillen MA. Hypothermia and acidosis worsen coagulopathy in the patient requiring massive transfusion. Am J Surg 1990;160:515–518.
61. Reed RL, Ciavarella D, Heimbach DM, et al. Prophylactic platelet administration during massive transfusion. Ann Surg 1986;203:40–48.
62. Harrigan C, Lucas CE, Ledgerwood AM. The effect of hemorrhagic shock on the clotting cascade in injured patients. J Trauma 1989;29: 1416–1422.
63. Ciavarella D, Reed RL, Counts RB, et al. Clotting factor levels and the risk of diffuse microvascular bleeding in the massively transfused patient. Br J Haematol 1987;67:365–368.
64. Lucas CE, Ledgerwood AM. Clinical significance of altered coagulation tests after massive transfusion for trauma. Am Surg 1981;47:125–130.
65. Counts RB, Haisch C, Simon TL, Maxwell NG, Heimbach DM, Carrico CJ. Hemostasis in massively transfused trauma patients. Ann Surg 1979;190:91–99.
66. Harrigan C, Lucas CE, Ledgerwood AM, Walz DA, Mammen EF. Serial changes in primary hemostasis after massive transfusion. Surgery 1985;98:836–844.
67. Villalobos TJ, Adelson E, Riley PA, Jr. A cause of the thrombocytopenia and leukopenia that occur in dogs during deep hypothermia. J Clin Invest 1958;37:1–7.
68. Johnston TD, Chen Y, Reed RL II. Functional equivalence of hypothermia to specific clotting factor deficiencies. J Trauma 1994;37: 413–417.
69. Reed RL, Bracey AW, Hudson JD, Miller TA, Fischer RP. Hypothermia and blood coagulation: dissociation between enzyme activity and clotting factor levels. Circ Shock 1990;32:141–152.
70. Reed RL, Johnston TD, Hudson JD, Fischer RP. The disparity between hypothermic coagulopathy and clotting studies. J Trauma 1992;33: 465–470.

Chapter 34

Hemorrhage in Pediatric Patients

RICHARD M. DSIDA
CHARLES J. COTÉ

INTRODUCTION

When caring for pediatric patients, consideration must be given to the anatomic and physiological differences between children and their adult counterparts. Pediatric surgical procedures, especially those addressing congenital problems, often provide unique challenges.

The size and age of the patient are major determinants of fluid and blood therapy. Fluid administration must include replacement of deficits, maintenance requirements, "third space," and blood losses (1) (Tables 34.1 and 34.2). Although the absolute blood volume may be small, children less than 1 year of age have a larger blood volume than adults when considered on the basis of weight. Preterm infants have an estimated blood volume (EBV) of 90–100 mL/kg, full-term newborns 80–90 mL/kg, and infants between 3 and 12 months of age 70–80 mL/kg. The blood volume of children older than 1 year of age is approximately 70 mL/kg.

Calculation of the patient's approximate blood volume and knowledge of the preoperative hematocrit enable the anesthesiologist to estimate the maximum allowable blood loss (MABL). The simplest means of calculating the MABL involves a simple proportion (2):

$$\text{MABL} = \frac{\text{EBV} \times (\text{Patient hematocrit} - \text{Minimum acceptable hematocrit})}{\text{Patient hematocrit}}$$

For example, a 3-year-old child weighing 20 kg with a starting hematocrit of 35% and a minimum acceptable hematocrit of 25%,

$$\text{MABL} = \frac{(20 \times 70) \times (35 - 25)}{35} = 400 \text{ mL}$$

In this example, 25% is used as the minimum acceptable hematocrit. The anesthesiologist may choose to accept a lower hematocrit in a patient who is healthy if further blood loss is not anticipated. If ongoing blood loss is expected or if the patient has significant pulmonary or cardiac disease, a higher value may be indicated to provide adequate oxygen-carrying capacity to meet physiological needs. Whatever the circumstance, it is necessary to maintain the circulating blood volume. If the MABL is exceeded, blood should be administered. To calculate the amount of blood to be transfused requires knowledge of the patient's blood volume, the patient's hematocrit, and the approximate hematocrit of the blood product to be transfused (3):

$$\text{Volume to transfuse} = \frac{\text{EBV} \times (\text{Desired hematocrit} - \text{Present hematocrit})}{\text{Hematocrit of blood product}}$$

For example, if the same 20-kg child now has a hematocrit of 20% and will be transfused with packed red cells with a hematocrit of 65%,

$$\text{Volume to transfuse} = \frac{1400 \times (30 - 20)}{65} = 215 \text{ mL}$$

The calculated volume to be transfused may be a fraction of 1 unit, especially in smaller children. However, the actual volume transfused from each unit should be maximized to decrease the likelihood of subsequent exposures to blood products.

Immaturity of the cardiovascular system may also have an impact on blood and fluid therapy. The neonatal ventricle is noncompliant and therefore does not have a normal Frank-Starling response to volume loading. Because of this, cardiac output is maintained by heart rate and filling pressure (4). Although hypotension is frequently due to hypovolemia, central venous pressure monitoring should be considered if large blood losses or fluid shifts are anticipated. The pediatric patient should not be denied the benefit of invasive monitoring simply because of size, age, or technical difficulty with placement.

Developmental aspects of the hematological system also merit consideration. Erythropoiesis begins during the third week of fetal life. The primary component of the red cell in the fetus and infant is fetal hemoglobin (HbF), comprising 80% at birth. In the fetus, the high oxygen affinity of HbF facilitates oxygen uptake at the placenta while still allowing delivery at the tissue level where oxygen tension is low. In the absence of hemoglobinopathies, the production of HbF ceases and erythropoiesis decreases profoundly at birth. As a result, hemoglobin levels decline in infants. Term newborns typically reach a nadir of 9–11 g/dL at 8–12 weeks of age. The hemoglobin concentration in preterm newborns generally decreases to a lower level at an earlier age. Although infants often present for elective surgery during this physiological nadir, they rarely require transfusion before anesthesia.

There are several unique elements of the coagulation system in neonates. Deficiencies in the vitamin K-dependent factors II, VII, IX, and X are usually corrected by routine administration of vitamin K at birth. After vitamin K, screening tests including the prothrombin time (PT), partial thromboplastin time (PTT), and fibrinogen levels generally reveal an abnormality in the PTT. This is most likely due to low levels of the contact factors XII and XI, prekallikrein, and high-molecular-weight kininogen (5). Platelet number and function should be adequate at birth in the absence of sepsis or maternal idiopathic thrombocytopenic purpura. Despite laboratory abnormalities, hemostasis in a healthy newborn is not usually a major clinical problem.

TABLE 34.1. HOURLY MAINTENANCE FLUID REQUIREMENTS

Weight (kg)	mL/kg
Newborns to 10 kg	4mL
10–20 kg	40 mL + 2 mL for each kg above 10 kg
>20 kg	60 mL + 1 mL for each kg above 20 kg

SPECIFIC PROBLEMS

TRAUMA

Trauma is the leading cause of death in children 14 years of age and under, representing almost half of the deaths in this age group. In the United States, 22,000 children die annually from accidental injuries (6). The leading cause of mortality and morbidity in injured children is prolonged deprivation of oxygen delivery to vital organs. Oxygen delivery is impaired if there is a decrease in cardiac output, hemoglobin concentration, or oxygen saturation. Appropriate airway management and maintenance of the circulating blood volume are critical in these patients.

Assessment of the need for volume resuscitation begins with the vital signs. Systolic blood pressure and heart rate are the most commonly used indicators of acute blood loss. Healthy children in the supine position typically maintain blood pressure even with the acute loss of 15–20% of their blood volume. Postural hypotension and/or a narrow pulse pressure may be more sensitive signs of hypovolemia. The index of suspicion for hypovolemia should always be high and the threshold for invasive monitoring should be low. It is unlikely for hypovolemic shock to occur in older children with an isolated closed-head or closed-extremity injury (7). Closed-head injury alone may, however, cause hemorrhagic shock in young children with open cranial sutures (8).

TABLE 34.2. FLUID REPLACEMENT

	Maintenance	Deficit	Third Space (mL/kg/hr)	Blood Loss (mL/mL blood)
First hour	See Table 34.1	1/2	2–15	2–3
Second hour	See Table 34.1	1/4	2–15	2–3
Third hour	See Table 34.1	1/4	2–15	2–3
Fourth hour	See Table 34.1	—	2–15	2–3

In select cases, 5% albumen can be substituted for lactated Ringer's solution to replace blood loss (mL for mL) and to reduce the clear fluid administered to make up for third-space losses to decrease edema formation.

Initial stabilization of the circulation should include large-bore venous access and intravenous administration of lactated Ringer's solution or normal saline (15–20 mL/kg). If signs of shock (low blood pressure, narrow pulse pressure, elevated heart rate, poor peripheral perfusion, or persistent metabolic acidosis) do not improve, additional boluses should be infused. If several fluid boluses are required, the patient probably requires red cell transfusion and should be evaluated for signs of ongoing blood loss. O-negative or type-specific blood, given in 10- to 20-mL/kg boluses, should be administered as circumstances dictate. If time permits, it is advisable to obtain a baseline hematocrit. It should be noted that a normal or near-normal value may be obtained in the face of significant blood loss if volume resuscitation has not yet begun. Frequent repeat measurements of hematocrit, assessment of acid/base status, and assessment of the color of the patient's mucous membranes are important to monitor the adequacy of red cell replacement.

Because the child with multiple injuries may require massive and rapid blood transfusion, a number of metabolical and hematological complications may occur. Children may be more susceptible to such complications because the ratio of the volume in a unit of blood product to their circulating blood volume is greater when compared with adults. Hypothermia, which is often present on arrival to the emergency room or operating room, may be exacerbated by the infusion of cold fluid and blood products. Hypothermia increases metabolic demands, may exacerbate coagulopathy, and is associated with decreased survival (9–11). A variety of methods for warming blood products and fluid are available and have been used safely. These include immersion of units in warm water, admixture with warm saline, and in-line warming (12). Fluids and blood from standard warmers lose heat by convection before entering the patient. Some recommendations for using warming devices take into account only the volume and the rate of infusion. However, the condition and size of the patient, especially in children, need to be factored into the decision of whether or not to warm blood products. For instance, 1–2 units of packed cells administered to a 70-kg teenager over several hours does not typically need to be warmed. The same volume given rapidly to a 20-kg child may result in serious problems if not warmed. Rapid transfusion devices with countercurrent heat exchangers provide the most efficient means of warming blood and fluids as they are administered to the patient (13).

Life-threatening electrolyte disturbances may also occur with rapid transfusion. The incidence of each disturbance will vary depending on the blood product transfused and the rate of transfusion (Table 34.3). Infused citrate binds ionized calcium. Ionized hypocalcemia and the resultant myocardial depression have been reported with rapid infusion of whole blood and fresh-frozen plasma (FFP) (14, 15). FFP contains the highest concentration of citrate per unit volume and therefore presents the greatest risk for acute ionized hypocalcemia. Caution should be exercised and prophylactic calcium administration considered when transfusion rates approach 1.5–2.0 mL/kg/min (Fig. 34.1) (14). This is particularly important in infants and small children. For example, a 10-kg child requires only 15–20 mL/min to develop clinically important hypocalcemia. The myocardial depressant effects of hypocalcemia may be magnified in patients anesthetized with volatile agents that have calcium channel blocking activity (16). Theoretically, there may also be added risk of myocardial depression with FFP or citrated whole blood administration via a central line versus a peripheral line because there is less time for mixing, dilution, and/or metabolism of citrate. Calcium chloride provides three times the ionized calcium when compared with calcium gluconate on a milligram basis. Ionization, however, occurs at the same rate and does not require hepatic metabolism of gluconate (5 mg calcium chloride is equivalent to 15 mg calcium gluconate) (17) (Fig. 34.2).

Hyperkalemia is a problem primarily associated with administration of whole blood but may rarely occur with very rapid infusion of packed red blood cells (18, 19). The plasma potassium concentration in blood products rises with increasing time of storage as a result of diffusion and hemolysis (Table 34.3). Although the plasma potassium concentration in packed cells is higher than similarly stored whole blood, the actual amount of potassium is less because of the smaller plasma volume contained in a unit of packed red cells. Infusion of *whole blood* at a rate of 1.5–2.0 mL/kg/min may result in clinically important increases in serum potassium. To reduce the risk of hyperkalemia, as well as toxicity from preservatives in neonates, the use of fresh packed cells and cell washing before infusion has been advocated for large-volume transfusions (more than 15 mL/kg) (19, 20). The need for repeated small volume transfusions may be met with older blood from split units (7–14 days storage) in an effort to minimize donor exposure (21).

Coagulation changes have long been recognized as a problem resulting from massive transfusion. Bleeding may result from a dilution of platelets, coagulation factors, or both, depending on the volume and type of blood products transfused. Dilutional effects may be compounded by shock and hypothermia (11). Most studies that implicate dilutional thrombocytopenia as the major reason for coagulopathy were carried out using whole blood or modified whole blood (22, 23). Levels of the labile factors V and VIII decrease in stored *whole* blood but remain adequate for hemostasis. Levels of all other coagulation factors, including fibrinogen, are minimally affected by storage as whole blood.

TABLE 34.3. COMPOSITION OF MAJOR BLOOD PRODUCTS

	Normal Whole Blood (In Vivo)	CPD Whole Blood		CPDA-1 Whole Blood		CPD PRBC[a]	CPDA-1 PRBC[a]		CPDAs + AS-1 PRBC[a]	FFP
Days Stored	—	0	21	0	35	14	0	35	49	—
pH	7.4	7.2	6.8	7.6	6.98	6.8	7.55	6.71	6.6	6.8
Potassium (mEq/L)	3.5–5.0	3.9	21	4.2	27	9–15	5.1	78	6.5	4–8
Citrate	None	4	4	4	4	2	2	2	1	8
2, 3-DPG (%)	Normal	100	21	100	<10	3	100	<10	<5	0
Factors 5 and 8	Normal	Normal	20–50%	Normal	20–50%	20–50%	Normal	20–50%	15–20%	Normal
Fibrinogen	Normal	Normal	Normal	Normal	Normal	Normal	Normal	Normal	60%	Normal
Platelets (/mm^3)	240–400,000	Normal	None	Normal	None	None	Minimal	None	None	None
Hematocrit (%)	35–45	35–45	35–45	35–45	35–45	60–70	60–70	60–70	50–60	0

[a] Although whole blood and packed cells have some similarities in their chemical composition and plasma components, the packed cells contain considerably less plasma volume than whole blood and thus represent a lesser total amount of these components.

CPD, citrate phosphate dextrose; CPDA-1, citrate phosphate dextrose-adenine-1; PRBC, packed red blood cells; AS–1, adenine-saline-1; 2,3–DPG, 2,3 diphosphoglycerate.

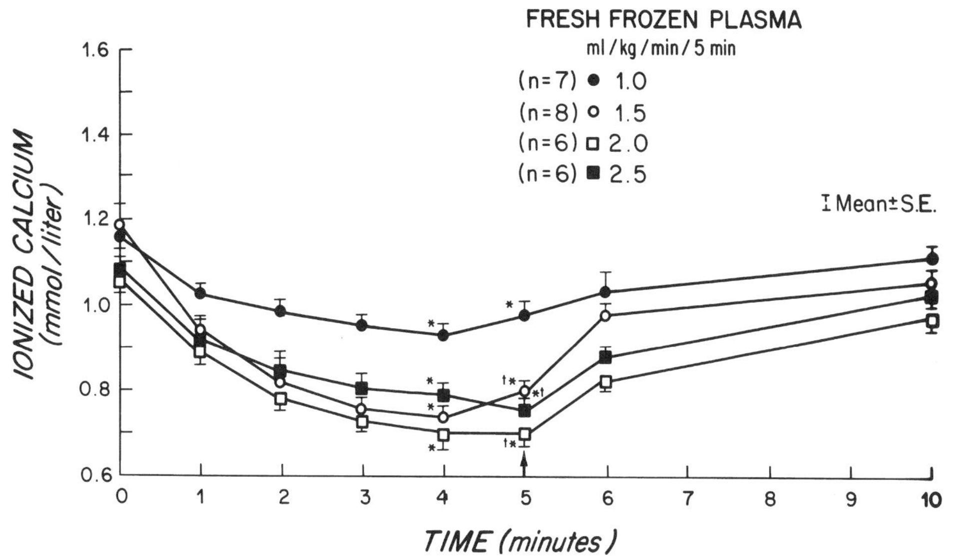

Figure 34.1. Changes in ionized calcium concentrations with various infusion rates of FFP in children with severe burns. Children without burns may exhibit larger changes because metabolic rate and hepatic blood flow are higher in the patient with burns. (Reprinted with permission from Coté CJ, Drop LJ, Hoaglin DC, Daniels AL, Young ET. Ionized hypocalcemia after fresh frozen plasma administration to thermally injured children. Anesth Analg 1988;67:152–160.)

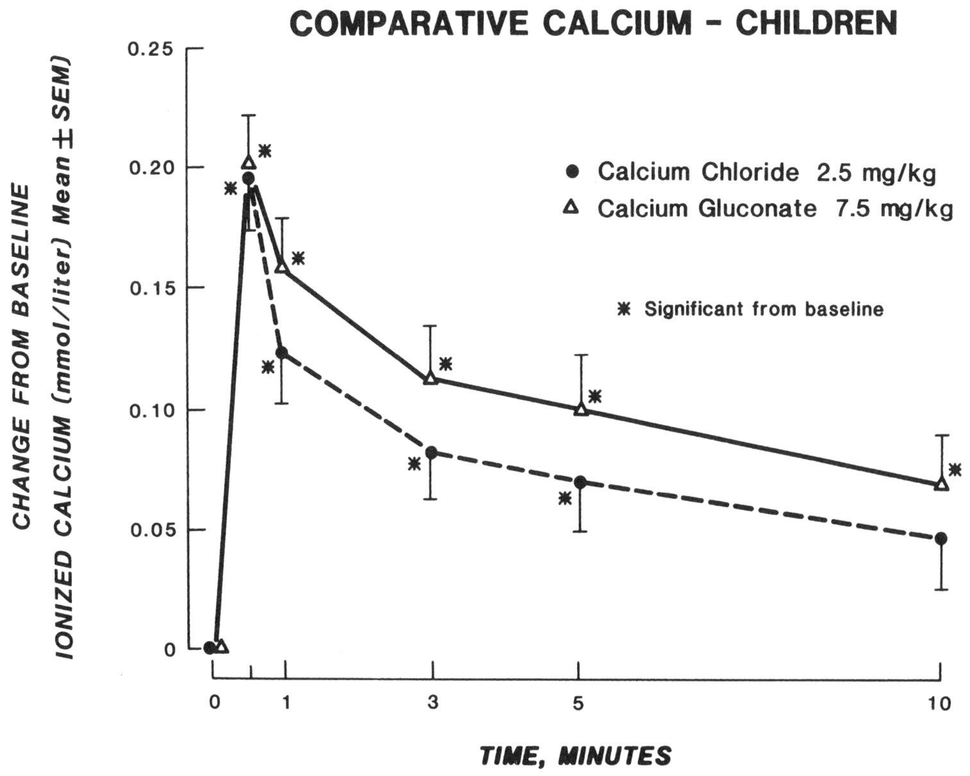

Figure 34.2. Changes from baseline in ionized calcium concentration (mean ± SEM) after calcium chloride (2.5 mg/kg) versus calcium gluconate (7.5 mg/kg) in 10 children. There was no significant difference in rate or degree of dissociation between calcium salts. (Reprinted with permission from Coté CJ, Drop LJ, Daniels AL, Hoaglin DC. Calcium chloride versus calcium gluconate: comparison of ionization and cardiovascular effects in children and dogs. Anesthesiology 1987;66:466–470.)

The extent of the dilution of platelets may be estimated by considering a logarithmic decay based on the initial platelet count and the number of blood volumes transfused (24). The actual platelet count tends to be slightly higher than calculated, possibly due to mobilization of platelets from extravascular sites (Fig. 34.3). Bleeding typically does not occur until a platelet count of less than 50,000/mm^3 is encountered and is unlikely to result from thrombocytopenia if the count is greater than 100,000/mm^3. If the starting platelet count is high (more than 500,000/mm^3), then the need for transfusion of platelets is unlikely even if blood loss exceeds three blood volumes (Fig. 34.4) (22).

Although replacement of massive acute blood loss with whole blood is still recommended (25), the use of whole blood has diminished since the advent of component therapy. However, data from massive transfusion exclusively with packed red blood cells are scant, particularly in children. These data come primarily from adults and adolescents undergoing scheduled procedures where hypothermia and shock are less likely to occur. Before the replacement of one blood volume with only packed red blood cells (no FFP), minimal changes in the PT and PTT occur. If the initial platelet count was normal (more than 250,000/mm^3), patients would be expected to have an adequate number of platelets for hemostasis even with this volume replaced. As the blood loss approaches 1.5 blood volumes in both children and adults, the platelet count generally remains adequate, but the dilution of clotting factors may become critical (26–28). The PT and PTT generally approach 1.5–2.0 times control values, and fibrinogen may decrease to less than 75 mg/dL, at which time FFP administration becomes necessary. From that point on, FFP, in a volume of 33% of further blood loss, should be infused to maintain adequate levels of coagulation factors.

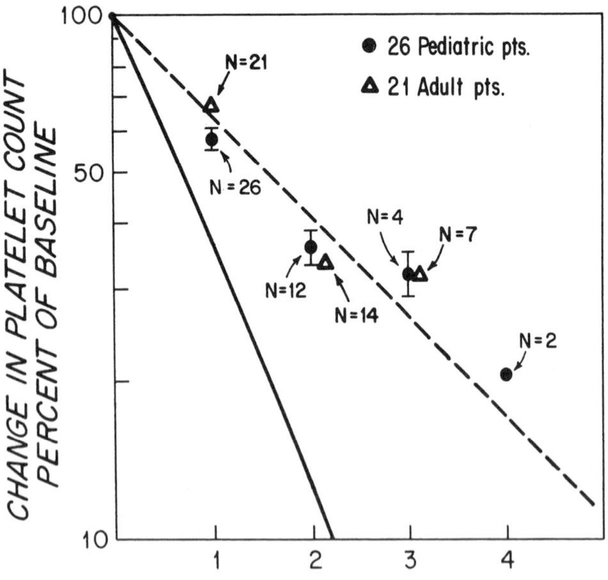

Figure 34.3. Change in platelet count with multiple blood volume transfusion. Adult data derived from study of adult combat victims (22). The broken line represents the observed changes; the solid line represents the predicted changes. The changes in platelet concentration during massive blood transfusion are similar in pediatric and adult patients when all data are correlated with estimated blood volumes transfused. (Reprinted with permission from Coté CJ, Liu LMP, Szyfelbein SK, Goudsouzian NG, Daniels AL. Changes in serial platelet counts following massive blood transfusion in pediatric patients. Anesthesiology 1985;62:197–201.)

GUIDELINES

1. Always consider massive transfusion in terms of the number of blood volumes replaced—not the number of units.
2. Platelet count decreases approximately 40% from baseline with one blood volume replaced, 60% with two blood volumes, and 70% with three. Administer platelets if the platelet count is less than 50,000/mm^3 or if further bleeding is expected and the platelet count is less than 100,000/mm^3. Transfuse 0.1–0.2 units/kg, observe for clinical signs of coagulopathy (oozing), and recheck platelet count. The manifestation of dilutional thrombocytopenia is dependent on the initial platelet count and the number of blood volumes replaced.
3. When transfusing exclusively whole blood, FFP is rarely necessary. With exclusive packed red blood cell transfusion, clinically important dilution of clotting factors occurs after replacement of approximately 1.5 blood volumes.

EAR, NOSE, AND THROAT (ENT) SURGERY

Although tonsillectomy is less frequently performed than in the past, it remains one of the most common operations in children. In 1992, approximately 80,000 tonsillectomies were performed (29), most frequently for upper airway obstruction and recurrent tonsillitis. The most common serious complication of tonsillectomy with or without adenoidectomy is postoperative hemorrhage. Early bleeding (in the first 24 hours) occurs in 0.14–2.1% of cases (30, 31). It is generally evident within the first 4–6 hours after surgery. Late bleeding, typically occurring on the fifth to seventh postoperative day, results from separation of the eschar from the tonsillar fossae and has been reported in 2.5–6.4% of cases (30, 32). Circulatory instability and acute airway obstruction may result from postoperative hemorrhage.

In an effort to minimize the potential for postoperative bleeding, preoperative history and laboratory screening have been used. A history of easy bruising or excessive bleeding with circumcision or dental procedures or a family history of

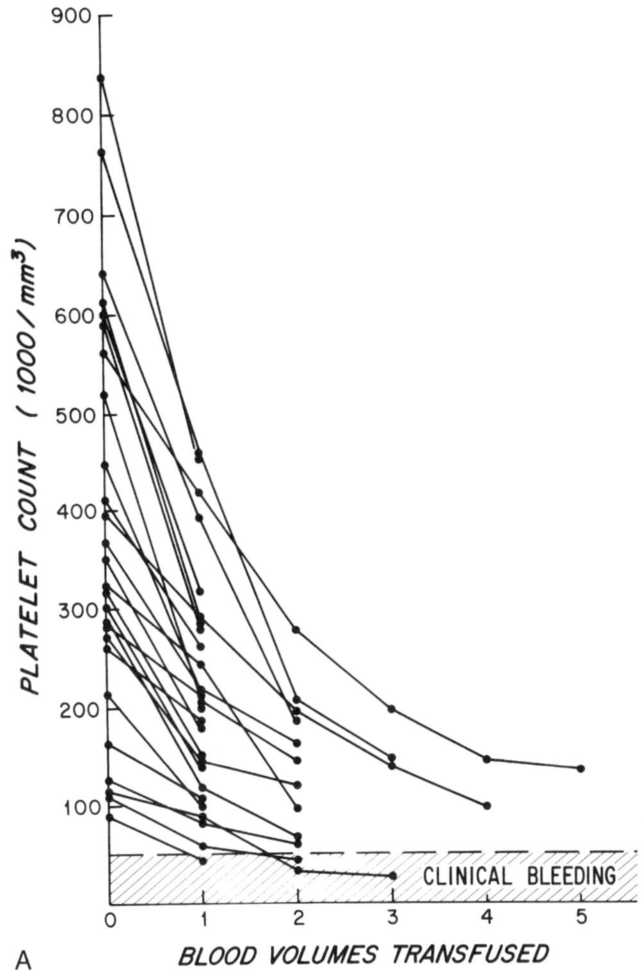

A

bleeding disorders should be sought. Some authors advocate routine laboratory screening because of the possibility of detecting inherited or acquired hemostatic disorders that may result in severe bleeding (30). Although commonly obtained, neither a bleeding history nor routine laboratory screening with PT, PTT, and bleeding time have been demonstrated to have a positive predictive value (33, 34). Although diagnosis of preexisting coagulopathy is important, meticulous surgical technique with particular attention to operative hemostasis is likely the most important factor in decreasing perioperative bleeding (30).

Because tonsillectomy is a procedure that can result in significant postoperative pain, a variety of modalities including local anesthetic infiltration, rectal acetaminophen, narcotics, and nonsteroidal anti-inflammatory drugs, including ketorolac, have been used. The effects of ketorolac on platelet function and clinical bleeding are concerns in this patient group. When administered at the beginning of the surgical procedure, ketorolac, when compared with acetaminophen, has led to statistically significant but not necessarily clinically significant increases in blood loss (2.67 mg/kg versus 1.44 mL/kg) (35). No patients in this study or another study of pediatric surgical patients, which included some for tonsillectomy and adenoidectomy, required reoperation for inadequate hemostasis (36). Furthermore, our experience in over 500 patients has demonstrated that ketorolac, used at the completion of the operation after the bulk of platelet activity is completed, is not associated with increased bleeding and provides prolonged analgesia.

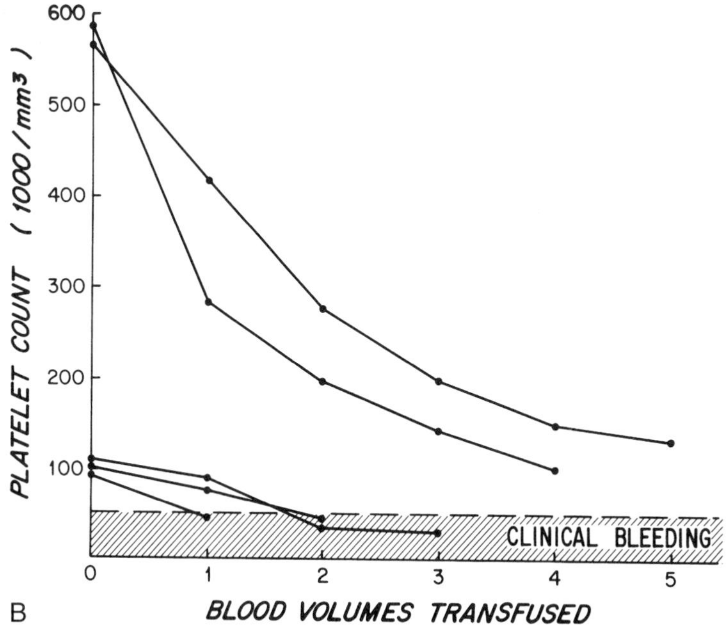

B

Figure 34.4. Changes in platelet count versus blood volumes transfused in 26 pediatric patients (**A**). Those patients requiring multiple blood volumes transfused who had a high initial platelet count did not require platelet transfusion. Those patients with low initial platelet count were more likely to require platelet transfusion (**B**). (Reprinted with permission from Coté CJ, Liu LMP, Szyfelbein SK, Goudsouzian NG, Daniels AL. Changes in serial platelet counts following massive blood transfusion in pediatric patients. Anesthesiology 1985;62:197–201.)

Treatment of postoperative hemorrhage includes repletion of circulating blood volume and obtaining hemostasis. Assessment of blood loss may be difficult because of the potential for a large volume of undetected swallowed blood in the stomach. If a coagulation screen was not previously performed, it should be done at this time. Adenoid bleeding may respond to topical vasoconstrictors and tonsillar bleeding to packing. However, some patients will require a second general anesthetic for exploration and operative hemostasis. Administration of blood products is necessary in 3–13% of these patients (0.06–0.35% of all tonsillectomies) (30, 31).

ORTHOPEDIC SURGERY

Spinal fusion, particularly posterior spinal fusion, is frequently associated with large amounts of blood loss (37). Excessive blood loss may increase morbidity because it can limit surgical exposure. It will also increase the patient's risk related to blood transfusions. Factors that affect blood loss include the extent of fusion, duration of surgery, and surgical and anesthetic techniques.

PREDONATION

Efforts to minimize perioperative homologous transfusion should begin with predonation of autologous units where feasible. Use of autologous blood limits infectious risk, antibody exposure, and transfusion reactions. In pediatric orthopedics, successful programs have included patients as small as 23 kg (38). Weekly donations of 1 unit of blood in larger children and fractions thereof in smaller children may be adjusted up or down depending on the patient's erythropoietic response. Refrigeration of blood with citrate, phosphate, dextrose, and adenine (shelf-life 35 days) or additive solutions such as Adsol, Nutricel, or Optisol (shelf-life 42 days) (39) allows for three to four donations before surgery. Limitations of this technique include very small patients, patients in poor medical condition, pain caused by repeated venipuncture, and inadequate erythropoietic response (40). Erythropoietic response should be augmented with iron supplementation (5 mg/kg orally two to three times daily [41]). Erythropoietin has been used successfully in autologous donors (42), but its cost and the need for weekly subcutaneous injections may limit its utility.

The issue of directed donation frequently arises before elective surgery where blood loss is likely. Directed donor programs exist because of legal and emotional reasons. No study has documented a medical benefit of directed donation in limiting the infectious complications of transfusion (43). Because many directed donors are donating for the first time and may have been asked by family members, it has been suggested that their blood may, in fact, be less safe than that received from repeat volunteer donors (44).

The use of directed donor blood from relatives increases the risk of transfusion-associated graft-versus-host disease. This occurs when viable lymphocytes are administered to a patient with a compromised immune system or to a patient with human lymphocyte antigen similarity to the donor. The donor T cells multiply and react against the recipient's tissue. Gamma irradiation of blood components before transfusion is used to prevent the lymphocytes from replicating. The American Association of Blood Banks recommends that blood and platelets be irradiated before transfusion in the following patients:

1. Recipients of donor units from blood relatives;
2. Immunocompromised patients;
3. Patients who have undergone bone marrow transplantation;
4. Fetuses receiving intrauterine transfusion (39).

The function of red cells and platelets is not affected by irradiation. Products such as FFP and cryoprecipitate, which contain no viable white blood cells, do not require irradiation.

Directed donor blood is often provided in the form of whole blood. The potential for hyperkalemia-induced cardiac arrhythmias is greater with whole blood than with packed red blood cells. Irradiation before storage may further elevate potassium levels in stored blood (45). These concerns raise additional questions about directed donations.

METHODS TO REDUCE BLOOD LOSS

POSITIONING

Limiting intraoperative blood loss begins with proper patient positioning. Pressure exerted on the anterior abdominal wall in the prone position can result in partial or complete obstruction of the inferior vena cava. Caval compression can lead to diversion of venous return to the vertebral venous plexus (46), resulting in increased blood loss during dissection. Appropriate positioning on a Relton-Hall frame or similar supports allows the abdomen to be free and thereby minimizes the potential for increased vertebral venous pressure and increased blood loss (47).

SURGICAL TECHNIQUE

The technical aspects of the procedure play an important role in the amount of blood lost. Before incision, the intradermal and subcutaneous areas are infiltrated with a dilute solution of epinephrine (1:500,000) (48). The vasoconstrictor response to epinephrine and the hydrostatic pressure exerted by the relatively large volume injected are thought to decrease venous blood loss during dissection. Digital compression of wound edges, packing of exposed bleeding surfaces, and subperiosteal dissection also limit bleeding (47). Because iliac crest donor sites may contribute significantly to blood loss, cadaveric bone graft may be used as an alternative (49). Laminar decortication should be performed as late as possible during the procedure to minimize the duration of uncontrolled bone bleeding (50).

DESMOPRESSIN

The effects of desmopressin (DDAVP) have been evaluated in patients undergoing spinal fusion. One study demonstrated a clinically important reduction in blood loss in patients with scoliosis of various etiologies (51). A subsequent study found no benefit in patients with idiopathic scoliosis (52). This suggests that DDAVP may be beneficial in patients with scoliosis of known etiology (e.g., neuromuscular). However, because DDAVP may cause hypotension on infusion and hyponatremia from water retention, it is not without risk. Its routine use in spinal surgery, therefore, cannot be advocated at this time.

HEMODILUTION

Acute normovolemic hemodilution is defined as the intraoperative removal of a predetermined volume of blood and its replacement with crystalloid or colloid solution. With this technique, blood lost during surgery has a lower hematocrit and proportionally fewer red blood cells are lost. The patient's own blood is then reinfused when hemostasis is obtained toward the completion of the procedure. Blood is withdrawn via the central venous or arterial catheter into a collection bag containing anticoagulant. The bag is weighed during filling to confirm the volume of blood removed. The desired patient hematocrit after withdrawal is generally 20–24% (53). The autologous blood volume to be withdrawn is calculated from the starting hematocrit, the target hematocrit, and the EBV using the equation for MABL.

Monitoring of ongoing blood loss, central venous pressure, and tissue perfusion are imperative. Blood should be used to maintain the hematocrit in an acceptable range. If it becomes apparent that the blood withdrawn intraoperatively will not meet the perioperative needs, blood donated preoperatively (autologous or homologous) should be given first. The blood withdrawn intraoperatively will provide the maximum benefit (platelets and coagulation factors) if administered later in the case. Extreme hemodilution has been used successfully on a very limited basis (54). In eight healthy patients, hemoglobin levels were reduced from 10 to 3.0 g/dL before spinal fusion. No patients developed significant complications. However, in the absence of continuous monitoring of end-organ oxygen supply and demand, routine use of hemodilution can only be recommended to a hematocrit of approximately 20% (55). Because of the smaller margin for error, this technique is usually limited to patients larger than 10 kg, although it has been used in patients as small as 3.1 kg (56). Acute normovolemic hemodilution is acceptable to some Jehovah's Witnesses. It has been successfully used with hypotensive anesthesia for spinal surgery (57), although the combined risks of these techniques dictate that they should rarely be used together, if at all (58).

CONTROLLED HYPOTENSION

Controlled hypotensive anesthesia may also be used to improve surgical conditions, shorten operative time, and decrease blood loss (59). Because the best technique for inducing controlled hypotension has not been determined, a variety of drugs, either alone or in combination, may be used. Volatile anesthetic agents have been used, but the myocardial depressant effects may not be readily reversible if acute blood loss and hypovolemia occur. Their utility is also limited because of their effects on somatosensory evoked potential monitoring and the prolongation of intraoperative wake-up tests. Vasodilators can effectively decrease blood pressure, but controversy exists over whether blood pressure or tissue blood flow determines surgical blood loss (60, 61). Sodium nitroprusside is a more effective hypotensive agent than nitroglycerine (61), but the effect on blood loss with these two agents has not been compared. Cyanide toxicity is also a risk with nitroprusside, especially if used at doses exceeding 10 μg/kg/min (62). β-Adrenergic blocking agents are frequently used with vasodilators to block reflex tachycardia and blunt the response of the renin-angiotensin system (63). Meticulous attention to maintaining normal Pa_{CO_2} and a constant circulating blood volume (stable central venous pressure (CVP) will reduce the potential for adverse effects on the cerebral circulation and wide fluctuations in blood pressure. In our experience, a narcotic-based anesthetic with a low-dose inhalation agent and a vasodilator when necessary provides an adequate degree of hypotension without undue depression of the myocardium or interference with neurological monitoring. This combination also reduces the amount of vasodilator needed to produce satisfactory hypotension (see Chapter 22).

RED BLOOD CELL SALVAGE

Intraoperative and postoperative red cell salvage may be used as an adjunct to the aforementioned techniques (64–66). Salvaged red blood cells are type-specific and devoid of transmissible infectious complications. Depending on the operation, this product may provide 50–100% of intraoperative needs. Because 250–350 mL of shed blood is necessary to fill a pediatric-sized centrifuge bowl (125–175 mL) and some time delay is inherent in processing, cell salvage should not be relied on as the sole source of red cells, particularly if intraoperative blood loss may be massive or unpredictable (67). The use of platelet transfusion and FFP must be considered as with any large-volume red blood cell transfusion (i.e., more than 1.0 blood volume) because platelets and coagulation factors are lost in processing.

BURNS

Every year in the United States, more than two million people sustain burn injuries. More than 100,000 burned patients are hospitalized, and children account for at least 30% of these patients (68). The replacement and maintenance of intravascular volume is a major challenge in the burned patient.

Volume resuscitation in the acute stage typically involves the replacement of intravascular fluid lost through the wound and into edematous tissue. Children are more susceptible to these shifts than adults because of their ratio of body surface area to weight. Adequate venous access for volume replacement and the insertion of a urinary catheter to assess the adequacy of volume resuscitation are mandatory. In the absence of associated injuries, blood and blood products are not typically necessary in the initial treatment. Although some controversy exists over the type of fluid to use, crystalloid is generally acceptable in the first 24 hours (e.g., the Parkland formula). Such formulas are useful guidelines, particularly in older patients, but may grossly underestimate the fluid requirements of children weighing less than 10 kg. After initial treatment has begun, placement of arterial, central venous, or pulmonary artery catheters should be considered.

Early wound excision and closure is advocated to control infection, improve cosmesis, and limit fluid and protein loss (69). Aggressive early surgical care can result in significant blood loss. The technique, extent, and timing of surgical excision will dictate the actual volume lost. Tangential excision involves the sequential removal of thin slices of the eschar until viable bleeding tissue is exposed for grafting. In all but the most minor burns, blood loss is rapid and massive (0.4 mL/cm^2 of surface area excised if performed within the first 24 hours after injury; 0.75 mL/cm^2 if excision occurs between days 2 and 14) (70). Fascial excision, which is used for large full-thickness injuries, results in less blood loss. The use of tourniquets, topical epinephrine, injected dilute epinephrine, topical thrombin, and local pressure may also limit blood loss.

Perioperative replacement is generally with packed red cells and lactated Ringer's solution. Central venous monitoring is particularly important because of the difficulty in assessing ongoing losses (71). Transfusion should be aimed at maintaining the hematocrit at 25–30% because of the increased metabolic rate in these patients. Ongoing hemolytic anemia, the inhibition of erythropoiesis, and frequent blood studies exacerbate operative losses (72, 73). FFP and platelet administration are limited to patients with documented coagulopathy. Consumption of platelets and clotting factors in the early stages gives way to elevated levels of factors V, VII, VIII, and fibrinogen and platelets later in the course of treatment (74). Platelet transfusion is rarely necessary in the absence of burn sepsis.

CARDIAC SURGERY

A variety of hemostatic abnormalities have been reported in patients with congenital heart disease. Included in these are thrombocytopenia (75, 76), platelet dysfunction (77), abnormalities in von Willebrand factor (78), primary fibrinolysis (76), disseminated intravascular coagulopathy (DIC) (79), and a number of clotting factor deficiencies (79, 80). In a recent study, 45 of 235 patients had some abnormality in their coagulation screening panel (platelet count, PT, PTT and activated PTT, or thrombin time) (80). Although abnormal values were common, increased intraoperative blood usage could not be predicted. More importantly, normal results did not rule out a major underlying bleeding diathesis.

Because of the conflicting nature of reports in this area, it appears that the coagulopathy associated with congenital heart disease is multifactorial in origin (81). Each child needs to be evaluated individually. Routine screening, although not always predictive, still appears to be the best available means to diagnose most clinically important abnormalities.

Patients with cyanotic lesions are most likely to have excessive bleeding. This appears to be related to the degree of hypoxemia and resultant polycythemia (75, 79). Hypoxemia affects platelet function and may prolong the bleeding time. Coagulation factor production may be decreased because of hepatic dysfunction resulting from chronic hepatic congestion. Consumption of factors may be increased from DIC. In addition, polycythemia decreases plasma volume and may artificially prolong the PTT if the volume of the anticoagulant used in sampling tubes is not adjusted. The high incidence of cerebral vascular accidents in these patients has led some to believe that polycythemia leads to a hypercoagulable state. A more likely explanation is that iron-deficient red cells are less deformable, causing increased viscosity and "sludging" (82, 83). This condition may improve with iron supplementation. Intraoperative bleeding can be decreased by preoperative phlebotomy coupled with volume expansion aimed at lowering the hematocrit to 55–60% (84, 85). Additional benefit may be derived from further hemodilution during cardiopulmonary bypass (CPB) (86).

Several operative factors increase the likelihood of blood transfusion in children undergoing open heart surgery. Increasingly complex procedures are performed in younger patients. Complex operations may require repeat sternotomy with resultant increased blood loss. Although younger patients generally have a higher blood volume relative to weight, the absolute volume involved may limit the use of certain methods of blood conservation. Smaller patients often require earlier and more frequent transfusion of multiple blood products.

CPB exposes many patients to homologous blood and adversely affects hemostasis. In infants, the relatively large volume of the pump prime compared with the child's blood volume causes profound dilution of platelets and coagulation factors (87). Efforts should be directed at reducing the extracorporeal circuit volume. This can reduce the dilution of clotting elements and the exposure to blood products (88). In addition, intraoperative autologous transfusion and hemodilution before and during CPB have been used. Children as young as 7 months and as small as 5.6 kg have been successfully hemodiluted for CPB to a hematocrit of 15% (89). Although this may be extreme, accepting a low hematocrit may decrease homologous blood requirement during bypass. Further work is necessary to quantify the extent of hemodilution that is safe with varying perfusion strategies. After bypass, reinfusion of pump blood that contains some functioning platelets and coagulation factors may better preserve hemostasis compared with transfusion of packed red cells alone.

Platelets are rendered less effective by CPB. Although the precise mechanism is unclear, platelets are activated by contact with synthetic surfaces and blood-gas and blood-tissue interfaces (90, 91). Aprotinin exerts a protective effect against platelet dysfunction apparently via preservation of platelet membrane-bound glycoprotein receptors (92). Experience with this drug, which has yet to be approved for use in children, is limited in pediatric cardiac surgery, and its effectiveness in decreasing blood loss and donor exposure in the perioperative period is not certain (93, 94).

Additional pharmacological efforts to minimize blood loss have focused on DDAVP. A reduction in blood loss with DDAVP in adults undergoing complex cardiac surgery has been demonstrated (95); however, in studies of children, no such benefit was evident (96, 97).

Because preoperative and intraoperative autologous donation may be limited because of the patient's size and medical condition, homologous blood transfusions are still necessary in most cases. Rather than relying on component therapy with multiple donor exposures, fresh whole blood has been effectively used (98). Time constraints for necessary screening and donor availability limit the use of fresh whole blood. Whole blood less than 48 hours old may be as effective as fresh whole blood and more effective than component therapy in limiting perioperative blood loss and blood exposure in children (99). This effect appears to be most profound in patients with complex heart disease who are less than 2 years of age. Although platelet function is known to deteriorate with refrigeration (100), the authors attribute the improvement in hemostasis to the infusion of functioning platelets in whole blood. Because the 24- to 48-hour-old whole blood provides red cells, coagulation factors, and platelets, it may be an alternative to component therapy. In addition, when component therapy is necessary, it should be remembered that platelet concentrates provide a large volume of plasma that may correct clotting factor deficiencies without requiring a separate exposure to FFP. This is particularly true for neonates and infants.

Cell separation and salvage during open heart surgery can yield a clinically important quantity of red blood cells. This is especially true if a large-volume circuit is used in a relatively small patient. Ultrafiltration of residual blood in the CPB circuit has been used effectively in pediatric patients (101). The product of ultrafiltration when compared with centrifugal techniques (Cell Saver) is superior with regard to platelet number and function and the concentration of plasma proteins, including fibrinogen (102–104). Because either process may result in heparin administration, repeat measurement of the activated clotting time is recommended after infusion of salvaged cells. Cell salvage has been successfully combined with hemodilution to limit or avoid homologous red cell transfusion (105, 106).

RENAL TRANSPLANTATION

Preoperative assessment of patients with renal disease typically reveals anemia and some degree of impaired hemostasis. Profound anemia (5–7 g/dL) commonly accompanies end-stage renal disease. Anemia results from relative deficiency of erythropoietin; accumulation in the serum of toxins that are inhibitors of erythropoiesis; decreased erythrocyte life span; blood loss through the gastrointestinal tract and with dialysis; and deficiencies of iron, folic acid, and other nutrients (107). Although chronic hemodialysis has been shown to lessen the degree of anemia in adults with end-stage renal disease, similar studies have not been carried out in children. Peritoneal dialysis, on the other hand, has reduced the severity of anemia in both adult and pediatric patients (108).

Recombinant human erythropoietin has been shown to be of some benefit for treatment of anemia (109). Preoperative transfusion is often considered because of the severity of anemia in some patients. However, chronic anemia in a euvolemic patient can generally be treated conservatively. Pretransplant blood transfusion has been used in the past to decrease the immune response and improve graft survival, but because of the advent of immune suppression therapy with cyclosporine, this is no longer seen as necessary (110). Thrombocytopenia and platelet dysfunction are common as well. Platelet number but not function may improve with dialysis.

Renal transplantation is an increasingly common procedure in pediatric centers. Data from the United Network for Organ Sharing show that 559 kidney transplants were carried out in the United States in children less than 18 years of age between October 1987 and January 1990. This accounts for approximately 5% of renal transplants performed. Although renal transplantation is not unique to pediatric patients, certain aspects are. Pediatric renal transplantation is characterized by expanding indications for younger patients. Patients as small as 5 kg and as young as 5 months of age may receive adult renal allografts. The adult donor kidney may sequester as much as 150–250 mL of blood. Release of clamps on renal vessels can mimic the acute loss of 25–40% of the recipient's blood volume. In addition, large femoral artery to vein shunts or grafts can lead to venous hypertension and diffuse intraabdominal or retroperitoneal bleeding that cannot be controlled until this vascular access system is clamped (111). Blood must be immediately available and is often administered to compensate for this sequestration and for blood loss due to anastomotic leak. Invasive hemodynamic monitoring of central venous pressure is helpful to guide the necessary volume expansion. Arterial access is not always necessary in older recipients, and avoidance may allow future use of arteries should hemodialysis again become necessary.

LIVER TRANSPLANTATION

Liver transplantation is now the treatment of choice for most infants and children with end-stage liver disease (112). As in adults, preexisting coagulopathy and multiple vascular anastomoses may result in rapid, massive blood loss. Chronic liver disease is associated with malabsorption of vitamin K, leading to decreased production of coagulation factors II, VII, IX, and X and the anticoagulants protein C and protein S (113). Thrombocytopenia is common and may result from bone marrow suppression, DIC, hypersplenism, or dilution (113). Preoperative treatment with vitamin K, clotting factors, and platelets is generally reserved for patients with severe coagulopathy (PT greater than 20 seconds, platelet count less than 20,000/mm^3) (113).

In contrast to adults, blood loss in pediatric transplantation does not correlate with routine preoperative coagulation tests (114, 115). Factors that do increase blood use include previous abdominal surgery (116), the use of reduced-sized liver transplant (117), and transplantation in infants (118).

Adequate venous access must be obtained before incision because of the possible need for massive blood and volume infusion. Large-bore intravenous lines are placed in the upper extremities to maintain access to the systemic circulation even if the inferior vena cava is cross-clamped. Arterial and central venous access are essential (119). Although venovenous bypass is common in adults, it is not generally used in children undergoing liver transplantation, because low-flow bypass without heparinization may pose a threat of pulmonary emboli (120).

The optimal system for intraoperative monitoring of hemoglobin, coagulation, and electrolytes has yet to be determined. Regardless of the system used, cooperation with and convenience to laboratory services are imperative with both pediatric and adult liver transplant procedures.

Coagulation monitoring generally includes some combination of PT, PTT, platelet count, and thromboelastography (TEG). Results of coagulation tests run in hospital laboratories are typically available in 15–60 minutes. Although generation of a complete thromboelastogram requires approximately 60 minutes, some useful information is available in 10–15 minutes. TEG, therefore, is often used as an adjunct to routine measures of coagulation. Children exhibit intraoperative coagulation changes similar to those of adults but to a lesser degree (121). This may be attributable to a lower incidence of hepatocellular disease.

Blood bank resources should be well organized before induction of anesthesia. Packed cells, FFP, platelet concentrates, and cryoprecipitate in suitable volumes, based on patient size, should be available. Rapid infusion devices and blood warmers are necessary. The possible metabolic derangements with large-volume transfusion discussed previously are exacerbated by the decreased ability of the recipient to metabolize citrate because of decreased or absent hepatic perfusion, underlying liver disease, and the need for rapid blood administration (122).

REFERENCES

1. Coté CJ. Blood, colloid, and crystalloid therapy. Anesthesiol Clin North Am 1991;9:865–884.
2. Kallos T, Smith TC. Replacement for intraoperative blood loss. Anesthesiology 1974;41:293–295.
3. Johnson KB. Hematology. In: Craven L, ed. The Harriet Lane handbook. 13th ed. St. Louis, MO: Mosby-Year Book, Inc., 1993:217–233.

4. Kenny J, Plappert T, Doubilet P, Salzman D, St. John Sutton MG. Effects of heart rate on ventricular size, stroke volume, and output in the normal fetus: a prospective Doppler echocardiographic study. Circulation 1987;76:52–58.
5. Andrew M, Paes B, Milner R, et al. Development of the human coagulation system in the full-term infant. Blood 1987;70:165–172.
6. Gotschall CS. Epidemiology of childhood injury. In: Craven L, ed. Pediatric trauma. Prevention, acute care, rehabilitation. St. Louis, MO: Mosby-Year Book, 1993:16–19.
7. Barlow B, Niemirska M, Gandhi R, Shelton M. Response to injury in children with closed femur fractures. J Trauma 1987;27:429–430.
8. Pascucci R, Walsh J. Evaluation and management of the injured child. In: Capan LM, Miller SM, Turndorf H, eds. Trauma anesthesia and intensive sare. Philadelphia: J. B. Lippincott Company, 1991:567–598.
9. Jurkovich GJ, Greiser WB, Luterman A, Curreri PW. Hypothermia in trauma victims: an ominous predictor of survival. J Trauma 1987;27: 1019–1024.
10. Luna GK, Maier RV, Pavlin EG, Anardi D, Copass MK, Oreskovich MR. Incidence and effect of hypothermia in seriously injured patients. J Trauma 1987;27:1014–1018.
11. Patt A, McCroskey BL, Moore EE. Hypothermia-induced coagulopathies in trauma. Surg Clin North Am 1988;68:775–785.
12. Iserson KV, Huestis DW. Blood warming: current applications and techniques. Transfusion 1991;31:558–571.
13. Uhl L, Pacini D, Kruskall MS. A comparative study of blood warmer performance. Anesthesiology 1992;77:1022–1028.
14. Coté CJ, Drop LJ, Hoaglin DC, Daniels AL, Young ET. Ionized hypocalcemia after fresh frozen plasma administration to thermally injured children: effects of infusion rate, duration, and treatment with calcium chloride. Anesth Analg 1988;67:152–160.
15. Stulz PM, Scheidegger D, Drop LJ, Lowenstein E, Laver MB. Ventricular pump performance during hypocalcemia. J Thorac Cardiovasc Surg 1979;78:185–194.
16. Coté CJ. Depth of halothane anesthesia potentiates citrate-induced ionized hypocalcemia and adverse cardiovascular events in dogs. Anesthesiology 1987;67:676–680.
17. Coté CJ, Drop LJ, Daniels AL, Hoaglin DC. Calcium chloride versus calcium gluconate: comparison of ionization and cardiovascular effects in children and dogs. Anesthesiology 1987;66:465–470.
18. Brown KA, Bissonnette B, MacDonald M, Poon AO. Hyperkalaemia during massive blood transfusion in paediatric craniofacial surgery. Can J Anaesth 1990;37:401–408.
19. Hall TL, Barnes A, Miller JR, Bethencourt DM, Nestor L. Neonatal mortality following transfusion of red cells with high plasma potassium levels. Transfusion 1993;33:606–609.
20. Luban NLC, Strauss RG, Hume HA. Commentary on the safety of red cells preserved in extended-storage media for neonatal transfusions. Transfusion 1991;31:229–235.
21. Cook S, Gunter J, Wissel M. Effective use of a strategy using assigned red cell units to limit donor exposure for neonatal patients. Transfusion 1993;33:379–383.
22. Miller RD, Robbins TO, Tong MJ, Barton SL. Coagulation defects associated with massive blood transfusions. Ann Surg 1971;174:794–801.
23. Counts RB, Haisch C, Simon TL, Maxwell NG, Heimbach DM, Carrico CJ. Hemostasis in massively transfused trauma patients. Ann Surg 1979;190:91–99.
24. Coté CJ, Liu LMP, Szyfelbein SK, Goudsouzian NG, Daniels AL. Changes in serial platelet counts following massive blood transfusion in pediatric patients. Anesthesiology 1985;62:197–201.
25. Consensus Conference. Fresh-frozen plasma. JAMA 1985;253: 551–553.
26. Murray DJ, Olson J, Strauss R, Tinker JH. Coagulation changes during packed red cell replacement of major blood loss. Anesthesiology 1988; 69:839–845.
27. Coté CJ, Coté MA. Changes in prothrombin and partial thromboplastin times during massive blood loss in children undergoing Harrington rod instrumentation. Presented at Spring Session, Section on Anesthesiology, American Academy of Pediatrics, 1988.
28. Murray DJ, Pennell BJ, Weinstein SL, Olson JD. Packed red cells in acute blood loss: dilutional coagulopathy as a cause of surgical bleeding. Anesth Analg 1995;80:336–342.
29. Graves EJ. 1992 Summary: National Hospital Discharge Survey. Advance data from vital and health statistics. Hyattsville, MD: National Center for Health Statistics 249, 1994.
30. Handler SD, Miller L, Richmond KH, Baranak CC. Post-tonsillectomy hemorrhage: incidence, prevention and management. Laryngoscope 1986;96:1243–1247.
31. Crysdale WS, Russel D. Complications of tonsillectomy and adenoidectomy in 9409 children observed overnight. Can Med Assoc J 1986;135:1139–1142.
32. Haberman RS, Shattuck TG, Dion NM. Is outpatient suction cautery tonsillectomy safe in a community hospital setting? Laryngoscope 1990;100:511–515.
33. Burk CD, Miller L, Handler SD, Cohen AR. Preoperative history and coagulation screening in children undergoing tonsillectomy. Pediatrics 1992;89:691–695.
34. Close HL, Kryzer TC, Nowlin JH, Alving BM. Hemostatic assessment of patients before tonsillectomy: a prospective study. Otolaryngol Head Neck Surg 1994;111:733–738.
35. Rusy LM, Houck CS, Sullivan LJ, et al. A double-blind evaluation of ketorolac tromethamine versus acetaminophen in pediatric tonsillectomy: analgesia and bleeding. Anesth Analg 1995;80:226–229.
36. Watcha MF, Jones MB, Lagueruela RG, Schweiger C, White PF. Comparison of ketorolac and morphine as adjuvants during pediatric surgery. Anesthesiology 1992;76:368–372.
37. McNeill TW, DeWald RL, Kuo KN, Bennett EJ, Salem MR. Controlled hypotensive anesthesia in scoliosis surgery. J Bone Joint Surg 1974;56-A:1167–1172.
38. Cowell HR, Swickard JW. Autotransfusion in children's orthopaedics. J Bone Joint Surg 1974;56-A:908–912.
39. American Association of Blood Banks. Standards for Blood Banks and Transfusion Services. 16th ed. Bethesda, MD: American Association of Blood Banks, 1994.
40. Goodnough LT, Wasman J, Corlucci K, Chernosky A. Limitations to donating adequate autologous blood prior to elective orthopedic surgery. Arch Surg 1989;124:494–496.
41. Bailey TE Jr, Flynn JC. Blood salvage. In: Weinstein SL, ed. The pediatric spine: principles and practice. New York: Raven Press, 1994: 1157–1167.
42. Kulier AH, Gombotz H, Fuchs G, Vuckovic U, Metzler H. Subcutaneous recombinant human erythropoietin and autologous blood donation before coronary artery bypass surgery. Anesth Analg 1993;76:102–106.
43. Strauss RG, Sacher RA. Directed donations for pediatric patients. Transfus Med Rev 1988;2:58–64.
44. Page PL. Controversies in transfusion medicine. Directed blood donations: Con. Transfusion 1989;29:65–74.
45. Rivet C, Baxter A, Rock G. Potassium levels in irradiated blood. Transfusion 1989;29:185.

46. Batson OV. The function of the vertebral veins and their role in the spread of metastases. Ann Surg 1940;112:138–149.
47. Relton JES, Hall JE. An operation frame for spinal fusion. A new apparatus designed to reduce haemorrhage during operation. J Bone Joint Surg 1967;49:327–332.
48. Bradford DS. Techniques of surgery. In: Bradford DS, Lonstein JE, Moe JH, Ogilvie JW, Winter RB, eds. Moe's textbook of scoliosis and other spinal deformities. 2nd ed. Philadelphia: WB Saunders, 1987: 135–190.
49. Montgomery DM, Aronson DD, Lee CL, LaMont RL. Posterior spinal fusion: allograft versus autograft bone. J Spinal Disord 1990;3: 370–375.
50. Phillips WA, Hensinger RN. Control of blood loss during scoliosis surgery. Clin Orthop 1988;229:88–93.
51. Kobrinsky NL, Letts RM, Patel LR, et al. 1-Desamino-8-d-arginine vasopressin (desmopressin) decreases operative blood loss in patients having Harrington rod spinal fusion surgery. A randomized, double-blinded, controlled trial. Ann Intern Med 1987;107:446–450.
52. Guay J, Reinberg C, Poitras B, et al. A trial of desmopressin to reduce blood loss in patients undergoing spinal fusion for idiopathic scoliosis. Anesth Analg 1992;75:405–410.
53. Kafer ER, Collins ML. Acute intraoperative hemodilution and perioperative blood salvage. Anesthesiol Clin North Am 1990;8:543–567.
54. Fontana JL, Welborn L, Mongan PD, Sturm P, Martin G, Bünger R. Oxygen consumption and cardiovascular function in children during profound intraoperative normovolemic hemodilution. Anesth Analg 1995;80:219–225.
55. Lindahl SGE. Thinner than blood. Anesth Analg 1995;80:217–218.
56. Schaller RT, Schaller J, Morgan A, Furman EB. Hemodilution anesthesia: a valuable aid to major cancer surgery in children. Am J Surg 1983;146:79–84.
57. Wong KC, Webster LR, Coleman SS, Dunn HK. Hemodilution and induced hypotension for insertion of a Harrington rod in a Jehovah's Witness patient. Clin Orthop 1980;152:237–240.
58. Brown RH, Schauble JF, Miller NR. Anemia and hypotension as contributors to perioperative loss of vision. Anesthesiology 1994;80: 222–226.
59. Patel NJ, Patel BS, Paskin S, Laufer S. Induced moderate hypotensive anesthesia for spinal fusion and Harrington-rod instrumentation. J Bone Joint Surg 1985;67-A:1384–1387.
60. Sivarajan M, Amory DW, Everett GB, Buffington C. Blood pressure, not cardiac output, determines blood bloss during induced hypotension. Anesth Analg 1980;59:203–206.
61. Yaster M, Simmons RS, Tolo VT, Pepple JM, Wetzel RC, Rogers MC. A comparison of nitroglycerin and nitroprusside for inducing hypotension in children: a double-blind study. Anesthesiology 1986;65: 175–179.
62. Bennett NR, Abbott TR. The use of sodium nitroprusside in children. Anaesthesia 1977;32:456–463.
63. Knight PR, Lane GA, Nicholls MG, et al. Hormonal and hemodynamic changes induced by pentolinium and propranolol during surgical correction of scoliosis. Anesthesiology 1980;53:127–134.
64. Kruger LM, Colbert JM. Intraoperative autologous transfusion in children undergoing spinal surgery. J Pediatr Orthop 1985;5:330–332.
65. Lennon RL, Hosking MP, Gray JR, Klassen RA, Popovsky MA, Warner MA. The effects of intraoperative blood salvage and induced hypotension on transfusion requirements during spinal surgical procedures. Mayo Clin Proc 1987;62:1090–1094.
66. Blevins FT, Shaw B, Valeri CR, Kasser J, Hall J. Reinfusion of shed blood after orthopaedic procedures in children and adolescents. J Bone Joint Surg 1993;75:363–371.
67. Salem MR, Klowden AJ. Anesthesia for orthopaedic surgery. In: Gregory GA, ed. Pediatric anesthesia. 3rd ed. New York: Churchill Livingstone, 1994:607–656.
68. Herndon DN, Thompson PB, Desai MH, Van Osten TJ. Treatment of burns in children. Pediatr Clin North Am 1985;32:1311–1332.
69. Herndon DN, Barrow RE, Rutan RL, Rutan TC, Desai MH, Abston S. A comparison of conservative versus early excision. Therapies in severely burned patients. Ann Surg 1989;209:547–553.
70. Desai MH, Herndon DN, Broemeling L, Barrow RE, Nichols RJ, Rutan RL. Early burn wound excision significantly reduces blood loss. Ann Surg 1990;211:753–762.
71. Budney PG, Regan PJ, Roberts AHN. The estimation of blood loss during burns surgery. Burns 1993;19:134–137.
72. Heideman M. The effect of thermal injury on hemodynamic, respiratory, and hematologic variables in relation to complement activation. J Trauma 1979;19:239–243.
73. Wallner SF, Vautrin R. The anemia of thermal injury: mechanism of inhibition of erythropoiesis (42236). Proc Soc Exp Biol Med 1986;181: 144–150.
74. Simon TL, Curreri PW, Harker LA. Kinetic characterization of hemostasis in thermal injury. J Lab Clin Med 1977;89:702–711.
75. Wedemeyer AL, Edson JR, Krivit W. Coagulation in cyanotic congenital heart disease. Am J Dis Child 1972;124:656–660.
76. Ekert H, Gilchrist GS, Stanton R, Hammond D. Hemostasis in cyanotic congenital heart disease. J Pediatr 1970;76:221–230.
77. Suarez CR, Menendez CE, Griffin AJ, Ow EP, Walenga JM, Fareed J. Cyanotic congenital heart disease in children: hemostatic disorders and relevance of molecular markers of hemostasis. Semin Thromb Hemost 1984;10:285–289.
78. Gill JC, Wilson AD, Endres-Brooks J, Montgomery RR. Loss of the largest von Willebrand factor multimers from the plasma of patients with congenital cardiac defects. Blood 1986;67:758–761.
79. Komp DM, Sparrow AW. Polycythemia in cyanotic heart disease—a study of altered coagulation. J Pediatr 1970;76:231–236.
80. Colón-Otero G, Gilchrist GS, Holcomb GR, Ilstrup DM, Bowie EJW. Preoperative evaluation of hemostasis in patients with congenital heart disease. Mayo Clin Proc 1987;62:379–385.
81. Stockman JA III, Ezekowitz A. Hematologic manifestations of systemic diseases. In: Nathan DG, Oski FA, eds. Hematology of infancy and childhood. 4th ed. Philadelphia: WB Saunders, 1993:1834–1873.
82. Card RT, Weintraub LR. Metabolic abnormalities of erythrocytes in severe iron deficiency. Blood 1971;37:725–732.
83. Martelle RR, Linde LM. Cerebrovascular accidents with tetralogy of Fallot. Am J Dis Child 1961;101:206–209.
84. Wedemeyer AL, Lewis JH. Improvement in hemostasis following phlebotomy in cyanotic patients with heart disease. J Pediatr 1973;83: 46–50.
85. Maurer HM, McCue CM, Robertson LW, Haggins JC. Correction of platelet dysfunction and bleeding in cyanotic congenital heart disease by simple red cell volume reduction. Am J Cardiol 1975;35:831–835.
86. Milam JD, Austin SF, Nihill MR, Keats AS, Cooley DA. Use of sufficient hemodilution to prevent coagulopathies following surgical correction of cyanotic heart disease. J Thorac Cardiovasc Surg 1985;89: 623–629.
87. Kern FH, Morana NJ, Sears JJ, Hickey PR. Coagulation defects in neonates during cardiopulmonary bypass. Ann Thorac Surg 1992; 54:541–546.

88. Kawaguchi A, Bergsland J, Subramanian S. Total bloodless open heart surgery in the pediatric age group. Circulation 1984;70(Suppl. I):I30–I37.
89. Rosen D, Rosen K, Bove E, Callow L, Wilton N. Hemodilution for heart surgery in children [abstract]. Anesthesiology 1987;73:A1241.
90. Campbell FW. The contribution of platelet dysfunction to postbypass bleeding. J Cardiothorac Vasc Anesth 1991;5:8–12.
91. Harker LA, Malpass TW, Branson HE, Hessel EA II, Slichter SJ. Mechanism of abnormal bleeding in patients undergoing cardiopulmonary bypass: acquired transient platelet dysfunction associated with selective α-granule release. Blood 1980;56:824–834.
92. van Oeveren W, Harder MP, Roozendaal KJ, Eijsman L, Wildevuur CRH. Aprotinin protects platelets against the initial effect of cardiopulmonary bypass. J Thorac Cardiovasc Surg 1990;99:788–797.
93. Herynkopf F, Lucchese F, Pereira E, Kalil R, Prates P, Nesralla IA. Aprotinin in children undergoing correction of congenital heart defects. A double-blind pilot study. J Thorac Cardiovasc Surg 1994;108: 517–521.
94. Boldt J, Knothe C, Zickmann B, Wege N, Dapper F, Hempelmann G. Aprotinin in pediatric cardiac operations: platelet function, blood loss, and use of homologous blood. Ann Thorac Surg 1993;55:1460–1466.
95. Salzman EW, Weinstein MJ, Weintraub RM, et al. Treatment with desmopressin acetate to reduce blood loss after cardiac surgery. A double-blind randomized trial. N Engl J Med 1986;314:1402–1406.
96. Reynolds LM, Nicolson SC, Jobes DR, et al. Desmopressin does not decrease bleeding after cardiac operation in young children. J Thorac Cardiovasc Surg 1993;106:954–958.
97. Seear MD, Wadsworth LD, Rogers PC, Sheps S, Ashmore PG. The effect of desmopressin acetate (DDAVP) on postoperative blood loss after cardiac operations in children. J Thorac Cardiovasc Surg 1989;98: 217–219.
98. Mohr R, Martinowitz U, Lavee J, Amroch D, Ramot B, Goor DA. The hemostatic effect of transfusing fresh whole blood versus platelet concentrates after cardiac operations. J Thorac Cardiovasc Surg 1988;96: 530–534.
99. Manno CS, Hedberg KW, Kim HC, et al. Comparison of the hemostatic effects of fresh-whole blood, stored whole blood, and components after open heart surgery in children. Blood 1991;77:930–936.
100. Murphy S, Gardner FH. Effects of storage temperature on maintenance of platelet viability—deleterious effect of refrigerated storage. N Engl J Med 1969;280:1094–1098.
101. Friesen RH, Tornabene MA, Coleman SP. Blood conservation during pediatric cardiac surgery: ultrafiltration of the extracorporeal circuit volume after cardiopulmonary bypass. Anesth Analg 1993;77: 702–707.
102. Boldt J, Kling D, von Bormann B, Züge M, Scheld H, Hempelmann G. Blood conservation in cardiac operations. J Thorac Cardiovasc Surg 1989;97:832–840.
103. Nakamura Y, Masuda M, Toshima Y, et al. Comparative study of cell saver and ultrafiltration nontransfusion in cardiac surgery. Ann Thorac Surg 1990;49:973–978.
104. Boldt J, Zickmann B, Czeke A, Herold C, Dapper F, Hempelmann G. Blood conservation techniques and platelet function in cardiac surgery. Anesthesiology 1991;75:426–432.
105. Valley RD, Freid EF, Norfleet EA, Calhoun P, Mill M, Wilcox B. Are blood conservation techniques useful in pediatric patients undergoing cardiopulmonary bypass [abstract]? Anesthesiology 1993;79:A11721.
106. Henling CE, Carmichael MJ, Keats AS, Cooley DA. Cardiac operation for congenital heart disease in children of Jehovah's Witnesses. J Thorac Cardiovasc Surg 1985;89:914–920.
107. Boineau FG, Fisher JW. Hematologic abnormalities in renal disease. In: Edelmann CM Jr, ed. Pediatric kidney disease. Boston: Little, Brown and Company, 1992:685–694.
108. Beckman BS, Brookins JW, Shadduck RK, Mangan KF, Deftos LJ, Fisher JW. Effect of different modes of dialysis on serum erythropoietin levels in pediatric patients. Pediatr Nephrol 1988;2:436–441.
109. Eschbach JW, Egrie JC, Downing MR, Browne JK, Adamson JW. Correction of the anemia of end-stage renal disease with recombinant human erythropoietin. Results of a combined phase I and II clinical trial. N Engl J Med 1987;316:73–78.
110. Potter DE, Portale AA, Melzer JS, et al. Are blood transfusions beneficial in the cyclosporine era? Pediatr Nephrol 1991;5:168–172.
111. Mauer SM, Nevins TE, Ascher N. Renal Transplantation in Children. In: Edelmann CM Jr, ed. Pediatric kidney disease. 2nd ed. Boston: Little, Brown and Company, 1992:941–981.
112. Anonymous. National Institutes of Health Consensus Development Conference statement: liver transplantation—June 20–23, 1983. Hepatology 1984;4:107S–110S.
113. Carton EG, Rettke SR, Plevak DJ, Geiger HJ, Kranner PW, Coursin DB. Perioperative care of the liver transplant patient: part 1. Anesth Analg 1994;78:120–133.
114. Borland LM, Roule M. The relation of preoperative coagulation function and diagnosis to blood usage in pediatric liver transplantation. Transplant Proc 1988;XX(N.1, Suppl. 1):533–535.
115. Bontempo FA, Lewis JH, Van Thiel DH, et al. The relation of preoperative coagulation findings to diagnosis, blood usage, and survival in adult liver transplantation. Transplantation 1985;39:532–536.
116. Carlier M, Van Obbergh LJ, Veyckemans F, et al. Hemostasis in children undergoing liver transplantation. Semin Thromb Hemost 1993; 19:218–222.
117. Kalayoglu M, D'Alessandro AM, Sollinger HW, Hoffman RM, Pirsch JD, Belzer FO. Experience with reduced-size liver transplantation. Surg Gynecol Obstet 1990;171:139–147.
118. Eckhoff DE, D'Alessandro AM, Knechtle SJ, et al. 100 consecutive liver transplants in infants and children: an 8-year experience. J Pediatr Surg 1994;29:1135–1140.
119. Castaldo P, Langnas AN, Stratta RJ, et al. Long-term central venous access in pediatric liver transplantation recipients: role of percutaneous insertion of subclavian broviac catheters. Transplant Proc 1991;23: 1991.
120. Kam I, Lynch S, Todo S, et al. Low flow venovenous bypasses in small dogs and pediatric patients undergoing replacement of the liver. Surg Gynecol Obstet 1986;163:33–36.
121. Kang Y, Borland LM, Picone J, Martin LK. Intraoperative coagulation changes in children undergoing liver transplantation. Anesthesiology 1989;71:44–47.
122. Jameson LC, Popic PM, Harms BA. Hyperkalemic death during use of a high-capacity fluid warmer for massive transfusion. Anesthesiology 1990;73:1050–1052.

Chapter 35

Transfusion Issues in Neurosurgery

MICK J. PEREZ-CRUET
RAYMOND SAWAYA

INTRODUCTION

To the neurosurgeon, hemostasis is paramount because the bony architecture of the skull and spine contain the central nervous system (CNS) within a fixed volume. Blood loss in the neurosurgical setting not only limits oxygen-carrying capacity to the CNS but also results in mass effect, leading to brain or spinal cord compression. Therefore, transfusion issues in neurosurgery should include methods of detecting and treating coagulopathic states, preoperative preparation to limit intraoperative bleeding, and methods of controlling bleeding during neurosurgical procedures.

HISTORY

Imhotep, physician to King Zoser, the first Pharoah of the third dynasty (2800 BC), was perhaps the first to note the existence of cerebral vessels and the pulsatile nature of the exposed brain during examination of a compound skull fracture with an underlying dural tear. Later, Alcmaeon of Croton (circa 450 BC), who studied medicine under Pythagoras, noted two types of blood vessels and the importance of blood for mental function. Herophylos of Chalcedon (circa 300–250 BC), who was a pupil of the Pythagoras School on the Island of Kos, further distinguished the arteries from the veins noting the arteries' pulsatile nature. Claudius Galen (AD 130–121), who was born in Pergamon in Asia Minor, studied medicine at the school in Alexandria and became the private physician of Emperor Marcus Aurelius. Galen's investigation of animals' cerebral blood flow, most notable in the pig, led to the understanding of arteries containing blood and the description of the rete mirabile, a network of vessels at the base of the brain not present in humans. Nevertheless, Galen's description of human cerebral vascular anatomy dominated anatomic thinking for the next 1500 years (1).

With the coming of the Renaissance, individuals began to question Galen's anatomic dogma. Andreas Vesalius (1514–1564) more accurately illustrated human cerebral circulation in his De Humani Corporis Fabrica (2). Mathaeus Realdus Columbus (1516–1580), an assistant to Vesalius, noted that the brain's pulsations were synchronous with those of the heart and arteries (3). Shortly after, Gabriel Fallopius (1523–1562) described the posterior arterial supply and the arterial circle at the base of the brain (4). It was William Harvey's (1578–1657) description of the blood circulation that transformed vascular anatomy into physiology (5). Later, Thomas Willis (1621–1675) published the first functional explanation of the arterial circle at the base of the brain that now bears his name (6). In the years to come, many investigations were made in understanding cerebral blood flow dynamics. A pioneer in the field was Adolf Fick (1829–1901), who was a physicist, mathematician, and quantitative physiologist. He contributed to our knowledge of cerebral blood flow and oxygen consumption (7).

CEREBROVASCULAR ANATOMIC OVERVIEW

Three major branches arise from the outer curve of the aortic arch and include the innominate, left common carotid, and left subclavian arteries. The innominate artery, also called the brachiocephalic trunk, is usually the first vessel off the aortic arch. It bifurcates into the right subclavian and right common carotid arteries. The major branches of the right subclavian are the right vertebral, internal mammary arteries, thyrocervical, and costocervical trunk vessels. The right common carotid arises from the proximal innominate artery or occasionally directly from the aortic arch itself. It bifurcates at the level of the third to fifth cervical vertebral body into the internal and external carotid arteries.

The second major vessel off the aortic arch is the left common carotid artery. This vessel can also arise from the innominate artery. It bifurcates into the internal and external carotid arteries. The last branch on the aortic arch is the left subclavian artery. The major branches of the left subclavian artery are the left vertebral artery, thyrocervical trunk, and the costocervical trunk. The left vertebral artery is usually dominant.

The external carotid artery supplies most extracranial areas of the head and neck. The branches of the external carotid are the superior thyroid artery, the ascending pharyngeal artery, the lingual artery, the facial artery, the occipital artery, the posterior auricular artery, the superficial temporal artery, and the internal maxillary artery.

The intracranial cavity is supplied by four vessels: the two internal carotid arteries located anterior and the two vertebral arteries located posterior. As the internal carotid ascends into the head, it is anatomically divided into four segments: the cervical, petrous, cavernous, and supraclinoidal segments. It then bifurcates into the anterior and middle cerebral arteries. The anterior cerebral artery is the smaller of the two and supplies the medial and anterior portions of the cerebral hemispheres. The larger middle cerebral artery courses through the sylvian fissure to supply much of the lateral portions of the cerebral hemispheres. Both arteries give off a number of branches that are not discussed.

The posterior circulation includes the vertebral arteries that pass through the foramina transversarium of the upper six cervical vertebrae and join at the level of the inferior anterior portion of the brainstem as the basilar artery. The basilar artery then continues upward along the anterior aspect of the brainstem, giving off branches, including the anterior inferior cerebellar arteries and superior cerebellar arteries. The basilar artery then bifurcates into the posterior cerebral arteries that supply the medial and posterior aspects of the cerebral hemispheres. The basilar artery and its branches supply the brainstem and posterior fossa structures, including the cerebellum.

The circle of Willis, located at the ventral surface of the midbrain, connects the anterior and posterior circulation via an interconnecting arterial polygon. It acts as a safeguard against cerebral ischemia. In the event that one or more of the four vessels leading to the intracranial cavity is occluded, blood from the remaining vessels can provide blood flow to the brain via the interconnecting circle of Willis.

Blood drains from the brain via a number of veins that empty into the venous sinuses. These sinuses can be injured during neurosurgical procedures and can lead to life-threatening blood loss. The superior sagittal sinus runs from the forehead to the occiput superiorly between the two cerebral hemispheres. It empties posteriorly into the torcula herophili or confluence of sinuses, which is also the intersection of the two transverse sinuses draining laterally, the straight sinus draining medially, and the occipital sinus draining inferiorly. Blood flows laterally through the transverse sinuses into the sigmoid sinuses and then down the jugular vein out of the cranial cavity.

The spinal cord is supplied anteriorly by an anterior spinal artery and posteriorly by two posterolateral arteries. Radicular arteries supply the spinal cord through its course with the largest radicular artery (the artery of Adamkiewicz), usually arising from the left side at a variable location in the lower thoracic to upper lumbar region.

CEREBRAL BLOOD FLOW

The total mean cerebral blood flow in humans is about 50 mL/100 g/min^{-1}. However, there are variations between the blood flow of the gray and white matter, which are about 80 and 20 mL/100 g/min^{-1}, respectively. Autoregulation of cerebral blood flow allows changes with varying levels of local metabolic activity.

MONITORING CEREBRAL BLOOD FLOW

The electroencephalogram (EEG) is useful in monitoring changes in cerebral blood flow during neurosurgical procedures such as carotid endarterectomy. Slowing of the EEG pattern has predictive value in the neurological outcome of patients (8). The EEG becomes slower when the cerebral blood flow drops below 20 mL/100 g/min^{-1} and becomes flat at or below 15 mL/100 g/min^{-1} at a temperature of 37°C. Blood flow below 15 mL/100 g/min^{-1} can result in irreversible neurological damage to the brain.

Spinal cord blood flow is similar to cerebral blood flow, with mean blood flows greatest in the lumbar region followed by the cervical and then the thoracic area (9).

MEASURING CEREBRAL BLOOD FLOW

A number of methods have been devised to measure cerebral blood flow, including radioactive xenon clearance. This method is based on the principle that the rate of xenon uptake and/or clearance is proportional to the blood flow in the tissue. The use of this radioactive tracer allows direct monitoring of tissue clearance by external detection using computed tomography. More recently, noninvasive techniques such as transcranial Doppler and magnetic resonance angiography with phase-contrast pulse sequences have been used to measure cerebral blood flow.

CONDITIONS THAT MAY INCREASE THE RISK OF INTRACRANIAL HEMORRHAGE

Most spontaneous intracerebral hemorrhages (ICHs) are caused by arterial hypertension (10). Intracranial hemorrhages can be grouped into primary or secondary hemorrhages. Primary hemorrhages are caused by hereditary defects in the hemostatic system, usually at the molecular or genetic level. Secondary hemorrhages are those caused by an acquired nontraumatic disorder, such as an embolic event or consumptive coagulopathy (11). A relatively low percentage (7.8%) of spontaneous intracranial hemorrhages are secondary to hemostatic disorders, coagulopathies, or the use of anticoagulants (12, 13).

PRIMARY (HEREDITARY) COAGULATION FACTOR DEFICIENCIES

Primary coagulation factor deficiencies resulting in ICH are relatively uncommon. When they do occur, they are most often caused by deficiencies of factors VIII and IX or von Willebrand factor (10, 14).

Factor VIII Deficiency

In this condition, patients have a prolongation of the partial thromboplastin time (PTT). Although spontaneous ICH can occur, most ICHs occur after direct trauma and are associated with a high mortality (15, 16). Treatment of factor VIII deficiency includes infusion of purified factor VIII or cryoprecipitate.

Factor IX Deficiency (Hemophilia B and Christmas Disease)

Spontaneous intracranial hemorrhage can occur with factor IX deficiency (17). An acquired factor IX deficiency is associated with the nephrotic syndrome (18). Patients with factor IX deficiency can be treated with fresh-frozen plasma or purified factor IX.

von Willebrand Factor Deficiency

von Willebrand factor deficiency is an autosomal dominant disorder with a high population frequency (14). However, spontaneous intracranial hemorrhage is probably less common than with factor VIII deficiency. Treatment for von Willebrand deficiency includes infusion of cryoprecipitate, which is the principal source of von Willebrand factor. Additionally, epsilon-aminocaproic acid and tranexamic acid are also used with cryoprecipitate. For minor surgical procedures in patients with type I von Willebrand disease, desmopressin (DDAVP) can be used to improve coagulation (11).

Factors I, VII, XII, XIII Deficiencies

Intracranial hemorrhages from factor VII or XIII deficiencies are unusual (11). However, recurrent subarachnoid hemorrhages have been reported for a patient with factor XII (Hageman factor) deficiency (19). Deficiencies of these factors can be associated with hepatic insufficiency. Factors VII and XIII deficiencies can be treated with fresh-frozen plasma and supplemented with parental vitamin K. Factor I (fibrinogen) deficiency can be treated with cryoprecipitate that contains a relatively high concentration of fibrinogen.

ACQUIRED COAGULOPATHIES

Idiopathic Thrombocytopenic Purpura

Idiopathic thrombocytopenic purpura (ITP) is an autoimmune disorder whereby platelets are destroyed in the reticuloendothelial system (20). ICHs occur in less than 5% of patients with ITP and can be life threatening (11). Treatment may include platelet transfusion, high-dose methylprednisolone, gamma globulin, and plasmapheresis (21). In patients with persistent hemorrhage, splenectomy can be performed (22).

Disseminated Intravascular Coagulation

Disseminated intravascular coagulation (DIC) is a consumptive coagulopathy in which thrombocytopenia, coagulation factor deficiencies, and increased fibrin split products exist, resulting in life-threatening hemorrhages. It has been associated with a number of conditions, including trauma, pregnancy, cancer, and infection (23–27). Besides increasing the neurological complications of neurosurgical procedures, DIC has been associated with subarachnoid hemorrhages, cortical and brainstem hemorrhages, infarcts, and cerebral vessel obstruction (26).

The mainstay of therapy is to treat the underlying cause of the DIC. Patients should be treated with platelet transfusion to maintain counts above 50,000/μL. Cryoprecipitate is used to provide fibrinogen, and fresh-frozen plasma infusion is used to treat the consumptive coagulopathy. Blood transfusions are given if anemia exists. The efficiency of treatment is monitored by checking the prothrombin time (PT) and PTT, fibrin split product, and platelet levels.

Thrombotic Thrombocytopenic Purpura

Thrombotic thrombocytopenic purpura (TTP) is associated with focal neurological findings, fever, renal insufficiency, thrombocytopenia, and microangiopathic hemolytic anemia. Intracranial hemorrhages occur in 5.9% of patients having TTP and coagulation abnormalities (11). Acute treatment for TTP includes plasma exchange with fresh-frozen plasma (28).

Uremia

Uremia from renal insufficiency is associated with platelet dysfunction leading to prolongation of bleeding time secondary to poor clot formation. Treatments include dialysis to remove urea nitrogens. In addition, cryoprecipitate and DDAVP may help reduce bleeding times (29, 30).

Hereditary Hemorrhagic Telangiectasia (Osler-Weber-Rendu Disease)

Osler-Weber-Rendu disease is an inherited autosomal dominant disorder characterized by angiodysplasia, including cerebral arterial venous malformations (31). These arteriovenous malformations can rupture, resulting in ICH. No specific treatment for this condition is currently used.

Amyloid Angiopathy

In cerebral amyloid angiopathy, amyloid beta protein is deposited in the walls of leptomeningeal and cortical arteries and arterioles (32). Because the arterial walls are weakened, spontaneous ICHs can occur in normotensive patients with cerebral amyloid angiopathy (33–35). These hemorrhages may be multiple, recurrent, and tend to be lobar in location (36, 37). The hemorrhagic diathesis may be caused by factor X activity, platelet dysfunction, or fibrin polymerization (38, 39). Neurosurgical evacuation of ICH in older individuals in poor neurological condition results in high mortality and morbidity, and therefore treatment should be restricted to supportive measures (40). Leblanc and coworkers (40) also recommend delayed surgery in patients in good condition, with meticulous attention to hemostasis to avoid rebleeding. Although there is no specific treatment for amyloid angiopathy, treating an underlying disorder such as chronic infection or dysproteinemia can be helpful (41).

LYMPHOPROLIFERATIVE OR MYELOPROLIFERATIVE DISORDERS

Multiple Myeloma

Multiple myeloma may produce bleeding diathesis by altering platelet function or survival (42). In addition, the accumulation of myeloma protein can result in coagulopathy (43, 44). Treatment includes plasmapheresis and cytoreduction.

Acute Promyelocytic Leukemia

Bleeding disorders leading to ICH are more common in acute promyelocytic than in acute myeloproliferative leukemia. The intracranial hemorrhages seen in leukemia result primarily from thrombocytopenia. In addition, the promyelocyte contains a tissue factor that is capable of causing DIC (45, 46). Treatment includes cytoreductive therapy, platelet transfusions, and the use of fresh-frozen plasma and cryoprecipitate when DIC exists.

Acute Myelogenous Leukemia

In this form of leukemia, thrombocytopenia and consumptive coagulopathy can occur (47). Platelet transfusions are frequently required.

MEDICAL CONDITIONS

Hypertension

Arterial hypertension accounts for 50–90% of spontaneous ICHs (48). A very high percentage (90–92%) of nontraumatic thalamic and putaminal hemorrhages are believed to result from arterial hypertension (10). Likewise, most cerebellar hemorrhages (86%) result from hypertension (49). The acute mortality is about 40% (50). The primary mechanism of ICH is a result of increase in flow (hemodynamic factor) and damage to penetrating blood vessels caused by chronic arterial hypertension (51). Antihypertensive therapy is effective at reducing the incidence of spontaneous ICH and recurrent hemorrhage (52, 53).

Sickle-Cell Disease

Neurological complications in sickle-cell disease occur in 6–34% of cases (54, 55). Of these cases, 75% are cerebral infarctions (56). ICH is the second most common cerebrovascular complication in sickle-cell disease and is estimated to occur in 2.7–20% of cases (57, 58). The preoperative management of patients with sickle cell disease undergoing craniotomy includes exchange transfusion with washed red blood cells, which reduces the proportion of hemoglobin S (59). Transfusion therapy has also been found to reduce the recurrence rate of stroke in patients with sickle-cell disease (60).

COCAINE ABUSE

Cocaine abuse is associated with a variety of CNS complications, including subarachnoid hemorrhage, vascular spasms, ICH, stroke, and possibly vasculitis (61–63). Jacobs and colleagues (64) showed that most patients with radiographic abnormalities and cocaine abuse had ischemic complications. The mechanisms for cocaine-induced cerebral ischemia may involve vasospasm (61, 65–67) or cerebral vasculitis (67). In addition, cocaine can affect hemostasis, leading to cerebral thrombosis due to enhanced platelet aggregation (68). Cocaine has been shown to affect arachidonic acid and thromboxane (68) and deplete antithrombin III and protein C (69). The best form of therapy is nonuse.

MEDICATIONS

Heparin

Heparin is used for acute short-term anticoagulation. It functions by binding to antithrombin III. Heparin then potentiates the inhibition of thrombin activity, resulting in reduced conversion of fibrinogen to fibrin. Its action can be reversed with protamine. Intracranial hemorrhages are the most common cause of fatal bleeding from anticoagulation therapy

(70, 71). In a large sample size of patients 40 years or older, the prevalence of spontaneous intracranial bleeding while on anticoagulant therapy was 6.7% (72). This same study found that the highest rate of ICH occurred within the first year of treatment. Excessive anticoagulation has been associated with an increased risk of spontaneous cerebral hematoma (73, 74).

Coumadin

Coumadin is given parenterally for long-term management of anticoagulation. It acts as a vitamin K antagonist by inhibiting the carboxylation of terminal glutamic acid residues of factors II, VII, IX, and X in the liver and reduces the plasma levels of protein C and S. The risk of ICH is increased 6- to 11-fold in patients taking oral anticoagulants compared with the general population (52, 74). To reduce the risk of intracranial hemorrhage, indications for starting anticoagulation therapy should be stringent, the duration of treatment should be as short as possible, and overtreatment should be avoided through careful monitoring (72).

Aspirin

Aspirin is often taken by older individuals to reduce the risk of embolic events. It acts by reducing platelet aggregation, which may cause blood oozing during surgical procedures. We recommend that patients discontinue taking aspirin at least 2 weeks before surgery. It takes 7–10 days before platelet function is back to normal after stopping aspirin.

Epsilon-Aminocaproic Acid

Epsilon-aminocaproic acid is an inhibitor of fibrinolysis and has been used to prevent rebleeding from ruptured cerebral aneurysms by preventing clot dissolution (75, 76). However, at higher doses, hemostatic studies have shown that epsilon-aminocaproic acid may actually increase the risk of bleeding by interfering with platelet function (77). Glick and coworkers (77) recommended that doses should not exceed 24 g/day and that patients should be evaluated with serial bleeding times to ensure normal platelet function. If the bleeding time is prolonged, the dosage should be lowered or the drug discontinued.

PREOPERATIVE EVALUATION

LABORATORY TEST

The preoperative laboratory evaluation for the neurosurgical patient generally does not differ drastically from that of other surgical specialties. Laboratory analysis generally includes hemoglobin and hematocrit levels, white blood cell count, platelet count, electrolytes, and urine analysis. Because complete hemostasis is imperative, a PT and PTT are ordered. In addition, some neurosurgeons request a bleeding time to assess platelet function, particularly for vascular cases, although no data exist that bleeding time can independently predict operating room hemorrhage (78). A chest x-ray and electrocardiogram are usually requested for patients over 40 years old or those with cardiac or pulmonary disease. If a bleeding disorder exists, hematological consultation is warranted for correction of the coagulopathic state before surgery.

INDICATION TO CROSS-MATCH BLOOD

Elective Laminectomy

For an elective laminectomy, a type and screen can be ordered rather than a type and cross match, which will help to reduce cost and waste. In the type and screen, the patient's red cells are typed for ABO-Rh and the serum is screened for irregular antibodies and is 99.99% compatible (79, 80). In a study of 10,000 patients undergoing one- or two-level laminectomy in community hospitals, 6.7% of patients with uncomplicated hospital stays received a blood transfusion. There was a significantly higher rate of blood transfusion (24%) in those patients having a complicated hospital stay (81). Sarma (82) found that in most patients needing a blood transfusion, after only a type and screen was ordered, there was sufficient time for the blood bank personnel to cross match the units before transfusion was started. In the remaining three cases not cross matched before receiving blood, no blood incompatibility occurred. The advantage of type and screen as opposed to type and cross match is that units of blood are not withheld for a specific patient, resulting in these units becoming outdated and discarded. On average, 2 to 3 units of blood were requested for each elective laminectomy (82). In a review of the literature, Sarma (82) reported that only 240 of 1512 (16%) laminectomy cases cross matched for blood actually required blood transfusion. Communication between blood bank personnel and surgical staff was the most important factor in reducing cost and waste by ordering a type and screen rather than a type and cross match for elective laminectomies.

Elective Craniotomy

In addition, some advocate type and screen for craniotomies because the ratio of used units cross matched versus actual units transfused is unacceptably high in most institutions. Generally, for every 5 units of blood ordered for elective craniotomies, only 1 unit is used (83). Type and cross match would be indicated in vascular neurosurgical cases such as aneurysm or arteriovenous malformation surgery.

Emergent Surgery

In emergent neurosurgical procedures such as severe head injury, patients should have a type and cross match performed upon arrival in the emergency room. Typically, these patients have already lost significant blood volume. Patients with scalp lacerations can lose many units of blood due to the highly vascular nature of the scalp. Indeed, patients may arrest from blood loss due to improper attention to scalp lacerations. In addition, trauma neurosurgery is very bloody because of the urgency needed to evacuate an intracranial mass lesion or because of the trauma-induced coagulopathic state of the patient. Complete hemostasis is often difficult, and large scalp and bone flaps add to the blood loss. These patients are often coagulopathic from dilution of clotting factors or develop trauma-related DIC. To replace clotting factors, fresh-frozen plasma can be given and a fresh-frozen plasma drip maintained during the operative procedure. Additional neurosurgical emergencies that would require immediate type and cross match for blood include ruptured cerebral aneurysm or arteriovenous malformation, removal of spontaneous ICH, and emergent pediatric neurosurgery.

NEURORADIOGRAPHIC APPEARANCE OF COAGULOPATHIES

Computed tomography has been helpful in defining those patients that may have an underlying coagulopathy associated with an ICH. A fluid-blood level in acute ICH is moderately sensitive in predicting the presence of a prolonged PT or PTT (84). Fluid-blood leveling within an intracerebral hematoma seen in coagulopathy is the result of insufficient clot formation resulting in large quantities of free serum (84–86). Pfleger and coworkers (84) reported a series of 199 cases of acute ICH. In 9% of the cases, imaging studies showed a fluid-blood layering in the hematoma. Of these cases, 82% had laboratory evidence of systemic coagulopathy with a prolonged PT or PTT. Identifying these patients earlier and before performing surgery can allow correction of the coagulopathic state and reduce mortality rates, which are estimated at 40%. Additionally, localized coagulopathy after traumatic brain injury has been documented, resulting in clotting abnormalities not manifested by prolongation of PT or PTT (87). In these patients, the radiographic fluid-blood layering may be the only evidence of a coagulopathic state. In a study of four patients, Hayman and coworkers (88) reported that extensive intraoperative bleeding and poor surgical outcome was encountered in patients taken to the operating room with intracerebral hematomas showing a radiographic fluid-blood layering. In contrast, patients with thrombocytopenia maintain fibrin mesh formation within the clot, and therefore fluid-blood layering is not seen (89).

PREOPERATIVE METHODS OF REDUCING INTRAOPERATIVE HEMORRHAGE

CEREBRAL EMBOLIZATION

Embolization techniques to reduce intraoperative blood loss from vascular lesions are becoming increasingly more popular as refinements of this technique develop. Cerebral lesions that are frequently embolized before surgical resection include arteriovenous malformations, meningiomas, and metastatic tumors (90–93).

Guglielmi coils are very flexible and thus easy to manage. By occluding major feeding vessels to arteriovenous malformations or tumors, the intraoperative blood loss can be significantly reduced. An additional advantage of platinum coils is that they can be removed and repositioned during the embolization procedure if their placement is not believed to be optimal.

Particulate material used for embolization has the advantage of conforming to the shape of the vessel lumen to achieve complete occlusion. Isobutyl-2-cyanoacrylate has been used for the preoperative embolization of cerebral arteriovenous malformations (93). Other embolization agents include gelatin, polyvinyl alcohol sponge, and microballoons. Microfibrillar collagen, another occlusive agent, has a very small particle size and causes occlusion of vessels ranging in size from 20 to 500 μm and thus may limit formation of collateral flow (94, 95).

SPINAL EMBOLIZATION

Surgery for spinal tumors can result in significant blood loss, requiring blood transfusion (96). The resection of metastatic renal cell carcinoma and large sacral tumors is usually very bloody, which limits their resection. Preoperative percutaneous arteriolar embolization can reduce the rate of blood loss and improve the ability to resect spinal tumors (94, 97). Broaddus and coworkers (94) reported on six patients who underwent this technique preoperatively. The tumors included metastatic renal carcinoma, metastatic thyroid carcinoma, metastatic melanoma, and giant cell tumor of the sacrum. The embolization technique used microfibrillar collagen, which allowed embolization of very small feeding vessels, preventing collateral flow to the tumor. In seven of nine procedures performed on these six patients, the estimated blood loss ranged from 400 to 800 mL and no blood transfusion was given. Without embolization, blood loss can range from 1500 to 3000 mL or greater (98).

INTRAOPERATIVE BLOOD SALVAGE

In neurosurgical cases, it is uncommon to use intraoperative blood salvage, most likely because of the relatively small volumes of blood loss. The largest neurosurgical series reported dates back to 1925 when Loyal Davis and Harvey Cushing used intraoperative blood salvage techniques on 23 cases (99). The reason for its lack of popularity is unclear. However, intraoperative blood salvage can be useful, particularly in the surgical management of vascular cerebral lesions such as arteriovenous malformation (100, 101). Additionally, situations that may justify the use of intraoperative blood salvage include the Jehovah's Witness patient. These patients will not accept blood transfusions but may accept intraoperative blood salvage. Relative contraindications include infection and malignancy, which could be spread to other organ systems.

INTRAOPERATIVE NEUROSURGICAL HEMOSTASIS

HEMOSTATIC NEUROSURGICAL INSTRUMENTS

The feature that most distinguishes neurosurgery as a specialty is control of hemorrhage without a ligature (102). The use of thermal energy to achieve hemostasis dates back to the time of ancient Egypt, where papyrus papers give reference to the use of cautery to achieve hemostasis. Galen also popularized the use of cautery. In the modern era, Cushing (103) popularized its use with electrocoagulation; currently, it is the most widely used form of hemostasis in neurosurgery. The advantage of electric cautery is that it causes tissue damage and hemostasis via induction, affecting a much smaller surface area than conductive cautery.

The Bovie electric scalpel can be used on a cutting mode, which makes a precision cut while coagulating the tissue, or on coagulation mode, which cauterizes a larger surface area. It is very effective in removing or cutting soft tissues while maintaining hemostasis.

The bipolar electrocautery was first developed by Greenberg in 1945. It delivers a more precise induction current between the two tips of a forceps. It is very effective in stopping bleeding from individual vessels or in a small working area such as at the bottom of a spinal incision or deep within the brain. Because it is a forceps, it can be used to place hemostatic agents such as Gelfoam or a cottonoid in the area of bleeding and coagulate at the same time. It is perhaps the most widely used instrument in the neurosurgical arena because of its versatility.

Lasers have recently come into vogue as effective instruments in removing tumors while maintaining hemostasis. Lasers cause hemostasis by exerting a thermal reaction with the tissue through excitation of rotational and vibrational qualities of matter (104). The neodymium:yttrium-aluminum-garnet laser causes its heating and coagulation effects by preferential absorption by heme-pigmented tissue, long extinction length, and decreased tissue absorption (104).

HEMOSTATIC AGENTS

Cushing introduced the first absorbable hemostatic agent to neurosurgery in 1911 by using skeletal muscle to stop capillary oozing (105).

Collagen-Derived Material

Microfibrillary collagen (Avitene; Avicon, Inc., Fort Worth, TX) is a fibrous web-like material. It is a water-insoluble natural collagen, consisting of fibers containing microcrystals made from purified bovine dermal collagen (106). Its mode of action is to provide a surface to which platelets can adhere, thereby accelerating platelet-mediated clot formation (107–109). It can be effective in treating lacerations of venous sinus that tend to bleed profusely and more briskly if coagulated. This material was more effective in treating sinus tears than Gelfoam soaked in thrombin (110). An excellent hemostatic agent, animal studies have shown this material to be safe and absorbed rapidly by inflammatory cells (111, 112). Resorption of collagen material is done principally by macrophages but also by granulocytes, which both contain collagenase (113).

Oxidized Cellulose

Oxidized cellulose (Surgicel; Johnson and Johnson, New Brunswick, NJ or Oxycel; Parke-Davis, Morris Plains, NJ) is an absorbable fabric consisting of cellulose in the form of cotton, gauze, or paper that is subjected to oxidation by nitrous oxide (114). The mechanism by which oxidized cellulose produces hemostasis is dependent on a chemical reaction. The major use of oxidized cellulose is to control blood oozing from broad surfaces such as the dura or brain surface. It is also used effectively in spinal operations for bleeding from the spinal cord where electrocautery hemostasis could lead to spinal cord damage. Surgicel has been used effectively to stop bleeding from an arterial tear at the neck of an aneurysm after clip placement. In this particular instance, small strips of Surgicel were carefully placed over and around the arterial tear, pressure applied with a cottonoid, and then an additional Surgicel pledget was placed over the surgicel to hold it in place.

An advantage of oxidized cellulose is its bactericidal activity that has been shown to affect over 20 pathological organisms (115). The bactericidal effect is caused in part by the acidic pH and can be reversed with base (116). The tissue reaction to oxidized cellulose is very mild and does not delay wound healing (117). The rate of absorption varies from 2 days to 6 weeks depending on the amount of agent used, the amount of blood present, and the degree of oxidation (118, 119).

Gelatin Foam

Gelatin sponge (Gelfoam; Upjohn Co., Kalamazoo, MI) is an absorbable gelatin material that has been specifically treated. It was first introduced in 1945 by Correll and Wise (120). Neurosurgeons frequently use Gelfoam because of its ease of application and hemostatic qualities. Typically, the Gelfoam-soaked sponge is used by first compressing the sponge to squeeze out excess thrombin, improving the hemostatic ability of the sponge, and then applying it to the wound and covered with a cotton pledget. A sucker is then applied to the cotton pledget. The sponge can be removed after 10 seconds or left in place. The gelatin sponge itself has no intrinsic hemostatic action, but after the addition of topical thrombin, it becomes a very effective hemostatic agent. The sponge is capable of absorbing 45 times its weight in blood (105). The pressure of the blood-soaked sponge and the large surface area produced by the pores in the sponge control oozing. However, because of the sponge's ability to absorb blood and expand, it should not be left in place in confined areas such as the spine where expansion could lead to nerve root or cord compression.

Studies have shown that the gelatin sponge material is usually absorbed completely within 20–45 days after implantation (121, 122). Because it is a foreign material, if left in place, it can increase the incidence of wound infection (123–125).

There are a number of neurosurgical applications for the gelatin sponge. It is very effective at controlling capillary bleeding from the brain. In spinal surgery, it is frequently used to control bleeding from the venous plexus during laminectomies. It has been used to control bleeding from cancellous bone during bone fusion and was found to reduce bleeding by 61–75% over control values (126, 127); at the same time, the gelatin sponge does not retard bone healing (126). Gelatin paste made by mixing 1 g of gelatin powder with normal saline was found to be more effective at controlling bone bleeding than Gelfoam (126, 128). The gelatin sponge is also effective at controlling venous sinus bleeding with no evidence of intravascular thrombus formation (125). In addition to its hemostatic applications, the gelatin sponge has also been used to repair dural defects and can be effective at sealing cerebral spinal fluid leaks (121). No significant difference in tissue reaction was seen in comparing brain tissue reaction with microfibrillar collagen and gelatin foam in canine brain lesions (129).

Hydrogen Peroxide

Hydrogen peroxide produces a chemical hemostasis. It is used by soaking cotton balls in 3% hydrogen peroxide. The soaked cotton balls are then packed into the oozing brain cavity and left in place for 5 minutes to produce hemostasis. The cotton ball is then gradually removed while irrigating slowly. Although using hydrogen peroxide on the brain is not encouraged by all neurosurgeons, no detrimental effect has been noted (130). This technique is especially effective in managing the oozing after evacuation of an intracerebral hematoma. Because of the expansion of hydrogen peroxide on exposure to blood, it should be instilled with caution in confined areas such as the subdural space to avoid brain compression (130). In addition to its hemostatic qualities, it also acts as a bactericidal agent.

Bone Wax

Invented by Horsley in 1892, bone wax has no adherent hemostatic properties. Bone wax prevents bleeding by its tamponade effect on bone bleeding (131).

Thrombin

Mellanby (132) first described the laboratory preparation of thrombin in 1933. Thrombin is a protein produced via a reaction in which bovine prothrombin is activated to thrombin by tissue thromboplastin in the presence of $CaCl_2$ (110). It is supplied as a powder and is made into a solution with normal saline. A commonly used and effective material for carrying thrombin is the gelatin sponge. Thrombin can be applied topically to control capillary oozing during operative procedures and has been found to shorten bleeding from puncture sites in heparinized patients (117). Thrombin begins to lose its activity within 8 hours at room temperature and within 48 hours if refrigerated (105).

Fibrin Glue

Fibrin glue is a topical hemostatic agent prepared by combining fibrinogen with thrombin to create a biological adhesive. Although commercial preparations are available, autologous fibrin glue carries less risk of transmitting infection. It is obtained by performing plasmapheresis collection or harvesting plasma from a unit of predonated blood and preparing cyroprecipitate (133). Fibrin glue has a number of applications in neurosurgery including controlling blood oozing; adhering muscle or fascial dural patch grafts; and preventing cerebral spinal fluid leakage after transsphenoidal, posterior fossa, or spinal surgery (134).

NEUROSURGICAL CASES FREQUENTLY MANAGED WITH BLOOD TRANSFUSIONS

VASOSPASM FROM SUBARACHNOID HEMORRHAGE

The most common cause of subarachnoid hemorrhage is a ruptured cerebral aneurysm. The amount of blood in the basal cistern within 4 days after a spontaneous subarachnoid hemorrhage, as seen by head computed tomography, is a good predictor of the severity of symptomatic intracranial cerebral vasospasm (135). Patients with ruptured aneurysms develop a reduction in circulating blood volume, and treatment is directed at restoring or elevating blood volume to reduce symptomatic vasospasm (136–138). Ischemic symptoms due to cerebral vasospasm after subarachnoid hemorrhage have been alleviated using intravascular volume expansion by blood transfusion, induced hypertension, increased cardiac output, and plasma expanders (139–142). The goal of this therapy is to improve regional cerebral oxygen delivery and therefore limit ischemic damage secondary to vasospasm. Autoregulation appears to be impaired in cerebral vasospasm after subarachnoid hemorrhage, and therefore cerebral blood flow in the ischemic brain is volume and pressure dependent (136, 143–145).

Protocols for treatment of vasospasm include intravascular volume expansion with whole blood or packed red blood cells, supplemented with plasma fractionate or albumin (146). Some neurosurgeons have advocated giving at least 400 mL of whole blood immediately after clipping a cerebral aneurysm even after conservative blood loss (147). These authors have reported improved clinical outcome and reduced symptomatic vasospasm after early blood transfusion at the time of operation (147, 148). Pritz and colleagues (141) reported a decreased incidence and severity of neurological deficits associated with postoperative vasospasm in patients who were "overtransfused" with 1–2 units of whole blood after aneurysm clipping. Therefore, they postulated that intraoperative volume depletion may play a role in vasospasm, particularly during the immediate postoperative period. Others have found that depleted red blood cell volume was more responsible for neurological deterioration than was a lowered plasma volume in patients with cerebral vasospasm after subarachnoid hemorrhage (147).

HEMORRHAGE CAUSED BY CNS NEOPLASMS

Brain Tumors

The incidence of spontaneous ICH from brain tumors has been reported to be 1.3–9.6% (149). There appears to be a correlation between tumor pathology and hemorrhage rates. Realization of possible tumor pathology based on clinical presentation, imaging techniques, and location of tumor before starting an operation can prepare the surgeon to take steps to minimize blood loss and the need for blood transfusions. Those tumors found to have the highest incidence of hemorrhage include metastatic melanoma (50%), mixed oligodendroglioma/astrocytomas (29.2%), and sarcomas (150). Tumors that are frequently associated with spontaneous hemorrhage include glioblastoma (151–153), tumors of neuroepithelial origin, oligodendroglioma (154), and renal cell carcinoma metastasis. Even though these tumors have a tendency to bleed spontaneously, their bleeding can generally be controlled during surgery. Additional tumor types that are prone to intratumoral hemorrhage include choriocarcinoma (155, 156), metastatic tumors (157), and pituitary adenomas (149). In contrast, meningiomas have a very low rate of spontaneous hemorrhage; however, their resection can be very bloody. A series of 310 cases of meningiomas reported only 4 having spontaneous hemorrhages (149). Intraoperative hemorrhage from meningiomas can be reduced by preoperative embolization and/or intraoperatively by coagulating the vascular pedicle to the tumor initially. Factors that may increased tumor hemorrhage rate include age, with children having a higher incidence of hemorrhage (149,158), and changes in intracranial pressure after placement of ventricular drainage, particularly in patients with posterior fossa tumors (159). Interestingly, hypertension and anticoagulant therapy do not appear to increase the incidence of spontaneous tumor hemorrhage (150).

Spinal Metastasis

Metastatic spinal tumors usually occur in individuals over 50 years of age and are more common in men than in women. In a series of 250 malignant extradural tumors, 68% were metastatic (160). Metastatic spinal neoplasms can be highly vascular, making resection difficult and bloody. Those metastatic tumors that are particularly vascular include renal carcinoma, thyroid carcinoma, and melanoma, which comprise roughly 9%, 6%, and 2% of metastatic tumors to the spine, respectively (161). As described in a previous section, preoperative arteriography and embolization of feeding vessels can significantly reduce intraoperative blood loss and enhance the ability to safely resect these lesions.

CRANIOSYNOSTOSIS SURGERY IN CHILDREN

The use of blood transfusion therapy is especially high in craniosynostosis surgery where a large portion of the scalp is peeled away from the skull, resulting in bone and scalp bleeding. Intraoperative blood loss has been estimated between 71% and 126% of estimated blood volume, with total fluid replacement ranging from 94% to 180% of the patient's estimated blood volume (162). Others have reported blood loss as being dependent on the suture operated upon. Kearney and coworkers (163) found that blood loss ranged from 24.1% of estimated blood volume for sagittal synostosis cases to 64.7% of estimated blood volume for bicoronal synostosis cases. In a multicenter study of craniosynostosis cases involving 793 cases, 5% of patients had more than one time their total estimated blood loss (164). Although attempts were made to limit blood loss during these operations, excessive blood loss has led some to condemn these operations as too risky. To dispel some of these concerns, Eaten and coworkers (165) conducted a retrospective analysis of surgery for craniosynostosis in young children in 73 consecutive cases to determine transfusion requirements, to document morbidity, and to identify variables associated with blood transfusion. They determined that the suture(s) being operated on is not the most important variable in determining blood loss, but that the neurosurgeon and more likely the anesthesiologist is the more causal variable in determining if the patient is to receive a blood transfusion. They reported that none of their patients experienced any transfusion-associated morbidity.

TRAUMATIC INJURIES

Gun Shot Wounds to the Head

There is a very high incidence of death (75–80%) with gun shot wounds to the head (166). Most patients with a gun shot wound to the head do not survive to make it to the neurosurgeon (167, 168). It is estimated that greater than 90% of patients shot in the head in civilian settings die, two-thirds at the scene of the crime (169). Surgical intervention can be extremely bloody. Frequently, the patient is coagulopathic from blood loss and hemodilution. An emergency type and cross match and a coagulation profile should be ordered upon arrival. Fresh-frozen plasma and platelets should be available intraoperatively. Not infrequently, a fresh-frozen plasma drip is started once the patient enters the operating room to improve coagulation.

NEUROGENIC SHOCK DUE TO HEAD TRAUMA

In addition to spinal cord injury, neurogenic shock can occur in the setting of head trauma with acutely elevated intracranial pressure (170). Patients with neurogenic shock after head injury are often treated using volume expanders such as whole blood, plasma, or crystalloid with or without vasoactive drugs such as dopamine. The efficacy of blood transfusion therapy has been questioned because animal studies have shown these products to be detrimental in the treatment of neurogenic shock due to brain injury (171). Rahimifar and coworkers (171) found that in the absence of hypovolemia, neurogenic shock due to raised intracranial pressure should be treated with dopamine and normal saline infusion but not blood transfusion. Transfusion of whole blood, packed cells, or plasma failed to improve hypotension due to neurogenic shock resulting from head injury and in fact caused further deterioration in the blood pressure. Because of neurogenically induced cardiac failure, they believed that blood transfusions may result in additional stress on the failing heart caused by increased cardiac preload.

Stab Wounds to the Head

Penetrating stab wounds to the brain can be best described as low-velocity wounds with a small area of impact. As many as one-third of these patients will have a vascular complication of some sort (172). Angiography is used to delineate vascular injury such as traumatic aneurysms, which occur in 12% of patients (173).

Dural Sinus Injuries

Lacerations of the dural sinuses either because of traumatic injury or during elective procedures can result in copious blood loss. The first step to controlling dural sinus lacerations is to gain an adequate exposure. This may involve tamponading the area with Gelfoam and a cottonoid while removing additional bone. Placing temporary clips can be helpful in controlling dural sinus lacerations; however, placing clips blindly may lead to further tearing of the sinus. Additionally, coagulation usually leads to increased bleeding because the dura shrinks away, widening the laceration. A Foley catheter tip can be inserted into the sinus and the balloon inflated to occlude the sinus while a bypass or graft is fashioned. However, most supratentorial sinuses, unless occluded slowly by a meningioma, cannot be occluded acutely without considerable risk (174). Additional techniques include primary closure of the laceration using a running suture; application of pericranium or fascial grafts; or the application of muscle, Gelfoam, or avitene to small dural lacerations. Raising the patient's head will help to reduce venous pressure and bleeding from a torn sinus.

Scalp Injuries

The scalp is very vascular and seemingly minor lacerations can result in possible life-threatening blood loss. Therefore, it is imperative that the patients who present with head trauma are adequately examined for scalp injuries. Injury to the superficial temporal or occipital arteries can result in hemodynamic instability and shock from blood loss. In patients with thick hair, shaving the head over the injured area is necessary to adequately examine the wound. Infants with cephalhematomas or blood located between the galia and skull can lose a significant blood volume. Cephalhematomas present with asymmetric swelling of the head and increase in frontal occipital circumference after head trauma. In these cases, the hemoglobin and hematocrit levels should be checked frequently.

Spinal Cord Injury

The rate of spinal cord blood flow does not differ significantly from cerebral blood flow; however, after spinal cord injury, animal models have shown a decline in the rate of spinal cord blood flow (175, 176). This decline is thought to be due to a loss of autoregulation at the level of injury (177, 178). A number of studies have investigated methods of reducing posttraumatic ischemia after spinal cord injury by improving spinal cord blood flow using whole blood transfusions and dextran (179). Although some studies have shown red blood cell transfusion is effective in reversing the postinjury hypotension by doubling the spinal cord blood flow rate (180), other studies using whole blood transfusion failed to show an increase in spinal cord blood flow. This lack of efficacy in the later case was explained on the basis of hemoconcentration (179).

TRANSFUSION IN BRAIN-DEAD PATIENTS FOR ORGAN DONATION

Maintaining hemodynamic stability is critical in the brain-dead patient if viable organs are to be harvested for transplantation. Although blood transfusions may be necessary, the administration of vasopressin and minimal dosage of epinephrine without transfusion have been successful in prolonging hemodynamic stability (181). In Yoshioka and coworkers' study (181), six brain-dead patients with severe head injury received arginine vasopressin at a constant rate of 1 or 2 units/hr (285 ± 45 units/kg/min) plus epinephrine to maintain systolic blood pressure above 90 mm Hg. This resulted in prolonging hemodynamic stability for a mean of 23.1 ± 19.1 days. Arginine vasopressin seemed to maintain a pressor response to epinephrine and vasomotor tone. These patients did not receive blood transfusions but rather lactated Ringer's solution to keep adequate venous pressure. Limiting blood transfusion reduces the risk of infectious transmission, such as hepatitis or human immunodeficiency virus, to donating organs.

TRANSFUSION IN HYPOTHERMIA

Hypothermia decreases the metabolic rate of the CNS and therefore has been investigated to reduce or prevent CNS damage after ischemic injury (182–184). Unfortunately, lower body temperatures can lead to coagulopathy and tissue damage. To avoid these complications and to sustain lower levels of hypothermia, Bailes and colleagues (185) investigated the use of blood substitution. Using a canine model, they lowered body temperature to near freezing point. In their pilot study, they were able to achieve complete exsanguination, blood replacement, and ultraprofound body temperatures using a continuous circulation of a blood substitute made of an aqueous, pH-adjusted, high-potassium solution containing electrolytes, plasma expander, and oxidizable substrate buffer. Continuous circulation and a core body temperature of 1.7°C was maintained for 2.5–3 hours. Of the eight animals, six survived the experiment, and five survived over a long period. None of the surviving dogs showed evidence of gross or microscopic ischemic injury to any CNS tissue.

JEHOVAH'S WITNESS NEUROSURGICAL PATIENT

To prevent the use of blood transfusions in Jehovah's Witness patients, whose religious beliefs deny use of blood products, erythropoietin therapy has been given to increase the hematocrit concentration before and after undergoing neurosurgical procedures (186). Erythropoietin therapy has improved blood counts in Jehovah's Witness patients undergoing cerebral hemispherectomy for epilepsy (187), skull base tumor resection (188), and spinal surgery (189). The typical dosage ranges from 100 to 300 units/kg given two to three times a week along with oral iron treatments (188). Additional techniques used to reduce blood loss in the Jehovah's Witness neurosurgical patient include preoperative embolization and staged procedures.

RECOGNIZING, TREATING, AND AVOIDING UNIQUE COMPLICATIONS

OPTIC NEUROPATHY

Ischemic optic neuropathy can result from intraoperative anemia and hypotension after uncomplicated lumbar spine surgery (190–192). Risk factors that may increase the incidence of ischemic optic neuropathy include hypertension, diabetes, smoking, and coronary artery disease. After an uneventful laminectomy with moderate blood losses, the patient typically reports decreased visual acuity. In Lee's (190) report of such a complication, the pre- and postoperative hematocrit fell from 15.6 to 11.4 g/dL, respectively. The patient awoke and reported poor vision and a central "dark spot" in his right eye. Although in this case vision could not be returned to baseline, early recognition by the surgeon of visual loss and prompt ophthalmologic consultation may be critical in preventing complete irreversible loss of vision. Partial return of vision has been reported with early, rapid, and aggressive blood transfusion to increase the patient's hematocrit and blood pressure (193).

DIALYSIS DISEQUILIBRIUM

Dialysis disequilibrium syndrome is characterized by nausea, vomiting, headache, visual disturbance, tremor, muscle twitching, disorientation, EEG abnormalities, and elevation of intracranial pressure (194). The rapid increase in intracranial pressure can be fatal after initiation of hemodialysis when an underlying intracranial lesion exists (195–197). The mortality rate is as high as 27% (195, 197) and is due to brain herniation. The intracranial pressure rises almost immediately after starting hemodialysis and reaches maximal values over 25 Torr in about 2 hours (194). Although the pathogenesis is unknown, the "reverse urea effect" is believed to be induced by an osmotic gradient that results when urea is cleared more slowly from the cerebral spinal fluid and the brain than from the blood, resulting in increased intracranial pressure (198, 199). Treatment includes intracranial pressure monitoring via a ventriculostomy that can drain cerebral spinal fluid to reduce intracranial pressure and the use of mannitol. The use of peritoneal dialysis can reduce the amount of intracranial pressure elevation (195). In addition, shorter, more frequent treatments using hemodialysis (200) and avoiding overhydration (196) can reduce dialysis disequilibrium complications.

OVERTRANSFUSION

Vasospasm

Complications can occur with overtransfusion of patients with vasospasm, and therefore it is important to determine that neurological deterioration is due to brain ischemia secondary to anemia and hypovolemia. Postoperative extradural hematoma has been reported in a patient receiving hypertensive therapy including blood transfusion for delayed cerebral ischemia after aneurysm clipping (201). In addition, hyponatremia, pulmonary edema, and coagulopathy can result from hypertensive hypervolemic therapy (146), leading to mental status changes. A marked increase in hemoglobin concentration can result in decreased blood viscosity and slugging, leading to infarction when vasospasm exists. In the unclipped aneurysm patients, this therapy can result in rerupture of the aneurysm. To ensure that neurological deterioration is secondary to vasospasm, serum electrolytes, electrocardiogram, chest x-ray, and head computed tomography should be checked if acute deterioration is noted. In addition, noninvasive techniques such as transcranial Doppler can predict the severity of vasospasm based on cerebral blood flow rate.

Pediatric Neurosurgery

In the pediatric population, because of relatively small blood volumes, excessive blood transfusion can occur and is associated with acute and delayed complications. Acute complications include hypocalcemia, hyperkalemia, and coagulation abnormalities (202). These complications, which are prevalent in patients who have lost more than half their blood volume, can be managed with therapies to replace lost electrolytes, thromboplastin, prothrombin, and the use of fresh-frozen plasma (203). Communication between the surgeon and anesthesiologist is important both preoperatively and intraoperatively. If a particularly bloody lesion is encountered, coagulopathic states can be avoided provided the anesthesiologist is prepared to handle excessive bleeding with blood, fresh-frozen plasma, and platelets on hand. Additionally, if the surgeon has difficulty controlling bleeding, a warning to the anesthesiologist or packing the wound and allowing the anesthesiologist to "catch up" will often avoid situations where the patient's blood volume and clotting factors become excessively low (204, 205).

REFERENCES

1. Bell BA. Early study of cerebral circulation and measurement of cerebral blood flow. In: Wood JH, ed. Cerebral blood flow. New York: McGraw-Hill, 1987:3–16.
2. Vesalius A. De Humani Corporis Fabrica. Basle: J Oporinus, 1543, libri VII.
3. Columbus MR. De Re Anatomica. Venice: N Beuilcqua, 1559, libri XV.
4. Fallopius G. Observationes Anatomicae. Venice: MA Ulmus, 1561, 1st ed., 1562, 2nd ed. 131–134.
5. Harvey W. Exercitatio Anatomica de Motu Cordis et Sanguinis in Animalibus. Francofurti: Fitzer, 1628.
6. Willis T. Cerebri Anatome: Cui Accessit Nervorum Descriptio et Usus. London: J Flesher, 1664.
7. Fick A. Ueber die Messung des Blutquantums in den Herzventrikeln. Sitz ber Physik-Med Ges Wurzburg 1870;2:16.
8. Sundt TM Jr, Sharbrough FW, Piepgras DG, Kearns TP, Messick JM Jr, O'Fallon WM. Correlation of cerebral blood flow and electroencephalographic changes during carotid endarterectomy with results of surgery and hemodynamics of cerebral ischemia. Mayo Clin Proc 1981;56:533–543.
9. Albin MS. Anesthesia for neurosurgical procedures. In: Grossman RG, Hamilton WJ, eds. Principles of neurosurgery. New York: Raven Press, 1991:1–19.
10. Weisberg LA, Stazio A, Shamsnia M, Elliott D. Nontraumatic parenchymal brain hemorrhages. Medicine 1990;69:277–295.
11. del Zoppo GJ, Mori E. Hematologic causes of intracerebral hemorrhage and their treatment. Neurosurg Clin North Am 1992;3:637–658.
12. Russell DS. Discussion: The pathology of spontaneous intracranial haemorrhage. Proc R Soc Med 1984;47:689.
13. Almaani W, Awidi A. Spontaneous intracranial bleeding in hemorrhage diathesis. Surg Neurol 1982;17:137–140.
14. Bloom AL. Inherited disorders of blood coagulation. In: Bloom AL, Thomas DP, eds. Haemostasis and thrombosis. Edinburgh: Churchill-Livingstone, 1987:393.
15. Eyster ME, Gill FM, Blatt PM, Hilgartner MW, Ballard JO, Kinney TR. Central nervous system bleeding in hemophilias. Blood 1978;51:1179–1188.
16. Kerr CB. Intracranial hemorrhage in hemophilia. J Neurol Neurosurg Psychiatry 1964;27:166.
17. Biggs R, Douglas AS, McFarlane RG, et al. Christmas disease: a condition previously mistaken for hemophilia. Br Med J 1952;2:1378.
18. Hendley DA, Lawrence JR. Factor IX deficiency in the nephrotic syndrome. Lancet 1967;1:1079–1081.
19. Kovalainen S, Myllyla VV, Tolonen U, Hokkanen E. Recurrent subarachnoid hemorrhage in patients with Hageman factor deficiency. Lancet 1979;1:1035–1036.
20. McMillan R. Chronic idiopathic thrombocytopenic purpura. N Engl J Med 1981;304:1135–1147.
21. Novak R, Wilimas J. Plasmapheresis in catastrophic complication of idiopathic thrombocytopenic purpura. J Pediatr 1978;92:434–436.
22. Berchtold P, McMillan R. Therapy of chronic idiopathic thrombocytopenic purpura in adults. Blood 1989;74:2309–2317.

23. Al-Mondhiry H. Disseminated intravascular coagulation: experience in a major cancer center. Thromb Diathes Haemorrh 1975;34:181–193.
24. Kelton JG, Neame PB, Gauldie J, Hirsh J. Elevated platelet-associated IgG in the thrombocytopenia of septicemia. N Engl J Med 1979;300:760–764.
25. Mant MJ, King EG. Severe, acute disseminated intravascular coagulation. Am J Med 1979;67:557–563.
26. Schwartzman RJ, Hill JB. Neurologic complications of disseminated intravascular coagulation. Neurology 1982;32:791–797.
27. Neame PB, Kelton JG, Walker IR, Stewart IO, Nossel HL, Hirsh J. Thrombocytopenia in septicemia: the role in disseminated intravascular coagulation. Blood 1980;56:88–92.
28. del Zoppo GJ, Harker LA. Thrombotic thrombocytopenic purpura. In: Bayless TM, Brain MC, Cherivak RM, eds. Current therapy in internal medicine. 2nd ed. Philadelphia: BC Decker, 1987:378.
29. Janson P, Jubelirer SJ, Weinstein MJ, Deykin D. Treatment of the bleeding tendency in uremia with cryoprecipitate. N Engl J Med 1980; 303:1318–1322.
30. Mannucci P, Remuzzi G, Pusineri F, et al. Deamino-8-delta-arginine vasopressin shortens the bleeding time in uremia. N Engl J Med 1983;308:8–12.
31. Adams HP, Subbiah B, Bosch EP. Neurologic aspects of hereditary hemorrhagic telangiectasia. Arch Neurol 1977;34:101–104.
32. Ulrich G, Taghavy A, Schmidt H. The nosology and etiology of congophylic angiopathy (shape of vessels of the cerebral amyloidosis). N Neurol 1973;206:39–59.
33. Filloux FM, Townsend JJ. Congophilic angiopathy with intracerebral hemorrhage. West J Med 1985;143:498–502.
34. Awasthi D, Voorhies RM, Eick J, Mitchell WT. Cerebral amyloid angiopathy presenting as multiple intracranial lesions on magnetic resonance imaging. J Neurosurg 1991;75:458–460.
35. Gilbert JJ, Vinters HV. Amyloid angiopathy: Incidence and complications in the aging brain. I. Cerebral hemorrhage. Stroke 1983;14:915–923.
36. Finelli PF, Kessimian N, Bernstein PW. Cerebral amyloid angiopathy manifesting as a recurrent intracerebral hemorrhage. Arch Neurol 1984; 41:330–333.
37. Ishii N, Nishihara Y, Horie A. Amyloid angiopathy and lobar cerebral haemorrhage. J Neurol Neurosurg Psychiatry 1984;47:1203–1210.
38. Shigekiyo T, Kosaka M, Shintani Y, Azuma H, Iisha Y, Saito S. Inhibition of fibrin monomer polymerization by Bence Jones protein in a patient with primary amyloidosis. Acta Haematol 1989;81:160–165.
39. Furie B, Voo L, McAdam KPWJ, Furie BC. Mechanism of factor X deficiency in systemic amyloidosis. N Engl J Med 1981;304:827–830.
40. Leblanc R, Preul M, Robitaille Y, Villemure J-G, Pokrupa R. Surgical considerations in cerebral amyloid angiopathy. Neurosurgery 1991; 29:712–718.
41. Rosenstein ED, Itzokowitz SH, Penziner AS, Cohen JI, Mornaghi RA. Resolution of factor X deficiency in primary amyloidosis following splenectomy. Arch Intern Med 1983;143:597–599.
42. Cortelazzo S, Barbui T, Bassan R, Dini E. Abnormal aggregation and increased size of platelets in myeloproliferative disorders. Thromb Haemost 1980;44:127–130.
43. Fritz E, Ludwig H, Scheithauer W, Sinzinger H. Shortened platelet half-life in multiple myeloma. Blood 1986;68:514–520.
44. Nilehn J, Nilsson IM. Coagulation studies in different types of myeloma. Acta Med Scand 1966;179:194–199.
45. Andoh K, Kubota T, Takada M, Tanaka H, Kobayashi N, Maekawa T. Tissue factor activity in leukemia cells. Special reference to disseminated intravascular coagulation. Cancer 1987;59:748–754.
46. Sakuragawa N, Takahashi K, Hoshiyama M, Jimbo C, Matsuoka M. Pathologic cells as precoagulant substance of disseminated intravascular coagulation syndrome in acute promyelocytic leukemia. Thromb Res 1976;8:263–273.
47. Leavy RA, Kahn SB, Brodshy I. Disseminated intravascular coagulation: a complication of chemotherapy in acute myelomonocytic leukemia. Cancer 1970;26:142–145.
48. Mohr JP, Caplan LR, Melski JW, et al. The Harvard Cooperative Stroke Registry: a prospective registry of patients hospitalized with stroke. Neurology 1978;28:754–762.
49. Little JR, Tubman DE, Ethier R: Cerebellar hemorrhage in adults. J Neurosurg 1978;48:575–579.
50. Douglas MA, Haerer AF. Long-term prognosis of hypertensive intracerebral hemorrhage. Stroke 1982;13:488–491.
51. Caplan L. Intracerebral hemorrhage revisited. Neurology 1988;38: 624–627.
52. Furlan AJ, Whisnant JP, Elveback LR. The decreasing incidence of primary intracerebral hemorrhage: a population study. Ann Neurol 1979; 5:367–373.
53. Lee KS, Bae HG, Yun IG. Recurrent intracerebral hemorrhage due to hypertension. Neurosurgery 1990;26:586–590.
54. Portnoy BA, Herion JC. Neurological manigestations in sickle-cell disease, with a review of the literature and emphasis on the prevalence of hemiplegia. Ann Intern Med 1972;76:643–652.
55. Adeloye A, Ogbeide MI, Odeku EL. Massive intracranial hemorrhage in sickle cell anemia. Neurology 1970;20:1165–1170.
56. Sarnaik SA, Lusher JM. Neurological complications of sickle cell anemia. Am J Pediatr Hematol Oncol 1982;4:386–394.
57. Powars D, Wilson B, Imbus C, Pegelow C, Allen J. The natural history of stroke in sickle cell anemia. Am J Med 1978;65:461–471.
58. Wood DH. Cerebrovascular complications of sickle cell anemia. Stroke 1978;9:73–75.
59. Anson JA, Koshy M, Ferguson L, Crowell RM. Subarachnoid hemorrhage in sickle-cell disease. J Neurosurg 1991;75:552–558.
60. Russell MO, Goldberg HI, Hodson A, et al. Effect of transfusion therapy on arteriographic abnormalities and on recurrence of stroke in sickle cell disease. Blood 1984;63:162–169.
61. Brown E, Prager J, Lee H-Y, Ramsey RG. CNS complications of cocaine abuse: prevalence, pathophysiology, and neuroradiology. AJR 1992;159:137–147.
62. Cregle LL, Mark H. Medical complications of cocaine abuse. N Engl J Med 1986;315:1495–1500.
63. Shick JFE, Senay EC. Diagnosis and management of cocaine abuse. In: Flack EF, ed. Directions in psychiatry. Vol. 7. New York: Hatherleigh Co., 1985:3–7.
64. Jacobs IG, Roszler MH, Kelly JK, Klein MA, Kling GA. Cocaine abuse: neurovascular complications. Radiology 1989;170:223–227.
65. Wang AM, Suojanen JN, Colucci VM, Arumbaugh CL, Hollenberg NK. Cocaine and methamphetamine-induced acute cerebral vasospasm: an angiographic study in rabbits. AJNR 1990;11:1141–1146.
66. Powers RH, Madden JA. Vasoconstrictive effects of cocaine, metabolites and structural analogs on cat cerebral arteries [abstract]. FASEB J 1990;4:A1095.
67. Kaye BR, Fainstat M. Cerebral vasculitis associated with cocaine abuse or subarachnoid hemorrhage. JAMA 1987;258:2104–2106.
68. Togna G, Tempesta E, Togna AR, Dolci N, Cebo B, Caprino L. Platelet responsiveness and biosynthesis of thromboxane and prostacyclin in response to in vitro cocaine treatment. Haemostasis 1985;15:100–107.
69. Isner JM, Chokshi SK. Cocaine and vasospasm. N Engl J Med 1989; 321:1604–1606.

70. Landefeld CS, Goldman L. Major bleeding in outpatients treated with warfarin: incidence and prediction by factors known at the start of outpatient therapy. Am J Med 1989;87:144–152.
71. Silverstein A. Neurological complications of anticoagulation therapy. Arch Intern Med 1979;139:217–220.
72. Fogelholm R, Eskola K, Kiminkinen T, Kunnamo I. Anticoagulant treatment as a risk factor for primary intracerebral haemorrhage. J Neurol Neurosurg Psychiatry 1992;55:1121–1124.
73. Kase CS, Robinson RK, Stein RW, et al. Anticoagulant-related intracerebral hemorrhage. Neurology 1985;35:943–948.
74. Wintzen AR, de Jonge H, Loeliger EA, Bots GTAM. The risk of intracerebral hemorrhage during oral anticoagulant treatment: a population study. Ann Neurol 1984;16:553–558.
75. Chowdhary UM, Carey PC, Hussein MM. Prevention of early recurrence of spontaneous subarachnoid haemorrhage by epsilon-aminocaproic acid. Lancet 1979;1:741–743.
76. Shucart WA, Hussain SK, Cooper PR. Epsilon-aminocaproic acid and recurrent subarachnoid hemorrhage. A clinical trial. J Neurosurg 1980;53:28–31.
77. Glick R, Green D, Ts'ao C, Witt WA, Yu AT, Raimondi AJ. High dose epsilon-aminocaproic acid prolongs the bleeding time and increases rebleeding and intraoperative hemorrhage in patients with subarachnoid hemorrhage. Neurosurgery 1981;9:398–401.
78. Rodgers RP, Levin J. A critical reappraisal of the bleeding time. Semin Thromb Hemost 1990;16:1–20.
79. Boral LI, Henry JB. The type and screen: a safe alternative and supplement in selected surgical procedures. Transfusion 1977;17:163–168.
80. Boyd PR, Sheedy KC, Henry JB. Type and screen: use and effectiveness in elective surgery. Am J Clin Pathol 1980;73:694–699.
81. Ramirez LF, Thisted R. Complications and demographic characteristics of patients undergoing lumbar discectomy in community hospitals. Neurosurgery 1989;25:226–230.
82. Sarma DP. Do we need to cross match blood for elective laminectomy? Neurosurgery 1983;13:569–571.
83. Sarma DP. Use of blood in elective surgery. JAMA 1980;243:1536–1538.
84. Pfleger MJ, Hardee EP, Contant CF, Hayman LA. Sensitivity and specificity of fluid-blood levels for coagulopathy in acute intracerebral hematomas. AJNR 1994;15:217–223.
85. Weisberg LA. Significance of the fluid-blood interface in intracranial hematoma in anticoagulated patients. Comput Radiol 1987;11:175–179.
86. Livoni JP, McGahan JP. Intracranial fluid-blood levels in the anticoagulated patient. Neuroradiology 1983;25:335–337.
87. Coccheri S, Testa C. Regional intravascular coagulation and microthrombosis in traumatic brain lacerations in man. In: Agnoti A, Fazio C, eds. Platelet aggregation in the pathogenesis of cerebrovascular disorders. Berlin: Springer-Verlag, 1977:121.
88. Hayman LA, Taber KH, Weisel JW, Nagaswami C, Northrup SR. Fluid/blood layering in intracerebral hematoma (ICH): an ominous sign of occult coagulopathy? (in press).
89. Pierce JN, Taber KH, Hayman LA. Acute intracranial hemorrhage secondary to thrombocytopenia: CT appearance unaffected by absence of clot retraction. AJNR 1994;15:213–215.
90. Djindjian R, Cophignon J, Theron J, Merland JJ, Houdart R. Embolization by superselective arteriography from the femoral route in neuroradiology. Review of 60 cases. 1. Technique, indications, complications. Neuroradiology 1973;6:20–26.
91. Hekster REM, Matricali B, Luyendijk W. Presurgical transfemoral catheter embolization to reduce operative blood loss. Technical note. J Neurosurg 1974;41:396–398.
92. Latchaw RE, Gold LHA. Polyvinyl foam embolization of vascular and neoplastic lesions of the head, neck and spine. Radiology 1979;131: 669–679.
93. Pelz DM, Fox AJ, Vinuela F, Drake CG, Ferguson GG. Preoperative embolization of brain AVM's with isobutyl-2 cyanoacrylate. AJNR 1988;9:757–764.
94. Broaddus WC, Grady MS, Delashaw JB Jr, Ferguson RDG, Jane JA. Preoperative superselective arteriolar embolization: a new approach to enhance resectability of spinal tumors. Neurosurgery 1990;27:755–759.
95. Diamond NG, Casarella WJ, Bachman DM, Wolf M. Microfibrillar collagen hemostat: a new transcatheter embolization agent. Radiology 1979;133:775–779.
96. Shikata J, Yamamuro T, Kotoura Y, Mikawa Y, Iida H, Maetani S. Total sacrectomy and reconstruction for primary tumors. J Bone Joint Surg [Am] 1988;70A:122.
97. Hilal SK, Michelsen WJ. Therapeutic percutaneous embolization for extra-axial vascular lesions of the head, neck, and spine. J Neurosurg 1975;43:275–287.
98. Carpenter PR, Ewing JW, Cook AJ, Kuster AH. Angiographic assessment and control of potential operative hemorrhage with pathologic fractures secondary to metastasis. Clin Orthop Rel Res 1977;123:6–8.
99. Davis LE, Cushing H. Experiences with blood replacement during or after major intracranial operations. Surg Gynecol Obstet 1925;40:310.
100. Williamson KR, Taswell HF. Intraoperative red cell salvage. In Pineda AP, Valbonesi M, Sniecinski IJ, ed. Donor hemapheresis. Milan: Wichtig Editore Srl, 1989:103.
101. Williamson KR, Taswell HF. Indications for intraoperative blood salvage. J Clin Apher 1990;5:100–103.
102. Light RU. Hemostasis in neurosurgery. J Neurosurg 1945;2:414.
103. Cushing H. Electro-surgery as an aid to the removal of intracranial tumors. Surg Gynecol Obstet 1928;47:752.
104. Tew JM Jr, Tobler WD. The laser: history, biophysics, and neurosurgical applications. Clin Neurosurg 1984;31:506–549.
105. Arand AG, Sawaya R. Intraoperative chemical hemostasis in neurosurgery. Neurosurgery 1986;18:223–233.
106. Battista OA, Erdi NZ, Ferraro CF, Karasisnski FJ. Novel microcrystals of polymers. Part II. J Appl Polymer Sci 1967;11:481.
107. Abbott WM, Austen WG. The effectiveness and mechanism of collagen-induced topical hemostasis. Surgery 1975;78:723–729.
108. Cowan DH. Platelet adherence to collagen: role of prostaglandin-thromboxane synthesis. Br J Haematol 1981;49:425–434.
109. Kay WW, Kurylo E, Chong G, Bharadwaj B. Inhibition and enhancement of platelet aggregation by collagen derivates. J Biomed Mater Res 1977;11:365–372.
110. Murphy DJ, Clough CA. A new microcrystalline collagen hemostatic agent. Surg Neurol 1974;2:77–79.
111. Voormolen JHC, Ringer J, Bots GTAM, van der Heide A, Hermans J. Hemostatic agents: brain tissue reaction and effectiveness. A comparative animal study using collagen fleece and oxidized cellulose. Neurosurgery 1987;20:702–709.
112. Chvapil M. The fate of natural tissue prosthesis. In: Williams WB, ed. Biocompatibility. Vol. 1. London: CTC Press, 1980:87–104.
113. Oronsky AL, Perper RJ, Schroder HC. Phagocytic release and activation of human leucocyte procollagenase. Nature 1973;246:417–419.
114. Yackel EC, Kenyon WO. The oxidation of cellulose by nitrous dioxide. J Am Chem Soc 1942;64:124.
115. Physicians' Desk Reference. 39th ed. Oradell, NJ: Medical Economics Co., Inc., 1985:613–614, 1044–1046, 1077, 1574–1575.

116. Dineen P. The effect of oxidized regenerated cellulose on experimental intravascular infection. Surgery 1977;82:576–579.
117. Scarff JE, Stookey B, Garcia F. The use of dry oxidized cellulose as a primary hemostatic agent in neurosurgery. J Neurosurg 1949;6:304.
118. Bennett DR, ed. AMA drug evaluation. 5th ed. Chicago: American Medical Association, 1984:869.
119. Frantz VK, Clarke HJ, Lattes R. Hemostasis with absorbable gauze (oxidized cellulose). Ann Surg 1944;120:181.
120. Correll JT, Wise EC. Certain properties of a new physiologically absorbable sponge. Proc Soc Exp Biol Med 1945;58:233.
121. Light RU, Prentice HR. Surgical investigation of a new absorbable sponge derived from gelatin for use in hemostasis. J Neurosurg 1945;2: 435.
122. Correll JT, Prentice HR, Wise EC. Biologic investigations of a new absorbable sponge. Surg Gynecol Obstet 1945;81:585.
123. Dineen P. Antibacterial activity of oxidized regenerated cellulose. Surg Gynecol Obstet 1976;142:481–486.
124. Hinman F Jr, Babcock KO. Local reaction to oxidized cellulose and gelatin hemostatic agents in experimentally contaminated renal wounds. Surgery 1949;26:633.
125. Lindstrom PA. Complications from the use of absorbable hemostatic sponges. Arch Surg 1956;73:133.
126. Harris WH, Crothers OD, Moyen BJ-L, Bourne RB. Topical hemostatic agents for bone bleeding in humans. J Bone Joint Surg [Am] 1978;60A:454.
127. Cobden RH, Thrasher EL, Harris WH. Topical hemostatic agents to reduce bleeding from cancellous bone. J Bone Joint Surg [AM] 1976; 58A:70.
128. Taheri ZE. Technical suggestions: the use of Gelfoam paste in anterior cervical fusion. J Neurosurg 1971;34:438.
129. Rybock JD, Long DM. Use of microfibrillar collagen as a topical hemostatic agent in brain tissue. J Neurosurg 1977;46:501–505.
130. Mawk JR. Hydrogen peroxide for hemostasis [letter]. Neurosurgery 1986;18:827.
131. Geary JR, Frantz VK: New absorbable bone wax: experimental and clinical studies. Ann Surg 1947;132:1128.
132. Mellanby J. Thrombase, its preparation and properties. Proc R Soc Lond Ser B, 1933;133:93–106.
133. Casali B, Rodeghiero F, Tosetto A, et al. Fibrin glue from single-donation autologous plasmapheresis. Transfusion 1992;32:641–643.
134. Shaffrey CI, Spotnitz WD, Shaffrey ME, Jane JA. Neurosurgical application of fibrin glue: augmentation of dural closure in 134 patients. Neurosurgery 1990;26:207–210.
135. Wilkins RH. Attempts at prevention or treatment of intracranial arterial spasm: an update. Neurosurgery 1986;18:808–825.
136. Maroon JC, Nelson PB. Hypovolemia in patients with subarachnoid hemorrhage. Therapeutic implications. Neurosurgery 1979;4:223–226.
137. Solomon RA, Post KD, McMurtry JG III. Depression of circulating blood volume in patients after subarachnoid hemorrhage: implications for the management of symptomatic vasospasm. Neurosurgery 1984;15:354–361.
138. Wijdicks EFM, Vermeulen M, Hijdra A, van Gijn J. Hyponatremia and cerebral infarction in patients with ruptured intracranial aneurysms: is fluid restriction harmful? Ann Neurol 1985;17:137–140.
139. Giannotta SL, McGillicuddy JE, Kindt GW. Diagnosis and treatment of postoperative cerebral vasospasm. Surg Neurol 1977;8:286–290.
140. Kosnik EJ, Hunt WE. Postoperative hypertension in the management of patients with intracranial arterial aneurysms. J Neurosurg 1976;45: 148–154.
141. Pritz MB, Giannotta SL, Kindt GW, McGillicuddy JE, Prager RL. Treatment of patients with neurological deficits associated with cerebral vasospasm by intravascular volume expansion. Neurosurgery 1978;3:364–368.
142. Sundt TM Jr. Management of ischemic complications after subarachnoid hemorrhage. J Neurosurg 1975;43:418–425.
143. Ishii R. Regional cerebral blood flow in patients with ruptured intracranial aneurysms. J Neurosurg 1979;50:587–594.
144. Kindt GW, Youmans JR, Albrand O. Factors influencing the autoregulation of the cerebral blood flow during hypotension and hypertension. J Neurosurg 1967;26:299–305.
145. Waltz AG. Effect of blood pressure on blood flow in ischemic and in nonischemic cerebral cortex. The phenomena of autoregulation and luxury perfusion. Neurology 1968;18:613–621.
146. Kassell NF, Peerless SJ, Durward QJ, Beck DW, Drake CG, Adams HP. Treatment of ischemic deficits from vasospasm with intravascular volume expansion and induced arterial hypertension. Neurosurgery 1982;11:337–343.
147. Kudo T, Suzuki S, Iwabuchi T. Importance of monitoring the circulating blood volume in patients with cerebral vasospasm after subarachnoid hemorrhage. Neurosurgery 1981;9:514–520.
148. Heilbrun MP. The relationship of neurological status and the angiographical evidence of spasm to prognosis in patients with ruptured intracranial saccular aneurysms. Stroke 1973;4:973–979.
149. Wakai S, Yamakawa K, Manaka S, Takakura K. Spontaneous intracranial hemorrhage caused by brain tumor: its incidence and clinical significance. Neurosurgery 1982;10:437–444.
150. Kondziolka D, Bernstein M, Resch L, et al. Significance of hemorrhage into brain tumors: clinicopathological study. J Neurosurg 1987;67:852–857.
151. DiMaio SM, DiMaio VJ, Kirkpatrick JB. Sudden, unexpected deaths due to primary intracranial neoplasms. Am J Forensic Med Pathol 1980;1:29–45.
152. Little JR, Dial B, Belanger G, Carpenter S. Brain hemorrhage from intracranial tumor. Stroke 1979;10:283–288.
153. Richardson RR, Siqueira EB, Cerullo LJ. Malignant glioma: its initial presentation as intrcranial haemorrhage. Acta Neurochir 1979;46:77–84.
154. Russell DS, Rubinstein LJ. Pathology of tumours of the nervous system. 4th ed. London: Edward Arnold, 1977:197.
155. Kothbauer P, Jellinger K, Flament H. Primary brain tumour presenting as spontaneous intracerebral haemorrhage. Acta Neurochir 1979;49:35–45.
156. Mandybur TI. Intracranial hemorrhage caused by metastatic tumors. Neurology 1977;27:650–655.
157. McCormick WF, Rosenfield DB. Massive brain hemorrhage: a review of 144 cases and an examination of their causes. Stroke 1973;4:946–954.
158. Laurent JP, Bruce DA, Schut L. Hemorrhagic brain tumours in pediatric patients. Child Brain 1981;8:263–270.
159. Vaquero J, Cabezudo JM, de Sola RG, Nombela L. Intratumoral hemorrhage in posterior fossa tumors after ventricular drainage: report of two cases. J Neurosurg 1981;54:406–408.
160. Torma T. Malignant tumors of the spine and spinal extradural space. Acta Surg Scand 1957;225(Suppl.):1.
161. Connolly ES. Spinal cord tumors in adults. In: Youmans JR, ed. Neurological surgery. 2nd ed. Vol. 5. Philadelphia: WB Saunders, 1982:3196–3214.
162. Loftness SL, Albin RE, O'Donnel RS, Hendee RW, Morrison JE. Perioperative management of craniofacial surgery in infants and children. In: Marchac D, ed. Craniofacial surgery. Berlin: Springer-Verlag, 1987:470.

163. Kearney RA, Rosales JK, Howes WJ. Craniosynostosis: an assessment of blood loss and transfusion practices. Can J Anaesth 1989;36:473–477.
164. Whitaker LA, Munro IR, Salyer KE, Jackson IT, Ortiz-Monasterio F, Marchac D. Combined report of problems and complications in 793 craniofacial operations. Plast Reconstr Surg 1979;63:198–203.
165. Eaton AC, Marsh JL, Pilgram TK. Transfusion requirements for craniosynostosis surgery in infants. Plast Reconstr Surg 1995;95:277–283.
166. Lee RK, Waxweiler RJ, Dobbins JG, Paschetag T. Incidence rates of firearm injuries in Galveston, Texas, 1979–1981. Am J Epidemiol 1991;134:511–521.
167. Kaufman HH, Makela ME, Lee KF, Haid RW Jr, Gildenberg PL. Gunshot wounds to the head—a perspective. Neurosurgery 1986;18: 689–695.
168. Kaufman HH, Loyola WP, Makela ME, et al. Civilian gunshot wounds: the limits of salvageability. Acta Neurochir (Wien) 1983;67: 115–125.
169. Kaufman HH. Civilian gunshot wounds to the head. Neurosurgery 1993;32:962–964.
170. Illingworth G, Jennett WB. The shocked head injury. Lancet 1965;2: 511.
171. Rahimifar M, Tator CH, Shanlin RJ, Sole MJ. Effect of blood transfusion, dopamine, or normal saline on neurogenic shock secondary to acutely raised intracranial pressure. J Neurosurg 1989;70:932–941.
172. Kieck CF, de Villiers JC. Vascular lesions due to transcranial stab wounds. J Neurosurg 1984;60:42–46.
173. du Trevou MD, van Dellen JR. Penetrating stab wound to the brain: the timing of angiography in patients presenting with the weapon already removed. Neurosurgery 1992;31:905–911.
174. Collins WF. Problematic intraoperative events. In: Appuzo MLJ, ed. Brain surgery complication avoidance and management. New York: Churchill Livingstone, 1993:91.
175. Senter HJ, Venes JL. Altered blood flow and secondary injury in experimental spinal cord trauma. J Neurosurg 1978;49:569–578.
176. Sandler AN, Tator CH. Regional spinal cord blood flow in primates. J Neurosurg 1976;45:638–659.
177. Palleske H. Experimental investigation on the regulation of the spinal cord circulation. III. The regulation of the blood flow in the spinal cord altered by oedema. Acta Neurochir 1969;21:319–327.
178. Senter HJ, Venes JL. Loss of autoregulation and post-traumatic ischemia following experimental spinal cord trauma. J Neurosurg 1979;50:198–206.
179. Wallace MC, Tator CH. Successful improvement of blood pressure, cardiac output, and spinal cord blood flow after experimental spinal cord injury. Neurosurgery 1987;20:710–715.
180. Dolan EJ, Tator CH. The effect of blood transfusion, dopamine, and gamma hydroxybutyrate on posttraumatic ischemia of the spinal cord. J Neurosurg 1982;56:350–358.
181. Yoshioka T, Sugimoto H, Uenishi M, et la. Prolonged hemodynamic maintenance by the combined administration of vasopressin and epinephrine in brain death: a clinical study. Neurosurgery 1986;18:565–567.
182. Baumgartner WA, Silverberg GD, Ream AK, Jamieson SW, Tarabek J, Reitz BA. Reappraisal of cardiopulmonary bypass with deep hypothermia and circulatory arrest for complex neurosurgical operations. Surgery 1983;94:242–249.
183. Busto R, Dietrich WD, Globus MYT, Valdes I, Scheinberg P, Ginsberg MD. Small differences in intraischemia brain temperature critically determine the extent of ischemic neuronal injury. J Cereb Blood Flow Metab 1987;7:729–738.
184. Natale JE, D'Alecy LG. Protection from cerebral ischemia by brain cooling without reduced lactate accumulation in dogs. Stroke 1989; 20:770–777.
185. Bailes JE, Leavitt ML, Teeple E Jr, et al. Utraprofound hypothermia with complete blood substitution in a canine model. J Neurosurg 1991;74:781–788.
186. Goodnough LT, Rudnick S, Price TH, et al. Increased preoperative collection of autologous blood with recombinant human erythropoietin therapy. N Engl J Med 1989;321:1163–1168.
187. Schiff DJ, Weinstein SL. Use of recombinant human erythropoietin to avoid blood transfusion in a Jehovah's Witness requiring hemispherectomy. Case report. J Neurosurg 1993;79:600–602.
188. Kantrowitz AB, Spallone A, Taylor W, Chi TL, Strack M, Feghali JG. Erythropoietin-augmented isovolemic hemodilution in skull-base surgery. J Neurosurg 1994;80:740–744.
189. Rothstein P, Roye D, Verdisco L, et al. Preoperative use of erythropoietin in an adolescent Jehovah's Witness. Anesthesiology 1990;73:568–570.
190. Lee A. Ischemic optic neuropathy following lumbar spine surgery: Case report. J Neurosurg 1995;83:348.
191. Katz DM, Trobe JD, Cornblath WT, Kline LB. Ischemic optic neuropathy after lumbar spine surgery. Arch Ophthalmol 1994;112: 925–931.
192. Brown RH, Schauble JF, Miller NR. Anemia and hypotension as contributors to perioperative loss of vision. Anesthesiology 1994;80: 222–226.
193. Connoly SE, Gordon KB, Horton JC. Salvage of vision after hypotension-induced ischemic optic neuropathy. Am J Ophthalmol 1994;117: 235–242.
194. Yoshida S, Tajika T, Yamasaki N, et al. Dialysis dysequilibrium syndrome in neurosurgical patients. Neurosurgery 1987;20:716–721.
195. Bertrand YM, Hermant A, Mahieu P, Roels J. Intracranial pressure changes in patients with head trauma during haemodialysis. Intensive Care Med 1983;9:321–323.
196. Kennedy AC. Dialysis disequilibrium syndrome. Electroencephalogr Clin Neurophysiol 1970;29:206–213.
197. Peterson HD, Swanson AG. Acute encephalopathy occurring during hemodialysis. The reverse urea effect. Arch Intern Med 1964;113:877.
198. Kennedy AC, Linton AL, Eaton JC. Urea levels in cerebrospinal fluid after haemodialysis. Lancet 1962;1:410.
199. Kennedy AC, Linton AL, Luke AG, Renfrew S, Dinwoodie A. The pathogenesis and prevention of cerebral dysfunction during dialysis. Lancet 1964;1:790.
200. Gilliland KG, Hegstrom RM. The effect of hemodialysis of cerebrospinal fluid pressure in uremic dogs. Trans Am Soc Artif Intern Organs 1963;9:44.
201. Gentleman D, Johnston RA. Postoperative extradural hematoma associated with induced hypertension. Neurosurgery 1985;17:105–106.
202. Furman EB, Roman DG, Lemmer LAS, Hairabet J, Jasinska M, Laver MB. Specific therapy in water, electrolyte and blood-volume replacement during pediatric surgery. Anesthesiology 1975;42:187–193.
203. Wilkinson E, Rieff J, Rekate HL, Beals S. Fluid, blood, and blood product management in the craniofacial patient. Pediatr Neurosurg 1992;18:48–52.
204. Baek S-M, Makabali GG, Bryan-Brown CW, Kusek JM, Shoemaker WC. Plasma expansion in surgical patients with high central venous pressure (CVP): the relationship of blood volume to hematocrit, CVP, pulmonary wedge pressure, and cardiorespiratory changes. Surgery 1975;78:304–315.
205. Collins RL, Al-Mondhiry H, Chernik NL, Posner JB. Neurologic manifestations of intravascular coagulation in patients with cancer. Neurology 1975;25:795–806.

Section VI
The Postoperative Transfusion Decision

Chapter 36

Anemia in the Postoperative Period

ROBERT S. HILLMAN

INTRODUCTION

Anemia in the postoperative period is a common problem and can present a challenge in terms of diagnosis and management. It is often a predictable complication based on an untreated preoperative anemia, the amount of blood loss during surgery, or a known sensitivity of the patient to increased red cell hemolysis. The development of a severe postoperative anemia can, however, come as a surprise. In the immediate postoperative period, major changes in fluid balance, undetected internal bleeding, or unexpected hemolysis may be responsible. Later in the recovery period, a persistent anemia can be a diagnostic challenge, requiring a full hematological evaluation to determine its cause.

A number of these issues are highlighted in the following discussion of postoperative anemia. This includes the patterns of response of the blood volume and the hemoglobin/hematocrit to surgical blood loss, the physiological response to acute anemia, the clinical evaluation of anemia severity as a foundation for transfusion decisions, the diagnosis of an anemia that persists after surgery, and a discussion of transfusion and pharmacological agents in the treatment of postoperative anemias.

HEMODYNAMIC RESPONSE TO SURGICAL BLOOD LOSS

Surgical blood loss like acute hemorrhage has an immediate impact on blood volume, cardiovascular performance, and tissue oxygen delivery. For many operative procedures, blood volume loss is anticipated and avoided by adequate perioperative volume replacement. Unexpected hemorrhage during or after a surgical procedure can, however, challenge the integrity of the vascular system, producing hypovolemia, cardiovascular collapse, and death.

The hemodynamic response of the average-sized adult to acute blood volume losses is summarized in Table 36.1 (1, 2). Sudden blood loss of up to 20% of the total blood volume should be compensated for by venospasm and contraction of the venous blood pool. However, this normal reflex mechanism may be absent in patients who are septic, poorly nourished, or elderly with advanced cardiovascular disease. Anesthesia may also interfere (3). When acute blood loss exceeds 20% of the blood volume, the patient will exhibit tachycardia and postural hypotension. With losses above 30%, signs of hypovolemic shock appear with a fall in supine blood pressure, an increase in pulse rate, and cool clammy skin. During the postoperative period, a patient with this much volume loss will appear confused, anxious, restless, and will often complain of being short of breath. Elderly patients are at high risk for myocardial ischemia and may complain of chest pain.

Left untreated, sudden blood volume losses in an adult are slow to resolve (4, 5). There are no ready reservoirs of albumin, the principal oncotic protein of plasma, so that compensatory expansion of the plasma volume is a relatively slow process, taking from 24 to 60 hours. It is important, therefore, to monitor the postoperative patient's volume status and respond to any signs and symptoms compatible with volume deficits with appropriate fluid replacement.

Depending on the rapidity and amount of blood loss, effective therapy will include appropriate infusions of electrolyte and/or colloid solutions (6). Standard electrolyte solutions such as normal saline or Ringer's lactate can be used as effective volume expanders. An infusion of 3–4 L will provide at least a 1-L expansion of the intravascular volume. Care must be exercised if very large volumes, more than 8 L, are administered to elderly patients or individuals with cardiovascular disease. There is a risk of producing significant

TABLE 36.1. HEMODYNAMIC RESPONSE TO BLOOD LOSS

Volume Lost		Symptoms/Signs
mL	%TBV[a]	
<1000	20	None or vasovagal reaction; postural hypotension in the ill or elderly
1000–1500	20–30	Anxiety, tachycardia, and postural hypotension
1500–2000	30–40	Hypovolemic shock with anxiety, confusion, tachycardia and fall in supine blood pressure
>2000	~50	Severe shock and death

[a]Total blood volume (TBV) assumed to be 5000 mL.

subcutaneous edema and precipitating congestive heart failure with pulmonary edema or, rarely, acute respiratory distress syndrome (7).

Colloid solutions such as 5% albumin solution, purified plasma protein fraction, and hydroxyethyl starch solution provide volume-for-volume intravascular expansion (8). They are of greatest value in patients with massive blood losses, where the required volume of electrolyte solution would be far too large. Fresh-frozen plasma (FFP) can also be used to replace volume losses. Although FFP has the advantage of simultaneously providing the patient with a number of coagulation factors, it can, however, cause an immediate acute sensitivity reaction with widespread urticaria, subcutaneous edema, and bronchospasm (9). This allergic reaction to FFP can even be severe enough to acutely reduce the plasma volume, the direct opposite result from that desired.

Successful management of volume replacement therapy can only be assessed from the bedside evaluation of the patient. Vital signs, urinary output, neck vein distention, and evidence of adequate peripheral perfusion are all useful. During acute blood loss, hemoglobin and hematocrit measurements are of little or no help. In fact, they can even be misleading. The rate of fall of these measurements depends on the rate of replacement of the plasma volume, because they reflect the ratio of red cell mass to total blood volume. When volume replacement falls behind the rate of blood loss, the hemoglobin and hematocrit will fail to reflect the true loss of red cell mass.

COMPENSATION FOR ANEMIA

Although the ability of the body to compensate for blood volume loss is limited, several mechanisms help dampen the impact of the loss of red blood cells from circulation (10). The most immediate compensatory mechanism is the ability of the individual red blood cell to self-regulate the amount of oxygen delivered to tissues (11). Whenever the number of red blood cells perfusing a tissue is significantly reduced, individual red cells respond with a shift in the hemoglobin-oxygen dissociation curve so as to release more oxygen to tissues (3). Initially, this is driven by the higher levels of tissue CO_2 and the acidic environment, a phenomenon known as the Bohr effect. Soon thereafter, the red cells increase the intracellular production of 2,3-DPG (diphosphoglycerate). This has the effect of maintaining the rightward shift of the dissociation curve, promoting oxygen release to tissues. Depending on the age and cardiovascular status of the patient, this will maintain relatively normal levels of tissue oxygen delivery despite losses of 30–40% of the circulating number of red blood cells.

With more severe anemia, mechanisms of cardiovascular compensation come into play (10). Both pulse rate and stroke volume increase to boost tissue blood flow. The fall in the hematocrit also helps by reducing whole blood viscosity. Redistribution of blood flow can help protect key organs. The very anemic patient will show reduced blood flow to skin and muscle, whereas flow to vital organs such as the brain, heart, and liver is increased.

In the days to weeks after surgical blood loss, the production of red blood cells increases to rebuild the red blood cell mass (12). The normal pattern of response of the erythron to a severe anemia is presented in Table 36.2 (13). The first step in the process is the detection of the reduction in red blood cell mass by the kidney and production of increased levels of erythropoietin (14). This unique cytokine stimulates erythroid marrow precursors to proliferate and mature, thereby increasing the number of red blood cells produced each day. The

TABLE 36.2. ERYTHRON RESPONSE TO BLOOD LOSS ANEMIA

Physiologic Response	Day	Day	Day
Post-bleed day	1–2	3–6	7–10
Erythropoietin	↑	↑	↑
Polychromasia	+	++	+++
E:G ratio	1:3	1:1	>1:1
Reticulocyte index	1	1–2	3–4
Hematocrit	—	—	↑ 0.5–2.0%/d

rapid rise in erythropoietin can be detected by direct measurement of the serum erythropoietin level or indirectly from the release of young marrow reticulocytes into circulation. The latter phenomenon is easily detected by simple inspection of the peripheral blood smear (polychromasia) or as a part of the automated measurement of the reticulocyte count.

The full proliferative response of the erythroid marrow occurs over several days. At first, it is reflected by a change of the marrow E:G ratio, the ratio of erythroid to granulocyte elements. The normal E:G ratio is approximately 1:3. After significant blood loss, the E:G ratio can increase to levels of 1:1 by the third to sixth day. The subsequent rise in the reticulocyte production index should be apparent by the 6th to 10th day after the development of the anemia. Depending on the nature of the blood loss, the severity of the anemia, and the adequacy of iron stores and iron supply to the marrow, the reticulocyte production index can reach levels of two to five times normal (15). This translates into rates of recovery of the hematocrit of from 0.5 to 2 percentage points per day, assuming the red blood cells remaining in circulation have a normal life span and there is no further blood loss.

The complexity of the marrow response needs to be recognized. A successful production response depends on the integrity of each of the key elements of erythropoiesis—the ability of the kidney to produce erythropoietin, the presence of normal numbers of erythroid marrow precursors in a healthy marrow, and an adequate iron supply (Fig. 36.1). Patients with compromised renal function can lose the peritubular cells required for erythropoietin production. Likewise, any damage to marrow stroma or erythroid marrow precursors by agents such as drugs, toxin exposures, or radiation will set clear limits to the proliferative response. Finally, iron supply plays a dominant role in setting the level of response (16). Iron-deficient patients will be unable to increase red cell production above basal levels. Patients with normal levels of reticuloendothelial iron stores will, in the face of surgical blood loss, be able to increase production two- to threefold. In contrast, the hemolytic anemia patient and, in some cases, patients who experience internal bleeding will be able to increase red blood cell production by four- to fivefold or more.

Several cytokines associated with systemic illness and acute tissue injury also play major roles in determining the red blood cell production response (Fig. 36.2) (16). Tumor necrosis factor (TNF), interleukin-1 (IL-1), and both gamma and beta interferon are capable of inhibiting the major components of erythropoiesis, including the erythropoietin response, the delivery of iron from the reticuloendothelial iron stores, and the stem cell proliferative response. Dramatic increases in TNF and beta interferon levels are associated with neoplasms and bacterial infections, whereas IL-1 and gamma interferon are the principal inhibitors of erythropoiesis in patients with chronic inflammatory states, especially connective tissue diseases.

The diagnostic pattern of cytokine suppression of erythropoiesis is summarized in Table 36.3. Typically, the patient exhibits a normocytic, normochromic anemia with a normal

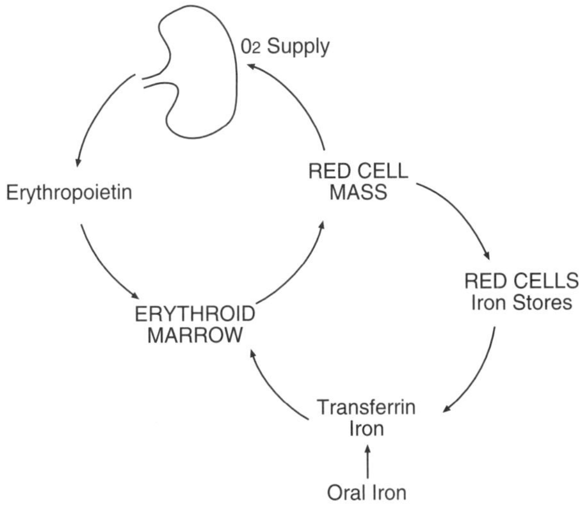

Figure 36.1. The maintenance of an appropriate red blood cell mass to supply oxygen to tissues depends on a number of key factors. This includes normal kidneys to provide an adequate erythropoietin response, a healthy bone marrow, and an adequate supply of iron. A disease that interferes with any one or several of these will produce an anemia.

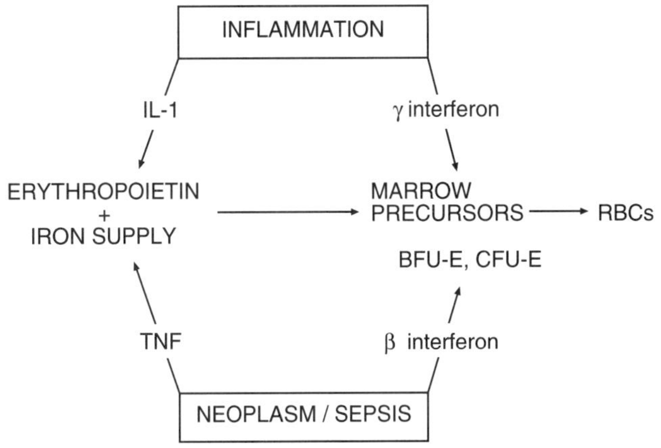

Figure 36.2. The principal elements of erythropoiesis—erythropoietin secretion, iron supply, and marrow precursor growth—are sensitive to the release of cytokines in patients with inflammatory states, sepsis, or neoplasm. Patients with chronic inflammatory states such as rheumatoid arthritis demonstrate a hypoproliferative anemia secondary to IL-1 inhibition of erythropoietin secretion and iron supply and through the release of gamma interferon the growth of marrow precursors. Patients with neoplasms or sepsis have a similar suppression of erythropoiesis via the release of TNF and beta interferon. RBC, red blood cell; BFU-E, blast-forming unit erythroid; CFU-E, cell-forming unit erythroid.

TABLE 36.3. ERYTHROPOIETIC PROFILE OF INFLAMMATORY ANEMIA

Laboratory Finding	Values
Hematocrit/hemoblobin	25–35%/8–11g/dL
Morphology/MCV	Normocytic, normochromic/80–90 fL
Marrow E:G ratio	1:3–1:2
Reticulocyte index	0.5–1.5
Serum iron	Decreased (<30 μg/dL)
TIBC	Decreased (<290 μg/dL)
Serum ferritin	Increased (20–200 μg/L)
Iron stores	Normal to increased

MCV, mean corpuscular volume.

RDW (reticulocyte dry weight) and little or no polychromasia, indicating a suppression of the erythropoietin response. The resulting failure in marrow proliferation is reflected in a normal E:G ratio (1:3) and a reticulocyte production index that is at or near basal levels. Measurements of serum iron and serum ferritin reveal a low serum iron, low total iron binding capacity (TIBC), and a moderately elevated serum ferritin level, a pattern that is the hallmark of cytokine-induced inhibition of the release of reticuloendothelial iron stores.

The importance of cytokine suppression of erythropoiesis as a cause of postoperative anemia must be emphasized. Patients with acute infections or chronic inflammatory states will present for surgery with an established inflammatory anemia and will demonstrate a poor marrow production response to worsening anemia during the postoperative period. Surgery, in and of itself, can be an inflammatory event. Iron studies performed during and immediately after surgery can show a fall in the serum iron, a reduction in the TIBC, and a rise in the serum ferritin level. Complications of surgery, especially tissue necrosis or postoperative wound infections, are invariably associated with cytokine suppression of erythropoiesis and the appearance of a full-blown inflammatory anemia.

Another example of the sensitivity of red blood cell production to surgery is the response of patients with hemolytic anemias. For example, sickle cell anemia patients demonstrate an increased rate of red cell hemolysis together with a reduction in red blood cell production in association with surgery. This can be correlated with the nature of the surgical procedure (17, 18). Studies of sickle cell patients undergoing elective cholecystectomy demonstrate a lower transfusion requirement when the procedure is performed by laparoscopy. This cannot be explained simply on the basis of the amount of blood lost. It reflects a significant difference between laparotomy and laparoscopic cholecystectomy in stimulating cytokine suppression of erythropoiesis.

Even in normal individuals, the nature of the surgery is a significant factor in determining not only the severity of postoperative anemia but also the rate of recovery. When a procedure results in a minimal or modest anemia, it is readily compensated for by a shift in the oxygen dissociation curve; erythropoietin levels and red blood cell production do not show dramatic increases (19). Any patient whose postoperative hematocrit is above 30–33% can be expected to exhibit this pattern of response. Furthermore, their recovery to baseline hematocrit can take many weeks and is not greatly accelerated by the administration of iron or vitamin supplements. This is true even when iron studies demonstrate a postoperative fall in the serum iron and TIBC levels.

Patients undergoing major elective surgery such as a hip replacement or coronary artery bypass graft (CABG) surgery can show a distinctly different response. First, a more severe anemia can result; hematocrits fall to levels below 25–30% as a result of greater loss of blood during surgery. This provides a strong stimulus for erythropoietin production with a response similar to that observed for phlebotomy-induced anemia (20). Red cell production as measured from the reticulocyte count and rate of hematocrit recovery is equally good. Data from a study of a group of elective CABG patients are shown in Figure 36.3 (21). After surgery, there was an immediate rise in erythropoietin and a reticulocyte hematocrit response, suggesting marrow production levels greater than two to three times basal.

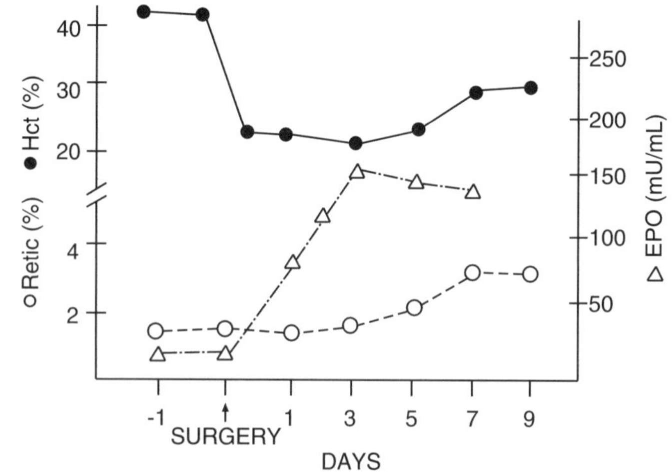

Figure 36.3. Measurements of serial hematocrits (●, Hct), reticulocyte counts (○, Retic), and serum erythropoietin levels (△, EPO) in the week after coronary artery bypass surgery demonstrate a brisk response of serum erythropoietin levels in the first 3–5 days after surgery. This is a response comparable with that observed in patients with moderately severe blood loss anemia.

CABG patients are able to repair their anemia after surgery despite evidence of cytokine-induced impairment of iron supply (3). Measurements of serum iron during the immediate postoperative period demonstrate a fall to iron-deficient levels (author's personal observation). How then does the marrow achieve a several-fold increase in production? The answer to this question may come from two clinical observations. First, therapeutic studies using recombinant erythropoietin in patients with inflammatory anemias have shown that the cytokine-induced block in iron supply can be overcome by very high levels of erythropoietin. A second explanation is that the bleeding into tissues during surgery, especially the loss of blood into the mediastinum, pleural, and pericardial cavities, may provide a unique source of iron to support erythropoiesis. Similar to the patient with a well-compensated hemolytic anemia, the internal breakdown of red blood cells may be a more effective source of iron than either reticuloendothelial iron stores or absorbed iron. As illustrated by patients with hereditary spherocytosis, red cell hemolysis by itself will drive an increased rate of red blood cell production even when the anemia is mild and erythropoietin levels are near basal levels.

EVALUATION OF ANEMIA SEVERITY

The decision to transfuse a patient for a postoperative anemia should ideally be based on a direct measure of oxygen supply to vital organs. Unfortunately, this is not clinically feasible. Rather, the clinician must evaluate the physiological responses of the patient to predict the need for red blood cell transfusion. As previously discussed, mild to moderate anemia is usually compensated for by a shift in the hemoglobin-oxygen dissociation curve (10, 11). The impact of more severe anemia may be modulated by increased tissue perfusion due to an increase in cardiac output, a decrease in peripheral vascular resistance, and a decrease in whole blood viscosity (22–24). However, there are recognized limits to this type of compensation according to the age and disease status of the patient.

To determine an individual patient's need for transfusion, the bedside evaluation should look carefully at both heart and brain function. Normally, the heart can adapt to anemia by increasing coronary blood flow, sufficient to support the extra work that goes into increases in stroke volume and rate (22–25). Myocardial oxygen consumption has been shown to increase in the face of anemia. Of course, there are limits to this response. In animal studies, electrocardiogram changes, including ST segment changes and increased myocardial lactate production, are observed when the hemoglobin falls below 5 g/dL (26). These changes can occur earlier (hemoglobin levels of 7–10 g/dL) in animals on beta blockers or who have experimental coronary stenoses. It makes sense, therefore, that patients with coronary artery disease, ventricular hypertrophy, or beta blockade will be less able to compensate for severe anemia and require earlier transfusion (26, 27).

Evaluation of tissue perfusion can be used to assess the adequacy of oxygen delivery. The patient's mental status examination is probably the best measure of oxygen supply to a vital organ. Significant changes in brain blood flow and blood oxygen content (anemia or hypoxia) result in increasing disorientation to the point of coma. With severe chronic anemia (hematocrits less than 15–20%), patients complain of throbbing headaches, inability to concentrate, insomnia, and nightmares. On physical examination, they can exhibit signs of brain edema, including papilledema and retinal hemorrhages.

Redistribution of blood flow to key organs is another sign of anemia severity. It is reflected by reduced perfusion of skin and distal extremities. Despite forceful bounding pulses, patients have cool pale extremities. Cyanosis of the distal extremities is not a sign of anemia. Even though the arterial venous oxygen difference dramatically widens as the patient becomes more anemic, the fall in the hemoglobin level and the increased rate of blood flow counterbalance the increase in deoxyhemoglobin levels.

Because of the complexity of the evaluation, clinicians have long looked for a recommended transfusion trigger for the surgical setting (24, 28–30). In past practice, a hemoglobin of 10 g/dL or hematocrit of 30% was commonly used as a threshold trigger for preoperative transfusion. This was carried over into the postoperative period where clinicians believed a higher hemoglobin level would translate into better wound healing (31). This concept of a "one shoe fits all" transfusion threshold is no longer acceptable. A number of clinical studies have now looked at postoperative mortality and morbidity in patients who are operated on with hematocrits below 30%. Perhaps the best was the study by Carson et al. (32) of 125 patients who refused blood transfusion for religious reasons. They found that healthy patients with preoperative hemoglobin levels above 8 g/dL and surgical blood losses below 500 mL did well without transfusion. At the same time, mortality increased significantly at lower hemoglobin levels. A third of patients with hemoglobins between 6 and 8 g/dL died and more than 60% of patients with preoperative hemoglobins below 6 g/dL did not survive. Therefore, a hemoglobin of 8 g/dL or hematocrit of 25% might be considered a better "lowest" threshold number for patients without comorbid illness, especially cardiovascular disease.

The concept of a threshold trigger must be modified when the patient is elderly or has other disease (33, 34). This applies both in the preparation of the patient for surgery and in the immediate postoperative period. Greatest emphasis needs to be given to factors such as the patient's age and the presence of pulmonary or cardiovascular disease. A number of the more important clinical findings that would set the transfusion trigger to a higher level are listed in Table 36.4 (30). These can be used together with the bedside evaluation of the patient to guide a transfusion decision.

DIAGNOSIS OF A PERSISTENT POSTOPERATIVE ANEMIA

Whereas the primary emphasis in the immediate postoperative period is to maintain tissue oxygen supply by appropriate transfusion, a persistent anemia in the weeks after surgery should be fully evaluated. Successful therapy will depend on identifying the specific cause of the anemia. The approach to the evaluation is best organized around the functional classification of anemia (13). This uses the complete blood count (CBC), reticulocyte count, and iron studies to determine whether the anemia is caused by a failure in marrow proliferation, a defect in erythroid marrow maturation, or increased adult red blood cell destruction. Based on this distinction, specific laboratory tests can be ordered to identify the underlying etiology.

The circumstance of the development of the anemia can be an obvious clue to its etiology. Patients who are otherwise healthy with a normal CBC before surgery would not be expected to demonstrate an increase in red blood cell hemolysis or the sudden reduction in red blood cell production (aplastic crisis) observed in patients with congenital hemolytic anemias. Instead, a persistent postoperative anemia most likely reflects a cytokine suppression erythropoiesis (an inflammatory anemia) or deficiency in a key nutrient such as iron or folic acid. The likelihood of an inflammatory anemia is obviously increased in the patient whose postoperative course is complicated by infection or marked tissue inflammation. Iron deficiency is likely in patients who experience losses of large volumes of blood and/or had limited iron stores before surgery. Children, adolescents, and women in general have lower levels of reticuloendothelial iron stores available for recovery. In fact, when surgical blood loss exceeds 500 mL, these individuals can be expected to develop iron-deficient erythropoiesis postoperatively. Patients with congenital hemolytic anemias—hereditary spherocytosis, sickle cell anemia, and thalassemia—are at risk of not only developing a more severe anemia immediately after surgery but also having a prolonged postoperative recovery. The most immediate threat is the combination of increased hemolysis of circulating red cells together with the cytokine suppression of new red blood cell production. If for any reason, the latter persists, the shortened survival of their circulating red blood cells will result in a severe anemia.

TABLE 36.4. CLINICAL FACTORS THAT SUPPORT TRANSFUSION TO A HIGHER HEMATOCRIT/HEMOGLOBIN

Transfusion trigger
Hematocrit/hemoglobin <25–30%/8–10 g/dL
Young age
Normal cardiovascular status
Absence of pulmonary disease
Hematocrit/hemoglobin >30–33%/10–11 g/dL
Older age
Cardiac disease, especially coronary artery disease, decreased ventricular function
Cerebrovascular disease
Pulmonary disease with hypoxia
Chronic illness with poor nutrition

A diagnostic algorithm for the laboratory evaluation of postoperative anemia is illustrated in Figure 36.4. The CBC, smear morphology, and reticulocyte count are used to separate those anemias that result from a failure in marrow proliferation or defect in precursor maturation from those with a high level of red blood cell production, typical of a hemolytic anemia. Iron studies, including measurements of the serum iron, TIBC, and serum ferritin, are then used to identify patients with iron deficiency secondary to blood loss or cytokine-induced inflammatory anemia. Similarly, measurements of serum folic acid and vitamin B_{12} can help identify the specific cause of a maturation disorder. In both situations, a bone marrow aspirate and biopsy can provide important information regarding marrow cellularity, cell development, and the status of reticuloendothelial iron stores. If marrow damage is suspected, the marrow biopsy is an essential part of the evaluation.

Several factors influence the success of an anemia workup. First, diagnostic changes in red blood cell morphology, reticulocyte production, and iron studies will depend on both the duration and severity of the anemia. Very mild anemias can be difficult to evaluate and, despite a full laboratory evaluation, can remain a diagnostic dilemma (35). At the same time, a severe anemia that is present for more than a week should show changes in these laboratory measurements. This is especially true for the most likely causes of postoperative anemia, including surgical blood loss, iron deficiency, and cytokine suppression of erythropoiesis (Fig. 36.4).

In those patients who have a protracted postoperative

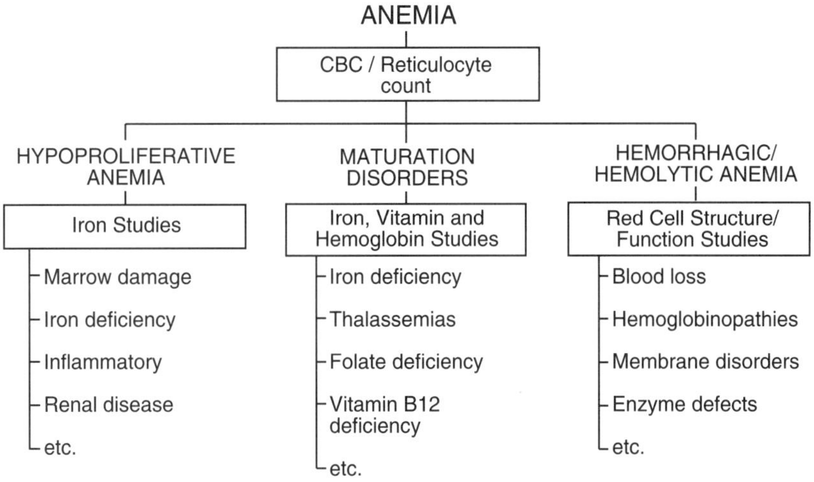

Figure 36.4. A severe anemia present for more than a week will show characteristic changes in a number of laboratory measurements. The CBC and reticulocyte count can be used to distinguish between those anemias that fall in the hypoproliferative category from anemias secondary to a maturation disorder, hemorrhage, or hemolysis. This then permits a further differential diagnosis using studies of iron supply, hemoglobin structure, vitamin supply, and red blood cell metabolism and membrane structure.

course complicated by infection and/or organ failure, other factors play a role in producing anemia (35). In this situation, the differential diagnosis widens to include increased red blood cell destruction and loss of erythropoietin production in patients with severe renal failure, ongoing blood loss, and a greater chance of iron and folic acid deficiency. In the latter case, patients with congenital hemolytic anemias are at high risk for the development of folic acid deficiency. Even though tube feedings and total parenteral nutrition (TPN) fluids are supplemented with folic acid, hemolytic anemia patients can require additional folate to support their very high levels of red blood cell production. In patients who are critically ill, repeated transfusion is usually required to keep the hematocrit above 30% to guarantee tissue oxygen delivery. This will, of course, tend to suppress the patient's physiological response to anemia. Moreover, the presence of large numbers of transfused cells in circulation will overshadow changes in red blood cell indices and cell morphology. This adds to the complexity of the evaluation.

Repeated transfusions can also be complicated by acute transfusion reactions or, in the occasional patient, the development of antibodies to minor blood group antigens. These may be detected as a part of the cross-matching procedure or as a result of a sudden drop in the patient's hematocrit secondary to rapid removal of the transfused cells from circulation. Even when antibodies are not detected, the critically ill patient may show a lower than predicted hematocrit increment after transfusion and a shortened survival of the transfused cells. Renal failure, sepsis, widespread malignancy, and severe tissue destruction are all associated with reductions in red blood cell life span of both the patient's own and transfused cells. Disseminated intravascular coagulation, in addition to encouraging additional blood loss, can result in fragmentation hemolysis of circulating cells.

Finally, the sensitivity of patients with congenital hemolytic anemias or inherited defects of red blood cell structure or metabolism needs to be kept in mind. Hereditary spherocytosis, elliptocytosis, thalassemia, sickle cell anemia, and other hemoglobinopathies and red cell enzyme deficiency states are the most common examples of inherited hemolytic anemias. Patients with autoimmune hemolytic anemias may also present with high levels of red blood cell production. All such patients are at risk for both increased red blood cell hemolysis and acute shutdown of red cell production with surgery. Glucose-6-phosphate dehydrogenase (G6PD) deficiency is another common inherited defect of red blood cell metabolism. The red blood cells of the G6PD-deficient individual are very sensitive to exposure to oxidant drugs or any acute systemic illness. Acute hemolysis with hematocrit falls of from 10 to 15% or more are commonly seen with acute illness, drug exposure, or surgery.

TREATMENT OF POSTOPERATIVE ANEMIAS

TRANSFUSION THERAPY

Management of anemia during the immediate postoperative period is targeted toward maintaining tissue oxygen delivery. Depending on the age and disease status of the patient, sufficient red blood cells should be transfused to increase the hematocrit to levels of 25–30% or higher (28, 30, 31, 33, 34). Young healthy individuals and patients with long-standing compensated anemias may tolerate hematocrits in the range of 20–25% if the postoperative course is uncomplicated. However, such patients should be closely monitored for evidence of poor tissue perfusion or cardiac decompensation.

Sickle cell anemia patients present a unique transfusion problem. Major surgery can be expected to not only increase the severity of their anemia but also bring on a severe, even life-threatening, sickle cell crisis (36). This reflects the exquisite sensitivity of these patients to worsening anemia, hypoxia, and acid base or fluid balance shifts. Any one or a combination of these factors will increase the number of circulating sickle cells and initiate vascular plugging, thrombosis, and even widespread disseminated intravascular coagulation. Vital organs including the lungs, kidneys, brain, and heart are at great risk of infarction during and after surgery.

To prevent the induction of a sickle cell crisis, homozygous sickle patients should be preoperatively transfused to increase the hematocrit to 35–40% (36). The dilution of circulating sickle cells with normal red blood cells has the effect of preventing the log-jamming of sickle cells in the microvasculature and will protect the patient from a sickle crisis. At the same time, the patient is still susceptible to an increased rate of red cell hemolysis after surgery together with a reduction in red blood cell production. It is important, therefore, to closely monitor the sickle cell anemia patient after surgery and to provide additional red blood cell transfusions to keep the hematocrit above 35%.

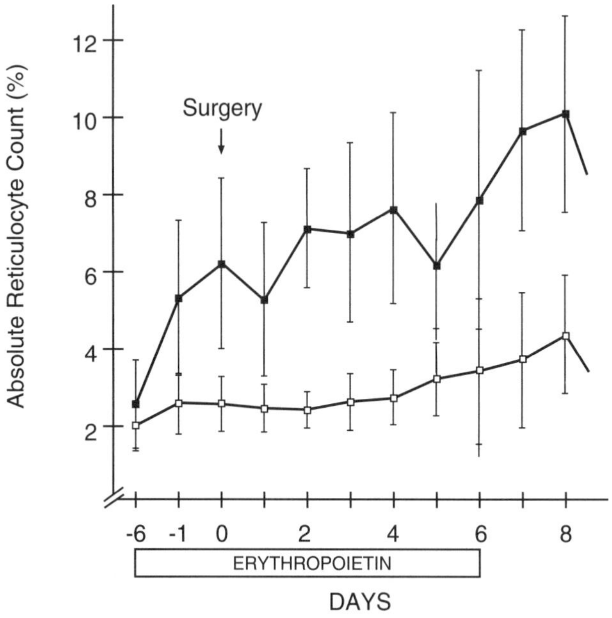

Figure 36.5. Serial reticulocyte count measurements in coronary bypass patients receiving recombinant erythropoietin perioperatively (■) demonstrate a significant increase in the absolute reticulocyte count both before and immediately after surgery. In contrast, control patients (□) demonstrate little change in the absolute reticulocyte count until 4–6 days postoperatively.

ERYTHROPOIETIN THERAPY

With the advent of recombinant erythropoietin as a pharmacological agent capable of stimulating erythropoiesis, a number of investigators have studied its use during the perioperative period. The principal target has been the ability to reduce the number of units of blood transfused during and after a major orthopedic or cardiovascular surgical procedure (21, 37, 38). Studies have also looked at the ability of erythropoietin to increase the storage of autologous blood in the weeks before elective surgery (39–42). Both models have shown the effectiveness of the hormone in stimulating erythropoiesis. At least two major studies of CABG patients have reported a reduction in the number of homologous red blood cell transfusions in individuals receiving recombinant erythropoietin perioperatively.

The impact of erythropoietin given during the perioperative period is illustrated in Figure 36.5. When given daily in a dose of 150–300 units/kg/day beginning the week before an elective procedure, there is a detectable rise in the reticulocyte count by the fourth day of therapy and a modest increase in the hematocrit by the day of surgery. If the erythropoietin is then continued during the first week to 10 days after surgery, the reticulocyte count continues to rise throughout the course of therapy. This is a different pattern from that seen in untreated patients. The latter demonstrate a decrease in the reticulocyte count immediately after surgery followed by a more gradual increase between days 5 and 10. The performance of the hematocrit in each group of patients correlates with the reticulocyte production measurement. Patients receiving erythropoietin exhibit less severe postoperative anemia and a 5–6% hematocrit rise by the 10th postoperative day. In contrast, control patients are more anemic with a somewhat slower hematocrit recovery despite the transfusion of 2 units of red blood cells on the average.

There are obvious limits to this use of erythropoietin. For proven effectiveness, it must be given for 5–7 days before surgery. This restricts its use to elective procedures where major blood loss is predictable. If erythropoietin administration is delayed until after surgery, there would appear to be little advantage over the natural stimulus of the severe anemia. In the CABG patient study, treated and untreated patients demonstrate comparable hematocrit recoveries by the fourth to sixth week. The cost of erythropoietin therapy is also an issue. Currently, a 10-day course of recombinant erythropoietin at a dose of 150 units/kg/day or higher would be considerably more expensive than the cost of red blood cell transfusion. If erythropoietin is used to improve the preoperative storage of autologous blood, the problem of increased cost will be even greater (43, 44).

IRON THERAPY

Attention must be given to the iron and vitamin requirements of the patient during the postoperative period (35). Faced with significant surgical blood loss, most patients, especially women and children, will require iron supplementation to support red blood cell production and guarantee a full hematocrit recovery. If the postoperative course is uncomplicated, oral iron supplementation with a standard oral iron preparation should be initiated once the patient has returned to a normal diet. If the anemia is severe (hematocrit less than 30%), a full dose of 150–200 mg (2–3 mg/kg) of elemental iron per day should be given to maximize iron delivery to the marrow. This dose can be reduced by half for children who weigh from 15 to 30 kg; infants and smaller children should receive a daily dose of 5 mg/kg. In the adult, this dose translates into a single tablet of ferrous sulfate three to four times a day taken between meals and at bedtime. Patients who are relatively iron deficient will absorb 20–30% of the administered dose, providing sufficient iron to support a red blood cell production level of two to three times normal.

Oral iron administration can be associated with significant side effects. A quarter or more of individuals given a full treatment dose will have gastrointestinal distress including abdominal pain, nausea, vomiting, constipation, or diarrhea. These symptoms can be severe enough to require a reduction in dosage or, in some cases, administration with meals, even though this reduces absorption efficiency. Once the patient's hematocrit increases to levels above 35%, the oral iron dose should be reduced to one tablet once or twice a day. This recognizes the fact that erythropoietin stimulation and red blood cell production naturally decline as the hematocrit/hemoglobin rises and that there is a concomitant reduction in iron absorption. The lower oral iron dose will have the added benefit of increasing compliance and guaranteeing the patient will remain on iron supplements for at least 6 months to rebuild reticuloendothelial iron stores.

Patients who have undergone gastric surgery or who are achlorhydric will demonstrate poor absorption of both food and medicinal iron. Some will be unable to remove the tablet coat and will pass the intact iron tablets in their stool. These patients will need to be placed on iron elixir or receive parenteral iron therapy. The latter is the preferred therapy in patients with severe gastric intolerance or malabsorption secondary to widespread small bowel disease. Parenteral iron is given as iron dextran injection (InFe D), a ferric hydroxide-dextran compound that is taken up by reticuloendothelial cells where it is digested to release the iron for transport to the marrow. Although iron dextran can be injected intramuscularly, the preferred route of administration is by bolus intravenous injection of from 500 to 2000 mg. The total amount required by the patient can be calculated using the formula body weight (kg) × 2.3 × (15 − patient's hemoglobin in g/dL + 500 mg (for stores) = total dose (mg).

Considerable care must be taken when using intravenous iron dextran. Patients who are allergic to the dextran portion of the compound can experience a life-threatening anaphylactic reaction. Therefore, the patient should be questioned regarding past exposure to parenteral iron or dextran and any infusion should be preceded by an initial test dose. If the patient is to receive a single treatment dose of 500–1000 mg or more, the iron dextran should be diluted in 250 mg of 0.9% sodium chloride solution for slow infusion over 60 minutes. At the beginning, the patient should be given less than 0.5 mL of this solution intravenously followed by a 10-minute period of close observation. The blood pressure should be monitored and the patient observed for any signs of itching, shortness of breath, chest pain, or back pain. If the patient tolerates the test dose, the infusion can be completed with continued close observation and frequent measurements of the blood pressure. If the patient becomes hypotensive or exhibits signs of cardiopulmonary distress, the infusion should be stopped immediately.

Although iron dextran can be given by intramuscular injection, it can result in significant skin staining and poor absorption. This is especially true for bedridden patients. Moreover, the intramuscular route does not avoid the issue of anaphylaxis or the serum sickness-like reaction seen in many patients as a late complication. In addition, intramuscular iron dextran can be administered only in 2-mL aliquots per injection site. Because the preparation contains 50 mg of elemental iron per mL, the intramuscular administration of 1000 mg of iron dextran will require 10 injections. Finally, it must be emphasized that two different parenteral iron injections are available. One contains 0.5% phenol for intramuscular use, whereas the other is phenol-free for intravenous administration. The phenol-containing preparation should never be given intravenously because it will be extremely painful and produce a local phlebitis.

VITAMIN THERAPY

Folic acid and vitamin B_{12} are two essential vitamins required by the erythroid marrow (35). Normal individuals have sufficient stores of both vitamins to sustain increased levels of red blood cell production for weeks if not months.

However, patients with gastrointestinal disorders, especially disorders of the small bowel that result in malabsorption, and patients with poor dietary intake (starvation, alcoholism, etc.) can present for surgery with such limited stores that they are at risk for developing a deficiency during the immediate postoperative period. Hemolytic anemia patients have an increased requirement for folic acid and therefore will develop folate deficiency within days of any decrease in dietary intake. These individuals require medicinal amounts of folic acid to sustain their high levels of red blood cell production.

Although a folic acid-deficiency anemia can be diagnosed from a measurement of the serum folate level, there is no "blood test" to measure the amount of liver folate stores. It is good practice, therefore, to anticipate and treat a possible deficiency in any patient who may be at risk. This includes all hemolytic anemia patients, alcoholics, starved or cachectic patients, or individuals with known small bowel disease. Folic acid can be given orally or by injection. If the patient is on TPN, folate supplementation is standard. However, the amount added to the TPN fluids may need to be increased if the patient has a very high level of red blood cell production, as seen with hemolytic anemias. Once the patient is back on a normal diet, the folate can be given as folic acid tablets as a single 1-mg tablet daily or for hemolytic anemia patients twice a day.

Vitamin B_{12} deficiency is of much less concern in younger otherwise healthy patients. However, similar to folic acid, vitamin B_{12} deficiency can occur in patients with autoantibodies to intrinsic factor (pernicious anemia), small bowel disease with ileal involvement, and as a result of gastric or small bowel surgery. Known pernicious anemia patients are at risk even if they are on what appears to be adequate vitamin B_{12} maintenance therapy. Surgery can represent an increased demand for vitamin B_{12} that exceeds the patient's maintenance therapy and available stores. Elderly patients undergoing surgery may, despite an apparent normal CBC, have little or no vitamin B_{12} stores. They will be at risk for deficiency state if the postoperative recovery is prolonged or there are complications.

The elderly and pernicious anemia patients should be evaluated for vitamin B_{12} deficiency if they develop a persistent anemia after surgery. Because the peripheral blood smear and marrow morphology is slow to evolve, measurements of serum vitamin B_{12} level and/or serum methylmalonic acid should be performed. If the suspicion is high, vitamin B_{12} therapy should not be delayed. It is better to err on the side of overtreatment than to allow the patient to run the risk of developing a more severe anemia or neurological signs of vitamin B_{12} deficiency. Therefore, once serum is collected to measure vitamin B_{12} and methylmalonic acid levels, a treatment dose of 100 μg of vitamin B_{12} should be administered by subcutaneous or intramuscular injection on a daily basis for 1–2 weeks.

Deficiencies of other vitamins or minerals are far less common. Pyridoxine deficiency is an issue in patients who receive the antituberculosis drugs, isoniazid and pyrazinamide. These patients should be routinely treated with a daily oral dose of 50 mg of pyridoxine. Interruption of the pyridoxine will result in the gradual evolution of a distal neuropathy and a ring sideroblastic anemia. Riboflavin deficiency has been reported in association with severe starvation and prolonged illness. It is very rare. Copper deficiency has been observed in patients who have undergone intestinal bypass surgery and in patients on high doses of zinc. It was observed early in the development of parenteral nutrition therapy and is the basis for the routine supplementation of TPN fluids with copper. Copper deficiency is associated with a microcytic anemia due to its role in iron transport and the formation of heme by mitochondria.

REFERENCES

1. Hillman RS. Acute blood loss anemia In: Beutler E, Lichtman MA, Coller BS, Kipps TJ, eds. Hematology. 5th ed. New York: McGraw-Hill, 1995:704–708.
2. Howarth S, Sharpey-Schafer EP. Low blood pressure phases following hemorrhage. Lancet 1947;1:19.
3. Theyl RA, Tuohy GF. Hemodynamics and blood volume during operation with ether anesthesia and unreplaced blood loss. Anesthesiology 1964;25:6.
4. Adamson J, Hillman RS. Blood volume and plasma protein replacement following acute blood loss in normal man. JAMA 1968;205:609–612.
5. Ebert RV, Stead EA Jr, Gibson JG II. Response of normal subjects to acute blood loss. Arch Intern Med 1941;68:578.
6. Maier RV, Carrico CJ. Developments in the resuscitation of critically ill surgical patients. Adv Surg 1986;19:271–328.
7. Shine KI, Kuhn M, Young LS, Tillisch JH. Aspects of the management of shock. Ann Intern Med 1980;93:723–734.
8. Lamke LO, Liljedal SO. Plasma volume changes after infusion of various plasma expanders. Resuscitation 1977;74:1486–1489.
9. Hutchison JL, Feedman JO, Richards BA, Burgen ASV. Plasma volume expansion and reactions after infusion of autologous and nonautologous plasma in mass. J Lab Clin Med 1960;50:734.
10. Finch CA, Lenfant C. Oxygen transport in man. N Engl J Med 1972; 286:407–415.
11. Torrance J, Jacobs P, Restrepo A. Intra-erythrocytic adaptation to anemia. N Engl J Med 1970;283:165–169.
12. Hillman RS. Characteristics of marrow production and reticulocyte maturation in normal man in response to anemia. J Clin Invest 1969; 48:443–453.
13. Hillman RS, Finch CA. Red cell manual. 7th ed. Philadelphia: FA Davis, 1996.
14. Krantz SB. Erythropoietin. Blood 1991;77:419–434.
15. Hillman RS, Henderson PA. Control of marrow production by the level of iron supply. J Clin Invest 1969;48:454–460.

16. Means RT, Krantz SB. Progress in understanding the pathogenesis of the anemia of chronic disease. Blood 1992;30:1639–1647.
17. Gibson TJ, O'Dell RF, Cathcart RS, Rambo WM. Treatment of cholethiasis in patients with sickle cell anemia. South Med J 1979;72:391–392.
18. Rudolph R, Williams JS. Cholecystectomy in patients with sickle cell disease: experience in a regional hospital in Georgia. J Natl Med Assoc 1992;84:692–696.
19. Levine EA, Rosen AL, Sehgal LR, et al. Erythropoietin deficiency after coronary artery bypass procedures. Ann Thorac Surg 1991;51:764–766.
20. Goodnough LT, Price TH, Parvin CA, et al. Erythropoietin response to anaemia is not altered by surgery or recombinant human erythropoietin therapy. Br J Haematol 1994;87:695–699.
21. D'Ambra MN, Finlayson DC, Gray R, et al. The effect of perioperative administration of recombinant human erythropoietin in coronary artery bypass graft patients: a multicenter double blind, placebo controlled trial. Anesthesiology 1992;77:A159.
22. Woodson RD, Auerbach S. Effect of increased oxygen affinity and anemia on cardiac output and its distribution. J. Appl Physiol 1982;53:1299–1306.
23. Murray JF, Escobar E, Rapaport E. Effects of blood viscosity on hemodynamic responses in acute normovolemic anemia. Am J Physiol 1969; 216:638–642.
24. Kowalyshyn TJ, Prager D, Young J. A review of the present status of preoperative hemoglobin requirements. Anesth Analg 1972;51:75–79.
25. Jan K, Shu C. Effect of hematocrit variations on coronary hemodynamics and oxygen utilization. Am J Physiol 1977;233:H106–113.
26. Brazier J, Cooper N, Maloney JV, et al. The adequacy of myocardial oxygen delivery in acute normovolemic anemia. Surgery 1974;75:508–516.
27. Hagl S, Heimisch W, Meisner H, et al. The effect of hemodilution on regional myocardial function in the presence of coronary stenosis. Basic Res Cardiol 1977;72:344–364.
28. Allen JB, Allen FB. The minimum acceptable level of hemoglobin. Int Anesthesiol Clin 1982;20:1–22.
29. Stehling LC, Ellison N, Faust RJ, Grotta AW, Moyers JR. A survey of transfusion practices among anesthesiologists. Vox Sang 1987;52:60–62.
30. Carson JL, Willett LR. Is a hemoglobin of 10 g/dL required for surgery. Med Clin North Am 1993;77:335–347.
31. Consensus conference. Perioperative red cell transfusion. JAMA 1988; 260:2700–2703.
32. Carson JL, Poses RM, Spence RK, et al. Anemia and surgery: The relationship between the severity of anemia and surgical mortality and morbidity. Lancet 1988;1:727–729.
33. Friedman BA, Burns TL, Schork MA. An analysis of blood transfusion of surgical patients by sex: a question for the transfusion triggers. Transfusion 1980;20:179–188.
34. Salem-Schatz SR, Avorn J, Soumerai SB. Influence of clinical knowledge, organizational context, and practice style on transfusion decision makeup. Implications for practice change strategies. JAMA 1990;264: 476–483.
35. Hillman RS, Ault KA. Hematology in clinical practice: a guide to diagnosis and management. New York: McGraw-Hill, 1994.
36. Steingart R. Management of patients with sickle cell disease. Med Clin North Am 1992;76:669–682.
37. Koyishi T, Ohbayashi T, Kaneko T, et al. Preoperative use of erythropoietin for cardiovascular operations in anemia. Ann Thorac Surg 1993; 56:101–103.
38. Canadian Orthopedic Perioperative Erythropoietin Group. Effectiveness of perioperative recombinant human erythropoietin in elective hip replacement. Lancet. 1993;341:1227–1232.
39. Goodnough LT, Rudnick S, Price TH, et al. Increased collection of autologous blood preoperative with recombinant human erythropoietin therapy. N Engl J Med 1989;321:1163–1168.
40. Goodnough LT, Price TH, Fiedman KD, et al. A phase III trial of recombinant human erythropoietin therapy in non-anemic orthopedic patients subjected to aggressive autologous blood phlebotomy: dose, response, toxicity, and efficacy. Transfusion 1994;34:66–71.
41. Mercuriali F, Gualtieri G, Swigaglia L, et al. Use of recombinant human erythropoietin to assist autologous blood donation by anemic rheumatoid arthritis patients undergoing major orthopaedic surgery. Transfusion 1994;34:501–506.
42. Hayashi J, Kumon K, Takamashi S, et al. Subcutaneous administration of recombinant human erythropoietin before cardiac surgery: a double-blind, multicenter trial in Japan. Transfusion 1994;34:142–146.
43. Birkmeyer JD, Aubuchon JP, Littenberg B, et al. The costs and benefits of preoperative autologous blood donation in elective coronary bypass surgery. Ann Thorac Surg 1994;57:161–168.
44. Birkmeyer JD, Goodnough LT, Aubuchon JP, Noordsij P, Littenberg B. The cost-effectiveness of preoperative autologous blood donation in total hip and knee replacement. Transfusion 1993;33:544–551.

Chapter 37

The Transfusion Decision

BRUCE D. SPIESS
RICHARD B. COUNTS
STEVEN A. GOULD

INTRODUCTION

The decision to transfuse a patient, with either a red cell product or coagulation component, should not be taken lightly. This constitutes a summary chapter, and the decision to transfuse an individual patient should involve a great deal of information from this text. Transfusion medicine is changing very rapidly. The risks of viral transmission are the lowest they have ever been in the history of blood banking (1–3). Yet they are not zero and never will be (1, 4–6). Allogeneic blood still carries a wide range of other potential problems and risks (7, 8). Therefore, although the blood supply is the safest it has ever been, there is little reason to liberalize transfusion practices. Transfusion, like all treatments in medicine, is the culmination of a risk:benefit ratio. The treating clinician must weigh the risks and assess the benefits before proceeding. All too often in the perioperative period, the patient has been rendered unable to participate in any part of the transfusion decision (due to anesthesia and sedation). Therefore, unlike many other therapeutic decisions, the perioperative transfusion decision may be made without patient input. Without such patient input, one would expect that the transfusion decision would be made only after considerable thought and contemplation. All too often, I have observed little thought involved in that decision.

THE RISKS

The risk:benefit ratio of transfusion has been extensively discussed in the chapters on infectious transmission and noninfectious risks of transfusion (chapters 3, 7, 37). These risks pertain to infectious risks to all allogeneic products that have not undergone heat treatment. Therefore, all red cell products, whole blood, fresh-frozen plasma (FFP), platelet units, and cryoprecipitate carry such risks. Some factor concentrates, antithrombin III, and human albumin may be virus-free, because they have undergone pasteurization. Additives to allogeneic units rendering them free of viral transmission are experimental.

The risks of viral transmission appear to be changing every year and as such they are improving. Greater than 90% of posttransfusion hepatitis is due to hepatitis C virus. In the 1980s, as many as 10% of transfusion recipients were sero-converting (9, 10). Today the per-unit incidence of hepatitis C virus sero-conversion is 0.03% (1). Those data are the best yet reported in the literature and come from Johns Hopkins Medical Center. No other reports have since been published either confirming or bettering that statistic. It may well be that the incidence is even lower because of the introduction of other surrogate testing for liver dysfunction. However, before practitioners are tempted to liberalize our transfusion triggers, some reality should be discussed. This is a single report. Pockets of higher exposure rate and thus early viremia may exist within the United States than what occurs in the donor population for this major academic medical center. Also, this report represents the best data from one of the finest health care centers in the world. The remainder of the world may not be able to match such statistics. At the recent World Congress of Anesthesiologists, reports on transmission of hepatitis virus and acquired immunodeficiency syndrome (AIDS) were forthcoming from central Africa and Australia, Western Europe, and the United States. The variability was astounding, and in some of the African countries, levels of viral transmission for hepatitis and AIDS may well exceed 40%. Therefore, those reading this textbook should not be hasty to judge that all blood sources have the same low risk for hepatitis as seen in the report from Johns Hopkins. That report alone should not trigger a liberalization of transfusion.

The risk of AIDS transmission has changed the way transfusion medicine is practiced worldwide. Its outbreak into the industrialized world has caused the lay public to pressure the medical community into enhanced testing for all viral illness in transfusion. Scandals in France have led to the imprisonment of officials from blood banks. Indeed, consumer confidence in Western Europe for transfusion products has created a crisis of scarcity of donors. This may not make rational sense, but it has occurred. Once again, the risks of viral transmission are the lowest they have ever been. Various reports over the last 5 years have set the risk of AIDS in the United States to be between 1 in 450,000 and 1 in 660,000. A most recent report puts that number at approximately 1 in 1,000,000 per unit of transfused blood (3, 4, 11, 12). But once again, even with other enhanced screening tests such as human immunodeficiency virus type 1 (HIV-1) antigen, parts of the world where HIV is prevalent should be at much higher risk for transmission of AIDS by blood transfusion.

These two viral entities, hepatitis and AIDS, may give the clinician an impression that the risk of viral transmission is so remote that in his or her individual patient they can be ignored and transfusion can go on without so much as a thought of such transmission. Indeed, some practitioners have voiced feelings that transfusion triggers could be liberalized. Some other statistics should be examined before embracing such thinking. Twenty-two million units of blood components are transfused per year in the United States (13). Probably 60% of these units are transfused in the perioperative period, with anesthesiologists and surgeons making the transfusion decision most often. The mean number of units transfused per patient is in excess of 5.4 units (14). Although that data may be somewhat dated by now, it probably holds true, or the number may be even higher as the driving force behind the ever-increasing use of blood components is the inception of extremely complex and hemorrhagic surgery such as hepatic transplantation.

With each patient receiving an excess of six donor exposures and the risk of viral transmission being 0.03%, mathematics alone would suggest that the risk per patient might be much higher. Some estimates would put the patient population at risk for new viral infection (hepatitis) to be between 20,000 and 60,000 individuals. Some 25–50% of those infected will develop symptoms that may complicate their hospital course, and that 20% may go on to develop chronic active hepatitis, whereas some 10% will go on to fulminant liver failure, death, or require hepatic transplantation (15). The prevention of these awesome statistics starts with each individual clinician at the time of the decision to transfuse. Any movement toward liberalization of a transfusion trigger will certainly increase these numbers for patients contracting hepatitis and therefore increase the eventual hepatic failure/transplantation requirement and death rate.

The most common viral transmission occurring in allogeneic blood is that of cytomegalovirus (CMV). Most healthy patients have a subclinical flu-like response or no response at all to CMV. However, in immunocompromised hosts such as those undergoing organ transplantation or those having surgery after some type of chemotherapy, CMV can be catastrophic. Once again, the exact statistics are not known, and most clinicians focus on the risks of hepatitis and HIV when thinking about transfusion risks. In the future, CMV may well become a major risk factor of allogeneic blood transfusion. Finding CMV-negative blood may not always be possible if the medical community begins to demand it for many or most transfusions. Perhaps other pathogens may enter the blood supply and may be discovered to be transmissible. Although the focus has been on viral disease transmission in the United States, in other parts of the world, parasitic diseases are extremely important, including malaria and babesiosis.

Noninfectious risks, unlike viral transmission, have not substantially changed since the increased public awareness of transfusion risks. Minor transfusion reaction including urticaria, fever, and malaise still occurs quite frequently (16). Blood units may be wasted, medications given, and even workups for transfusion reaction begun because of such reactions. No one has studied the cost of such minor reactions. Under anesthesia, during surgery, and often in the immediate postoperative period, patients are not able to express the sensory complaints associated with these reactions. Hives may be noticed by the observant anesthesiologist or surgeon, but more often than not, the patient is draped and large segments of skin are not readily available for inspection. Fever and hypotension, also nonspecific markers of transfusion reaction, are not infrequent and nonspecific events during anesthesia and surgery and may or may not create a link in the clinician's mind with transfusion. If the anesthesiologists and surgeons do make a temporal link between a blood transfusion and changes in the vital signs, very often the blood transfusion will be halted. There are no data on how often this results in aborted surgery or other interventions. However, in awake nonoperated patients, the incidence of febrile or minor transfusion reaction may be as high as 10%. Nonhemolytic (1–5%) and the feared event of hemolytic transfusion reaction (1–6000 to 1–33,000) can be difficult to discern in the anesthetized or heavily sedated patient (16, 17). Vital signs change and hematuria may be unreliable or caused by a wide range of events unlinked to transfusion.

Immunosuppression is almost certainly a response to allogeneic transfusion (8, 18–21). The data still garner some controversy, and the extent of its impact on immediate hospital course, prevalence of other opportunistic infections, and recurrence of cancer is still debated (22, 23). However, it does appear that white cell transmission in red cell products and particularly platelets may be an etiology for the resulting immunosuppression. Clearly, higher rates of other infections have occurred in matched randomized studies using either allogeneic or autologous blood. Those receiving autologous blood had lower incidence of infection (19). All data gathered to date regarding reduction in viral transmission have no impact on the incidence of immunosuppression. The use of white cell filtering of red cell products may decrease the risk of immunosuppression in the future, but that technology is still being investigated, and indications and cost-effectiveness studies have not been done in enough situations to allow the medical community to widely embrace the technology.

Practices today are changing in response to market forces relating to costs. Blood transfusion may be costly, and modification of perioperative transfusion strategies can therefore influence costs. Data on the costs of components are now available. The per-unit cost of a red cell transfusion exceeds $155–260 (24–26). This takes into account not only the unit charge, but also risks of transfusion. We have no way of estimating the costs of personnel time for administration, vigilance of complications, and workup. With an estimated 12 million red cell units transfused in the United States per year, that means a cost of over 2 billion dollars annually. The number could be easily twice that, and the cost of other components including coagulation components may be in the range of 1–2 billion dollars. Those are estimates of the cost of components alone. Other added costs such as intravenous sets, saline, blood warmers, medications to treat febrile reactions, works for blood reactions, and so on are not even attempted to be analyzed. Attempts at understanding the long-term cost impact of transfusion based on the risk of hepatitis and HIV transmission have put the added cost at roughly $5–10 per unit (26). This may seem small, but it is based solely on the latest and best statistics from the Johns Hopkins report. It is also based on a number of assumptions and may not include the costs of liver transplantation or terminal care for the few thousand patients who will require that in the future. Also, such analysis does not even attempt to comprehend the economic impact of lost wages, home health care, loss of insurance, divorce, or other lifestyle changes required by the acquisition of a chronic disease. So the estimates of added hidden amortized health care costs for hepatitis and HIV are woefully inadequate. Most importantly, these estimates of cost simply avoid analyzing any cost that they consider controversial, such as the cost of immunosuppression. It may well be that immunosuppression, by contributing to length of hospital stay, secondary adverse outcome, and some mortality, is by far the most costly to our medical economy. If, for example, we accept the data from orthopedic surgery and find that postoperative infection is three times as prevalent in patients transfused allogeneic blood as autologous blood, then it is entirely reasonable to consider that allogeneic blood transfusion may be a significant cause of morbidity in these total joint patients (19). The costs of CMV infection have not been estimated or investigated and they may be substantial because more transfusions are used for transplantations and immunocompromised host. So with 22 million units of blood components transfused per year and costs from blood acquisition, transfusion, infection, and so on, it may be that the true cost of transfusion in health care today is between 25 and 50 billion dollars annually.

The United States is not self-sufficient in its blood supply (27). Some 2% of blood is imported, primarily from Western Europe. With approximately 285,000 units per year being "purchased," assuming an acquisition cost of $50.00 (my best estimate) per unit, that represents a 14.5 million dollar overseas expenditure just to support the United States' blood needs. In other nations where blood is a paid donation, the cost to the economy may be high as well.

In today's capitated care environment, the expenses for blood transfusion come directly from the total reimbursement fee paid to the hospital and physicians. Therefore, attention to truly indicated cost effective and necessary transfusion is one method of saving a hospital or practice considerable financial resources.

THE BENEFITS

The above discussion has summarized some data on risks of transfusion and costs. As stated at the beginning of the chapter, the transfusion decision is a risk:benefit ratio. On one side, there are (yet incomplete and constantly changing) data regarding the risks of transfusion. However, surprisingly little of the benefits of transfusion are known. To most clinicians, it might seem intuitive that when needed, patients appropriately transfused have improved outcomes. Yet any literature in support of such claims is hard to find. Transfusions are given to prevent anticipated adverse events. For coagulation components, the prevention or treatment of excess coagulopathic bleeding is a very viable rationale for administration. However, the rationale for administration of red cells, although intuitively obvious, is very hard to prove.

The threat of diminished oxygen-carrying capacity and its physiological consequences were discussed in Chapters 3 and 21. Tissue oxygen delivery is dependent on cardiac output and blood oxygen-carrying capacity (a product of hemoglobin and its saturation plus physically dissolved oxygen in plasma). When reading historical literature regarding transfusion and outcome, the reader must be quite careful to separate hypovolemia from isolated euvolemic anemia. There is no doubt that anemia in the presence of hypovolemia is extremely detrimental. But anemia in the presence of normovolemia may be quite surprisingly tolerated (27–31). The lower limit of human tolerance for normovolemic anemia may be one definition of a transfusion trigger.

Unfortunately, the transfusion trigger (as just defined, the lower limit of euvolemic anemia) is not only not established in healthy humans but also probably extremely variable depending on disease states. In studies of acute anemia, the myocardium does not change its lactate flux until levels below 6g/dL are reached (31, 32). Heart failure does not occur until the hematocrit drops below 10% (3.3 g/dL hemoglobin) (33). In animal models with varying models of coronary artery stenosis, the lactate flux reaction to anemia is extremely variable. Levels of 17–47% hematocrit have demonstrated myocardial ischemia in animal models (34, 35). This author has experience with two patients, both young and healthy before surgery, who experienced extremely low levels of hematocrit and survived (one reached a hematocrit of 9% and the other, 3.6%). Both were Jehovah's Witnesses and refused blood transfusion, but with modern intensive care capabilities (surface cooling, mechanical respiration, extensive sedation, and muscle paralysis), neither developed myocardial, renal, or hepatic long-term sequelae of their severe euvolemic hemodilution. Therefore, what is the correct red cell transfusion trigger?

Clinical series with Jehovah's Witnesses and case reports show that levels of 6–8 g/dL of hemoglobin are routinely tolerated without any increase in mortality (28, 36, 37). In a review of multiple series of Jehovah's Witnesses involving some 1404 operations, lack of blood and exsanguination caused only 8 deaths or 0.6% and contributed to death in another 12 or 0.9% (28). That is a surprisingly small number. One might argue that those were all preventable by transfusion, but what we do not know is what other possible complications caused by transfusion were avoided in these 1404 operations (28). Another statistical analysis of the outcome of Jehovah's Witness operations found that hemoglobin was not a significant predictor of outcome unless it was below 3 g/dL (38). Yet another article reviewing some 61 independent reports of Jehovah's Witnesses found 23 deaths due to anemia (0.48%) (27). Compare that with the suspected and computed risk of hepatitis transfusion in all patients transfused (perhaps 0.1–1%). If withholding all blood transfusion causes a mortality rate of about 0.5% and using blood in those as presently used causes hepatitis in 0.1–1%, with multiple other morbidities and largely unknown mortalities, the issue of what is the appropriate transfusion trigger becomes even cloudier.

Patients with coronary artery disease or undergoing coronary artery bypass surgery might be considered to be at high risk for adverse outcomes of anemia and thus transfusion at a higher hematocrit than for healthy patients would therefore be warranted. One retrospective study with 27 patients (a small number) reveals that those undergoing peripheral vascular surgery were found to have a higher incidence of morbid events if their hematocrit dropped below 28% (14 patients) (39). Yet the group that had these events was older and underwent longer and more complex surgery than the other 13 patients without such events. Therefore, we are not able to conclude that in this high-risk patient group, a 28% or above hematocrit is necessarily the appropriate transfusion trigger. Another study of 30 patients who had multiple organ dysfunctions perioperatively showed no impact on oxygen consumption if their hemoglobin dropped below 10 g/dL (40).

Recent data from 2,202 patients undergoing coronary artery bypass grafting at 25 different centers throughout the United States actually showed a decrease in morbidity, myocardial infarction, and severe left ventricular dysfunction if their hematocrit was lower (less than 24%) on entry to the intensive care unit (41). Indeed intensive care unit entry hematocrit was the most important single variable in predicting adverse outcome in these patients, yet it was not confounded by patient risk or transfusion behavior. Also, in those with unstable angina, emergency surgery and reoperative coronary artery bypass (a high-risk group) showed substantially higher mortalities if their hematocrits were allowed to rise to 34% or greater as compared with 24% or below. Perhaps oxygen-carrying capacity and tissue oxygen delivery are not the only part of the story; rheology, platelet endothelial interactions, and other complex mechanisms may be at work. Once again, we are left with the question of when is it appropriate to transfuse and where should the transfusion trigger be in patients with preexisting disease. Various authors have discussed the state of the art in transfusion in subspecialty areas, and there are unique considerations in each of these presented. Yet not one can give a definitive answer of what is the appropriate transfusion trigger.

Indeed, to my knowledge, there is not a single publication in the world's literature supporting improved outcome with any given level of transfusion. There are no obvious clinical benefits that have been proven to transfusion, yet it seems so intuitively necessary. Wound healing has been promoted as better with transfusion and higher hematocrits, yet fibroblast activity requires only a very low oxygen content and perfusion has been shown to be what is necessary, not any prescribed level of hemoglobin or hematocrit. Subjective patient complaints of weakness or improved energy after transfusion have also been proposed in support of transfusion. However, where is the objective evidence? Any attempt to do a study regarding subjective feelings of wellness is fraught with inability to blind patients to receiving a transfusion. Transfusion carries such an emotional context with it that any patient infused with a red fluid might well feel better. Blood has widely been promoted as "the life-giving force" in an attempt to stir the public to donate. Therefore, if one is in the hospital and receiving of "the life-giving force," how can any study be objective regarding a subjective assessment of "feeling better." In the end, we are left with no objective data that transfusion of red cells at any one hematocrit improves outcome.

Yet 12 million red cell transfusions are given each year, some 60% of which are in the perioperative period. The decision-making process to transfuse should be based on a risk:benefit ratio for an individual patient. We know only some of the risks; we have no proven (objectively) benefits. Therefore, the decision must be made on an individual patient basis, guided by the best understanding of that patient's physiology.

Some organizations have tried to help in the guidance of the transfusion decision. In the 1980s, the National Institutes of Health (NIH) tried to change the practice and the nation by convening consensus conferences on red cell transfusion, platelet therapy, and the administration of FFP (42–44). In 1984, the American College of Obstetricians and Gynecologists published its recommendations regarding blood therapy (45). In 1990, the American Association of Blood Banks issued guidelines for blood therapy in patients undergoing coronary artery bypass grafting (46). In 1992, the American College of Physicians published red cell transfusion guidelines, and in 1994, the American College of Pathologists published guidelines for the usage of FFP, cryoprecipitate, and platelet transfusions (47, 48). A supplement to the *American Journal of Surgery* in December of 1995 contained the proceedings and conclusion of a consensus conference on blood management. Also in 1994, the American Association of Blood Banks published guidelines for appropriate review of blood utilization and also published consensus conferences on the use of autologous blood (49, 50). Most recently, and appropriate for perioperative transfusion, the American Society of Anesthesiology has published its guidelines for blood component therapy (51). Indeed, there is a tremendous response from organized medicine in trying to guide the practitioner regarding transfusion decisions. All agree that the old transfusion trigger of 10 g/dL hemoglobin is outdated and incorrect. All seem to point toward individualization of the indication for transfusion and most agree that levels of 7 g/dL are well tolerated in otherwise healthy individuals.

The transfusion decision might be subcategorized into different clinical scenarios. Patients requiring in excess of 5 units and tending toward or requiring massive transfusion (1 blood volume) clearly need a transfusion. There would be no argument and probably a great deal of survival data to suggest that blood improves outcome in this group. But no study will ever be done in support of that because it is immoral to conceive of not transfusing such patients. However, volume resuscitation is more important than hemoglobin, and once some transfusion has taken place, there is no need to expect better outcome with hematocrits in excess of 30%. Massive transfusions are relatively rare even in centers that perform hepatic transplantation, major complex cardiovascular surgery, or level 1 trauma (51). It is not so rare that they do not occur, but in one center doing level 1 trauma with more than 10,000 operations per year, the incidence of massive transfusion was only 125 times per year (51).

In patients transfused with somewhat less than 5 units, perhaps 2–5 units, the transfusion trigger and requirements become considerably more difficult to discern. Most clinicians may still agree that a transfusion was wise in these cases, but once again there may be more disagreement on how many units and what hematocrit to target either the beginning or end of transfusion. Again, one should be careful not to exceed 30% hematocrit because there is no indication for that.

Those patients receiving 2 or fewer units of transfusion might constitute an extremely large group of surgical patients. With a unit of red cells expected to increase hematocrit by approximately 3%, one has to wonder if there is any scientific expectation that morbidity or mortality would be improved at all in this group of patients. Perhaps this subgroup of patients might experience only the risk side of the transfusion equation. Once again, there are no data to examine such a question. The individual surgeon or anesthesiologist transfusing such a patient should take the greatest time and thought in examining exactly what is to be accomplished with a transfusion.

There is absolutely no support for an old transfusion guideline that if you are going to transfuse 1 unit, you should give 2 units. Clearly, 2 units represent twice the donor exposure and risk of 1 unit. However, if a unit of red cells can be expected to increase a normal patient (not on cardiopulmonary bypass) hematocrit by only 3%, one has to wonder when that single unit could truly improve oxygen-carrying capacity to the point of improving outcome. Once again, the individual clinician must ask the questions: What is to be accomplished by transfusing this single unit of blood? Is it to be given to increase a reserve of hematocrit in the anticipation of ongoing or future bleeding risk?

The indications for autologous blood harvest and transfusion are less clear. As the transfusion of choice, autologous blood avoids the risks of viral transmission, alloimmunization, and immunosuppression. But it is not totally risk-free, because of septicemia and clerical error. Because the risks to the patient from transfusion of autologous blood are reduced, it does make sense that this subtype of red cell transfusion should have different criteria for usage. Opinion differs on that subject, and some members of the NIH consensus panel voiced opinions that its indications should be the same as those for allogeneic blood. Perhaps the greatest risk is that a patient selected to be transfused and having only a portion of available units as autologous will receive allogeneic blood when his or her autologous blood is present. This does happen even in the best systems with checks and security measures. If a transfusion reaction, viral transmission, or other adverse event occurred in such a case, the event would seem particularly sad if the transfusion was triggered because of a liberalized transfusion trigger in anticipation of administering an autologous unit.

That is a hypothetical situation, but in the face of little data supporting the efficacy of transfusion one has to argue how can we liberalize transfusion triggers for autologous blood. If we support the liberalization of transfusion triggers, then we should be able to show or anticipate improved outcome in those with the more liberalized transfusion trigger. There are no published data to date to suggest that those patients receiving their autologous units do better than patients with a lower hematocrit/hemoglobin for like surgeries who did not receive any allogeneic blood. Perhaps it is easier on a case-by-case basis to face patients and families and explain that they received their autologous blood and therefore the added expense was not "wasted." Time and considerably more research will have to be done to settle the question of whether this practice of a liberalized transfusion trigger is correct for autologous blood.

With all of this production of august opinion and guidelines for therapy, there still exists an increasing demand for blood products. More astoundingly, there is a wide variability in practice. Nowhere is it more apparent than in cardiopulmonary bypass. In the early 1990s, data from 18 centers showed transfusion occurring in coronary artery bypass graft patients from 17–100% (52). A recent study in over 2000 patients at 25 centers showed that matching chest tube output to transfusion utilization had inappropriately high transfusion in 27% of patients (53). When surveyed by the American Association of Blood Banks, some 57% of physicians would have made inappropriate transfusion decisions (54). Physicians who were older or more removed from their training (residency) had a higher incidence of inappropriate transfusion decision-making. The literature is vast, and the recommendations are there regarding proper blood transfusion decisions. The public is demanding reform, and in Europe, officials are imprisoned for less than acceptable (in the public's view) decisions. Blood transfusion decision-making is serious business. It is made by the individual physician attaching the individual unit of blood to and infusion device or intravenous line. Each decision should be made with extreme care.

REFERENCES

1. Donahue JG, Munoz A, Ness PM, et al. The declining risk of post-transfusion hepatitis C virus infection. N Engl J Med 1992;327:369–373.
2. Aach RD, Szmuness W, Mosley JW, et al. Serum alanine aminotransferase of donors in relation to the risk of non-A, non-B hepatitis in recipients: the transfusion-transmitted viruses study. N Engl J Med 1981;304: 989–994.
3. Lackritz E, Satten GA, Aberle-Grasse J, et al. Estimated risk of transmission of the human immunodeficiency virus by screened blood in the United States. N Engl J Med 1995;333:1721–1725.
4. Busch MP, Lee LL, Satten GA, et al. Time course of detection of viral and serologic markers preceding human immunodeficiency virus type 1 seroconversion: implications for screening of blood and tissue donors. Transfusion 1995;35:91–97.
5. LePont F, Costagliola D, Rouzioux C, Valleron AJ. How much would the safety of blood transfusion be improved by including p24 antigen in the battery of tests? Transfusion 1995;35:542–547.
6. Zuck TF. Greetings—a final look back with comments about a policy of zero-risk blood supply [editorial]. Transfusion 1987;27:447–448.
7. Sazama K. Reports of 355 transfusion associated deaths: 1976 through 1985. Transfusion 1990;30:583–590.
8. Klein HG. Immunologic aspects of blood transfusion. Semin Oncol 1994;21:16–20.
9. Alter HJ, Purcell RH, Shih JW, et al. Detection of antibody to hepatitis C virus in prospectively followed transfusion recipients with acute and chronic non-A, non-B hepatitis. N Engl J Med 1989;321:1494–1500.
10. Warner MW, Faust RJ. Risks of transfusion in hemorrhagic disorders. Anesthesiol Clin North Am 1990;8:501–517.
11. Schreiber GB, Busch MP, Kleinman SH, Korelitz JJ, the Retrovirus Epidemiology Donor Study. The risk of transfusion-transmitted viral infections. N Engl J Med 1996;334:1685–1690.
12. Korelitz JJ, Busch MP, Williams AE. The retrovirus epidemiology donor study. Transfusion 1996;36:203–208.
13. Wallace EL, Surgenor DM, Hao HS, An J, Chapman RH, Churchill WH. Collection and transfusion of blood and blood components in the United States, 1989. Transfusion 1993;33:139–144.
14. Cumming PD, Wallace EL, Schorr JB, Dodd RY. Exposure of patients to human immunodeficiency virus through the transfusion of blood components that test antibody-negative. N Engl J Med 1989;321:941–946.
15. Alter MJ, Margolis HS, Krawczynski K, et al. The natural history of community-acquired hepatitis C in the United States. N Engl J Med 1992;327:1899–1905.
16. Office of Medical Applications of Research, National Institutes of Health. Perioperative red cell transfusion. JAMA 1988;260:2700–2703.
17. Linden JV, Kaplan HS. Transfusion errors: causes and effects. Transfus Med Rev 1994;8:169–183.
18. Blumberg N, Chuang-Stein C, Heal JM. The relationship of blood transfusion, tumor staging, and cancer recurrence. Transfusion 1990;30: 291–294.
19. Mezrow CK, Bergstein I, Tartter PI. Postoperative infections following autologous and homologous blood transfusions. Transfusion 1992;32: 27–30.

20. Murphy P, Heal JM, Blumberg N. Infection or suspected infection after hip replacement surgery with autologous or homologous blood transfusions. Transfusion 1991;31:212–217.
21. Edna TH, Bjerkeset T. Association between blood transfusion and infection in injured patients. J Trauma 1992;33:659–661.
22. Vamvakas EC, Moore SB. Blood transfusion and postoperative septic complications. Transfusion 1994;34:714–727.
23. Vamvakas EC, Moore SB, Cabanela M. Blood transfusion and septic complications after hip replacement surgery. Transfusion 1995;35:150–156.
24. Lubarsky DA, Hahn C, Bennett DH, et al. The hospital cost (fiscal year 1991/1992) of a simple perioperative allogeneic red blood cell transfusion during elective surgery at Duke University. Anesth Analg 1994;79: 629–637.
25. Forbes JM, Anderson MD, Anderson GF, Bleecker GC, Rossi EC, Moss GS. Blood transfusion costs: a multicenter study. Transfusion 1991;31:318–323.
26. Birkmeyer JD, AuBuchon JP, Littenberg B, et al. Cost-effectiveness of preoperative autologous donation in coronary artery bypass grafting. Ann Thorac Surg 1994;57:161–169.
27. Viele MK, Weiskopf RB. What can we learn about the need for transfusion from patients who refuse blood? The experience with Jehovah's Witnesses. Transfusion 1994;34:396–401.
28. Kitchens CS. Are transfusions overrated? Surgical outcome of Jehovah's Witnesses. Am J Med 1993;94:117–119.
29. Messmer K, Sunder-Plassmann L, Jesch F, Görnandt L, Sinagowitz E, Kessler M. Oxygen supply to the tissues during limited normovolemic hemodilution. Res Exp Med Berl 1973;159:152–166.
30. Czer LS, Shoemaker WC. Optimal hematocrit value in critically ill postoperative patients. Surg Gynecol Obstet 1978;147:363–368.
31. Doak GJ, Hall RI. Does hemoglobin concentration affect perioperative myocardial lactate flux in patients undergoing coronary artery bypass surgery? Anesth Analg 1995;80:910–916.
32. Mathru M, Kleinman B, Blakeman B, Sullivan H, Kumar P, Dries DJ. Myocardial metabolism and adaptation during extreme hemodilution in humans after coronary revascularization. Crit Care Med 1992;20:1420–1425.
33. Case RB, Berglund E, Sarcroft SJ. Ventricular function VIII. Changes in coronary resistance and ventricular function resulting from acutely induced anemia and the effect thereon of coronary stenosis. Am J Med 1955;18:397–405.
34. Yoshikawa H, Powell WJ, Bland JH, Lowenstein E. Effect of acute anemia on experimental myocardial ischemia. Am J Cardiol 1973;32: 670–678.
35. Most AS, Ruocco NA, Gewirtz H. Effect of a reduction in blood viscosity on maximal myocardial oxygen delivery distal to a moderate coronary stenosis. Circulation 1986;74:1085–1092.
36. Spence RK, Alexander JB, DelRossi AJ, et al. Transfusion guidelines for cardiovascular surgery: lessons learned from operations in Jehovah's Witnesses. J Vasc Surg 1992;16:825–829.
37. Carson JL, Poses RM, Spence RK, Bonavita G. Severity of anaemia and operative mortality and morbidity. Lancet 1988;1:727–729.
38. Spence RK, Costabile JP, Young GS, et al. Is hemoglobin level alone a reliable predictor of outcome in the severely anemic surgical patient? Am Surg 1992;58:92–95.
39. Nelson AH, Fleisher LA, Rosenbaum SH. Relationship between postoperative anemia and cardiac morbidity in high-risk vascular patients in the intensive care unit. Crit Care Med 1993;21:860–866.
40. Babineau TJ, Dzik WH, Borlase BC, Baxter JK, Bistrian BR, Benotti PN. Reevaluation of current transfusion practices in patients in surgical intensive care units. Am J Surg 1992;164:22–25.
41. Spiess BD, Kapitan S, Body S, et al. ICU entry hematocrit does influence the risk of perioperative myocardial infarction (MI) in coronary artery bypass graft surgery [abstract]. Anesth Analg 1995;80:SCAA47.
42. Office of Medical Applications of Research, National Institutes of Health. Fresh frozen plasma: indications and risks. JAMA 1983;253: 551–553.
43. Office of Medical Applications of Research, National Institutes of Health. Platelet transfusion therapy. JAMA 1987;257:1777–1780.
44. Office of Medical Applications of Research, National Institutes of Health. Perioperative red blood cell transfusion. JAMA 1988;260: 2700–2703.
45. American College of Obstetricians and Gynecologists. Blood component therapy. Technical Bulletin no. 78. Washington, DC: American College of Obstetricians and Gynecologists, 1984.
46. Goodnough LT, Johnston MF, Ramsey G, et al. Guidelines for transfusion support in patients undergoing coronary artery bypass grafting. Ann Thorac Surg 1990;50:675–683.
47. American College of Physicians. Practice strategies for elective red blood cell transfusion. Ann Intern Med 1992;116:403–406.
48. College of American Pathologists. Practice parameter for the use of fresh frozen plasma, cryoprecipitate, and platelets. JAMA 1994;271: 777–781.
49. Stehling L, Luban NL, Anderson KC, et al. Guidelines for blood utilization review. Transfusion 1994;34:438–448.
50. Maffei LM, Thurer RL, eds. American Association of Blood Banks. Autologous blood transfusion: current issues. Transcribed proceedings of a national conference and issues forum. Arlington, VA: AABB, 1988.
51. Task Force on Blood Component Therapy. Practice guidelines for blood component therapy: a report by the American Society of Anesthesiologists Task Force on Blood Component Therapy. Anesthesiology 1996;84:732–747.
52. Goodnough LT, Johnston MF, Toy PT, et al. The variability of transfusion practice in coronary artery bypass surgery. JAMA 1991;265:86–90.
53. Stover EP, Siegel LC, Parks R, McSPI Research Group. Variability in transfusion practice for coronary artery bypass surgery persists despite national consensus guidelines [abstract]. Anesthesiology 1994;81:A1224.
54. Salen-Schatz SR, Aworn J, Soumerai SB. Influence of clinical knowledge, organizational context, and practice style on transfusion decision making: Implications for practice change strategies. JAMA 1990; 264:476–483.

Index

Page numbers in *italics* denote illustrations; those followed by a "t" denote tables.

F